Family Practice Guidelines

Jill C. Cash, MSN, APRN, FNP-BC, a family nurse practitioner for over 20 years, currently practices as a family nurse practitioner at the Vanderbilt Medical Group, Westhaven Family Practice, in Franklin, Tennessee. Her past experience includes teaching as an instructor for the School of Nursing, Southern Illinois University in Edwardsville and Carbondale, Illinois, in the undergraduate BSN program and the graduate NP program. She has been a clinical preceptor for a variety of programs. Her previous experience includes high risk obstetrics as a clinical nurse specialist in maternal–fetal medicine at Vanderbilt University Medical Center, rheumatology in the outpatient setting, women's health in the outpatient setting, and providing wound care in skilled nursing facilities. She has served as a member and officer on numerous boards which include Hospice of Southern Illinois, the Marion Memorial Health Foundation, the American Cancer Society, and Women for Health and Wellness in Southern Illinois. Ms. Cash has authored several chapters in other textbooks and is the co-author of *Family Practice Guidelines*, first, second, third, and fourth editions, and *Adult-Gerontology Practice Guidelines*. Most recently, she was awarded the 2017 AANP Nurse Practitioner State Award for Excellence from Illinois.

Cheryl A. Glass, MSN, WHNP, RN-BC, is a women's health nurse practitioner who currently practices as a clinical research specialist for KEPRO in TennCare's Medical Solutions Unit in Nashville, Tennessee. She is also adjunct faculty at Vanderbilt University School of Nursing. Previously, Ms. Glass was a clinical trainer and trainer manager for Healthways. Her previous nurse practitioner practice was as a clinical research coordinator on pharmaceutical clinical trials at Nashville Clinical Research. She also worked in a collaborative clinical obstetrics practice with the director and assistant directors of maternal–fetal medicine at Vanderbilt University Medical Center Department of Obstetrics–Gynecology. Ms. Glass is the author of several book chapters and is coauthor of *Family Practice Guidelines*, second, third, and fourth editions, and *Adult-Gerontology Practice Guidelines*. She has published five refereed journal articles. In 1999, Ms. Glass was named Nurse of the Year by the Tennessee chapter of the Association of Women's Health, Obstetric and Neonatal Nurses.

Family Practice Guidelines

Fourth Edition

Jill C. Cash, MSN, APRN, FNP-BC
Cheryl A. Glass, MSN, WHNP, RN-BC
Editors

SPRINGER PUBLISHING COMPANY
NEW YORK

Springer Publishing Company, LLC
11 West 42nd Street
New York, NY 10036
www.springerpub.com

Acquisitions Editor: Margaret Zuccarini
Compositor: Newgen KnowledgeWorks

ISBN: 978-0-8261-7711-7
e-book ISBN: 978-0-8261-7712-4
Patient Teaching Guide: 978-0-8261-7713-1

Patient Teaching Guides are available for download at springerpub.com/familypracticeguidelines4e

17 18 19 20 / 5 4 3 2 1

The author and the publisher of this Work have made every effort to use sources believed to be reliable to provide information that is accurate and compatible with the standards generally accepted at the time of publication. Because medical science is continually advancing, our knowledge base continues to expand. Therefore, as new information becomes available, changes in procedures become necessary. We recommend that the reader always consult current research and specific institutional policies before performing any clinical procedure. The author and publisher shall not be liable for any special, consequential, or exemplary damages resulting, in whole or in part, from the readers' use of, or reliance on, the information contained in this book. The publisher has no responsibility for the persistence or accuracy of URLs for external or third-party Internet websites referred to in this publication and does not guarantee that any content on such websites is, or will remain, accurate or appropriate.

Library of Congress Cataloging-in-Publication Data
Names: Cash, Jill C., editor. | Glass, Cheryl A. (Cheryl Anne), editor.
Title: Family practice guidelines/[edited by] Jill C. Cash, Cheryl A. Glass.
Description: Fourth edition. | Danvers, MA: Springer Publishing Company, LLC, [2017] | Includes bibliographical references and index.
Identifiers: LCCN 2016048484 | ISBN 9780826177117 (paperback) | ISBN 9780826177124 (e-book)
Subjects: | MESH: Family Practice—methods | Primary Nursing—methods | Diagnostic Techniques and Procedures | Nurse Practitioners | Physician Assistants | Handbooks
Classification: LCC RT120.F34 | NLM WY 49 | DDC 610.73—dc23
LC record available at https://lccn.loc.gov/2016048484

Printed in the United States of America by Bradford & Bigelow.

This book is dedicated to all of our families, friends, and colleagues who have influenced our lives, careers, and dreams. We greatly appreciate our colleagues, Margaret Zuccarini and Joanne Jay at Springer Publishing, and Ashita Shah and the Newgen KnowledgeWorks staff for keeping us on track for deadlines and understanding that life happens!

Jill C. Cash and Cheryl A. Glass

Contents

5. Eye Guidelines

6. Ear Guidelines

7. Nasal Guidelines

8. Throat and Mouth Guidelines

9. Respiratory Guidelines

10. Cardiovascular Guidelines

11. Gastrointestinal Guidelines

12. Genitourinary Guidelines

13. Obstetrics Guidelines

ANTEPARTUM

POSTPARTUM

14. Gynecologic Guidelines

15. Sexually Transmitted Infections Guidelines

16. Infectious Disease Guidelines

17. Systemic Disorders Guidelines

18. Musculoskeletal Guidelines

19. Neurologic Guidelines

20. Endocrine Guidelines

21. Rheumatological Guidelines

22. Psychiatric Guidelines

23. Assessment Guide for Sport Participation

II. PROCEDURES

III. PATIENT TEACHING GUIDES

Contributors

Julie Adkins, DNP, APN, FNP-BC, FAANP
Certified Family Nurse Practitioner
Adkins Family Practice, LLC
West Frankfort, Illinois

Rhonda Arthur, DNP, CNM, WHNP-BC, FNP-BC, CNE
Associate Professor
Frontier Nursing University
Hyden, Kentucky

Amy C. Bruggemann, MSN, APRN-BC, CWS
Director of Clinical Operations
Specialized Wound Management
Chesterfield, Missouri

Beverly R. Byram, MSN, FNP
Clinical Instructor
Vanderbilt University School of Nursing
Director, Ryan White Part D
Comprehensive Care Center
Nashville, Tennessee

Jill C. Cash, MSN, APN, FNP-BC
Vanderbilt Medical Group Westhaven Family Practice
Franklin, Tennessee; and
Vanderbilt University Medical Center
Nashville, Tennessee

Moya Cook, APN, CNP
Morthland College Health Services
West Frankfort, Illinois

Susan Drummond, RN, MSN, C-EFM
Associate in Obstetrics
Department of Obstetrics and Gynecology
Vanderbilt University Medical Center
Nashville, Tennessee

Cheryl A. Glass, MSN, WHNP, RN-BC
Clinical Research Specialist
KEPRO Peer Review
Medical Solutions Unit
Nashville, Tennessee

Debbie Gunter, APRN, FNP-BC, ACHPN
Nurse Practitioner
Emory University
Atlanta, Georgia

Mellisa A. Hall, DNP, APN-BC, FNP-BC, ACHPN
University of Southern Indiana
Evansville, Indiana

Audra C. Malone, DNP, FNP-BC
Assistant Professor
Frontier Nursing University
Hyden, Kentucky

Robertson Nash, PhD, ACNP, BC
Director, PATHways Clinic
Nurse Practitioner, Medicine/Infectious Diseases
Comprehensive Care Clinic
Vanderbilt University Medical Center
Nashville, Tennessee

Laura A. Petty, MSN, GNP-BC
Gerontological Nurse Practitioner
Lebanon, Tennessee

Bunny Pounds, DNP, FNP, BC
Frontier Nursing University
Hyden, Kentucky

Angelito Tacderas, APN
Marion, Illinois

Nancy Pesta Walsh, DNP, CNP
Frontier Nursing University
Hyden, Kentucky

Kimberly D. Waltrip, PhD(c), APRN-BC
Instructor of Nursing
Southeast Missouri State University
Cape Girardeau, Missouri

Alyson Wolz, DNP, APN, PMHCNS, BC
Harrisburg Medical Center
Harrisburg, Illinois

Reviewers for the Third and Fourth Editions

Julie Adkins, DNP, APN, FNP-BC, FAANP
Certified Family Nurse Practitioner
Adkins Family Practice, LLC
West Frankfort, Illinois

Rhonda Arthur, DNP, CNM, WHNP-BC, FNP-BC, CNE
Associate Professor
Frontier Nursing University
Hyden, Kentucky

Leanne Busby, DSN, RN, FAANP
Certified Nurse Practitioner
Adjunct Faculty
Gordon E. Inman School of Health Sciences and Nursing
Belmont University
Nashville, Tennessee

Andrew W. Hull, PA-C
Director, Chair, and Assistant Professor of Physician Assistant Studies
Milligan College Physician Assistant Program
Milligan College, Tennessee

Heather C. Justice, MSPAP, PA-C
Assistant Professor
Milligan College
Milligan College, Tennessee

David Knechtel, PA-C
Johnson City, Tennessee

Maureen Knechtel, MPAS, PA-C
Assistant Professor of Physician Assistant Studies
Milligan College
Milligan College, Tennessee

Keith A. Lafferty, MD, FAAEM
Codirector of Emergency Medicine
Gulf Coast Regional Medical Center
Atlanticare Regional Medical Center
Atlantic City, New Jersey

Ethel M. Robertson, EdD, FNP-BC, WCC
Certified Nurse Practitioner
Harmony Family Health Care/Physicians Services
Nashville, Tennessee

Lucy WacheraKibe, DrPH, MS, MHS, PA-C
Director of Doctoral Education
Assistant Professor
Department of Physician Assistant Medicine
School of Graduate Health Sciences
Lynchburg College
Lynchburg, Virginia

Preface

We are excited to collaborate again on the new fourth edition of *Family Practice Guidelines*. The guidelines have been written and updated by experienced nurse practitioners in their fields of expertise. This valuable resource is designed to assist novice and experienced nurse practitioners in organizing and using the content in a quick-reference format. Emphasis is placed on history taking, physical examination, and key elements of the diagnosis. Useful website links have also been incorporated, along with updated patient teaching guides to offer to patients.

This book is organized into chapters using a body-system format. The disorders included within each chapter are organized in alphabetical sequence for easy access. Disorders that are more commonly seen in the primary care setting are included. Patient teaching guides are also organized in alphabetical order. Bold text or italic text highlights *alerts* for practitioners and educational *clinical pearls* are easily found.

Organization

The book is now organized into three major sections:

- *Section I: Guidelines* presents 23 chapters containing the individual disorder guidelines.
- *Section II: Procedures* presents procedures that commonly are conducted within the office or clinic setting.
- *Section III: Patient Teaching Guides* presents patient teaching guides that are easy to distribute to patients as a take-home teaching guide. The teaching guidelines are arranged in alphabetical order for ease of reference and the pages are perforated for easy pull-out and photocopying. **The Patient Teaching Guides are also available for download at springerpub.com/familypracticeguidelines4e**

New to This Edition

New guidelines have been added to the fourth edition, and include the following:

- The newest up-to-date Centers for Disease Control and Prevention (CDC) guidelines on health maintenance and immunization schedules for adults and children.
- An entire chapter is dedicated to the sports preparticipation examination.
- A new chapter on Public Health Guidelines, including the subchapter Homelessness.
- The Dermatology Guidelines include the newest guidelines for wound care management.
- The Respiratory Guidelines include a new subchapter on shortness of breath and the newest updated treatment guidelines for chronic obstructive pulmonary disease (COPD) and pneumonia.
- The Cardiovascular chapter includes the newest guidelines for heart failure and hypertension.
- The Genitourinary Guidelines include an updated subchapter on erectile dysfunction and a new subchapter on premature ejaculation.
- The Gynecologic Guidelines have been updated with a new subchapter, female sexual dysfunction.
- New subchapters have been added to the Infectious Disease chapter, including the new CDC guidelines for the Zika virus.
- Updated guidelines are included in the Neurologic chapter, together with the newest treatment options for stroke and trigeminal neuralgia.
- A brand new Rheumatological Guidelines chapter includes the most common rheumatic conditions encountered in primary care, including fibromyalgia, psoriatic arthritis, gout, and many others.
- The section concludes with the newest treatment recommendations in psychiatric conditions including the new subchapters bipolar disorder, depression, sleep disorders, and others.

New Patient Teaching Guides

- Chapter 4, Dermatology Guidelines: Wound Care: Lower Extremity Ulcers; Wound Care: Pressure Ulcers; Wound Care: Wounds
- Chapter 6, Ear Guidelines: Tinnitus
- Chapter 10, Cardiovascular Guidelines: Atrial Fibrillation, Chronic Venous Insufficiency, Superficial Thrombophlebitis, and Varicose Veins
- Chapter 12, Genitourinary Guidelines: Kidney Disease: Chronic

- Chapter 19, Neurologic Guidelines: Migraine Headache
- Chapter 22, Psychiatric Guidelines: Sleep Disorders/ Insomnia

Procedures

Three of the procedures have been updated: Clock-Draw Test, Cystometry, and Prostatic Massage Technique: 2-Glass Test.

We hope you find this fourth edition of *Family Practice Guidelines* easy to access and a valuable resource during your clinical practice. We appreciate your support for our first three editions and hope you find the fourth edition as rewarding as the others.

Jill C. Cash
Cheryl A. Glass

I Guidelines

1. Health Maintenance Guidelines
2. Public Health Guidelines
3. Pain Management Guidelines
4. Dermatology Guidelines
5. Eye Guidelines
6. Ear Guidelines
7. Nasal Guidelines
8. Throat and Mouth Guidelines
9. Respiratory Guidelines
10. Cardiovascular Guidelines
11. Gastrointestinal Guidelines
12. Genitourinary Guidelines
13. Obstetrics Guidelines
14. Gynecologic Guidelines
15. Sexually Transmitted Infections Guidelines
16. Infectious Disease Guidelines
17. Systemic Disorders Guidelines
18. Musculoskeletal Guidelines
19. Neurologic Guidelines
20. Endocrine Guidelines
21. Rheumatological Guidelines
22. Psychiatric Guidelines
23. Assessment Guide for Sport Participation

1 Health Maintenance Guidelines

Cultural Diversity and Sensitivity

Angelito Tacderas

Culture is more than nationality or race. Culture influences a person's reasoning, decisions, and actions. It is the accumulation of learned beliefs, values, habits, and practices. Culture influences decision making, thoughts, what is approved or disapproved, what is normal or not, which are all acquired from close personal relations (family/members of society) over time.

Cultural diversity exists when groups of different cultures must coexist within an environmental area (family, neighborhood, township, city, or country). Knowing that there are differences in cultures and not assigning values among different cultures reflects cultural sensitivity. However, significant differences may exist in the way health care is perceived and practiced because of the differing values and beliefs regarding health and illness inherent among people of varying cultural backgrounds.

Factors Contributing to Cultural Diversity

- Fewer White non-Hispanic children
- Increase in immigration
- Efficiency in transportation and travel
- Increase in the homeless and the poor populations
- Increase in divorce rate
- Increase in single parenting
- Grandparents raising grandchildren
- Substance abuse
- Violence
- Transgender sex changes
- Homosexual acceptance
- Information explosion/high technology
- Illiteracy
- Increase in non-English-proficient health care providers
- Federal regulations

Cultural sensitivity is the responsibility of all health care providers. Each office visit is an opportunity to gain more knowledge about a client's health beliefs and practices. Inadequate awareness of the client's health beliefs and practices influenced by culture may lead to mistrust. This may result in barriers, including inappropriate delivery of care, increased cost, noncompliance, and seeking care elsewhere. Thus, this may eventually lead to even more barriers to health care access, resulting in unfavorable health care outcomes. Title VI of the Civil Rights Act is very specific about providing services that are less than the existing standard of care to anyone based on race, age, sex, or financial status. According to this document, "No person in the United States shall, on the grounds of race, color or national origin be excluded in the participation in, be denied the benefits of, or be discriminated under any programs or activity receiving federal financing assistance" (U.S. Department of Justice [USDJ], n.d.).

Thoughtful Consideration

Providing care without being sensitive to the cultural needs of a client may suggest that the health care provider's values and beliefs are superior to those of the client and may lead to disparity of care. The limited patient involvement in care may result in noncompliance, placing patients at greater risk of health-related complications. The delay in provision of health care can result in life-threatening complications.

Numerous cultural resources are available throughout the literature and the Internet. Preference as to which educational/assessment tools to use are within the health care provider's prerogative.

The following are guidelines for promoting cultural sensitivity in the clinical setting:

A. Provide a cultural diversity self-assessment/practice organization.

1. Consult online Internet self-assessment tools, for example, Centers for Disease Control and Prevention (CDC) website (see the next section).

2. Download self-assessment tools from public sites (see Exhibit 1.1).

3. Use existing self-assessment tools and make necessary changes to fit the need of your community (see Exhibit 1.1).

B. Identify the need of the population served.

1. Understand the community and its health status.

2. Evaluate resources, attitudes, and barriers inside the community and practice location.

a. Access to resources

b. Notification of assistance

c. Range of assistance options

i. Transportation

ii. Communication; consider an interpreter (personal vs. automated)

1) Identify bilingual staff.

2) Use family members or personal acquaintances as interpreters (adults only).

3) Provide multilingual written materials.

iii. Education (meaningful/multilingual)

1) User friendly

2) Friendly technology

C. Educate staff to cultural diversities.

1. Assessments should include the patient's health values and beliefs (see Exhibit 1.2).

2. Communication should be meaningful.

a. Be precise and clear.

b. Maintain eye contact when speaking.

c. Use plain language.

d. Observe facial expressions and body language.

e. Use short sentences to explain lengthy information.

f. Avoid medical jargon

g. Use repetition for emphasis

h. Ask questions to confirm understanding

D. Schedule longer appointments if needed.

E. Health care providers should clarify the limitations of a health care provider's role.

F. Clearly identify alternatives offered by health care provider.

EXHIBIT 1.1 Cultural Diversity and Sensitivity Self-Evaluation Form

Using a scale of 1 to 5, with 1 = never and 5 = always, please answer the following questions:

Question	Response Value
1. I am comfortable with my culture and can compromise on situations without sacrificing my integrity.	
2. I think about what I say and how it may affect people with different beliefs and practices.	
3. I am aware that others may stereotype me, and I am willing to proactively get involved and share my beliefs and practices.	
4. I evaluate what the real reasons are when I encounter a conflict with persons of a different culture.	
5. I am aware of sensitive issues when I am around women and persons of different beliefs and races.	
6. I ask for clarification when I do not understand what others mean.	
7. I am aware of my assumptions about others who are culturally or racially different from me and I am okay with it.	
8. I object when others tell ethnic jokes.	
9. I listen without interrupting when someone is speaking.	
10. I am comfortable forming friendships with people of different cultures.	
11. I find ways to learn more about different cultures and to communicate effectively.	
12. I realize that flexibility and empathy allow me to evaluate persons of different cultures without imposing any judgments, which allows me to collaborate effectively.	
13. I recognize that there are other ways to do things than mine.	
14. I accept people for who they are regardless of color, educational achievement, financial status, or gender.	
15. I do not mind apologizing if I have wronged or offended someone.	
16. I respect that others may have a different interpretation of personal space than I do.	
17. I treat people differently than suggested by the biases and prejudices of members of my culture.	
18. I do not look down on people who do not speak English fluently or may have an accent.	
19. I understand that there are other ways to communicate than I do.	
20. I use simple and common phrases when around someone of diverse culture who may not speak my language proficiently.	
Add up all of the numbers to get a total score.	

Total score:
Outstanding: 95–100
Good: 85–94
Average: 75–84
Needs improvement: 74 or less
(This tool is intended for personal use only. It is designed to be performed as a personal self-assessment. No reliability test that measures stability, equivalence, and homogeneity has been performed.)

Source: American Academy of Family Physicians, American Academy of Pediatrics, American College of Sports Medicine, American Medical Society for Sports Medicine (2010). Copyright © 2010 American Academy of Pediatrics. Reproduced with permission.

EXHIBIT 1.2 Sample History Form

Client: Personal, Social, and Family Information

Name ____________________
DOB ____________________
1. Today's date ____________________ 2. Age ____________________
3. Gender: M or F
Is your answer to question number 3 based on a transgender sexual change?
If no sexual change has taken place, skip questions 4 and 5.
4. Date of procedure ____________________ 5. Type of procedure ____________________
Medications prescribed ____________________
____
Sexual orientation: heterosexual ________ gay/lesbian ________ other ________
Proficient in speaking English YES NO
Proficient in reading English YES NO
Ability to read lips YES NO
Preferred spoken language ____________________
Most comfortable language when speaking ____________________
Most comfortable language when reading ____________________
Preferred greeting Mr. Mrs. Ms. First name ____________________
Type of nonverbal communication used ____________________
Eye contact ____________________
Need of interpreter ____________________
Relation to interpreter ____________________
Quiet/use of silence ____________________
Use and definition of time ____________________
Use of any common signs (okay, pain, clapping) ____________________
Use of comfort space ____________________
Tactile use ____________________
Use of cultural jargon or slang that may affect evaluation
____
____
Perception of pain ____________________
Culture ____________________ Ethnicity ____________________
Family role and function ____________________
Work ____________________
Leisure activities ____________________
Friends ____________________ Others ____________________
Country of origin ____________________
Country of birth ____________________
Years in United States ____________________
Did you grow up in a city ________ town ________ suburb ________ rural ________
Ethnicity ____________________
Major support group ____________________
Dominant members of the family ____________________
Decision makers for the family ____________________
Previous work history ____________________
Present work history ____________________
Education ____________________
Describe importance of religion ____________________
Religious beliefs/practices ____________________
Religious association ____________________
Cultural/religious practices/restrictions ____________________
____
Meaning and use of religious symbols ____________________
Interaction with family/significant other—describe ____________________
____
Role of father ____________________ Role of mother ____________________
Role of elder sibling/siblings ____________________
Grandparents' role ____________________

(*continued*)

EXHIBIT 1.2 **Sample History Form (*continued*)**

Expectation from this visit ______
Food preferences ______
Beliefs on health promotion ______
______
Family history ______
______
Skin color/hair structure ______

Reason for Visit

Chief complaint ______
Perceived cause ______
Reasons for cause ______
Symptoms of illness ______
______
Onset and severity (pain scale) ______
Effects of illness on activities of daily living (ADLs) ______
Fear of the unknown about illness ______
Treatment expectations and results ______
Beliefs/practices about illness ______
Health promotion beliefs and practice ______
______
Types of healing practices ______
Client's appearance ______
Common diseases and disorders ______
Beliefs and practices regarding traumatic events ______
______
Beliefs and practices for preventive health ______
______
Surgical history ______
Other medical history ______
______
Any additional information that may improve client care ______

Source: American Academy of Family Physicians, American Academy of Pediatrics, American College of Sports Medicine, American Medical Society for Sports Medicine (2010).

Health Maintenance During the Life Span

Jill C. Cash and Debbie Gunter

Health maintenance involves identifying individuals who are at risk of health problems and encouraging behaviors that reduce these risks. An important aspect of health maintenance is patient education, including teaching individuals about their risk factors for disease and ways to modify their behaviors to reduce their risks of comorbidities. This book contains Patient Teaching Guides that the practitioner may use for patient education; these forms are found in Section III: Patient Teaching Guides. They may be photocopied by the practitioner, filled in according to the patient's evaluation and needs, and given to the patient.

This chapter describes tools that the practitioner can use in preventive health care assessment, which include websites, screening guidelines, and suggestions for patient education and counseling.

Pediatric Well-Child Evaluation

The Well-Child Care chart (Exhibit 1.3) is designed for use with newborns and young children up to 5 to 6 years old. When complications arise, a detailed Subjective, Objective, Assessment, and Plan (SOAP) note is required for documentation. The documentation should be kept in the front of the child's chart for easy reference.

The growth charts for children are available in English; metric versions and charts in multiple languages, including Spanish and French, are available on the Centers for Disease Control and Prevention (CDC) website (www.cdc.gov/growthcharts).

Anticipatory Guidance by Age

The anticipatory guidance tool (Exhibit 1.4) provides a quick reference for the practitioner from the child's initial visit at 1 month throughout his or her well-child visits until age 15 years. It lists topics that the practitioner should discuss with the caregiver. This information should be supplemented with booklets, teaching guides, and brochures for the caregiver.

EXHIBIT 1.3 **Well-Child Care**

Name ______ DOB ______ Chart# ______

BIRTH HISTORY:

Mother's name ______; Age ______; G ______; P ______; Gestational age at delivery ______ weeks; Birth weight ______ pounds ______ ounces.

Apgar scores: 5 min ______ 10 min ______.

Delivery: Vaginal delivery or cesarean ______. Pregnancy/delivery complications ______

	Initial Visit	2 Wk	2 Mo	4 Mo	6 Mo	9 Mo	12 Mo	15 Mo	18 Mo	24 Mo	3 Y	4 Y	5 Y
Date													
Height percentile													
Weight percentile													
Head circ. percentile													
Vital signs													
Labs													
Immunize													
Hepatitis B (HepB) (Initial at birth)			#2		#3								
Diphtheria, tetanus, and acellular pertussis (DTaP)			#1	#2	#3			#4				#5	
Inactivated poliovirus (IPV)/oral poliovirus (OPV)			#1	#2				#3				#4	
Measles, mumps, rubella (MMR)							#1					#2	
Varicella (VAR)							#1					#2	
Rotavirus (RV)			#1	#2	#3								
Haemophilus influenza B			#1	#2	#3		#4						
Pneumococcal													
Influenza							#1			#2	#3	#4	#5

(*continued*)

EXHIBIT 1.3 **Well-Child Care (*continued*)**

	Initial Visit	2 Wk	2 Mo	4 Mo	6 Mo	9 Mo	12 Mo	15 Mo	18 Mo	24 Mo	3 Y	4 Y	5 Y
Hepatitis A (HepA)							#1						
Feedings													
Denver Development Screening Tool													
Physical examination date													
General appearance													
Skin													
Head/neck													
Eyes/ears													
Nose/throat													
Mouth/teeth													
Heart/lungs													
Abdomen													
Extremities													
Back													
Genitalia													
Neurologic													
Medication review													
Assessment plan													
Follow-up													

Source: American Academy of Family Physicians, American Academy of Pediatrics, American College of Sports Medicine, American Medical Society for Sports Medicine (2010).

EXHIBIT 1.4 Anticipatory Guidance

Immunizations: Please see the Centers for Disease Control and Prevention (CDC) Immunization chart for the recommended vaccination schedule for each visit: www.cdc.gov/vaccines/schedules.

Initial Visit: 2 Weeks to 1 Month

A. *Safety*
1. Review sleeping position: Back or side-lying.
2. Avoid placing newborn on top of tables, counters, bed, and so forth. Discuss risk of fall.
3. Avoid toys, pillows in crib.
4. *Discuss car seat safety.* Use rear-facing car seat.

B. *Nutrition*
1. Breast/bottle feeding
2. Feeding patterns/frequency
3. Regurgitation
4. Avoid propping bottles

C. *Development*
1. Handling fussy periods
2. Soothing techniques: Music, reading
3. Reaction to pain

D. *Health Care Management*
1. Use of thermometer
2. Fever
3. Vomiting
4. Diarrhea
5. Skin: Sun protection

E. *Family Dynamics*
1. The new role of parenting
2. Exhaustion
3. Sleeping patterns of the newborn and parents
4. Sibling reactions, anticipated jealousy

2 Months

A. *Safety*
1. Review sleeping habits.
2. Use rails on cribs.
3. Do not leave child unattended on bed, changing table, and so on.
4. Discuss car seat safety.

B. *Nutrition*
1. *See Section III: Patient Teaching Guide for this chapter, "Infant Nutrition"*
2. Breastfeeding/formula intake

C. *Development*
1. Head control
2. Eyes follow moving object to midline

D. *Health Care Management*
1. Skin care, infant acne
2. Use of thermometer

E. *Family Dynamics*
1. Child care
2. Relaxation and personal time for the parents
3. Sleeping patterns of infant and parents
4. Sibling rivalry/relationships

4 Months

A. *Safety*
1. Car seat safety
2. Choking, suffocation
3. Ways to assist in an emergency
4. Water safety: Tubs, buckets, pools, and so on
5. Use of safety gates
6. Poison control: Provide poison control number for parent
7. Covering electrical outlets

B. *Nutrition*
1. Begin solids (infant cereal)
2. Breastfeeding/formula intake

C. *Development*
1. Sits with support
2. Follows moving object past midline
3. Social smile, squeals
4. Lifts head up
5. Rolls over supine to prone

D. *Health Care Management*
1. Patterns of sleep
2. Digestive changes

E. *Family Dynamics*
1. Parents' time away
2. Child care
3. Sibling rivalry

6 Months

A. *Safety*
1. Review of 4-month information
2. Car seat safety
3. Reinforce home safety
4. Security of chemicals, toxins, detergents
5. Use of cabinet and door locks, or gates for stairs
6. High-chair safety
7. Poison control phone number

B. *Nutrition*
1. Breastfeeding/formula intake
2. Cereals/fruits/vegetable introduction

C. *Development*
1. No head lag
2. Turns to rattle noise
3. Reaches toward object
4. Sits without support
5. Transfers object from hand to hand
6. Rolls over prone to supine
7. Shows stranger anxiety

D. *Health Care Management*
1. Dental care
2. Footwear
3. Laboratory: Hematocrit/hemoglobin

E. *Family Dynamics*
1. Parents' time away
2. Child care
3. Sibling rivalry

9 Months

A. *Safety*
1. Childproofing the home
2. Use of gates, locks, cabinet locks
3. Poison control phone number

B. *Nutrition*
1. *See Section III: Patient Teaching Guide for this chapter, "Childhood Nutrition"*
2. Breastfeeding/formula intake
3. Solid foods and choking hazards
4. Easy snacks (Cheerios, crackers)

C. *Development*
1. Takes two cubes, pincer grasp
2. Verbalizes "mama"
3. Crawls, cruises

(*continued*)

EXHIBIT 1.4 **Anticipatory Guidance (*continued*)**

4. Weight-bearing legs
5. Imitates sound
6. Setting limits with "no"

D. *Health Care Management*
1. Elimination patterns
2. Sleeping habits
3. Dental care

E. *Family Dynamics*
1. Sibling interactions
2. Child care

12 Months

A. *Safety*
1. Accident prevention (poison control, windows, outlets, water)
2. Poison control phone number

B. *Nutrition*
1. Introduction to cow's milk
2. Use of cup
3. Solid food intake

C. *Development*
1. Read books with caregiver
2. Playtime
3. Praising behavior
4. Stranger and separation anxiety
5. Encourage speech
6. Walking

D. *Health Care Management*
1. Exercise
2. Elimination patterns
3. Sleeping habits
4. Dental care

E. *Family Dynamics*
1. Sibling relationships
2. Child care

15 Months

A. *Safety*
1. Accident prevention review
2. Water safety
3. Choking hazards
4. Plastic bags
5. Electrical safety

B. *Nutrition*
1. Feeding patterns and habits
2. Dental care

C. *Development*
1. Socialization skills changing
2. Goes up steps in childlike manner
3. Bedtime routines
4. Looking/reading books
5. Establishing hand preference

D. *Health Care Management*
1. Treating small injuries at home (abrasions, falls, etc.)
2. Exercising/activities
3. Elimination patterns
4. Sleeping habits

E. *Family Dynamics*
1. Child care
2. Parent relaxation/time alone
3. Extended family

18 Months

A. *Safety*
1. Review 12 months
2. Window safety
3. Falls

B. *Nutrition*
1. Feeding patterns and habits
2. Dental care

C. *Development*
1. Pretend play
2. Temper tantrums
3. Reinforce self-care
4. Self-comforting behavior
5. Peer interactions/sharing skills
6. Kick, throw a ball

D. *Health Care Management*
1. Exercise/activity
2. Sleeping habits
3. Elimination patterns

E. *Family Dynamics*
1. Child care
2. Parent relaxation/time alone
3. Extended family

24 Months

A. *Safety*
1. Review 12 months
2. Crib-to-bed transition
3. Car seat and helmet safety
4. Water safety
5. Storage of hazardous household supplies
6. Poison control
7. Street safety
8. Playground (slides, swings, bikes, and so on)
9. Firearm safety
10. Climbing
11. Lighters and matches
12. Motorized toys

B. *Nutrition*
1. Fun foods to eat
2. Feeding habits/daily intake
3. Dental care

C. *Development*
1. Peer interaction
2. Toileting habits
3. Common routines for eating
4. Bedtime routines
5. Story time
6. Praising good behavior
7. Two-word sentences, knowledge of approximately 250 words

D. *Health Care Management*
1. Laboratory studies: Hematocrit/hemoglobin
2. Urinalysis
3. Lead screening
4. Skin care
5. Elimination and voiding habits

E. *Family Dynamics*
1. Day care/child care
2. Extended family interactions
3. Sibling rivalry

3 to 4 Years

A. *Safety*
1. See topics at 24 months

B. *Nutrition*
1. Daily dietary intake
2. Healthy snacks

(*continued*)

EXHIBIT 1.4 Anticipatory Guidance (*continued*)

C. *Development*
  1. Pretend play
  2. Fears
  3. Fantasy
  4. Sleeping habits (night terrors)
  5. Setting realistic limits
  6. Praising good behavior
  7. Reading
  8. Music
  9. Child care

D. *Health Care Management*
  1. Dental
  2. Vision
  3. Hearing
  4. Speech evaluation
  5. Laboratory studies: Hematocrit/hemoglobin
  6. Tuberculosis (TB) skin test
  7. Lead screen

E. *Family Dynamics*
  1. Sibling rivalry
  2. Child care
  3. Parent time alone/relaxation

5 to 6 Years

A. *Safety*
  1. Review as discussed at previous visits
  2. Safety with strangers

B. *Nutrition*
  1. Healthy eating habits
  2. Healthy snacks

C. *Development*
  1. School readiness
  2. Sexual curiosity
  3. Peer interactions
  4. Good health habits (dental, diet, exercise, sleep)
  5. Praise good behavior
  6. Adult role models
  7. Fears
  8. Lying

D. *Health Care Management*
  1. Dental
  2. Vision
  3. Hearing

E. *Family Dynamics*
  1. Family traditions
  2. Changes in the family household (pets, moving, divorce)
  3. Sibling rivalry
  4. Extended family interactions

10 Years

A. *Safety*
  1. Car and cycle safety
  2. Pedestrian safety

B. *Nutrition*
  1. Daily intake
  2. Healthy snacks
  3. Healthy nutrition for athletes

C. *Development*
  1. School adjustments
  2. Social interactions
  3. Communications skills
  4. Health habits (same topics as ages 5–6)

D. *Health Care Management*
  1. Laboratory studies: Hemoglobin, hematocrit, urinalysis
  2. Vision
  3. Hearing
  4. Scoliosis
  5. TB skin test

E. *Family Dynamics*
  1. Sibling rivalry
  2. Extended family
  3. Parenting
  4. Family responsibilities/chores
  5. Family rituals
  6. Changes in family household (pets, moving, divorce)

15 Years

A. *Safety*
  1. Stranger awareness
  2. Car and cycle safety

B. *Nutrition*
  1. Diet, healthy habits
  2. *See Section III: Patient Teaching Guide for this chapter, "Adolescent Nutrition"*

C. *Development*
  1. Relationships with peers
  2. Body image
  3. Sexuality
  4. Self-esteem
  5. Peer pressure
  6. Decision making
  7. Role models
  8. School adjustments
  9. Extracurricular activities: Sports, hobbies, exercise
  10. Drug, alcohol, tobacco use
  11. Suicide

D. *Health Care Management*
  1. Cardiopulmonary resuscitation (CPR)
  2. Emergency numbers
  3. Skin care
  4. Vision
  5. Hearing
  6. Scoliosis
  7. TB skin test
  8. Hemoglobin, hematocrit

E. *Family Dynamics*
  1. Change in family household (pets, moving, divorce)
  2. Family responsibilities/chores
  3. Identifying role models
  4. Family events
  5. Earning an allowance

Source: American Academy of Family Physicians, American Academy of Pediatrics, American College of Sports Medicine, American Medical Society for Sports Medicine (2010). Copyright © 2010 American Academy of Pediatrics. Reproduced with permission.

Nutrition

Proper nutrition is an essential part of maintaining health and preventing diseases. Promote well-balanced diets for all patients with an emphasis on the prevention of obesity. Diet modification is an important part of disease or disorder management. The U.S. Department of Agriculture (USDA) provides a variety of interactive educational tools on nutrition, weight management, and physical activity. It is recommended that patients use these tools for family education on healthy diet and lifestyle. Diet information is found in Appendix B: Diet Recommendations (see also Tables 1.1–1.3 for more specific information).

TABLE 1.1 Nutrition for Kids: Guidelines for a Healthy Diet

	Daily Guidelines for Ages 2–3 Years	Daily Guidelines for Ages 4–8 Years		Daily Guidelines for Ages 9–13 Years		Daily Guidelines for Ages 14–18 Years	
	Girls and Boys	Girls	Boys	Girls	Boys	Girls	Boys
Calories dependent on growth and activity level	1,000–1,400	1,200–1,800	1,200–2,000	1,400–2,200	1,600–2,600	1,800–2,400	2,000–3,200
Protein	2–4 ounces	3–5 ounces	3–5.5 ounces	4–6 ounces	5–6.5 ounces	5–6.5 ounces	5.5–7 ounces
Fruits	1–1.5 cups	1–1.5 cups	1–2 cups	1.5–2 cups	1.5–2 cups	1.5–2 cups	2–2.5 cups
Vegetables	1–1.5 cups	1.5–2.5 cups	1.5–2.5 cups	1.5–3 cups	2–3.5 cups	2.5–3 cups	2.5–4 cups
Grains	3–5 ounces	4–6 ounces	4–6 ounces	5–7 ounces	5–9 ounces	6–8 ounces	6–10 ounces
Dairy	2–2.5 cups	2.5–3 cups	2.5–3 cups	2.5–3 cups	3 cups	3 cups	3 cups

Protein: Choose seafood, lean meat and poultry, eggs, beans, peas, soy products, and unsalted nuts and seeds.
Fruits: Encourage your child to eat a variety of fresh, canned, frozen, or dried fruits.
Vegetables: Serve a variety of fresh, canned, or frozen vegetables—especially dark green, red, and orange vegetables; beans; and peas.
Grains: Choose whole grains, such as whole-wheat bread, oatmeal, popcorn, quinoa, or brown or wild rice.
Dairy: Encourage your child to eat and drink fat-free or low-fat dairy products, such as milk, yogurt, cheese, or fortified soy beverages.

Source: Reprinted with permission from the Mayo Foundation for Medical Education and Research (2016) (www.mayoclinic.com/health/nutrition-for-kids/NU00606). All rights reserved.

TABLE 1.2 Recommended Number of Food Servings per Day

	Children			Teens		Adults			
	2–3 Years	4–8 Years	9–13 Years	14–18 Years		19–50 Years		51+ Years	
	Girls and Boys			Female	Male	Female	Male	Female	Male
Vegetables and fruits	4	5	6	7	8	7–8	8–10	7	7
Grain products	3	4	6	6	7	6–7	8	6	7
Milk and alternatives	2	2	3–4	3–4	2	2	3	3	3
Meat and alternatives	1	1	1–2	2	3	2	3	2	3

Source: Health Canada (www.hc-sc.gc.ca/fn-an/food-guide-aliment/order-commander/eating_well_bien_manger-eng.php).

TABLE 1.3 Food Sources for Common Vitamin and Mineral Deficiencies

Common Nutritional Deficiencies	Food Sources
Calcium	Dairy sources of calcium include, yogurt, and cheese.
	Nondairy sources of calcium are vegetables, including kale, broccoli, and Chinese cabbage.
	Calcium is also found in fortified sources, including breakfast cereals, fruit juices, and tofu.
Folate	Found naturally in vegetables (especially dark green leafy vegetables), fruits, fruit juices, nuts, beans, peas, dairy products, poultry and meat, eggs, seafood, and grains.
	In January 1998, the U.S. Food and Drug Administration began requiring manufacturers to add folic acid to enriched breads, cereals, flours, cornmeal, pasta, rice, and other grain products.
Iron	Heme iron is found in animal foods that originally contained hemoglobin, including red meat, fish, and poultry.
	Nonheme iron is found in plant foods, including lentils and beans.
	Iron is also found in fortified ready-to-eat cereals.
Magnesium	Widely distributed in plant and animal foods, including green leafy vegetables, legumes, nuts (almonds, peanuts, and cashews), seeds, and whole grains.
	Magnesium is also found in fortified breakfast cereals.

(*continued*)

TABLE 1.3 Food Sources for Common Vitamin and Mineral Deficiencies (*continued*)

Common Nutritional Deficiencies	Food Sources
Vitamin A	Concentrations of preformed vitamin A are highest in liver, fish oils, leafy green vegetables, orange and yellow vegetables, tomato products, fruits, and some vegetable oils.
	Vitamin A is also found in fortified breakfast cereals.
Vitamin B_6	Richest sources include fish; beef, liver, and other organ meats; potatoes and other starchy vegetables such as chickpeas; and fruit (except for citrus).
	Vitamin B_6 is also found in fortified breakfast cereals.
Vitamin B_{12}	Found naturally in animal products, including fish, meat, poultry, eggs, and milk and milk products.
	Generally not present in plant foods.
	Vitamin B_{12} is found in fortified breakfast cereals.
Vitamin D	Very few foods in nature contain vitamin D; it is found primarily in fortified foods.
	Almost all of the U.S. milk supply is voluntarily fortified with vitamin D.
	Both the United States and Canada mandate the fortification of infant formula with vitamin D.
Vitamin E	Found in nuts and seeds (sunflower seeds, almonds, hazelnuts, and peanuts), green leafy vegetables, and vegetable oils.
	Vitamin E is found in fortified breakfast cereals.
Zinc	Red meat and poultry provide the majority of zinc in American diets; however, oysters contain more zinc per serving than any other food. Other food sources include beans, nuts, seafood (crab and lobster), and dairy products.
	Zinc is also found in fortified breakfast cereals.

Source: National Institutes of Health, Office of Dietary Supplements (2015) (https://ods.od.nih.gov/factsheets/Mvms-HealthProfessional).

The obesity epidemic is the responsibility of all health care providers. Each office visit is an opportunity to evaluate the patient's weight and to discuss exercise programs. As the pain assessment becomes the "fifth vital sign" in the hospital setting, the body mass index (BMI) becomes the fifth vital sign in the outpatient setting.

Teaching parents the correct serving sizes for children will help guide their children's eating habits for life. Dr. Debby Demory-Luce (2004) notes the rule of thumb for measuring portion sizes for fruits and vegetables is "one tablespoon per year of life" for children aged 1 to 6 years. Serving sizes for older children and adults are based on the food pyramids. Use the food pyramid to teach and reinforce proper nutrition. Some helpful websites about nutrition are as follows:

A. The USDA resources for nutrition and health are located at www.choosemyplate.gov

B. My Plate kids' place is located at https://www.choosemyplate.gov/kids

C. Nutrition Expedition Games for children are available at www.nutritionexplorations.org/kids.php

D. The Childhood Nutrition website is located at www.nourishinteractive.com. This informative website gives helpful information such as:

1. Controlling portion sizes
2. Parent tips tool
3. Interactive nutrition tools
4. A fun area for children with interactive nutrition games
5. Healthy living tips ready to print

Height and weight are used to calculate BMI. The mathematical calculation is BMI = kg/m^2; however, the Internet provides easy-to-use BMI calculators.

A. The National Heart, Lung, and Blood Institute (NHLBI, n.d.) includes a calculator in its Obesity Education Initiative: www.nhlbi.nih.gov/health/educational/lose_wt/BMI/bmicalc.htm. This support site also includes patient information on risk assessment, weight control, and helpful recipes.

B. The CDC provides an online source for the calculation of BMI for children and teens: https://nccd.cdc.gov/dnpabmi/calculator.aspx

The CDC's website also provides information on weight loss, physical activity, and parental tips.

Malnutrition and vitamin and mineral deficiency are commonly seen in the elderly population. Vitamins B_6, B_{12}, D, E, folic acid, zinc, calcium, and iron are often deficient in the elderly diet, along with protein and calorie deficiencies. Using Zawada's (1996) acronym WEIGHT LOSS can help you easily identify common causes of weight loss in the elderly.

W: Wandering and not eating, because of forgetting to take time to eat
E: Emotional problems, including depression
I: Impecuniosity (finances do not meet the needs to buy food and other things)
G: Gut problems
H: Hyperthyroidism or other endocrine abnormalities
T: Tremor or neurologic problems that make eating and holding utensils difficult
L: Low-salt, low-cholesterol diets avoided, often because of disliking the taste of recommended diets

O: Oral problems: edentulous, poor dental care, dentures not fitting, mouth disorders such as oral ulcers

S: Swallowing problems, difficulty swallowing or chewing food because of stroke or other impairment

S: Shopping or food preparation barriers, inability to purchase or prepare food, and no resources for assistance

Identification of factor(s) contributing to an elderly patient's malnutrition assists you, the patient, and the patient's family in resolving them. Utilize your state's Area Agencies on Aging (AAA) for information on elder care resources in your area (websites not provided because they are state specific).

Exercise

Physical exercise is a vital component of health maintenance. Exercise provides cardiovascular fitness and weight control, prevents osteoporosis through weight-bearing exercise, and decreases lipids. Exercise is important for flexibility, strength, and coordination. Exercise can also be used for both weight control and reduction. Approximately 3,500 calories must be burned to lose 1 pound of fat. Therefore, along with exercise, caloric intake must remain the same or decrease to result in weight loss.

Planning an Exercise Program

Exercise plans should be started after a health provider screens a patient, because heavy physical exertion may trigger an acute myocardial infarction. Factors most likely to influence risk are age, medical conditions, hypertension, and the intensity of the exercise planned. The medical history screening identifies individual and family history of problems such as coronary heart disease, hypertension, and diabetes. Review health habits such as previous exercise or sedentary lifestyle, diet, and smoking.

Providers need to evaluate the patient using screening tests before prescribing an exercise program. Consider the patient's age and all comorbidities for additional tests.

A. Complete blood count
B. Blood glucose
C. Cholesterol screening
D. EKG (in patients older than 40 years)
E. Holter monitoring for arrhythmias

Persons with a heart murmur or other abnormal physical finding should defer exercise until the full nature of the disorder is evaluated. The best measure of an exercise work capacity is the determination of oxygen consumption at maximal activity, which is measured with a stress test. Hypertension, elevated resting blood pressures, and chronic obstructive lung disease are other factors that require attention before participation in exercise. Persons with hypertension should undergo a thorough evaluation, have antihypertensive agent(s) prescribed, and be monitored periodically during their prescribed graded exercise program.

Physical exercise should be strictly monitored in the following conditions and may need to be curtailed, or even stopped, based on the condition:

A. **Congestive heart failure**
B. **Uncontrolled hypertension**
C. **Uncontrolled epilepsy**
D. **Uncontrolled diabetes**
E. **Atrioventricular (AV) heart block**
F. **Aneurysms**
G. **Ventricular instability**
H. **Aortic valve disease**

Measurement of the heart rate during exercise is an easy and inexpensive method to evaluate cardiovascular fitness. Target heart rates vary by physical condition and a person's age. The following formula is used to evaluate target heart/aerobic activity level:

[220 – (age of individual)] × 0.65 = Maximum heart rate range

Maximum heart rate × 0.65 = Minimum aerobic effect

Maximum heart rate × 0.85 = Maximum aerobic effect

Patient Education Before Exercise

All exercise program prescriptions should include frequency, duration, intensity, and time to abort the exercise. Persons should be educated on the signs and symptoms of heat exhaustion and should be advised when to seek first aid.

Exercise programs with aerobic activity at least three times a week on nonconsecutive days is the minimal amount of exercise individuals should set as a goal. The target heart rate should be sustained for 20 to 30 minutes for maximal cardiovascular effect.

Women engaged in regular physical exercise before pregnancy may safely continue exercise throughout pregnancy. The target heart rate for a pregnant woman during exercise should not exceed 140 beats per minute. Activities should also be limited to low-impact aerobics and activities that do not require agility, because a woman's center of balance changes throughout pregnancy, leaving the woman at risk of falling and injury.

Swimming is ideal for upper and lower body conditioning, with low impact on joints. Swimming is not well suited for women at risk of osteoporosis, because it is not a weight-bearing exercise. Examples of weight-bearing exercise to help prevent osteoporosis include dancing, impact aerobics, and resistance training.

For exercise to benefit individuals, it must be continued lifelong. The health care provider should evaluate individual lifestyle and preferences in designing an exercise program. One exercise program can become boring over a period and probably will not be continued. A variety of activities, class participation, and positive reinforcement help to keep physical activity fun as an integral part of a health maintenance program. *See Section III: Patient Teaching Guide for this chapter, "Exercise."* ◀

Health care professionals who will be monitoring and prescribing exercise plans for large numbers of individuals are encouraged to seek special training and certification. The American College of Sports Medicine has a program that includes training for health care professionals.

Other Collaborating Providers

Jill C. Cash and Debbie Gunter

The role of the primary care provider is to ensure that the patient becomes a partner in preventive health measures to avoid disease comorbidities. The practitioner should refer the patient to other health care providers to continue health maintenance.

A. Dental care
   1. Dental care should be routinely discussed.
   2. Once teeth emerge, brushing should begin with a small soft brush.
   3. In children, dental care should begin with soft, rubber brushes for gum care.
   4. Encourage the child to brush teeth twice daily to promote healthy habits.
   5. Refer the patient to a dentist at 3 years, unless problems arise earlier.
   6. Older child should be encouraged to use mouth guards with contact sports.
   7. Encourage flossing when the child has the cognitive and developmental dexterity to use dental floss.

B. Vision care
   1. Begin initial vision screening for children at 3 years of age using the age-appropriate eye chart.
   2. School screening should include a vision-screening component.
   3. Refer patients to an optometrist for routine evaluation.

Adult Risk Assessment Form

Jill C. Cash and Debbie Gunter

The Adult Risk Assessment Form (Exhibit 1.5) should be used for all adult patients. It is used to evaluate a patient's

EXHIBIT 1.5 **Adult Risk Assessment Form**

Name __________ DOB __________ Chart # __________

Allergies ______________________________

Occupation ______________________________

Assess the patient for the following risk factors:

Family History First-degree relatives with remarkable diseases (e.g., hypertension, diabetes mellitus, coronary artery disease [CAD], cancer, and thyroid)	
1.	6.
2.	7.
3.	8.
4.	9.
5.	10.

A. Coronary heart disease
   1. High-fat/high-cholesterol diet
   2. Obese
   3. Elevated cholesterol level
   4. Stroke
   5. Hypertension
   6. Tobacco use

B. Lung cancer
   1. High-fat/high-cholesterol diet
   2. Tobacco use

C. Cervical cancer
   1. Early age of first intercourse
   2. Multiple sexual partners

D. Breast cancer
   1. Nulliparous
   2. Primigravida after age 35 years
   3. High-fat diet

E. Colon cancer
   1. History of polyps
   2. High-fat diet

F. Osteoporosis
   1. Less than 1 g of calcium per day
   2. History of tobacco or alcohol use
   3. Sedentary lifestyle
   4. Thin, Caucasian
   5. Female gender

G. Glaucoma/visual impairment
   1. Family history of glaucoma
   2. Diabetes mellitus

H. Sexually transmitted infections (STIs)/HIV
   1. Alcohol and drug use or abuse
   2. Multiple sexual partners
   3. Homosexual or bisexual partner
   4. History of intravenous drug use
   5. History of blood transfusion
   6. Exposed to or past history of STI

I. Substance abuse
   1. Alcohol or drug use history
   2. Family history of substance abuse
   3. Stress or poor coping mechanisms
   4. Administer the *CAGE* assessment:
      Have you ever tried to Cut down on your alcohol/drug use?
      Do you get Annoyed if someone mentions your use is a problem?
      Do you ever feel Guilty about your use?
      Do you ever have an "Eye-opener" first thing in the morning after you have been drinking or using the night before?

J. Accidents and suicide
   1. Family history of suicide
   2. Alcohol or tobacco use
   3. History of depression
   4. High-stress or "hot-reactor" personality
   5. Male gender
   6. Alcohol use
   7. Previous suicide attempt
   8. Poor coping mechanisms or stress

K. Safety
   1. Does not use seat belt or car seat
   2. Drinks and drives
   3. Drives over the speed limit
   4. Does not wear safety helmet if driving motorcycle
   5. Inadequate number of smoke detectors or none in the home
   6. Firearms in the home
   7. Feels safe at home/at risk for domestic violence

risk for particular diseases. The practitioner should interview the patient, assessing for the risk factors listed on the Risk Assessment Form. The family history of first-degree relatives (parents, siblings, and children) should also be discussed, as many diseases are related to genetic factors. Keep a copy of the Risk Assessment Form in the front of the patient's chart, and update yearly or as needed. When complete, this tool can guide the practitioner in determining the assessment needs of each patient.

Adult Preventive Health Care

Jill C. Cash and Debbie Gunter

The flow sheet given in Exhibit 1.6 helps the practitioner identify changes in the adult patient's risk factor status, make recommendations for health maintenance (e.g., immunizations, laboratory work, physical examinations), and educate patients in prevention (Exhibit 1.7). Screening guidelines for each of these can be found in the associated chapters in this book, according to the national association recommendations (e.g., screening recommendations for mammograms were obtained from the American Cancer Society). The Adult Health Maintenance Guide in Exhibit 1.7 can be used as a quick reference for the practitioner to evaluate the patient's adherence to preventive measures. Keep a copy of this flow sheet and guide in the front of the patient's chart where they can be reviewed routinely and updated as necessary. If using electronic medical records, a special section should be identified as routine health maintenance.

EXHIBIT 1.6 Adult Preventive Health Care Flow Sheet

Immunization Schedule				
Immunization	**Date**	**Date**	**Date**	**Date**
Tetanus/diphtheria				
Measles, mumps, rubella (MMR)				
Tuberculosis (TB; yearly)				
Hepatitis B (HepB)				
Influenza (yearly)				
Pneumonococcal				
Zoster vaccine				
Other				

Assess patients for the following behaviors:

Risk Assessment				
Examination	**Date**	**Date**	**Date**	**Date**
Tobacco, amount				
Alcohol, amount				
Substance use				
Domestic violence				
Depression screening				

Patients should be educated about any behavior modifications that can reduce their risk factors for health problems. The practitioner should note the date as well as the type of counseling given to a patient.

Patient Education				
Behavior Modification	**Date**	**Date**	**Date**	**Date**
Diet/exercise				
Tobacco/alcohol				
Injury prevention				
Skin protection				
Hormone replacement therapy				
Sexual practices				
Occupational hazards				
Self-examination: Breast/testicular				

EXHIBIT 1.7 **Adult Health Maintenance Guide**

Name ______________ DOB ______________ Chart # ______________

Allergies ______________ Occupation ______________

The following tests should be performed according to the individual patient's risk factors, as part of preventive health care. The practitioner should fill in the date and result of each test and highlight any remarkable results. This list is not exhaustive and special populations may need additional screenings. www.uspreventiveservicestaskforce.org/BrowseRec/Index/browse-recommendations

Test	Date	Result	Date	Result	Date	Result	Date	Result
Height								
Weight								
Body mass index (BMI)								
Blood pressure (B/P)								
Skin examination								
Oral cavity examination								
EKG								
Thyroid-stimulating hormone (TSH)								
Lipid profile								
Urinalysis								
Rectal examination								
Hemoccult								
Chest x-ray (lung cancer screening)								
Colonoscopy								
Prostate-specific antigen (PSA)								
Testicular examination								
Pelvic examination/Pap smear								
Breast examination								
Mammogram								
Bone mineral density								
Sexually transmitted disease (STD)/HIV								
Additionally, the practitioner should ensure that the patient receives other health care as needed. Assess the patient's adherence to other preventive health care examinations:								
Dental examination								
Vision/glaucoma examination								

Immunizations

The CDC is the primary source for the current immunization schedules. Consult the CDC's website for pocket-sized schedules, printable versions, and versions for mobile devices. The download information for your smartphone is available on the CDC website at www.cdc.gov/vaccines/schedules/hcp/child-adolescent.html

Immunizations for Travel

The CDC recommends certain vaccines to protect travelers from illnesses present in other parts of the world and to protect others on return to the United States. The CDC's Travelers' Health website is located at www.cdc.gov; it is an interactive website to individualize the needs of travelers to their specific destination. Vaccinations required are dependent on several factors:

A. Travel destination
B. Travel season
C. Age
D. Pregnancy or breastfeeding
E. Traveling with infants or children
F. Immunocompetent secondary to diabetes or HIV

The CDC also has a Health Education sheet for travelers at www.cdc.gov/travel/page/traveler-information-center

Immunization Links: 2016

- Recommended immunization schedule for persons aged 0 through 18 years—2016 is available at: www.cdc.gov/vaccines/schedules/downloads/child/0-18yrs-schedule-bw.pdf
- Catchup immunization schedule for persons aged 4 months through 18 years who started late or who are more than 1 month behind—United States—2016 is available at: www.cdc.gov/vaccines/schedules/downloads/child/catchup-schedule-bw.pdf
- Recommended adult immunization schedule—United States—2016 is available at: www.cdc.gov/vaccines/schedules/downloads/adult/adult-schedule-bw.pdf
- Recommended vaccination of persons with primary and secondary immunodeficiencies is available at: www.cdc.gov/mmwr/preview/mmwrhtml/rr6002a1.htm; www.cdc.gov/vaccines/schedules/hcp/imz/child-adolescent.html; www.cdc.gov/vaccines/schedules/hcp/imz/catchup.html

Beers Criteria for Medication Use in Older Adults

Check the Beers list for harmful drugs in the geriatric population. The 2015 American Geriatrics Society Updated Beers Criteria for Potentially Inappropriate Medication Use in Older Adults is available at https://www.guideline.gov/summaries/summary/49933/american-geriatrics-society-2015-updated-beers-criteria-for-potentially-inappropriate-medication-use-in-older-adults.

Bibliography

Allender, J. A., Rector, C., & Warner, K. D. (2013). *Community health nursing* (8th ed.). Philadelphia, PA: Kluwer/Lippincott Williams & Wilkins.

American Academy of Family Physicians, American Academy of Pediatrics, American College of Sports Medicine, American Medical Society for Sports Medicine. (2010). *Preparticipation physical evaluation* (4th ed.). Elk Grove Village, IL: American Academy of Pediatrics.

Andrews, M. M., & Boyle, J. S. (2015). *Transcultural concepts in nursing care* (7th ed.). Philadelphia, PA: Lippincott Williams & Wilkins.

Benton, J. (2003). Making schools safer and healthier for lesbian, gay, bisexual, and questioning students. *Journal of School Nursing: The Official Publication of the National Association of School Nurses, 19*(5), 251–259.

Bernhardt, D. T. (2015). Concussion. *Medscape.* Retrieved from www.medscape.com

Centers for Disease Control and Prevention. (2015, March 11). Cultural competence. Retrieved from https://npin.cdc.gov/pages/cultural-competence

Centers for Disease Control and Prevention. (2016a). CDC catchup immunization schedule for persons aged 4 months through 18 years who start late or who are more than 1 month behind—United States 2016. Retrieved from https://www.cdc.gov/vaccines/schedules/hcp/imz/catchup.html

Centers for Disease Control and Prevention. (2016b). CDC recommended adult immunization schedule—United States 2016. Retrieved from https://www.cdc.gov/vaccines/schedules/hcp/adult.html

Centers for Disease Control and Prevention (CDC). (2016c). CDC recommended immunization schedule for persons aged 0 through 6 years—United States 2016. Retrieved from https://www.cdc.gov/vaccines/schedules/hcp/imz/child-adolescent.html

Centers for Disease Control and Prevention. (2016d). Information for travelers. Retrieved from www.cdc.gov/travel/page/traveler-information-center

Centers for Disease Control and Prevention. (n.d.a). BMI percentile calculator for child and teen: English version Retrieved from https://nccd.cdc.gov/dnpabmi/calculator.aspx

Centers for Disease Control and Prevention. (n.d.b). Growth charts. Retrieved from https://www.cdc.gov/growthcharts

Centers for Disease Control and Prevention. (n.d. c). Immunization applications for PC/handhelds. Retrieved from https://www.cdc.gov/vaccines/pubs/vis/vis-downloads.htm

Childhood Nutrition. (n.d.). Serving sizes. Retrieved from http://www.nourishinteractive.com/parents_area/healthy_family_nutrition_newsletter/portion_control_childhood_easy_weight_management_tips_reducing_kids_food_serving_sizes

Douglas, M. K., Rosenkoetter, M., Pacquiao, D. F., Callister, L. C., Hattar-Pollara, M., Lauderdale, J., . . . Purnell, L. (2014). Guidelines for implementing culturally competent nursing care. *Journal of Transcultural Nursing: Official Journal of the Transcultural Nursing Society/Transcultural Nursing Society, 25*(2), 109–121.

Health Canada. (2007). How much food you need every day. Retrieved from http://www.hc-sc.gc.ca/fn-an/food-guide-aliment/basics-base/quantit-eng.php

Huber, D. L. (2013). *Leadership and nursing care management* (5th ed.). St. Louis, MO: Saunders.

Mayo Foundation for Medical Education and Research. (2016, January). Nutrition for kids: Guidelines for a healthy diet. Retrieved from http://www.mayoclinic.com/health/nutrition-for-kids/NU00606

Miller, N., Reicks, M., Redden, J. P., Mann, T., Mykerezi, E., & Vickers, Z. (2015). Increasing portion sizes of fruits and vegetables in an elementary school lunch program can increase fruit and vegetable consumption. *Appetite, 91*, 426–430.

Mirabelli, M. H., Devine, M. J., Singh, J., & Mendoza, M. (2015). The preparticipation sports evaluation. *American Family Physician, 92*(5), 371–376.

Muronda, V. (2016, July). The culturally diverse nursing student: A review of the literature. *Journal of Transcultural Nursing, 4*, 400–412.

National Heart Lung and Blood Institute. (n.d.). Obesity education initiative: BMI calculator. Retrieved from http://www.nhlbi.nih.gov/health/educational/lose_wt/BMI/bmicalc.htm

National Institutes of Health, Office of Dietary Supplements. (2015). Food sources for common vitamin and mineral deficiencies. Retrieved from https://ods.od.nih.gov/factsheets/Mvms-HealthProfessional/

Pigozi, P. L., & Jones Bartoli, A. (2016). School nurses' experiences in dealing with bullying situations among students. *Journal of School Nursing: The Official Publication of the National Association of School Nurses, 32*(3), 177–185.

Purnell, L. D., & Paulanka, B. J. (2013). *Transcultural health care: A culturally competent approach* (4th ed.). Philadelphia, PA: F. A. Davis.

Ritchie, C. (2015, October 22). Geriatric nutrition: Nutritional issues in older adults. *UpToDate.* Retrieved from http://www.uptodate.com/contents/geriatric-nutrition-nutritional-issues-in-older-adults

Sanders, B., Blackburn, T. A., & Boucher, B. (2013). Preparticipation screening: The sports physical therapy perspective. *International Journal of Sports Physical Therapy, 8*(2), 180–193.

Sharma, S., Merghani, A., & Gati, S. (2015). Cardiac screening of young athletes prior to participation in sports: Difficulties in detecting the fatally flawed among the fabulously fit. *JAMA Internal Medicine, 175*(1), 125–127.

Spector, R. E. (2012). *Cultural diversity in health and illness* (8th ed.). Upper Saddle River, NJ: Prentice-Hall.

Stepler, R. (2016). *World's centenarian population projected to grow eightfold by 2050.* Washington, DC: *Pew Research Center.* Retrieved from http://www.pewresearch.org/fact-tank/2016/04/21/worlds-centenarian-population-projected-to-grow-eightfold-by-2050

U.S. Census. (n.d.). Quickfacts. Retrieved from https://quickfacts.census.gov/qfd/staes/oooo.html

U.S. Department of Agriculture. (n.d.). Food pyramid. Retrieved from https//:www.choosemyplate.gov

U.S. Department of Agriculture. (n.d.). My Plate kids' place. Retrieved from https://www.choosemyplate.gov/kids

Zawada, E. (1996). Malnutrition in the elderly: Is it simply a matter of not eating enough? *Postgraduate Medicine, 100(1)*, 208.

2 Public Health Guidelines

Homelessness

Robertson Nash

Overview

Homelessness is a multifaceted structural problem that has a syndemic effect on people. The term *syndemic* refers to situations in which the net effect of multiple physical and social comorbidities is worse than the sum of the individual effects (Merrill, 2009). In the case of people experiencing homelessness, consider all of the possible interactions among unmanaged chronic diseases (diabetes mellitus type 2, hypertension, hyperlipidemia), multiple caries and gingival abscesses, chronic soft tissue infections, and untreated depression and anxiety. For people without the support of stable housing and nutrition, these interactions can be overwhelming. Data show that, on average, people who are chronically homeless live approximately 20 years less than their housed peers.

Definition (Federal)

A. The U.S. Department of Housing and Urban Development (HUD) is responsible for defining the criteria by which an individual's housing status is assessed. The required criteria for the determination of homelessness include the following (HUD, 2011):

1. Individuals and families who lack a fixed, regular, and adequate nighttime residence OR an individual residing in an emergency shelter or place not fit for human habitation OR an individual exiting an institution that provided temporary residence

2. Individuals and families at imminent risk of losing their primary nighttime residence

3. Unaccompanied youth and families with children not otherwise qualifying as homeless

4. Individuals and families fleeing or attempting to flee dating/domestic violence, sexual assault, stalking, or other dangerous or life-threatening situations

B. In order to meet the criteria of "chronically homeless," an individual has to be determined to have been homeless either continuously for at least 12 months, or on at least four separate occasions in the past 3 years, with a total experience of homelessness greater than 12 months. Both families and individuals may meet this definition (HUD, 2015).

Incidence

A. According to data published by the HUD, on a given night in January 2013, an estimated 610,042 people were homeless. Of these, an estimated 394,698 were sheltered and 215, 344 were unsheltered (Henry, Cortes, & Morris, 2013). According to this same source, total homelessness in the United States has declined by more than 9% between 2007 and 2013 (Henry et al., 2013).

Pathogenesis

A. Homelessness is a catastrophic experience at the individual level. However, most of the factors that contribute to homelessness are structural in nature and are beyond the control of any one patient or provider. For example, cities with an inadequate supply of Section 8 housing will not be able to provide people experiencing homelessness with a place to live. Furthermore, the disparity between federal and state minimum wages and the living wage translate into people who work 40 or more hours a week who are often unable to secure housing.

Predisposing Factors

A. Chronic illnesses: People who are homeless suffer from chronic illnesses at rates that exceed those in the general population. In many cases, overlapping and negatively interacting manifestations of illness exacerbate each other, leading to several complicated comorbidities whose management may tax the resources available to both patient and provider.

Common Complaints

A. Cough/upper respiratory infection
B. Sinusitis
C. Soft tissue infections
D. Dental abscesses/gingivitis
E. Tinea pedis
F. Pest infestations
G. Mental health-related complaints

Other Signs and Symptoms

A. Does the patient smell of smoke, as if he or she has been sleeping outdoors by a fire? If so, this would trigger a chest x-ray and detailed pulmonary examination.

B. Does the patient smell of urine, suggesting a possible urinary tract infection? If so, this would trigger a genitourinary skin examination, urinalysis, and social work consult regarding access to clean clothing.

C. Unilateral lower extremity pitting edema, pain, and tenderness suggest the presence of a deep vein thrombosis, which is considered a medical emergency.

D. Bilateral lower extremity pitting edema may be a sign of heart failure. This finding would trigger a thorough clinical examination for the following: S3, S4 heart sounds, jugular venous pulse, and jugular venous distension.
E. Brawny edema and venous stasis ulcerations would trigger a thorough peripheral vascular examination and a sensory examination of the plantar surfaces of both feet.
F. Itchiness suggests pest infestation, needs treatment, shower, wash cloth, new clothes, and contact shelter to treat the environment
G. Unusual behavior; for example, hallucination, visible depression, intoxication and so on refer to mental health

Subjective Data: Factors to Consider When Evaluating People Experiencing Homelessness

A. Where did the patient sleep last? Does the patient have a safe place to sleep tonight?
B. When was the last time the patient was able to bathe?
C. When was the last time the patient ate?
D. Is the patient able to find bathrooms when needed?
E. Are symptoms of depression and anxiety interfering with survival?
F. Is the patient being physically, sexually, or emotionally abused?
G. Is the patient being forced to engage in behaviors against his or her will in exchange for food and shelter?
H. Does the patient have a safe way to manage medications on the street, such as, insulin?
▶ **I.** Assess/discuss current substance abuse. *See Section III: Patient Teaching Guide for this chapter, "Alcohol and Drug Dependence."*

Physical Examination

Providers should be aware that, due to past trauma, many people experiencing homelessness are reluctant to touch. Take your time with the physical examination, ask permission for each step of the physical examination, and explain what you are doing and why.
A. Check temperature, pulse, respirations, and blood pressure.
B. Inspect
 1. Scalp—assess for nits.
 2. Oral cavity—assess for caries, or active oral abscesses.
 3. Assess skin for burns, abrasions, trauma, and evidence of accidental or intentional injury. Visualize both feet for infection and trauma.
C. Palpate the abdomen for tenderness or masses. Perform pelvic examination as appropriate. This may not be possible on the first examination. For some females, intentionally poor hygiene is viewed as protection against male assault.
D. Auscultate heart, lungs, and abdomen.
E. Neurologic examination
 1. Assess for neuropathy in feet.
 2. Assess hearing and vision, as these faculties are central to survival when living on the street.
F. Mental health examination
 1. Perform depression/anxiety screening. See depression/anxiety in Chapter 22: Psychiatric Guidelines, for screening.
 2. Evaluate suicidal ideation. See Chapter 22: Psychiatric Guidelines, for assessment/screening.
 3. Assess for active audio/visual hallucinations.
 4. Assess for paranoia.

Diagnostic Tests

A. Complete blood count (CBC)
B. Comprehensive metabolic panel (CMP)
C. B_{12}/folate
D. Urine: Urinalysis for protein/glucose and *Neisseria gonorrhea*/Chlamydia
E. Rapid plasma reagin (RPR)
F. HIV
G. HAV/HBV profile, hepatitis C virus antibody
H. Glycosylated hemoglobin A1c
I. Purified protein derivative (PPD)/T-SPOT

Differential Diagnoses

A. Homelessness
B. Substance use/abuse
C. Depression
D. Malnutrition
E. Schizophrenia

Plan

A. General interventions
 1. There are no disease-based standards of care that specifically address people who are homeless. Rather, providers must be creative and resourceful, working with patients toward higher levels of self-efficacy within the resource bounds imposed on the situation by society at large.
 2. Community-based care: No single provider or ancillary service organization (ASO) can provide all of the care needed for people experiencing homelessness. In order to maximize care, providers should make an effort to identify and be in communication with their local ASOs before a crisis, so that resources can be coordinated and maximized when acute issues arise.
 3. Identifying and assisting the patient with current health needs is imperative. In addition to addressing homelessness, the patient may have other acute and chronic health conditions that should be addressed and treated as appropriate.
B. Patient teaching
 1. Lifestyle modifications, focusing on diet, exercise, and smoking cessation, form the cornerstone of advanced practice nurse (APN) patient teaching for chronic disease management. The following principles should be used to guide the teaching of these principles in this population:
  a. People experiencing homelessness rarely have access to exercise facilities. In addition, they often lack a safe place to store their belongings while they exercise.
  b. People experiencing homelessness have little to no control over their food selection. Dependence on volunteer-driven, charity-led food banks and meal programs is a significant impediment to healthy eating, as many of these programs assume

that a high-carbohydrate, calorie-dense meal, such as spaghetti and bread, is what people experiencing homelessness like and want to eat.

c. The prevalence of poor dentition among the homeless greatly exceeds that of the stably housed, employed population. Accordingly, people experiencing homelessness may not be able to eat fresh fruits and vegetables.

d. The rates of substance abuse among the chronically homeless exceed those in the general population. Some people may be successfully clean and sober from alcohol, some yet continue to smoke tobacco. Although this is not ideal, focus on patient strengths, praise sobriety, and acknowledge that smoking cessation is perceived as being more difficult than sobriety from alcohol and may need to have a lower priority in a patient's overall plan of care.

e. Blanket dietary and exercise recommendations developed around stably housed, fully employed people will likely not translate well to people experiencing homelessness. Failure to account for the unique challenges of people experiencing homelessness will exacerbate feelings of depression, low self-worth, and decreased self-efficacy.

f. Caring for individuals experiencing homelessness requires a team approach. Successful teams include clinicians, social workers, behavioral health providers, psychiatric providers, and also nursing staff. No one provider or discipline can address all of the needs of people experiencing homelessness. It is also critical that the care team work well together and prioritize the work of building rapport with the patient, whose life experiences have likely reinforced his/her distrust of the systems that we all depend on to deliver care.

Follow-Up

A. One of the primary challenges facing providers of those experiencing homelessness is the deep-seated lack of trust that these people have in the health care system within which most providers operate. In order to encourage people to return to the clinic for appropriate follow-up care, every effort must be made during the first visit to establish a true therapeutic relationship with the patient. Providers should attempt to work with patients to identify and address concerns that are important to the patient. Providers should remember that topics, such as smoking cessation and sobriety from alcohol may best be deferred during an initial visit. All clinic staff should be trained to treat all patients with a professional, welcoming, and empathetic manner.

Consultation/Referral

A. Referring patients to specialists is an everyday part of primary care, and advanced practice nurses serve important screening and gatekeeper functions in this role. However, the insurance-based system that we rely on for care is not available to most people experiencing homelessness, as they lack health insurance. Should insurance be available, then providers must still identify specialists willing to take specific insurances and work with people experiencing homelessness. Effective providers will identify specialists in their local communities and seek to build relationships that will facilitate referrals. Given the lack of access to transportation in this population, it is important to set an expectation that a missed appointment does not mean that the patient does not want or need care, and that specialists may need to be flexible regarding missed appointments with people in this population.

Individual Considerations

A. Pediatrics/minors: According to data published by the National Association for the Education of Homeless Children and Youth (NAEHCY, www.naehcy.org), there are between 1.6 and 1.7 million children experiencing homelessness every year in the United States. The majority of these children have been physically and/or sexually abused. Providers are strongly encouraged to review related content on the NAEHCY website. Additionally, providers should make contact with their community YMCA/YWCA resources to develop a referral plan should a homeless minor present for care. Please remember that homeless youth are likely to be extremely mistrustful of medical, social work, and law enforcement professionals.

B. Pregnancy: All pregnant women who are experiencing homeless and present for care should be seen by a social worker before leaving the site. In cases where abuse is suspected, law enforcement must be notified.

Elderly: All people older than 60 years of age who are experiencing homeless and present for care should be seen by a social worker before leaving the site. In cases where abuse is suspected, law enforcement must be notified.

Resources

Federal

HUD exchange: Homelessness assistance: www.hudexchange.info
National Coalition to End Homelessness: www.nationalhomeless.org
National Health Care for the Homeless Council: www.nhchc.org

State

Providers should use the Internet search engine of choice to locate emergency shelters and care for people experiencing homelessness in their locale. There is no centralized database of state/local shelters. Many larger shelters will have a list of local places for people to find food and community assistance, and this information can be invaluable for providers to keep on hand.

Classic Texts

King, T. E, Jr., & Wheeler, M. E. (Eds.). (2007). *Medical management of vulnerable and underserved populations*. New York, NY: McGraw-Hill.
O'Connell, J. J. (Ed.). (2004). *The health care of homeless persons*. Boston, MA: Boston Healthcare for the Homeless Program.

Obesity

Angelito Tacderas and Bunny Pounds

Definition

A. Obesity is a multifactorial disease with physical, psychological, and social consequences. The body mass index (BMI) is a standard measuring tool. The BMI is calculated by using the formula: Weight in kilograms divided by height in meters squared (weight [kg]/height [m]^2). In adults, obesity is defined as a BMI greater than 30 kg/m^2.

TABLE 2.1 Childhood Obesity by Percentiles

Childhood Obesity Category	BMI Definitions by Percentiles
Underweight	Less than the fifth percentile
Healthy weight	Fifth to less than 85th percentile
Overweight	85th to less than 95th percentile
Obese	Equal to or greater than 95th percentile

BMI, body mass index.

TABLE 2.2 Adult Obesity by BMI

Classification of Adult Obesity by BMI	BMI (kg/m²)
Underweight	<18.5
Normal	18.5–24.9
Overweight (preobese)	25.0–29.9
Obesity	30.0–34.9
Severely obese	>40.0
Morbidly obese	40.0–49.9
Super obese	>50.0
Super-super obese (SSO)	≥60.0

BMI, body mass index.

B. The BMI for children is calculated the same way as for adults, but is interpreted using age- and gender-specific percentages (BMI-for-age) clinical charts (see Tables 2.1 and 2.2). The Centers for Disease Control and Prevention (CDC) defines childhood obesity by percentiles. Charts for children are available on the CDC website at www.cdc.gov/growthcharts

Incidence

A. More than two thirds of the U.S. population is overweight (BMI of 27) and of those, one third of the adults are obese, along with 17% of U.S. children (ages 2–19 years). Obesity rates cross all groups in society, regardless of age, sex, race, ethnicity, socioeconomic status, educational level, or geographic group.

Pathogenesis

Numerous factors contribute to the development of obesity, including:

A. Imbalance between energy intake and energy output
B. Genetics (40%–70% presumed explanation)
C. Environmental factors
D. Drug-induced obesity
  1. Antidepressants (amitriptyline, doxepin, imipramine, mirtazapine, nortriptyline, paroxetine, phenelzine)
  2. Antihistamines (cyproheptadine)
  3. Antipsychotics (clozapine, haloperidol, olanzapine, quetiapine, risperidone, thioridazine)
  4. Antidiabetics (insulin, sulfonylureas, thiazolidinediones)
  5. Anticonvulsants (sodium valproate, carbamazepine, gabapentin)
  6. Steroids (contraceptives, glucocorticoids, progestational steroids)
  7. Beta- or alpha-adrenergic blockers (propranolol, doxazosin)
E. Sleep disturbance-induced obesity

Predisposing Factors

A. Consuming too many calories/high-fat diet
B. Poor dietary choices
C. Readily available food sources, especially fast foods
D. Lack of exercise/sedentary lifestyle
E. Decreased/elimination of physical education requirements in public schools
F. Television, computer, and hand-held game use more than 3 hours a day
G. Increased leisure time
H. Lack of funding and planning for community parks and recreation areas
I. Ethnic background: African American, Hispanic
J. Family history of obesity
K. Poverty
L. Insomnia, difficulty staying asleep and frequent wakefulness

Common Complaints

A. Difficulties with activities of daily living (ADLs) or functional impairment
B. Lack of interest/inability to tolerate exercise
C. Shortness of breath and/or asthma exacerbations
D. Difficulty with personal hygiene
E. Urinary incontinence
F. Desire to lose weight

Other Signs and Symptoms

A. Obstructive sleep apnea (OSA)
B. Increased asthma symptoms
C. Infertility/Polycystic ovary syndrome (PCOS)
D. Symptoms associated with cholelithiasis
E. Hypertension
F. Early sexual maturity in girls
G. Joint pain (OA)

Subjective Data

A. Review the onset of weight gain and duration of obesity. Identify when the patient first noticed the weight gain.
B. Ask the patient about other symptoms secondary to obesity.
C. Review full medical history.
D. Review medications, including over-the-counter (OTC) herbals and diet products.
E. Review the patient's previous history of weight-loss attempts.
F. Assess activities of daily living (ADLs) and functional limitations and the presence of exercise intolerance.
G. Elicit history of sleep disorders (i.e., snoring and obstruction, sleep apnea).

H. Review 24-hour dietary recall. Review the patient's normal average meals per day, including snacks.
I. Review consumption of high-calorie drinks and alcohol intake.
J. Assess for history of binge eating, purging, night eating syndrome, lack of satiety, food-seeking behaviors, and other abnormal feeding habits.
K. Assess for depression.
L. Assess for readiness and commitment for weight loss. People who voluntarily enroll in a weight-loss program generally lose weight.
M. Ask the patient to describe his or her activity level, exercise routine, and daily activity (work activity).
N. Ask about screen time.
O. Ask about family history of obesity.
P. Ask about possible biopsychosocial and behavioral risk factors for weight gain such as starting a new medication, change in occupation or marital status, recent illness, pregnancy, menopause, stressful events, or smoking cessation.

Physical Examination

A. Check pulse, respirations, and blood pressure: Supine, sitting, and standing
B. Measurements:
- **1.** Determine height and weight to calculate BMI.
- **2.** Measure waist and hip circumferences to calculate the waist-to-hip circumference ratio. The waist-to-hip ratio is the strongest anthropometric measure that is associated with myocardial infarction risk and is a better predictor than BMI. A waist-to-hip ratio that is greater than 0.8% usually has some form of premetabolic syndrome or insulin resistance.

C. Inspect
- **1.** Observe the overall appearance and note body fat distribution.
- **2.** Examine the skin.
- **3.** Mouth and teeth: Assess dental enamel for signs of purging.

D. Auscultate
- **1.** Heart
- **2.** Lungs
- **3.** Carotid arteries
- **4.** Abdomen

E. Palpate
- **1.** Neck and thyroid
- **2.** Extremities—noting edema
- **3.** Abdomen for masses, tenderness, rebound tenderness

Diagnostic Tests

A. Thyroid function
B. Lipid panel
C. Liver enzymes
D. Complete blood count
E. 25-hydroxy vitamin D test
F. Pregnancy test
G. Fasting blood sugar/3-hour glucose tolerance test (GTT)
H. Consider fasting insulin level
I. Sleep study (if indicated)
J. Consider genetic testing
K. Nocturnal hypoxemia study

Differential Diagnoses

A. Obesity
B. Pseudo tumor cerebri
C. Binge eating
D. Genetic syndrome (e.g., Prader–Willi syndrome)
E. Cushing's syndrome
F. Diabetes mellitus
G. Insulin resistance syndrome
H. Primary pulmonary hypertension

Plan

Manage obesity as a chronic relapsing disease, including the comanagement of other diseases secondary to obesity (i.e., diabetes, hypertension).

A. General interventions
- **1.** Treat any underlying cause of obesity.
- **2.** Reinforce the positive impact that weight loss measures (diet, exercise) can have and the overall health benefits of weight loss. Weight loss of even 5% to 15% can provide a significant reduction in obesity-related complications.
- **3.** Identify and monitor any cardiovascular complications.
- **4.** Behavior modification: Intensive behavior therapy has been shown to lead to better success with weight loss and sustainable weight loss for longer periods of time. Behavior therapy includes weekly meetings with health care professionals for at least 6 to 8 weeks.
  - **a.** Dietary plan
    - **i.** Consume 500 to 1,000 fewer calories per day for 1- to 2-pound-per-week weight loss.
    - **ii.** Most diets have good short-term efficacy but limited sustainability.
    - **iii.** Diets shown to be effective include portion control, low-fat, Mediterranean, low-carbohydrate, low glycemic index, and commercial weight-loss diets.
    - **iv.** Increase water intake, particularly drinking 500 mL of water before meals
    - **v.** Protein-dense and high fiber foods increase satiety with less calories
  - **b.** Exercise: Both children and adults
    - **i.** Approximately 150 minutes of moderate intensity exercise is recommended per week for adults, 155 to 180 minutes per week for children.
    - **ii.** Multiple short sessions (four 10-minute sessions per day, 5 days per week) may have the same benefit as fewer longer sessions (one 40-minute session, 5 days per week).
    - **iii.** Walking 30 minutes per day has been shown to prevent weight gain; higher amounts of exercise promote weight loss.
    - **iv.** The combination of exercise and diet is more effective than either alone.

c. Wide range of benefits of exercise and weight loss

i. Helps lower blood pressure
ii. Improves cholesterol count
iii. Helps lower hemoglobin A1c in diabetes
iv. Helps strengthen bones
v. Promotes weight loss
vi. Improves depression
vii. Boosts immune system
viii. Reduces stress
ix. Improves sense of well-being
x. Believed to be a major driving force in lifestyle change
xi. Improves joint pain

d. Obtain counseling on stimulus control, goal setting, self-monitoring, and contracts that reward behaviors.

e. Contraindication to exercise: There are several contraindications for beginning exercise:

i. Individuals with recent myocardial infarction (2 weeks)
ii. Unstable angina
iii. Severe aortic stenosis
iv. Decompensated congestive heart failure (low ejection fraction)
v. Left ventricular outflow obstruction
vi. Uncontrolled dysrhythmias
vii. Uncontrolled diabetes or diabetic complications
viii. Uncontrolled hypertension
ix. Uncontrolled respiratory conditions such as asthma and COPD

B. Patient teaching on obesity treatment modalities

1. Advise the patient to keep a food diary to identify food triggers and for accountability. Patients who maintain a food diary have been shown to have as much as 90% more weight loss than those who do not keep a diary.

2. Counsel patients about pharmaceutical therapy drug side effects and the lack of long-term safety data. Stress to the patient the temporary nature of the weight-loss medication. Typical weight loss is modest, less than 5 kg (10–11 lb) at 1 year.

3. Teach patients how to read food labels.

C. Pharmaceutical therapy

1. After an adequate trial (minimum of 6 months) of diet and exercise therapy, consider adding pharmaceutical therapy. Pharmacological intervention is not covered by some health plans. State statutes should be considered before prescribing weight-control products.

2. Studies lack evidence to support whether one drug is more efficacious than another; the literature does not support the use of combination therapy for increased weight loss.

3. The choice of a pharmaceutical agent depends on the side-effect profile of the drug and tolerance of the side effects.

4. The Food and Drug Administration (FDA) has not approved any weight-loss medication for use beyond 2 years in adults. Appetite suppressants that are FDA approved:

a. Qsymia, phentermine, diethylpropion, benzphetamine, and phendimetrazine are approved for short-term (12 weeks) use.

b. Sibutramine (Meridia, Reductil) is FDA approved for 1-year use.

c. Orlistat (Xenical) is FDA approved for 2-year use.

5. Appetite suppressants

a. Qsymia (phentermine and topiramate extended release). Start with 3.75/23 mg extended release per day for initial BMI greater than 30 kg/m^2, or BMI greater than 27 kg/m^2 in the presence of risk factors. May gradually increase dose to 15/92 mg.

i. Avoid evening dose.
ii. Not to be taken by adolescents younger than 16 years of age.
iii. Avoid in pregnancy.
iv. Monitor for hypersensitivity to phentermine and topamax.
v. These drugs are not recommended in the presence of hypertension, hyperthyroidism, cardiovascular disease, and drug or alcohol abuse.
vi. Do not use if a history of glaucoma or hyperthyroidism is present, or within 14 days of use of monoamine oxidase inhibitors (MAOIs).

b. Phentermine (Adipex-P) 37.5 mg orally once daily before or 1 to 2 hours after breakfast, or 18.75 mg one to two times per day for initial BMI greater than 30 kg/m^2, or BMI greater than 27 kg/m^2 in the presence of risk factors such as controlled elevated blood pressure, diabetes, and high cholesterol.

i. Avoid late-evening dosing.
ii. Not recommended for children younger than 16 years.
iii. Not recommended in the presence of hypertension, hyperthyroidism, cardiovascular disease, and drug or alcohol abuse.
iv. Do not prescribe during or within 14 days of MAOIs.

c. Benzphetamine (Didrex) 25 to 50 mg orally initially in the midmorning or midafternoon. Increase if needed to 25 to 50 mg one to three times a day.

i. Not recommended in children or adolescents.
ii. Not recommended in the presence of hypertension, hyperthyroidism, cardiovascular disease, and drug or alcohol abuse.
iii. Not to be prescribed during or within 14 days of MAOIs.
iv. Pregnancy category X: Known to cause fetal abnormalities or toxicity in animal and human studies.

d. Diethylpropion (Tenuate) 25 mg 1 tablet every 8 hours, 1 hour before meals. May add one additional dose for night hunger. Half-life of 4 to 6 hours.

i. Avoid late-evening dosing.

ii. Not recommended for children younger than 16 years.
iii. Not recommended in the presence of hypertension, hyperthyroidism, cardiovascular disease, and drug or alcohol abuse.
iv. Do not prescribe during or within 14 days of MAOIs.

e. Phendimetrazine (Bontril PDM) 35 mg orally two or three times daily 1 hour before meals. May reduce to 17.5 mg/dose. Maximum dose 210 mg/d in three evenly divided doses. Also available in slow-release 105 mg in the morning 30 to 60 minutes before breakfast.
i. Not recommended in children or adolescents.
ii. Not recommended in the presence of hypertension, hyperthyroidism, cardiovascular disease, and drug or alcohol abuse.
iii. Not to be prescribed during or within 14 days of MAOIs.

f. Sibutramine (Meridia) 10 mg orally once a day. After 4 weeks, may titrate to 15 mg once a day.
i. Not recommended in children or adolescents younger than 16 years.
ii. FDA approved for use up to 2 years.
iii. Not recommended for nursing mothers.
iv. Blood pressure and pulse should be monitored regularly during therapy. Consider discontinuing sibutramine with sustained blood pressure and pulse increases.
v. Not recommended with severe renal or hepatic dysfunction or with a history of narrow-angle glaucoma.

6. Lipase inhibitor
a. Orlistat (Xenical) for use with a low-fat diet. Recommend 30% of calories spread over three main meals.
i. Take one 120-mg capsule orally during or up to 1 hour after main meals up to three times per day.
ii. If a meal is missed or had no fat, skip dosage.
iii. May decrease absorption of fat-soluble vitamins and beta-carotene.
iv. Orlistat carries an FDA warning regarding safety and efficacy for use in patients younger than 12 years and in pregnancy and lactation as it interferes with the absorption of fat-soluble vitamins.
v. Supplement diet with a multivitamin.
vi. FDA approved for up to 2 years' use in adults.
vii. Gastrointestinal side effects include fatty/oily stools, oily spotting, flatus with discharge, fecal urgency, and fecal incontinence.
viii. Contraindicated in chronic malabsorption syndrome and cholestasis.
ix. May affect doses for antidiabetic medications.
x. Monitor warfarin and cyclosporine levels.

b. Alli, a lipase inhibitor, is the only FDA-approved OTC weight-loss product.

7. Glucagon-like peptide-1 (GLP-1) receptor agonist
a. Saxenda subcutaneous was FDA approved for chronic weight management as an adjunct to a reduced-calorie diet and increased physical exercise in December of 2014 for use in adults with BMI of 30 kg/m^2 or greater or 27 kg/m^2 or greater with at least one weight-related comorbidity.
i. Start with 0.6 mg once daily for a week; may increase by 0.6 mg daily at weekly intervals up to 3 mg once daily.
ii. Delay dose increase if tolerance is an issue.
iii. If 3 mg once daily is not tolerated, discontinue drug. Efficacy has not been established for lower doses.
iv. Evaluate at 16 weeks of therapy; discontinue if at least 4% of baseline body weight loss has not been achieved.
v. Pregnancy category X; contraindicated in patients with multiple endocrine neoplasia syndrome type 2 (MEN2).

8. Off-label medications used for obesity: These medications are not FDA approved for weight loss. The patient should be counseled regarding this and use at discretion.
a. Metformin (Glucophage) is used to decrease central adiposity in weight loss, lower insulin levels, and slow down the process of gluconeogenesis.
i. Start Metformin 500 mg at the evening meal. The dosage can be increased by 500 mg/wk in divided doses up to the maximum of 2,000 mg/d.
ii. Titrate slowly because of the gastrointestinal side effects.
iii. Check a metabolic panel before and every 3 to 6 months to evaluate for lactic acidosis.
iv. Metformin is contraindicated in patients with renal impairment; assess renal function before instituting metformin and monitor regularly.
v. Metformin must be stopped before any procedure with radiographic dye.
vi. May be used in children with central adiposity, especially those with signs of premetabolic syndrome.
vii. May be used on a patient with a waist-to-hip ratio greater than 0.8%.

b. Topiramate (Topamax) is used to treat seizures and several types of headache. In small doses, it can be used alone or as adjunct with phentermine to suppress appetite longer. Be familiar with the risks associated with the use of Topamax.
i. If used alone, the drug may start at 25 mg every day in the morning. Increase up to two or three times a day. Topamax has a long half-life of 19 to 25 hours.
ii. May be used as adjunct with phentermine. Start patient at 18.75 mg of phentermine and 12.5 mg of Topamax. Then gradually increase the dose to 37.5 mg of phentermine and 25 mg of Topamax.

iii. Always give the phentermine in the morning, preferably 30 minutes before meals. Topamax should be dosed in the afternoon or evening.
iv. Phentermine (Adipex-P) 37.5 mg orally once daily before or 1 to 2 hours after breakfast, or 18.75 mg one to two times per day for initial BMI greater than 30 kg/m^2, or BMI greater than 27 kg/m^2 in the presence of risk factors such as controlled elevated blood pressure, diabetes, or high cholesterol.
v. Avoid late evening dosing.
vi. Not recommended for children younger than 16 years.
vii. Not recommended in the presence of hypertension, hyperthyroidism, cardiovascular disease, and drug or alcohol abuse.
viii. Do not prescribe during or within 14 days of MAOIs.

Follow-Up

A. Reevaluate the patient every week for 6 to 8 weeks, then monthly if pharmaceutical therapy is used until goal is achieved.
B. Maintain the recommended schedule for comorbid conditions.
C. If the patient is a candidate for bariatric surgery, follow recommended pretreatment/reauthorization guidelines required by the payer and bariatric center.

Consultation/Referral

A. Refer to a nutritionist/registered dietitian for consultation.
B. Consider a referral to a bariatric center/surgical consultation and evaluation of bariatric surgery.
C. Consider a psychology consultation (may be required before bariatric surgery).
D. If the family is eligible, refer to the Women, Infant, and Children (WIC) program. Referral to some commercial weight loss programs may be beneficial. See www.fns.usda.gov/wic/women-infants-and-children-wic

Individual Considerations

A. Pregnancy
1. Benzphetamine (Didrex) is a category X drug. Avoid use during pregnancy.
2. Weight loss should never be a goal during pregnancy.
3. Counsel patients regarding appropriate weight gain and healthy eating habits during pregnancy.
B. Pediatrics
1. The cornerstone for management of obesity in children is modification of dietary and exercise habits.
2. The first step for overweight children older than 2 years is maintenance of baseline weight if there is no secondary complication of obesity (i.e., diabetes and hypertension). Any dietary modification must ensure adequate nutrients for the growing child (see chapter on pediatrics).
3. The weight-loss goal should be approximately 1 pound per month for a BMI below the 85th percentile.
4. Decrease sedentary behaviors (i.e., watching TV, surfing the Internet, and playing video games).
5. Increase physical activity and incorporate exercise into family time.
6. Long-term safety and effectiveness of low-carbohydrate, high-protein diets, such as the Atkins diet, have not been adequately studied in children.
7. Use of pharmacotherapies in children and adolescents requires further research, unless previously noted under drug therapies.
C. Geriatrics
1. All adults should avoid inactivity. Some exercise is better than none. Any dietary modification must ensure adequate nutrients for the aging adult (refer to geriatric chapter).

Resources

American Heart Association: www.heart.org/HEARTORG
American Heart Association Go Red for Women: https://www.goredforwomen.org
Centers for Disease Control and Prevention (CDC). Overweight and obesity: www.cdc.gov/obesity/index.html
Exercise: A guide from the National Institute on Aging: www.nia.nih.gov/HealthInformation/Publications/ExerciseGuide
National Institutes of Health (NIH) Senior Health: Exercise and physical activity for older adults: nihseniorhealth.gov/exerciseforolderadults/healthbenefits/01.html
President's Council on Fitness, Sports & Nutrition: www.fitness.gov
The Obesity Society: www.obesity.org/home
SHAPE America, Society for Health and Physical Educators: http://www.shapeamerica.org/

Post–Bariatric Surgery Long-Term Follow-Up

Cheryl A. Glass and Bunny Pounds

Definition

A. The number of obese people in the United States has more than doubled in the past 50 years, with severe obesity increasing more rapidly than nonsevere obesity. The traditional management of obesity, a combination of diet, exercise, and behavioral modification, often results in moderate success with limited sustainability. Increasing prevalence of obesity combined with improvements in surgical weight-loss procedures and improved insurance coverage has resulted in exponential growth of the number of people opting for surgical management. Patients who undergo surgical weight-loss procedures have unique health care needs and require lifelong follow-up. Although the bariatric treatment team is the ideal source of follow-up and monitoring, primary care providers can play a critical role and need to be cognizant of the unique needs of this population.
B. The primary mechanism of action for surgical weight-loss procedures is either restriction or a combination of restriction and malabsorption (see Table 2.3). All procedures have some form of restriction that reduces the volume of food that can be ingested. Restriction can occur by means of a physical barrier such as a laparoscopic adjustable gastric band (LAGB; see Figure 2.1) or by removing a portion of the digestive tract such as with the gastric sleeve (GS; see Figure 2.2). Malabsorptive procedures cause

TABLE 2.3 Surgical Weight Loss Procedures and Mechanism of Action

Procedure	Mechanism of Action	Advantages	Disadvantages
Laparoscopic adjustable gastric band (LAGB); Figure 2.1	Restriction	No cutting or rerouting of digestive tract Reversible and adjustable Lowest risk of nutritional deficiencies	Slower (more gradual) weight loss Greater chance of failure to lose 50% of excess weight Foreign device in body; slippage and erosion possible Highest rate of reoperation
Gastric sleeve (GS); Figure 2.2	Restriction and some malabsorption	No rerouting Hormonal hunger suppression, appetite reduction, and increased satiety	Not reversible Potential for nutrient deficiencies Higher complication rate than LAGB
Roux-en-Y gastric bypass (RYGB); Figure 2.3	Restriction and malabsorption	Reduces appetite, enhances satiety Better initial and long-term weight loss compared with LAGB	Long-term nutritional-deficiency risk Lifelong adherence to diet and supplementation required Higher complication rate compared with LAGB and GS
Biliopancreatic diversion with duodenal switch (BPD/DS)	Malabsorption and some restriction	Greatest weight loss overall Reduces appetite, improves satiety Most effective for treatment of diabetes mellitus	Greatest risk of nutritional deficiencies Strict lifetime adherence to diet and supplements Highest complication rate
Vertical banded gastroplasty: No longer performed			

weight loss by changing the way nutrients are absorbed, which is accomplished by removing portions of the stomach and/or small intestine and sometimes by rerouting the digestive tract (Roux-en-Y; see Figure 2.3). The success of surgical weight loss is defined by initial weight loss, maintenance of weight loss, and prevention of complications. Success is directly related to the aftercare a person receives.

Incidence

A. According to the 2009 to 2010 National Health and Nutrition Examination Survey, more than one third (35.7%) of the adults in the United States are obese. The American Society for Metabolic and Bariatric Surgery (ASMBS) reports an estimated 200,000 weight-loss operations were performed in 2009. About 90% of surgical weight-loss procedures are performed laparoscopically now. The most common procedures performed today include the gastric bypass, gastric sleeve, adjustable gastric band, and biliopancreatic diversion with duodenal switch.

Pathogenesis

A. The pathogenesis of obesity is reviewed under "Obesity" in this chapter. Significant improvements in the safety of surgical weight-loss procedures in recent years result from improved surgical techniques, accreditation, and the use of laparoscopy. The overall mortality rate is about 0.1% and the risk of major complications about 4.3%. The incidences of complications vary by surgical procedure. Postoperative complications may occur immediately or may occur many years after surgery. Nutritional deficiencies are by far the most common long-term complication.

Predisposing Factors

A. Higher body mass index (BMI)
B. Noncompliance with bariatric diet and exercise
C. Lack of follow-up with health care professionals
D. Obesity-related health problems:
  1. Sleep apnea
  2. Diabetes
  3. Arthritis
  4. Hypertension
  5. GERD

E. Complexity and type of surgery

Common Complaints

Functional and Nutritional

A. Dumping syndrome usually occurs within 30 minutes of eating high fat/high sugar foods and involves flushing, sweating, lightheadedness, tachycardia, palpitations, nausea, diarrhea, cramping.
B. Hypoglycemia occurs 1 to 3 hours after eating high-carb meals and involves shakiness, anxiety, sweating, chills, clamminess, confusion, rapid heart rate, dizziness, hunger, and nausea.
C. New or exacerbated reflux is more common with a gastric sleeve.
D. Vitamin deficiencies or toxicities. Refer to Table 2.4.
  1. Most common
    a. Iron deficiency—fatigue, lethargy, pica, food cravings
    b. Iron toxicity—gastrointestinal irritation, nausea, vomiting, indigestion, constipation, diarrhea
    c. Protein deficiency—weakness, decreased muscle mass, brittle hair, generalized edema

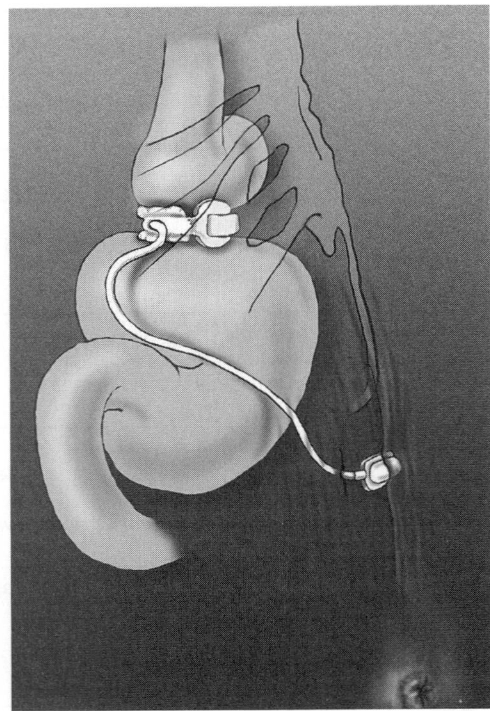

FIGURE 2.1 Laparoscopic adjustable gastric band (LAGB).
Source: Reprinted with permission from the American Society of Metabolic and Bariatric Surgery. Copyright 2013, all rights reserved.

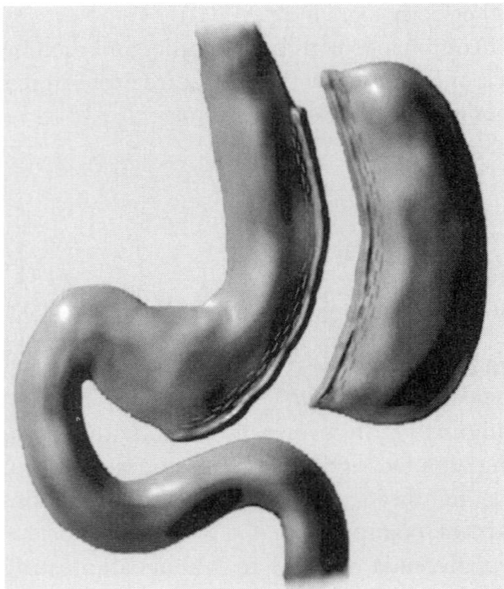

FIGURE 2.2 Sleeve bypass procedure with stomach resection.
Source: Reprinted with permission from Smith, Schauer, and Nguyen (2008).

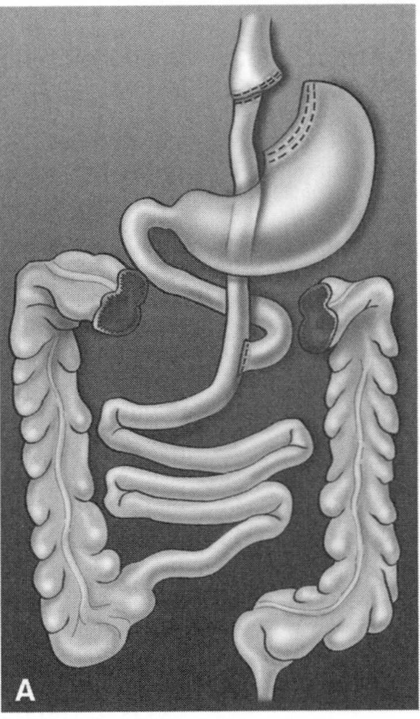

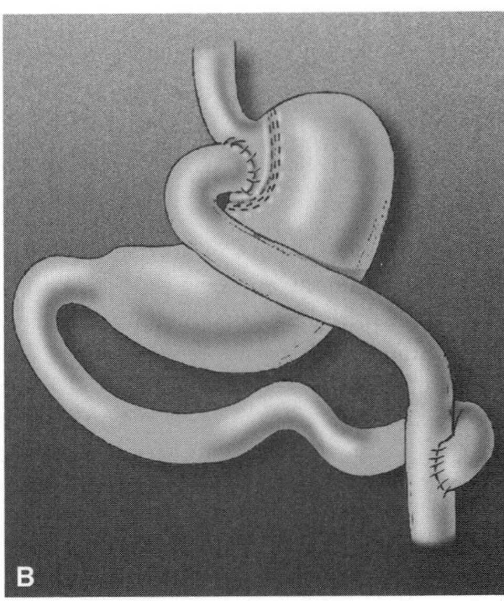

FIGURE 2.3 (A, B) Roux-en-Y gastric bypass (RYGB).
Source: Reprinted with permission from the American Society of Metabolic and Bariatric Surgery. Copyright 2013, all rights reserved.

d. Folate deficiency—fatigue, palpitations, sore tongue, diarrhea, restless legs
e. Calcium deficiency—usually silent, hyperpara thryoidism
f. Calcium toxicity—constipation, nausea, vomiting, dry mouth, loss of appetite
g. Vitamin D deficiency—spasms/twitching of eyes, burning in mouth, sweating, weakness
h. Vitamin B_{12} deficiency—fatigue, burning lips/mouth, rapid heart rate, palpitations, sore tongue, weakness, mood changes, neurologic changes

2. Less common
   a. Thiamine (B_1) deficiency—usually in first 3 months postop, often a result of vomiting, blurred or double vision, difficulty swallowing, rapid heart rate, fatigue, confusion, memory loss, burning feet, leg weakness, amnesia
   b. Zinc deficiency—loss of smell, diminished sense of taste, poor wound healing, skin rashes

TABLE 2.4 Most Common Nutrient Deficiencies

Nutrient	Protein	Iron	Folate	Calcium	Vitamin B_{12}	Vitamin D
Assay	Serum albumin <3.5 mg/dL May need prealbumin and serum creatinine levels also	Iron saturation <10% Serum ferritin <10 ng/mL or iron saturation <7% regardless of ferritin value	Serum folic acid	Total and ionized calcium Phosphorus 24-hr urinary calcium excretion Intact serum parathyroid hormone Bone density	Serum B_{12} level May need methylmalonic acid level also	25 (OH)D_3 <30 ng/mL
Incidence	18%–25% after malabsorptive procedures	6%–50%	1%–10%	10%–25%	5%–25%	Up to 63%
Complications and symptoms	Anemia Edema Alopecia Asthenia (weakness, decreased muscle mass, brittle hair, generalized edema)	Microcytic, hypochromic anemia (pallor, fatigue, poor capillary refill, palpitations, pica, brittle hair)	Megaloblastic or macrocytic anemia (palpitations; fatigue; diarrhea; smooth, sore tongue) Neural tube defects May aggravate B_{12} deficiency	Secondary hyperparathyroidism Enhanced bone loss Metabolic bone disease (tetany, tingling, cramping)	Megaloblastic anemia with macrocytosis Neuropathy Cognitive dysfunction (glossitis, constipation, diarrhea, neurologic changes, depression, dementia)	Myopathy Secondary hypocalcemia
Recommended daily amount for prevention	1.1–1.5 g/kg ideal body weight/day 10%–35% of total energy intake should be from protein	45–60 mg/d from multivitamins and iron supplements for malabsorptive procedures Menstruating women may need more	400 mcg/d	1,200–1,500 mg/d of calcium citrate from food and supplements	500 mcg/d oral for band 1,000 mcg/d oral for malabsorptive procedures; may need 500–1,000 mcg/mo intramuscular	At least 3,000 IU of oral D_3 daily, better to titrate to therapeutic level
Treatment dosing	If previous options are not effective, may need parenteral nutrition	150–200 mg of elemental iron twice daily, preferably with vitamin C	1,000 mcg/d for 3 months	2,000 mg/d with adequate vitamin D supplementation	Depends on the level of deficiency Recheck levels after 3–6 months of repletion	6,000–10,000 IU/d or 50,000 IU/wk up to 50,000 IU/d Recheck level every 3 months

Source: Adapted from Becker, Balcer, and Galetta (2012); Handzlik-Orlik, Holecki, Orlik, Wylezol, and Dulawa (2015); and Kerner (2014).

or roughness, hair loss, poor appetite, lethargy, grooved or deformed nails, canker sores

c. Magnesium deficiency—hyperexcitability, cramps, tremors, fasciculation, spasms, fatigue, loss of appetite, apathy, confusion, insomnia, irritability, poor memory

d. Selenium deficiency (very rare)—signs of hypothyroidism (selenium is necessary for conversion of thyroxine into its active form, triiodothyronine)

e. Selenium toxicity (rare)—hair loss, abnormal nails, dermatitis, peripheral neuropathy, nausea, diarrhea, fatigue, irritability, garlic odor of breath

E. Surgical complications

1. Short term

a. Anastomic leak—less than 4.4% with Roux-en-Y gastric bypass (RYGB), but has a mortality of up to 30% when it does happen; presenting symptom is tachycardia

b. Bleeding—less than 4% after RYGB, 0.1% after LAGB

c. Wound infection—2.9% of laparoscopic cases, 6.6% of open cases

d. Thromboembolism—deep vein thrombosis up to 1.3%, pulmonary embolism up to 1.1% after RYGB, lower with LAGB

e. Anastomotic strictures—2% to 16% after RYGB, typically within first 3 months, nausea and/or vomiting

2. Long term

a. Band slippage—15% to 20% of LAGB patients—abdominal pain, acid reflux, regurgitation, or dysphagia

b. Band erosion—up to 4% of LAGB patients—may be asymptomatic, abdominal pain, gastrointestinal bleeding, weight loss, abdominal sepsis

c. Intestinal obstruction—4.4% after RYGB, caused by internal hernias, adhesions, and anastomotic stenosis—colicky central abdominal pain, nausea, vomiting, abdominal distention, absolute constipation

d. Hepatobiliary complications—rapid weight loss is associated with gallstone formation; 13% to 36% of patients develop this within 6 months of surgery

e. Gastrointestinal bleeding—rare and usually caused by ulceration

f. Marginal ulcers—0.7% to 5.1% after RYGB—abdominal pain, vomiting, bleeding, or anemia

Other Signs and Symptoms

A. Expected weight loss

1. LAGB—Initial loss of 40% to 50% of excess body weight in 3 to 5 years. Expected maintenance <50%.

2. GS—Initial loss of >50% of excess body weight in 3 to 5 years. Expected maintenance >50%.

3. RYGB—Initial loss of 60% to 80% of excess body weight in 1 year. Expected maintenance >50%.

4. Biliopancreatic diversion with duodenal switch (BPD/DS)—Initial loss of 60% to 70% of excess body weight in 1 year. Expected maintenance of 60% to 70%.

B. Weight regain of up to 20 pounds is common after 2 years.

C. Constipation and/or diarrhea may occur, depending on the procedure.

D. Weight loss of less than 25% of excess body weight is considered a surgical failure and may be revised.

E. Even if weight loss is adequate, patients may express disappointment and/or depression related to rate or amount of weight lost.

F. Nausea and vomiting after LAGB may indicate need for band adjustment.

Subjective Data

A. Review onset and duration of symptoms.

B. Elicit the date of surgery, type of surgery, and any reoperations or complications.

C. Review previous highest weight and amount of excess weight lost since surgery.

D. Evaluate the location and level of pain/discomfort.

E. Evaluate the overall psychosocial changes since surgery.

F. Review a 24-hour food recall, choices of healthy foods, skipping meals, food aversion (e.g., red meat), and intolerance.

G. Review medications and supplement use

Physical Examination

A. Check height, weight, waist and hip circumference. Calculate body mass index (BMI), waist/hip ratio, pulse, respirations, and blood pressure. Check temperature if infection is suspected.

B. Inspect

1. Examine the skin, evaluate surgical site(s), evaluate redness and tenderness.

2. Oral/dental examination.

3. Evaluate for dehydration.

4. Eye examination: Evaluate eye movement (thiamine deficiency).

5. Evaluate gait.

6. General overview of personal presence and affect.

C. Auscultate

1. Auscultate the heart and lungs.

2. Auscultate the abdomen for bowel sounds.

D. Palpate abdomen.

1. Evaluate for the presence of tenderness.

2. Evaluate for masses.

E. Neurologic examination

1. Perform neurologic examination, including checking deep tendon reflexes (DTRs), sense of smell, and Babinski reflex (vitamin B_{12} deficiency).

Diagnostic Tests

A. Annual recommended laboratory testing for all procedures

1. Complete blood count (CBC) with differential
2. Liver function tests
3. Glucose
4. Creatinine
5. Electrolytes

B. Annual laboratory testing suggested for LAGB, recommended for all other procedures

1. Iron/ferritin
2. Vitamin B_{12}
3. Folate
4. Calcium
5. Intact parathyroid hormone (PTH)
6. 25-hydroxy vitamin D
7. Albumin/prealbumin

C. Optional labs that may be required based on symptoms

1. Zinc
2. Copper
3. Vitamin B_1
4. Vitamin B_6
5. Vitamin A

D. Other labs as appropriate for condition and prevention

1. Monitor HgA1c and blood glucose closely in patients with diabetes. Diabetes has resolved after bariatric surgery in some patients.

2. Lipid profile

E. Abdominal ultrasound

F. CT scan abdomen

G. Doppler ultrasound of limb for suspected deep vein thrombosis (DVT)

H. Pulmonary ventilation/perfusion scan for suspected pulmonary embolus

I. Bone mineral density (dual-energy x-ray absorptiometry [DEXA]) scan: Recommended annually until stable after malabsorptive procedures
J. Endoscopy as needed for abdominal complaints

Differential Diagnoses

A. Postoperative surgical complication(s)
B. Infection
C. Abdominal pain
D. Fascial dehiscence
E. DVT
F. Bowel obstruction
G. Band slippage
H. Anastomosis leakage
I. Stomal stenosis/stricture
J. Cholecystitis
K. Dumping syndrome
L. Food intolerance
M. Gastric ulcer
N. Gastroenteritis
O. Vitamin deficiency
P. Malnutrition/protein deficiency
Q. Incisional hernia
R. Osteoporosis

Plan

A. General interventions
  1. Lifelong follow-up is required after bariatric surgery. Ideally, patients should follow up with their surgical group, but many do not. Primary care providers are well positioned to capture those lost to follow-up. Continuous reinforcement of good nutritional habits is important.
B. Patient teaching: Many complications can be prevented by adhering to diet and lifestyle recommendations.
  1. Supplements are required lifelong; strict adherence will prevent deficiencies.
  2. Dumping syndrome can be prevented by avoiding foods that trigger it such as high sugar and/or high-fat foods. Patients can keep food diaries to identify triggers.
  3. Hypoglycemia can usually be prevented by careful monitoring of carbohydrate intake.
  4. Surgery does not replace the need for a balanced diet or exercise. Approximately 150 minutes of moderate activity each week is recommended, though safety and tolerance differs so exercise recommendations should be individualized. Any activity is better than none.
  5. Food should be chewed thoroughly and consumed slowly. Liquids should be avoided 30 minutes before and after meals. Avoid eating and drinking liquids simultaneously.
  6. Protein is important for maintaining muscle mass during rapid weight loss and avoiding hunger during maintenance. Between 60 and 100 g of protein daily is recommended. Limit carbohydrate intake to 50 g per day or less. Limiting carbohydrate intake reduces risk of weight regain by preventing rebound hunger.
  7. To prevent dehydration, as well as reduce the risk of kidney stones and constipation, encourage 64 ounces of fluids daily.
  8. Stress, boredom, and emotions often affect eating habits. Identifying problems and seeking help early are important.
  9. Support groups can be a vital source of education and social support, both of which are key to weight loss and maintenance.
  10. Weight plateaus are common and normal. This is the body's way of trying to establish a new set point. Do not be discouraged by plateaus. Consistency is key to overcoming them.
  11. Adequate sleep and successful stress management are also key to successful weight loss and maintenance.
C. Pharmaceutical therapy
  1. Medication absorption can be altered after bariatric surgery. Evaluate need for adjustments of medication dosing, especially diabetic, psychiatric, and antihypertensive medications as well as any medica tion with a narrow therapeutic window.
  2. Patients may require alternate formulations of medications, including crushed, chewable, liquid, patches, intramuscular, or subcutaneous. Long-acting, extended-release, or enteric coated medications may not be absorbed as well and may need to be switched to immediate release.
  3. Refer to Table 2.5.
  4. Recommended supplementations:
    a. Multivitamin plus mineral
      i. LAGB: One daily
      ii. All other procedures: Two daily
    b. Calcium: (all procedures) 1,200 to 1,500 mg daily from food and calcium citrate in divided doses
    c. Vitamin D: (all procedures) 3,000 IU daily, titrate to therapeutic level
    d. Iron
      i. LAGB: Not usually necessary
      ii. All other procedures: 45 to 60 mg daily from multivitamin plus additional supplementation
    e. Vitamin B_{12}
      i. LAGB: Not usually necessary
      ii. All other procedures: As needed to maintain levels in the form best tolerated
    f. Long-term anticoagulation may be needed for DVT/ pulmonary embolism (PE) prophylaxis.
    g. Nonsteroidal anti-inflammatory drugs (NSAIDs) and corticosteroids should be avoided to reduce the risk of marginal ulcers.
D. Psychosocial changes: Bariatric surgery often results in dramatic lifestyle and body changes and may require significant psychosocial adjustments for the patient as well as his or her friends and family.
  1. Monitor for depression/anxiety, body image concerns, and social support.
  2. Alcoholism can be a concern after bariatric surgery. Less alcohol is needed to elevate blood alcohol

TABLE 2.5 Routine Supplementation Based on Type of Gastric Bypass Surgery

Supplement	Gastric Band	Gastric Sleeve	Gastric Bypass	BPD/DS
Multivitamin plus mineral	One daily	Two daily	Two daily	Two daily
Calcium	1,200–1,500 mg daily from food and calcium citrate divided doses	1,200–1,500 mg daily from food and calcium citrate divided doses	1,200–1,500 mg daily from food and calcium citrate divided doses	1,200–1,500 mg daily from food and calcium citrate divided doses
Vitamin D	3,000 IU daily Titrate to therapeutic level	3,000 IU daily Titrate to therapeutic level	3,000 IU daily Titrate to therapeutic level	3,000 IU daily Titrate to therapeutic level
Iron	Not usually necessary	45–60 mg/d from multivitamin plus additional supplement	45–60 mg/d from multivitamin plus additional supplement	45–60 mg/d from multivitamin plus additional supplement
Vitamin B_{12}	Not usually necessary	As needed to maintain levels in the form best tolerated	As needed to maintain levels in the form best tolerated	As needed to maintain levels in the form best tolerated

BPD/DS, biliopancreatic diversion with duodenal switch.
Source: Adapted from Kerner (2014); Shannon, Gervasoni, and Williams (2013).

TABLE 2.6 Recommended Annual Laboratory Monitoring for Bypass Patients

	Gastric Band	Gastric Sleeve	Gastric Bypass	BPD/DS
Complete blood count	X	X	X	X
Liver function tests	X	X	X	X
Glucose	X	X	X	X
Creatinine	X	X	X	X
Electrolytes	X	X	X	X
Iron/ferritin	Suggested	X	X	X
Vitamin B_{12}	Suggested	X	X	X
Folate	Suggested	X	X	X
Calcium	Suggested	X	X	X
Intact PTH	Suggested	X	X	X
Vitamin D 25-OH	Suggested	X	X	X
Albumin/prealbumin	Suggested	X	X	X
Bone mineral density		X	X	X
Zinc		Optional	Optional	Optional
Vitamin B_1		Optional	Optional	Optional
Vitamin A		Optional 24 months and beyond	Optional 24 months and beyond	Optional 24 months and beyond

BPD/DS, biliopancreatic diversion with duodenal switch; PTH, parathyroid hormone.
*Source:*Adapted from Heber, Greenway, Kaplan, Livingston, Salvador, and Still (2010).

levels and blood alcohol levels are sustained longer after bariatric surgery.

Follow-Up

A. Bariatric surgery requires lifelong follow-up, ideally by a multidisciplinary team of health care providers. Initial follow-up schedules are set by the surgeon. Long-term follow-up (after the first 2 years) is usually provided for by the bariatric surgery program, but research has shown that follow-up is often poor, which leads to poor outcomes and substandard patient care.

B. Laboratory and diagnostic testing is required as listed in Table 2.6. Early recognition of nutritional deficiencies can prevent permanent damage and even death.

C. Chronic disease management (particularly diabetes, lipids, and bone disease) can be simpler or more complex after bariatric surgery, depending on the patient's adherence to lifestyle and nutritional recommendations.

Consultation/Referral

A. Bariatric surgeon for surgical complications, revisions

B. Surgeon for cholecystectomy (preferably bariatric surgeon or general/GI surgeon experienced in the care of bariatric patients)

C. Gastroenterology consult
D. Nutrition consultation and/or counseling
E. Psychologist consultation
F. Physical therapy/exercise specialist
G. Support group

Individual Considerations

A. Women
a. All women of childbearing age should receive adequate folate supplementation and be given contraception and preconception counseling.
b. Oral contraceptives (OCPs) may not be as effective after bariatric surgery because of changes in absorption.
B. Pregnancy
a. Pregnancy should be delayed for 12 to 18 months after bariatric surgery or however long it takes for weight loss to stabilize.
b. Bariatric surgeon consult may be required.
c. Increased folic acid may be needed preconception to reduce risk of neural tube defects.
d. Increased vitamin supplementation may be necessary during pregnancy. Vitamin A should be limited to 5,000 IU daily.
e. Gastric band may need to be adjusted during pregnancy.
f. Serial ultrasounds may need to be done to follow fetal growth.

Substance Use Disorders

Moya Cook and Robertson Nash

Definition

With the publication of the fifth edition of the *Diagnostic and Statistical Manual of Mental Disorders* (*DSM-5*; American Psychiatric Association [APA], 2013), there has been a significant shift in the classification of substance use disorders and their categorization. Previously, the *Diagnostic and Statistical Manual of Mental Disorders,* fourth edition (*DSM–IV*; APA, 1994) provided distinct groups of substance use, listed as follows:
A. Substance abuse: A maladaptive pattern of substance use leading to clinically significant impairment or distress, as manifested by one (or more) specific symptoms, occurring within a 12-month period.
B. Substance intoxication: The development of a reversible substance-specific syndrome caused by recent ingestion of (or exposure to) a substance.
C. Substance dependence: A maladaptive pattern of substance use, leading to clinically significant impairment or distress, as manifested by three (or more) specific symptoms, occurring at any time in the same 12-month period.
D. Substance withdrawal: The development of a substance-specific syndrome caused by the cessation of (or reduction in) substance use that has been heavy and prolonged.

The *DSM-5* states that diagnosis of a substance use disorder should be based on a pathologic pattern of behaviors related to the use of the substance. The *DSM-5* notes that an underlying characteristic of substance use disorders is changes in brain circuitry that may persist beyond detoxification. Manifestations of those changes include intense drug craving and relapse. Those patterns of behavior have been categorized into four groups, listed in the following:
E. Impaired control
1. Use of a substance in larger amounts or for a longer time than originally intended
2. Repeated unsuccessful attempts to cut down use of substance
3. A great deal of time spent obtaining, using, and recovering from the substance
4. Intense desire for the substance, especially in an environment in which it was previously used.
F. Social impairment
1. Recurrent substance use leading to a failure to meet personal and social obligations
2. Continued substance use, in spite of significant, ongoing social problems caused or exacerbated by the substance
3. Abandoning important personal and social goals because of substance use
G. Risky use
1. Recurrent substance use in environments in which it is dangerous to use the substance
2. Continued substance use in spite of knowledge of persistent/recurrent physical/psychological problems caused by the substance.
H. Pharmacological criteria
1. Requirement for a markedly increased dose to achieve desired effect or markedly reduced effect at standard dose
2. Desire to consume the substance as a means to mitigate withdrawal symptoms

As a modifier, use severity is assessed across three categories, listed as follows. It is important to note that the word *addiction* has been removed from the *DSM-5* because of its vague definition and possible negative connotation.
A. Mild—two or three of the symptoms listed as follows are present;
B. Moderate—four to five symptoms listed as follows are present;
C. Severe—six or more symptoms listed as follows are present.

Incidence

A. Statistics indicate that the most commonly used legal substances are caffeine, alcohol, and nicotine. According to the National Institute on Drug Abuse (NIDA), tobacco use is the leading preventable cause of disease, disability, and death in the United States. According to the Centers for Disease Control and Prevention (CDC), approximately one in five premature deaths in the United States every year is the result of cigarette smoking.

B. The most commonly used illicit drugs are marijuana and cocaine. In 2013, an estimated 24.6 million Americans aged 12 years or older had used an illicit substance in the past 30 days. NIDA reports usage for the most commonly abused drugs (see Table 2.7).

C. NIDA notes that in 2013 approximately 6.5 million Americans (aged 12 years or older) used prescription drugs for a nonmedical reason in the past 30 days (see Table 2.8). Opioids, central nervous system (CNS) depressants, and stimulants are the most abused prescription drugs.

D. Studies indicate that 8% of adults in the United States had a substance use disorder in the past 12 months. Approximately 40% of hospital admissions are related to substance abuse or related to the effects of using substances.

E. Approximately 88% of the American population consumes some alcohol (at one time or another). In 2009, the Drug Abuse Warning Network (DAWN) reported 4.6 million drug-related emergency department encounters, 32% of which involved alcohol alone or in combination with another substance; 5% to 7% of Americans have alcoholism in a given year, and 13% will have it sometime during their lifetime. Prevalence rates of alcoholism are 5% to 6% for men and 1% to 2% for women. Alcoholism is highest in men aged 18 to 64 years and women aged 18 to 24 years.

F. Approximately 21% of Americans use tobacco products. One study states that there is a link between early nicotine use and alcohol abuse and depression. Smoking before the age of 13 years significantly increases the risk of drug dependence.

G. It is estimated that 37% of the population aged 12 years or older has used an illicit psychoactive drug at least once.

A substance abuse problem is recognized in as few as 1 in 20 substance-abusing patients seeking medical attention.

Pathogenesis

A. No single gene has been identified as the culprit in the predisposition to substance dependence. Certain biological features seem to be inherited by first-degree relatives (particularly males) of alcoholics, for example, a resistance to intoxication, a subnormal cortisol rise after drinking, and a subnormal epinephrine release following stress.

B. Some theories postulate alterations in metabolism of alcohol and drugs in people who are dependent. Studies pertaining to alcohol have included research into genetic heritability, flawed metabolism of alcohol by alcoholics, insensitivity to alcohol inherited by alcoholics (thus tending to increase tolerance or ability to know when to stop), and alterations in brain waves in alcoholics.

C. Although much of the research is specific to only one drug, much of what we know about the research can be applied to other drugs. There appears to be a higher rate of substance dependence, not limited to alcohol, in children of alcoholics.

Predisposing Factors

Factors vary among individuals, and no one factor can account entirely for the risk of substance abuse. Studies indicate a high correlation between substance use and the presence of psychiatric disorders, especially anxiety disorders, depression, schizophrenia, and, in women, eating disorders.

A. Genetic
B. Familial
C. Environmental
D. Occupational
E. Socioeconomic
F. Cultural
G. Personality
H. Life stress
I. Psychiatric comorbidity
J. Biological
K. Social learning and behavioral conditioning

Common Complaints

Patients' complaints will be focused on the symptoms of the problem rather than the substance dependence. The problem itself will be avoided through the use of denial, minimization, blaming, and projection (all signs of the disease of substance dependence).

A. Chronic anxiety and tension
B. Insomnia
C. Chronic depression
D. Headaches and/or back pain

Consider patients who present frequently with somatic complaints, such as back pain or headache, as "drug seeking," especially when the patient knows what drugs work best or asks for specific narcotic analgesics.

E. Blackouts
F. Gastrointestinal problems
G. Tachycardia/palpitations
H. Frequent falls or minor injuries

Substance abuse should be suspected in all patients who present with accidents or signs of repeated trauma, especially to the head.

I. Problems with a loved one, problems at work, or with friends

Other Signs and Symptoms

A. Defensiveness about alcohol/drug use or vagueness with answers

B. History of problems with family life, marital relationships, work, finances, and physical health

C. Change in spiritual beliefs (stops attending religious services)

D. Unexplained job changes and multiple traffic accidents

E. History of impulsive behavior, fighting, or unexplained falls

F. Arrest for public drunkenness, driving under the influence, or illegal activity when alcohol/drugs were involved

G. Tremors (shakes)

TABLE 2.7 Commonly Abused Drugs

Substances: Category and Name	Examples of Commercial and Street Names	DEA Schedule[a]/How Administered[b]	Acute Effects/Health Risks
Tobacco			Increased blood pressure and heart rate/ chronic lung disease; cardiovascular disease; stroke; cancers of the mouth, pharynx, larynx, esophagus, stomach, pancreas, cervix, kidney, bladder, and acute myeloid leukemia; adverse pregnancy outcomes; addiction
Nicotine	Found in cigarettes, cigars, bidis, and smokeless tobacco (snuff, spit tobacco, chew)	Not scheduled/ smoked, snorted, chewed	
Alcohol			In low doses, euphoria, mild stimulation, relaxation, lowered inhibitions; in higher doses, drowsiness, slurred speech, nausea, emotional volatility, loss of coordination, visual distortions, impaired memory, sexual dysfunction, loss of consciousness/increased risk of injuries, violence, fetal damage (in pregnant women); depression; neurologic deficits; hypertension; liver and heart disease; addiction; fatal overdose
Alcohol (ethyl alcohol)	Found in liquor, beer, and wine	Not scheduled/ swallowed	
Cannabinoids			Euphoria; relaxation; slowed reaction time; distorted sensory perception; impaired balance and coordination; increased heart rate and appetite; impaired learning, memory; anxiety; panic attacks; psychosis/cough; frequent respiratory infections; possible mental health decline; addiction
Marijuana	Blunt, dope, ganja, grass, herb, joint, bud, Mary Jane, pot, reefer, green, trees, smoke, sinsemilla, skunk, weed	I/smoked, swallowed	
Hashish	Boom, gangster, hash, hash oil, hemp	I/smoked, swallowed	
Opioids			Euphoria; drowsiness; impaired coordination; dizziness; confusion; nausea; sedation; feeling of heaviness in the body; slowed or arrested breathing; constipation; endocarditis; hepatitis; HIV; addiction; fatal overdose
Heroin	Diacetylmorphine: Smack, horse, brown sugar, dope, H, junk, skag, skunk, white horse, China white; cheese (with OTC cold medicine and antihistamine)	I/injected, smoked, snorted	
Opium	Laudanum, paregoric: Big O, black stuff, block, gum, hop	II, III, V/swallowed, smoked	
Stimulants			Increased heart rate, blood pressure, body temperature, metabolism; feelings of exhilaration; increased energy, mental alertness; tremors; reduced appetite; irritability; anxiety; panic; paranoia; violent behavior; psychosis/weight loss; insomnia; cardiac or cardiovascular complications; stroke; seizures; addiction Also, for cocaine—nasal damage from snorting Also, for methamphetamine—severe dental problems
Cocaine	Cocaine hydrochloride: Blow, bump, C, candy, Charlie, coke, crack, flake, rock, snow, toot	II/snorted, smoked, injected	
Amphetamine	Biphetamine, dexedrine: Bennies, black beauties, crosses, hearts, LA turnaround speed, truck drivers, uppers	II/swallowed, snorted, smoked, injected	
Methamphetamine	Desoxyn: Meth, ice, crank, chalk, crystal, fire, glass, go fast, speed	II/swallowed, snorted, smoked, injected	
Club Drugs			MDMA—mild hallucinogenic effects; increased tactile sensitivity, empathic feelings; lowered inhibition; anxiety; chills; sweating; teeth clenching; muscle cramping/sleep disturbances; depression; impaired memory; hyperthermia; addiction Flunitrazepam—sedation; muscle relaxation; confusion; memory loss; dizziness; impaired coordination/addiction GHB—drowsiness; nausea; headache; disorientation; loss of coordination; memory loss/ unconsciousness; seizures; coma
MDMA	Ecstasy, Adam, clarity, Eve, lover's speed, peace, uppers	I/swallowed, snorted, injected	
Flunitrazepam[c]	Rohypnol: Forget-me pill, Mexican Valium, R2, roach, Roche, roofies, roofinol, rope, rophies	IV/swallowed, snorted	
GHB[c]	Gamma-hydroxybutyrate: G, Georgia home boy, grievous bodily harm, liquid ecstasy, soap, scoop, goop, liquid X	I/swallowed	

(*continued*)

TABLE 2.7 Commonly Abused Drugs (*continued*)

Substances: Category and Name	Examples of Commercial and Street Names	DEA Schedule[a]/How Administered[b]	Acute Effects/Health Risks
Dissociative Drugs			Feelings of being separate from one's body and environment, impaired motor function/ anxiety, tremors, numbness, memory loss, nausea Also for ketamine—analgesia, impaired memory, delirium, respiratory depression and arrest, death Also for PCP and analogs—analgesia, psychosis, aggression, violence, slurred speech, loss of coordination, hallucinations Also for DXM—euphoria, slurred speech, confusion, dizziness, distorted visual perceptions
Ketamine	Ketalar SV: Cat Valium, K, Special K, vitamin K	III/injected, snorted, smoked	
PCP and analogs	Phencyclidine: Angel dust, boat, hog, love boat, peace pill	I, II/swallowed, smoked, injected	
Salvia divinorum	Salvia, Shepherdess's Herb, Maria Pastora, magic mint, Sally-D	Not scheduled/ chewed, swallowed, smoked	
Dextromethorphan (DXM)	Found in some cough and cold medications: Robotripping, Robo, Triple C	Not scheduled/ swallowed	
Hallucinogens			Altered states of perception and feeling; hallucinations; nausea Also for LSD and mescaline—increased body temperature, heart rate, blood pressure; loss of appetite; sweating; sleeplessness; numbness; dizziness; weakness; tremors; impulsive behavior; rapid shifts in emotion Also for LSD—flashbacks, hallucinogen persisting perception disorder Also for psilocybin—nervousness; paranoia; panic
Lysergic acid diethylamide (LSD)	LSD: Acid, blotter, cubes, microdot, yellow sunshine, blue heaven	I/swallowed, absorbed through mouth tissues	
Mescaline	Buttons, cactus, mesc, peyote	I/swallowed, smoked	
Psilocybin	Magic mushrooms, purple passion, shrooms, little smoke	I/swallowed	
Other Compounds			Steroids—no intoxicating effects/hypertension; blood clotting and cholesterol changes; liver cysts; hostility and aggression; acne; in adolescents—premature stoppage of growth; in males—prostate cancer, reduced sperm production, shrunken testicles, breast enlargement; in females—menstrual irregularities, development of beard and other masculine characteristics Inhalants (varies by chemical)—stimulation; loss of inhibition; headache; nausea or vomiting; slurred speech; loss of motor coordination; wheezing/cramps; muscle weakness; depression; memory impairment; damage to cardiovascular and nervous systems; unconsciousness; sudden death
Anabolic steroids	Anadrol, Oxandrin, Durabolin, Depo-Testosterone, Equipoise: Roids, juice, gym candy, pumpers	III/injected, swallowed, applied to skin	
Inhalants	Solvents (paint thinners, gasoline, glues); gases (butane, propane, aerosol propellants, nitrous oxide); nitrites (isoamyl, isobutyl, cyclohexyl): Laughing gas, poppers, snappers, whippets	Not scheduled/inhaled through nose or mouth	
Prescription Medications			
CNS depressants	For more information on prescription medications, please visit www.nida.nih.gov/DrugPages/PrescripDrugsChart.html		
Stimulants			
Opioid pain relievers			

CNS, central nervous system; DEA, Drug Enforcement Administration; GHB, gamma-hydroxybutyric acid; MDMA, methylenedioxymethamphetamine; OTC, over the counter.; PCP, phenylcyclidine.

[a]Schedule I and II drugs have a high potential for abuse. They require greater storage security and have a quota on manufacturing, among other restrictions. Schedule I drugs are available for research only and have no approved medical use; Schedule II drugs are available only by prescription (unrefillable) and require a form for ordering. Schedule III and IV drugs are available by prescription, may have five refills in 6 months, and may be ordered orally. Some Schedule V drugs are available OTC.

[b]Some of the health risks are directly related to the route of drug administration. For example, injection drug use can increase the risk of infection through needle contamination with staphylococci, HIV, hepatitis, and other organisms.

[c]Associated with sexual assaults.

Source: National Institute on Drug Abuse (NIDA): Visit NIDA at www.drugabuse.gov; National Institutes of Health (NIH); U.S. Department of Health and Human Services; NIH: Turning Discovery Into Health.

(*continued*)

TABLE 2.7 Commonly Abused Drugs (*continued*)

Principles of Drug Addiction Treatment

More than three decades of scientific research show that treatment can help drug-addicted individuals stop drug use, avoid relapse, and successfully recover their lives. Based on this research, 13 fundamental principles that characterize effective drug abuse treatment have been developed. These principles are detailed in NIDA's *Principles of Drug Addiction Treatment: A Research-Based Guide*. The guide also describes different types of science-based treatments and provides answers to commonly asked questions.

1. **Addiction is a complex but treatable disease that affects brain function and behavior**. Drugs alter the brain's structure and how it functions, resulting in changes that persist long after drug use has ceased. This may help explain why abusers are at risk of relapse even after long periods of abstinence.
2. **No single treatment is appropriate for everyone**. Matching treatment settings, interventions, and services to an individual's particular problems and needs is critical to his or her ultimate success.
3. **Treatment needs to be readily available**. Because drug-addicted individuals may be uncertain about entering treatment, taking advantage of available services the moment people are ready for treatment is critical. Potential patients can be lost if treatment is not immediately available or readily accessible.
4. **Effective treatment attends to multiple needs of the individual, not just his or her drug abuse**. To be effective, treatment must address the individual's drug abuse and any associated medical, psychological, social, vocational, and legal problems.
5. **Remaining in treatment for an adequate period of time is critical**. The appropriate duration for an individual depends on the type and degree of his or her problems and needs. Research indicates that most addicted individuals need at least 3 months in treatment to significantly reduce or stop their drug use and that the best outcomes occur with longer durations of treatment.
6. **Counseling—individual and/or group—and other behavioral therapies are the most commonly used forms of drug abuse treatment**. Behavioral therapies vary in their focus and may involve addressing a patient's motivations to change, building skills to resist drug use, replacing drug-using activities with constructive and rewarding activities, improving problem-solving skills, and facilitating better interpersonal relationships.
7. **Medications are an important element of treatment for many patients, especially when combined with counseling and other behavioral therapies**. For example, methadone and buprenorphine are effective in helping individuals addicted to heroin or other opioids stabilize their lives and reduce their illicit drug use. Also, for persons addicted to nicotine, a nicotine replacement product (nicotine patches or gum) or an oral medication (bupropion or varenicline), can be an effective component of treatment when part of a comprehensive behavioral treatment program.
8. **An individual's treatment and services plan must be assessed continually and modified as necessary to ensure it meets his or her changing needs**. A patient may require varying combinations of services and treatment components during the course of treatment and recovery. In addition to counseling or psychotherapy, a patient may require medication, medical services, family therapy, parenting instruction, vocational rehabilitation, and/or social and legal services. For many patients, a continuing care approach provides the best results, with treatment intensity varying according to a person's changing needs.
9. **Many drug-addicted individuals also have other mental disorders**. Because drug abuse and addiction—both of which are mental disorders—often co-occur with other mental illnesses, patients presenting with one condition should be assessed for the other(s). And when these problems co-occur, treatment should address both (or all), including the use of medications as appropriate.
10. **Medically assisted detoxification is only the first stage of addiction treatment and by itself does little to change long-term drug abuse**. Although medically assisted detoxification can safely manage the acute physical symptoms of withdrawal, detoxification alone is rarely sufficient to help addicted individuals achieve long-term abstinence. Thus, patients should be encouraged to continue drug treatment following detoxification.
11. **Treatment does not need to be voluntary to be effective**. Sanctions or enticements from family, employment settings, and/or the criminal justice system can significantly increase treatment entry, retention rates, and the ultimate success of drug treatment interventions.
12. **Drug use during treatment must be monitored continuously, as lapses during treatment do occur**. Knowing their drug use is being monitored can be a powerful incentive for patients and can help them withstand urges to use drugs. Monitoring also provides an early indication of a return to drug use, signaling a possible need to adjust an individual's treatment plan to better meet his or her needs.
13. **Treatment programs should assess patients for the presence of HIV/AIDS, hepatitis B and C, tuberculosis, and other infectious diseases, as well as provide targeted risk-reduction counseling to help patients modify or change behaviors that place them at risk of contracting or spreading infectious diseases**. Targeted counseling specifically focused on reducing infectious disease risk can help patients further reduce or avoid substance-related and other high-risk behaviors. Treatment providers should encourage and support HIV screening and inform patients in whom highly active antiretroviral therapy (HAART) has proven effective in combating HIV, including among drug-abusing populations.

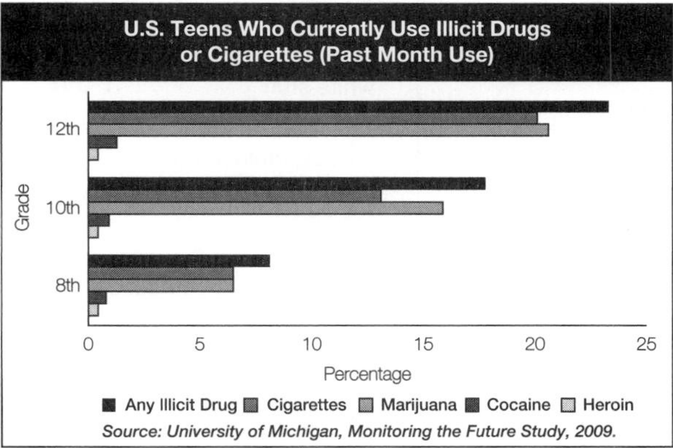

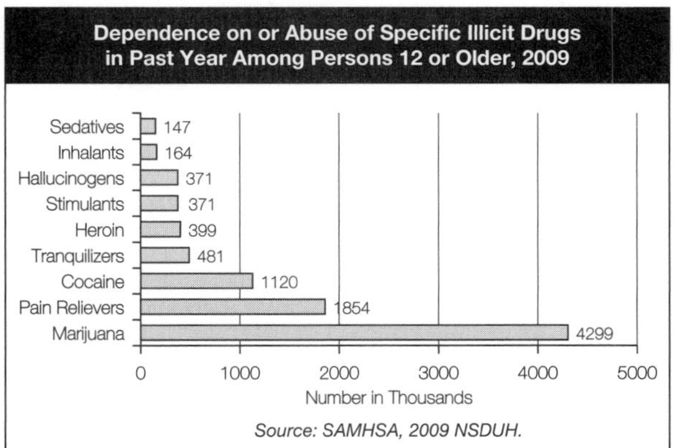

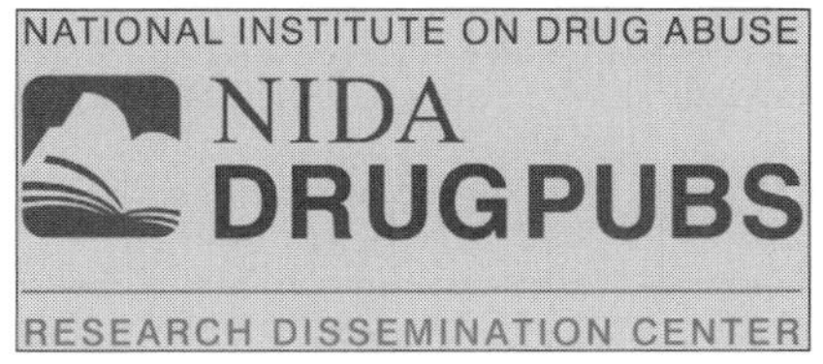

TABLE 2.8 Commonly Abused Prescription Drugs

Substances: Category and Name	Examples of Commercial and Street Names	DEA Schedule[a]/How Administered	Intoxication Effects/Health Risks
Depressants			Sedation/drowsiness; reduced anxiety; feelings of well-being; lowered inhibitions; slurred speech; poor concentration; confusion; dizziness; impaired coordination and memory/slowed pulse; lowered blood pressure; slowed breathing; tolerance; withdrawal; addiction; increased risk of respiratory distress and death when combined with alcohol For barbiturates—euphoria; unusual excitement; fever; irritability/life-threatening withdrawal in chronic users
Barbiturates	*Amytal, Nembutal, Seconal, Phenobarbital*: Barbs, reds, red birds, phennies, tooies, yellows, yellow jackets	II, III, IV/injected, swallowed	
Benzodiazepines	*Ativan, Halcion, Librium, Valium, Xanax, Klonopin*: Candy, downers, sleeping pills, tranks	IV/swallowed	
Sleep medications	*Ambien (zolpidem), Sonata (zaleplon), Lunesta (eszopiclone)*	IV/swallowed	
Opioids and Morphine Derivatives[b]			Pain relief; euphoria; drowsiness; sedation; weakness; dizziness; nausea; impaired coordination; confusion; dry mouth; itching; sweating; clammy skin; constipation/slowed or arrested breathing; lowered pulse and blood pressure; tolerance; addiction; unconsciousness; coma; death. Risk of death increased when combined with alcohol or other CNS depressants For fentanyl—80 to 100 times more potent analgesic than morphine For oxycodone—muscle relaxation/twice as potent analgesic as morphine; high abuse potential For codeine—less analgesia, sedation, and respiratory depression than morphine For methadone—used to treat opioid addiction and pain; significant overdose risk when used improperly
Codeine	*Empirin with Codeine, Fiorinal with Codeine, Robitussin A-C, Tylenol with Codeine:* Captain Cody, Cody, schoolboy; (with glutethimide: Doors & fours, loads, pancakes, and syrup)	II, III, IV/injected, swallowed	
Morphine	*Roxanol, Duramorph:* M, Miss Emma, monkey, white stuff	II, III/injected, swallowed, smoked	
Methadone	*Methadone, Dolophine:* Fizzies, amidone (with MDMA: Chocolate chip cookies)	II/swallowed, injected	
Fentanyl and analogs	*Actiq, Duragesic, Sublimaze:* Apache, China girl, dance fever, friend, good-fella, jackpot, murder 8, TNT, Tango and Cash	II/injected, smoked, snorted	
Other opioid pain relievers: Oxycodone HCL, hydrocodone bitartrate, hydromorphone, oxymorphone, meperidine, propoxyphene	*Tylox, Oxycontin, Percodan, Percocet:* Oxy, O.C., oxycontin, oxycet, hillbilly heroin, percs; *Vicodin, Lortab, Lorcet:* Vike, Watson-387; *Dilaudid:*Juice, smack, D, footballs, dillies; *Opana, Numorphan, Numorphone:* Biscuits, blue heaven, blues, Mrs. O, octagons, stop signs, O Bomb; *Demerol, meperidine hydrochloride:* Demmies, pain killer; *Darvon, Darvocet*	II, III, IV/chewed, swallowed, snorted, injected, suppositories	
Stimulants			Feelings of exhilaration; increased energy; mental alertness/increased heart rate; blood pressure; and metabolism; reduced appetite; weight loss; nervousness; insomnia; seizures; heart attack; stroke For amphetamines—rapid breathing; tremor, loss of coordination; irritability; anxiousness; restlessness/delirium; panic; paranoia; hallucinations; impulsive behavior; aggressiveness; tolerance; addiction For methylphenidate—increase or decrease in blood pressure; digestive problems; loss of appetite; weight loss
Amphetamines	*Biphetamine, Dexedrine, Adderall:* Bennies, black beauties, crosses, hearts, LA turnaround, speed, truck drivers, uppers	II/injected, swallowed, smoked, snorted	
Methylphenidate	*Concerta, Ritalin:* JIF, MPH, R-ball, Skippy, the smart drug, vitamin R	II/injected, swallowed, snorted	

(*continued*)

TABLE 2.8 Commonly Abused Prescription Drugs (*continued*)

Substances: Category and Name	Examples of Commercial and Street Names	DEA Schedule[a]/How Administered	Intoxication Effects/Health Risks
Other Compounds			Euphoria; slurred speech/increased heart rate and blood pressure; dizziness; nausea; vomiting; confusion; paranoia; distorted visual perceptions; impaired motor function
Dextromethorphan (DXM)	Found in some cough and cold medications: Robotripping, Robo, Triple C	Not scheduled/ swallowed	

CNS, central nervous system; DEA, Drug Enforcement Administration; HCl, hydrochloride; MDMA, methylenedioxymethamphetamine.
[a]Schedule I and II drugs have a high potential for abuse. They require greater storage security and have a quota on manufacturing, among other restrictions. Schedule I drugs are available for research only and have no approved medical use. Schedule II drugs are available only by prescription and require a new prescription for each refill. Schedule III and IV drugs are available by prescription, may have five refills in 6 months, and may be ordered orally. Most Schedule V drugs are available OTC.
[b]Taking drugs by injection can increase the risk of infection through needle contamination with staphylococci, HIV, hepatitis, and other organisms. Injection is a more common practice for opioids, but risks apply to any medication taken by injection.
Source: National Institute on Drug Abuse (NIDA): Visit NIDA at www.drugabuse.gov; National Institutes of Health (NIH); U.S. Department of Health and Human Services; NIH: Turning Discovery Into Health.

H. Delirium tremens (DTs)
I. Seizures related to drugs
J. Hallucinations
K. History of chronic family chaos and instability
L. Physical indications of chronic alcohol/drug use include spider angiomas, ruddy nose and face, nasal lesions, bruxism, swollen features, bruises, needle marks/tracks, cutaneous abscesses, malnourishment, anemia, jaundice, and severe dental problems such as "meth mouth."
M. Active withdrawal symptoms include nausea and vomiting, malaise, weakness, tachycardia, diaphoresis, tremors, lightheadedness or dizziness, insomnia, irritability, confusion, perceptual abnormalities or hallucinations (auditory, visual, or tactile), paresthesia, blurred vision, diarrhea, anorexia, abdominal cramps, severe depression, severe anxiety, piloerection, fasciculation (muscle twitching), rhinorrhea, fever, elevated blood pressure and pulse, tinnitus, nystagmus, delirium, or seizures.
N. Overdose symptoms related to drug(s) include seizures, cardiovascular depression/collapse, and respiratory depression/collapse. Be prepared to provide cardiovascular and respiratory support and supportive care until transport.

Subjective Data

A. Review the onset, duration, and course of presenting complaints.
B. The U.S. Preventive Services Task Force (USPSTF) recommends that all adults be screened in primary care for alcohol and drug use.
C. Question the patient regarding relatives with a history of alcohol, tobacco, or drug use or problems pertaining to use.
D. When questioning the patient, assume some use, for example, "At what age did you first start drinking?" Start with the least invasive questions first: Cigarettes, over-the-counter (OTC) medications, prescription medications, then alcohol, marijuana, stimulants, opiates, sedatives, hypnotics, benzodiazepines, barbiturates, hallucinogens, inhalants, steroids, and other drugs.
E. Review use of the following drugs concerning quantity and type (if cigarettes, brand smoked; if alcohol, type of alcohol: Beer, wine, hard liquor), and age at initiation. Query regarding previous attempts to stop use.
F. Start with the past and proceed to the present with use; include first use of the mood-altering substance, amounts, and the last use of the particular substance and amount.
G. Follow the CAGE test. The **CAGE** (two out of four) is highly predictive of addiction.

1. Have you ever tried to **cut** down on your alcohol/drug use?
2. Do you get **annoyed** if someone mentions your use is a problem?
3. Do you ever feel **guilty** about your use?
4. Do you ever have an **"eye-opener"** first thing in the morning after you've been drinking or using the night before?

H. If patient admits drinking or drug use, ascertain specific amounts and last use of each substance.
I. Establish usual weight and recent loss and in what length of time.
J. Determine whether patient experiences suicidal ideation and whether there is a history of past attempts (see Chapter 22, Psychiatric Guidelines, Suicide).

Physical Examination

A. Check temperature, pulse, respirations, blood pressure, and weight.
B. Inspect

1. Observe general appearance, dress, grooming, breath odor, wasted appearance, attitude, sad affect, psychomotor retardation, or tremors.
2. Conduct a dermal examination for spider angiomas, bruises, track marks, color, pallor, rash, jaundice, petechiae, and gynecomastia in men (hallucinogens).

3. Examine the eyes for sclera color and features, pupil size, and reactivity.
4. Inspect the nasal mucosa for erythema, edema, spider telangiectasis, and discharge; look for septal lesions or perforation, deviation, and polyps.
5. Inspect the mouth/pharynx: Oral lesions, poor dental hygiene, erythema, and teeth for uneven surfaces, tooth decay, and gum erosion.

C. Palpate
1. Palpate the neck and thyroid.
2. Palpate the axilla and groin for lymphadenopathy.
3. Palpate the abdomen; note hepatomegaly/tenderness.

D. Percuss
1. Percuss the chest; note pulmonary consolidation.
2. Percuss the abdomen for hepatosplenomegaly.

E. Auscultate
1. Auscultate the heart for murmur, new S4 gallop, single S2, and arrhythmias.
2. Auscultate the lungs for rales, effusion, and consolidation.

F. Perform neurologic examination/mental status.

Diagnostic Tests

A. Blood alcohol level
B. Cotinine level (nicotine); (where available)
C. Urine drug screen
D. Complete blood count (CBC) with differential
E. Platelet count
F. HIV or hepatitis

Intravenous drug use contributes strongly to the spread of AIDS, hepatitis B and hepatitis C, and other infectious diseases. Consider evaluation for sexually transmitted infections.

G. Antinuclear antibody, erythrocyte sedimentation rate, and rheumatoid factor
H. Electrolytes
I. Liver panel
1. Elevated liver enzymes can also be attributed to overuse of acetaminophen (Tylenol), found in combination with opiates.

J. Blood cultures (fever)
K. Bone density studies
1. Patients who have been drinking for years should have bone density studies done because alcohol increases the risk for osteoporosis.

Differential Diagnoses

A. Substance use disorder
B. Chronic pain syndrome
C. Anxiety
D. Depression

Plan

A. General interventions
1. Discuss your concerns about alcohol, nicotine, or drug use and discuss addiction treatment with the patient (refer to the NIDA Principles of Drug Addiction Treatment mentioned earlier in the chapter).
2. At each office visit, provide support to help prevent relapse. If relapse occurs, encourage the patient to try again immediately.
3. Consider signing a contract with the patient to stop smoking, drinking, or using drugs.
4. Assess potential for suicide with every office visit.
5. If possible, obtain confirmation of the patient's abstinence from a family member.
6. Stress the importance of 12-step meetings such as Alcoholics Anonymous (AA), Cocaine Anonymous (CA), and Narcotics Anonymous (NA).
7. Have the patient sign a written release of information so that you can speak with a rehabilitation counselor. If the patient is willing, refer to an alcohol and drug treatment facility or smoking-cessation program, after initial assessment and differential diagnosis is made.
8. Treat physical/laboratory findings as indicated.
9. Identify potential withdrawal symptoms from the cessation of stimulants, such as caffeine intake reduction, alcohol, and drug use.
10. If malnourished, discuss dietary needs and treatment.

B. Patient teaching; *See Section III: Patient Teaching Guide for this chapter, "Alcohol and Drug Dependence."* ◀
1. Educate the patient about the impact of alcohol, tobacco, and drugs on physical/emotional health. Provide information for the patient to read at home.

C. Pharmaceutical therapy
1. Consider nicotine replacement for those who smoke more than one pack of cigarettes per day or who smoke their first cigarette within 30 minutes of waking. Stress that there is *no smoking* while using the nicotine patch. The FDA has changed this warning www.fda.gov/ForConsumers/ConsumerUpdates/ucm345087 .htm
2. Nicoderm (dosing based on more than 10 cigarettes/d habit)
   a. 21 mg/qD for 6 weeks (14 mg qD × 6 weeks for less than 10 cigarettes/d) *then*
   b. 14 mg/qD for 2 weeks (7 mg qD × 6 weeks for less than 10 cigarettes/d) *then*
   c. 7 mg/qD for 2 weeks (only for more than 10 cigarettes/d habit)
3. Nonnicotine therapy: Adults—Bupropion (Zyban, Wellbutrin) 150 extended release (ER) mg daily for 3 days, then increase to 150 mg ER twice daily. Treat for 7 to 12 weeks. The patient may continue to smoke during the first 2 weeks of starting medication. This medication should not be given to patients with seizure disorders.
4. Varenicline (Chantix): Start at 0.5 mg/d for the first 3 days, then for the next 4 days, 0.5 mg twice

daily. After the first 7 days the dose is 1 mg twice daily × 11 weeks.

a. Encourage the patient to choose a stop date for smoking and start the Chantix 1 to 2 weeks before this stop date.

b. Patients should be encouraged to quit even if they have relapses.

c. Instruct patients that the most common side effects of Chantix are insomnia, vivid or strange dreams, and nausea. Advise that side effects are usually transient.

d. Warn the patient regarding potential side effects of mood swings, aggression, homicidal thoughts, psychosis, anxiety, and panic disorder, which may occur on rare occasions.

e. See package inserts or the *Physicians' Desk Reference* for detailed instructions.

5. Detoxification and methadone maintenance: Should be performed by specially licensed and trained professionals.

6. Disulfiram (Antabuse) therapy is not recommended. Patients who consume alcohol after taking Antabuse can become extremely ill.

7. Refer the patient to a physician or specialist if the patient is experiencing withdrawal; consider admission to rehabilitation center for detoxification and treatment.

Follow-Up

A. Make a follow-up appointment weekly. Make contact with the referral source (smoking cessation program, alcohol/drug rehabilitation program) before the next follow-up visit to check on the patient's progress. At the weekly visit, question the patient regarding compliance.

B. Order blood alcohol, urine drug screen, or nicotine level (as appropriate) with every office visit while in outpatient treatment and throughout the year following treatment.

C. Once positive change is seen, the patient can be seen monthly. Discuss changes the patient has made, past relapses, circumstances under which they occurred, and any special concerns.

D. Refer to the medical diagnosis for other applicable follow-up recommendations.

Consultation/Referral

A. Refer patients with drug and/or alcohol dependence to a community mental health center that has an outpatient alcohol/drug rehabilitation program or to a specialist in the community who deals frequently with substance abuse/dependence.

B. Planning a family meeting to confront the patient is best done with the help of an experienced mental health professional.

C. Have referral numbers at close hand, so that the patient's moment of motivation is not lost.

Individual Considerations

A. Pregnancy

1. Substance-dependent pregnant women frequently avoid early prenatal care for fear of identification and reprisal.

2. Cocaine use is associated with abruptio placenta and preterm labor. Consider drug screen for emergent admissions for patients in preterm labor and abruption.

3. Notify the hospital nursery personnel/neonatologist before delivery to closely monitor the newborn for withdrawal and seizure precautions.

4. Nicotine/smoking use is associated with intrauterine growth restriction, preterm delivery, and bleeding in pregnancy.

5. Nicotine-dependent pregnant women should be encouraged to stop smoking without pharmacological treatment. The nicotine patch should be used during pregnancy only if the increased likelihood of smoking cessation, with its potential benefits, outweighs the risk of nicotine replacement and potential concomitant smoking. Similar factors should be considered in lactating women.

6. Pregnant women who use alcohol, tobacco, or drugs should always be classified as substance dependent rather than substance abusive.

B. Pediatrics

1. Infants of smokers have increased risk of sudden infant death syndrome (SIDS).

2. The diagnosis of substance dependence is more difficult to make in children younger than 18 years. If there is any indication of substance dependence, children should be referred to a pediatrician who deals specifically with this problem.

3. Consider drug use when alienation of friends and family, falling grades, and isolation occur.

4. "Huffing" is common with gasoline, glues, aerosol sprays, and spray paints.

5. The use of synthetic cannabinoid products is on the rise in the adolescent population. K2, Spice, and bath salts and others are available in tobacco stores, gas stations, over the Internet, and in other small shops. These products can be very harmful. They are not detected on routine toxicology drug screens. Be aware of illicit drug use if patients present with change in behavior, depression, paranoid delusion, and aggressive behaviors. Educate the patient and family regarding the toxic use of these OTC substances. Stress to the patient that these are abusive substances that can potentially be fatal. Stress cessation of use and refer to specialist.

C. Adults

1. With women, tolerance can be established by asking the question, "How many drinks does it take to make you high?" More than two drinks indicates some tolerance.

2. In considering a diagnosis of alcohol dependence, consider the following diagnostic findings: Hypertension; nonspecific EKG changes; cardiomyopathy; palpitations; increased mean cell volume; decreased red blood cell count; low platelet count; increased alanine aminotransferase (ALT), aspartate aminotransferase (AST), lactic dehydrogenase, gamma-glutamyl transpeptidase, alkaline phosphatase; type IV hyperlipoproteinemia; gout; and adult-onset diabetes mellitus.

D. Geriatrics
   1. In this population, consumption of as little as 1 oz/d can indicate a problem.
   2. Pain medications and benzodiazepines, along with multiple medications for health problems, may create a substance abuse problem.
E. Partners/family members
   1. For fear of retribution, the family may remain silent about the problem, even if accompanying the patient to the health care visit.
   2. Some studies by corporate business show that, per capita, business spends more money on the care of family members of substance-dependent patients than on the employee.
   3. Refer family members of alcoholics/drug addicts to Al-Anon, Nar-Anon, Co-dependents Anonymous, or Adult Children of Alcoholics (ACOA) meetings.

Resources

American Society of Metabolic and Bariatric Surgery: www.info@asmbs.org
National Institute on Drug Abuse (NIDA): www.drugabuse.gov; NIDA for Teens: https://teens.drugabuse.gov
Substance Abuse and Mental Health Services Administration (SAMSHA): http://www. samsha.gov

References

American Psychiatric Association. (1994). *Diagnostic and statistical manual of mental disorders* (4th ed.). Washington, DC: American Psychiatric Press.
American Psychiatric Association. (2013). *Diagnostic and statistical manual of mental disorders* (5th ed.). Arlington, VA: American Psychiatric Publishing.

Violence

Moya Cook and Robertson Nash

Children

Definition

The definitions of *sexual abuse, childhood abuse*, and the age of children included in statistics changes with each state in the United States. Any family member, friend, or stranger can perpetrate abuse; however, fathers, mothers' boyfriends, female babysitters, and mothers are the most common perpetrators of abuse. Nonaccidental injury/abuse may result in serious physical or emotional harm and may result in failure to thrive (FTT), delayed developmental progress, or death.

A. Physical abuse: Infliction of pain/harm producing injuries, including skeletal fractures, skin (i.e., burns), and CNS injuries (i.e., abusive head trauma [AHT] and shaken baby syndrome [SBS]/shaking-impact syndrome)
B. Sexual abuse: Inappropriate exposure; fondling; sexual stimulation; coercion; oral, genital, buttock, breast contact; anal or vaginal penetration; foreign-body insertion; and making use of child pornography
C. Emotional abuse: Rejection, lack of affection or stimulation, ignoring, dominating, intimidating, describing the child negatively, blaming the child, and verbal abuse (belittle, yell, threats of severe punishment) abuse, resulting in impaired psychological growth and development
D. Child neglect: Isolation; starvation; lack of medical care; inadequate supervision; failure to provide love, affection, and emotional support; and failure to enroll/attend school

Incidence

A. Childhood abuse occurs worldwide; the exact incidence is not known. It occurs across all cultures and at all racial, socioeconomic, and educational levels.
B. Approximately one million cases of child abuse and/or neglect are reported annually by child protective services (CPS).
C. Sexual abuse is underreported, underrecognized, and undertreated.
D. Approximately one in six boys is sexually abused before the age of 16 years.
E. Greater than 15 million children live with families in which partner violence occurs at least once a year. Seven million children live in families in which severe partner violence occurs. Witnessing domestic violence is associated with experiencing physical abuse and witnessing physical abuse of a sibling.

Pathogenesis

A. Society, lack of parenting skills, the home environment substance abuse, and untreated mental illness are all factors that contribute to abuse.

Predisposing Factors

A. Child victims
   1. Minority children
   2. Disabled or medically fragile children
      a. Congenital anomalies
      b. Mental retardation
      c. Handicapped
      d. Chronic medical illness
      e. Hyperactive
      f. Adopted children/stepchildren
      g. Poor bonding
   3. Age of children (physical abuse)
      a. Younger than 1 year (67%)
      b. Children younger than 3 years (80%)
B. Parental factors
   1. Young or single parents
   2. Distant or absent extended family
   3. Low educational level of parents
   4. Few role boundaries
   5. Acute or chronic instability and stress in the family
      a. Loss of employment
      b. Divorce/death
      c. Drug/alcohol abuse
      d. Parents with a history of abuse/neglect as a child (learned behavior)
      e. Presence of psychiatric illness
      f. Poverty
      g. Criminal history

C. Sexual abuse risk factors
  1. Male
    a. Younger than 13 years
    b. Non-White
    c. Low socioeconomic status
    d. Not living with the biological father
    e. Disabled
  2. Female
    a. Young age between 7 and 14 years
    b. Absence of a parent
    c. Appearance of isolation, depression, or loneliness

Common Complaints

A. Oral/facial injuries
  1. Oropharyngeal sexually transmitted infections: Sexual abuse
  2. Black eyes
  3. Nasal perforation/septal deviation
  4. Skull fracture
  5. Traumatic alopecia
  6. Retinal hemorrhage
  7. Hearing loss/tympanic injury
B. Burns (6%–20% of injuries)
  1. Cigarette burns (pathognomonic for child abuse)
  2. Scalding/immersion
  3. Caustic exposure
  4. Branding
  5. Microwave burns
  6. Stun-gun burns
C. Fractures (second most common injury)
D. Bruises (most common type of injury)
E. Lacerations
F. Bites
G. Force feeding "bottle jamming"/forced ingestion (water, salt, pepper, poisons)
H. Starvation
I. Sexual abuse
  1. Difficulty with bowel movements
  2. Urinary tract infections
  3. Vaginal infections, itching, or discharge
  4. Complains of stomachaches
  5. Headaches
  6. Vaginal or rectal bleeding
  7. Difficulty walking or sitting
J. Behavioral signs
  1. Loss of appetite/eating disorder
  2. Clinging, withdrawn, or aggressive
  3. Nightmares, disturbed sleep pattern, and fear of the dark
  4. Regression (i.e., bedwetting, thumb sucking, crying)
  5. Poor grades/school attendance
  6. Expression of interest or affection inappropriate for the child's age
  7. Intercourse or masturbation or other sexual acting out
  8. Self-injurious behavior (i.e., cutting, biting, pulling out hair)

Other Signs and Symptoms

A. A caregiver's refusal to allow an interview of the child alone in the examination room is considered a "red flag" for abuse.
B. The history is inconsistent, changes with repeated questioning, conflicts with other family members/caregivers who are interviewed, is implausible, or there is a total lack of history (i.e., "I don't know how it happened").
C. History is inconsistent with the child's developmental ability/stage.
D. Caregiver behaviors that may indicate abuse include delay in seeking care, argumentativeness, lack of emotional response, inappropriateness, or violence.
E. Radiographs should be obtained for a history of "soft," easily broken bones.
F. The child exhibits inappropriate behavior for his or her developmental age.

Subjective Data

A. Use open-ended questions during the history to evaluate how injuries were sustained. As the interview continues, ask specific questions related to responses. If the child can talk, direct questions to him or her before the caregiver.
B. If this is the first clinic visit, ask whether the child had routine health care, including immunizations.

Physical Examination

The physical examination should be performed with the child totally unclothed; however, clothing can be removed as the physical progresses from head to toe (i.e., upper body, torso, lower body, lastly perineum/rectum). Detailed documentation of history is essential.

A. Check blood pressure, pulse, and respirations, and temperature if indicated.
B. A forensic examination requires thorough documentation of injuries.
  1. Use color photographs before any treatment is started.
  2. Photograph damaged clothing.
  3. Take at least one full-body photograph and a facial photograph.
  4. Take close-up photographs of all injuries.
  5. Use a ruler to identify/document the size of injuries.
  6. Documentation on the back of the photographs should include the patient's name, date, photographer's name, as well as any witnesses to the examination. The photographer should also sign each photograph.
C. General observation
  1. Observe the interactions between the caregiver and the child. Is the child fearful or reluctant to have the examination? Are there signs of discomfort during the examination with movement such as range of motion (ROM)?
  2. Evaluate the child's overall appearance: Is the child clean and are his or her clothes appropriate for the

season? Observe for poor hygiene, body odor, malnourishment, dehydration, depression, violence, withdrawn, behavioral compliance even during a painful examination of the rectum/genitalia, and level of consciousness.

3. Dermal examination: Evaluate from head to toe, including the palms, soles of the feet, and between toes; observe for injuries in different stages of healing and new trauma, including burns, lesions, swelling, bruises, and signs of pinching. Evaluate the corner of the mouth for signs of being gagged. Examine the head for alopecia from hair pulling. Evaluate bruises and burns for the characteristics of shapes (i.e., iron, handprints, long belt marks, loops, bite marks, ligature marks).

4. Eye examination: Observe for retinal hemorrhages, black eyes, periorbital edema, and papilledema (indicates increased intracranial pressure).

5. Ear examination: Evaluate hearing, hemotympanum or possible laceration to the external canal, and insertion of foreign objects.

6. Nasal examination: Evaluate the presence of blood, swelling, and foreign objects.

7. Mouth and throat: Evaluate the presence of caustic ingestion; observe for ligature marks and cry/voice quality.

D. Auscultate

1. Heart

2. Lungs

3. Abdomen in all four quadrants

4. Over the globes of the eyes if warranted (bruit may indicate traumatic carotid cavernous fistula)

5. The carotid arteries bilaterally if warranted (bruit may indicate carotid dissection)

E. Palpate

1. Examine for facial fractures; palpate for instability of the facial bones, including the zygomatic arch.

2. Palpate abdomen in all four quadrants for guarding, tenderness, and masses (hematoma).

3. Examine for any trauma to the spine.

F. Neurologic examination

1. Assess mental status and memory: Determine whether the patient is awake, alert, cooperative, and oriented (to person, place, time, and situation). Temporary impairment of memory is one of the most common deficits after a head injury.

2. Assess cranial nerve function.

a. Opthalmoscopic/visual examination (cranial nerve II)

b. Pupillary response (cranial nerve III)

c. Extraocular movements (cranial nerves III, IV, VI)

d. Facial sensation and muscles of mastication (cranial nerve V)

e. Facial expression and taste (cranial nerve VII)

3. Perform a motor examination on all four extremities.

4. Perform a sensory examination on all four extremities.

G. Genital/rectal examination

1. Evaluate genitals/anal area for redness, swelling, bruising, hematomas, abrasions, or lacerations.

2. Evaluate for evidence of sperm.

3. Evaluate for presence of condyloma.

4. Evaluate for presence of foreign bodies.

Diagnostic Tests

Diagnostic tests and x-rays are ordered dependent on the type of presenting complaints and physical examination.

A. Complete blood count (CBC) with differential and peripheral smear; bleeding evaluation, including prothrombin time/partial thromboplastin time (PT/PTT), alanine aminotransferase (ALT), and aspartate aminotransferase (AST), to evaluate injury to the liver, serum amylase, or lipase to rule out pancreatic injury

B. Urinalysis

C. Drug screen/toxicology (urine and serum)

D. Obtain forensic DNA samples from the skin, under nails, vagina, rectum, and saliva from bite marks using sterile cotton-tipped applicators that have been moistened with sterile saline. These should be sent to a crime laboratory as soon as possible.

E. Test for sexually transmitted infections/HIV.

F. Pregnancy test (age appropriate)

G. Radiographs: Facial injury, anteroposterior (AP) and lateral radiograph for any areas of bone tenderness, swelling, deformity, or limited ROM

H. Neuroimaging CT/MRI for any suspected nonaccidental head injury (i.e., head trauma, history of shaking, and scalp hematoma)

Differential Diagnoses

A. Child abuse (physical, sexual, emotional, and/or neglect)

B. Congenital syphilis

C. Rickets

D. Osteogenesis imperfecta (OI)

E. Mongolian spots

F. Impetigo

G. Dermatitis herpetiformis

H. Folk-healing practices

I. Immune thrombocytopenia (ITP)

J. Malignancy

K. Meningitis: Neurologic signs

Plan

A. General interventions

1. Each state may have a requirement for parental permission before taking any photographs.

B. Safety planning is the first priority. Contact (states differ on reporting).

C. Increase public awareness.

D. Failure to report a suspected case of sexual abuse may incur criminal charges.

Patient Teaching

A. Reinforce that abuse/neglect is not the victim's fault.

B. Help is available.

Pharmaceutical Therapy

A. Prescribe antibiotics to treat sexually transmitted infections or wounds.

B. Antidepressant therapy may be appropriate.

Follow-Up

A. Each state mandates reporting of child abuse. Refer to your state requirements or laws. CPS is responsible for investigations. Depending on your locality, police involvement may be mandatory. The Child Abuse Prevention Services (CAPS) website lists individual state abuse hotlines: www.capsli.org/reporting-abuse/individual-state-hotlines

B. Hospitalization may be required, depending on physical findings, child safety, and parental observation.

C. Child victims are at high risk of depression, anxiety, eating disorders, discipline problems, drug/alcohol use, runaway tendencies, and low self-esteem. Therapy and follow-up vary for each individual child. Family participation in a recommended treatment program is helpful. The goal of treatment is to help the child regain his or her prior state of mental and psychological health. Neglect is the major reason that children are removed from a home, especially when the parents have drug/alcohol problems.

Consultation/Referral

A. Consult with other health care providers who have greater experience with abuse (i.e., CPS, physician, psychiatrist or psychologist, social worker).

B. Refer for a nurse in-home assessment if available/indicated.

C. Specialty consultations

- **1.** Genetic consultation: OI
- **2.** Orthopedic consultation
- **3.** Plastic surgeon
- **4.** Child psychiatrist
- **5.** Ophthalmology

Resources

Childhelp Prevention and Treatment of Child Abuse: www.childhelp.org
National Child Abuse Hotline: 1-800-422-4453
Rape, Abuse & Incest National Network (RAINN): 1-800-656-HOPE
Stop It Now: 1-888-PREVENT (1-888-773-8368)

Intimate Partner Violence

Definition

A. *Intimate partner violence (IPV)* is defined as intentional control or victimization of a person with whom the abuser has had or is currently in an intimate, romantic, or spousal relationship. Domestic IPV crosses all cultures and economic boundaries; it encompasses violence between both genders, including gay and lesbian relationships. Abusive behaviors can occur in a single event, sporadically, or continually. The following is a list of the many forms through which IPV may manifest itself:

B. Physical abuse, sexual assault, coercion, social isolation, emotional abuse, economic control, and deprivation are associated with IPV. There is no typical abuser, although all abusers tend to be violent in the home setting and their behavior at work is normal.

C. Forms of physical violence include threatening or assaulting with weapons, pushing, shoving, slapping, punching, choking, kicking, holding, throwing objects, and binding.

D. Psychological abuse includes threats of physical harm to the victim or others, humiliations, intimidation, degradation, ridicule, false accusation, isolation, and deprivation of food, money, access to health care, and transportation.

E. Psychological abuse in lesbian, gay, bisexual, and transgender (LGBT) relationships includes the threat to "out" their partner as well as threats related to custody of coparent children.

F. Cyberstalking is psychological abuse via the Internet or texting. Intimate partner stalking can occur during a relationship or after the relationship ends.

- **1.** Monitoring cell phone and Internet activity
- **2.** Posting photographs or other types of humiliation on social media

G. Sexual abuse is nonconsensual (unwanted kissing or touching) or painful sexual acts.

H. Reproductive coercion is another form of IPV.

- **1.** Partner sabotage of safe-sex practices (i.e., refusal to use condoms, exposing the patient to sexually transmitted infections)
- **2.** Refusal/control of contraception
- **3.** Forcing the woman to have an abortion, or utilizing physical violence to endanger a pregnancy
- **4.** Controlling access to health care

Incidence

> *The exact incidence of IPV is unknown because of the lack of reporting. The United Nations estimates that more than 600 million women live in countries where domestic violence is not considered a crime. The most significant reason for missing the diagnosis of IPV is failure to ask the patient.*

A. Domestic violence is the leading cause of homicide in women globally.

B. Up to 75% of domestic assaults occur after separation; women are most likely to be murdered when reporting abuse or attempting to leave an abusive relationship.

C. An estimated 81% of women stalked by an intimate partner also suffer physical assault. Stalking by an intimate partner is estimated at 1 million women and 317,000 men per year.

D. An estimated 4% to 15% of women presenting in emergency rooms have situations related to domestic violence.

E. Women who separate have a risk of violence approximately three times that of divorced women.

- **1.** More than half of the children who witness domestic violence intervene in some way, including yelling to the abuser to stop, calling for help, and trying to get away.

F. The incidence of abused men is estimated as one in three. Men are also victims of attempted or complete rape, at approximately 3% during their lifetime.

G. Pregnancy has an increased incidence of violence.

- **1.** One in five young women and 35% of women overall have experienced pregnancy coercion.
- **2.** 53% of young women have experienced birth control sabotage.
- **3.** It is estimated that 5% to 20% of intimate partner abuse occurs against pregnant women.

H. Sexual violence, rape, physical assault, or stalking by an intimate partner occurs in 11% of lesbians and in 15% of men with male partners.

I. Among college women, 20% to 30% report violence during a date.

J. Physical, emotional, or verbal abuse is estimated in one in three adolescent girls from a dating partner in the United States.

  1. The tween population (ages 11 to 14 years) reports that half of their friends have experienced dating violence.

  2. Tween population reports that their friends are victims of verbal abuse.

  3. Teen victims are more likely to smoke, use drugs, and have other risky behaviors.

K. Women in the military are recognized as a vulnerable population susceptible to abuse because of geographical location away from family and friends and the social isolation within the military culture.

  1. In 2012, the Department of Defense (DoD) estimated that 26,000 instances of unwanted sexual contact occurred in the U.S. military.

    a. Only 2,949 (approximately 7%) were reported.

  2. One in three convicted military sex offenders remain in the military.

  3. The highest rates of abuse occur in the Army, followed by the Marines and then the Navy; the Air Force has the lowest rate of abuse of the branches of the service.

Pathogenesis

Intrapartner violence is not associated with an underlying medical condition. The cycle of abuse has three phases.

A. Tension building, in which the victim tries to avoid violence and is described as "walking on eggs," unsure what will trigger an abusive incident

B. Explosion and acute battering occur

C. "Honeymoon phase," noted for the absence of tension and reconciliation

D. Victims stay with their partners for multiple reasons, including fear, shame, denial, religious reasons, lack of resources, custody issues and other legal issues, fear of being "outed," and family pressures.

Predisposing Factors

A. Gender: Victims are predominantly female.

B. Race: African American, American Indians, Hispanic women, and Alaskan Natives

C. Higher incidence in interracial couples

D. Pregnancy

E. History of violence

  1. Violence present in family of origin

  2. Abuse as a child: 50% report abuse as an adult

F. History of drug use

G. Posttraumatic stress disorder (PTSD)

H. Lack of social support systems

I. Impulse control disorders

J. Poor economic status

K. Lesbian, gay, bisexual, and transgender (LGBT)

Common Complaints

A. Vague complaints

B. Sexual problems

C. Depression

D. Chronic pain inconsistent with organic disease

E. Chronic headaches/migraines

F. Stress

  1. Anxiety

  2. Panic attacks

G. Alcohol or drug abuse (the batterer, victim, or both)

H. Current or past self-mutilation

I. Gynecologic and obstetric complaints

  1. Dyspareunia

  2. Frequent vaginal or urinary tract infections

  3. Pelvic pain/infection

  4. Recurrent sexually transmitted infections

  5. Unintended pregnancy

  6. Late prenatal care

  7. Miscarriage

  8. Preterm bleeding/delivery

J. Complaints of falls and other recurrent accidents

K. Eating disorders

L. Gastrointestinal complaints/irritable bowel syndrome

M. Musculoskeletal complaints

Other Signs and Symptoms

A. Multiple prior visits to the emergency room for traumatic and nontraumatic complaints

B. A delay between injury and office visits (may result from lack of transportation or the inability to leave the house)

C. Noncompliance with the treatment or missed appointments (lack of access to money or telephones)

D. Suicide attempt (25% higher in women with IPV)

E. A partner who accompanies the patient at all visits

Subjective Data

The "gold standard" research method to document the prevalence of women's exposure to violence includes conducting the interview one on one, in private, and asking specific direct questions.

A. The batterer often refuses to leave the patient alone and may answer questions for the patient. Translators should not be a member of the patient's or suspected abuser's family.

B. Use direct questions: Women-validated Partner Violence Screen (PVS).

  1. Have you been hit, punched, kicked, or otherwise hurt by someone in the past year? If yes, by whom and were you injured?

  2. Do you feel safe in your current relationship?

  3. Is a partner from a previous relationship making you feel unsafe now?

  4. Are you here today because of injuries from a partner?

  5. Are you here today because of illness or stress related to threats, violent behavior, or fears of a partner?

C. Assess whether the patient has ever told family or friends, called hotlines, or attempted to leave the abuser.

D. Has the patient sought help with law enforcement or legal help, that is, filed a criminal complaint or got an order of protection?
E. Are there any weapons in the home?
  1. Has the abuser ever threatened or tried to kill you?
  2. Are you thinking of suicide? Have you ever considered or attempted to commit suicide because of problems in your relationship?
  3. Have you ever considered or attempted killing your batterer?
  4. Do you have a plan?

Physical Examination

A. Enforce the need to interview and conduct physical examinations in private. Do a full-body examination, including the head/scalp.
  1. Most injuries are to the central (breast, chest, and abdomen) area, which is easily concealed by clothing.
  2. Other frequent sites of injury include the head, face, throat, and genitals.
  3. Explain the physical examination and touch with permission.
  4. Forensic examinations need thorough documentation of injuries.
    a. Use color photographs before any treatment is started.
    b. Photograph damaged clothing.
    c. Take at least one full-body photograph and a facial photograph.
    d. Take close-up photographs of all injuries.
    e. Use a ruler to identify/document the size of injuries.
    f. Documentation on the back of the photographs should include the patient's name, date, and photographer's name, as well as any witnesses to the examination. The photographer should also sign each photograph.
    g. Use direct quotes of the patient's history of the violence.
B. Check blood pressure, pulse, and respirations.
C. General observation: Observe for depression/withdrawn, or flat affect, anxiousness, fearfulness, evasiveness, poor eye contact, and wearing heavy makeup or clothing to conceal signs of abuse. Evaluate voice changes: Dysphonia and aphonia. Observe for difficulty breathing.
D. Inspect
  1. Dermal examination for the presence of cigarette burns, impression marks, rope burns, welts, abrasions, scratch marks, claw marks, bite marks, ligature marks, petechiae, and contusions at multiple sites (e.g., back, legs, buttocks).
  2. Eye examination
    a. Observe subconjunctival hemorrhages from strangulation/struggle.
    b. Perform a funduscopic examination (if indicated secondary to trauma).
  3. Evaluate the genitals for lacerations and hematomas of the vagina or labia.
E. Auscultate
  1. All lung fields.
  2. The bowel sounds in all four quadrants of the abdomen.
F. Palpate
  1. Evaluate skull/facial trauma to the maxillofacial area, eye orbits, mandible, and nasal bones. Facial injuries are reported in 94% of victims.
  2. Evaluate for dislocations, fractures (including spiral fractures), sprains, and contusions to the wrists and forearms, and shoulders.
G. Percuss abdomen, chest, and areas of injury (if indicated secondary to trauma).
H. Perform a neurologic examination (if indicated secondary to trauma).
I. Genital/rectal examination
  1. Evaluate genitals/anus area for redness, swelling, bruising, hematomas, abrasions, or lacerations.
  2. Perform bimanual examination (females).
  3. Order an anoscopy (if indicated).
  4. Evaluate for evidence of sperm (recto/vaginal).
  5. Evaluate for the presence of condyloma (perineum, rectum, vagina).
  6. Evaluate for the presence of foreign bodies (recto/vaginal).

Diagnostic Tests

Diagnostic tests and x-rays are ordered dependent on the type of presenting complaints and physical examination.
A. Administer a domestic abuse assessment screening tool and have the victim mark a body map of injuries (see Figure 2.4).
B. CBC with differential and peripheral smear, bleeding evaluation, including PT/PTT, ALT, and AST, to evaluate injury to the liver, serum amylase, or lipase to rule out pancreatic injury.
C. Urinalysis
D. Drug/toxicology screen (urine and blood)
E. Obtain forensic DNA samples from the skin, under nails, vagina, rectum, and saliva from bite marks using sterile cotton-tipped applicators that have been moistened with sterile saline. These should be sent to a crime laboratory as soon as possible.
F. Test for sexually transmitted infections/HIV.
G. Pregnancy test (if indicated)
H. Radiographs: Facial injury, AP, and lateral radiograph for any areas of bone tenderness, swelling, deformity, or limited ROM
I. Ultrasounds as indicated
J. Neuroimaging CT/MRI may be used for any suspected nonaccidental head injury (i.e., head trauma, or scalp hematoma)

Differential Diagnoses

A. Domestic violence
  1. Intimate partner abuse
  2. Elder abuse
  3. Child abuse
B. Rape
C. Other: Related to presenting symptoms

ABUSE ASSESSMENT SCREEN

1. Have you ever been emotionally or physically abused by your partner or someone important to you?
   Yes ☐ No ☐
   If yes, by whom? ___________
   Total number of times ___________
2. Within the last year, have you been hit, slapped, kicked, or otherwise physically hurt by someone?
   Yes ☐ No ☐
   If yes, by whom? ___________
   Total number of times ___________
3. Since you've been pregnant, have you been hit, slapped, kicked, or otherwise physically hurt by someone?
   Yes ☐ No ☐
   If yes, by whom? ___________
   Total number of times ___________
4. Within the last year, has anyone forced you to engage in sexual activity?
   Yes ☐ No ☐
   If yes, by whom? ___________
   Total number of times ___________
5. Are you afraid of your partner or anyone you listed previously?
   Yes ☐ No ☐

MARK THE AREA OF INJURY ON A BODY MAP AND SCORE EACH INCIDENT ACCORDING TO THE FOLLOWING SCALE

If any of the descriptions for the higher number apply, use the higher number.

1 = Threats of abuse, including use of a weapon
2 = Slapping, pushing; no injury and/or lasting pain
3 = Punching, kicking, bruises, cuts, and/or continuing pain
4 = Beating up, severe contusions, burns, broken bones
5 = Head injury, internal injury, permanent injury
6 = Use of weapon; wound from weapon

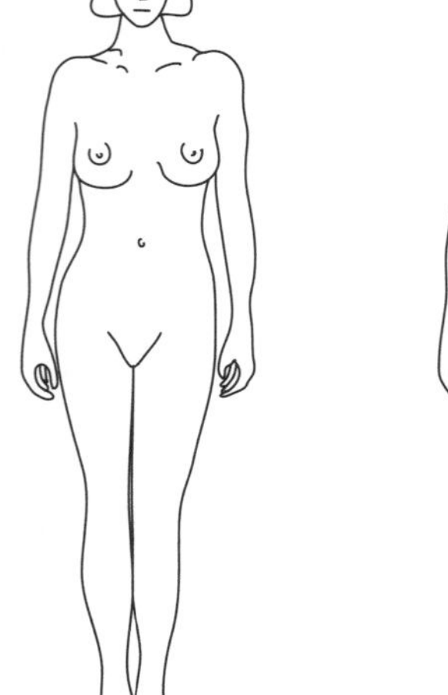
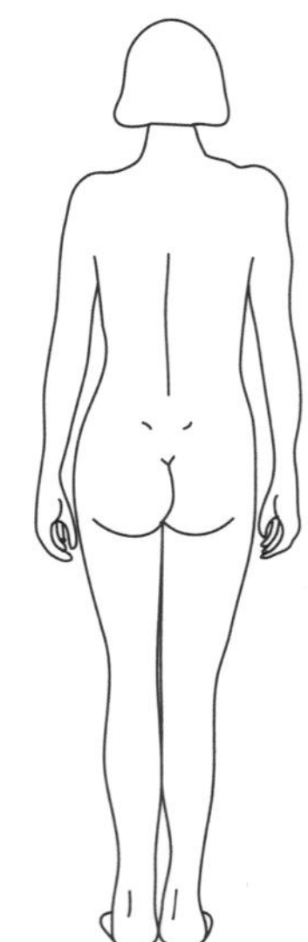
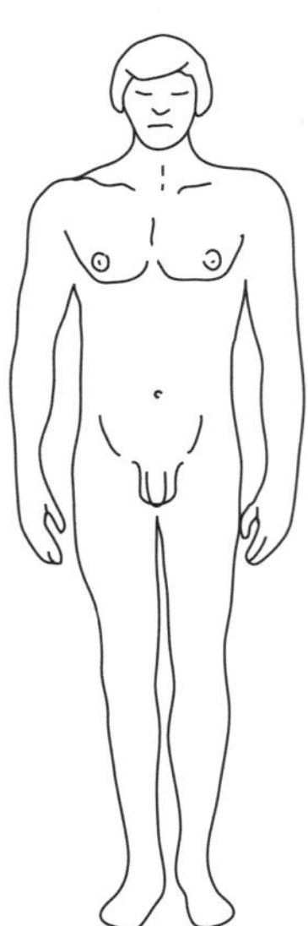
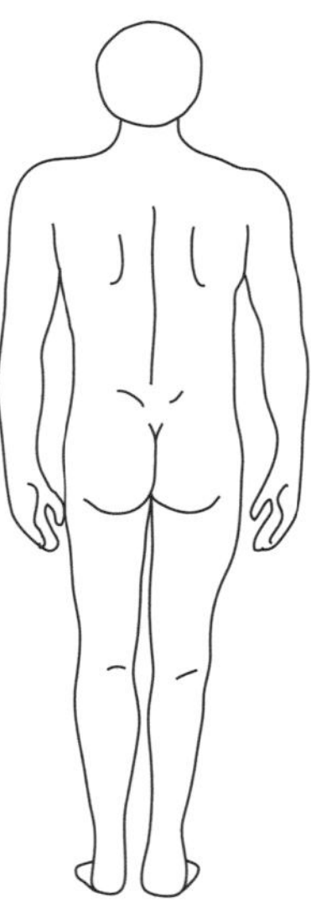

FIGURE 2.4 Abuse assessment screening tool with body map.
Source: Reprinted with permission from Futures Without Violence: www.futureswithoutviolence.org

Plan

A. Provide a safe environment. Assess for immediate danger.
B. Clearly document the history, physical findings, and interventions.
C. Determine the risk to the victim and any children.
D. Evaluate the need for emergency room/hospital admission.
E. Battery is a crime; assess the victim's readiness for police intervention and need for a court order of protection.
F. Help develop a safety plan.
G. Assess readiness to leave: Signs include collection important papers (e.g., birth certificates, custody papers, divorce papers, and legal agreements, address book, copies of restraining orders), access to money/credit cards, and telling family and friends.
H. Provide contact numbers for shelters. Have the patient hide information in her shoes.
I. Counsel that violence may escalate.

Patient Teaching

A. Reinforce that the violence is not the victim's fault. IPV is very common and the victims do not deserve to be abused. Discuss the cycle of abuse.
B. Violence increases in frequency and severity.
C. Help is available.
D. The DoD has a self-help phone app created by the Rape, Abuse, & Incest National Network (RAINN) for sexual assault survivors to create a customized self-care plan. This app is available through the iTunes store. The app is a resource for Active Duty, National Guard, and Reserve service members.

Pharmaceutical Therapy

A. Prescriptions are related to physical injuries.
B. Provide treatment may be offered for sexually transmitted infections in the oral anal genital areas.
C. Tranquilizers may impair the victim's ability to flee or defend herself/himself and should not be prescribed.

Follow-Up

A. Develop a follow-up plan.
  1. What type of help does the patient want?
  2. Does the patient have a plan for returning? Is the batterer home? Does she think it is safe?
  3. Does she have a place to stay with family or friends; or does she want to go to a shelter?
  4. Give the telephone numbers for shelters and crises hotlines.
B. Screen the patient for abuse at all subsequent visits.
C. Mandatory reporting
  1. States require reporting when domestic violence involves a child younger than 18 years and abuse or neglect of the child is suspected.
  2. Abuse of a disabled person must be reported to the Disabled Persons Protection Commission.
  3. Reporting elder abuse may be mandatory in your state.
D. Your state may mandate reporting and intervention with law enforcement. Refer to the Domestic Violence, Sexual Assault, and Stalking Data Resource Center. www.jrsa.org/dvsa-drc/st-summary.shtml
E. The 2013 National Protocol for Sexual Assault Medical Forensic Examination for Adults and Adolescents is available at https://ncjrs.gov/pdffiles1/ovw/241903.pdf

Consultation/Referral

A. Facilitate referrals to a shelter, counseling, and legal services.
B. Contact a Sexual Assault Nurse Examiner (SANE)-qualified health care provider if indicated.
C. Refer to community or private support groups and agencies.
D. Refer for a consultation with a psychiatrist if the victim is homicidal or suicidal.
E. Refer for a neurologic or neurosurgical consultation for intracranial injuries or focal neurologic findings.
F. Refer for an orthopedic consultation for fractures.

Individual Considerations

A. Pregnancy is a known period of increased risk of violence.
  1. The genitals, breast, and abdomen are common sites targeted for trauma.
  2. Women may present with a miscarriage or premature labor.
  3. Blunt trauma is a common injury in pregnancy.
  4. Perform universal screening at each trimester and postpartum as abuse often begins during pregnancy.

Resources

Dating Abuse Stops Here: www.datingabusestopshere.com
Domestic Violence, Sexual Assault and Stalking Data Resource Center: http://www.jrsa.org/dvsa-drc/st-summary.shtml
Futures Without Violence (*Formerly Family Violence Prevention Fund*): www.futureswithoutviolence.org
National Domestic Violence Hotline: 1-800-799-7233
National TEEN Dating Abuse Helpline: 1-866-311-9474
Rape Abuse & Incest National Network (RAINN) Hotline: 1-800-656-4673: www.domesticviolence.org

Older Adults

Definition

Abuse in older individuals, defined as older than age 65, is associated with loss of functional capacity, depression, cognitive impairment, and increased morbidity and mortality. Perpetrators include partners, and family members (of all ages), as well as strangers. There are several types of maltreatment in this population.
A. Physical abuse: Willful unnecessary restraint, the infliction of physical pain, or injury
B. Sexual abuse: Nonconsensual sexual contact
C. Psychological abuse: Infliction of emotional harm, bullying, ridicule, verbal abuse, and terrorizing
D. Neglect: Failing to provide for needs and protection of a vulnerable adult
E. Self-neglect: FTT of the elder as a subset of neglect
F. Abandonment: Desertion
G. Financial exploitation: Misappropriation of resources
H. Health care fraud and abuse: Not providing care, but charging for services, overmedicating or undermedicating

Incidence

A. In 2011, the population of those aged 65 years and older was estimated to be 41.4 million. It is estimated that one in every eight people in the United States is an older person (65+ years). By 2040, the population of 85+ years is projected to be 14.1 million.
B. The exact incidence of elder abuse, neglect, exploitation, and self-neglect is unknown; however, it is believed to be common. The incidence is underreported because of the reluctance to report abuse, fear of implicating family members, and fear of being removed from the home.
C. Abuse is not uncommon in the institutional setting.
D. The highest rate of abuse is among elderly women older than age 80, with the abuser being the spouse or adult child. In the case of cognitive impairment, the victim may not remember or recognize abuse.

Pathogenesis

Maltreatment of vulnerable adults occurs by people who have an ongoing relationship with the older person when there is an expectation of responsibility: these include sons/daughters, spouses/intimate partners, other family members such as grandchildren, and others, including paid and unpaid caregivers. There have been several identifying psychopathologies in the abuser.

A. Physical frailty and mental impairment of the victim plays an indirect role. The victim may have a decreased ability to defend or escape.

B. Caregiver stressors from caring for the elderly patient, including the patient's physical and verbal demands. Psychosocial factors of the caregiver, mental illness, and alcohol or drug abuse contribute.

C. The child who was once abused may continue the cycle of violence transferred to the parent.

Predisposing Factors

A. Age: 65 years and older (some studies indicate age 60 years)

B. Institutionalized

C. Cognitive impairment/diminished capacity

D. Decreased capacity for performing activities of daily living (ADLs)

- **1.** Difficulty feeding themselves
- **2.** Difficulty bathing and dressing themselves
- **3.** Difficulty going to the toilet and performing personal hygiene

E. Decreased capacity performing instrumental activities of daily living (IADLs)

- **1.** Ability to prepare meals
- **2.** Ability to do household chores
- **3.** Ability to use the telephone
- **4.** Ability to manage personal finances

F. Females have a higher incidence of physical/sexual abuse.

G. Male gender is associated with self-neglect associated with impaired ADLs and IADLs.

H. Family stressors involving the caretaker

Common Complaints

A. Depression

B. Falls

C. History of hip fracture

D. Pressure ulcers

E. Bruises, lacerations, and burns

Other Signs and Symptoms

A. Indications of healing spiral fractures on x-ray

B. Poor nutrition: Lack of resources/transportation to obtain food; caregiver not providing adequate nutrition/withholding food

C. Multiple hospitalizations

D. Recurrent urinary tract infections

E. Noncompliance: May not be able to pay for medications; medications may be withheld, or even given in excess by the caregiver.

F. Complaints of sexual abuse

- **1.** Pain or soreness in the genital area
- **2.** Bruises or lacerations on the perineum/rectum
- **3.** Vaginal or rectal bleeding

G. Traumatic tooth and/or hair loss

H. Sedation from overmedicating

I. Changes in personality

Subjective Data

A. The caregiver often refuses to leave the patient alone and may answer questions for the patient.

B. The caregiver has a different explanation of the injury.

C. Ask the patient directly about abuse, neglect, or exploitation.

- **1.** Has anyone at home threatened or ever hurt you?
- **2.** Are you afraid of anyone at home?
- **3.** Are you left alone for long periods of time?
- **4.** Who cooks your meals? How often and what amounts of food do you eat?
- **5.** Who handles your financial business? Have you signed any documents that you did not understand?

D. Assess the patient's living arrangements. Has the patient ever told family or friends of his or her concerns, called hotlines, or attempted to leave the caregiver?

Physical Examination

A. Assessment

- **1.** Observation: If abuse is suspected, enforce the need to do the physical examination in private. Do a full-body examination.
  - **a.** Forensic examinations need thorough documentation of injuries.
    - **i.** Use color photographs before any treatment is started.
    - **ii.** Take at least one full-body photograph and a facial photograph.
    - **iii.** Take close-up photographs of all injuries.
    - **iv.** Use a ruler to identify/document the size of the injuries.
    - **v.** Documentation on the back of the photographs should include the patient's name, date, and photographer's name, as well as any witness to the examination. The photographer should also sign each photograph.
    - **vi.** Use direct quotes of the victim's history.
- **2.** Check blood pressure, pulse, respirations, and weight.
- **3.** General observation: Observe for depression, withdrawal demeanor, flat affect, fearfulness, poor eye contact, inappropriate dress, and signs of malnutrition.
- **4.** Observe for poor hygiene, presence of urine and feces, matted or lice-infected hair, odors, dirty nails and skin, and soiled clothing.
- **5.** Assess cognitive abilities, depression, and functional ability of ADLs and IADLs.

B. Inspect

- **1.** Dermal examination for signs of burns, tears, lacerations, impression marks, and bruises in different stages of healing. Frequent areas of the body involved are the neck, arms, and/or legs. Evaluate for the presence of decubitus/pressure ulcers. Signs of dehydration include dry fragile skin, dry sore mouth, and mental confusion.

2. Oral examination for poor oral hygiene, absence of dentures, and dry mucous membranes.
3. Evaluate breasts and genitals for lacerations, and hematomas of the vagina or labia.

C. Auscultate
1. All lung fields
2. Bowel sounds in all four quadrants of the abdomen

D. Palpate: Evaluate for dislocation, fractures, sprains, and contusions to the wrists, forearms, and shoulders.

E. Percuss abdomen and chest (if indicated).

F. Genital/rectal examination
1. Evaluate genitals/anus for redness, swelling, bruising, hematomas, abrasions, or lacerations.
2. Evaluate for evidence of sperm.
3. Evaluate for the presence of foreign bodies.

Diagnostic Tests

A. Diagnostic tests and x-rays are ordered dependent on the type of presenting complaints.

B. Obtain a CT for evaluation of injuries to the head and assault to the face, neck, or head. A CT or Doppler ultrasound may be ordered for abdominal injuries.

C. Order laboratory testing to evaluate dehydration, malnutrition, electrolyte imbalance, and medication/substance abuse.
1. CBC
2. Chemistry-7
3. Urinalysis
4. Calcium, magnesium, and phosphorus
5. Drug/alcohol screen
6. Serum levels for relevant medications

D. Obtain DNA samples if sexual abuse is present.

Differential Diagnoses

A. Elder abuse
B. Depression
C. Abdominal trauma
D. Sexual assault
E. Gait disturbance/fall
F. Pathologic fracture
G. Epidural/subdural hematoma

Plan

A. Provide a safe environment.

B. Clearly document the history, physical findings, and interventions.

C. Determine the perpetrator(s).

D. Evaluate the need for emergency room/hospital admission.

Patient Teaching

A. Reinforce that abuse/neglect is not the victim's fault. Elder abuse is very common.

B. Help is available.

Pharmaceutical Therapy

A. Ensure prescriptions are related to physical injuries.

B. Recommend treatment for sexually transmitted infections in the oral anal genital areas.

Follow-Up

A. Develop a follow-up plan. All states have legislation protecting against abuse, neglect, and exploitation of the older population.

B. Know whether your state has mandatory requirements to report any suspicion of elder mistreatment.

C. Abuse of a disabled person must be reported to the Disabled Person Protection Commission.

D. Know whether your state has additional regulations related to self-neglect. Contact adult protective services or law enforcement agencies.

E. At the present time, there is no recommendation for universal screening of all older adult patients except in nursing facilities.

Consultation/Referral

A. Schedule a social Order a social work consultation to coordinate an in-home geriatric assessment visit.

B. Facilitate referrals to a shelter, counseling, and legal services.

C. Contact a SANE qualified health care provider if indicated.

D. Refer to the community Area Agency on Aging for assistance.

E. Refer for a psychiatric consultation if indicated.

F. Refer for a neurologic or neurosurgical consultation for intracranial injuries or focal neurologic findings.

G. Refer for an orthopedic consultation for fractures.

Resources

American Association of Retired Persons (AARP): www.aarp.org

Clearinghouse on Abuse and Neglect of the Elderly (CANE): www.cane.udel.edu

Help Hotline for suspected elder abuse, neglect, or exploitation: 1-800-677-1116

National Adult Protective Services Association (NAPSA): www.napsa-now.org

National Center on Elder Abuse Administration on Aging (NCEA): www.ncea.aoa.gov

Bibliography

Administration on Aging Administration for Community Living, U.S. Department of Health and Human Services. (2015). A profile of older Americans: 2015. Retrieved from https://aoa.acl.gov/Aging_Statistics/Profile/2015/docs/2015-Profile.pdf

American College of Obstetricians and Gynecologists. (2012, February). Intimate partner violence. *Committee Opinion, 518,* 1–5.

American Psychiatric Association. (2013). *Diagnostic and statistical manual of mental disorders* (5th ed.). Arlington, VA: American Psychiatric Publishing.

American Society for Metabolic and Bariatric Surgery. (2014). Approved procedures. Retrieved from https://asmbs.org

Angstman, K. B., Pietruszewski, P., Rasmussen, N. H., Wilkinson, J. M., & Katzelnick, D. J. (2012). Depression remission after six months of collaborative care management: Role of initial severity of depression in outcome. *Mental Health in Family Medicine, 9*(2), 99–106.

Beck, A. T., Ward, C. H., Mendelson, M., Mock, J., & Erbaugh, J. (1961). An inventory for measuring depression. *Archives of General Psychiatry, 4,* 561–571.

Becker, D. A., Balcer, L. J., & Galetta, S. L. (2012). The neurological complications of nutritional deficiency following bariatric surgery. *Journal of Obesity, 2012.* doi:10.1155/2012/608534

Cahoo, C. G. (2012). Depression in older adults. *American Journal of Nursing, 112*(11), 22–31.

Centers for Disease Control and Prevention. (2014). Adult obesity facts. Retrieved from https://www.cdc.gov/obesity/data/adult.html

Centers for Disease Control and Prevention. (2015). Overweight & obesity. Retrieved from https://www.cdc.gov/obesity/index.html
Dating Abuse Stops Here. (n.d.). Create a safety plan. Retrieved from www.datingabusestopshere.com/create-a-safety-plan/
Dating Abuse Stops Here. (n.d.). Warning signs in depth. Retrieved from www.datingabusestopshere.com/warning-signs/warning-signs-in-depth
Devries, K. M., Mak, J. Y. T., Garcia-Moreno, C., Petzold, M., Child, J. C., Falder, G., . . . Watts, C. H. (2013, June 30). The global prevalence of intimate partner violence against women. *Sciencexpress*. Retrieved from http://www.sciencemag.org/content/early/recent
Domestic Abuse Intervention Project. (n.d.). Abuse of children wheel. Retrieved from www.theduluthmodel.org/pdf/Abuse%20of%20Children.pdf
Domestic Abuse Intervention Project. (n.d.). Power and control wheel. Retrieved from www.theduluthmodel.org/pdf/powerandcontrol.pdf
Domestic Violence, Sexual Assault and Stalking Data Resource Center. (n.d*.).* State summaries. Retrieved from http://www.jrsa.org/dvsa-drc/state-summaries.shtml
domesticviolence.org. Personalized safety plan-domestic violence. (n.d.). Retrieved from www.dynamed.com/topics/dmp-AN-T115009/Obesity-in-adults
DynaMed Plus. (2016, March 8). Obesity in adults. Ipswich, MA: EBSCO Information Services. Retrieved from https://www.dynamed.com/topics/dmp-AN-T115009/Obesity-in-adults
Ewing, J. A. (1984). Detecting alcoholism. The CAGE questionnaire. *The Journal of the American Medical Association, 252*(14), 1905–1907.
Futures Without Violence, Formerly Family Violence Prevention Fund. (n.d.). The facts on children's exposure to intimate partner violence. Retrieved from https://www.futureswithoutviolence.org/the-facts-on-childrens-exposure-to-intimate-partner-violence
Futures Without Violence, Formerly Family Violence Prevention Fund. (n.d.). The facts on the military and violence against women. Retrieved from https://www.futureswithoutviolence.org/userfiles/file/Children_and_Families/Military.pdf
Giardino, A. P. (2013, April 1). Physical child abuse. *Medscape*. Retrieved from http://emedicine.medscape.com/article/915664-overview
Gupta, A. K. (2016, February 19). Obesity and weight loss (adult). *Essentials Evidence Plus*. Retrieved from www.essentialevidenceplus.com
Handzlik-Orlik, G., Holecki, M., Orlik, B., Wylezol, M., & Dulawa, J. (2015). Nutrition management of the post-bariatric surgery patient. *Nutrition in Clinical Practice: Official Publication of the American Society for Parenteral and Enteral Nutrition, 30*(3), 383–392.
Hamdan, K., Somers, S., & Chand, M. (2011). Management of late post-operative complications of bariatric surgery. *British Journal of Surgery, 98*(10), 1345–1355.
Hardy, S. (2013). Prevention and management of depression in primary care. *Nursing Standard (Royal College of Nursing (Great Britain): 1987), 27*(26), 51–56; quiz 58.
Healthy Place America's Mental Health Channel. (n.d.). Abuse test: Woman abuse screening tool. Retrieved from http://www.healthyplace.com/psychological-tests/woman-abuse-screening-tool
Heber, D., Greenway, F. L., Kaplan, L. M., Livingston, E., Salvador, J., & Still, C.; Endocrine Society. (2010). Endocrine and nutritional management of the post-bariatric surgery patient: An Endocrine Society Clinical Practice Guideline. *Journal of Clinical Endocrinology and Metabolism, 95*(11), 4823–4843.
HelpGuide.org. (n.d.). Child abuse and neglect: Recognizing, preventing, and reporting child abuse. Retrieved from www.helpguide.org/mental_abuse_physical_emoional_sexual_neglect.htm
HelpGuide.org. (n.d.). Domestic violence and abuse: Signs of abuse and abusive relationships. Retrieved from www.helpguide.org/mental/domestic_violence_abuse_types_signs_causes_effects.htm
HelpGuide.org. (n.d.). Elder abuse and neglect: Warning signs, risk factors, prevention, help. Retrieved from www.helpguide.org/mental/elder_abuse_physical_emotional_sexual_neglect.htm
HelpGuide.org. (n.d.). Help for abused men: Escaping domestic violence by women or domestic partners. Retrieved from www.helpguide.org/mental/domestic-violence-men-abused-by-women.htm
Henry, M., Cortes, A., & Morris, S. (2013). *The 2013 Annual Homeless Assessment Report (AHAR) to Congress*. Washington, DC: U.S. Department of Housing and Urban Development.
Jensen, M. D., Ryan, D. H., Donato, K. A., Apovian, C. M., Ard, J. D., Comuzzie A. G., . . . Yanovski, S. Z. (2014). Special issue: Guidelines (2013) for managing overweight and obesity in adults. *Obesity, 22* (S2), i–xvi, S1–S410.
Kerner, J. (2014). Nutrition support after bariatric surgery. *Support Line, 36*(3), 9–20.
Liraglutide. (2016). Retrieved from www.drugs .com/cdi/liraglutide.html
Merrill, S. (2009). *Introducing syndemics: A critical systems approach to public and community health*. San Francisco, CA: Jossey-Bass.
Moyer, V. A.; U.S. Preventive Services Task Force. (2013). Screening for intimate partner violence and abuse of elderly and vulnerable adults: U.S. Preventive Services Task Force recommendation statement. *Annals of Internal Medicine, 158*(6), 478–486.
National Committee for the Prevention of Elder Abuse. (2008). Elder abuse. Retrieved from www.preventelderabuse.org/elderabuse
National Committee for the Prevention of Elder Abuse. (n.d.). Domestic violence. Retrieved from http://www.preventelderabuse.org/elderabuse/domestic.html
National Committee for the Prevention of Elder Abuse. (n.d.). Financial abuse. Retrieved from http://www.preventelderabuse.org/elderabuse/fin_abuse.html
National Committee for the Prevention of Elder Abuse. (n.d.). Neglect. Retrieved from http://www.preventelderabuse.org/elderabuse/neglect.html
National Committee for the Prevention of Elder Abuse. (n.d.). Physical abuse. Retrieved from http://www.preventelderabuse.org/elderabuse/physical.html
National Committee for the Prevention of Elder Abuse. (n.d.). Psychological abuse. Retrieved from http://www.preventelderabuse.org/elderabuse/psychological.html
National Committee for the Prevention of Elder Abuse. (n.d.). Sexual abuse. Retrieved from http://www.preventelderabuse.org/elderabuse/s_abuse.html
National Institute on Drug Abuse. (2011, March). Commonly abused drugs chart. Retrieved from www.drugabuse.gov/drugs-abuse/commonly-abused-drugs/commonly-abused-drugs-chart
National Institute on Drug Abuse. (2016, January). Commonly abused prescription drug chart. Retrieved from www.drugabuse.gov/drugs-abuse/commonly-abused-drugs-charts
O'Malley, P. A. (2012). Baby boomers and substance abuse: The curse of youth again in old age: Implications for the clinical nurse specialist. *Clinical Nurse Specialist, 26*(6), 305–307.
Pounds, B. P. (2015). *Improving primary care provider knowledge regarding malabsorptive nutritional deficiencies after bariatric surgery*. Unpublished manuscript, Frontier Nursing University, Hyden, KY.
Prevent Child Abuse America. (n.d.). Fact sheet: Sexual abuse of boys. Retrieved from www.preventchildabuse.org/images/docs/sexualabuseofboys.pdf
Prevent Child Abuse America. (n.d.). Fact sheet: The relationship between parental alcohol or other drug problems and child maltreatment. Retrieved from www.preventchildabuse.org/images/docs/therelationshipbetweenparentalalcoholandotherdrugproblemsandchildmaltreatment.pdf
Prevent Child Abuse America. (2016, February). Fact sheet: Emotional child-abuse. Retrieved from www.preventchildabuse.org/images/docs/emotionalchildabuse.pdf
Prevent Child Abuse America. (2016, February). Fact sheet: Maltreatment of children with disabilities. Retrieved from http://www.preventchildabuse.org/images/docs/maltreatmentofchildrenwithdisabilities.pdf
Prevent Child Abuse America. (2016, February). Fact sheet: Sexual abuse of children. Retrieved from www.preventchildabuse.org/resource/sexual-abuse-of-children-fact-sheet
Prevent Child Abuse America. (2016, February). Recognizing child abuse: What parents should know. Retrieved from www.preventchildabuse.org/images/docs/recognizingchildabuse-whatparentsshouldknow.pdf
Rape, Abuse & Incest National Network. (n.d.). State resources. Retrieved from https://www.rainn.org/state-resources
Rape, Abuse & Incest Rational Network. (n.d.). Victims of sexual violence: Statistics Retrieved from http://www.rainn.org/get-information/statistics/sexual-assault-victims
Richardson, L., & Puskar, K. (2012, June). Screening assessment for anxiety and depression in primary care. *Journal for Nurse Practitioners, 8*(6), 475–481.
Ross, R., Roller, C., Rusk, T., Martsolf, D., & Draucker, C. (2009). The SATELLITE sexual violence assessment and care guide for perinatal

patients. *Women's Health Care: A Practical Journal for Nurse Practitioners, 8*(11), 25–31.

Saha, S., Deanne Wilson, J., & Adger, R. J. (2012). K2, spice, and bath salts drugs of abuse commercially available. *Contemporary Pediatrics, 29*(10), 22–28.

Shannon, C., Gervasoni, A., & Williams, T. (2013). The bariatric surgery patient–nutrition considerations. *Australian Family Physician, 42*(8), 547–552.

Smith, M. (2013). Care of adolescents who have mental health and substance misuse problems. *Mental Health Practice, 1*(5), 32–36.

U.S. Department of Defense. (2012, September 17). New DOD safe helpline mobile app now available [News release]. Retrieved from www.115fw.ang.af.mil/shared/media/document/AFD-121013-016.pdf

U.S. Department of Health and Human Services, National Institute of Diabetes and Digestive and Kidney Diseases. (2012). Overweight and obesity statistics (NIH Publication No. 04-4158). Retrieved from win.niddk.nih.gov/statistics

U.S. Department of Housing and Urban Development. (2011). Homeless emergency assistance and rapid transition to housing. Retrieved from https://www.hudexchange.info/homelessness-assistance/hearth-act

U.S. Department of Justice, Office on Violence Against Women. (2013). *A national protocol for sexual assault medical forensic examinations: Adults/adolescents* (2nd ed.). Washington, D.C.: Author. Retrieved from https://www.ncjrs .gov/pdffiles1/ovw/241903.pdf

U.S. Food and Drug Administration. (2016). Find information about a drug. Retrieved from www.fda.gov/Drugs/ResourcesForYou/Consumers /ucm450624.htm

Wendell, A. D. (2013). Overview and epidemiology of substance abuse in pregnancy. *Clinical Obstetrics and Gynecology, 56*(1), 91–96.

World Health Organization. (2011). Intimate partner violence during pregnancy. Retrieved from http://apps.who.int/iris/bitstream/10665/70764/1/WHO_RHR_11.35_eng.pdf

World Health Organization. (2013). Gender and women's mental health. Retrieved from www.who.int/mental_health/prevention/genderwomen/en

3 Pain Management Guidelines

Acute Pain

Moya Cook

Definition

A. *Acute pain* is defined as pain of a short, limited duration, usually the result of an injury, surgery, or medical illness that generally results from tissue injury; however, it may be experienced even with no identifiable cause. Acute pain usually resolves when the tissue injury improves with the healing process. Most acute pain resolves in less than 6 weeks.

Incidence

A. Acute pain is the most common reason for self-medication and presentation for treatment in the health care system. Acute pain is very individual, and if not treated properly it can have devastating physiological and psychological effects. Because pain is very subjective, the patient care plan needs to be individualized to meet the patient's needs. Proper treatment of acute pain could prevent the development of some types of chronic pain syndromes.

Pathogenesis

A. Acute pain is usually the result of stimulation of the sympathetic nervous system.

Common Complaints

A. Pain at the specific site
B. Increased heart rate
C. Increased respiratory rate
D. Elevated blood pressure (B/P)
E. Sweating
F. Nausea

Other Signs and Symptoms

A. Urinary retention
B. Dilated pupils
C. Pallor

Subjective Data

A. Elicit location of pain.
B. Note effects of pain on activities of daily living (ADLs).
C. Note intensity of pain at rest and during activity.
D. List precipitating factors.
E. Identify alleviating factors.
F. Note the quality of pain.
G. Is there radiation of pain?
H. Rate pain on a pain scale (usually on the 1–10 scale, with 1 being the least and 10 being the worst).

Adaptations need to be made to the assessment tool using the Faces scale in children. Incapacitated or cognitively impaired patients may also need special consideration to evaluate their pain.

Physical Examination

A. Check temperature, pulse, respiration, and blood pressure.
B. Inspect
  1. Observe overall appearance.
  2. Note affect and ability to express self and pain.
  3. Note facial grimaces with movement.
  4. Note gait, stance, and movements.
  5. Inspect area at pain site.
C. Auscultate
  1. Auscultate heart and lungs.
  2. Auscultate neck and abdomen.
D. Palpate: Palpate affected area of pain.
E. Percuss
  1. Percuss chest.
  2. Percuss abdomen.
F. Perform musculoskeletal examination.

When performing a musculoskeletal examination, identify the location of pain, presence of trigger points, evidence of injury or trauma, edema, erythema, warmth, heat, lesions, petechiae, tenderness, decreased range of motion, pain with movement, crepitus, laxity of ligaments or cords, spasms, or guarding.

  1. Perform complete musculoskeletal examination, concentrating on the area of pain.
  2. Assess deep tendon reflexes (DTRs).
G. Neurologic examination
  1. Perform complete neurologic examination.
  2. Identify change in sensory function, skin tenderness, weakness, muscle atrophy, and/or loss of DTRs.

Diagnostic Tests

A. No diagnostic testing is required unless clearly indicated to rule out organic cause of pain. If organic disease is suspected, diagnostic testing may include:
  1. CT imaging
  2. MRI
  3. Blood chemistries
  4. Radiographic x-ray
  5. Lumbar puncture
  6. Ultrasound
  7. Electrocardiogram (EKG)/echocardiogram

Differential Diagnoses

The differential diagnoses depend on the location of the acute pain.

A. Head
   1. Migraine
   2. Cluster headache/migraine headache
   3. Temporal arteritis
   4. Intracranial bleeding or stroke
   5. Sinusitis
   6. Dental abscess

B. Neck
   1. Meningitis
   2. Muscle strain/sprain
   3. Whiplash injury
   4. Thyroiditis

C. Chest
   1. Pulmonary emboli
   2. Myocardial infarction
   3. Pneumonia
   4. Costochondritis
   5. Angina
   6. Gastroesophageal reflux disease/esophagitis

D. Abdomen
   1. Peritonitis
   2. Appendicitis
   3. Ectopic pregnancy/uterine pregnancy
   4. Endometriosis
   5. Pelvic inflammatory disease
   6. Peptic ulcer
   7. Cholelithiasis
   8. Colitis/diverticulitis
   9. Constipation
   10. Gastroenteritis
   11. Irritable bowel syndrome
   12. Urinary tract infection, kidney stone, pyelonephritis
   13. Prostatitis
   14. Malignancies

E. Musculoskeletal
   1. Muscle sprain/strain/tear
   2. Skeletal fracture
   3. Viral infection
   4. Gout
   5. Vitamin D deficiency

Plan

A. General interventions
   1. Acute pain is a symptom, not a diagnosis.
   2. Identify the cause or source of the acute pain depending on the location. If the pain is organic in nature, make the appropriate referral.
   3. Overall goal is to treat the acute pain appropriately.

B. Patient teaching
   1. The pain management plan must include patient and family education regarding preventing and controlling pain, potential medication side effects, and how to prevent the side effects.
   2. Discussion must include addiction concerns.
   3. The newest recommendation from the Centers for Disease Control and Prevention (CDC) is the lowest possible dose of narcotics for pain for no longer than 3 to 5 days before reevaluation. Explain that risk of addiction is low when medication is used as directed for a short duration. Explain that complete pain relief may not be achievable initially, but the overall goal is to decrease the pain, thus allowing some daily activities at home to begin recovery.

C. Pharmaceutical therapy
   1. *Visceral pain*: Treatment of choice is corticosteroids, intraspinal local anesthetics, nonsteroidal anti-inflammatory drugs (NSAIDs), and opioids.
   2. *Somatic pain*: Acetaminophen, cold packs, corticosteroids, localized anesthetics, NSAIDs, opioids, and tactile stimulation.
   3. *Neuropathic pain*: Tricyclic antidepressants (TCAs), using amitriptyline are the fi rst- line treatment for neuropathic pain. Anticonvulsants like carbamazepine (Tegretol), phenytoin (Dilantin), and valproic acid (Depakene) can be useful in treating neuropathic pain. Other treatments include local anesthetics, tramadol (Ultram), and glucocorticoids.

> *Know each medication's mechanism of action, potential adverse side effects, half-life, and drug–drug interaction potential. Always document that you have advised on the potential for sedation, suggested no driving/machinery use, or no alcohol while taking medication with these potential adverse side effects. The Food and Drug Administration (FDA) advises extreme caution when using NSAIDs with patients with cardiovascular disease due to the increased risk of heart attack and stroke.*

Follow-Up

A. Once organic cause of pain has been ruled out, initial follow-up is 48 to 72 hours after onset.

B. Ensure that the patient has access to care on a regular schedule.

Consultation/Referral

A. If the acute pain is organic, make the appropriate referral to a specialist.

Individual Considerations

A. Geriatrics
   1. Physiologic changes that occur in the elderly, such as decreased body mass, hepatic dysfunction, and renal dysfunction may cause increased serum drug concentrations of pain medication. Use caution when prescribing pain medication to this population.
   2. Antiinflammatories are not recommended for the elderly as a general rule due to the effects of the medication on the kidneys.

Chronic Pain

Moya Cook

Definition

A. *Chronic pain* is defined as an alteration in comfort that persists longer than 6 weeks (or longer than the anticipated healing time).The pain may be continuous or recurrent and of sufficient duration and intensity. Legitimate chronic pain interferes with a patient's ability to function with normal daily activities and decreases quality of life.

Incidence

Pain syndromes are commonly seen in clinical practice and are the third most widespread health problem in the United States. Chronic pain costs the American people about $65 billion a year in health care expenses, disability costs, and lost productivity. The Centers for Disease Control and Prevention (CDC) found that 11.2% of adults state that they have pain daily. Chronic pain patients have a better than 50% chance of becoming addicted to prescription pain medications. As the U.S. population continues to age and the average life expectancy is increasing, the primary care provider will be providing care for more chronic diseases and handling more chronic pain patients.

A. Women are affected more than men by two to one.
B. Onset is usually in the fourth, fifth, or sixth decades and is often associated with marked functional disability.

Pathogenesis

A. *Skeletal muscle pain* occurs in the soft tissue involving the neck, shoulders, trunk, arms, low back, hips, and lower extremities. *Myofascial pain syndrome* relates to the fascia surrounding the muscle tissue.
B. *Inflammatory pain* is caused by chemicals, such as prostaglandins, leading to the stimulation of the pain receptors. Examples include arthritis, infection, tissue injury, and postoperative pain.
C. *Mechanical/compressive pain* is the direct result of the muscle, ligament, and tendon causing strain, leading to the stimulation of the pain receptors. Diagnosis may be based on diagnostic imaging results, which may include fracture, obstruction, dislocation, or compression of tissue by a tumor, cyst, or bony structure.
D. *Neuropathic pain* involves dysfunction of the somatosensory system. The most common types are diabetic neuropathy, sciatica from nerve root compression, trigeminal neuralgia, and postherpetic neuralgia.
E. *Nociceptive pain* is caused by nociceptors, a type of sensory neuron that receives the pain signal. Mechanical/compressive pain and inflammatory pain are examples of this type of pain. They both respond well to opioids, with the exception of arthritis.

Predisposing Factors

A. Age 30 to 50 years
B. Female gender
C. History of having seen many physicians
D. Frequent use of several nonspecific medications
E. Depression
F. Personality, including moods, fears, expectations, coping efforts, and resources

Common Complaints

A. Specific to site of pain
B. Emotional distress related to fear, maladaptive or inadequate support systems, and other coping resources
C. Treatment-induced complications
D. Overuse of drugs
E. Inability to work
F. Financial complications
G. Disruption of usual activities
H. Sleep disturbances
I. Pain becomes primary life focus

Other Signs and Symptoms

A. Pain lasts longer than 6 months.
B. There may be anger and loss of faith or trust in the health care system. This type of patient frequently takes too many medications, spends a great deal of time in bed, sees many physicians, and experiences little joy in either work or play.

Subjective Data

A. Elicit a clear description of the onset, location, quality, intensity, and time course of pain and any factors that aggravate or relieve it. Use the acronym OLD CARTS-U. O = onset, L = location, D = duration, C = characteristics, A = aggravating triggers, R = relieving triggers, T = timing, S = severity, U = YOU. What do YOU think is going on? What have YOU done to relieve it?
B. *Self-reporting pain assessment tools* should be used early in the process of patient evaluation. Use the tool at each office visit to see progression or regression. Lack of pain assessment is a barrier to good pain control. Consider the age of the patient; his or her physical, emotional, and cognitive status; and preference when choosing the self-reporting pain assessment tool.

   1. Verbal rating scales rate pain as mild, moderate, or severe.
   2. Numeric rating scales rate pain intensity from 0 to 10. They are patient friendly and quick to complete.
   3. The Faces scale is useful for pediatric and cognitively impaired patients. Multicultural translations may be downloaded at www.wongbakerfaces.org

C. Determine the extent to which the patient is suffering, disabled, and unable to enjoy usual activity. It is important to inquire about activities of daily living (ADLs) and functional limitations.
D. Obtain a complete review of systems, including nausea, numbness, weakness, insomnia, loss of appetite, dysphoria, malaise, fatigue, or depression signs and symptoms.
E. Obtain a complete family and social history. Address spiritual and cultural issues. History of chemical dependency is of interest in this patient population.
F. Obtain the patient's medical history relevant to the pain, including diagnosis, testing, treatments, and outcomes.
G. Obtain a pain history to identify the patient's attitudes, beliefs, level of knowledge, and previous experiences with pain. Are previously used methods for pain control helpful? What is the patient's attitude toward the use of certain pain medications? Often, the patient discusses certain adverse side effects or allergies from undesired pain medication.

Physical Examination

A. Check temperature, pulse, respirations, and blood pressure.

B. Inspect
  1. Observe overall appearance.
  2. Note affect and ability to express self and pain.
  3. Note facial grimaces with movement.
  4. Note gait, stance, and movements.
  5. Inspect area at pain site.
C. Auscultate
  1. Heart and lungs
  2. Neck and abdomen
D. Palpate the affected area of pain.
E. Percuss
  1. Chest
  2. Abdomen
F. Perform musculoskeletal examination.

When performing musculoskeletal examination, identify the location of pain, presence of trigger points, evidence of injury or trauma, edema, erythema, warmth, heat, lesions, petechiae, tenderness, decreased range of motion, pain with movement, crepitus, laxity of ligaments or cords, spasms, or guarding.

  1. Perform a complete musculoskeletal examination, concentrating on the area of pain.
  2. Note limitations in range of motion.
G. Neurologic examination
  1. Perform complete neurologic examination.
  2. Note the patient's affect and mood. Is the patient cooperative during examination?
  3. Identify change in sensory function, skin tenderness, weakness, muscle atrophy, and/or loss of deep tendon reflexes (DTRs).
H. Functional assessment
  1. The baseline functional assessment provides objective measurable data on a patient's physical abilities and limitations. It can be used to determine if the patient's efforts are valid and complaints are reliable.
  2. The information may be used to identify areas of impairment, establish specific functional goals, and measure the effectiveness of treatment interventions.
  3. These objective data may be used in worker compensation cases, returning-to-work status, federal disability, and motor vehicle accident lawsuits.
  4. Know the resources in your area that are trained to perform functional assessments. Physical therapists and occupational therapists are the best qualified to perform the assessments.

Diagnostic Tests

A. None is required unless clearly indicated to rule out the organic cause of pain.
  1. Remember that pain previously diagnosed as chronic pain syndrome can be organic and vice versa. Organic causes must always be evaluated and excluded.
  2. Plain radiography should be ordered first for muscle, inflammatory, or skeletal pain. Plain radiography will diagnose a fracture. Additional studies may be recommended by the radiologist if a lesion/abnormality is seen on plain radiography.
  3. MRI and CT are ordered if the plain radiograph is negative and the patient continues to complain of pain.
  4. Electromyography and nerve conduction studies are used to evaluate neuropathic pain. Numerous serum and urine studies should also be considered if the neuropathic pain is undiagnosed.
B. Depression screening tool: Consider using a depression assessment tool such as the Beck Depression Inventory or Patient Health Questionnaire 9 (PHQ9). These tools can be administered at a subsequent appointment to follow the patient's symptoms.

Differential Diagnosies

A. Pain disorder
B. Pain related to a disease with no cure/malignancy
C. Somatization disorder
D. Conversion disorder
E. Hypochondriasis
F. Depression
G. Chemical dependency
H. Fibromyalgia

Plan

A. General interventions
  1. Treatment is multidimensional and should not be focused on pharmacological treatment alone.
  2. Offer hope and potential for improvement of pain control and improvement of function but *not* cure.
  3. The pain is real to the patient, and acceptance of the problem must occur before a mutually agreed-on treatment plan can be initiated.
  4. Depression is a common emotional disturbance in chronic pain patients and is treatable.
  5. Identify specific and realistic goals for therapy such as having a good night's sleep, going shopping, or returning to work. Patient discussion needs to include the idea that the goal may be decreasing pain intensity, not eliminating pain.
  6. Carefully assess the level of pain using available tools such as a daily pain diary or other pain assessment scales.
  7. Avoid pain reinforcement such as sympathy and attention to pain. Provide positive response to productive activities. Improving activity tolerance assists in desensitizing the patient to pain.
  8. Shift the focus from the pain to accomplishing daily assigned self-help tasks. The accomplishment of these tasks functions as positive reinforcement.
B. Patient teaching: *See Section III: Patient Teaching Guide for this chapter, "Chronic Pain."* ◀
C. Pharmaceutical interventions
  1. Skeletal muscle pain: Treatment should focus on physical rehabilitation and behavioral management. Tricyclic antidepressants (TCAs) and muscle relaxants (cyclobenzaprine) may be used. Research is lacking regarding the need for opioids.

2. Inflammatory pain: Nonsteroidal anti-inflammatory drugs (NSAIDs) and corticosteroids are first-line pharmaceutical interventions. Topical creams and solutions have been used in treating arthritis pain.

3. Mechanical/compressive pain: Opioids may be used to manage these symptoms while other measures are being taken.

4. Neuropathic pain

a. Gabapentin (Neurontin) and pregabalin (Lyrica) have become first-choice treatments in recent years for diabetic neuropathy and postherpetic neuralgia.

b. TCAs are extremely useful. Patients who are not depressed obtain excellent pain relief with TCAs such as amitriptyline and doxepin.

c. Selective serotonin reuptake inhibitors (SSRIs) are also effective for chronic pain control. Duloxetine (Cymbalta) has been approved for chronic pain as monotherapy or in conjunction with TCAs.

d. Anticonvulsants are useful in controlling some neuropathic pain: Carbamazepine (Tegretol), phenytoin (Dilantin), and valproic acid (Depakene). **Patients need to be monitored monthly for hepatic dysfunction and hematopoietic suppression.**

e. Topical agents: Capsaicin applied three to four times per day can reduce pain without significant systemic effects. Topical lidocaine 5% patches are approved for postherpetic neuralgia.

f. Carbamazepine is used as the first-line treatment for trigeminal neuralgia.

g. Opioids: Tramadol is considered to be a good choice if an opioid is indicated. In addition to pain control, tramadol also causes serotonin reuptake inhibition similar to that seen with the TCAs.

5. All therapies need a 2- to 3-week trial period to adequately evaluate therapy. Some medications take longer than that to evaluate.

6. NSAIDs should be used for flare-ups of mild to moderate inflammatory or nonneuropathic pain.

7. Opioids require careful patient selection, titration, and monitoring. Avoid long-term, daily treatment with short-acting opioids (Vicodin, Norco, and Percocet). For as-needed use, prescribe small quantities.

8. Smiths Medical received Food and Drug Administration (FDA) approval in February 2013 to market ambulatory infusion pumps in the United States. These pumps can be programmed to administer pain management medication continuously, intermittently, tapered, or patient controlled.

9. Benzodiazepines and barbiturates are not advised for treatment of chronic pain due to the high risk of substance abuse.

10. Addiction risk interventions when considering opioids: A checklist for prescribing opioids can be found at www.cdc.gov/drugoverdose/pdf/PDO_Checklist-a.pdf

a. Check your state's prescription monitoring program (PMP) before prescribing controlled substances, as needed, and at least annually. PMPs are state-run electronic databases that track dispensing of controlled substances. PMPs provide clinicians with critical information about patient narcotic prescription history and identify drug-seeking behavior patterns.

b. Contact the patient's pharmacy for a list of current medications. The PMP is not in real time, and all current patient prescriptions are available from the pharmacy.

c. Perform urine drug screen before prescribing controlled substances initially, as needed, and annually. National guidelines recommend the enzyme immunoassay (EIA) and gas chromatography/mass spectroscopy urine screen. Depending on the results of urine drug screening, the provider may seek additional consultation, change medication therapy, refer for substance abuse, or discharge the patient.

d. A written controlled substance treatment agreement among patient, provider, and clinic is recommended. Include expectations of the patient: No other controlled substances will be prescribed by any other provider. One pharmacy only should be used. Medication must be taken as prescribed. These are no early refills on controlled substances. The patient must agree to random drug screens and may be called to report to the clinic for random drug screens and/or pill counts.

e. Utilize tools such as the Addiction Behavior Checklist, Diagnosis, Intractability, Risk, Efficacy (DIRE) score, or CAGE (have you ever tried to *c*ut down on your alcohol/drug use? Do you get *a*nnoyed if someone mentions your use is a problem? Do you ever feel *g*uilty about your use? Do you ever have an "*e*ye-opener" first thing in the morning after you have been drinking or using the night before?) assessment.

f. Red flags for misuse, abuse, addiction, and diversion with opioids include:

i. Psychiatric illness

ii. Personal history of alcohol or drug abuse

iii. Family history of alcohol or drug abuse

D. Alternative interventions

1. Cognitive behavioral training: Examples of cognitive behavioral training include problem solving, guided imagery, hypnosis, controlled breathing exercises, attention diversion, meditation, and yoga exercises; progressive muscle relaxation (PMR) is recommended to help relax major muscle groups. Randomized controlled trials showed significant reduction in pain with alternative interventions such as music, relaxation, distraction, and massage use.

2. Exercise: Examples of exercise include yoga exercises and PMR. PMR is recommended to help relax major muscle groups. Research indicates that yoga decreases bothersome pain after 12 weeks of regular exercise. The benefits of yoga exercise include improved strength, balance, coordination, range of motion, and reduced anxiety. Yoga instruction by a qualified teacher is a low-cost intervention. Yoga is an effective form of self-care and is an affordable way to alleviate pain. Always advise patients to start slowly and be prepared for an approach to pain management that may take several weeks of therapy.

3. Alternative therapies: Randomized controlled trials showed significant reduction in pain with alternative interventions such as music, relaxation, distraction, acupuncture, myofascial release treatments, and massage use.
4. Occupational therapy
5. Vocational therapy
6. Physical therapy such as noninvasive techniques, transcutaneous electrical nerve stimulation, hot or cold therapy, hydrotherapy, traction, massage, bracing, and exercise
7. Individual and family therapy or counseling
8. Aesthetic or neurosurgical procedures
9. Patients will inquire about the use of herbal products to treat chronic pain. Advise patients that these products are not regulated by the FDA. Advise them that these herbal products may interact with current medications and cause complications. Advise them to research all herbal products on reputable medically based websites, not blogs or chat rooms. Caution patients regarding devil's claw, feverfew, willow bark, glucosamine, and chondroitin. Discourage any use of dimethylsulfoxide.

Follow-Up

A. See patients every 4 to 6 weeks for evaluation.
B. Ensure that the patient has access to care on a regular schedule.
C. These brief visits should be regular so that care is not perceived to be dependent on escalation of symptoms.

Consultation/Referral

A. Consider patient referral to a pain management clinic if pain control is not adequate. Interventions commonly performed at the specialty clinic include facet joint injections, percutaneous radiofrequency neurotomy, epidural corticosteroid injections, transforaminal epidural injections, and sacroiliac joint injections.
B. Consult with a physician if referral is needed for psychological counseling or if substance abuse is suspected.
C. Refer to a certified pain specialist physician if the patient is taking high doses of opioids and detoxification is indicated. Buprenorphine (Suboxone) is the most common medication prescribed by a certified pain specialist physician.
D. Consider rheumatology consult if indicated.

Lower Back Pain

Moya Cook

Definition

Painful conditions of the lower back may be categorized as follows:

A. Potentially serious disorders: Acute fractures, tumor, progressive neurologic deficit, nerve root compression, and cauda equina syndrome
B. Degenerative disorders: Aging or repetitive use, degenerative disease, and osteoarthritis
C. Nonspecific disorders: Benign and self-limiting with unclear etiology

Incidence

A. Lower back pain is commonly seen in patients from ages 20 to 40 years.
B. Approximately 70% to 80% of people experience back pain at one point in their lifetime.

Pathogenesis

A. Pain arises from fracture, tumor, nerve root compression, a degenerative disc, osteoarthritis, and strain of the ligaments and musculature of the lumbosacral area.

Predisposing Factors

A. Trauma causing ligament tearing; stretching of vertebra, muscles, tendons, ligaments, or fascia
B. Repetitive mechanical stress
C. Tumor
D. Exaggerated lumbar lordosis
E. Abnormal, forward-tipped pelvis
F. Uneven leg length
G. Chronic poor posture due to inadequate conditioning of muscle strength and flexibility, improper lifting techniques causing excessive strain, and poor body mechanics
H. Inadequate rest
I. Emotional depression

Common Complaint

A. Pain in the lower back area may range from discomfort to severe back pain, with or without radiation.

Other Signs and Symptoms

A. Ambulating with a limp
B. Limited range of motion
C. Posture normal to guarded

Subjective Data

A. Ask the patient to discuss the origin of pain. How has the pain progressed or changed since the initial injury?
B. Ask the patient to point to an area where pain is felt.
C. Have the patient describe the pain. Is it radiating, with sharp, shooting pain down to the lower leg and feet?
D. Ask: What makes the pain worse or better? Does activity make the pain worse or better? Have the patient list current medications or therapies used for pain, noting results of treatment.
E. Investigate occurrence of systemic symptoms such as fever and weight loss.
F. Explore the patient's past medical history. Note previous trauma or overuse, tuberculosis, arthritis, cancer, and osteoporosis.
G. Inquire about symptoms such as dysuria, bowel or bladder incontinence, muscle weakness, paresthesia, and loss of sensation. **Bowel or bladder dysfunction, bilateral sciatica, and saddle compression may be symptoms of severe compression of the cauda equina that necessitate an urgent workup and referral.**
H. Ask the patient about precipitating factors such as athletics, heavy lifting, driving, yard work, occupation, sleep habits, or systemic disease.
I. Use a pain scale to describe the worst pain and the best pain levels.

Physical Examination

A. Check temperature, pulse, blood pressure, and respiration.
B. Inspect
  1. Observe general appearance; note discomfort and grimacing on movement and/or examination.
  2. Distraction may distinguish pain behavior from actual pathology.
  3. Note evidence of trauma with bruises, cuts, and fractures.
  4. Note posture and gait.
C. Palpate
  1. Palpate spine and paravertebral structures, noting point tenderness and muscle spasm. Palpation elicits paravertebral tenderness and generalized tenderness over the lower back to upper buttocks.
  2. Examine abdomen for masses.
  3. Extremities: Palpate peripheral pulses.
D. Perform neurologic examination
  1. Identify sensation and pain distribution.
  2. Determine motor strength and evaluate whether muscle strength is symmetrical: Upper extremity resistance is equal bilaterally.
  3. Test deep tendon reflexes (DTRs) and dorsiflexion of the big toes.
E. Check sensation of perineum to rule out cauda equina syndrome.
F. Perform traction tests: Straight leg raises, crossed leg raises, Yeoman Guying, Patrick's test. Musculoskeletal findings include the following:
  1. Straight leg raising and dorsiflexion of foot on the affected side may reduce lower back discomfort.
  2. Elevate each leg passively with flexion at the hip and extension of the knee. Positive straight leg raise gives radicular pain when the leg is raised 30° to 60°.
  3. Crossed leg raises: Test is positive when pain occurs in the leg not being raised.
  4. Yeoman Guying: Unilateral hyperextension in prone position identifies lumbosacral mechanical disorder.
  5. Patrick's test: Place heel on opposite knee and apply lateral force; check for hip or sacroiliac disease.
  6. Range of motion: Increased pain with extension often indicates osteoarthritis. Increased pain with flexion often indicates strain or injured disk.
G. Pelvic examination: Consider pelvic and rectal examination, if indicated. If the patient has fallen on the coccyx, a rectal examination is needed to check for stability.

Diagnostic Tests

A. Laboratory: Complete blood count, erythrocyte sedimentation rate, serum calcium, alkaline phosphatase, urinalysis, and serum immunoelectrophoresis when inflammatory, neoplastic, diffuse bone disease, or renal disease is suspected
B. Radiography of spine
C. Consider the following tests
  1. MRI to rule out disk disease and tumors
  2. Bone scan to rule out cancer

Differential Diagnoses

A. Back pain secondary to musculoskeletal pain
B. Herniated intervertebral disease
C. Sciatica
D. Fracture
E. Ankylosing spondylitis
F. Malignancy/tumor
G. Abdominal aneurysm
H. Pyelonephritis
I. Metabolic bone disease
J. Gynecologic disease
K. Peripheral neuropathy
L. Depression
M. Prostatitis
N. Spinal stenosis
O. Osteoarthritis
P. Osteoporosis

Plan

A. General interventions
  1. The patient should continue physical activity as tolerated.
  2. For acute muscle strain, have the patient apply local cold packs 20 to 30 minutes several times a day for the first 24 hours. Heat packs are recommended after the initial 24 hours of injury.
  3. Chronic or recurrent pain may be treated with either ice or heat applications, whichever gives relief.
B. Patient teaching
  1. Give accurate information on the prognosis for quick recovery such as continuing light physical activity, performing back-strengthening exercises, and avoiding overuse of medications.
  2. Improvement occurs in most cases in a few weeks, although mild symptoms may persist.
  3. Joint guidelines by the American College of Physicians and the American Pain Society recommend rehabilitative therapies for patients who do not improve after medications and self-care recommendations. Rehabilitative therapies include exercise therapy, acupuncture, massage therapy, spinal manipulation, cognitive behavioral therapy, and yoga.
  4. Provide educational handouts on back exercises; *see Section III: Patient Teaching Guide for this chapter, "Back Stretches."* ◀
  5. After intense pain abates, the patient may perform low-back exercises for range of motion and strengthening, and isometric tightening exercises of abdominal and gluteal muscles.
  6. Teach patient knee–chest exercises. Recommend to the patient to place his or her back against the wall and contract abdominal and gluteal muscles with 5 to 10 repetitions four to six times per day.
  7. Research indicates that yoga is beneficial for many types of back pain. Types of back pain benefited by yoga include musculoskeletal injury, herniated disc, spinal stenosis, spondylolisthesis, piriformis syndrome, arthritis, and sacroiliac joint derangement.
  8. Encourage the patient to perform walking exercise daily.
  9. Teach relaxation techniques.

10. Encourage the patient to modify work hours and job tasks.

11. Refer the patient for therapeutic massage or physical therapy as needed.

12. Obesity is often related to decreased exercise and poor physical fitness with reduced trunk muscle strength and endurance. Obese patients may experience back pain with normal activity.

C. Pharmaceutical therapy

1. Analgesics: Acetaminophen 350 to 650 mg every 4 to 6 hours. Maximum dose is 4,000 mg a day. Inquire of any other current medications and/or over-the-counter preparations containing acetaminophen.

2. Nonsteroidal anti-inflammatory drugs (NSAIDs): Unless contraindicated due to gastrointestinal symptoms or cardiovascular disease

a. Aspirin: 325 to 650 mg every 4 to 6 hours

b. Ibuprofen: 200 to 800 mg every 6 to 8 hours; maximum dose is 3.2 g a day under the care of the provider, otherwise 1.2 g a day

c. Naproxen: 500 mg initially, followed by 250 mg every 6 to 8 hours

d. Piroxicam (Feldene): 20 mg every day

e. Meloxicam (Mobic): 7.5 to 15 mg daily

f. Celebrex: 100 to 200 mg twice a day

3. Muscle relaxants

a. Cyclobenzaprine Hcl (Flexeril): 10 mg three times daily

b. Carisoprodol (Soma): 350 mg four times daily—use with extreme caution due to risk of addiction

c. Methocarbamol (Robaxin): 1.5 g every day initially, and then 750 to 1,000 mg every day

d. Orphenadrine citrate (Norflex): 100 mg twice a day

e. Metaxalone (Skelaxin): 800 mg three to four times a day

Follow-Up

A. If pain is severe or unimproved, follow up in 24 hours.

B. If pain is moderate, reevaluate the patient in 7 to 10 days.

C. See the patient in 2 to 4 weeks to reevaluate his or her condition and behavioral changes.

D. Recurrences are not uncommon but do not indicate a chronic or worsening case.

Consultation/Referral

A. Consult with a physician when considering red-flag diagnoses such as cauda equina syndrome, herniated disk, widespread neurologic involvement, carcinoma, or significant trauma.

B. Referral to a physician is needed for patients who note significant morning stiffness with a gradual onset prior to age 40 years, with continuing spinal movements in all directions, and involving some peripheral joints, iritis, skin rashes indicating inflammatory disorders such as ankylosing spondylitis and related disorders.

Individual Considerations

A. Pregnancy: Pregnancy is often associated with low-back discomfort. This is due to the redistribution of body weight. As weight increases in the abdominal area with the growing fetus, patients tend to compensate by changing posture and tilting the spine back.

B. Adults

1. For patients older than 50 years presenting with no prior history of backache, consider a differential diagnosis of neoplasm. The most common metastasis seen is secondary to the primary site of breast cancer, prostate cancer, or multiple myeloma. Pain most prominent in a recumbent position rarely radiates into the buttock or leg.

2. Men and women in their early adulthood (ages 20–45 years) who present with chronic back pain that improves with activity should be further evaluated for ankylosing spondylitis.

Bibliography

Centers for Disease Control and Prevention. (2016, March 15). CDC guidelines for prescribing opioids for chronic pain—United States, 2016. *Morbidity and Mortality Weekly Reports.* Retrieved from https://www.cdc.gov/mmwr/volumes/65/rr/rr6501e1.htm

Centers for Disease Control and Prevention. (2016, March 22). Checklist for prescribing opioids for chronic pain. Retrieved from https://www.cdc.gov/drugoverdose/pdf/PDO_Checklist-a.pdf

Chronic Pain Perspectives. (2013). Ambulatory infusion system gets FDA clearance. Retrieved from https://www.google.com/webhp?sourceid=chrome-instant&ion=1&espv=2&ie=UTF-8#q=Ambulatory+infusion+system+gets+FDA+clearance

Costead, L., & Banasik, J. (2012). *Pathophysiology* (5th ed.). St. Louis, MO: Elsevier Saunders.

Dunphy, L., Brown, J., Porter, B., & Thomas, D. (2015). *Primary care: The art and science of advanced practice nursing* (4th ed.). Philadelphia, PA: F. A. Davis.

Fishman, L. (2012). Efficacy and application of yoga for back pain. *Chronic Pain Perspectives.* Retrieved from http://chronicpainperspectives.com/articles/feature-article/article/efficacy-and-application-of-yoga-for-back-pain/8c51fc8df7a517da1a5e8baa1f28d7e8.html

Goertz, M., Thorson, D., Bonsell, J., Bonte, B., Campbell, R., Haake, B., ... Timming, R. (2012). *Health care guideline: Adult acute and subacute low back pain* (15th ed.). Bloomington, MN: Institute for Clinical Systems Improvement. Retrieved from https://www.icsi.org/_asset/bjvqrj/LBP.pdf

Hooten, W. M., Timming, R., Belgrade, M., Gaul, J., Goertz, M., Haake, B., ... Walker, N. (2013). *Health care guideline: Assessment and management of chronic pain* (6th ed.). Bloomington, MN: Institute for Clinical Systems Improvement. Retrieved from https://pdfs.semanticscholar.org/e1f7/c26a36d83686607ad89ee835daa3c9db3f4c.pdf

Michigan Quality Improvement Consortium. (n.d.). Management of acute low back pain. Retrieved from https://www.guidelines.gov

National Guideline Clearinghouse. (2011a). *Guideline summary: Guideline for the evidence-informed primary care management of low back pain.* Rockville, MD: Agency for Healthcare Research and Quality. Retrieved from https://www.guideline.gov/content.aspx?id=37954&search=chronic+low+back+pain+and+acute+low+back+pain+and+assessment+and+management+of+pain

National Guideline Clearinghouse. (2011b). *Guideline summary: Managing chronic non-terminal pain in adults including prescribing controlled substances.* Rockville, MD: Agency for Healthcare Research and Quality.Retrieved from https://www.guideline.gov/summaries/summary/25657/managing-chronic-nonterminal-pain-in-adults-including-prescribing-controlled-substances?q=Managing+chronic+nonterminal+pain+including+prescribing+controlled+substances

National Guideline Clearinghouse. (2013, November). *Guideline summary: Assessment and management of chronic pain.* Rockville, MD: Agency for Healthcare Research and Quality. Retrieved from https://www.guideline.gov/summaries/summary/47646

Rosenquist, E. (2016). Evaluation of chronic pain in adults. In T. W. Post & M. Aronson (Eds.), *UpToDate.* Retrieved from https://www.uptodate.com/contents/evaluation-of-chronic-pain-in-adults?source=search_result&search=chronic+pain&selectedTitle=3%7E150

4 Dermatology Guidelines

Acne Rosacea

Jill C. Cash and Amy C. Bruggemann

Definition

A. A multifactorial vascular skin disorder, acne rosacea is characterized by chronic inflammatory processes in which flushing and dilation of the blood vessels occur on the face. It is manifested in four stages of pathologic events.

Incidence

A. Acne rosacea affects approximately 13 million people in the United States.

Pathogenesis

A. Rosacea is a functional vascular anomaly with a tendency toward recurrent dilation and flushing of the face. This results in inflammatory mediator release, extravasation of inflammatory cells, and the formation of inflammatory papules and pustules.

Predisposing Factors

A. Tendency to flush frequently
B. Exposure to heat, cold, or sunlight
C. Consumption of hot or spicy foods and alcoholic beverages
D. Some topical medications, astringents, or toners

Common Complaints

A. Papules, pustules, and nodules. Hallmarks for diagnosis are the small papules and papulopustules. Many presenting erythematous papules have a tiny pustule at the crest. No comedones are present.
B. Periodic reddening or flushing of face
C. Increase in skin temperature of face
D. Face flushing in response to heat stimuli (hot liquids) in mouth

Other Signs and Symptoms

A. Periorbital erythema
B. Telangiectasia, paranasally and on cheeks
C. Rhinophyma
D. Blepharoconjunctivitis with erythematous eyelid margins
E. Conjunctivitis: Diffuse hyperemic type or nodular
F. Keratitis: Lower portion of cornea, associated with pain, photophobia, and foreign-body sensation

Subjective Data

A. Ask the patient to describe the location and the onset. Was the onset sudden or gradual? How have the symptoms continued to develop?
B. Assess if the skin is itchy or painful.
C. Assess for any associated discharge (blood or pus).
D. Complete a drug history. Has the patient recently taken any antibiotics or other medications?
E. Determine whether the patient has used any topical medications, astringents, toners, or new skin-care products.
F. Rule out any possible exposure to industrial or domestic toxins, insect bites, and possible contact with venereal disease or HIV.
G. Ask the patient about close contact with others with skin disorders.
H. Identify whether exposure to heat, cold, or sunlight provokes the symptoms.
I. Ask whether eating or drinking hot or spicy foods or consumption of alcoholic beverages provokes the symptoms.

Physical Examination

A. Check temperature, pulse, and blood pressure.
B. Inspect
  1. Skin, focusing on face and scalp
  2. Nose and paranasal structures
  3. Eyes, eyelids, conjunctiva, and cornea. **An ocular manifestation, rosacea keratitis, may cause corneal ulcers to develop.**

Diagnostic Tests

A. Consider skin biopsy to rule out lupus, sarcoidosis, or other possible causes if history and physical exam findings warrant further testing.

Differential Diagnoses

A. Acne rosacea
B. Acne vulgaris
C. Steroid-induced acne
D. Perioral dermatitis
E. Seborrheic dermatitis
F. Lupus erythematosus
G. Cutaneous sarcoidosis

Plan

A. General interventions: Identify any causative or provocative factors—heat, cold, hot or spicy foods, alcoholic beverages, sunlight.

1. Advise washing face with a mild cleanser such as Cetaphil or Cerave in the morning and at night.

2. Avoid direct sunlight exposure by wearing protective clothing/hats when outdoors. Suggest using a sunscreen of sun protection factor (SPF)-30 when exposed to sunlight.

▶ **B.** Patient teaching: *See Section III: Patient Teaching Guide for this chapter, "Acne Rosacea."*

C. Pharmaceutical therapy

1. Drug of choice: Tetracycline 500 to 1,000 mg twice to four times daily for 2 to 4 weeks.

2. Others: Erythromycin 500 mg twice daily until clear, minocycline (Minocin), 50 to 200 mg daily divided into two doses, doxycycline (Vibramycin) 100 mg daily, Amoxil, and metronidazole (Flagyl, Protostat). Start at a higher dose and taper to the maintenance dose.

a. Topical antibiotics. Apply topical Metrogel twice daily after cleansing skin.

b. Do not use topical steroids. Topical steroids may worsen irritation.

c. Other topical antibiotics: Clindamycin (Cleocin T), erythromycin twice daily.

3. Refractory cases may respond to isotretinoin (Accutane).

Follow-Up

A. Follow up in 2 weeks to evaluate therapy.

B. See patients monthly for evaluation until maintenance is reached.

C. Relapses are common following discontinuance of antibiotics; repeat treatment.

Consultation/Referral

A. Consult or refer the patient to a dermatologist if there is no improvement, or if the patient is unable to reach maintenance.

B. Provide an immediate referral to an ophthalmologist for treatment and follow up if the eye is involved.

Individual Consideration

A. Adults: Tinted sulfacetamide (Sulfacet-R) lotion may be used by fair-skinned patients to cover erythema.

Acne Vulgaris

Jill C. Cash and Amy C. Bruggemann

Definition

A. Acne vulgaris is a disorder of the sebaceous glands and hair follicles of the skin that are most numerous on the face, back, and chest. The sebaceous glands become inflamed and form papules, pustules, cysts, open or closed comedones, and/or nodules on an erythemic base. In severe cases, scarring can result.

Incidence

A. Acne is the most common skin disorder in the United States, affecting 40 to 50 million persons of all ages and races. Nearly 80% to 90% of all adults experience acne during their lifetime. Acne vulgaris, commonly seen in adolescence, may even extend into the third or fourth decade of life.

Pathogenesis

A. Sebum is overproduced and collects in the sebaceous gland. Sebum, keratinized cells, and hair collect in the follicle. With *Propionibacterium acnes* present, the duct becomes clogged, and lesions (noninflammatory and/or inflammatory) evolve.

Predisposing Factors

A. Age (adolescence)

B. External irritants to skin (makeup, oils, equipment contact on skin)

C. Hormones (oral contraceptives with high progestin content)

D. Medications (lithium, halides, hydantoin derivatives, rifampin)

E. Hot, humid weather

Common Complaints

A. Outbreak of pimples on face, chest, shoulders, and back that do not resolve with over-the-counter (OTC) treatment.

B. Acne rosacea: Telangiectasia, flushing, and rhinophyma present

Other Signs and Symptoms

A. Mild: Comedones open (blackhead) and closed (whitehead)

B. Moderate: Comedones with papules and pustules

C. Severe: Nodules, cysts, and scars

Subjective Data

A. Elicit the age of onset of outbreak, duration, and course of symptoms.

B. Determine what makes the lesions worse or better.

C. Ask whether there are certain times of the month or year when lesions are better or worse.

D. Identify the patient's current method of cleanser or moisturizer treatment.

E. Ask if the patient has ever been treated by a provider for this problem. If so, determine the treatment and results of the treatment.

F. Assess whether other family members have this same problem.

G. Ask the patient for a description of his or her environment and occupation.

H. Explore with the patient any current stress factors in his or her life.

Physical Examination

A. Inspect

1. Observe skin for location and severity of lesions.

2. Rate severity of lesions as mild, moderate, or severe.

a. Mild: Few papules/pustules, no nodules
b. Moderate: Several papules/pustules, rare nodules
c. Severe: Many papules/pustules with many nodules

3. Take a picture of areas of affected skin for chart and document date. Use this for future appointments as a reference to compare results for follow-up visits.

Diagnostic Tests

A. No tests are generally required.
B. Culture lesions to rule out gram-negative folliculitis with patients on antibiotics.
C. Consider hormone testing if other primary causes of acne are taken into account (follicle-stimulating hormone, luteinizing hormone, testosterone levels).

Differential Diagnoses

A. Acne vulgaris
B. Acne rosacea
C. Steroid rosacea
D. Folliculitis
E. Perioral acne
F. Drug-induced acne

Plan

A. General interventions
1. Document location and severity of lesions. Assess quality of improvement at each office visit.
2. The primary goal of treatment is prevention of scarring. Good control of lesions during puberty and early adulthood is required for best results. Anticipate ups and downs during the normal course of treatment.

B. Patient teaching
1. *See Section III: Patient Teaching Guide for this chapter: "Acne Vulgaris."*
2. Instruct the patient on proper cleansing routine. The patient should wash affected areas with a mild soap (Purpose, Cetaphil) twice a day and apply medications as directed.
3. Warn the patient that washing the face more than two to three times a day can decrease oil production and cause drying.
4. Discuss current stressors in the patient's life and discuss treatment options.
5. Recommend an exercise routine 3 to 5 days a week.
6. Recommend oil-free sunscreens.

C. Pharmaceutical therapy: **It may take 1 to 3 months before results are visible when using these medications.**
1. Mild: Treatment of choice is topical. Use one of the following:
a. Benzoyl peroxide, 2.5%, 5%, 10%; begin with 2.5% at bedtime. May graduate to 5% or 10% twice daily, if needed, as tolerated.
b. T-Stat: Apply to dried areas twice daily. Avoid eyes, nose, and mouth creases.
c. Topical tretinoin 0.1% (Retin-A Micro); use at bedtime.
i. With Retin-A use, the patient may see rapid turnover of keratin plugs.
ii. Instruct the patient to avoid abrasive soaps.
iii. Warn the patient regarding photosensitivity.
iv. Warn the patient regarding increased dryness. May apply a moisturizer such as Cerave or Cetaphil if needed.
d. Desquam E: Use at bedtime. Wash face with soap and then apply Desquam E.
2. Moderate: Use one of the aforementioned topical medications in addition to one of the following oral medications:
a. Tetracycline 500 mg twice daily for 3 to 6 weeks, for adolescents older than 14 years. As condition improves, begin tapering medication to 250 mg twice daily for 6 weeks, then to daily or to every other day.
i. Instruct the patient to take tetracycline on an empty stomach and to avoid dairy products, antacids, and iron.
ii. Warn the patient about photosensitivity. This medication may be used as a maintenance dose at 250 mg daily or every other day for those patients who break out after discontinuing antibiotic therapy. No drug resistance is seen with tetracycline.
b. Erythromycin 250 mg four times per day after meals or topical erythromycin 2%, solution or gel, twice daily, or clindamycin (Cleocin T) solution, pads, or gel, twice daily. Erythromycin resistance has been seen.
c. Minocycline 100 mg twice daily. When this is effective, taper to 50 mg twice daily.
i. Have the patient drink plenty of fluids.
ii. Central nervous system (CNS) side effects (headaches) have been seen.
d. Bactrim single strength twice daily, if the aforementioned regimens do not work well. Bactrim works well if others fail because it is effective for Gram-negative folliculitis.
e. Oral contraceptives with higher doses of estrogen have also been effective for girls.
f. Doxycycline
g. Spironolactone
3. Severe: Medications as prescribed by the dermatologist.

Follow-Up

See patients every 6 to 8 weeks for evaluation.
A. Mild: Adjust dose depending on local irritation.
B. Moderate (oral and topical medications)
1. Adjust dose according to irritation.
2. Taper oral antibiotics with discretion and/or continue topical medications.
3. Oral antibiotics may be tapered and discontinued when inflammatory lesions have resolved.
C. Severe: Recommend referral to dermatology and follow-up with the specialty.

Consultation/Referral

A. Consult with a physician if treatment is unsuccessful after 10 to 12 weeks of therapy or if acne is severe.
B. The patient may need dermatology consultation.

Individual Considerations

A. Pregnancy
   1. Acne may flare up or improve during pregnancy.
   2. Medications preferred during pregnancy are topical agents.
   3. **Teratogens include tretinoin, tetracycline, and minocycline.**
      a. **When using teratogenic medications, contraception must be practiced to avoid pregnancy to prevent severe fetal malformations.**
      b. **Begin contraception 1 month before starting the medication and continue contraception 1 month after finishing the medication.**

Animal Bites, Mammalian

Jill C. Cash and Amy C. Bruggemann

Definition

A. Bites of any mammalian animal to the human can be potentially dangerous. Human bites are included.

Incidence

A. Account for 1 to 3.5 million emergency room (ER) visits each year.
B. About 80% to 90% of bites are dog bites.
C. About 6% of bites are cat bites.
D. From 1% to 15% are human bites.
E. Children and the elderly are especially prone.

Pathogenesis

A. Mechanical trauma and break to skin and/or underlying structures
B. Infection from transmission of bacteria
   1. *Pasteurella multocida* is primarily associated with cat bites but may also be associated with dog bites.
   2. *Staphylococcus aureus*, *Staphylococcus epidermis*, and *Enterobacter* species can be transmitted by dog and cat bites.
   3. *Streptobacillus moniliformis* can be transmitted by rat and mice bites.
   4. *Streptococcus, Staphylococcus,* and *Eikenella* can be transmitted by human bites.
   5. Human bites can transmit diseases: Actinomycosis, syphilis, tuberculosis, hepatitis B, and potentially HIV.

C. Rabies, an acute viral infection, may be transmitted by means of infected saliva or by an infected animal licking mucosa of an open wound. It is rarely contracted by means of airborne transmission, but this has been reported to occur in bat-infested caves.

Predisposing Factors

A. Entering an animal's territorial space and/or surprising an animal

Common Complaints

A. Bitten
B. Pain
C. Redness
D. Swelling

Other Signs and Symptoms

A. Normal: Mild redness and swelling, sero-sanguinous oozing, discomfort
B. Abnormal: Erythema, fever, pus, red streaks, pain, loss of sensation

Subjective Data

A. What person or type of animal bit the patient?
B. Was this a provoked or an unprovoked attack?
C. Did the patient identify and contact the owner of the animal?
D. What was the behavior of the animal: Unusual, strange, or ill appearing?
E. How much time elapsed from being bitten to seeking treatment?
F. Did the patient start any self-treatment?
G. What is the patient's tetanus immunization status?
H. Review history for any prior rabies immunizations.
I. Does the patient know if the animal was a domestic animal? Is the animal's vaccination status known?
J. If the bite is of human origin, determine if it is a closed-fist injury or plain bite.

Physical Examination

A. Check blood pressure, pulse, and respirations, and observe overall respiratory status.
B. See Table 4.1.

Diagnostic Test

A. Refer to Table 4.1.

Differential Diagnoses

A. Animal bite: Dog, cat, human, and so forth
   1. Cat bites more frequently become infected.
   2. Bites on the hand have the highest infection rates. Bites on the face have the lowest infection rates.

B. Cellulitis and abscesses
C. High-risk potential for rabies from the following:
   1. Skunks, foxes, raccoons, and bats are primary carriers.
   2. Rabbits, squirrels, chipmunks, rats, and mice are seldom infective for rabies.
   3. Properly vaccinated animals seldom are infective.

Plan

A. General interventions
   1. Control bleeding.
   2. Perform wound care.
      a. Immediately wash wound copiously with soap and water.
      b. Irrigate wound with saline using a 20-gauge or larger catheter.
      c. Use 150 to 1,000 mL of solution.
      d. Direct saline stream on the entire wound surface.
      e. Scrub entire surrounding area.
      f. Debride all wounds.
      g. Trim any jagged edges to prevent cosmetic and/or functional complications.
      h. Cover with dry dressing.
   3. Do not suture wounds with high risk of infection:
      a. Hand bites, closed-fist injuries
      b. Bites older than 6 hours

TABLE 4.1 Bites

Animal	Signs and Symptoms	Physical Examination: Check Patient Temperature for All Animal Bites	Diagnostic Tests
Dog	Crush injury, lacerations, and abrasions	Inspect site; underlying structures; and distal neurovascular, motor, and sensory functions. Palpate area. If wound is more than 24 hours old, check for any signs of cellulitis or lymphangitis.	If infected—Laboratory: Complete blood count (CBC), culture and sensitivity for anaerobes and aerobes
Cat	Puncture wounds, may be deep	Determine depth and extent of wound. Check for foreign bodies. If wound is more than 24 hours old, check for any signs of cellulitis or lymphangitis.	If sepsis suspected—Laboratory: CBC, culture and sensitivity of abscess/tissue site
Rat and squirrel	Laceration, abrasions; more superficial in nature	Check for signs of infection if wound is more than 24 hours old. Check for any signs of cellulitis or lymphangitis.	
Human	Crush injury, laceration; wound of hand (closed-fist wound)	Check for signs of infection if wound is more than 24 hours old. Check for any signs of cellulitis or lymphangitis. Also, examine for fractures, air in the joint, subchondral bone defects, and osteomyelitis. Examine for full range of interphalangeal and metacarpophalangeal joints.	If infected—Laboratory: CBC, culture and sensitivity Also, take an x-ray film of structures underlying the bite

c. Deep or puncture wounds

d. Bites with extensive injury of surface or underlying structures

4. Rabies control measures:

a. Consult with the local health department regarding the risk of rabies in the area.

b. The domestic animal should be identified, caught, and confined for 10 days of observation. If the animal develops any signs of rabies, it should be destroyed and its brain tissue analyzed. No treatment is necessary if results are negative.

c. The wild animal should be caught and destroyed for brain tissue analysis. No treatment is necessary if results are negative.

d. If the bat or wild carnivore cannot be found, rabies prophylaxis is instituted.

B. Patient teaching

1. Stress the importance of keeping the site free from infection. Instruct the patient on how to keep the site free from infection such as teaching cleaning techniques, good handwashing, and using medications as prescribed.

2. Discuss symptoms to report to the provider if signs of infection begin (erythema, swelling, drainage, and tenderness).

C. Pharmaceutical therapy

1. Antibiotic prophylaxis is controversial, but it is generally recommended for wounds involving subcutaneous tissues and deeper structures.

a. Amoxicillin/clavulanic acid (Augmentin) 875 mg every 12 hours; for children, prescribe 25 to 45 mg/kg/dose in two divided doses for 3 to 7 days. Available as 200 mg/5 mL and 400 mg/5 mL liquid.

b. Alternatively, prescribe doxycycline 100 mg twice per day for 3 to 7 days; for children, prescribe clindamycin 10 to 25 mg per kg divided every 6 to 8 hours plus trimethoprim/sulfamethoxazole 8 to 10 mg per kg (trimethoprim component) divided every 12 hours for 3 to 7 days.

2. Tetanus prophylaxis

3. Rabies prophylaxis

a. Active immunization: Human diploid cell vaccine (HDCV), 1 mL, is given intramuscularly (IM) on the first day of treatment, and repeat doses are administered on days 3, 7, 14, and 28.

b. Passive immunization: Rabies immunoglobulin; (human) should be used simultaneously with the first dose of HDCV; the recommended dose of RIG is 20 IU/kg. Approximately one half of RIG is infiltrated into the wound, and the remainder is given IM.

Follow-Up

A. Evaluate wound and change dressing in 24 to 48 hours.

B. Reevaluate as indicated. If the patient is on immunoprophylaxis and has no signs of infection, see the patient in 1 week.

C. Instruct the patient to return immediately in case of any signs of infection.

Consultation/Referral

A. Refer all patients with bites of the ears, face, genitalia, hands, and feet.

B. Consult with a doctor if suspicion of rabies is involved.
C. Contact the local health department.
D. Wounds involving tendon, joint, or bone require hospitalization and surgical consultation.

Individual Consideration

A. Pregnancy: Use appropriate antibiotic management.
B. Pediatrics: Children are more prone to animal bites.
C. Geriatrics: The elderly population is more prone to animal bites.

Benign Skin Lesions

Jill C. Cash and Amy C. Bruggemann

Definition

A benign skin lesion is a cutaneous growth with no harmful effects to the body. Benign lesions must be distinguished from the following:
A. Basal cell carcinoma (BCC): Nodular tumor with pearly surface, telangiectasia on surface, and depressed center or rolled edge
B. Squamous cell carcinoma (SCC): Irregular papule, with scaly, friable, bleeding surface
C. Malignant melanoma: Asymmetric papule, with irregular border, of two or more colors, and size varies

Incidence

A. Benign lesions are common to all races, and they are seen primarily in the adult and elderly populations.

Pathogenesis

A. The course varies, depending on the specific type of lesion.

Predisposing Factors

A. Sun exposure in the adult and elderly populations
B. Dermatosis papulosa nigra: Common in African Americans and Asians

Common Complaint

A. New lesion of the skin

Other Signs and Symptoms

A. Seborrheic keratosis: Waxy papule with a stuck-on appearance is seen in adults; they appear symmetric, 0.2 to 3.0 cm in size, with a well-demarcated border and a variety of colors (tan, black, and brown).
B. Dermatosis papulosa nigra: Hyperpigmented mole located on face or neck; a pedunculated papule that is symmetric, 1 to 3 mm in diameter.
C. Cherry angioma: Vascular papule, red to purple, located on trunk in adults; begins in early adulthood; 1- to 3-mm diameter papules that do not blanch.
D. Solar lentigines (liver spots): Tan maculae on sun-exposed areas in elders, especially on face and hands; border is irregular, and the size varies.
E. Sebaceous hyperplasia: Enlarged sebaceous glands that appear as yellow papules on sun-exposed areas, especially on the face in elders; papules have central umbilication, and their size varies.
F. Actinic keratoses: Rough, scaly patch on your skin that develops from years of exposure to the sun. They are most commonly found on your face, lips, ears, back of your hands, forearms, scalp, or neck. These areas should be monitored closely as they can become cancerous.

Subjective Data

A. Identify when the patient first discovered the lesion.
B. Determine whether the lesion has changed in size, shape, or color.
C. Ask if the patient has discovered more lesions.
D. Elicit information regarding a family history of skin lesions or cancer.

Physical Examination

A. Inspect
  1. Observe skin; note all lesions and evaluate each for asymmetry, border, color, diameter, evolving changes, and/or elevation change.
  2. Note the patient's skin type.

Diagnostic Tests

A. Benign lesions do not require any tests.
B. If unsure regarding possible malignancy, a biopsy is recommended.

Differential Diagnoses

A. Benign skin lesion
  1. Seborrheic keratosis
  2. Dermatosis papulosa nigra
  3. Cherry angioma
  4. Solar lentigines
  5. Senile sebaceous hyperplasia
  6. Keratoacanthoma

Plan

A. General interventions
  1. Reassure the patient that lesions are benign. No treatment is required unless the patient chooses to have the lesion removed for cosmetic purposes.
  2. Benign skin lesions may be removed using cryotherapy if they are bothersome for the patient.
B. Patient teaching: *See Section III: Patient Teaching Guide for this chapter, "Skin Care Assessment."* ◀
C. Pharmaceutical therapy
  1. Medications are not recommended for treatment.

Follow-Up

A. Routine skin examinations should be performed yearly.

Consultation/Referral

A. Immediately refer the patient to a dermatologist if malignancy is suspected or confirmed by biopsy.

Individual Considerations

A. Adults: Skin lesions begin to appear in early adulthood. Encourage patients to monitor lesions over time.
B. Geriatrics: Benign lesions are commonly seen in the elderly population.

Candidiasis

Jill C. Cash and Amy C. Bruggemann

Definition

A. A fungal infection of the mucous membranes and/or skin, candidiasis is caused by the *Candida albicans* fungus.

Incidence

A. It occurs frequently in women, children, and the elderly population.

Pathogenesis

A. An overgrowth of *C. albicans* occurs when mucous membranes and/or skin are exposed to moisture, warmth, and an alteration in the membrane barrier.

Predisposing Factors

A. Immunosuppression
B. Use of antibiotics
C. Hyperglycemia
D. Chronic use of steroid
E. Frequent douching by women
F. Adults wearing dentures

Common Complaints

A. Oral: A persistent white patch on the tongue or roof of mouth may be slightly reddened with or without crevices on the tongue
B. Vaginal: Thick, white, "cottage-cheese-like" vaginal discharge with or without vaginal itching
C. Genital: Bright red rash with well-demarcated satellite lesions advancing to pustules or erosions in genital or diaper area
D. Males: Erythemic rash that may advance to erosions seen on male genitalia; scrotum is perhaps involved

Subjective Data

A. Question the patient about onset, duration, and location of lesions.
B. Determine whether the patient has a history of previous infections.
C. Inquire into medical history and current medications.
D. Rule out the presence of any other current medical conditions.

Physical Examination

A. Inspect
- **1.** Assess skin and mucous membranes for discharge and lesions.
- **2.** Observe location and severity of lesions.

B. Palpate: Palpate lymph nodes in neck and groin.

Diagnostic Tests

A. Vaginal and genital infections need to be evaluated for sexually transmitted infections (STIs), especially if the patient is sexually active with multiple partners. Vaginal/genital culture specimen should be sent for gonorrhea/chlamydia testing.
B. Other specimens to consider include wet prep/potassium hydroxide (KOH) 10% solution, Gram stain vaginal culture for *Candida*.

Differential Diagnoses

A. Oral candidiasis
- **1.** Leukoplakia
- **2.** Stomatitis
- **3.** Formula (for newborns)

B. Diaper area
- **1.** Candidiasis
- **2.** Contact dermatitis
- **3.** Bacterial infection

C. Genital area
- **1.** Candidiasis
- **2.** Bacterial infection
- **3.** Bacterial vaginosis
- **4.** Chlamydia
- **5.** Gonorrhea
- **6.** Trichomoniasis

Plan

A. General interventions
- **1.** Treatment can be successful with good hygiene and medications.
- **2.** Stress to the patient to keep the affected area cool and dry. Frequent changes of clothing may be necessary to keep the area cool and dry to avoid damp conditions.
- **3.** Diaper area will need to be changed more frequently; suggest using cloth diapers and allowing skin to be exposed to air for short periods.

B. Patient teaching
- **1.** Use medication on the skin to help with symptoms.
- **2.** Do not scratch. Keep fingernails short.

C. Pharmaceutical therapy: Choose *one* of the following pharmaceutical therapies:
- **1.** Oral
  - **a.** Nystatin (Mycostatin) oral suspension 100,000 U/mL, 2 mL for infants and 4 to 6 mL for older children and adults, four times daily for 7 to 10 days
  - **b.** Gentian violet aqueous solution, 1% for infants and 2% for adults, one to two times per day
  - **c.** Lotrimin buccal troches, five times per day for 2 weeks, only for adults
- **2.** Diaper
  - **a.** Nystatin cream, three to four times per day for 7 to 10 days
  - **b.** Mycolog II; apply sparingly to skin twice daily until resolved
- **3.** Vaginal
  - **a.** Clotrimazole 1% cream, 5 g intravaginally for 7 to 14 days
  - **b.** Miconazole 2% cream, 5 g intravaginally for 7 days (over the counter [OTC])
  - **c.** Terconazole 0.8% cream, 5 g intravaginally for 3 days
  - **d.** Terconazole 80 mg vaginal suppository, at bedtime for 3 days
  - **e.** Fluconazole (Diflucan) 150 mg, oral tablet one time
  - **f.** Other preparations available in stronger or weaker doses

Follow-Up

A. None indicated unless not resolved or complications arise.

Consultation/Referral

A. Consult a physician if not resolved within 2 weeks.

Individual Considerations

A. Pregnancy
   1. Most effective medications for pregnant women are clotrimazole, miconazole, and terconazole.
   2. Recommend a full 7-day course of treatment during pregnancy.
B. Adults
   1. Consider immunosuppression in all adults with oral candidiasis (HIV, diabetes, chemotherapy, leukemia).
   2. Adults with oral lesions need to be assessed for leukoplakia, especially if the patient has a history of smoking or chewing tobacco.

Contact Dermatitis

Jill C. Cash and Amy C. Bruggemann

Definition

A. Contact dermatitis is a cutaneous response to direct exposure of the skin to irritants (irritant contact dermatitis) or allergens (allergic contact dermatitis).
   1. Irritant contact dermatitis is a nonimmunologic response of the epidermis.
   2. Allergic contact dermatitis is an immunologic response after one or more exposures to a particular agent.

Incidence

A. Occurs in all ages. People who work with chemicals daily and wash their hands numerous times a day have a higher incidence of irritant dermatitis. Irritant contact dermatitis is seen in the elderly because of dry skin.

Pathogenesis

A. Irritant contact dermatitis is caused by an alteration of the outer layer of the dermis caused by exposure to chemicals; lotions; cold, dry air; soaps; detergents; or organic solvents.

B. Allergic contact dermatitis is caused by an alteration in the epidermis when, after exposure to an allergen, the immune system responds by producing inflammation of the cutaneous tissue. Common allergens include poison ivy, poison oak, sumac, nickel jewelry, hair dye, rubber and leather chemicals (latex gloves), cleaning supplies, harsh soaps, detergents, and topical medicines.

Predisposing Factors

A. Occupation (hairdresser, nurse, housecleaner, etc.)
B. Jewelry
C. Activities in yard or woods

Common Complaints

A. Irritation of the skin, ranging from redness to pruritic inflammation, with possible progression of blisters.
   1. Poison oak, ivy, and sumac induce classic presentation: Lesions (vesicles) and papules on an erythemic base presenting in a linear fashion with sharp margins.
   2. Diffuse pattern with erythema may be seen when oleoresin is contacted from pets or smoke from burning fire.

B. Exposure to some type of irritant known to the patient. Round or annular lesions may have an internal cause such as a drug reaction.

Other Signs and Symptoms

A. Chronic
   1. Erythema with thickening
   2. Scaling
   3. Fissures
   4. Inflammation; with chronic dermatitis, lichenification may occur with scales and fissures.

B. Diaper dermatitis: Prominent red, shiny rash on buttocks and genitalia

C. Candidiasis diaper rash
   1. Bright red rash with satellite lesions at margins
   2. Inflammation and excoriations present
   3. Creases may be involved.

Subjective Data

A. Ask the patient when irritation began and how it has progressed.
B. Elicit history of exposure to allergens.
C. Question the patient regarding activity and skin contact with irritants before outbreak (cleaning agents, walking in woods, hobbies, change in soap/laundry detergent, shaving cream, lotions, etc.).
D. List occupation and family history of allergens.
E. Review medication list, including prescription, over-the-counter (OTC), and herbal medicines, to evaluate an interaction.
F. List medications used to relieve symptoms and results.

Physical Examination

A. Check temperature (if indicated).
B. Inspect
   1. Inspect skin, noting types of lesions and location of lesions. **Note the pattern of inflammation. The shape of irritation may mimic the shape of the irritant, such as the skin under a ring or watch, for example.**
   2. Determine progression of lesions.
   3. Differentiate between primary and secondary lesions.

Diagnostic Tests

A. Consider none if source is known.
B. Wet mount (potassium hydroxide [KOH], saline) to rule out fungal infection if candida is suspected
C. Culture/sensitivity of pustules
D. Patch test to rule out allergic contact dermatitis

Differential Diagnoses

A. Irritant contact dermatitis
B. Allergic contact dermatitis
C. Diaper dermatitis
D. Candida
E. Tinea pedis, corporis, cruris
F. Drug reactions
G. Pityriasis rosea
H. Scabies

Plan

A. General interventions
1. Irritant contact dermatitis: Removal of irritating agent
a. Use topical soaks with saline or Burow's solution (1:40 dilution) for weeping areas.
b. Suggest lukewarm baths (not hot); or oatmeal (Aveeno) baths, as needed.
c. For dry erythematous skin, use recommend Eucerin or Aquaphor ointments to rehydrate skin.
d. Remind the patient to avoid scratching skin and to keep nails short.
e. Suggest use of mild soaps and cleansers.
2. Allergic contact dermatitis
a. Instruct the patient to avoid contact with the causative agent.
b. Have the patient wash the affected area with cool water immediately after exposure.
c. Recommend lukewarm baths with oatmeal (Aveeno) three to four times per day.
d. Tell the patient to apply calamine lotion after baths.
3. Diaper dermatitis
a. Instruct the caretaker to change the patient's diaper frequently, cleaning with water only, and allow skin to air dry 15 to 30 minutes four times a day. Tell the parent not to use lotions or powders, but to apply zinc oxide (Desitin ointment or powder, or Happy Hiney) with each diaper change.
b. If candidiasis diaper rash presents, for treatment refer to the "Candidiasis" section in this chapter.

▶ **B.** Patient teaching: *See Section III: Patient Teaching Guide for this chapter, "Dermatitis."*

C. Pharmaceutical therapy
1. Irritant contact dermatitis: Hydrocortisone 2.5% ointment three to four times per day for 2 weeks
2. Allergic contact dermatitis
a. Low-dose topical steroids: Hydrocortisone 2.5% ointment three to four times per day for 1 to 2 weeks after blistering stage. Triamcinolone acetonide 0.025% (Kenalog) ointment/cream twice daily.
b. Intermediate-dose topical steroids: Triamcinolone acetonide 0.1% (Kenalog) cream twice daily. Cream/ointment should not be used longer than 2 weeks at a time.
c. High-potent topical steroids: Fluocinonide 0.05% (Lidex) ointment three to four times per day; not to be used on face or skin folds. Cream/ointment should not be used longer than 2 weeks at a time.
d. Hydroxyzine 25 to 50 mg four times daily, diphenhydramine Hcl (Benadryl) 25 to 50 mg four times daily. For children, 0.5 mg/kg/dose three times daily as needed.
e. If the rash is severe (face, eyes, genitalia, mucous membranes), consider prednisone 60 to 80 mg/d to start and taper over 10 to 14 days.
f. Triamcinolone acetonide (Kenalog) 40 to 60 mg by intramuscular (IM) injection
3. Secondary bacterial infections: Erythromycin 250 mg four times daily or amoxicillin/clavulanic acid (Augmentin) 875 mg twice daily for 10 days
4. Candidiasis
a. Use miconazole nitrate 2% cream, miconazole powder, or nystatin cream.
b. Use clotrimazole (Lotrimin) or ketoconazole (Nizoral) cream three to four times per day for 10 days.
c. If inflammation is present along with yeast, use Mycolog II.
d. If secondary bacterial infection is present, use mupirocin (Bactroban) ointment three times daily for 7 to 10 days.

Follow-Up

A. None required if case is mild.
B. See the patient again in 2 to 3 days for severe cases, or phone to assess progress.

Consultation/Referral

A. Consult with a physician when steroid treatment is necessary or if worsening symptoms develop despite adequate therapy.

Individual Considerations

A. Pregnancy: If medications are necessary during pregnancy, consider the gestational age of the fetus and category of medication.
B. Pediatrics: For infants and children, consider hydroxyzine (Atarax) 0.5 mg/kg/dose three times daily as needed for severe pruritus.
C. Elderly: Patients may only exhibit scaling as the prominent irritation rather than erythema and inflammation. Topical medications (neomycin, vitamin E, lanolin) and acrylate adhesives are common causes of contact dermatitis.

Eczema or Atopic Dermatitis

Jill C. Cash and Amy C. Bruggemann

Definition

A. This pattern of skin inflammation has clinical features of erythema, itching, scaling, lichenification, papules, and vesicles in various combinations. Currently, the term *eczema* is used interchangeably with *dermatitis.* Most common variants are atopic dermatitis and atopic eczema. Classification is done by cause, either endogenous or exogenous.

Incidence

A. Overall prevalence of all forms of eczema is about 18 in 1,000 in the United States.
B. With atopic dermatitis, 60% of those affected become afflicted between infancy and 12 years of age. It is more common in boys. Approximately 20% of children and 3% of adults are affected.

Pathogenesis

A. Eczema is characterized by a lymphohistiocytic infiltration around the upper dermal vessels. Epidermal spongiosis or intercellular epidermal edema and inflammation are seen.

Predisposing Factors

A. Family history of atopic triad: Dermatitis, asthma, and allergic rhinitis

B. Exposure to allergens

1. Common foods: Cow's milk, nuts, wheat, soy, and fish

2. Common environmental allergens: Dust, mold, cat dander, and low humidity (dry air)

C. Exposure to topical medications, most commonly neomycin, lanolin, and topical anesthetics like benzocaine

D. Skin irritants: Harsh soaps, skin-care products with perfumes, chemicals and alcohol, fabrics containing wool, tight clothing

E. Stress

Common Complaints

Skin changes

A. Itching, impossible to relieve

B. Dryness

C. Discoloration, lichenification, and scaling

D. Skin thickening

E. Associated bleeding and oozing skin

Other Signs and Symptoms

A. Primary lesions, papules, and pustules that may lead to excoriation

B. Lesions commonly seen on trunk, face, and antecubital and popliteal fossae of children. Adults will have lesions on the face, trunk, neck, and genital area.

C. Other common features include infraorbital fold (Dennie sign), increased palmar creases, facial erythema, and scaling.

Subjective Data

A. Determine whether the onset was sudden or gradual.

B. Ask the patient if the skin is itchy or painful.

C. Assess if there is any associated discharge (blood or pus).

D. Ask if the patient has recently taken any antibiotics, other oral drugs, or topical medications.

E. Ask the patient about use of soaps, creams, or lotions.

F. Assess for any preceding systemic symptoms (fever, sore throat, anorexia, vaginal discharge).

G. Ask the patient about recent travel abroad.

H. Rule out insect bites.

I. Rule out any possible exposure to industrial or domestic toxins.

J. Elicit what precipitates itching.

K. Evaluate for increased stress level at home, work, in relationships, and so on.

Physical Examination

A. Check temperature (if indicated).

B. Inspect

1. Inspect skin for lesions.

2. Recognize bacteria-infected eczema; *Staphylococcus aureus* is the most common pathogen. It appears with acute weeping dermatitis; crusted, and small, superficial pustules.

Diagnostic Tests

A. Culture skin lesions to determine viral, bacterial, or fungal etiology.

B. Blood work: Serum immunoglobulin E (IgE) is elevated with atopic dermatitis.

Differential Diagnoses

A. Atopic dermatitis, acute or chronic

B. Contact dermatitis, acute or chronic

C. Seborrheic dermatitis

D. Ichthyosis vulgaris

E. Bacterial/fungal infections

F. Neoplastic disease

G. Immunologic and metabolic disorders

Plan

A. General interventions

1. Frequently treat the dry skin with emollients (Aquaphor, Eucerin).

2. Pat, do not rub skin.

3. Children: Only bathe every two to three nights. Avoid excessive use of soap and water when bathing Use gentle cleansers such as Cetaphil or Cerave when bathing.

4. Avoid wool products and lanolin preparations.

5. Keep fingernails cut short to prevent scratching/scarring skin.

6. May need to treat secondary bacterial infections as appropriate.

7. Eliminate trigger foods one at a time for 1 month at a time to see improvement. Begin with eliminating cow's milk products. Consider soy-based foods instead.

8. Allergy testing may be considered if symptoms continue.

9. Ointments are usually recommended over creams for moisturizing.

B. Patient teaching: *See Section III: Patient Teaching Guide for this chapter, "Eczema."* ◀

C. Pharmaceutical therapy

1. Atopic: Acute, adult

a. Wet dressings with Burow's solution and change every 2 to 3 hours

b. Potent topical corticosteroid: Betamethasone valerate 0.1% two to three times daily for up to 2 to 3 weeks

c. Antihistamine of choice: Cetirizine Hcl (Zyrtec) or diphenhydramine Hcl (Benadryl)

d. Severe cases: Oral steroid: Prednisone 1 mg/kg (40–60 mg/d) tapered over 2 to 3 weeks

2. Atopic: Acute; occurs in infants and children

a. Hydrocortisone: Infants and children—2.5% ointment twice daily; 1% on face and intertriginous areas

b. Adolescents: Triamcinolone acetonide 0.1% (Aristocort) ointment; apply thinly twice daily for 2 to 3 weeks. **Precautions should be given regarding possibility of hypopigmentation of skin even with short-term use of steroids on skin.**

c. Antihistamines for itching

i. Infants and children: May use hydroxyzine (Atarax) 0.5 mg/kg/dose three times daily as needed or diphenhydramine Hcl (Benadryl). For those 2 to 6 years: 6.25 mg every 4 to 6 hours. For those 6 to 12 years: 12.5 to 25 mg every 4 to 6 hours.

ii. Adolescents: May use hydroxyzine 25 to 50 mg/dose every 4 to 6 hours or diphenhydramine Hcl (Benadryl).
iii. Atopic: Chronic, adult—short course of potent topical corticosteroid betamethasone dipropionate (Diprolene) or clobetasol propionate (temovate) twice daily for 7 days.

3. Antibacterial treatments for secondary bacterial infections: *S. aureus*
 a. Adults:
  i. Augmentin 875 mg by mouth twice a day for 10 to 14 days
  ii. Keflex 500 mg by mouth four times a day for 10 to 14 days
  iii. Erythromycin 500 mg by mouth four times a day for 10 to 14 days *or*
  iv. Dicloxacillin 250 mg every 6 hours for 10 days
 b. Children:
  i. Augmentin 25 to 45 mg/kg/d by mouth in two divided doses for 10 days
  ii. Erythromycin 30 to 50 mg/kg/d by mouth in two, three, or four evenly divided doses for 10 days
  iii. Omnicef (cefdinir): Not recommended for children younger than 6 months; 6 to 12 months: 7 mg/kg every 12 hours for 10 days

Follow-Up

A. See patient in office in 1 to 2 weeks and then every month until condition is stabilized.
B. Monitor the patient for superimposed staphylococcal infection; may use oral erythromycin or dicloxacillin.
C. Patient may be seen every 3 to 6 months thereafter for patient education updates.

Consultation/Referral

A. Eczema herpeticum (herpes simplex type 1) may progress rapidly. Refer the patient to a dermatologist.
B. Refer the patient to a dermatologist if skin eruptions are severe or fail to respond to conservative treatment.

Individual Considerations

A. Pregnancy: Avoid oral steroids.
B. Children: Teach patients to apply emollients when they have an itch rather than scratching. The goal is to control the rash and symptoms.
C. Young adults and elderly: Nummular eczema is commonly seen, characterized by coin-shaped vesicles and papules seen on extremities and/or trunk.

Erythema Multiforme

Jill C. Cash and Amy C. Bruggemann

Definition

A. This dermal and epidermal inflammatory process is characterized by symmetric eruption of erythematous, iris-shaped papules ("target" lesions), and vesiculobullous lesions.

Incidence

A. Erythema multiforme accounts for up to 1% of dermatology outpatient visits.
B. Children younger than 3 years and adults older than 50 years are rarely affected.
C. It may occur in seasonal epidemics.
D. Approximately 90% of cases of erythema multiforme minor follow a recent outbreak of herpes simplex virus (HSV)-1 or mycoplasma infection.

Pathogenesis

A. The disorder is thought to be an immunologic reaction in the skin, possibly triggered by circulating immune complexes.

Predisposing Factors

A. Infections: Recurrent HSV, mycoplasmal infections, and adenoviral infections
B. Drugs: Sulfonamides, phenytoin, barbiturates, phenylbutazone, penicillin
C. Idiopathic: Greater than 50%; consider occult malignancy

Common Complaints

A. Rash with intense pruritus
B. Nonspecific upper respiratory infection followed by rash
C. General malaise, body aches, and joint pain
D. Fever

Other Signs and Symptoms

A. Primary: Macules, papules, and plaques
B. Secondary: Erythema, dull red target-like lesions blanch to pressure; distribution is symmetric, primarily on flexor surfaces. **Classic target lesions develop abruptly and symmetrically and are heaviest peripherally; they often involve palms and soles.**
C. Swelling of hands and feet
D. Painful oral lesions
E. Eye discomfort (redness, itching, burning, pain, visual changes)

Subjective Data

A. Ask if the patient has ever been diagnosed with erythema multiforme.
B. Determine whether the onset of symptoms was sudden or gradual.
C. Assess for any associated discharge (blood or pus).
D. Identify the location of the symptoms.
E. Complete a drug history. Has the patient recently taken any antibiotics or other drugs? Question the patient regarding use of any topical medications.
F. Determine the presence of any preceding systemic symptoms (fever, sore throat, anorexia, or vaginal discharge).
G. Rule out any possible exposure to industrial or domestic toxins.
H. Question the patient concerning any possible contact with venereal disease.
I. Ask the patient about any close physical contact with others with skin disorders.

J. Elicit information concerning any possible exposure to HIV.
K. Rule out sources of chronic infection, neoplasia, or connective tissue disease.

Physical Examination

A. Check temperature, pulse, respirations, and blood pressure.
B. Inspect
  1. Skin for lesions
  2. Mouth and mucous membranes for lesions
C. Palpate abdomen for masses and tenderness.
D. Auscultate heart, lungs, and abdomen.
E. Neurologic examination

Diagnostic Tests

A. Punch biopsy of skin
B. Complete blood count (CBC)
C. Urinalysis

Differential Diagnoses

A. Erythema multiforme
  1. Erythema multiforme minor: Pruritus, swelling of hands and feet, painful oral lesions
  2. Erythema multiforme major: Fever, arthralgias, myalgias, cough, oral erosions with severe pain
B. Urticaria
C. Viral exanthems
D. Stevens–Johnson syndrome (SJS): **SJS is a severe, life-threatening, systemic reaction with fever, malaise, cough, sore throat, chest pain, vomiting, diarrhea, myalgia, arthralgia, and severe skin manifestations with painful bullous lesions on mucous membranes.**
E. Pemphigus vulgaris
F. Bullous pemphigoid
G. Other bullous diseases
H. Staphylococcal scalded skin syndrome
I. Vasculitis

Plan

A. General interventions
  1. Identify and treat precipitating causes or triggers.
  2. Burow's solution or warm compresses may be used for mild cases as needed.
  3. Oral lesions may be treated with saline solution, warm salt water, and/or Mary's mouthwash (Benadryl, lidocaine, and Kaopectate).
  4. Discontinue any medications suspected of precipitating symptoms.
  5. Provide adequate pain relief if skin or oral lesions are painful. Lesions remain fixed at least 7 days.
  6. Maintain nutrition and fluid replacement for this hypercatabolic state.
  7. Consider chronic viral suppression therapy for recurrent herpes simplex viral infections.
▶ **B.** Patient teaching: *See Section III: Patient Teaching Guide for this chapter, "Erythema Multiforme."*
C. Pharmaceutical therapy
  1. Antihistamines, such as Benadryl or Claritin, may be used for itching.
  2. Acetaminophen may be used to reduce fever and for general discomfort/pain.
  3. Potent topical corticosteroids: Betamethasone dipropionate 0.05% or clobetasol propionate 0.05% twice daily for up to 2 weeks. Avoid use on face and groin.
  4. Open lesions should be treated like open burn wounds. Stop offending medications that may cause blistering of wounds and treat with steroids.
  5. Oral antibiotics may be needed to control secondary bacterial skin infection.
  6. Hospitalization for severe cases. Intravenous immunoglobulins may be needed.

Follow-Up

A. See the patient in the office in 1 to 2 days to evaluate initial treatment.

Consultation/Referral

A. If the patient has recurrent or chronic infection, refer him or her to a physician.
B. Immediate consultation and/or hospital admission is critical if SJS is suspected.

Individual Consideration

A. Pediatrics: Systemic corticosteroids may increase the risk of infection and prolong healing. Use low- to mid-potency topical corticosteroids.

Folliculitis

Jill C. Cash and Amy C. Bruggemann

Definition

A. Folliculitis is a bacterial infection of the hair follicle.
B. Malassezia folliculitis, also known as pityrosporum, is an inflammatory skin disorder of the hair follicle triggered by yeast. This is often confused with acne vulgaris; the defining difference is itch.

Incidence

A. A very common disorder, folliculitis occurs in all ages and is seen more frequently in males.
B. Malassezia folliculitis is commonly seen in patients with immunosuppression, diabetes, and antibiotic use.

Pathogenesis

A. Bacterial organisms (most commonly *Staphylococcus aureus*) invade the follicle wall and cause an infectious process.
B. For malassezia folliculitis, fungal organisms invade the follicle walls and cause a fungal infection that causes a pruritic rash.

Predisposing Factors

A. Break in the skin tissue
B. Use of razors on skin
C. Poor hygiene
D. Diabetes

Common Complaint

A. Outbreak of pustules on the face, scalp, or extremities that do not resolve despite proper hygiene and care.

Other Signs and Symptoms

A. Tenderness and itching at the site
B. Furuncle (abscess): A deep pustule, tender, firm or fluctuant, found in groin, axilla, waistline, or buttocks
C. Carbuncle: A group of follicles coalescing into one larger, painful, infected area; fever and chills possible.
D. Excoriated folliculitis: Chronic thickened, excoriated papules or nodules

Subjective Data

A. Elicit the initial outbreak of lesions and onset and progression of lesions.
B. Identify what makes the lesions better or worse.
C. Ask the patient what medications, soaps, or lotions have been used on the lesions.
D. Complete a medical history. Ask if the patient has had an outbreak similar to this before.
E. Describe systemic symptoms if they have occurred (fever, chills, etc.).
F. Does the patient have a beard, shave his face, or use a razor frequently?
G. Is there a recent history of use of a hot tub? (Commonly seen 1–4 days after use of hot tub, whirlpool, or swimming pool.)
H. Does the patient wear tight pants/jeans or use oils that clog pores in the groin area?
I. Is the patient currently being treated with antibiotics for acne? (May see flare of gram-negative folliculitis with chronic use of antibiotics.)

Physical Examination

A. Check temperature, pulse, respirations, and blood pressure.
B. Inspect: Assess skin for lesions and describe.
C. Palpate: Palpate lesions and associated lymph nodes.

Diagnostic Tests

A. Culture and sensitivity to verify appropriate antibiotic coverage
B. Gram stain
C. Potassium hydroxide (KOH)/wet prep
D. Fungal culture hair if fungi suspected (tinea of scalp)
E. Skin biopsy for the diagnosis of malassezia folliculitis

Differential Diagnoses

A. Folliculitis
B. Acne vulgaris
C. Ingrown hair follicle
D. Keratosis pilaris
E. Contact dermatitis

Plan

A. General interventions
  1. Apply warm, moist compresses to site for comfort.
B. Patient teaching:
  ▶ **1.** *See Section III: Patient Teaching Guide for this chapter, "Folliculitis."*
  2. If razors are used on the area, have the patient use clean, sharp razors, throw old razors away, and not share razors. Avoid use of irritating creams or lotions on affected area.
  3. Encourage proper hygiene, with frequent washing of hands and skin with an antibacterial soap.
  4. Warm compresses three to four times a day are encouraged at the site for 15 to 20 minutes.
  5. Bleach bath (0.5–1 cup of bleach to 20 L water) reduces spread of *Staphylococcus* infection.
C. Pharmaceutical therapy
  1. Mild cases: Apply mupirocin (Bactroban) ointment to affected area three times daily until resolved.
  2. *S. aureus*
    a. Dicloxacillin (Dynapen) 250 mg by mouth four times daily for 10 to 14 days
    b. Erythromycin 250 mg by mouth four times daily for 10 to 14 days
    c. Cephalexin (Keflex) 500 mg by mouth for 10 to 14 days
  3. *Pseudomonas aeruginosa*
    a. Ciprofloxacin (Cipro) 500 mg by mouth twice daily for 10 days
    b. Ofloxacin 400 mg by mouth twice daily for 10 days
  4. Antistaphylococcal antibiotics
    a. Cephalexin 250 to 500 mg four times a day (children: 25–50 mg/kg/d given in two divided doses)
    b. Clindamycin 150 to 300 mg four times a day (children: 8–16 mg/kg/d in three to four doses/d)
    c. Dicloxacillin 125 to 500 mg four times a day (children: 12.5 mg/kg/d four times a day)
    d. Erythromycin 250 to 500 mg four times a day (children: 30–50 mg/kg/d four times a day)
  5. Bacterial infections caused by organisms other than *Staphylococcus* may be treated for an extended period, 4 to 8 weeks. These areas may include axilla, chest, back, beard, and groin.
  6. Methicillin-resistant *Staphylococcus aureus* (MRSA)
    a. Bactrim DS 160/800 twice a day (children: 8–10 mg/kg/d divide and give q12h)
    b. Doxycycline 100 mg twice daily for 1 day and then once a day for the remainder of the duration (children: 2.2 mg/kg twice daily for 1 day and then for the remainder of the duration once a day)
  7. Severe cases may be treated with oral antibiotics with topical permethrin every 12 hours every other night for a 6-week period or itraconazole 400 mg daily, isotretinoin 0.5 mg/kg/d for up to 4 to 5 months with ultraviolet B (UVB) light therapy. Consider dermatology referral for severe cases.
  8. Treatment for malessezia folliculitis is as follows:
    a. Antifungal treatment: Oral antifungal medications (itraconazole, fluconazole, or ketoconazole) should be prescribed for at least 4 weeks for treatment (Rubenstein & Malerich, 2014).

Follow-Up

A. If not resolved in 2 weeks, further evaluation is needed.
B. Severe cases, in which carbuncles are not improved with antibiotic therapy, warrant incision and drainage and referral to dermatology.
C. Continue to follow every 2 weeks until resolved.
D. Test for diabetes mellitus in severe cases.

Consultation/Referral

A. Refer the patient to a physician for testing for immunodeficiency if severe cases occur or if resistance is seen.
B. Dermatology referral.

Hand, Foot, and Mouth Syndrome

Jill C. Cash and Amy C. Bruggemann

Definition

A. This is a viral infection caused by coxsackievirus A16, with vesicular lesions present on the hands, feet, and oral mucosa.

Incidence

A. Hand, foot, and mouth syndrome is most commonly seen in preschool children.

Pathogenesis

A. Enteroviruses invade the intestinal tract of humans and are spread to others by fecal–oral and/or oral–oral (respiratory) routes. The incubation period is approximately 4 to 6 days.

Predisposing Factors

A. Childhood
B. Confined households or day care centers, camps
C. Seasonal: Summer and fall most common

Common Complaints

A. Generalized rash, with lesions on the tongue, gums, and roof of the mouth
B. Lesions (vesicles) also present on the hands, feet, and buttocks

Other Signs and Symptoms

A. Fever
B. Sore throat
C. Some enteroviruses have been associated with severe consequences such as meningitis, encephalitis, and others. The family should monitor symptoms carefully.

Subjective Data

A. Question the patient regarding onset, duration, and progression of symptoms and lesions.
B. Determine whether any family member or other contact person had similar symptoms.
C. Identify areas where the child comes in contact with numerous children (child care facility, nurseries at church, school, etc.).
D. If not noted in the presenting symptoms, ask the patient about his or her upper respiratory symptoms (sore throat, fever, headache, runny nose, cough, etc.).

Physical Examination

A. Check temperature, pulse, respirations, and blood pressure.
B. Inspect skin, ears, nose, and oral cavity for lesions.
C. Palpate
  1. Palpate abdomen and lymph nodes in neck.
  2. Assess for meningism.
D. Auscultate lungs and heart.

Diagnostic Test

A. Usually none; consider cultures of oral lesions if secondary bacterial infection is suspected.

Differential Diagnoses

A. Hand, foot, and mouth syndrome
B. Pharyngitis
C. Pneumonia
D. Meningitis
E. Meningococcemia: Exanthem, petechial rash

Plan

A. General interventions: Supportive treatment—warm saline gargles, acetaminophen (Tylenol) as needed for discomfort, and increased fluids. Popsicles are useful to soothe the oral lesions, especially for small children.
B. Patient teaching: Reinforce good oral and body hygiene. The virus may be harbored in the gastrointestinal tract for long periods.
C. Pharmaceutical therapy
  1. None is recommended.
  2. Acetaminophen (Tylenol) as needed for fever and malaise.

Follow-Up

A. None is recommended unless symptoms worsen or do not resolve in 7 to 10 days.

Consultation/Referral

A. Refer to physician for any symptoms related to meningitis or encephalitis.

Individual Consideration

A. Pediatrics: Seen primarily in the pediatric population

Herpes Simplex Virus Type 1

Jill C. Cash and Amy C. Bruggemann

Definition

Herpes simplex virus (HSV)-1 viral infection of the cutaneous tissue manifests itself by vesicular lesions on the mucous membranes and skin. HSV-1 is most often associated with oral lesions (mouth and lips), and HSV-2 is associated with genital lesions. The virus appears in three stages:
A. Primary
B. Latent
C. Recurrent infections

Incidence

A. HSV-1 is seen in patients of all ages and in equal numbers of males and females.
B. There are approximately 776,000 new cases of herpes diagnosed annually in the United States.

Pathogenesis

A. Viral infection can be transmitted from a vesicular lesion or fluid (saliva) containing the virus to the skin or mucosa of another person by direct contact, with an incubation period of 2 to 14 days. Trigeminal ganglia are the host of the oral virus. The virus can be reactivated, whereupon it travels along the affected nerve route and produces recurrent lesions. Common sites of infection are the lips, face, buccal mucosa, and throat.

Predisposing Factors

A. Immunocompromised patients
B. Prior HSV infections
C. Exposure to virus

Common Complaint

A. Painful lips, gums, and oral mucosa

Other Signs and Symptoms

A. Primary lesion: Fever, blisters on lips, malaise, and tender gums
B. Recurrent episodes: Fever blisters with prodrome of itching, burning, and tingling sensation at the site before vesicles appear

Subjective Data

A. Ask questions regarding location, onset, and duration of lesions.
B. Elicit description of prodromal symptoms.
C. Ask the patient if systemic symptoms occur with vesicular outbreak.
D. Determine when the initial outbreak of lesions occurred (commonly seen in childhood).
E. Inquire whether the patient has been exposed to anyone with similar lesions.
F. If the lesion(s) is recurrent, ask the patient if stress, skin trauma, or sun exposure stimulates an outbreak of fever blisters.

Physical Examination

A. Inspect the skin and note location, appearance, and stage of vesicles.
B. Palpate lymph nodes for lymphadenopathy.

Diagnostic Test

A. Viral cultures

Differential Diagnoses

A. HSV-1
B. Impetigo: Appears as amber-colored vesicular lesions with crusting.
C. Stomatitis: Appears as erythemic or erosion lesions in the mouth and lips.
D. Herpes zoster: Causes vesicles that run along a single dermatome.
E. Stevens–Johnson syndrome (SJS)
F. Herpangina: Vesicles can be noted on the soft palate, tonsillary area, and uvula area; usually caused by the coxsackievirus.

Plan

A. General interventions
  1. Comfort measures. Ice may be used to reduce swelling as needed.
  2. Vaseline or other lip ointments may be applied as needed and lip ointment with sun protection factor (SPF)-30 or greater may be applied when exposed to sunlight.
B. Patient teaching
  1. Educate the patient regarding the disease process of HSV-1.
  2. Instruct the patient to wash hands frequently.
  3. Suggest proper care of lips to prevent drying and to reduce pain.
  4. Educate regarding transmission of virus to others.
  5. Teach the patient to expect recurrences at variable times.
C. Pharmaceutical therapy: Precautions should be used when administering medication to patients who are immunocompromised and who have a history of renal insufficiency.
  1. Lidocaine 2% as needed for comfort.
  2. Diphenhydramine (Benadryl) elixir may be used to rinse mouth as needed.
  3. Acetaminophen (Tylenol) as needed for pain.
  4. Campho-Phenique application as needed.
  5. Initial episode: Acyclovir 200 mg by mouth five times per day for 7 to 10 days or until resolved.
  6. Recurrent episodes: Begin one of the following when prodrome begins or within 2 days of onset of lesions to get maximum effect
    a. Acyclovir 200 mg by mouth five times per day for 5 days
    b. Acyclovir 800 mg by mouth twice daily for 5 days
  7. Other alternative antivirals: Dosage depends on renal function
    a. Famciclovir (Famvir)
    b. Valacyclovir (Valtrex)
  8. Suppressive therapy
    a. Acyclovir 200 mg by mouth two to five times per day for 1 year
    b. Acyclovir 400 mg by mouth twice daily for 1 year

Follow-Up

A. None needed if resolved without complications

Consultation/Referral

A. Refer the patient to a physician if treatment is unsuccessful or further complications arise.

Individual Considerations

A. Pediatrics
  1. Initial outbreak commonly occurs in childhood.
B. Adolescents/adults
  1. HSV-1 can also be transmitted sexually when having oral sex. Educate teens/adults regarding transmitting the virus during sexual contact. Transmission is possible if having sexual relations with partners; avoid contact when lesions are present.
  2. Advise using a dental dam during oral sex to prevent transmission.
  3. Avoid sharing toothbrushes and eating utensils.

Herpes Zoster or Shingles

Jill C. Cash and Amy C. Bruggemann

Definition

A. Herpes zoster is a viral infection manifested by painful, vesicular lesions on the skin, limited to one side of the body, following one body dermatome.

Incidence

A. Infection may occur at any age; however, it is more common in older adults and the elderly. It occurs in 10% to 20% of the U.S. population.

Pathogenesis

A. After the primary episode of chickenpox (varicella zoster), the virus remains dormant in the body. Herpes zoster occurs when the varicella virus has been stimulated and reactivated in the dorsal root ganglia, producing the clinical manifestations of herpes zoster as discussed in the following. Duration of infection usually lasts 14 to 21 days, but may be longer in elderly or debilitated patients.

Predisposing Factors

A. Adulthood
B. Immunocompromised patients
C. Spinal cord trauma or injury

Common Complaints

A. Prodrome: Itching, burning, tingling, or painful sensation at lesion sites
B. Active: Malaise, fever, headache, or pruritic rash on the skin

Other Signs and Symptoms

A. Lesions: Clusters of vesicles on an erythemic base that burst and produce crusted lesions. These are most commonly found on the chest and back area, but they may also occur on the head and neck area or extremities. Distribution of lesions typically appears along a single dermatome.
B. Motor weakness (may be seen in approximately 5% of patients)

Subjective Data

A. Determine onset, location, and progression of rash.
B. Ask the patient about prodromal symptoms: Burning, itching, tingling, or painful sensation at the site before lesions break out.
C. Evaluate patient status regarding immunosuppressive agents, diseases, and so forth.

Physical Examination

A. Check temperature, pulse, respiration, and blood pressure.
B. Inspect
  1. Observe skin for lesions, noting characteristics and distribution.
  2. Inspect ears, nose, and throat.
C. Auscultate heart and lungs.

Diagnostic Tests

A. Usually none
B. Culture vesicular lesions
C. Consider Tzanck smear
D. Young patients with herpes zoster: Consider test for HIV

Differential Diagnoses

A. Herpes zoster
B. Varicella
C. Poison ivy
D. Herpes simplex virus (HSV)
E. Contact dermatitis
F. Coxsackievirus
G. Postherpetic neuralgia

Plan

A. General interventions
  1. Comfort measures. Instruct the patient to apply wet dressings (Burow's solution) on the site for 30 to 60 minutes at least four times a day. Calamine lotions may be used as needed; oatmeal (Aveeno) bath may be used for comfort; acetaminophen (Tylenol) is taken as needed for malaise, temperature, and comfort.
B. Patient teaching:
  1. *See Section III: Patient Teaching Guide for this chapter, "Herpes Zoster, or Shingles."* ◀
  2. Tell the patient that the rash usually lasts approximately 2 to 3 weeks.
  3. Instruct the patient to monitor for signs/symptoms of postherpetic neuralgia.
  4. Instruct the patient to call if symptoms worsen or do not improve, or signs of bacterial infection occur.
  5. Emphasize to the patient that the virus is easily transmitted to vulnerable persons.
C. Pharmaceutical therapy
  1. Antiviral medications should be initiated within 24 to 48 hours after outbreak.
    a. Acyclovir (Zovirax) 800 mg every 4 hours while awake for 7 to 10 days
    b. Famciclovir (Famvir) 500 to 750 mg by mouth three times daily for 7 days
    c. Valacyclovir (Valtrex) 1,000 mg by mouth three times daily for 7 days
  2. Acetaminophen (Tylenol) or ibuprofen as needed for pain or discomfort.
  3. Narcotics may be used for severe pain as needed.
  4. Postherpetic neuralgia
    a. Postherpetic neuralgia may be treated with narcotics or other pain-relieving medications.
    b. Long-term medications may be needed for control of pain.
      i. Gabapentin 100 to 600 mg three times daily
      ii. Amitriptyline 25 mg every bedtime or other low-dose tricyclic antidepressants
      iii. Lyrica: Start 150 mg/d orally (PO) divided twice (BID) a day to three times a day (TID), may be increased to 300 mg/d PO divided BID–TID within 1 week, and then may be

increased to 600 mg/d PO divided BID–TID after another 2 to 4 weeks; maximum 600 mg/d; taper dose over at least 1 week to discontinue medication.

5. If secondary bacterial infection of the skin occurs, apply silver sulfadiazine (Silvadene) topically to the site until resolved.

6. Use of steroids is controversial. Corticosteroids may be used with caution. May increase risk of dissemination.

Follow-Up

A. As needed for complications.

B. Monitor the patient for complications: Postherpetic neuralgia, Guillain–Barré syndrome, motor weakness, secondary infection, meningoencephalitis, ophthalmic and facial palsy, corneal ulceration, and so forth.

Consultation/Referral

A. Ramsay Hunt syndrome occurs when a shingles outbreak affects the facial nerve near one of the ears. This can cause facial paralysis and hearing loss in the affected ear. Consult a physician.

B. Hutchinson's sign refers to vesicles in the peri-orbital region. These patients require an ophthamologist referral.

C. Consult with a physician if secondary infection occurs or if secondary complications arise.

Individual Considerations

A. Pregnancy: Acyclovir falls under category C drug classification. The safety and efficacy of the use of the antiviral medications during pregnancy need to be considered.

B. Pediatrics: Shingles is rarely seen in children.

C. Elderly

1. Postherpetic neuralgia occurs in approximately 15% of patients. It is commonly seen in elderly patients.

2. The Centers for Disease Control and Prevention (CDC) recommends the shingles vaccine Zostavax for all patients 60 years of age and older, irrespective of whether they have had the chickenpox or shingles infection in the past. For those who have had a recent shingles outbreak, it is recommended that resolution of the rash be complete before administering the Zostavax vaccination.

3. The virus is contagious for those who have not had chickenpox.

Impetigo

Jill C. Cash and Amy C. Bruggemann

Definition

A. Impetigo is a bacterial infection of the skin, most commonly caused by *Staphylococcus aureus* or *Streptococcus pyogenes,* or both.

Incidence

A. It occurs equally in males and females and is most commonly seen in children, especially those 2 to 5 years of age.

Pathogenesis

A. An alteration in the skin integrity allows bacterial invasion into the epidermis, causing an infection. Small, moist vesicles ranging from red macules to honey-colored crusts or erosions occur singly or grouped together. Most common organisms are *S. aureus* and Group A beta-hemolytic *S. pyogenes.*

Predisposing Factors

A. Poor hygiene

B. Warm climate

C. Break in the skin

Common Complaint

A. Tender sores around the mouth and nose area in which the lesions continue to spread and worsen, despite over-the-counter (OTC) medication treatment.

Subjective Data

A. Elicit onset, progression, duration, and location of lesions.

B. Ask the patient whether he or she has had contact with any other child or person with similar lesions.

C. Assess whether the patient exhibits any other symptoms, especially systemic symptoms (fever, malaise, etc.).

D. Elicit what treatment has been tried, if any.

Physical Examination

A. Check temperature.

B. Inspect

1. Examine skin, noting types of lesions and skin involvement.

2. Examine ears, nose, mouth, and throat.

C. Auscultate lungs and heart.

Diagnostic Tests

A. None required

B. May perform culture if recurrent or resistant to treatment

Differential Diagnoses

A. Impetigo

B. Varicella

C. Folliculitis

D. Erysipelas

E. Herpes simplex

F. Second-degree burns

G. Pharyngitis or tonsillitis: Throat erythema, with tonsillary hypertrophy and exudate present; lymph nodes: Adenopathy of anterior cervical chain

H. Ecthyma: Severe case of impetigo with lymphadenitis

I. Insect bites

J. Necrotizing fasciitis

K. Contact dermatitis

L. Scabies

Plan

A. General interventions

1. Crusted lesions may be removed with thorough, gentle washing with mild soap three to four times daily.

2. Impetigo must be adequately treated and resolved to prevent postinfection complications such as the following: Poststreptococcal acute glomerulonephritis, cellulitis, ecthyma, and bacteremia.

B. Patient teaching: Encourage good handwashing and hygiene to reduce spreading infection.

C. Pharmaceutical therapy

1. If few lesions are noted without involvement of face or cellulitis: Mupirocin (Bactroban) ointment—to site four times daily for 10 days
2. Systemic antibiotics
   - a. Children older than 3 months: Amoxicillin/clavulanate 40 mg/kg/d divided every 12 hours
   - b. Adults: Amoxicillin/clavulanate 875/125 mg every 12 hours
   - c. Children: Cephalexin 30 mg/kg/d po divided every 12 hours
   - d. Adults: Cephalexin 500 mg every 12 hours
3. Other effective antibiotics include cefaclor, cephradine, cefadroxil, clindamycin, and amoxicillin.

Follow-Up

A. Schedule appointment in 10 to 14 days to determine resolution of infection.

Consultation/Referral

A. Consult a physician if complications arise or if resolution is not complete with antibiotic therapy.

Insect Bites and Stings

Jill C. Cash and Amy C. Bruggemann

Definition

A. Bites and/or stings on the skin come from commonly encountered insects: Bees, hornets, wasps, mosquitoes, chiggers, ticks, fleas, fire ants, and bedbugs

Incidence

A. Bites are seen in all age groups, more common in summer months.

Pathogenesis

A. Some bites elicit local tissue inflammation and destruction because of proteins and enzymes in the poison or venom of the insect.

B. Immunoglobulin E (IgE)-mediated allergic reactions (immediate or delayed) may occur.

C. Serum-sickness reaction may appear 10 to 14 days after a sting with venom. Toxic reactions can also occur from multiple stings yielding large inoculation of poison or venom.

D. With tick bites, exposure to Rocky Mountain spotted fever, Lyme disease, ehrlichiosis, and babesiosis disease may occur.

Predisposing Factors

A. Exposure to areas of heavy insect infestations

B. Warm-weather months

C. Outdoor exposure with barefeet, bright clothes

D. Use of perfumes and/or colognes

E. Previous sensitization

Common Complaints

A. Local reaction: Pain, swelling, and redness at the site after insect bite

B. Toxic reaction: Local reaction plus headache, vertigo, gastrointestinal symptoms (nausea, vomiting, diarrhea), syncope, convulsions, and/or fever

Subjective Data

A. Did the patient see what bit or stung him or her?

B. If the patient felt the bite or sting, was he or she bitten or stung once or multiple times?

C. How long ago did it occur?

D. Where was the patient when the injury occurred (environment)?

E. Has the patient ever been bitten or stung before? If so, did he or she have any reaction then? If so, what was the treatment?

Physical Examination

A. Check temperature, pulse, respiration, and blood pressure. Observe overall respiratory status.

B. Inspect

1. Inspect site of injury for local reaction; note erythema, rash, or edema.
2. Perform ear, nose, and throat examination.

C. Auscultate: Assess heart and lungs.

D. Palpate

1. Palpate injured site.
2. Assess nodes for lymphadenopathy.
3. Perform abdominal examination, if appropriate.

Diagnostic Tests

A. None is required.

B. Consider taking skin scrapings to evaluate under a microscope.

C. Consider culture if infection is suspected.

Differential Diagnoses

A. Insect bite

1. Bees, hornets, wasps, bedbugs: Local pain, redness, pruritus, and swelling occur at the site. Red papules and wheals appear, enlarge, and then subside within hours. Delayed hypersensitivity occurs within 7 days with enlarged, local reaction, with fever, malaise, headache, arthralgias, and lymphadenopathy. Toxicity can occur. Anaphylaxis may be seen with generalized warmth and urticaria, erythema, angioedema, intestinal cramping, bronchospasm, laryngospasm, shock, and collapse.
2. Ticks: Local redness, swelling, itching; Enlarged area of redness and swelling may occur.
3. Mosquitoes and chiggers: Local redness, swelling, and itching occur. Delayed reaction can include edema and burning sensation.
4. Fleas: Local redness, swelling, and itching occur. Usually papules noted in a zigzag pattern, especially

on legs and waist. Note hemorrhagic puncta surrounded by erythematous and urticarial patches.

5. Body lice: Small noninflammatory red spots, intensely pruritic, are found on waist, shoulders, axilla, and neck. Note linear scratch marks. Note secondary infection.

6. Scabies: Pruritus is the dominant symptom. Note inflammation and burrows in skin with papules and vesicles, especially in the webs of the hands and feet.

7. Fire ants: Papules appear and turn to pustules within 6 to 24 hours after bite. Watch for localized necrosis with scarring. Urticaria and angioedema can occur.

B. Allergic reaction

Plan

A. General interventions. Anaphylaxis: Activate emergency medical services (EMS) immediately.

1. With all bites and stings, treat anaphylaxis first.

2. Local reactions: Treat with analgesic of choice. Apply ice packs to the site for approximately 10 minutes. Elevate affected extremities.

3. Delayed reactions: Administer antihistamines as needed. Consider corticosteroid use.

4. Routine wound care: Cleanse wound. Remove stinger. If it is a painful sting, apply a cotton ball soaked in meat tenderizer or sodium bicarbonate paste.

5. Debride as necessary.

6. For embedded insects, apply petroleum jelly, nail polish, or alcohol over site for 30 minutes and wait for insect or tick to withdraw.

7. Referral to allergist-immunologist is recommended for patients with a severe systemic reaction for skin testing and to evaluate for candidacy of venom immunotherapy treatment.

8. Hospitalize the patient for severe reactions.

▶ **B.** *See Section III: Patient Teaching Guide for this chapter, "Insect Bites and Stings."*

C. Pharmaceutical therapy

1. Antihistamines

a. Children

i. Younger child:2 to 6 years: Diphenhydramine 6.25 mg every 4 to 6 hours

ii. Older child: 6 to 12 years: Diphenhydramine 12.5 to 25 mg every 4 to 6 hours

b. Adult: Diphenhydramine (Benadryl) 50 mg every 6 hours as needed

2. Mild anaphylaxis

a. Epinephrine 1:1,000 (aqueous) administered subcutaneously. Usual dose is as follows:

i. Children: 0.01 mg/kg; may repeat in 4 hours if needed

ii. Adults: 0.3 mg intramuscular (IM); may repeat if needed

3. Oral antihistamines for next 24 hours (Atarax)

a. Children: Hydroxyzine hydrochloride (Atarax) 2 to 4 mg/kg/d divided into three doses

b. Adults: Hydroxyzine hydrochloride (Atarax) 10 to 25 mg four times daily

4. Severe anaphylaxis

a. Epinephrine 1:1,000 (aqueous), given subcutaneously (see mild anaphylaxis, mentioned earlier)

b. Oxygen 2 to 4 L as needed

c. Albuterol (Ventolin) 5 mg/mL per dose by nebulizer

i. Children: 0.1 to 0.15 mg/kg in 2 mL of saline

ii. Adults: 2.5 mg (0.5 mL of 0.5% solution) in 2 mL saline

5. Self-treatment for anaphylaxis (emergency treatment kits)

a. Ana-Kit contains a preloaded syringe.

b. Epipen and Epipen Junior Auto-Injectors are spring-loaded automatic injectors. Children: 0.01 mg/kg IM in thigh. Adults: 0.3 mg IM in thigh.

Follow-Up

A. Follow up in 2 weeks to evaluate effectiveness of treatment. If symptoms worsen before this, reevaluation is needed.

Consultation/Referral

A. Consult with a physician when anaphylaxis occurs.

Individual Considerations

A. Pediatrics: Children are at a higher risk than adults for complications of a reaction.

B. Geriatrics: Elderly adults are at high risk for complications of reactions.

Lice (Pediculosis)

Jill C. Cash and Amy C. Bruggemann

Definition

Pediculosis (lice) is an infestation of the louse on human beings in one of three areas:

A. Head (*Pediculosis capitis*)

B. Pubic area (*Pthirus pubis*)

C. Body (*Pediculosis corporis*)

Incidence

A. *Pediculosis capitis* is most common in children. It is estimated that head lice infestations occur in the school systems anywhere from 10% to 40% of the time.

B. They are more commonly found in girls than boys.

C. *Phthirus pubis* infestation is more common in adults.

D. Lice affect all demographics; all social, racial, and economic groups get lice.

Pathogenesis

A. Head and body lice are transmitted by direct contact from person to person, that is, through sharing hats, combs, brushes, and so forth. The parasite hatches from an egg, or nit. Once hatched, the lice live on humans by sucking blood through the skin. The average adult louse lives 9 to 10 days. The nits appear as small white eggs on the hair shaft. Nits are very difficult to remove and survive up to 3 weeks after removal from the host. Body lice lay nits in the seams of clothing.

B. Pubic lice are found at the base of the hair shaft, where they lay nits. Pubic lice are transmitted through sexual contact.

Predisposing Factors

A. Head and body lice: Exposure to crowded public areas, such as schools; inability to clean and launder clothing, bed linens, and so forth

B. Pubic lice: Sexual contact with infected people

C. Poor hygiene

Common Complaints

A. Head lice: Severe itching and scratching of the head, neck area, and commonly behind the ears

B. Body lice: Severe itching on the body, which may lead to secondary infections of the skin

C. Pubic lice: Severe itching of genital area

Other Signs and Symptoms

A. Excoriated skin from intense scratching.

B. Visible lice or nits in hair, body, or clothing.

C. Papules with an erythemic base may develop on the genital area, axilla, chest, beard, or eyelashes.

D. *Phthirus pubis* or nits or lice are found on eyelashes of children.

Subjective Data

A. Inquire as to exposure to anyone known to have lice.

B. Identify whether the patient attends a crowded environment such as school, day care, and so forth.

C. Ask if lice and nits have been seen by the patient or guardian.

D. Determine onset, duration, and course of symptoms. Ask: When were lice or nits first discovered?

E. Assess whether the patient has been symptomatic (itching, scratching).

F. Inquire about social habits of cleaning, laundry, and so forth.

Physical Examination

A. Check temperature to rule out any secondary infection.

B. Inspect

- **1.** Inspect hair, body, pubic area, and clothing seams for nits or lice.
- **2.** Note excoriation of skin.
- **3.** Examine eyelashes of children.
- **4.** Examine skin for secondary bacterial infection.

Diagnostic Tests

A. None

B. Culture excoriated area if secondary bacterial infection suspected

Differential Diagnoses

A. Lice

B. Scabies

Plan

A. General interventions

- **1.** Treat immediately with appropriate pediculicides (see Pharmaceutical therapy, in the following).
- **2.** After treatment, it is imperative to remove each nit and louse; use fine-tooth comb for nit removal.
- **3.** Evaluate entire family for lice.
- **4.** Treat secondary bacterial infection as needed.

B. Patient teaching

- **1.** *See Section III: Patient Teaching Guide for this chapter, "Lice (Pediculosis)."* ◀
- **2.** Specific instructions need to be given to clients on how to get rid of lice and nits.
- **3.** Reinforce good hygiene; teach children not to share combs, brushes, hats, and hair accessories.

C. Pharmaceutical therapy

- **1.** Malathion lotion 0.5% (Ovide): Pediculicidal and partially ovicidal
- **2.** Permethrin lotion 1% (Nix): Pediculicidal only. Available over the counter (OTC) for treatment.
- **3.** Synergized pyrethrins (Rid 0.3%; Available OTC).
- **4.** Apply, repeat in 24 hours, and then again in 1 week.
- **5.** Do not use a shampoo/conditioner or conditioner before using head lice treatments. Do not wash hair for 1 to 2 days after using lice treatment regimen.
- **6.** *Pthirus pubis:* Lindane (Kwell) or permethrin (Nix); apply to pubic area as directed.
- **7. Lindane (Kwell) toxicity may occur from ingestion or overuse and is exhibited by headaches, dizziness, and convulsions.**
- **8.** Eyelash manifestation: After removing nits, apply petroleum jelly to lashes three to four times a day for 8 to 10 days. **Eyelashes should never be treated with pediculicides.**

Follow-Up

A. None recommended

B. Some schools and institutions require follow-up to evaluate whether infestation is resolved before admitting the child back into the classroom.

Consultation/Referral

A. If lice are a repeated problem, contact social services or the health department to have a visiting nurse or aide visit the home to evaluate home conditions and to teach the family how to prevent infestations.

Individual Considerations

A. Pregnancy: Lindane (Kwell) is contraindicated during pregnancy.

B. Pediatrics

- **1.** Head lice is commonly seen in school-aged children.
- **2.** Lindane (Kwell) should not be used in infants. The American Academy of Pediatrics does not recommend lindane as a first-line treatment for head lice for children secondary to the toxic effects of the brain and central nervous system (CNS).

Lichen Planus

Jill C. Cash and Amy C. Bruggemann

Definition

A. Lichen planus is a relatively common acute or chronic inflammatory dermatosis. It affects skin and mucous membranes with characteristic flat-topped, shiny, violaceous (purplish color) pruritic papules with lacy lines on the skin, and milky-white papules in the mouth.

Incidence

A. Lichen planus accounts for 0.1% to 1.2% of office visits to dermatologists.
B. It exhibits no racial preference.

Pathogenesis

A. Etiology is unknown, although it is possibly a cell-mediated immune response. Most cases remit within 7 years. Lesions may heal with significant post-inflammatory hyperpigmentation.

Predisposing Factors

A. Severe emotional stress
B. Drugs may induce lichenoid plaques.

Common Complaints

A. Rash with or without pruritus
B. Primary lesions: Small, flat-topped papules that are polygonal, lightly scaly, and violaceous.
C. Secondary lesions: Erythema, scales, and erosions

Other Signs and Symptoms

A. Distribution: Volar aspect of wrists, ankles, mouth, genitalia, and lumbar region
B. Wickham's striae (white, lacelike pattern on surface)
C. Scalp: Atrophic skin with alopecia
D. Nails: Destruction of nail fold and bed, especially in the large toe
E. Men: Lesions of glans penis
F. Women: Erosive lesions of labia and vulva

Subjective Data

A. Determine whether the onset was sudden or gradual.
B. Ask the patient to describe if the skin is itchy or painful.
C. Assess lesions for any associated discharge (blood or pus).
D. Identify the location(s) of the problem.
E. Complete a drug history. Ask the patient if he or she has recently taken any antibiotics or other drugs. Ask if he or she has used any topical medications, lotions, or other creams.
F. Determine the presence of any preceding systemic symptoms (fever, sore throat, anorexia, or vaginal discharge).
G. Rule out insect bites.
H. Identify any possible exposure to industrial toxins, domestic toxins, or color-film-developing chemicals.
I. Ask if the patient has had any possible sexual contact with persons with HIV or sexually transmitted infections (STIs).
J. Ask if the patient has had close physical contact with others with skin disorders.

Physical Examination

A. Inspect
  1. Inspect skin and note lesion distribution.
  2. Inspect mucous membranes: Buccal mucosa, tongue, and lips.
  3. Examine hair and nails.
  4. Observe genitalia.

Diagnostic Tests

A. A drop of mineral oil accentuates the papule
B. If necessary to confirm diagnosis, deep shave or punch biopsy of developed lesions
C. HIV or STI testing if indicated
D. Hepatitis testing should be completed to assess for hepatitis C as lichen planus has been shown to have a correlation.

Differential Diagnoses

A. Lichen planus
B. Lichenoid drug eruptions
C. Leukoplakia
D. Chronic graft-versus-host disease
E. Candidiasis (thrush)
F. Lupus erythematosus
G. Contact dermatitis
H. Bite trauma
I. Secondary syphilis

Plan

A. General interventions: Discontinue any suspected drug agent.
B. Patient teaching: *See Section III: Patient Teaching Guide for this chapter, "Lichen Planus."* ◀
  1. Instruct patients that the disease may be chronic; most cases resolve spontaneously.
  2. Encourage the patient to avoid severe emotional stress.
  3. Encourage the patient to avoid scratching and prevent secondary infection.
  4. Reassure the patient that lichen planus is not contagious.
C. Pharmaceutical therapy
  1. Oral antihistamines: Hydroxyzine hydrochloride 10 to 50 mg four times daily as needed for pruritus, or cetirizine Hcl (Zyrtec) 10 mg daily
  2. Medium- to high-potency topical corticosteroids
    a. Mouth lesions: Fluocinonide 0.05%, ointment or gel, two or three times daily
    b. Body lesions: Betamethasone dipropionate (Diprolene) 0.05%, triamcinolone (Kenalog), clobetasol (Temovate, Cormax) 0.05%, or other class 1 cream or ointment, two times daily for 2 to 3 weeks and then stop use. **Caution patients about steroid atrophy.**
    c. Genital lesions: Desonide cream 0.05% twice daily initially, although higher potency creams may be necessary. Topical corticosteroids should be used on genitalia in short bursts only.
    d. Hypertrophic lesions: Intralesional injections, such as injecting triamcinolone 5 to 10 mg/mL,

0.5 to 1 mL per 2-cm lesion, are helpful for pruritus relief. Use cautiously in dark-skinned patients because of risk of hypopigmentation.
3. Oral prednisone is rarely used, but if necessary use with a short course only and taper.

Follow-Up

A. See the patient in 1 week for evaluation of treatment.

Consultation/Referral

A. Refer the patient to a dermatologist if there is no response to initial treatment.

Individual Considerations

A. Pregnancy: Use caution with medications prescribed.
B. Pediatrics: For severe itching, consider oral antihistamine.

Pityriasis Rosea

Jill C. Cash and Amy C. Bruggemann

Definition

A. Pityriasis rosea is an acute, self-limiting, benign skin eruption characterized by a preceding "herald patch" that is followed by widespread papulosquamous lesions.

Incidence

A. Pityriasis rosea is relatively common, with more than 75% of cases in individuals from 10 to 35 years of age.
B. Incidence is slightly higher in women than in men.
C. Incidence is higher during the spring and autumn.

Pathogenesis

A. Disease is idiopathic; some evidence exists to support a viral origin or autoimmune disorder.

Predisposing Factor

A. Recent acute infection

Common Complaints

A. Rash: Salmon, pink, or tawny-colored lesions generally are concentrated in the trunk, but may develop on arms, legs, and rarely on the face.
B. Mild pruritus

Other Signs and Symptoms

A. Earliest lesions may be papular but may progress to 1- to 2-cm oval plaques.
B. Long axes of oval lesions run parallel to each other, hence the term "Christmas tree distribution."
C. Preceding herald patch (2–10 cm with central clearing) closely resembles ringworm; usually appears abruptly a few days to several weeks before the generalized eruptive phase.

Subjective Data

A. Elicit information about occurrence of initial, single, 2- to 10-cm round to oval lesion.
B. Question the patient as to known contact with similar symptoms. Small epidemics have been identified in fraternity houses and military bases.

Physical Examination

A. Check temperature to rule out any infection.
B. Inspect
1. Examine all body surfaces with patient unclothed.
2. Look for characteristic lesions and distribution.
3. Check the mucous surfaces, palms, and soles, which are usually spared by pityriasis rosea.

Diagnostic Tests

A. Generally none required; however, potassium hydroxide (KOH) wet preparation may be useful to distinguish a herald patch from tinea corporis.
B. Serology to rule out syphilis, if applicable.
C. If unable to identify herald patch, a serologic test for syphilis should be ordered because syphilis may be clinically indistinguishable from pityriasis rosea.
D. White blood count (WBC) normal; no specific laboratory markers for pityriasis rosea.

Differential Diagnoses

A. Pityriasis rosea
B. Nummular eczema
C. Tinea corporis
D. Tinea versicolor
E. Viral exanthems
F. Drug eruptions
1. Captopril
2. Bismuth
3. Barbiturates
4. Clonidine
5. Metronidazole
G. Secondary syphilis
H. Lichen planus

Plan

A. General interventions
1. Direct sunlight to the point of minimal erythema hastens the disappearance of lesions and decreases itching. Ultraviolet B (UVB) light in five consecutive daily exposures can decrease pruritus and shorten rash, particularly if administered within the first week of eruption.
2. Not proven to be contagious and relatively harmless, so isolation is not required.
B. Patient teaching
1. *See Section III: Patient Teaching Guide for this chapter, "Pityriasis Rosea."* ◀
2. Advise patients that the disease is self-limiting and clears spontaneously in 1 to 3 months.
C. Pharmaceutical therapy
1. Generally none is required, but for itching the following recommendations exist: Group V topical steroids and oral antihistamines as per usual dosing.
2. Prednisone 20 mg twice daily for 1 to 2 weeks in rare cases of intense itching.

Follow-Up

A. None is required unless secondary infection (impetigo) develops. Disease may recur in approximately 2% of patients.

Consultation/Referral

A. Consult or refer the patient to a physician when disease persists beyond 3 months.

Individual Considerations

A. Pregnancy: Disease has not been shown to affect fetus.
B. Pediatrics: Rash more frequently affects face and distal extremities. Impetigo may result from scratching or poor hygiene.
C. Geriatrics: Disease is rarely seen in geriatric patients. Strongly consider other differential diagnoses, particularly drug reactions.

Precancerous or Cancerous Skin Lesions

Jill C. Cash and Amy C. Bruggemann

Definition

A. Potentially malignant or malignant cutaneous cells form precancerous or cancerous skin lesions, respectively.

Incidence

A. There are approximately 700,000 new cases of basal cell carcinomas (BCC) and squamous cell carcinomas (SCC) reported each year in the United States. Approximately 32,000 of these cases per year are found to be malignant melanoma.
   1. SCC accounts for 20% of all skin cancers, and it occurs mostly in the middle-aged and elderly populations.
   2. BCC is the most common form of skin cancer, with approximately 400,000 new cases per year in the United States. It is often seen in the sixth or seventh decade of life.
   3. Malignant melanoma accounts for less than 5% of all skin cancers and is responsible for more than 60% of deaths because of skin cancer. Melanoma is frequently seen in younger people, with the median age being in the low 40s.

Pathogenesis

A. SCC: Abnormal cells of the epidermis penetrate the basement membrane of the epidermis and move into the dermis, producing SCC. This often begins as actinic keratosis that undergoes malignant change.
B. BCC: Abnormal cells of the basal layer of the epidermis expand. The surrounding stroma supports the basal cell growth. Ultraviolet rays (sunlight) are the major contributor to BCC. BCC is a slow-growing tumor that rarely metastasizes.
C. Malignant melanoma: Abnormal cells proliferate from the melanocyte system. Initially, the cells grow superficially and laterally into the epidermis and papillary dermis. After a period, the cells begin growing up into the reticular dermis and subcutaneous fat. Malignant tumors occur because of the inability of the damaged cells to protect themselves from the long-term exposure of the ultraviolet rays.
D. Keratoacanthoma: Sun-exposed-area lesion that at first appears as a smooth, skin-colored, or reddish dome-shaped papule that may then grow to 1 to 2 cm in a few weeks, with crusted interior.

Predisposing Factors

A. Advanced age (older than age 50 years)
B. Median age of 40 years for malignant melanoma
C. Exposure to ultraviolet light (sun exposure)
D. Fair complexion
E. Smokers (damaged lips)
F. Skin damaged by burns and/or chronic inflammation
G. History of blistering sunburns before 18 years of age increases risk

Common Complaints

A. New lesions found on the skin
B. Ulcer that does not heal

Other Signs and Symptoms

A. SCC: Skin lesions seen in sun-exposed areas or skin damaged by burns or chronic inflammation; lower lip lesions common; firm, irregular papules with scaly, bleeding, friable surface like sandpaper; grows rapidly
B. BCC: Tumor seen on face and neck; nodules greater than 1 cm that appear shiny, pearly color with telangiectasia; center caves in
C. Malignant melanoma: Asymmetrical tumor of skin with irregular border, variation in color, and greater than 6 mm in diameter; can metastasize to any organ
D. Bowen's disease (SCC in situ): Chronic, nonhealing erythemic patch with sharp, irregular borders; occurs on skin and/or the mucocutaneous tissue; resembles eczema but does not respond to steroids

Subjective Data

A. Have the patient identify when lesion was first noted.
B. Ask the patient to describe any changes in size, color, or shape of the lesion.
C. Determine whether the patient has noted any new lesions.
D. Ascertain any family history of malignant melanoma.
E. Determine the patient's history of skin exposure to the sun or any other ultraviolet rays.
F. Ask the patient about smoking history. If the patient smokes, ask how many packs per day.
G. Ask if patient is up to date on routine cancer screenings.

Physical Examination

A. Inspect
   1. Perform full body exam of the skin for lesions
   2. Note surface, size, shape, border, color, and diameter of lesion.

Diagnostic Test

A. Biopsy suspicious lesions.

Differential Diagnoses

A. SCC
B. BCC
C. Malignant melanoma
D. Actinic keratosis
E. Solar lentigo
F. Seborrheic keratosis
G. Common nevus
H. Leukoplakia

Plan

A. General interventions
  1. Monitor progress/change of lesions detected.
  2. Biopsy any suspicious lesions. Excise lesion with narrow margins, making sure to include all margins. If biopsy results of specimen are inadequate for accurate histologic diagnosis or staging, repeat biopsy. Include all clinical history information on the pathology report with the specimen when sending to pathology.

B. Patient teaching
  1. *See Section III: Patient Teaching Guide for this chapter, "Skin Care Assessment."*
  2. Educate patients regarding importance of early identification of lesions and monthly assessment of skin.

C. Pharmaceutical therapy: None indicated.

Follow-Up

A. If diagnosis is made, follow up with examination every month for 3 months, twice a year for 5 years, then yearly.

Consultation/Referral

A. Refer all patients to the dermatologist if skin cancer is suspected.

Individual Considerations

A. Pediatrics: Teach parents to use sun protection factor (SPF) 30 or greater on pediatric patients exposed to the sun.

B. Geriatrics: The elderly are at high risk of skin lesions. Monitor them closely.

Psoriasis

Jill C. Cash and Amy C. Bruggemann

Definition

A. A common benign, chronic, inflammatory skin disorder, psoriasis is characterized by whitish scaly patches commonly seen on the scalp, knees, and elbows.

Incidence

A. Disease occurs in about 2% of the world population.

B. Psoriasis affects 2 to 8 million people in the United States.

C. It occurs at any age.
  1. Peaks of onset seen in young adults aged 15 to 30 years.
  2. May also be seen in adults aged 57 to 60 years.

Pathogenesis

A. Etiology is unknown; this is a multifactorial disease with a definite genetic component. Hyperproliferation of the epidermis and inflammation of the epidermis and dermis are seen, with epidermal transit time rapidly increased (six- to ninefold). A T-lymphocyte-mediated dermal immune response may occur because of microbial antigen or autoimmune process.

Predisposing Factors

A. Family history

B. Drugs that exacerbate condition
  1. Lithium
  2. Beta-blockers
  3. Nonsteroidal anti-inflammatory drugs
  4. Anti-malarial
  5. Sudden withdrawal of systemic or potent topical corticosteroids

C. Stress (common triggering factor)

D. Local trauma or irritation

E. Recent streptococcal infection

F. Alcohol use

G. Tobacco use

H. HIV association; suspected if onset is abrupt

Common Complaint

A. Dry scaly rash

Other Signs and Symptoms

A. Pruritic and/or painful lesions

B. Silvery scales on discrete erythematous plaques
  1. Onset commonly occurs as a guttate form with small, scattered, teardrop-shaped papules and plaques after a streptococcal infection in a child or young adult.
  2. Larger, chronic plaques occur later in life.

C. Lesions commonly seen on the scalp, elbows, and knees, but may involve any area of the body.

D. Glossitis or geographic tongue: Small pits or yellow-brown spots (oil spots)

E. Positive Auspitz sign: Punctate bleeding points with removal of scale

F. Onycholysis

G. Stippled nails and pitting; approximately 50% of patients have nail involvement

H. Periarticular swelling of small joints of fingers and toes. **Joint pain and involvement signals psoriatic arthritis.**

I. Pustular variant with predominant involvement of hands and/or feet, including nails

Subjective Data

A. Question the patient regarding any predisposing factors listed earlier to identify risk factors.

B. Ask the patient if there have been changes in the course of symptoms.

C. Ascertain whether the symptoms worsen in winter and improve in summer.

D. Determine the site of the lesion and whether the onset is sudden and/or painful.

E. Ask the patient to describe the skin, whether it is itchy or painful.

F. Assess lesions for any associated discharge (blood or pus).

G. Ask if the patient is using any new soaps, creams, or lotions.

H. Rule out any exposure to industrial or domestic toxins.

I. Ask the patient about any possible contact with venereal disease (sexually transmitted diseases [STDs]).

J. Review whether there has been any close physical contact with others with skin disorders.

K. Elicit information regarding any preceding systemic symptoms (fever, sore throat, and anorexia).

Physical Examination

A. Check temperature (if indicated).

B. Inspect
1. Inspect skin; note type of lesion and distribution. Assess oral mucosa, nails, and nail beds.
2. Assess joints.
C. Palpate joints for tenderness.

Diagnostic Tests

A. None is indicated unless HIV infection is suspected; if so, order HIV test.
B. If joint inflammation is present, consider rheumatoid factor, erythrocyte sedimentation rate, and uric acid.
C. If there is a history of streptococcal infection, order antistreptolysin O titer.

Differential Diagnoses

A. Psoriasis
B. Scalp: Seborrheic dermatitis
C. Body folds: Candidiasis
D. Trunk: Pityriasis rosea, tinea corporis
E. Hand dermatitis
F. SCC
G. Cutaneous lupus erythematosus

Plan

A. General interventions
1. This is a chronic disorder that requires long-term treatment, a high degree of patient involvement, and therapy that is simple and inexpensive.
2. Aim of treatment is control, not cure.
3. Exposure to sunlight may be beneficial. However, symptoms worsen in a small percentage of patients with exposure to sunlight.
4. Mild to moderate disease may be treated with phototherapy if allowable because of cost.
5. Sequence of agents for involvement of less than 20% body surface is as follows:
a. Emollients (Eucerin cream or Aquaphor cream)
b. Keratolytic agents (salicylic acid gel or ointment)
c. Topical corticosteroids: Use lowest potency to control disease.
d. Calcipotriene ointment: Vitamin D analogue (calcipotriene ointment 0.005%)
e. Anthralin: Use as short-contact therapy 1% to 3%.
f. Coal tar (Estar, PsoriGel): Use in conjunction with topical steroids or anthralin. May apply at bedtime or in the morning for 15 minutes and then shower off.
g. Medicated shampoos: Useful for scalp psoriasis, in conjunction with topical steroids and other treatments.
B. Patient teaching
▶ **1.** *See Section III: Patient Teaching Guide for this chapter, "Psoriasis."*
2. Help the patient understand the chronic nature of this disease characterized by flares and remission. Teach stress monitoring and control. Assist with coping techniques.
3. A trial of a gluten-free diet may be tried to help symptoms. See Appendix B: "Gluten-Free Diet."
4. If phototherapy is not effective, systemic agents are recommended.
C. Pharmaceutical therapy: If the disease is not controlled with the first agent, then an alternative agent may be tried.
1. Mild to moderate disease: Topical steroids as first-line therapy.
2. Emollients to start treatment (e.g., Eucerin Plus lotion or cream, Lubriderm Moisture Plus, Moisturel)
3. Scalp: Use coal tar shampoo (Zetar, T/Gel, Pentrax) in place of regular shampoo two times per week.
a. Apply lather to scalp, allow to soak for 5 minutes, and then rinse.
b. If plaques are very thick, use P and S Liquid (over the counter [OTC]). Massage in at night and wash out in the morning.
4. For additional treatment as needed, apply triamcinolone acetonide 0.1% (Kenalog 0.1%) lotion or equivalent to scaly, stubborn areas once or twice daily until controlled. **Avoid face.**
5. Dovonex scalp solution: Apply on dry scalp as directed.
6. Face and skin folds: Hydrocortisone cream 1%, apply sparingly up to 4 weeks, preferably no more than 2 weeks. If lesions are unresponsive, consider increasing to 2.5% and taper quickly with improvement.
7. Body, arms, and legs: Use triamcinolone acetonide 0.025% (Aristocort A) cream twice daily up to 2 weeks. **Avoid normal skin.**
8. For thick plaques, try Keralyt gel (6% salicylic acid), then corticosteroids.
9. Use coal tar (Estar gel) once or twice daily in combination with corticosteroids.
10. Anthralin (Dritho-Creme) is beneficial as an alternate to steroid lotion for scalp psoriasis. **Avoid sunlight.**
11. Vitamin D_3 analogue: (Calcipotriol), twice daily up to 8 weeks, is comparable to midpotency corticosteroids. **Avoid face and skin folds.**
12. Systemic agents for moderate to severe psoriasis may be used if other measures fail. Systemic agents should be prescribed by a dermatology specialist; these medications include retinoids, methotrexate, cyclosporine, and apremilast. These medications should be monitored closely for liver/ kidney function changes.

Follow-Up

A. See patients in 2 to 3 weeks to evaluate treatment.
B. Follow up in 2 months to monitor side effects.
C. Follow-up must be individualized for each patient.

Consultation/Referral

A. Medical management: For involvement greater than 20% of body, refer the patient to a dermatologist for the following:
1. Light therapy with ultraviolet A (UVA) or UVB. UVB light therapy is often used in conjunction with keratolytic agents.
2. Synthetic retinoids: Etretinate or acitretin are options.
3. Low-dose cyclosporine or Azulfidine can be effective.
B. Refer patients with extensive disease, psoriatic arthritis, or inflammatory disease to a rheumatologist. New medications, called biologics, are used to suppress the

immune system's response, which include adalimumab (Humira), alefacept (Amevive), etanercept (Enbrel), infliximab (Remicade), and ustekinuman (Stelara).

C. Cases of generalized pustular psoriasis of exfoliative erythroderma should be referred immediately to a dermatologist.

D. All systemic therapies should be given under supervision of a dermatologist or rheumatologist.

Individual Considerations

A. Adults

1. Patients with moderate to severe disease that is not well controlled should be referred to a dermatology specialist for systemic treatment.

Scabies

Jill C. Cash and Amy C. Bruggemann

Definition

A. Scabies is a contagious skin infestation by the mite *Sarcoptes scabiei.*

Incidence

A. Scabies occurs mainly in individuals in close contact with many other individuals such as schoolchildren or nursing-home residents. It is rare among African Americans.

Pathogenesis

A. Scabies is transmitted through close contact with an individual who is infested with the mite *S. scabiei.* Transmission may occur through sexual contact or contact with mite-infested clothing or sheets. The fertilized female mite burrows into the stratum corneum of a host and deposits eggs and fecal pellets. Larvae hatch, mature, and repeat the cycle.

B. A hypersensitivity reaction is responsible for the intense pruritus.

Predisposing Factors

A. Close contact with large numbers of individuals

B. Institutionalized

C. Poverty

D. Sexual promiscuity

Common Complaints

A. Intense itching, worse at night

B. Skin excoriation

C. Generalized pruritus

D. Rash

Other Signs and Symptoms

A. Mites burrow in finger webs, at wrists, in the sides of hands and feet, at the axilla buttocks, and in the penis and scrotum in males.

B. Discrete vesicles and papules, distributed in linear fashion.

C. Erythema is a symptom.

D. Secondary infections caused by scratching or infection (pustules and pinpoint erosions).

E. Nodules in covered areas (buttocks, groin, scrotum, penis, and axilla), which may have slightly eroded surfaces that persist for months after mites have been eradicated

F. Diffuse eruption that spare the face.

Subjective Data

A. Elicit information regarding housing conditions, close contact, or sexual contact with potentially infected individuals.

B. Question the patient regarding onset, duration, and location of itching.

Physical Examination

A. Check temperature.

B. Inspect

1. Examine all body surfaces with patient unclothed.

2. Use a magnifying lens to identify characteristic burrows in finger webs, wrists, and penis.

3. Inspect adult pubic area for lesions.

Diagnostic Tests

A. Three findings are diagnostic of scabies:

1. Microscopic identification of *S. scabiei* mites

2. Eggs

3. Fecal pellets (scybala)

B. Burrow identification: Ink the suspected area with a blue or black felt-tipped pen, then wipe with an alcohol swab. The burrow absorbs the ink, while the surface ink is wiped clean.

C. A tiny black dot may be seen at the end of a burrow, which represents the mite, ova, or feces, and can be transferred by means of a 25-gauge hypodermic needle to immersion oil on a slide for microscopic identification.

D. Place a drop of mineral oil on a suspected lesion, scrape the lesion with a #15 blade, and transfer the shaved material to a microscope slide for direct examination of the mite under low power.

Differential Diagnoses

A. Scabies

B. Atopic dermatitis

C. Insect bites

D. Pityriasis rosea

E. Eczema

F. Seborrheic dermatitis

G. Syphilis

H. Pediculosis

I. Allergic or irritant contact dermatitis

Plan

A. General interventions

1. Implement comfort measures to reduce pruritus.

2. Treat secondary infection(s) with antibiotics.

3. Household members should be treated simultaneously as a prophylactic measure and to reduce the chance of reinfection.

4. The patient should be advised that pruritus may continue for up to a week even with a successful treatment because of local irritation.

B. Patient teaching: *See Section III: Patient Teaching Guide for this chapter, "Scabies."* ◀

C. Pharmaceutical therapy

1. First line of therapy, because of its low toxicity, is 5% permethrin (Elimite cream) applied to all body areas from the neck down and washed off in 8 to

14 hours. One application is highly effective, but some dermatologists recommend retreatment in 1 week.
2. Alternative therapy is lindane (Kwell) cream, applied to all skin surfaces from the neck down and washed off in 8 to 12 hours. Some dermatologists retreat in 1 week.
3. A single oral dose of the anthelmintic agent ivermectin (200 mcg/kg) has been shown to be effective and to rapidly control pruritus in healthy patients and HIV patients.
4. Diphenhydramine (Benadryl) 25 to 50 mg may be given by mouth every 4 to 6 hours if indicated for pruritus. Other nonsedating antihistamines may be used. Toxicity is usually a result of patient overtreatment (failure to follow prescribed regimen). Advise the patient of this danger.

Follow-Up

A. Follow up in 2 weeks to assess treatment response.

Consultation/Referral

A. Consult or refer the patient to the physician if, at 2-week follow-up, pharmaceutical therapy has been ineffective.

Individual Considerations

A. Pregnancy
1. Permethrin is preferred to lindane in pregnant and/or lactating women because of decreased toxicity.
2. Patient should be warned of its potential to cause neurotoxicity and convulsions with overuse (more than two treatments).
B. Pediatrics
1. Infants and toddlers often have more widespread involvement that can include the face and scalp.
2. Vesicular lesions on palms and soles are more commonly seen.
3. Drug of choice is permethrin 5% cream; apply over the head, neck, and body, avoiding the eyes. The cream should be removed by bathing within 8 to 14 hours.
4. Lindane should not be used in infants and toddlers.
5. Infants and children with underlying cutaneous disease, malnutrition, prematurity, or a history of seizure disorders should be treated with special caution because of their increased risk of toxicity.
C. Partners: All intimate contacts within the past month and close household and family members should be treated.
D. Geriatrics
1. The elderly tend to have more severe pruritus despite fewer lesions.
2. They are at risk of extensive infections because of age-related decline in immunity.
3. The excoriations may become severe and may be complicated by cellulitis.

Seborrheic Dermatitis

Jill C. Cash and Amy C. Bruggemann

Definition

A. A common chronic, erythematous, scaling dermatosis, seborrheic dermatitis occurs in areas of the most active sebaceous glands such as the face and scalp, body folds, and presternal region.

Incidence

A. Seborrheic dermatitis is very common.
B. Incidence is higher in HIV-infected individuals.

Pathogenesis

A. Etiology is unknown. There is a possibility that it is hormonally dependent, has a fungal (*Pityrosporum ovale* or *Candida albicans*) component, is neurogenic, or may reflect a nutritional deficiency.
B. Currently, it is identified as an inflammatory disorder that most probably results from a dysfunction of sebaceous glands.

Predisposing Factors

A. Possible link between infantile and adult forms
B. Possible familial trend
C. High association with HIV-infected individuals

Common Complaints

A. Infants: “Cradle cap”
B. Adults: “Dandruff,” dry flaky scalp
C. Rash with “sticky flakes”

Often no presenting complaints are found on a routine physical examination.

Other Signs and Symptoms

A. Variable pruritus, often increasing with perspiration and in winter
B. Oily, flaking skin on erythemic base around ears, nose, eyebrows, and eyelids
C. Red, cracking skin in body folds; axilla; groin; or anogenital, submammary, or umbilical areas
D. Primary lesions: Plaques
E. Secondary lesions: Erythema, scales, fissures, exudate, and symmetric eyelid involvement
F. Lesions with drainage or crusting may indicate secondary bacterial infection
G. Distribution pattern in infants: Scalp and diaper area
H. Distribution area in adults: Scalp, eyebrows, paranasal area, nasolabial fold, chin, behind ears, chest, and groin
I. Secondary impetigo in children

Subjective Data

A. Identify location, onset, and progression of symptoms.
B. Ask the patient to describe symptoms. Ask if the skin is itchy or painful.
C. Assess lesions for any associated discharge (blood or pus).
D. Elicit information regarding use of topical medications, soaps, creams, or lotions. Quiz the patient regarding any oral medications being taken.
E. Determine whether there were any preceding systemic symptoms (fever, sore throat, anorexia, or vaginal discharge).
F. Rule out any possible exposure to industrial or domestic toxins.

G. Ask the patient to identify what improves or worsens this condition.

Physical Examination

A. Inspect

1. Inspect skin; note areas of lesions and distribution.

2. Assess eyes for blepharitis.

3. Inspect ears and nose.

B. Palpate skin, noting texture and moisture.

Diagnostic Tests

A. None required.

B. Consider fungal culture in children and adolescents to rule out a fungal infection.

C. Consider possible skin biopsy to rule out other conditions.

Differential Diagnoses

A. Seborrheic dermatitis

B. Atopic dermatitis

C. Candidiasis

D. Dermatophytosis

E. Histiocytosis X

F. Psoriasis vulgaris

G. Rosacea

H. Systemic lupus erythematosus

I. Tinea capitis

J. Tinea versicolor

K. Vitamin deficiency

L. Impetigo

M. Eczema

Plan

A. General interventions

1. Shampooing is the foundation of treatment.

a. Infants: Rub petroleum jelly into scalp to soften crusts 20 to 30 minutes before shampooing.

b. Shampoo daily with baby shampoo using a soft brush.

c. Toddlers or adolescents: Shampoo every other day with antiseborrheic shampoo (Selsun Blue, Exsel, or Nizoral).

2. If skin does not clear after 1 to 2 weeks of treatment, it is appropriate to use ketoconazole 2% cream.

3. Seborrheic blepharitis

a. Hot compresses plus gentle debridement with cotton-tipped applicator and baby shampoo twice a day

b. For secondary bacterial infection, sulfacetamide sodium 10% (ophthalmic Sodium Sulamyd)

4. Continue treatment for several days after lesions disappear.

▶ **B.** Patient teaching: *See Section III: Patient Teaching Guide for this chapter, "Seborrheic Dermatitis."*

C. Pharmaceutical therapy

1. Most shampoos should be used two times per week. Those with coal tar can be used three times per week.

2. Medicated shampoos

a. Coal tar (Denorex, T/Gel, Pentrax, Tegrin) shampoo, apply as directed.

b. Salicylic acid (Ionil Plus, P and S) shampoo, apply as directed.

c. Selenium sulfide (Exsel, Selsun Blue) shampoo, use daily.

d. Ketoconazole 2% (Nizoral) cream, apply to affected area twice daily for 4 to 6 weeks.

e. Combination shampoos: Coal tar and salicylic acid (T/Sal); salicylic acid and sulfur (Sebulex). These shampoos may be used one to two times a week, alternating with other shampoos during the week. Always apply corticosteroids in a thin layer only; avoid the eyes.

3. Topical corticosteroid lotions or solutions: Use in combination with medicated shampoo if 2 to 3 weeks of treatment with shampoo alone fails.

4. Adults: Scalp

a. Start with medium potency, for example, betamethasone valerate 0.1% lotion twice daily.

b. If treatment is not effective in 2 weeks, increase potency, for example, fluocinonide 0.05% solution twice daily, or fluocinolone acetonide 0.01% oil 120 mL nightly with shower cap.

c. As dermatitis is controlled, decrease to mild potency, for example, hydrocortisone 1% to 2.5% lotion once or twice daily.

5. Adults: Face or groin

a. Low-potency agents, for example, hydrocortisone 1% cream or desonide 0.05% cream once or twice daily

b. Consider lotion for eyebrows for easier application.

c. Metronidazole 1% gel on face once or twice daily

6. Recalcitrant disease

a. Add ketoconazole 2% cream (15, 30, or 60 g) every day.

b. Use sulfacetamide sodium 10%, with sulfur 5%, lotion 25 g once or twice daily.

Follow-Up

A. Tell the patient to call the office in 5 to 6 days to report progress.

B. Have the patient return to the office if no improvement is seen.

Consultation/Referral

A. Refer the patient to a dermatologist if the condition does not clear in 10 to 14 days.

Individual Considerations

A. Pregnancy: Ketoconazole is not recommended.

B. Pediatrics

1. Avoid using tar preparations on infants.

2. Use baby shampoo only.

3. If lesions are inflammatory, use topical steroids no stronger than hydrocortisone 0.5% to 1.0% twice daily.

4. Betamethasone valerate (Valisone) lotion may be used daily for scalp only if other treatments fail.

5. Be aware of potential for emotional distress in adolescents.
6. Treat with antiseborrheic shampoo every other day for adolescents.

Tinea Corporis (Ringworm)

Jill C. Cash and Amy C. Bruggemann

Definition

A. Tinea corporis (ringworm) is a fungal infection of the skin tissue (keratin) commonly seen on the face, trunk, and extremities.

Incidence

A. Ringworm is a fairly common fungal infection seen in adults and children.

Pathogenesis

A. The causative fungal species varies, depending on the location of the infection. Three common organisms are *Epidermophyton, Microsporum*, and *Trichophyton.*
B. The infection can be obtained from other people, animals (puppies, kittens), and the soil.

Predisposing Factors

A. Exposure to person or facilities (e.g., locker rooms) infected with the fungus
B. Poor nutrition
C. Poor health
D. Poor hygiene
E. Warm climates
F. Immunosuppression

Common Complaint

A. Scaly, itchy patch of skin, often circular in shape

Other Signs and Symptoms

A. Tinea capitis: Erythema, scaling of scalp, with hair loss at site asymptomatic
B. Tinea corporis: Circular, erythematous, well-demarcated lesion on the skin with hypopigmentation in center of lesion; usually pruritic
C. Tinea cruris: Well-demarcated scaling lesions on groin (not scrotum) or thigh; usually pruritic
D. Tinea pedis: Scaly, erythemic vesicles on feet, between toes, and in arch, with extreme pruritus
E. Tinea unguium (onychomycosis): Thickening and yellowing of toenail or fingernail, often with other fungal infection or alone

Subjective Data

A. Ask the patient about onset, duration, and progression of the patch or rash on the skin.
B. Assess the patient about other areas of skin involvement.
C. Ask if the lesion is pruritic.
D. Inquire as to the patient's exposure to anyone with similar symptoms.
E. Determine whether the patient has a history of similar lesions.
F. Query the patient regarding predisposing factors.
G. Review with the patient what remedies were used and with what results.

Physical Examination

A. Check temperature (if indicated).
B. Inspect
   1. Examine all areas of skin.
   2. Note type of lesions present.

Diagnostic Tests

A. Obtain scrapings of the border of the lesion for evaluation.
   1. Potassium hydroxide (KOH)
   2. Wet prep
   3. Fungal cultures

Differential Diagnoses

A. Tinea corporis
B. Dermatitis
C. Alopecia areata
D. Psoriasis
E. Contact dermatitis
F. Atopic eczema

Plan

A. General interventions
   1. Identify type of lesion.
   2. Identify other infected family members or sexual partners for treatment.
B. Patient teaching
   1. *See Section III: Patient Teaching Guide for this chapter, "Ringworm Tinea."* ◀
   2. Reinforce medication regimen for 4- to 8-week period for resolution.
C. Pharmaceutical therapy
   1. Tinea capitis
      a. Adults: Griseofulvin 500 mg by mouth per day for 4 to 8 weeks
      b. Children: Griseofulvin 10 to 20 mg/kg/d for 4 to 8 weeks. **Griseofulvin is best absorbed with high-fat foods.**
      c. Ketoconazole (Nizoral) may also be used.
   2. Tinea corporis, pedis, and cruris: Use wet dressings with Burow's solution along with one of the following:
      a. Clotrimazole 1% (Lotrimin) cream, or econazole nitrate 1% cream, twice daily for 14 to 28 days
      b. Terbinafine 1% cream (Lamisil), topical, apply once or twice daily for 1 to 4 weeks. Not recommended for children.
   3. Onychomycosis: Successful treatment is difficult.
      a. Itraconazole (Sporanox) 100 mg, two tablets by mouth twice daily for 7 days. Repeat in 1 month, then repeat again in 1 more month.

> *Monitor liver function tests (LFTs) at 6 weeks after starting medication.*

      b. Terbinafine 1% cream (Lamisil)
         i. Fingernail: 250 mg once daily for 6 weeks
         ii. Toenail: 250 mg daily for 12 weeks

c. Home cure: Apply Vicks VapoRub on toenail bed every night at bedtime for approximately 4 to 6 months or until resolved. This treatment offers a safe, cost-effective alternative to oral medications.

Follow-Up

A. A 2- to 4-week follow-up is recommended to evaluate progress.
B. Monitor LFT at 6 weeks and if itraconazole (Sporanox) is continued longer.

Consultation/Referral

A. Consult a physician if the infection has not improved.

Individual Considerations

A. Pregnancy: Oral antifungal medications are not recommended during pregnancy.
B. Pediatrics
1. Tinea capitis is common in children 2 to 10 years old. When hair has been lost, regrowth takes time.
2. Tinea pedis is common in adolescents.
3. Tinea unguium is common in adolescents, but rare in children.
C. Adults
1. Tinea capitis is rare in adults.
2. Tinea cruris is more common in obese males, but rare in females.
3. Tinea pedis is common in adults.
4. Tinea unguium is seen in adults.

Tinea Versicolor

Jill C. Cash and Amy C. Bruggemann

Definition

A. Tinea versicolor is a fungal infection of the skin, which may be chronic in nature. It is most commonly seen on the upper trunk; however, it may spread to extremities.

Incidence

A. Tinea versicolor is seen most frequently in adolescents and young adults.

Pathogenesis

A. Tinea versicolor is a fungal infection of the skin caused by an overgrowth of *Pityrosporum orbiculare,* part of the normal skin flora.
B. Discoloration of the skin is seen, forming round or oval maculae, which may become confluent.
C. Maculae range from 1 cm to very large, greater than 30 cm.

Predisposing Factors

A. Immunosuppressive therapy
B. Pregnancy
C. Warm temperatures
D. Corticosteroid therapy

Common Complaint

A. Scaly rash on the upper trunk with occasional mild itching

Other Signs and Symptoms

A. Annular maculae with mild scaling
B. Asymptomatic or pruritic
C. Pink-, white-, or brown-colored rash

Subjective Data

A. Ascertain when and where the rash began.
B. Have the patient describe how the rash has changed.
C. Assess the patient for any associated symptoms with the rash such as itching and burning.
D. Identify what products the patient has used on the skin to treat rash and with what results.
E. Elicit information regarding a history of similar rashes.
F. Query the patient regarding current medications.
G. Review any medical history for comorbid conditions.

Physical Examination

A. Inspect
1. Inspect skin and note type of lesion.
2. Examine other areas of skin for similar lesions.

Diagnostic Tests

A. Wet prep/potassium hydroxide (KOH)
B. Wood's lamp: Wood's lamp is useful in examining skin to determine the extent of infection. Inspection of fine scales with Wood's lamp reveals scales with a pale yellow-green fluorescence that contains the fungus.
C. Culture lesion: When obtaining a sample scraping, obtain the sample from the edge of the lesion for the best sample of hyphae. (Hyphae and spores have a "spaghetti and meatball" appearance.)

Differential Diagnoses

A. Tinea versicolor
B. Tinea corporis
C. Pityriasis alba
D. Pityriasis rosea: Herald patch is clue to diagnosis
E. Seborrheic dermatitis
F. Vitiligo

Plan

A. General interventions: Apply medication as directed.
B. Patient teaching
1. *See Section III: Patient Teaching Guide for this chapter, "Tinea Versicolor."* ◀
2. These causative species are a normal inhabitant of skin flora; recurrence is possible.
3. Skin pigmentation returns after infection is cleared up. This may take several months to resolve.
C. Pharmaceutical therapy
1. Selenium sulfide 2.5% (Selsun Blue)
a. Apply to skin at bedtime one time. Shower off in the morning.
b. For 12 days, apply Selsun Blue to skin lesions, wait 30 minutes, and then shower off.

c. Treatment may be needed monthly until desired results are obtained. Encourage use of Selsun Blue on entire body surface except for face and head.

2. Other medications used
   a. Clotrimazole 1% cream twice daily for 4 weeks
   b. Ketoconazole (Nizoral) cream daily for 14 days
   c. Ketoconazole (Nizoral) 200 mg by mouth once daily for 3 days, for adults only. When using ketoconazole (Nizoral) as treatment, caution the patient regarding liver damage with toxicity.

Follow-Up
A. None is required if resolution occurs.
B. Monitor liver function tests (LFTs) every 6 weeks if patient is on ketoconazole.

Consultation/Referral
A. Consult with a physician if current treatment is unsuccessful.

Individual Considerations
A. Pediatrics: Commonly seen in adolescents
B. Adults: Commonly seen in young adults

Warts

Jill C. Cash and Amy C. Bruggemann

Definition
A. A wart is an elevation of the epidermal layer of the skin (skin tumor). Warts are caused by the papillomavirus.

Incidence
A. Warts occur in people of all ages, more common in children and during early adulthood.
B. By adulthood, 90% of all people have positive antibodies to the virus.
C. Warts are seen more frequently in females than in males.

Pathogenesis
A. A circumscribed mass develops on the skin that is limited to the epidermal layer. The virus, papillomavirus, is located within the nucleus of the cell.
B. The virus may be transmitted by touch and is commonly seen on the hands and feet.
C. Most warts resolve without treatment within 12 to 24 months.

Predisposing Factors
A. Skin trauma
B. Immunosuppression
C. Exposure to public showers, pools, locker rooms, and so forth

Common Complaints
A. Bump on the skin or specific area of the body (hands, feet, arms, and legs)
B. Usually painless unless present on the bottom of the foot

Other Signs and Symptoms
A. Common wart (verruca vulgaris): Flesh-colored, irregular lesion with rough surface; black dots in center of lesion occasionally seen, which is thrombosed capillaries; can occur on any body part
B. Filiform wart (verruca filiformis): Thin, threadlike, projected papule on face, lips, nose, or eyelids
C. Flat wart (verruca plana): Flat-topped, flesh-colored papule, 1 to 3 mm in diameter, with smooth surface; seen in clusters or in a line, on face and extremities
D. Plantar wart (verruca plantaris): Firm papula, 2 to 3 cm in diameter, indented into skin with verrucous surface; painful with ambulation, when placed on ball or heel of foot
E. Genital warts: See Chapter 15: Sexually Transmitted Infections Guidelines.

Subjective Data
A. Determine onset, location, and duration of tumor.
B. Elicit information regarding a history of previous warts.
C. Identify with the patient what treatment has been used in the past and what the results were. Question the patient regarding length of time over-the-counter (OTC) medications were used, and how aggressive he or she was with the treatment.

Physical Examination
A. Inspect
   1. Assess skin for lesions, noting location, appearance, size, and surface texture of tumor.
   2. Examine the entire body for other lesions.

Diagnostic Test
A. None indicated

Differential Diagnoses
A. Wart
   1. Verruca vulgaris
   2. Verruca filiformis
   3. Verruca plana
   4. Verruca plantaris
B. Seborrheic keratosis
C. Callus
D. Molluscum contagiosum: Flesh-colored group of firm papules found on the face, trunk, and/or extremities. A white core may be expressed from the lesion. Lesion may be successfully removed by curettage or cryotherapy.

Plan
A. General interventions
   1. Identify the type of wart.
   2. Conservative treatment is recommended for children.
B. Patient teaching: *See Section III: Patient Teaching Guide for this chapter, "Warts."* ◀
C. Pharmaceutical therapy
   1. Common wart: After soaking and filing wart with a nail file, apply one of these:
      a. Salicylic acid 17% (Compound W) gel twice daily for up to 12 weeks, if needed. Keep site covered with adhesive.

b. Apply duct tape to site after treatment. Repeat this treatment every night for up to 12 weeks or until resolved.
c. Cryotherapy with liquid nitrogen to site. Repeat every 3 to 4 weeks until resolved. Apply adhesive tape over site and keep covered.
2. Flat wart or filiform wart
a. Retinoic acid; apply to site twice daily for 4 to 6 weeks.
b. Aldara (imiquimod) 5% cream may be applied by the patient at home. Although the labeled use is for genital warts, the patient may consider off-label use at bedtime and wash off after 6 to 8 hours every other day until resolved. Precautions should be stressed regarding the caustic nature of the cream to healthy skin.
3. Plantar wart: Salicylic acid 40% (Mediplast), apply over wart. Remove in 24 to 48 hours, and remove dead skin with a pumice stone or by scraping or using a nail file. Repeat every 24 to 48 hours until wart is removed. May take up to 6 to 8 weeks.
4. Educate the patient to throw away the emory board nail file after each use. If using a nail file, after each use, cleanse with alcohol.

Follow-Up
A. Follow the patient every 4 to 6 weeks until resolved.

Consultation/Referral
A. If diagnosis is unclear, refer the patient to a dermatologist for surgical excision and biopsy.

Individual Consideration
A. Pediatrics: Warts are commonly seen in young school-aged children.

Wound Care

Lower Extremity Ulcer

Amy C. Bruggemann

Definition
A. Vascular ulcer
1. Arterial/ischemic ulcer
a. Skin ulcers usually found on the medial or lateral foot or ankle; ulcers are nonhealing because of inadequate arterial flow.
2. Venous ulcer
a. Chronic skin and subcutaneous lesions are usually found on the lower extremity between the ankle and knee, thought to occur from intracellular edema or inflammatory processes.
B. Diabetic foot ulcer
1. Skin ulcers are usually found on the plantar surface of the foot, most commonly occurring from trauma or plantar pressure.

Incidence
A. Diabetic foot ulcers precede more than 80% of lower extremity amputations in the United States.
B. The financial burden of venous ulcers is estimated to be $2 billion per year in the United States.
C. Up to 20% of lower extremity ulcers have been shown to have mixed etiology disease.

Pathogenesis
A. An ulcer that is found between the knees and toes constitutes a lower extremity ulcer, and guidelines are based according to the etiology. The thing to remember with lower extremity ulcers is that they may have more than one cause. The most common etiologies are venous insufficiency, arterial insufficiency, diabetic foot ulcer, and/or pressure of time.

Predisposing Factors
A. Arterial insufficiency
B. Congestive heart failure
C. Coronary artery disease
D. Diabetes
E. Edema
F. Hyperlipidemia
G. Obesity
H. Age: Older than 65 years
I. Venous insufficiency
J. Peripheral neuropathy

Common Complaints
A. Lower extremity or foot pain
B. Bleeding
C. Drainage
D. Hyperglycemia

Subjective Data
A. Ask the patient to describe the location and onset. What does he or she think may have been the cause? Was the onset sudden or gradual? How have the symptoms continued to develop?
B. Assess if the area is itchy or painful. Does the patient feel the area?
C. Assess for any associated drainage. Ask about the color and if any odor is noted.
D. Complete a drug history. Ask the patient if he or she is taking any steroids or anticoagulants.
E. Has the patient been treated in this location location before? If so, describe.
F. Determine whether the patient has attempted to treat this at home. If yes, with what?
G. Does the patient have any numbness or tingling in the lower extremities? Does the patient wake up at night with pain? Does he or she have any pain with ambulation? Does he or she have sensation in the feet?
H. Rule out any possible exposure to industrial or domestic toxins, or insect bites.
I. Assess for iodine and sulfa allergies before starting treatment.

Physical Examination
A. Check temperature, pulse, respiration, and blood pressure.
B. Inspect
1. Assess the lower extremities, feet, and toes.
a. Color of the skin:
i. Assess skin; begin at the top of the legs, move down the legs to the toes looking for changes in color that may exhibit signs of ischemia.

ii. Hemosiderin staining may exhibit venous insufficiency.

2. Inspect the ulcer.
   a. Measure length × width × depth:
      i. Undermining: Measure and note location, using the face of a clock to document the site of undermining: 12 o'clock, 3 o'clock, 6 o'clock, or 9 o'clock.
      ii. Tunneling: Measure and note the location, using the face of a clock to document the site of tunneling: 12 o'clock, 3 o'clock, 6 o'clock, or 9 o'clock.
   b. Describe the wound bed.
      i. Tissue in the wound bed
         1) Necrotic tissue, granulation tissue, or epithelial tissue
      ii. Color of the tissue (percentage to equal 100%, i.e., 80% pink, 20% yellow)
         1) Red, pink, yellow, brown, tan, or black
      iii. Drainage
         1) Amount
            a) None, scant, moderate, or copious
         2) Color
            a) Serous, sanguineous, purulent, yellow, serosanguineous, or green
      iv. Odor
      v. Periwound
         1) Intact
         2) Not intact
            a) Describe periwound: Note erythema, fever, induration, maceration, excoriation, calloused, or epiboly

C. Palpate
   1. Note temperature of the skin.
   2. Assess sensation of the skin.
   3. Check capillary refill.
   4. Assess pulses in bilateral extremities.

Diagnostic Tests

A. Ankle brachial index (ABI)
B. Arterial Doppler
C. Bone scan
D. CBC
E. Hemoglobin A1c (Hgb A1c)
F. MRI
G. Wound culture
H. Wound biopsy
I. Venous Doppler
J. X-ray

Differential Diagnoses

A. Vascular ulcer
   1. Arterial/ischemic ulcer
   2. Venous ulcer
B. Diabetic foot ulcer
C. Abscess
D. Atypical ulcers
E. Dermatological disorder
F. Necrotizing fasciitis
G. Skin cancers
H. Pressure ulcer
I. Trauma
J. Pyoderma gangrenosum

Plan

General Interventions

A. Vascular ulcers
   1. Arterial ulcer
      a. Refer to vascular surgery for assessment to improve arterial flow.
      b. Refer to wound care specialist.
   2. Venous ulcer
      a. Establish arterial flow.
         i. Refer to vascular surgeon if deficiency found.
      b. For signs and symptoms of infection, treat the infection first with tissue culture and sensitivity. Treat per pharmaceutical recommendations. Treat with silver alginate to the site for moderate drainage and silver gel to the site for scant drainage.
      c. Once arterial flow has been established as sufficient and infection has been ruled out, compression therapy is the mainstay of treatment for venous ulcers. Compression therapy recommendations:
         i. ABI: 0.8 to 1.0 full compression
            1) Pro-fore
               a) Change in 3 days; if tolerating, then change weekly.
         ii. ABI: 0.6 to 0.8 Light compression
            1) Pro-fore lite
            2) Apply calcium alginate to ulcer, then wrap with a Unna Boot, and then cover with a coban wrap.
               a) Change in 3 days; if tolerating well, then change weekly.

B. Diabetic foot ulcer
   1. Establish arterial flow.
      a. Refer to a vascular surgeon if deficiency found.
   2. For signs and symptoms of infection, use a sterile culturette to obtain a tissue culture and sensitivity first to assess what organism is present and to determine sensitivities. Treat per pharmaceutical recommendations. Treat with silver alginate to the site for moderate drainage, and silver gel to the site for scant drainage.
   3. Initiate offloading to site.
      a. Refer to an orthotist for assessment if devices are required.
   4. Treatment options
      a. To debride: Cleanse with normal saline (NS), apply Santyl, and change dressing daily and as needed.
      b. To granulate an ulcer with scant drainage: Cleanse with NS, apply hydrogel, and change dressing daily and as needed.
      c. To granulate an ulcer with moderate drainage: Cleanse with NS, apply calcium alginate, and change dressing daily as needed.

C. Patient teaching
1. *See Section III: Patient Teaching Guide for this chapter, "Wound Care: Lower Extremity Ulcers."*

D. Pharmaceutical therapy
1. If culture and sensitivity are performed, antibiotics may be used as recommended per sensitivity.

Follow-Up

A. Follow up in 1 to 2 weeks to evaluate therapy.

B. See patients every 1 to 2 weeks until healing well; then patient may reduce to 2- to 4-week evaluation until complete closure.

Consultation/Referral

A. Consult or refer the patient to a wound care specialist when the patient has:
1. Extensive ulcer that you are not comfortable with
   a. Visible bone, muscle, or tendon
2. Multiple medical comorbidities (especially diabetes)
3. Not responded to treatment of 2 to 4 weeks
4. Ulcer showing decline on follow-up visit
5. Infection present

Individual Considerations

A. Adults
1. Ischemic ulcers warrant immediate referral
2. Complaints of severe pain, lack of pulse, cool digit, or new onset of purplish/bluish discolorations to the feet require immediate workup for arterial clot to lower extremity.

Pressure Ulcers

Amy C. Bruggemann

Definition

A. "A pressure ulcer is localized damage to the skin and/or underlying soft tissue, usually over a bony prominence, or related to a medical or other device. The injury can present as intact skin or related to a medical or other device. The injury occurs as a result of intense pressure in combination with shear. The tolerance of soft tissue for pressure and shear may also be affected by microclimate, nutrition, perfusion, comorbidities and condition of the soft tissue" (Diagnosis; used with permission from the National Pressure Ulcer Advisory Panel [NPUAP], 2016).

Incidence

A. Acute care: 0.4% to 38%

B. Long-term care: 2.2% to 23.9%

C. Home care: 0% to 17%

Pathogenesis

A. Pressure ulcers occur when an area of tissue remains in surface contact for a period of time. This contact causes occlusion of microvascular vessels, which leads to tissue hypoxia and eventually may cause ischemia. Over time, a pressure ulcer develops. The amount of time this takes is patient dependent and can be altered by physical and/or environmental factors of time.

Predisposing Factors

A. Acute illness

B. Fecal/urinary incontinence

C. Malnutrition

D. Weight loss

E. Failure or inability to offload
1. For example, fracture, elevation of head of bed (HOB), lack of education, or noncompliance

Common Complaints

A. Pain

B. Bleeding

Subjective Data

A. Ask the patient to describe the location and onset. What did he or she think may have been the cause? Was the onset sudden or gradual? How have the symptoms continued to develop?

B. Assess if the area is itchy or painful.

C. Assess for any associated drainage. Ask about the color and if any odor is noted.

D. Complete a drug history. Ask the patient if he or she is taking any steroids or anticoagulants.

E. Has the patient been treated in this location before? If so, describe.

F. Determine whether the patient has attempted to treat this problem at home. If yes, ask with what.

G. Rule out any possible exposure to industrial or domestic toxins, or insect bites.

H. Assess for iodine and sulfa allergies before starting treatment.

Physical Examination

A. Check temperature, pulse, respirations, and blood pressure.

B. Inspect the pressure ulcer.
1. Measure length × width × depth.
   a. Undermining: Measure and note location, using the face of a clock to document the site of undermining: 12 o'clock, 3 o'clock, 6 o'clock, or 9 o'clock. Undermining is documented as from one time to another.
   b. Tunneling: Measure and note location, using the face of a clock to document the site of tunneling. Tunneling is documented at one point of time per the clock face
2. Describe the wound bed:
   a. Tissue in the wound bed
      i. Necrotic tissue, slough tissue, granulation tissue, or epithelial tissue
   b. Color of the tissue (percentage to equal 100%, i.e., 80% pink, 20% yellow):
      i. Red, pink, yellow, brown, tan, or black
   c. Drainage
      i. Amount
         1) None, scant, moderate, or copious
      ii. Color
         1) Serous, sanguineous, purulent, yellow, serosanguineous, or green
   d. Odor
   e. Periwound
      i. Intact

ii. Not intact
1) Erythema, fever, induration, maceration, excoriation, calloused, or epiboly

Diagnostic Tests

A. CBC
B. Wound culture
C. Wound biopsy
D. X-ray
E. MRI
F. Bone scan

Diagnosis

A. Stage 1: Pressure injury—Nonblanchable erythema of intact skin
1. Definition: Intact skin with localized area of nonblanchable erythema, which may appear differently in darkly pigmented skin. Presence of blanchable erythema or changes in sensation, temperature, or firmness may precede visual changes. Color changes do not include purple or maroon discoloration; these may indicate deep tissue injury.
B. Stage 2: Pressure injury—Partial-thickness skin with exposed dermis
1. Definition: Partial-thickness loss of skin with exposed dermis. The wound bed is visible, pink or red, moist, and may also present as an intact or ruptured serum-filled blister. Adipose (fat) is not visible and deeper tissues are not visible. Granulation tissue, slough, and eschar are not present. These injuries commonly result from adverse microclimate and shear in the skin over the pelvis and shear in the heel. This stage should not be used to describe moisture-associated skin damage (MASD) including incontinence-associated dermatitis (IAD), intertriginous dermatitis (ITD), medical adhesive-related skin injury (MARSI), or traumatic wounds (skin tears, burns, abrasions).
C. Stage 3: Pressure injury—Full-thickness skin loss
1. Definition: Full-thickness loss of skin, in which adipose (fat) is visible in the ulcer and granulation tissue and epibole (rolled wound edges) are often present. Slough and/or eschar may be visible. The depth of tissue damage varies by anatomical location; areas of significant adiposity can develop deep wounds. Undermining and tunneling may occur. Fascia, muscle, tendon, ligament, cartilage, and/or bone are not exposed. If slough or eschar obscures the extent of tissue loss, this is an unstageable pressure injury.
D. Stage 4: Pressure injury—Full-thickness skin and tissue loss
1. Definition: Full-thickness skin and tissue loss with exposed or directly palpable fascia, muscle, tendon, ligament, cartilage, or bone in the ulcer. Slough and/or eschar may be visible. Epibole (rolled edges), undermining, and/or tunneling often occur. Depth varies by anatomical location. If slough or eschar obscures the extent of tissue loss, this is an unstageable pressure injury.
E. Unstageable pressure injury: Obscured full-thickness skin and tissue loss
1. Definition: Full-thickness skin and tissue loss in which the extent of tissue damage within the ulcer cannot be confirmed because it is obscured by slough or eschar. If slough or eschar is removed, a Stage 3 or Stage 4 pressure injury will be revealed. Stable eschar (i.e., dry, adherent, intact without erythema, or fluctuance) on an ischemic limb or the heel(s) should not be removed.
F. Deep tissue pressure injury (DTPI): Persistent nonblanchable deep-red, maroon, or purple discoloration
1. Definition: Intact or nonintact skin with localized area of persistent nonblanchable deep-red, maroon, purple discoloration, or epidermal separation revealing a dark wound bed or blood-filled blister. Pain and temperature change of skin precede skin color changes. Discoloration may appear differently in darkly pigmented skin. This injury results from intense and/or prolonged pressure and shear forces at the bone–muscle interface. The wound may evolve rapidly to reveal the actual extent of tissue injury, or may resolve without tissue loss. If necrotic tissue, subcutaneous tissue, granulation tissue, fascia, muscle, or other underlying structures are visible, this indicates a full-thickness pressure injury (unstageable, Stage 3, or Stage 4). Do not use DTPI to describe vascular, traumatic, neuropathic, or dermatologic conditions.
H. Additional pressure injury definitions: This describes an etiology. Use the staging system to stage:
1. Medical device–related pressure injury: This describes the etiology of the injury. Medical device-related pressure injuries result from the use of devices designed and applied for diagnostic or therapeutic purposes. The resultant pressure injury generally conforms to the pattern or shape of the device. The injury should be staged using the staging system.
2. Mucosal membrane pressure injury: Mucosal membrane pressure injury is found on mucous membranes with a history of a medical device in use at the location of the injury. Due to the anatomy of the tissue, these injuries cannot be staged.

Differential Diagnoses

A. Abscess
B. Trauma
C. Skin cancer
D. Vascular ulcer
E. Diabetic foot ulcers
F. Dermatological disorder
G. Venous ulcer

Plan

A. General interventions
1. Identify the cause of pressure and alleviate.
2. Steps taken to debride ulcer: Cleanse with normal saline (NS), apply Santyl, and change dressing daily and as needed.

3. Steps taken to granulate an ulcer with scant drainage: Cleanse with NS, apply hydrogel, and change dressing daily and as needed.
4. Steps taken to granulate an ulcer with moderate drainage: Cleanse with NS, apply calcium alginate, and change dressing daily as needed.

B. Patient teaching
1. Educate patient and family regarding the treatment plans for the pressure ulcer.
2. Stress importance of alleviating pressure to the site. Depending on location of the ulcer, provide suggestions to alleviate/offload pressure to the area.

C. Pharmaceutical therapy
1. Unless bacterial infection is present, oral antibiotics are not indicated with initial wound treatment.

Follow-Up

A. Follow up in 1 to 2 weeks to evaluate therapy.
B. See patients every 1 to 2 weeks until healing well; then patient may reduce to 2- to 4-week evaluation until complete closure.

Consultation/Referral

A. Consult or refer the patient to a wound care specialist for the following:
1. Extensive ulcer that you are not comfortable treating
2. Patient with multiple medical comorbidities (especially diabetes)
3. Patient not responding to treatment of 2 to 4 weeks
4. Ulcer showing decline on follow-up visit
5. Infection present needing alternative treatment

Individual Consideration

A. Adults
1. Patients at end-of-life may develop pressure ulcers related to the dying process, referred to as Kennedy terminal ulcers. These patients are treated for comfort.

Wounds of the Skin

Jill C. Cash and Amy C. Bruggemann

Definition

A. Wounds are breaks in the external surface of the body.

Pathogenesis

A. Wounds can be caused by any one of the innumerable objects that breach the skin. Lacerations and abrasions typically heal by a three-stage process of clotting, inflammation, and skin cell proliferation. The most common pathogens of wound infections are *Staphylococcus aureus* and beta-hemolytic streptococcus.

Predisposing Factors

A. Exposure to accidental or intentional injury
B. Accident prevention failure
C. High-risk behaviors
D. Conditions that predispose to poor wound healing
1. Diabetes
2. Corticosteroid therapy
3. Immunodeficiency
4. Advanced age
5. Undernourishment

Common Complaints

A. Bleeding
B. Pain
C. “Cut” in the skin integrity

Other Signs and Symptoms

A. Signs and symptoms of infection: Deep wounds and dirty wounds have increased risk for infection.
B. Soft-tissue damage: Wounds with tissue necrosis have increased risk for infection.

Subjective Data

A. Elicit the patient’s description of how the wound occurred, including where and when the injury was sustained.
B. Ascertain how much time elapsed until treatment. If 6 hours have elapsed, bacterial multiplication is likely.
C. Ask if the patient is currently immunized for tetanus.
D. Complete a drug history; include any allergies to medications, anesthetics, or dressings.
E. Ask if the patient is taking any medications, especially steroids, or anticoagulants.
F. Assess iodine and sulfa drug allergies before starting treatment.
G. Review with the patient whether anything significant in the past medical history may interfere with the healing process (e.g., immunodeficiency, diabetes, etc.).

Physical Examination

A. Check temperature, pulse, respirations, and blood pressure.
B. Inspect
1. Inspect wound.
2. Measure wound for size: Length, width, and depth. Wounds with untidy edges may heal more slowly and with disfigurement.
3. Assess underlying bony structures.
4. Inspect for foreign objects.

C. Palpate
1. Palpate extremities for neurovascular function and sensation.
2. Palpate tissue distal to wound.
3. Palpate lymph nodes surrounding injured area.

D. Neurologic examination: Assess motor function distal to wound.

Diagnostic Tests

A. Culture wound site if suspicious of infection.
B. Take x-ray films for deep or crushing wounds.

Differential Diagnoses

A. Wound, minor
B. Nonaccidental self-inflicted injury
C. Self-inflicted injury
D. Domestic violence

Plan

A. General interventions
1. Wounds that require open-wound management
a. Abrasions and superficial lacerations
b. Wounds with great amount of tissue damage
c. Wounds more than 6 hours old
d. Contaminated wounds
e. Large area of superficial skin denudation
f. Puncture wounds
2. For wounds that do not require sutures:
a. Cleanse wound well with normal saline (NS); remove all dirt and foreign bodies.
b. Forceful irrigation may be needed; use fine-pore sponge (Optipore) with a surfactant such as poloxamer 188 (Shur-Clens). If wound edges easily approximate, apply Steri-Strips.
c. Dry, sterile dressings (Telfa, Duoderm, or Opsite) may be used.
3. If inflammation is present, soak and wash for 15 to 20 minutes three to four times per day. Cover with clean, dry dressing. **Do not use Steri-Strips.**
4. For wounds that require sutures:
a. Irrigate with sterile saline solution.
b. Anesthetize with 1% to 2% lidocaine (Xylocaine). Do not use solution with epinephrine at fingertips, nose, or ears. Probe wound for any remaining foreign bodies. Approximate wound edges.
c. Suture with technique appropriate to site:
i. Skin sutures: Nonabsorbable material (e.g., nylon, Prolene, or silk)
ii. Subcutaneous and mucosal sutures: Absorbable material (e.g., Dexon, Vicryl, or plain or chromic gut)
iii. Extremities: 4-0 nylon
iv. Soles of feet: 2-–0 nylon
d. Cover with clean, dry dressing; change after first 24 hours.
e. Suture removal is based on location:
i. Head and trunk: 5 to 7 days
ii. Extremities: 7 to 10 days
iii. Soles and palms: 7 to 10 days
iv. Distal extremities: 10 to 14 days
f. Tetanus prophylaxis (see Chapter 1, Health Maintenance Guidelines)

▶ B. Patient teaching: *See Section III: Patient Teaching Guide for this chapter, "Wound Care: Pressure Ulcers."*

C. Pharmaceutical therapy
1. Control pain with acetaminophen (Tylenol) as needed.
2. Topical antibiotic ointments: Bacitracin and mupirocin
3. Oral antibiotics for prophylaxis
a. Amoxicillin, clavulanic acid (Augmentin)
i. Adolescents: 250 to 500 mg twice daily
ii. Children: 25 to 45 mg/kg/d twice daily for 7 to 10 days; available as 200 mg/5 mL or 400 mg/5 mL liquid
b. With penicillin allergy, use erythromycin
i. Adolescents: (E-Mycin) 250 mg four times daily for 7 to 10 days
ii. Children: (Eryped) 30 to 60 mg/kg/d four times daily for 7 to 10 days; available as 200 mg/5 mL or 400 mg/5 mL liquid.
4. Other alternatives: Cephalexin (Keflex), cefadroxil (Duricef), ciprofloxacin
5. Tetanus toxoid 0.5 mL by intramuscular (IM) injection in deltoid, if no booster has been administered in the last 5 years

Follow-Up

A. Have the patient return for evaluation and dressing change in 24 to 48 hours.

Consultation/Referral

Refer the patient to a physician for wounds of the type listed here.

A. Facial wounds
B. Subcutaneous tissue penetration
C. Functional disturbance of tendons, ligaments, vessels, or nerves
D. Grossly contaminated wounds
E. Wounds requiring hospitalization or aggressive antimicrobial therapy for evidence of pyogenic abscess, cellulitis, and ascending lymphangitis
F. Wounds diagnosed with methicillin-resistant *S. aureus* should be treated with the following oral antibiotics: Trimethoprim sulfamethoxazole (Bactrim), minocycline or doxycycline, clindamycin, rifampin (should be used in combination with one of the previous antibiotics), and linezolid. Antibiotics that are not recommended because of high resistance include: Beta lactams, fluoroquinolones, dicloxacillin, and cephalexin. Treating the nares with Bactroban ointment twice a day and having the patient use Hibiclens soap for showering will help to prevent recurrent infections. For severe cases of infection, the patient requires hospitalization for aggressive antibiotic treatment.

Individual Consideration

A. Adults with chronic conditions, such as diabetes or immune deficiency, should be monitored closely for infection and delayed wound healing.

Xerosis (Winter Itch)

Jill C. Cash and Amy C. Bruggemann

Definition

A. Xerosis, often called "winter itch," is dry skin.

Incidence

A. Xerosis occurs in 48% to 98% of patients with atopic dermatitis.
B. It occurs more frequently in elderly patients.

Pathogenesis

A. Dry skin may fissure, appear shiny and cracked, and leave subsequent inflammatory changes.

Predisposing Factors

A. Frequent bathing with hot water and harsh soaps
B. Cold air
C. Low humidity
D. Central heating or cooling
E. Alcohol use
F. Poor nutrition
G. Cholesterol-lowering drugs
H. Systemic disease manifested by thyroid, renal, or hepatic disease; anemia; diabetes; or malignancy

Common Complaint

A. Dry, rough skin, especially on legs

Other Signs and Symptoms

A. Pruritic, scaling skin, particularly on legs, with cracks and/or fissures
B. Pruritus may be associated with systematic disorders or other infections. **Itching of scabies is particularly intense at night.**
C. Plaques 2 to 5 cm in diameter
D. Erythema
E. Wheal-and-flare response typical of urticaria

Subjective Data

A. Obtain the patient's description of the onset of symptoms and whether it was sudden or gradual.
B. Ask the patient to identify any discomfort. Ask if the skin is itchy or painful.
C. Assess lesions for any associated discharge (blood or pus).
D. Determine whether the patient has recently ingested any new medicines (antibiotics, cholesterol-lowering medications, or other drugs), alcohol, or new foods.
E. Ask the patient about use of any topical medications.
F. Identify any preceding systemic symptoms (fever, sore throat, anorexia, or vaginal discharge).
G. Ask the patient about bathing in hot water and if patient is bathing regularly.
H. Review the patient's full medication history for comorbid conditions.

Physical Examination

A. Inspect: Inspect skin for lesions, noting texture of skin.
B. Palpate
   1. Palpate abdomen for masses and hepatosplenomegaly.
   2. Palpate lymph nodes.

Diagnostic Test

A. There are no diagnostic tests for xerosis.

Differential Diagnoses

A. Xerosis
B. Scabies
C. Atopic dermatitis

Plan

A. General interventions
   1. Hydrate and lubricate the skin.
   2. Assess for and treat secondary infection.

B. Patient teaching
   1. *See Section III: Patient Teaching Guide for this chapter, "Xerosis (Winter Itch)."*
   2. Avoid alkaline soaps: Use Dove, Basis, mild soap, or soap substitute such as Cetaphil or Aquanil.

C. Pharmaceutical therapy
   1. Apply emollient cream or lotion (Sarna, Lac-Hydrin, or Eucerin).
   2. Use over-the-counter (OTC) skin lubricants (petroleum jelly, mineral oil, or cold cream).
   3. Topical corticosteroid
      a. Triamcinolone 0.025% two to four times daily or 0.1% two to three times daily; apply sparingly.
      b. Hydrocortisone 1% or 2.5% two to four times daily; apply thin film, avoid face.
   4. Systemic antihistamine is used to control pruritus, such as diphenhydramine (Benadryl) 25 to 50 mg every 4 to 6 hours as needed

Follow-Up

A. Follow up as indicated until resolved.

Consultation/Referral

A. Consult or refer the patient to a dermatologist if no improvement is seen.

Individual Considerations

A. Pediatrics: Avoid corticosteroid preparation or use low-potency corticosteroid only.
B. Geriatrics: Monitor the patient for possible skin breakdown and/or ulceration.

Bibliography

Aziz, H., Rhee, P., Pandit, V., Tang, A., Gries, L., & Joseph, B. (2015). The current concepts in management of animal (dog, cat, snake, scorpion) and human bite wounds. *Journal of Trauma and Acute Care Surgery, 78*(3), 641–648.

Baranoski, S., & Ayello, E. (2015). *Wound care essentials: Practice principle.* Philadelphia, PA: Lippincott Williams, and Wilkins.

Blereau, R. P. (2012). Acneiform folliculitis. *Consultant* (00107069), *52*(6), 469.

Brackenbury, J. (2016). Recommended topical treatments for managing adult acne in women. *Nurse Prescribing, 14*(3), 126–129.

Centers for Disease Control and Prevention. (2013). Genital herpes—CDC fact sheet. Retrieved from https://www.cdc.gov/std/herpes/STDFact-Herpes.htm

Centers for Disease Control and Prevention. (2016, August 19). Shingles (herpes zoster). Retrieved from https://www.cdc.gov/shingles

Clancy, C. J., & Nguyen, M. H. (2012). The end of an era in defining the optimal treatment of invasive candidiasis. *Clinical Infectious Diseases, 54*(8), 1123–1125.

Collins, L., & Seraj, S. (2010). Diagnosis and treatment of venous ulcers. *American Family Physician, 81*(8), 989–996.

Derby, R., Rohal, P., Jackson, C., Beutler, A., & Olsen, C. (2011). Novel treatment of onychomycosis using over-the-counter mentholated ointment: A clinical case series. *Journal of the American Board of Family Medicine, 24*(1), 69–74.

Eichenfield, L. F., Tom, W. L., Berger, T. G., Krol, A., Paller, A. S., Schwarzenberger, K., . . . Sidbury, R. (2014). Guidelines of care for the management of atopic dermatitis: Section 2. Management and treatment of atopic dermatitis with topical therapies. *Journal of the American Academy of Dermatology, 71*(1), 116–132.

Ellis, R., & Ellis, C. (2014). Dog and cat bites. *American Family Physician, 90*(4), 239–243.

Ely, J. W., Rosenfeld, S., & Seabury Stone, M. (2014). Diagnosis and management of tinea infections. *American Family Physician, 90*(10), 702–710.

Gagliardi, A. M. Z., Andriolo, B. N. G., Torloni, M. R., & Soares, B. G. O. (2016). Vaccines for preventing herpes zoster in older adults. *Cochrane Database of Systematic Reviews, 2016*(3). doi/:10.1002/14651858. CD008858.pub3

Gaston, R., & Lewis, D. R. (2010). Animal bites to the hand. *Current Orthopaedic Practice, 21*(6), 559–563.

Gunning, K., Pippitt, K., Kiraly, B., & Sayler, M. (2012). Pediculosis and scabies: Treatment update. *American Family Physician, 86*(6), 535–541.

Habif, T. P. (Ed.). (2011). *Skin disease diagnosis and treatment* (3rd ed.). Philadelphia, PA: Saunders Elsevier.

Hartman-Adams, H., Banvard, C., & Juckett, G. (2014). Impetigo: Diagnosis and treatment. *American Family Physician, 90*(4), 229–235.

Iavazzo, C., Gkegkes, I. D., Zarkada, I. M., & Falagas, M. E. (2011). Boric acid for recurrent vulvovaginal candidiasis: The clinical evidence. *Journal of Women's Health (2002), 20*(8), 1245–1255.

Kennedy, K. (2016). *Understanding the Kennedy terminal ulcer.* Retrieved from http:// www.kennedyterminalulcer.com

Martinez-Diaz, G., & Mancini, A. (2010). CNE series. Head lice: Diagnosis and therapy. *Dermatology Nursing, 22*(4), 2–8.

Monroe, J. (2012). Papules and plaques from head to foot. *Journal of the American Academy of Physician Assistants, 25*(9), 16.

Moore, S. J., Mordue Luntz, A. J., & Logan, J. G. (2012). Insect bite prevention. *Infectious Disease Clinics of North America, 26*(3), 655–673.

Mounsey, K. E., & McCarthy, J. S. (2013). Treatment and control of scabies. *Current Opinion in Infectious Diseases, 26*(2), 133–139.

National Clearing House Guidelines. (2001). *Guidelines of care for the management of primary cutaneous melanoma* (revised 2011 November) NGC:009038. Rockville, MD: American Academy of Dermatology-Medical Specialty Society.

National Pressure Ulcer Advisory Panel. (2016, April 13). Pressure injury staging. Retrieved from http://www.npuap.org/resources/educational-and-clinical-resources/npuap-pressure-injury-stages

National Pressure Ulcer Advisory Panel and European Pressure Ulcer Advisory Panel. (2009). *Prevention and treatment of pressure ulcers; clinical practice guideline.* Washington, DC: Author.

Nutten, S. (2015). Atopic dermatitis: Global epidemiology and risk factors. *Annals of Nutrition & Metabolism, 66*(Suppl. 1), 8–16.

Oge, L. K., Muncie, L. H., & Phillips, A. R. (2015). Rosacea: Diagnosis and treatment. *American Family Physician, 92*(3) 187–196.

Plaza, J. A., & Prieto, V. G. (2013). Erythema multiforme. *Medscape* Retrieved from http://emedicine.medscape.com/article/1122915-overview

Radley, K. (2015). The management and treatment of acnes. *Primary Health Care, 25*(4), 34–41.

Reddy, M., Gill, S. S., & Rochon, P. A. (2006). Preventing pressure ulcers: A systematic review. *The Journal of the American Medical Association, 296*(8), 974–984.

Rubenstein, R., & Malerich, S. (2014). Malassezia (pityrosporum) folliculitis. *Journal of Clinical Aesthetic Dermatology,* 7(4), 37–41.

Sankararaman, S., & Velayuthan, S. (2014). Multiple recurrences in pityriasis rosea—A case report with review of the literature. *Indian Journal of Dermatology, 59*(3), 316.

Selden, S. (2012). Seborrheic dermatitis. *Medscape.* Retrieved from http://emedicine.medscape.com/article/1108312-overview

Shah, J., Sheffield, P., & Fife, C. (2011). *Wound care certification: Study guide.* Flagstaff, AZ: Best Publishing.

Sokumbi, O., & Wetter, D. A. (2012). Clinical features, diagnosis, and treatment of erythema multiforme: A review for the practicing dermatologist. *International Journal of Dermatology, 51*(8), 889–902.

Thakral, G., La Fontaine, J., Kim, P., Najafi, B., Nichols, A., & Lavery, L. A. (2015). Treatment options for venous leg ulcers: Effectiveness of vascular surgery, bioengineered tissue, and electrical stimulation. *Advances in Skin & Wound Care, 28*(4), 164–172.

Thompson, D. L., & Thompson, M. J. (2014). Knowledge, instruction and behavioural change: Building a framework for effective eczema education in clinical practice. *Journal of Advanced Nursing, 70*(11), 2483–2494.

Titus, S., & Hodge, J. (2012). Diagnosis and treatment of acne. *American Family Physician, 86*(8), 734–740.

Van Onselen, J. (2012). Rosacea: Symptoms and support. *British Journal of Nursing (Mark Allen Publishing), 21*(21), 1252–1255.

Vandiver, A., & Cohe, B. A. (2016). Vesicular rash in an infant with eczema. *Contemporary Pediatrics, 33*(6), 38–40.

Watkins, J. (2010). Treating shingles (herpes zoster) in the older person. *British Journal of Community Nursing, 15*(9), 420, 422, 424 passim.

Watkins, J. (2011). Eczema diagnosis and management in the community. *British Journal of Community Nursing, 16*(9), 418, 420, 422.

Watkins, J. (2012). Problems with acne vulgaris in adolescence. *Practice Nursing, 23*(11), 562–565.

Weigle, N., & McBane, S. (2013). Psoriasis. *American Family Physician, 87*(9), 626–633.

Williams, H. C., Dellavalle, R. P., & Garner, S. (2012). Acne vulgaris. *Lancet (London, England), 379*(9813), 361–372.

Wilson, J. F. (2011). In the clinic. Herpes zoster. *Annals of Internal Medicine, 154*(5), ITC31–15; quiz ITC316.

Wyndham, M. (2011). Pityriasis rosea. *Practice Nurse, 41*(1), 41.

5 Eye Guidelines

Amblyopia

Jill C. Cash and Nancy Pesta Walsh

Definition

A. Amblyopia is a decrease in the visual acuity of one eye. It is commonly seen in young children and cannot be corrected with either glasses or contact lenses.

Incidence

A. Amblyopia is most commonly diagnosed in children and occurs in approximately 2.5% of the population.
B. Most common cause of childhood vision loss.

Pathogenesis

Amblyopia has numerous causes, including:
A. Congenital defect
B. Develops from a corneal scar or cataract
C. Occurs from an uncorrected high refractive error, which causes visual blurring
D. Develops when each eye has a different refractive error that leads to blurred vision
E. Strabismic amblyopia may also occur due to the loss of vision in the eye that turns inward or outward.

Predisposing Factors

A. One parent with amblyopia
B. Prematurity
C. Small for gestational dates
D. Maternal smoking or alcohol use

Common Complaints

A. Decreased vision—complains of sitting close to the TV, sitting in the front row of a classroom, having trouble seeing the ball in sports, and so on
B. Vision that is not corrected with either glasses or contact lenses
C. Wandering eye and frequent eye squinting

Other Signs and Symptoms

A. Frequent rubbing of the eyes
B. Tired eyes

Subjective Data

A. Elicit the onset of visual changes, noting course of symptoms and severity.
B. Assess for pain or any new injury or trauma to the eye.
C. Inquire about new events or changes in health history, including contact lenses, glasses, illnesses, and cataracts.
D. Review patient and family history of amblyopia.

Physical Examination

A. Inspect eyes
   1. Note extraocular movements (EOMs) of eyes.
   2. Examine sclera, pupil, iris, and fundus.
   3. Examine eyes for red reflex.
B. Assess vision based on age, using LEA SYMBOLS®, Sloan letters, Sloan numerals, Tumbling E, and the HOTV. The Kindergarten Eye Chart and the Snellen chart are less preferred methods, as they do not meet the World Health Organization/Committee on Vision Standards.
C. Visual fields may be assessed with a parent holding the child in his or her lap.

Diagnostic Test

A. None

Differential Diagnoses

A. Amblyopia
B. Organic brain lesion

Plan

A. General interventions
   1. All children need to have a visual examination prior to starting school.
   2. Recommend examination by an ophthalmologist for children with strabismus and for those with a family history of amblyopia.
   3. Measures for refractive correction or patching of the stronger eye are usually performed to encourage the weak eye to develop.
   4. Surgery may be required for abnormal positioning of the eye.

Follow-Up

A. Follow-up with an ophthalmologist.

Consultation/Referral

A. Refer the patient to an ophthalmologist for evaluation and treatment.

Individual Consideration

A. None

Blepharitis

Jill C. Cash and Nancy Pesta Walsh

Definition

A. Blepharitis is dryness and flaking of the eyelashes, resulting from an inflammatory response of the eyelid.

Incidence

A. The exact incidence is not known; however, blepharitis is one of the most commonly seen eye conditions.

Pathogenesis

A. Seborrheic: Excessive shedding of skin cells and blockage of glands
B. *Staphylococcus:* Most common bacteria found, responsible for bacterial infection of lid margin
C. Commonly seen with inadequate flow of oil and mucus into the tear duct

Predisposing Factors

A. Diabetes
B. Candida
C. Seborrheic dermatitis
D. Acne rosacea

Common Complaints

A. Burning and itching
B. Lacrimal tearing
C. Photophobia
D. Recurrent eye infections, styes, or chalazions
E. Dry, flaky secretions on lid margins and eyelashes
F. Dry eyes

Other Signs and Symptoms

A. Seborrheic blepharitis: Lid margin swelling and erythema, flaking, nasolabial erythema, and scaling
B. *Staphylococcus aureus* blepharitis: Erythema/edema, scaling, burning, tearing, itching, and recurrent stye or chalazia
C. Meibomian gland dysfunction: Prominent blood vessels crossing the mucocutaneous junction, frothy discharge along eyelid margin, thick discharge, and chalazion; may have rosacea or seborrheic dermatitis
D. May have dandruff of scalp and eyebrows

Subjective Data

A. Elicit onset and duration of signs and symptoms.
B. Note sensations of itching, burning, or pain in the eye.
C. Ask: What makes signs and symptoms worse? What makes signs and symptoms better?
D. Any change in soaps, creams, lotions, or shampoos?
E. Has the patient had similar signs and symptoms in the past?
F. Note any visual change or pain since the last eye examination.
G. Note contributing factors involved, if present.

Physical Examination

A. Inspection
- **1.** Inspect eyes, noting extraocular movements (EOMs) of eyes.
- **2.** Examine sclera, pupil, iris, and fundus.
- **3.** Examine eyes for red reflex.
- **4.** Note erythema or edema on lid margin; note dryness, scaling, and flakes.
- **5.** Assess vision based on age, using Snellen chart for children older than 3 years.
- **6.** Visual fields may be assessed with a parent holding the child in his or her lap.

Diagnostic Test

A. None

Differential Diagnoses

A. Blepharitis
- **1.** *S. aureus*
- **2.** Seborrheic
- **3.** Meibomian gland dysfunction

B. Conjunctivitis
C. Squamous cell carcinoma
D. Stye
E. Upper respiratory infection
F. Sinusitis

Plan

A. General interventions
- **1.** Assess patient and rule out bacterial infection and vision changes.
- **2.** When examining a child, notify the parent of diagnosis and educate the parent regarding findings.
- **3.** Patients with recurrent blepharitis need further follow-up.

B. Patient teaching
- **1.** Wash eye with antibacterial soap and water. May use gentle baby shampoo.
- **2.** Apply warm compresses to the eye for comfort daily for approximately 10 to 20 minutes.
- **3.** Stop use of contacts until the eye is healed.
- **4.** Encourage good hygiene for prevention of recurrent episodes.

C. Pharmaceutical therapy
- **1.** Apply bacitracin or erythromycin ophthalmic ointment to the margin of the eye at bedtime, taking care not to contaminate the medication bottle.
- **2.** Oral antibiotics: Tetracycline 250 mg by mouth, four times a day, or doxycycline 100 mg by mouth, twice a day, tapering after clinical improvement, for a total of 2 to 6 weeks. Alternative: Erythromycin 250 to 500 mg daily or azithromycin 250 to 500 mg one to three times a week for 3 weeks.
- **3.** Consider long-term treatment with doxycycline, if infections reoccur.

Follow-Up

A. Recommend follow-up with a primary provider in 1 to 2 weeks.
B. Consider referral to an eye specialist for recurrent episodes of blepharitis and for slit-lamp examination.

Individual Considerations

A. Pediatrics: Tetracycline is not recommended for children younger than 8 years.

B. Pregnant or lactating women: Tetracycline is not recommended.
C. Azithromycin may lead to abnormalities of heart electrical rhythm; use with caution in patients with a high risk of cardiovascular disease.

Cataracts

Jill C. Cash and Nancy Pesta Walsh

Definition

A. A cataract, opacity of the crystalline lens of the eye, causes progressive, painless loss of vision (functional impairment). Presenile and senile cataract formation is painless and progresses throughout months and years. Cataracts are frequently associated with intraocular inflammation and glaucoma.

Incidence

A. Cataracts are the most common cause of blindness in the world.
B. Ninety-five percent of people older than 60 years have cataracts without visual disturbance.
C. Fifty percent of people older than 40 years have significant visual loss due to cataracts.

Pathogenesis

A. Age-related changes of the lens of the eye result from protein accumulation, which produces a fibrous thickened lens that obscures vision.

Predisposing Factors

A. Age
B. Trauma
C. Medications (e.g., topical or systemic steroids, major tranquilizers, or some diuretics)
D. Medical diseases (e.g., diabetes mellitus, Wilson's disease, hypoparathyroidism, glaucoma, congenital rubella syndrome, chronic anteri, or uveitis)
E. Chronic exposure to ultraviolet (UV) B light
F. Alcohol use
G. Family history
H. Prior intraocular surgery
I. Obesity
J. Smoking

Common Complaints

A. Decreased vision
B. Blurred or foggy vision, "ghost" images
C. Inability to drive at night

Other Signs and Symptoms

A. Initial visual event can be a shift toward nearsightedness.
B. Visual impairment can be more marked at distances, with abnormal visual acuity examinations.
C. Severe difficulty with glare can occur.
D. Altered color perception may be noticed.
E. Frequent falls or injuries may occur.

Subjective Data

A. Review the onset, course, and duration of visual changes, including altered day or night vision and nearsighted versus farsighted vision.
B. Assess whether involvement is in one or both eyes.
C. Determine what improves vision—use of glasses or use of extra light.
D. Review the patient's medical history and current medications.
E. Review the patient's history for traumatic injury.
F. Discuss the patient's occupation and leisure activities to determine exposure to UV rays.

Physical Examination

A. Inspect
  1. Conduct a funduscopic examination.
    a. Check red reflex and opacity.
      i. A bright red reflex is seen in the normal eye.
      ii. Cataract formation is seen by the disruption of the red reflex.
      iii. Lens opacities appear as dark areas against the background of the red-orange reflex.
    b. Examine color of opacity. For brunescent cataracts, the nucleus acquires a yellow-brown coloration and becomes progressively more opaque.
    c. Check retinal abnormalities, hemorrhage, scarring, and drusen (small yellow deposits).

Diagnostic Tests

A. Perform visual acuity examination.
B. Perform peripheral vision examination.
C. Perform slit-lamp examination to determine the exact location and type of cataract.
D. Dilated eye examination.

Differential Diagnoses

A. Cataracts
B. Glaucoma
C. Age-related macular degeneration (macular degeneration causes vision loss that is symptomatically similar to cataracts)
D. Diabetic retinopathy
E. Temporal arteritis

Plan

A. General interventions
  1. Monitor the patient for increased interference of visual impairment on his or her lifestyle.
  2. Cataracts do not need to be removed unless there is impairment of normal, everyday activities.
  3. Surgery is the definitive treatment; however, modification of glasses may improve vision adequately to defer surgery. Contact lenses are optically superior to glasses.
B. Patient teaching
  1. Prevention is important. Teach the patient to use protective eyewear to prevent trauma.
  2. Use sunglasses to prevent the penetration of UV B rays.
  3. Wear a hat with a visor to protect eyes when outdoors.

Follow-Up

A. Surgical removal is indicated if the visual disturbance is interfering with the patient's life, such as causing falls or prohibiting reading.

Consultation/Referral

A. Refer patient for ophthalmologic consultation.
B. Patients should be followed by an ophthalmologist to monitor the cataract for increased size and progressive visual impairment.
C. Contact a social worker or community resources as needed.

Chalazion

Jill C. Cash and Nancy Pesta Walsh

Definition

A. Chalazion is a chronic lipogranulomatous inflammation of a meibomian gland located in the eyelid margin. Inflammation occurs from occlusion of the ducts.

Incidence

A. Commonly seen, though the incidence is unknown.

Pathogenesis

A. Meibomian glands secrete the oil layer of the tear film that covers the eye. When the glands become blocked, the oil or lipid extrudes into the surrounding tissue, causing the formation of a nodule.

Predisposing Factor

A. Chalazion may occur as a secondary infection of the surrounding tissues.

Common Complaints

A. Swelling, nontender palpable nodule, usually pea-sized, inside lid margin or eye
B. Discomfort or irritation due to swelling

Other Signs and Symptoms

A. Tearing
B. Feeling of a foreign body in the eye
C. If infection is present, the entire lid becomes painfully swollen

Subjective Data

A. Review the onset of symptoms, their course and duration, and any concurrent visual disturbance.
B. Question the patient regarding possible foreign body or trauma to the eye.
C. Elicit the quality of pain or tenderness of the eyelid.
D. Review the past eye problems and the treatment received.

Physical Examination

A. Temperature
B. Inspect
   1. Inspect the eye, sclera, and conjunctiva for a foreign body.
   2. Check for red- or gray-colored subconjunctival mass.
C. Palpate
   1. Palpate the eyelid for masses and tenderness. Usually a hard, nontender nodule is found on the middle portion of the tarsus, away from the lid border; it may develop on the lid margin if the opening of the duct is involved. Some chalazia continue to increase in size and can cause astigmatism by putting pressure on the eye globe.
   2. Chalazia may become acutely tender; however, note the difference between the chalazia and the stye, which is found on the lid margin.
   3. Check for preauricular adenopathy.

Diagnostic Test

A. Perform visual acuity examination.

Differential Diagnoses

A. Chalazion
B. Chronic dacryocystitis
C. Hordeolum (Stye)
D. Blepharitis
E. Xanthelasma
F. Cellulitis of the eyelid

Plan

A. General interventions
   1. Small chalazia, usually, do not require treatment.
   2. Warm, moist compresses may be applied for 15 minutes four times a day.
B. Patient teaching: Instruct patient regarding compresses and handwashing.
C. Pharmaceutical therapy
   1. Sulfacetamide sodium (Sulamyd) ophthalmic ointment 10%, four times daily, for 7 days for bacterial infection
   2. Tobradex ophthalmic drops: 1 to 2 drops every 2 hours for first 24 to 48 hours, then every 4 to 6 hours. Reduce dose as the condition improves. Treat for 5 to 7 days as needed. Not recommended in children younger than 2 years.
   3. Intrachalazion corticosteroid injection is performed by an ophthalmologist.

Follow-Up

A. For large infected chalazia, follow up with patient in 1 week and then evaluate the patient every 2 to 4 weeks.

Consultation/Referral

A. If the chalazion does not resolve spontaneously, incision and curettage by an ophthalmologist may be necessary.

Conjunctivitis

Jill C. Cash and Nancy Pesta Walsh

Definition

A. Conjunctivitis is inflammation of the conjunctiva.

Incidence

A. Viral conjunctivitis is the most common type; conjunctivitis occurs in 1% to 12% of newborns.

Pathogenesis

Primarily three types of conjunctivitis are seen:
A. Bacterial (*Haemophilus influenzae*, *Streptococcus pneumoniae*, *Streptococcus aureus*, *Neisseria gonorrhoeae*, and *Chlamydia*)

B. Viral (adenovirus, coxsackievirus, and enteric cytopathic human orphan [ECHO] viruses)
C. Allergic (seasonal pollens or allergic exposure)

Predisposing Factors

A. Contact with another person with the diagnosis of conjunctivitis
B. Exposure to sexually transmitted infection (STI)
C. Other atopic conditions (allergies)

Common Complaints

A. Red eyes
B. Eye drainage
C. Itching (with allergic conjunctivitis)

Other Signs and Symptoms

A. Bacterial
- **1.** Fast onset, 12 to 24 hours of copious purulent or mucopurulent discharge
- **2.** Burning, stinging, or gritty sensation in eyes
- **3.** Crusted eyelids upon awakening, with swelling of eyelid
- **4.** Usually starts out unilaterally; may progress to bacterial infection
- **5.** Bacterial conjunctivitis may present as beefy red conjunctiva

B. Viral
- **1.** Symptoms may begin in one eye and progress to both eyes
- **2.** Tearing of eyes
- **3.** Sensation of foreign body
- **4.** Systemic symptoms of upper respiratory infection (runny nose, sore throat, sneezing, fever)
- **5.** Preauricular or submandibular lymphadenopathy
- **6.** Photophobia, impaired vision
- **7.** Primary herpetic infection: Vesicular skin lesion, corneal epithelial defect in form of dendrite, uveitis

C. Allergic
- **1.** Itchy, watery eyes, bilateral
- **2.** Seasonal symptoms
- **3.** Edema of eyelids without visual change
- **4.** With allergic conjunctivitis, hyperemia of eyes is always bilateral and giant papillae on tarsa may be seen.
- **5.** May also see eczema, urticaria, and asthma flare

Subjective Data

A. Elicit the onset, duration, and course of symptoms.
B. Question patient regarding the presence of discharge upon awakening.
C. Elicit changes in vision since symptoms began.
D. Determine whether there has been any injury or trauma to the eye.
E. Assess whether these symptoms have appeared before.
F. Rule out exposure to anyone with conjunctivitis.
G. Ask patient about any new events, such as use of contact lenses or change in contact lenses or solutions.
H. Review patient and family history of allergies.

Physical Examination

A. Check temperature.
B. Inspect
- **1.** Observe eyes for color and foreign objects. Perform complete eye examination.
- **2.** Note lid edema.
- **3.** Assess pupillary reflexes.
- **4.** Examine skin.
- **5.** Inspect ears, nose, and throat.

C. Auscultate
- **1.** Auscultate heart and lungs.

D. Palpate
- **1.** Palpate preauricular lymph nodes and anterior and posterior cervical chain lymph nodes.

Diagnostic Tests

A. Gram stain testing for discharge/exudate extracted from eyes if gonococcal infection is suspected and/or all neonates.
B. Culture for chlamydia, if suspected.
C. Perform fluorescein stain of eye if foreign body is suspected or corneal abrasion/ulceration is suspected.
D. Test visual acuity with the Snellen chart. Assess peripheral vision and EOMs.

Differential Diagnoses

A. Conjunctivitis
B. Corneal abrasion
C. Blepharitis
D. Drug-related conjunctivitis
E. Herpetic keratoconjunctivitis
F. Iritis
G. Gonococcal or chlamydial conjunctivitis

Plan

A. General interventions
- **1.** Distinguish among bacterial, allergic, or viral infection.
- **2.** Consider other diagnoses if eye pain is noted.

B. Patient education: *See Section III: Patient Teaching Guide for this chapter, "Eye Medication Administration."* ◀
- **1.** Cool compresses to the affected eye should be applied several times a day.
- **2.** Clean eyes with warm, moist cloth from inner to outer canthus to prevent spreading infection.
- **3.** Encourage good handwashing technique with antibacterial soap.
- **4.** Instruct on the proper method of instilling medication into eye. Give patient the teaching guide on "How to Administer Eye Medications."
- **5.** Instruct the female patient to discard all eye makeup, including mascara, eyeliner, and eye shadow, worn at the time of the infection.
- **6.** Teach the patient/parent the difference among bacterial, allergic, and viral infections. Educate according to appropriate diagnosis.
- **7.** If using aminoglycoside or neomycin ointments or drops, use caution and monitor closely for reactive keratoconjunctivitis.
- **8.** Bacterial conjunctivitis is contagious until 24 hours after beginning medication.
- **9.** Viral conjunctivitis is contagious for 48 to 72 hours, but it may last up to 2 weeks. This is typically self-limiting, and does not require antibiotic treatment.

C. Pharmaceutical therapy

1. Bacterial

a. Aminoglycosides: Gentamicin 0.3%: Severe infections: 2 gtts every hour on day 1, then 1 to 2 gtts every 4 hours for 5 to 7 days. Mild/moderate infections: 1 to 2 gtts every 4 hours for 5 to 7 days

b. Tobramycin 0.3%; severe infections: 2 gtts every hour on day 1, then 1 to 2 gtts four times a day for 5 to 7 days. Mild- to- moderate infections: 1 to 2 gtts four times a day for 5 to 7 days

c. Polymyxin B: Trimethoprim/polymyxin B sulfate (Polytrim) ophthalmic ointment in each eye four times daily for 7 days. Polymyxin B/bacitracin (Polysporin) drops may also be used, 1 gtt every 3 hours for 7 to 10 days

d. Macrolides: Erythromycin (Ilotycin) ophthalmic ointment 0.5% in each eye four times daily for 7 days

e. Fluoroquinolones: Ciprofloxacin 0.3%: 1 to 2 gtts every 2 hours for 2 days, then every 4 hours for 5 days. Moxifloxacin (Vigamox) 0.5% 1 gtt three times a day for 7 days

2. Viral

a. Antiviral medications

i. Trifluridine 1% drops: 1 drop every 2 hours while awake; no more than 9 drops per day. May then alter to 1 drop every 4 hours for 7 days. Not recommended for children younger than 6 years.

ii. Oral antiviral medications (trifluridine, valacyclovir) may be used for herpes simplex keratitis. Herpes zoster ophthalmicus is often treated with acyclovir, famciclovir, or valacyclovir and lessens symptoms if started within 72 hours of onset of symptoms.

3. Allergic

a. Topical antihistamines/mast cell stabilizer

i. Azelastine HCl (Optivar): Not recommended for those younger than 3 years. For those older than 3 years, 1 drop to the affected eye twice a day.

ii. Olopatadine HCl (Pataday) 0.2%: Not recommended for those younger than 3 years. For those older than 3 years, 1 drop to the affected eye daily.

iii. Olopatadine HCl (Patanol) 0.1%: Not recommended for those younger than 3 years. For those older than 3 years, 1 drop twice a day to the affected eye.

b. Mast cell stabilizer

i. Cromolyn sodium (Crolom) ophthalmic solution for children older than 4 years, 1 to 2 drops four to six times daily.

c. Topical nonsteroidal anti-inflammatory drug (NSAID)

i. Ketorolac tromethamine (Acular) 0.5%: Not for use in children younger than 3 years: 1 drop four times a day. This is used for severe symptoms of atopic keratoconjunctivitis.

d. Artificial tears four to five times daily

e. Oral antihistamines may be used in severe cases (loratadine or diphenhydramine HCl).

4. Concurrent conjunctivitis and otitis media should be treated with a systemic antibiotic; no topical eye antibiotic is needed.

Follow-Up

A. If resolution occurs within 5 to 7 days after proper treatment, follow-up is not needed.

B. If patient continues to have symptoms or if different symptoms appear, then follow-up with the primary provider is recommended.

Consultation/Referral

A. Consult or refer patient to a physician if patient is not responding to treatment.

B. Refer if patient is suspected of having periorbital cellulitis.

C. Refer to eye specialist if patient has vision change or eye pain, or is not responding to treatment.

Individual Considerations

A. Pediatrics: In neonates, consider gonococcal and chlamydial conjunctivitis. Perform culture if suspected.

B. Partners: Check partners for gonorrhea and chlamydia when adolescent or adult presents with gonococcal or chlamydial conjunctivitis.

Corneal Abrasion

Jill C. Cash and Nancy Pesta Walsh

Definition

A. A corneal abrasion is the loss of epithelial tissue, either superficial or deep, from trauma to the eye.

Incidence

A. In the United States, approximately 2.4 million eye injuries occur annually.

B. Corneal abrasions account for approximately 10% of new admissions to eye emergency units.

Pathogenesis

A. Trauma occurs to the epithelial tissue of the cornea.

Predisposing Factors

A. Trauma to the eye caused by a human fingernail, tree branches, wood particles, children's toys, and sports injuries

B. A history of surgical trauma, causing globe weakening.

Common Complaints

A. Sudden onset of eye pain

B. Foreign-body sensation in the eye

C. Watery eye

D. Mild photophobia

E. Blurred vision

F. Headache

Other Signs and Symptoms

A. Change in vision

B. Redness, swelling, inability to open the eye

Subjective Data

A. Elicit the onset, duration, and course of symptoms; note any past history of similar symptoms.
B. Question the patient regarding visual changes (blurred, double, or lost vision, or loss of a portion of the visual field).
C. Question the patient regarding the mechanism of injury and how much time has elapsed since the injury (minutes, hours, or days). Ask: What is his or her occupation, and what sports are involved? Were goggles being worn and are they routinely worn during the sport or activity?
D. Review the patient's history of exposure to herpetic outbreaks.
E. Determine the degree of pain, if any; headache; photophobia; redness; itching; or tearing.
F. Ascertain whether the patient wears contact lenses or glasses and for what length of time.
G. Ask if the patient has tried any treatments before presentation to the office. If so, what?
H. Rule out the presence of any other infections, such as sinus infection. **Conjunctival discharge signifies an infectious etiology.**

Physical Examination

A. Vital signs: Temperature
B. Inspect
  1. Observe *both* eyes.
  2. Test visual acuity and pupil reactivity and symmetry.
  3. Observe the corneal surface with direct illumination, noting any shadow on the surface of the iris.
  4. Perform funduscopic examination.
  5. Evert eyelids for cornea inspection.
  6. Inspect for foreign body and remove if indicated.
  7. Fluorescein stain to visualize changes in epithelial lining. Cobalt blue light or Wood's lamp should be used for visualization.

Diagnostic Test

A. Perform fluorescein stain test: An epithelial defect that stains with fluorescein is the hallmark symptom.

Differential Diagnoses

A. Corneal abrasion
B. Corneal foreign body
C. Acute-angle glaucoma
D. Herpetic infection (herpes simplex virus [HSV]):HSV is associated with decreased corneal sensation.
E. Recurrent corneal ulceration
F. Ulcerative keratitis
G. Corneal erosion

Plan

A. General interventions
  1. Superficial corneal abrasions do not need patching.
  2. For deeper abrasions, apply a patch that prevents lid motion for 24 to 48 hours.
  3. Pressure patch is no longer recommended.
B. Patient teaching
  1. Discuss the use of protective eyewear and prevention of future ocular trauma for the patient with a history of use of power tools or hammering.
  2. *See Section III: Patient Teaching Guide for this chapter, "Eye Medication Administration."* ◀
  3. Advise that the patient should not use/wear contact lenses until the eye is completely healed.
C. Pharmaceutical therapy
  1. Antibiotic drops or ointment. Ointments are suggested over drops as they provide lubrication for the eye. Never instill antibiotic ointment if there is a possibility of a perforation. Patch the eye and refer the patient to a physician or ophthalmologist.
    a. Adults and children: Sulfacetamide sodium ophthalmic solution 10% (Sulamyd), 1 to 2 drops instilled into the lower conjunctival sac every 2 to 3 hours during the day; may instill every 6 hours during the night × 5 to 7 days.
    b. Sulfacetamide's sodium (Sulamyd) ophthalmic solution or ointment interacts with gentamicin. Avoid using them together.
    c. Para-aminobenzoic acid (PABA) derivatives decrease sulfacetamide's action. Wait 0.5 to 1 hour before instilling sulfacetamide.
    d. Sulfacetamide precipitates when used with silver preparations. Avoid using them together.
  2. Adults and children: Polymyxin B sulfate (Polytrim) 10,000 U/g, bacitracin zinc 500 U/g ophthalmic ointment (Polysporin), a small ribbon of ointment applied into the conjunctival sac one or more times daily or as needed.
  3. Adults and children: Erythromycin ophthalmic ointment 0.5% (Ilotycin), 1-cm ribbon of ointment applied into the conjunctival sac up to four to six times daily, depending on the severity of infection.
  4. Bacitracin 500 U/g ointment, 1/2-inch ribbon twice a day to four times a day for 7 days.
  5. Contact lens wearers are often colonized with *Pseudomonas*, and should be treated with either a fluoroquinolone or an aminoglycoside. Ciprofloxacin 0.3% solution, 1 to 2 drops four times a day, for 3 to 5 days; gentamycin 0.3% solution 1 to 2 drops, four times a day, for 3 to 5 days; or tobramycin (Tobrex) ointment or drops, four times a day for 3 to 5 days.
  6. Analgesics: Topical analgesics should be used sparingly. Diclofenac (Voltaren) 0.1% solution to eye four times a day as needed, or ketorolac (Acular) 0.5% solution in eye four times a day as needed.
  7. Avoid use of home prescriptions that will interfere with the healing process.
  8. Avoid the use of medications containing steroids. These products may increase the risk of superinfection and may slow down the healing process.

Follow-Up

A. Reevaluate the patient within 24 hours. The cornea usually heals within 24 to 48 hours.

B. Ophthalmic ointment or drops should be continued for 4 days after reepithelialization occurs to help in the healing process.
C. If the patient is still symptomatic in 48 hours, consider referral to an ophthalmologist.

Consultation/Referral

> *Immediate referral to an ophthalmologist is required for large or central lesions, or deep or penetrating wounds.*

Individual Considerations

A. Pregnancy: Retinal detachment should be considered as a source of eye pain and visual loss, especially in a woman with severe pregnancy-induced hypertension.
B. Pediatrics: The use of ointments is suggested over the use of eye drops due to the lubricating effect. Blurry vision may be experienced; therefore, apply the ointment at nap time and bedtime. Eye drops commonly burn/sting.
 1. Pressure patches are not recommended for children. Children commonly pull patches off and this counteracts the purpose of the use of a pressure patch.
 2. Preventive precautions include encouraging the use of protective eyewear for contact sports, including hockey, soccer, baseball, and basketball.

Dacryocystitis

Jill C. Cash and Nancy Pesta Walsh

Definition

A. Infection or inflammation of the lacrimal sac, or dacryocystitis, can be acute or chronic.
B. Dacryocystitis is usually secondary to obstruction.

Incidence

A. The incidence is unknown.

Pathogenesis

A. Bacterial infection of the lacrimal sac usually is caused by *Staphylococcus* or *Streptococcus.*

Predisposing Factors

A. Nasal trauma
B. Deviated septum
C. Nasal polyps
D. Congenital dacryostenosis
E. Inferior turbinate hypertrophy

Common Complaints

A. Pain in the eye
B. Redness
C. Swelling
D. Fever
E. Tearing

Other Signs and Symptoms

A. Purulent exudate may be expressed from the lacrimal duct.

Subjective Data

A. Elicit the onset, course, and duration of symptoms. Are symptoms bilateral or unilateral?
B. Review the patient's activity when the symptoms began to determine if etiology is chemical, traumatic, or infectious.
C. Review other presenting symptoms such as fever and discharge.
D. Review the patient's history for previous episodes. Note treatments used in past.
E. Review history for a recent HSV or fever blister.
F. Review ophthalmologic history.
G. Review medications.

Physical Examination

A. Check temperature, pulse, and blood pressure.
B. Inspect
 1. Assess both eyes.
 2. Check peripheral fields of vision, and sclera.
 3. Evaluate conjunctiva for distribution of redness, ciliary flush, and foreign bodies.
 4. Inspect lid margins: Evaluate for crusting, ulceration, and masses.
C. Palpate: Palpate lacrimal duct. Discharge can be expressed from the tear duct with the application of pressure.

Diagnostic Tests

A. Check visual acuity.
B. Culture discharge for *Neisseria* if suspected.

Differential Diagnoses

A. Dacryocystitis
B. Chalazion
C. Blepharitis
D. Xanthoma
E. Bacterial conjunctivitis
F. Hordeolum
G. Foreign body
H. Cellulitis

Plan

A. General interventions
 1. Apply warm, moist compresses at least four times per day.
 2. Instruct female patients to discard old makeup, including mascara, eyeliner, and eye shadow, used before infection.
B. Patient teaching: Application of compresses, handwashing, and proper cleaning. *See Section III: Patient Teaching Guide for this chapter, "Eye Medication Administration."* See Figure 5.1: How to instill eye drops into the eye. ◀
C. Pharmaceutical therapy
 1. Dicloxacillin 250 mg by mouth four times daily for 7 days
 2. Erythromycin 250 mg by mouth four times daily for 7 days

Follow-Up

A. Follow up in 2 weeks if symptoms are not resolved.

Consultation/Referral

A. Refer the patient to an ophthalmologist for irrigation and probing if needed.
B. Lab studies are generally performed by an ophthalmologist.

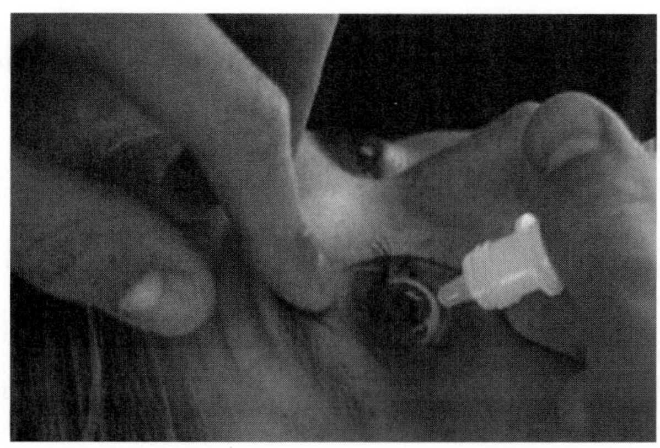

FIGURE 5.1 How to instill eye drops into the eye.

Dry Eyes

Jill C. Cash and Nancy Pesta Walsh

Definition

A. Insufficient lubrication of the eye, or dry eyes, is caused by a deficiency of any one of the major components of the tear film.
B. Defects in tear production are uncommon but may occur in conjunction with systemic disease. Presence of systemic disease should be evaluated.

Incidence

A. Increased incidence of dry eyes in the elderly is due to decreased rate of lacrimal gland secretions.

Pathogenesis

A. Decreased production of one or more components of the tear film results in dry eyes. The tear film comprises three layers:
  1. An outermost lipid layer, excreted by the lid meibomian glands
  2. A middle aqueous layer, secreted by the main and accessory lacrimal glands
  3. An innermost mucinous layer, secreted by conjunctival goblet cells
B. A defect in production of the aqueous phase by lacrimal glands causes dry eyes or keratoconjunctivitis sicca. The condition most often occurs as a physiological consequence of aging, and it is commonly exacerbated by dry environmental factors. It may also develop in patients with connective tissue disease.
C. In Sjögren's syndrome, the lacrimal glands become involved in immune-mediated inflammation.
D. Mucin production may decline with vitamin A deficiency.
E. Loss of goblet cells can occur secondary to chemical burns.

Predisposing Factors

A. History of severe conjunctivitis
B. Eyelid defects such as fifth or seventh cranial nerve palsy, incomplete blinking, exophthalmos, and lid movement hindered by scar formation
C. Drug-induced conditions, including the use of anticholinergic agents
  1. Phenothiazine
  2. Tricyclic antidepressants
  3. Antihistamines
  4. Diuretics
  5. Isotretinoin (Accutane)
D. Systemic disease such as rheumatoid disease, Sjögren's syndrome, and neurologic disease
E. Environmental factors such as heat (wood, coal, and gas), air conditioners, winter air, and tobacco smoke
F. Use of contacts
G. Increasing age
H. Lipid abnormalities

Common Complaints

A. Ocular fatigue
B. Foreign-body sensation in the eye
C. Itching, burning, irritation, or dry sensation in the eye
D. Redness
E. Eye discharge

Other Signs and Symptoms

A. Photophobia
B. Cloudy, blurred vision
C. Rainbow of color around lights. Acute angle-closure glaucoma can present with a red, painful eye; cloudy, blurred vision and a rainbow of color around lights; dilatation of the pupil; nausea and vomiting
D. Bell's palsy, signs of stroke, or other conditions that affect the blinking mechanism

Subjective Data

A. Elicit the onset, duration, and frequency of symptoms.
B. Note factors that worsen or alleviate symptoms.
C. Note medical history for systemic conditions and strokes.
D. List current medications, noting anticholinergic drugs and isotretinoin (Accutane) use.
E. Note whether the patient wears contact lenses or glasses, and ask for what length of time.
F. Review occupational and home exposure to irritants and allergens.
G. Assess whether the patient produces tears. Note eye drainage amount, color, and frequency.
H. Review history of any previous ocular disease, surgeries, and so forth.

Physical Examination

A. Check temperature, pulse, respirations, and blood pressure.
B. Inspect
  1. Observe and evaluate *both* eyes.
  2. Conduct a detailed eye examination: Check the eye, lid, and conjunctiva for masses and redness.

3. Check pupil reactivity and corneal clarity. The corneal reflex should be checked if there is concern about a neuroparalytic keratitis or facial nerve palsy.
4. Complete a funduscopic examination. Check for completeness of lid closure as well as position of eyelashes.
5. Examine mouth for dryness.
6. Inspect skin for butterfly rash.

C. Palpate
1. Palpate lacrimal ducts for drainage.
2. Invert upper lid and check for foreign body or chalazion.
3. Check sinuses for tenderness.
4. Palpate thyroid.
5. Palpate joints for warmth and redness or inflammation.

Diagnostic Test

A. Perform Schirmer's test. Use Whatman no. 41 filter paper, 5 mm by 35 mm. A folded end of filter paper is hooked over the lower lid nasally, and the patient is instructed to keep his or her eyes lightly closed during the test. Wetting is measured after 5 minutes; less than 5 mm is usually abnormal. More than 10 mm is normal.

Differential Diagnoses

A. Dry eyes
B. Stevens–Johnson syndrome
C. Sjögren's syndrome: Chronic dry mouth, dry eyes, and arthritis triad suggest Sjögren's syndrome. Facial telangiectasias, parotid enlargement, Raynaud's phenomenon, and dental caries are associated features. Patients complain first of burning and a sandy, gritty, foreign-body sensation, particularly later in the day.
D. Systemic lupus erythematosus
E. Scleroderma
F. Ocular pterygium
G. Superficial pemphigoid
H. Vitamin A deficiency

Plan

A. General interventions
1. If no ocular disease is present, reduce environmental dryness by use of a room humidifier for a 2-week trial.
2. Apply artificial tear substitutes and nonprescription drops.
3. Consider stopping medications being used that may be contributing to the source of dry eye symptoms.
4. Caution should be used when using over-the-counter (OTC) allergy medications, if allergy is a contributing cause. Topical antihistamines may exacerbate the condition over time.

▶ **B.** Patient teaching: *See Section III: Patient Teaching Guide for this chapter, "Eye Medication Administration."*

C. Pharmaceutical therapy
1. Topical artificial tears 1 or 2 drops four times daily, preferably one without preservatives (i.e., Thera-tears, Dry Eye Therapy, Tears Naturale).
2. Drops may be instilled as often as desired.

Follow-Up

A. Determined by the severity of the issue. Reevaluate the patient in 2 weeks.

Consultation/Referral

A. Refer the patient to an ophthalmologist if symptoms are unrelieved at the 2-week follow-up.
B. Make an immediate referral for red eye, visual disturbance, or eye pain.

Individual Consideration

A. Geriatrics: The rate of lacrimal gland secretions diminishes with age; therefore, the elderly are at an increased risk for developing dry eye.
B. ACE inhibitors may reduce the risk of dry eye syndrome in some patients. Consider treatment with ACE inhibitors for hypertension as appropriate in clients.

Excessive Tears

Jill C. Cash and Nancy Pesta Walsh

Definition

A. Excessive tears disorder is an overproduction of tears. Complaints vary from watery eyes to overflowing tears that run down the cheeks, a condition known as *epiphora.*

Incidence

A. The incidence is unknown.

Pathogenesis

A. The most common cause is reflex overproduction of tears (as occurs in the elderly) due to a deficiency of the tear film.
B. Lacrimal pump failure and obstruction of the nasolacrimal outflow system are other causes of excessive tears.
C. Canalicular infections may be caused by *Actinomyces israelii* (Streptothrix) and *Candida.*

Predisposing Factors

A. Blepharitis (inflammation of the eyelid)
B. Allergic conjunctivitis (infectious or foreign body)
C. Exposure to cold, air conditioning, or dry environment
D. Lid problems: Impaired pumping action of the lid motion due to seventh nerve palsy or conditions that stiffen the lids such as scars or scleroderma
E. Lid laxity from aging or ectropion (sagging of the lower lid)
F. Sinusitis
G. Atopy
H. Age: Increased incidence in the elderly due to an overproduction of tears by the lacrimal gland
I. Congenital obstruction

Common Complaints

A. Watery eyes or tears running down cheeks are common complaints.

Other Signs and Symptoms

A. Unilateral tearing: Obstructive etiology
B. Bilateral tearing: Environmental irritants

Subjective Data

A. Inquire about onset, course, and duration of symptoms. Note frequency of excessive tearing.
B. Ascertain whether this is a new symptom or whether the patient has a past history of similar complaints. Ask how it was treated, and what was the response to treatment(s).
C. Determine severity. Do the tears run down the cheek?
D. Ascertain whether tearing is unilateral or bilateral.
E. Review common environmental predisposing factors.
F. Question the patient regarding vision changes.
G. Review medical history.
H. Review recent history for sinus infections or drainage, facial fractures, and surgery.

Physical Examination

A. Inspect
  1. Evaluate *both* eyes.
  2. Observe the lid structure and motion.
  3. Conduct a dermal examination to rule out butterfly rash.
B. Palpate
  1. Apply gentle pressure over the lacrimal sac to check drainage.
  2. Invert upper lid to check for foreign body.
  3. Palpate face for sinus tenderness.

Diagnostic Test

A. Culture any drainage expressed from the lacrimal sacs.

Differential Diagnoses

A. Excessive tears
B. Dendritic ulcer: Early symptoms are tears running down cheeks associated with a foreign-body sensation.
C. Congenital glaucoma
D. Dacryocystitis (purulent discharge)
E. Reflex tearing caused by dry eye
F. Blepharitis

Plan

A. General interventions
  1. Eliminate identifiable irritants.
  2. Treatment is mainly aimed at the underlying condition (i.e., ocular infection).
  3. Dacryocystitis is treated with hot compresses at least four times a day and systemic antibiotics.
B. Patient teaching: Instruct the patient on the application of compresses.
C. Pharmaceutical therapy
  1. None is required for diagnosis of excessive tears without infectious pathology.
  2. Dacryocystitis
    a. Erythromycin 250 mg four times daily for 7 days
    b. Dicloxacillin 250 mg four times daily for 7 days

Follow-Up

A. See patient in 48 to 72 hours to evaluate symptoms, especially if antibiotic therapy was needed.

Consultation/Referral

A. Patients unresponsive to treatment should be promptly referred to an ophthalmologist.
B. Consider referral for lid malposition or nasolacrimal duct obstructions.

Individual Consideration

A. Pediatrics: Nasolacrimal duct obstruction. Approximately 6% of newborns are diagnosed with a congenital obstruction within the first weeks of life. With moist heat and massage, many resolve spontaneously.

Eye Pain

Jill C. Cash and Nancy Pesta Walsh

Definition

A. Sensation of pain may affect the eyelid, conjunctiva, or cornea.

Incidence

A. Unknown. Pain in the eye is most often produced by conditions that do not threaten vision.

Pathogenesis

A. The external ocular surfaces and the uveal tract are richly innervated with pain receptors. As a result, lesions or disease processes affecting these surfaces can be acutely painful.
B. Pathology confined to the vitreous, retina, or optic nerve is rarely a source of pain.

Predisposing Factors

A. Eyelids: Inflammation such as hordeolum (stye), trichiasis (in-turned lash), and tarsal foreign bodies
B. Conjunctiva: Viral and bacterial conjunctivitis or allergic conjunctivitis; toxic, chemical, and mechanical injuries
C. Cornea: Keratitis (inflammation of the cornea) accompanying trauma, infection, exposure, vascular disease, or decreased lacrimation; microbial keratitis from contact use. If blood vessels invade the normally avascular corneal stroma, vision may become cloudy. Severe pain is a prominent symptom; movement of the lid typically exacerbates symptoms.

Common Complaints

A. Eye pain (sharp, dull, deep): The quality of the pain needs to be considered. Deep pain is suggestive of an intraocular problem. Inflammation and rapidly expanding mass lesions may cause deep pain. Displacement of the globe and diplopia may ensue.
B. Eye movement may cause sharp pain due to meningeal inflammation (the extraocular rectus muscles insert along the dura of the nerve sheath at the orbital apex). Most cases are idiopathic, but 10% to 15% are associated with multiple sclerosis.
C. Headache

Other Signs and Symptoms

These symptoms may be unilateral or bilateral.
A. Eyelids
  1. Tenderness
  2. Sensation of foreign body

3. Redness
4. Edema

B. Conjunctiva
1. Mild burning
2. Sensation of foreign body
3. Itching (allergic)

C. Cornea
1. Burning
2. Foreign-body sensation
3. Considerable discomfort
4. Reflex photophobic tearing
5. Blinking exacerbates pain
6. Pain relieved with pressure (i.e.,holding the lid shut). With a foreign body or a corneal lesion, pain is exacerbated by lid movement and relieved by cessation of lid motion.

D. Sclera: Redness

E. Uveal tract (uveitis or iritis)
1. Dull, deep-seated ache and photophobia
2. Profound ocular and orbital pain radiating to the frontal and temporal regions accompanying sudden elevation of pressure (acute angle-closure glaucoma)
3. Vagal stimulation with high pressure may result in nausea and vomiting.
4. Usual history of mild intermittent episodes of blurred vision preceding onset of throbbing pain, nausea, vomiting, and decreased visual acuity
5. Halos around light

F. Orbit
1. Deep pain with inflammation and rapidly expanding mass lesions
2. Eye movement causing sharp pain due to meningeal inflammation

G. Sinusitis: Secondary orbital inflammation and tenderness on extremes of eye movement

Subjective Data

A. Review the onset, duration, and course of symptoms. Inquire regarding the quality of pain.

B. Review any predisposing factors such as trauma or a foreign object. Ask: Was the onset sudden or gradual?

C. Note reported changes in visual acuity or color vision.

D. Note aggravating or alleviating factors.

E. Determine whether the eye pain is bilateral or unilateral.

F. Review history for herpes, infections, and toxic or chemical irritants.

G. Review history for glaucoma and previous eye surgeries or treatments.

H. Assess the patient for any other symptoms such as migraine headache, sinusitis, or tooth abscess.

I. Inquire whether the patient has lost a large amount of sleep.

J. Inquire whether he or she has been exposed to a large amount of ultraviolet (UV) light or sunlight (vacation, tanning beds).

K. Review history for any other medical problems such as lupus, sarcoidosis, or inflammatory bowel disease.

Physical Examination

A. Inspect
1. Evaluate *both* eyes.
2. Test visual acuity and color vision.
3. Observe for EOMs.
4. Check the eye, lid, and conjunctiva for masses and redness.
5. Check pupil reactivity and corneal clarity.
6. Conduct a funduscopic examination for disc abnormalities.
7. Perform ear, nose, and throat examination.

B. Palpate
1. Palpate lacrimal ducts for drainage.
2. Palpate sinus for tenderness.
3. Invert upper lid and check for foreign body or chalazion.

Diagnostic Tests

A. Fluorescein stain

B. Measurement of intraocular pressure (IOP)

Differential Diagnoses

A. Eye pain

B. Hordeolum

C. Chalazion

D. Acute dacryocystitis

E. Irritant exposure

F. Conjunctival infection

G. Corneal abrasion

H. Foreign body

I. Ulcers

J. Ingrown lashes

K. Contact lens abuse

L. Scleritis

M. Acute angle-closure glaucoma; may present with fixed, midposition pupil, redness, and a hazy cornea

N. Uveitis

O. Referred pain from extraocular sources such as sinusitis, tooth abscess, tension headache, temporal arteritis, and prodrome of herpes zoster

Plan

A. General interventions
1. The initial task is to be sure that there is no threat to vision.
2. Treatment modality depends on the underlying cause of eye pain.

B. Patient teaching: *See Section III: Patient Teaching Guide for this chapter, "Eye Medication Administration."* See Figure 5.1: How to instill eye drops into the eye.

C. Pharmaceutical therapy: Medication depends on the underlying cause.

Follow-Up

A. Follow-up depends on the underlying cause.

Consultation/Referral

A. Any change in visual acuity or color vision requires an urgent ophthalmologic consultation.

Glaucoma, Acute Angle-Closure

Jill C. Cash and Nancy Pesta Walsh

Definition

A. This ocular emergency is caused by elevations in intraocular pressure (IOP) that damage the optic nerve, leading to loss of peripheral fields of vision; it can lead to loss of central vision and result in blindness.

Incidence

A. Acute angle closure glaucoma is the second leading cause of blindness in the United States. Approximately 5% to 15% of the patient population develops glaucoma.

Pathogenesis

A. The essential pathophysiologic feature of glaucoma is an IOP that is too high for the optic nerve. Increased IOP increases vascular resistance, causing decreased vascular perfusion of the optic nerve and ischemia. Light dilates the pupil, causing the iris to relax and bow forward. As the iris bows forward, it comes into contact with the trabecular meshwork and occludes the outflow of aqueous humor, resulting in increased IOP.

Predisposing Factors

A. Narrow anterior ocular chamber
B. Prolonged periods of darkness
C. Drugs that dilate the pupils (i.e., anticholinergics)
D. Advancing age: Greater than 60 years
E. African American heritage
F. Family history
G. Trauma
H. Neoplasm
I. Corticosteroid therapy
J. Neovascularization
K. Female sex

Common Complaints

A. Ocular pain
B. Blurred vision, decreased visual acuity, "cloudiness" of vision
C. "Halos" around lights at night
D. Neurologic complaints (headache, nausea, or vomiting)

Other Signs and Symptoms

A. Red eye with ciliary flush
B. "Silent blinder" causes extensive damage before the patient is aware of visual field loss
C. Dilated pupil
D. Hard orbital globe
E. No pupillary response to light
F. Increase IOP (normal IOP is 10–20 mmHg).

Subjective Data

A. Review the onset, course, and duration of symptoms; note visual changes in one or both eyes.
B. Review medical history and medications.
C. Review family history of glaucoma.
D. Determine whether there has been any difficulty with peripheral vision, any headache photophobia, or any visual blurring.
E. In children, ask about rubbing of eyes, refusal to open eyes, and tearing.
F. Rule out presence of any chemical, trauma, or foreign bodies in the eye.
G. Review any recent history of herpes outbreak.
H. Ask the patient whether this has ever occurred before, and if so, how it was treated.

Physical Examination

A. Blood pressure
B. Inspect
  1. Examine both eyes.
  2. Rule out foreign body.
  3. Inspect for redness, inflammation, and discharge.
  4. Check pupillary response to light.
  5. Redness noted around iris, pupil is dilated, and cornea appears cloudy.
  6. Inspect anterior chamber of eye by holding penlight laterally and direct toward nasal area. Shallow chamber will cast a shadow on the nasal side of the iris.

C. Palpate: Palpate the globe of the eye, which will feel firm on palpation.
D. Funduscopic examination: This may reveal notching of the cup and a difference in cup-to-disc ratio between the two eyes.

Diagnostic Tests

A. Check visual acuity and peripheral fields of vision.
B. Measure IOP with a tonometer. Normal level is 10 to 21 mmHg; acute angle closure glaucoma IOP is greater than 50 mmHg. Tonometer examination is not recommended if external infection is present.
C. Slit-lamp examination: Edematous and/or cloudy cornea

Differential Diagnoses

A. Acute angle-closure glaucoma
B. Acute iritis
C. Acute bacterial conjunctivitis
D. Iridocyclitis
E. Corneal injury
F. Foreign body
G. Herpetic keratitis

Plan

A. General interventions
  1. Severe attacks can cause blindness in 2 to 3 days. Seek medical attention immediately to prevent permanent vision loss.
  2. Frequency of attacks is unpredictable.

B. Patient teaching: *See Section III: Patient Teaching Guide for this chapter, "Eye Medication Administration."* ◀
C. Pharmaceutical therapy: Must be instituted by an ophthalmologist.
  1. Acetazolamide (Diamox) 250 mg orally
  2. Pilocarpine (Pilocar) 4% every 15 minutes during acute attack

D. Surgical intervention
  1. Surgery is indicated if IOP is not maintained within normal limits with medications or if there

is progressive visual field loss with optic nerve damage.

2. Surgical treatment of choice is peripheral iridectomy—excision of a small portion of the iris whereby the aqueous humor can bypass the pupil.

Follow-Up

A. Annual eye examinations by an ophthalmologist are necessary to monitor IOP and treatment efficacy.

Consultation/Referral

A. All patients should be referred to an ophthalmologist *immediately* for measurement of IOP, acute management, and possible surgical intervention (laser peripheral iridectomy).

Individual Considerations

A. Pediatrics: Infants with tearing, rubbing of eyes, and refusal to open eyes should be referred to a pediatric ophthalmologist for immediate care.

B. Adults

1. Women normally have slightly higher IOPs than men.
2. Asians may have higher IOPs than African Americans and Caucasians.
3. Individuals older than age 40 years should have their IOP measured periodically. Every 3 to 5 years is sufficient after a stable baseline is established for the patient.

C. Geriatrics: Incidence increases with age, usually in those older than 60 years.

Hordeolum (Stye)

Jill C. Cash and Nancy Pesta Walsh

Definition

A. Hordeolum is an infection of the glands of the eyelids (follicle of an eyelash or the associated gland of Zeis [sebaceous] or Moll's gland [apocrine sweat gland]), usually caused by *Staphylococcus aureus.*

B. If swelling is under the conjunctival side of the eyelid, it is an internal hordeolum.

C. If swelling is under the skin of the eyelid, it is an external hordeolum.

Incidence

A. The incidence is unknown; it is more common in children and adolescents than in adults.

Pathogenesis

A. Acute bacterial infection of the meibomian gland (internal hordeolum) or of the eyelash follicle (external hordeolum) is usually caused by *S. aureus.*

Predisposing Factor

A. Age: More common in the pediatric population

Common Complaints

A. Eye tenderness

B. Sudden onset of a purulent discharge

Other Signs and Symptoms

A. Redness and swelling of the eye

Subjective Data

A. Review the onset, course, and duration of symptoms.

B. Determine whether there is any visual disturbance.

C. Note whether this is the first occurrence. If not, ask how it was treated before.

D. Evaluate how much pain or discomfort the patient is experiencing.

E. Review the patient's history for chemical, foreign body, and/or trauma etiology.

F. Review the patient's medical history and medications.

Physical Examination

A. Inspect

1. Examine both eyes; note redness, site of swelling, and amount and color of discharge.
2. Evert the lid and check for pointing.
3. Assess sclera and conjunctivae for abnormalities.
4. Inspect ears, nose, and throat.

B. Palpate

1. Palpate eye for hardness and expression of discharge.
2. Evaluate for preauricular adenopathy.

Diagnostic Tests

A. Test visual acuity.

B. Discharge can be cultured but is usually treated presumptively.

Differential Diagnoses

A. Hordeolum

B. Chalazion: The main differential diagnosis is chalazia, which point on the conjunctival side of the eyelid and do not usually affect the margin of the eyelid.

C. Blepharitis

D. Xanthoma

E. Bacterial conjunctivitis

F. Foreign body

Plan

A. General interventions: Contain the infecting pathogen. Crops occur when the infectious agent spreads from one hair follicle to another.

B. Patient teaching

1. *See Section III: Patient Teaching Guide for this chapter, "Eye Medication Administration."* See Figure 5.1: How to instill eye drops into the eye. ◀
2. Reinforce good handwashing.
3. Instruct on proper eyelid hygiene.
4. Patients should discard all eye makeup, including mascara, eyeliner, and eye shadow.

C. Pharmaceutical therapy

1. Sulfacetamide sodium (Sulamyd) ophthalmic ointment 10%; 0.5 to 1.0 cm placed in the conjunctival sac four times daily for 7 days
2. Sulfacetamide sodium (Sulamyd) 10% ophthalmic drops; 2 drops instilled every 3 to 4 hours for 7 days
3. Polymyxin B sulfate and bacitracin zinc (Polysporin) ophthalmic ointment; 0.5 to 1.0 cm placed in the conjunctival sac four times daily for 7 days

4. If crops of styes occur, some clinicians recommend a course of tetracycline to stop recurrences (consult with a physician).

Follow-Up

A. Have patient telephone or visit the office in 48 hours to check response.
B. If crops occur, diabetes mellitus must be excluded. Perform blood glucose evaluation.

Consultation/Referral

A. Hordeolum may produce a diffuse superficial lid infection known as *preseptal cellulitis* that requires referral to an ophthalmologist.
B. If hordeolum does not respond to topical antimicrobial treatment, refer the patient to an ophthalmologist.

Individual Consideration

A. None

Strabismus

Jill C. Cash and Nancy Pesta Walsh

Definition

Strabismus is an eye disorder in which the optic axes cannot be directed toward the same object due to a deficit in muscular coordination. It can be nonparalytic or paralytic.
A. *Esotropia* is a nonparalytic strabismus in which the eyes cross inward.
B. *Exotropia* is a nonparalytic strabismus in which the eyes drift outward. Exotropia may be intermittent or constant.
C. Pseudostrabismus gives a false appearance of deviation in the visual axes.

Incidence

A. Strabismus occurs in approximately 3% of the population.
B. Esotropia (nonparalytic strabismus) is the most common ocular misalignment, representing more than half of all ocular deviations in the pediatric population. Accommodative esotropia typically occurs between 1 and 3 years of age, with an average age of 2.5 years, and it may be intermittent or constant.
C. Intermittent exotropia is the most common type of exotropic strabismus and is characterized by an outward drift of one eye, most often occurring when a child is fixating at distance.

Pathogenesis

A. *Paralytic strabismus* is related to paralysis or paresis of a specific extraocular muscle. *Nonparalytic strabismus* is related to a congenital imbalance of normal eye muscle tone, causing focusing difficulties, unilateral refractive error, nonfusion, or anatomical difference in the eyes.

Predisposing Factors

A. Familial tendencies
B. Congenital defects

Common Complaints

A. Crossing of the eyes
B. Turning in of the eyes
C. Photophobia
D. Diplopia

Other Signs and Symptoms

A. The patient's head or chin tilts or the patient closes one eye to focus on objects.

Subjective Data

A. Describe the onset, duration, and progression of symptoms.
B. Review any history of eye problems. Ask: How were they corrected?
C. Determine whether the patient, if a child, has reached the age-appropriate milestones in development.
D. Does the patient make faces or move his or her head to see better (tilting the head or chin to improve acuity or to correct diplopia)?
E. Rule out any eye damage, surgery, and so forth.

Physical Examination

A. Inspect: Observe alignment of lids, sclera, conjunctiva, and cornea.
B. Check pupillary response to light, size, shape, and equality.
C. Check the red reflex.

Diagnostic Tests

A. Test visual acuity.
B. Perform the cover–uncover test: In this test, the "lazy eye" drifts out of position and snaps back quickly when uncovered.
C. Corneal light reflex (Hirschberg's) test: Perform the Hirschberg's test for symmetry of the pupillary light reflexes to help detect strabismus. Normally, the light reflexes are in the same position on each pupil, but not with strabismus (positive Hirschberg's test).
D. Test EOMs: If a nerve supplying an extraocular muscle has been interrupted or the muscle itself has become weakened, the eye fails to move in the direction of the damaged muscle. If the right sixth nerve is damaged, the right eye does not move temporally. This is paralytic strabismus.

Differential Diagnoses

A. Strabismus
B. Pseudostrabismus
C. Ocular trauma
D. Congenital defect

Plan

A. General interventions
   1. When poor fixation is present, patch the stronger, dominant eye to promote vision and muscle strengthening in the weaker eye.
B. Patient teaching: Reinforce the need to consistently wear an eye patch, especially with children.
C. Pharmaceutical therapy: None.

Follow-Up

A. Monitor progress with eye patch.
B. Surgical intervention depends on the degree of deviation.

Consultation/Referral

A. Additional testing should be done by an ophthalmologist.

B. Pseudostrabismus (a false appearance of strabismus when visual axes are really in alignment) is one of the most common reasons a pediatric ophthalmologist is asked to evaluate an infant.

Individual Considerations

A. Pediatrics

1. Use the tumbling or illiterate E to test children; for preschoolers, use the Allen picture cards.

2. In very young children, test visual acuity by assessing developmental milestones: Looking at mother's face, responsive smile, reaching for objects. By 3 to 5 years of age, most children can cooperate for performance of accurate visual acuity screening tests.

3. The eyes of the newborn are *rarely aligned* during the first few weeks of life. By the age of 3 months, normal oculomotor behavior is usually established, and an experienced examiner may be able to document the existence of abnormal alignment by that time.

Subconjunctival Hemorrhage

Jill C. Cash and Nancy Pesta Walsh

Definition

A. Subconjunctival hemorrhage presents as blood patches in the bulbar conjunctiva.

Incidence

A. Frequently seen in newborns, subconjunctival hemorrhage may also be seen in adults after forceful exertion (coughing, sneezing, childbirth, strenuous lifting).

Pathogenesis

A. This disorder is believed to be secondary to increased intrathoracic pressure that may occur during labor and delivery or with physical exertion.

Predisposing Factors

A. Local trauma
B. Systemic hypertension
C. Acute conjunctivitis
D. Vaginal delivery (pushing during delivery)
E. Severe coughing
F. Severe vomiting

Common Complaint

A. Red-eyed appearance without pain

Other Signs and Symptoms

A. Bright red blood in plane between the conjunctiva and sclera
B. Usually unilateral
C. Normal vision

Subjective Data

A. Identify onset and duration of symptoms.
B. Elicit information about trauma to the eye; is it due to severe coughing or vomiting?
C. Identify history of conjunctivitis or hypertension.

Physical Examination

A. Check temperature, pulse, respirations, and blood pressure (rule out hypertension).

B. Inspect

1. Observe eyes.
2. Inspect ears, nose, and mouth.
3. Inspect skin for bruises or other trauma.
4. Assess for signs of trauma or abuse. Blood in the anterior chamber (hyphema) can result from injury or abuse.

C. Other physical examination components are dependent on etiology.

Diagnostic Tests

A. Perform visual screening.
B. Test EOMs and peripheral vision.

Differential Diagnoses

A. Subconjunctival hemorrhage
B. Systemic hypertension
C. Blood dyscrasia
D. Trauma to eye
E. Conjunctivitis
F. Hyphema
G. Abuse

Plan

A. General interventions: Reassure the patient. The hemorrhage is not damaging to the eye or vision, and the blood reabsorbs on its own over several weeks.
B. Teach safety to prevent trauma to the eye.
C. Pharmaceutical therapy: None.

Follow-Up

A. If subconjunctival hemorrhage recurs, evaluate the patient further for systemic hypertension or blood dyscrasia.

Consultation/Referral

A. Consult or refer the patient to a physician if hyphema is noted, if glaucoma is suspected, or if the patient has additional eye injuries.

Individual Considerations

A. Pediatrics: Hemorrhage is common in newborns after vaginal delivery.

B. Adults: Always measure blood pressure to rule out systemic hypertension.

C. Geriatrics

1. Always measure blood pressure to rule out systemic hypertension.
2. Consider evaluation for blood dyscrasia.
3. Check clotting times if patient is taking warfarin (Coumadin).

Uveitis

Jill C. Cash and Nancy Pesta Walsh

Definition

A. Uveitis, also known as *iritis,* is inflammation of the uveal tract (iris, ciliary body, and choroid) and is usually accompanied by a dull ache and photophobia resulting from the irritative spasm of the pupillary sphincter.

Incidence

A. The true incidence is unknown. Approximately 15% of patients with sarcoidosis present with uveitis.

Pathogenesis

A. The cause is unknown. Underlying causes include infections, viruses, and arthritis.

Predisposing Factors

A. Collagen disorders
B. Autoimmune disorders
C. Ankylosing spondylitis
D. Sarcoidosis
E. Juvenile rheumatoid arthritis
F. Lupus
G. Reiter's syndrome
H. Behcet's syndrome
I. Syphilis
J. Tuberculosis
K. AIDS
L. Crohn's disease

Common Complaints

A. Eye pain: Painless to deep-seated ache
B. Photophobia
C. Blurred vision with decreased visual acuity
D. Black spots
E. Eye redness

Other Signs and Symptoms

A. Unilateral or bilateral symptoms
- **1.** Unilateral: The pupil is smaller than that of the other eye because of spasm.

B. Ciliary flush
C. Pupillary contraction
D. Nausea and vomiting with vagal stimulation
E. Halos around lights
F. Hypopyon (pus in anterior chamber)
G. Limbal flush with small pupil

Subjective Data

A. Elicit the onset, course, duration, and frequency of symptoms. Are symptoms bilateral or unilateral?
B. Identify the possible causal activity or agent (chemical, traumatic, or infectious etiologies).
C. Review the patient's history of previous uveitis and other ophthalmologic disorders.
D. Review any associated fever, rash, weight loss, joint pain, back pain, oral ulcers, or genital ulcers.
E. Review full medical history for comorbid conditions.

Physical Examination

A. Check temperature, pulse, respirations, and blood pressure.
B. Inspect
- **1.** Assess both eyes for visual acuity and peripheral fields of vision.
- **2.** Check sclera and conjunctiva.

C. Other physical components need to be completed related to comorbid conditions.

Diagnostic Tests

A. Slit-lamp test: Slit-lamp examination reveals cells in the anterior chamber and "flare," representing increased aqueous humor protein. Inflammatory cells, called *keratic precipitates,* can collect in clusters on the posterior cornea.
B. Penlight examination: Flashlight examination shows a slightly cloudy anterior chamber in the uveitic eye.

Differential Diagnoses

A. Uveitis: Uveitis is usually idiopathic, but it may be associated with many systemic and ocular diseases.
B. Acute angle closure glaucoma
C. Retinal detachment
D. Central retinal artery occlusion
E. Endophthalmitis

Plan

A. General interventions
- **1.** Treat underlying cause as indicated.
- **2.** Provide immediate referral to an ophthalmologist due to possible complications of cataracts and blindness.

B. Patient teaching: Inform the patient that recurrent attacks are common and also require immediate attention.
C. Pharmaceutical therapy
- **1.** Medications are given per ophthalmologist.
- **2.** Uveitis and colitis often flare simultaneously; oral steroids are effective for both.

Follow-Up

A. The patient with uveitis needs a follow-up with an ophthalmologist.

Consultation/Referral

A. The patient should be referred *immediately* to an ophthalmologist for evaluation and intervention.

Individual Considerations

A. Recurrent uveitis may be a sign of another systemic condition. Other conditions to consider: Infections (bacterial, spirochetal, viral, fungal, and parasitic infections); inflammatory diseases, including spondyloarthropathies (ankylosing spondylitis, psoriatic arthritis, reactive arthritis); inflammatory bowel disease; multiple sclerosis; and the use of new medications. Further workup should be performed for recurrent uveitis.

Resources

American Academy of Ophthalmology
P.O. Box 7424
San Francisco, CA 94120–7424
415-561-8500
Fax: +1 415-561-8533
E-mail: member_services@aao.org

American Council of the Blind
1703 N. Beauregard St.
Suite 420
Arlington, VA 22201
Phone: 202-467-508, 1 800-424-8666
Fax: 703-465-5085
E-mail: info@acb.org

American Foundation of the Blind
2 Penn Plaza, Suite 1102
New York, NY 10121
Phone: 212-502-7600
Fax: 888-545-8331
E-mail: afbinfo@afb.net

American Printing House for the Blind
1839 Frankfort Avenue
P.O. Box 6085
Louisville, KY 40206–6085
Phone: 800-223-1839; 502-895-2405
Fax: 502-899-2284
E-mail: info@aph.org

Books on Tape
Phone: 800-733-3000

Glaucoma Research Foundation
251 Post Street, Suite 600
San Francisco, CA 94198
Phone: 415-986-3162
800-826-6693
E-mail: questions@glaucoma.org

Guide Dog Foundation for the Blind
371 E Jerico Turnpike
Smithtown, NY 11787
Phone: 631-930-9000; 800-548-4337
Fax: 631-930-9009
9 a.m. to 5 p.m. (Eastern Standard Time),
Monday through Friday, E-mail: info@guidedog.org

National Service for the Blind and Physically Handicapped
National Library of Congress
1291 Taylor Street NW
Washington, DC 20542
Phone: 800-424-8567; 202-707-5100; TDD 202-707-0744;
Fax: 202-707-07128 a.m. to 4:30 p.m. (Eastern Standard Time),
Monday through Friday
E-mail: nls@loc.gov

National Society to Prevent Blindness
Prevent Blindness America
211 West Wacker Drive
Suite 1700
Chicago, IL 60606
www.preventblindness.org/contact-us
800-331-2020

Bibliography

American Academy of Ophthalmology. (2013a, October). Blepharitis PPP 2013. Retrieved from https://www.aao.org/preferred-practice-pattern/blepharitis-ppp--2013

American Academy of Ophthalmology. (2013b, October). Conjunctivitis PPP 2013. Retrieved from https://www.aao.org/preferred-practice-pattern/conjunctivitis-ppp--2013

American Academy of Ophthalmology. (2013c, October). Dry eye syndrome PPP 2013. Retrieved from https://www.aao.org/preferred-practice-pattern/dry-eye-syndrome-ppp--2013

American Academy of Ophthalmology. (2015, November). Conjunctivitis summary benchmark 2015. Retrieved from https://www.aao.org/summarybenchmarkdetail/conjunctivitissummarybenchmark--october-2012

Carlisle, R. T., & Digiovanni, J. (2015). Differential diagnosis of the swollen red eyelid. *American Family Physician, 15*(92), 106–112.

Centers for Disease Control and Prevention. (2015, September). Vision quest initiative. Retrieved from https://www.cdc.gov/visionhealth/faq.htm

Dohm, K. D. (2015, January). Practice pearls for managing anterior uveitis. *Review of Optometry, 2015*(1), 58–63.

Gunton, W. B., Wasserman, B. N., & DeBenedictis, C. (2015). Strabismus. *Primary Care: Clinics in Office Practice, 2*(3), 393–407.

Swaminathan, A., Otterness, K., Milne, K., & Rezaie, S. (2015). The safety of topical anesthetics in the treatment of corneal abrasions: A review. *Journal of Emergency Medicine, 49*(5), 810–815.

Wipperman, J. L., & Dorsch, J. N. (2015). Evaluation and management of corneal abrasions. *American Family Physician, 87*(2), 114–120.

6 Ear Guidelines

Acute Otitis Media

Jill C. Cash and Moya Cook

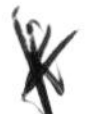

Definition

A. Acute otitis media (AOM) is inflammation of the middle ear associated with an acute bacterial infection of the middle ear.

Incidence

A. AOM may occur at any age. It is most commonly seen in children.
B. Over two thirds of children have had at least one episode of otitis media by 3 years of age.
C. One third of children have had three or more episodes by 3 years of age.
D. One third of all pediatric visits are for otitis media.

Pathogenesis

A. Obstruction of the Eustachian tube can lead to a middle-ear effusion and infection. Contamination of this middle-ear fluid often results from a backup of nasopharyngeal secretions. The most common bacterial pathogens are *Streptococcus pneumoniae*, *Haemophilus influenzae*, and *Moraxella catarrhalis.*

Predisposing Factors

A. Age less than 12 months
B. Recurrent otitis media (three or more episodes in the last 6 months)
C. Previous episode of otitis media within the last month
D. Medical condition that predisposes to otitis media (i.e., Down syndrome, AIDS, cystic fibrosis, cleft palate, and craniofacial abnormalities)
E. Native American heritage
F. Exposure to tobacco smoke and air pollution
G. Day-care attendance
H. Bottle propping
I. Family history of allergies
J. Pacifier use

Common Complaints

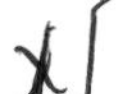

A. Ear pain
B. Pulling ears
C. Fever may or may not be present

Other Signs and Symptoms

A. Sleeplessness within past 48 hours
B. Decreased appetite
C. Increased fussiness
D. Acute hearing loss
E. Upper respiratory infection (URI) symptoms
F. Mastoiditis presenting with a swollen and red mastoid
G. Perforated tympanic membrane (sudden severe pain followed by immediate relief of pain with fluid drainage from the ear)
H. Cholesteatoma (saclike structure in the middle ear accompanied by white, shiny, greasy debris)

Subjective Data

A. Elicit onset and duration of symptoms.
B. Inquire whether the patient recently had (or has concurrently) a URI.
C. Determine whether the patient has any change in hearing.
D. Assess the patient for any drainage from the ear(s).
E. Question the patient or his or her caregiver regarding risk factors.
F. Identify the patient's history of otitis media.

Physical Examination

A. Check temperature, pulse, respirations, and blood pressure.
B. Inspect
  1. Observe the canal and auricle for redness, deformity, drainage, or foreign body.
  2. Inspect the tympanic membrane position to determine if it is neutral and whether landmarks are visible, retracted, full, or bulging.
  3. Observe ears for decreased or absent tympanic membrane mobility.
  4. Inspect nose, mouth, and throat.
C. Auscultate heart and lungs.

Diagnostic Tests

A. Tympanogram shows flat or type B curve.
B. Hearing test should be done in patients with persistent otitis media (greater or equal to 3 months' duration).
C. Consider complete blood count if the patient appears toxic with a high fever.

Differential Diagnoses

A. AOM
B. Otitis media with effusion (OME)

C. Red tympanic membrane secondary to crying (differentiated from AOM by mobility with pneumatic otoscopy)
D. URI
E. Mastoiditis
F. Foreign body in the ear
G. Otitis externa

Plan

A. General intervention: Pain relief with acetaminophen or ibuprofen. Auralgan may be used for a topical pain relief in children older than 3 years.
B. Patient teaching
  1. *See Section III: Patient Teaching Guide for this chapter, "Acute Otitis Media."*
  2. Educate parents and care providers that children should avoid smoke exposure. Smoke-filled rooms increase the risk of frequent ear infections in children.
  3. For young children who use a bottle for feeding, stress the importance of NOT propping bottles at any time for feeding. Propping bottles increases the risk of ear infections.
C. Pharmaceutical therapy
  1. Drug of choice: Amoxicillin 90 mg/kg/d divided into two daily doses for 10 days, up to a maximum of 3 g/d.
  2. For concerns of amoxicillin resistance, treatment failure, recent use of antibiotic in the previous 30 days, and/or concurrent other infections, use an antibiotic with beta-lactamase activity such as amoxicillin-clavulanate (Augmentin). Other alternatives include cefdinir, cefpodoxime, cefuroxime, and ceftriaxone.
  3. For penicillin allergy: Cefdinir 14 mg/kg/d in one to two doses, maximum dose 600 mg/d. Cefpodoxime 10 mg/kg/d, once daily, maximum dose 800 mg/d. Cefuroxime susp, 30 mg/kg/d in two divided doses, maximum dose 1 g/d. Capsules: 250 mg every 12 hours.
  4. Alternative: One dose of ceftriaxone 50 mg/kg intramuscularly (IM). If clinically improved in 48 hours, no further treatment is recommended. If signs/symptoms continue, administer the second dose of ceftriaxone in 48 hours.
  5. Other alternatives: Macrolides
    a. Erythromycin plus sulfisoxazole (Pediazole): 50 to 150 mg/kg/d of erythromycin divided into four doses/d for 10 days; maximum dose 2 g erythromycin or 6 g sulfisoxazole/d. **Do not use in children younger than 2 months.**
    b. Azithromycin 10 mg/kg/d, maximum dose 500 mg/d as single dose on day 1, then 5 mg/kg/d, maximum dose of 250 mg/d on days 2 to 5 for 10 days
    c. Clarithromycin 15 mg/kg/d divided into two doses, maximum dose 1 g/d.
    d. Trimethoprim with sulfamethoxazole 8 mg/kg/d of trimethoprim (40 mg/kg/d of sulfamethoxazole) divided into two daily doses for 10 days
  6. Children younger than 2 years should be treated with antibiotic therapy for 10 days. Children older than 2 years, without a previous history of otitis media, may be treated for 5 to 7 days. Erythromycin with sulfisoxazole 40 mg/kg/d (150 mg/kg/d of sulfisoxazole [Pediazole]) divided into four daily doses for 10 days. **Do not use in children younger than 2 months.**
  7. If the patient is asymptomatic and AOM is found on examination, consider observation without antibiotics only if child is older than 2 years. Recommend follow-up examination in 48 hours.
  8. Other antibiotics (if first-line antibiotic fails): Amoxicillin and clavulanic acid (Augmentin), cefixime (Suprax), azithromycin (Zithromax), and cefprozil (Cefzil).
  9. For persistent otitis media (3 months or longer), consider using an antibiotic for 21 days. **Residual otitis media may need treatment with additional amoxicillin or beta-lactamase-resistant antibiotic.**

Follow-Up

A. Check the patient in 2 to 4 weeks or if fever and complaints persist for more than 48 hours after the antibiotic is begun. Documentation of the resolution of the ear infection is valuable information if recurrent infections occur.

Consultation/Referral

A. Consult or refer the patient to a physician if he or she is less than 6 weeks of age, appears septic, or has mastoiditis.
B. A patient with persistent otitis media with a hearing loss of 20 dB or more should be referred to an otolaryngologist.

Individual Considerations

A. Pregnancy: Do not use sulfa medications (sulfonamides) in pregnant patients, clients at gestation.
B. Pediatrics
  1. Children 6 weeks old or younger: Consider a blood culture and lumbar puncture if septicemia is suspected. The patient may need intravenous (IV) antibiotics depending on culture results. Do not use sulfa medications (sulfonamides) in children younger than 2 months.
  2. The American Academy of Pediatrics does not recommend the use of over-the-counter (OTC) cough and cold medications for children younger than 6 years. In older children, consider decongestants for nasal congestion. Antihistamines are not recommended.
C. Geriatrics: Elderly patients may present with OME and/or otitis media secondary to a blocked Eustachian tube and/or URI.

Cerumen Impaction (Earwax)

Jill C. Cash and Moya Cook

Definition

A. Cerumen impaction, or earwax buildup, can cause conductive hearing loss or discomfort.

Incidence

A. Cerumen impaction occurs in patients of all ages. It is commonly seen in the elderly. The incidence in nursing home patients is 40%.

Pathogenesis

A. Wax builds up in the external canal. With age, the normal self-cleaning mechanisms of the ear fail. Cilia, which have become stiff, cannot remove cerumen and dirt from the ear canal. The pushing of cotton swabs, paper clips, bobby pins, and so forth, into the ear canal may also impact cerumen.

Predisposing Factors

A. Aging (decreased function of ear cilia)
B. Use of hearing aids
C. Use of cotton swabs to clean ear canals

Common Complaints

A. Dryness and itching of ear canal
B. Dizziness
C. Ear pain
D. Hearing loss

Subjective Data

A. Elicit onset and duration of symptoms.
B. Elicit history of cerumen impaction.
C. Question the patient regarding the method of cleaning ears.

Physical Examination

A. Check temperature, pulse, respirations, and blood pressure.
B. Inspect
  1. Observe ears for thick, light- to dark-brown wax occluding the auditory canal.
  2. Observe the tympanic membrane if possible. A perforated tympanic membrane is associated with otitis media.
  3. Inspect the nose and throat.
C. Auscultation: Auscultate heart and lungs.

Diagnostic Tests

A. Conductive hearing loss of 35 to 40 dB
B. Perform Rinne and Weber tests.
  1. The Rinne tuning-fork test reveals bone conduction greater than air conduction in the affected ear (abnormal). The Rinne test is performed by placing the struck tuning fork against the mastoid bone. Begin counting or timing the interval from the start to when the patient can no longer hear. Continue counting or timing the interval to determine the length of time sound is heard by air conduction. Air-conducted sound should be heard twice as long as bone-conducted sound after bone conduction stops.
  2. The Weber test reveals conductive hearing loss when sound travels toward the poor ear. Sensorineural hearing loss is present when sound travels toward the good ear. This is performed by striking a tuning fork and then placing it on the middle of the head. The patient should be asked where sound is being heard: from the left ear, the right ear, or equal in both ears. Normal results are reflected by sound being heard equally in both ears.

Differential Diagnoses

A. Cerumen impaction
B. Foreign body in the ear canal
C. Otitis externa: White, mucus-like ear discharge associated with otitis externa

Plan

A. General interventions
  1. Remove impaction by means of lavage or curettage. Be sure to inspect the canal and tympanic membrane after removal of the cerumen.
  2. Document the patient's hearing before and after removal of cerumen.
B. Patient teaching
  1. *See Section III: Patient Teaching Guide for this chapter, "Cerumen Impaction (Earwax)."* ◀
  2. Instruct the patient not to clean ears with cotton swabs, bobby pins, and so forth. Using these devices pushes the wax further into the ear canal and can worsen symptoms.
C. Pharmaceutical therapy
  1. Drug of choice: Debrox, mineral oil, or olive oil two to three drops in the ear every day for 1 week to loosen the cerumen before lavage or curettage. **Do not use Debrox if perforation of tympanic membrane is suspected.**
  2. For prevention, have the patient use the aforementioned softeners for 2 to 3 days. Then have him or her use one capful of hydrogen peroxide in the ear twice daily, allow it to bubble for 5 to 10 minutes, then turn head to allow it to run out.

Follow-Up

A. No follow-up is needed unless indicated. Recurrence is common.

Consultation/Referral

A. Consult or refer the patient to a physician when cerumen cannot be cleared.

Individual Considerations

A. Geriatrics
  1. Cerumen impaction is very common in the elderly due to atrophic cilia and dry epithelium in the ear canal.
  2. The use of hearing aids also can contribute to wax buildup and cause wax to be pushed further into the canal. Persons with hearing aids should be evaluated for wax buildup as indicated.

Hearing Loss

Jill C. Cash and Moya Cook

Definition

Impaired hearing (complete or partial hearing loss) results from interference with the conduction of sound, its conversion to electrical impulses, or its transmission through the nervous system. There are three types of hearing loss:

A. Conductive hearing loss
B. Sensorineural hearing loss
C. Combined conductive and sensorineural loss

Incidence

A. Hearing loss is present in 10% to 15% of patients; approximately 30 million Americans have some degree of hearing impairment.

Pathogenesis

A. *Conductive hearing loss* presents with a diminution of volume, particularly low tones and vowels. It may be caused by one of the following:

1. Otosclerosis disorder of the architecture of the bony labyrinth fixes the footplate of the stapes in the oval window.
2. Exostoses are bony excrescences of the external auditory canal.
3. Glomus tumors are benign, highly vascular tumors derived from normally occurring glomera of the middle ear and jugular bulb.

B. *Sensorineural hearing loss* characteristically produces impairment of the high-tone perception. Affected patients can hear people speaking, but they have difficulty deciphering words because discrimination is poor. It may be caused by one of the following:

1. Presbycusis is hearing loss associated with aging and is the most common cause of diminished hearing in the elderly; onset is bilateral, symmetric, and gradual.
2. Noise-induced hearing loss is due to chronic exposure to sound levels in excess of 85 to 90 dB.
3. Drug-induced hearing loss can be caused by aminoglycoside antibiotics, furosemide, ethacrynic acid, quinidine, and aspirin.
4. Ménière's disease produces a fluctuating, unilateral, low-frequency impairment usually associated with tinnitus, a sensation of fullness in the ear, and intermittent episodes of vertigo.
5. Acoustic neuroma is a benign tumor of the eighth cranial nerve (rare).
6. Sensorineural hearing loss is generally bilateral and symmetric, and it may be genetically determined.
7. Sudden deafness can derive from head trauma, skull fracture, meningitis, otitis media, scarlet fever, mumps, congenital syphilis, multiple sclerosis, and perilymph leaks or fistulas.

Predisposing Factors

A. Acoustic or physical trauma
B. Ototoxic medications (such as gentamicin and aspirin)
C. Changes in barometric pressures
D. Recent upper respiratory infection (URI)
E. Pregnancy
F. Otosclerosis
G. Nasopharyngeal cancer
H. Serous otitis media
I. Cerumen impaction
J. Foreign body in the ear

Common Complaints

A. Partial hearing loss
B. Total hearing loss
C. Difficulty understanding the television, phone conversations, and people talking

Other Signs and Symptoms

A. Unilateral or bilateral hearing loss
B. Hearing noises as "ringing," "buzzing," and so forth
C. Fullness in ear(s)

Subjective Data

A. Elicit the onset, duration, progression, and severity of symptoms. Note whether symptoms are bilateral or unilateral.
B. Obtain the patient's history of past or recent trauma.
C. Review the patient's occupational and recreational exposure to risk factors.
D. Review the patient's medical history and medications, including OTC drugs and prescriptions.
E. Review the patient's history for recent URI or ear infections, especially for chronic ear infections.
F. Elicit data about any previous hearing loss, how it was treated, and how it affected daily activities. There is often a history of previous ear disease with conductive hearing loss.
G. Review the patient's other symptoms such as dizziness, fullness or pressure in the ears, and noises.
H. Review what causes difficulty with hearing, high tones versus low frequencies. Can the patient hear people talking, the television at normal volume, doorbells ringing, telephone ringing, and watch ticking?

Physical Examination

A. Temperature
B. Inspect

1. Examine both ears for comparison.
2. Externally inspect ears for discharge; note color and odor. Obstruction of the auditory canal by impacted cerumen, a foreign body, exostoses, external otitis, OME, or scarring or perforation of the eardrum due to chronic otitis may be present.
3. Conduct otoscopic examination to observe the auditory canal for cerumen impaction or foreign body.
4. Examine tympanic membrane for color, landmarks, contour, perforation, and acute otitis media (AOM). A reddish mass visible through the intact tympanic membrane may indicate a high-riding jugular bulb, an aberrant internal carotid artery, or a glomus tumor.

C. Palpate

1. Palpate auricle and mastoid area for tenderness, swelling, or nodules.
2. Check lymph nodes if infection is suspected.

D. Neurologic testing

1. Weber test

a. Perform a Weber screen. The Weber test reveals conductive hearing loss when sound travels toward the poor ear. Sensorineural hearing loss is present when sound travels toward the good ear. This is performed by striking a tuning fork and then placing it on the middle of the head. The patient should be asked where sound is being heard from, the left ear, the right ear, or equal in both ears. Normal results are reflected by sound being heard equally in both ears.

2. Rinne screen
   a. The Rinne tuning-fork test reveals bone conduction greater than air conduction in the affected ear (abnormal). The Rinne test is performed by placing the struck tuning fork against the mastoid bone. Begin counting or timing the interval from the start to when the patient can no longer hear. Continue counting or timing the interval to determine the length of time sound is heard by air conduction. Air-conducted sound should be heard twice as long as bone-conducted sound after bone conduction stops.

Diagnostic Tests

A. Audiogram in primary setting
B. Air insufflation for tympanic membrane mobility
C. Tympanometry brainstem-evoked response audiogram
D. CT or MRI after consultation with an otolaryngologist

Differential Diagnoses

A. Congenital hearing loss
B. Traumatic hearing loss
C. Ototoxicity
D. Presbycusis
E. Ménière's syndrome
F. Acoustic neuroma
G. Cholesteatoma
H. Infection
I. Cerumen impaction
J. Otitis externa
K. Foreign body in the ear
L. Tumors
M. Otosclerosis
N. Perforation of tympanic membrane
O. Serous otitis media
P. Hypothyroidism
Q. Paget's disease

Plan

A. General interventions
   1. Treat any primary cause (i.e., remove impacted cerumen).
   2. Inform the patient regarding results of screening and indications for further testing.

B. Patient teaching
   1. Discuss avoiding loud noises, using earplugs, and so forth.
   2. Instruct the patient not to insert small objects into the ear.

C. Pharmaceutical therapy: Treat primary condition if applicable.

Follow-Up

A. If the primary cause of hearing loss is not identified, refer the patient to a physician.

Consultation/Referral

A. The patient should be referred to an otolaryngologist for an extensive workup when the primary cause cannot be identified.
B. Referral should be made to a hearing aid specialist for hearing evaluation and treatment as indicated (i.e., hearing aids).

Individual Considerations

A. Pediatrics
   1. Most children are able to respond to a test of gross hearing using a small bell. To determine the patient's hearing ability, note if the child stops moving when the bell is rung and if the child turns his or her head toward the sound.
   2. When examining children, pull the pinna back and slightly upward to straighten the canal.

B. Adults
   1. The external auditory canal in the adult can best be exposed by pulling the earlobe upward and backward.

C. Geriatrics
   1. Impaired hearing among the elderly is common and can lower the quality of life.
   2. People with seriously impaired hearing often become withdrawn or appear confused.
   3. Subtle hearing loss may go unrecognized.
   4. Impacted cerumen is very common in the elderly.

Otitis Externa

Jill C. Cash and Moya Cook

Definition

A. Otitis externa is a common, acute, self-limiting inflammation or infection of the external auditory canal and auricle.

Incidence

A. Otitis externa is seen in patients of all ages. Incidence is higher during summer months. All varieties (with exception of necrotizing otitis externa) are common.

Pathogenesis

A. Acute diffuse otitis externa (swimmer's ear): *Pseudomonas* is the most common bacterial infection (67%), followed by *Staphylococcus* and *Streptococcus*. Infection can also be fungal (*Aspergillus*, 90%). Bacterial or fungal invasion is usually preceded by trauma to the ear canal, aggressive cleaning of the naturally bactericidal cerumen, or frequent submersion in water (swimming).
B. Chronic otitis externa: Condition generally results from a persistent, low-grade infection and inflammation with *Pseudomonas*.
C. Eczematous otitis externa: Otitis externa associated with primary coexistent skin disorder such as atopic dermatitis, seborrheic dermatitis, and psoriasis.
D. Necrotizing or malignant otitis externa: Invasive *Pseudomonas* infection results in skull base osteomyelitis.

It is most commonly seen in the immunocompromised or diabetic geriatric patient.

Predisposing Factors

A. Ear trauma from scratching with a foreign object or fingernail, overly vigorous cleaning of cerumen from canal
B. Humid climate
C. Frequent swimming
D. Use of a hearing aid
E. Eczema (eczematous otitis externa)
F. Debilitating disease (necrotizing otitis externa)

Common Complaints

A. Otalgia
B. Itching
C. Erythematous and swollen external canal
D. Purulent discharge
E. Hearing loss from edema and obstruction of canal with drainage

Other Signs and Symptoms

A. Plugged ear sensation (aural fullness)
B. Tenderness to palpation (tragus)

Subjective Data

A. Elicit the onset, duration, and intensity of ear discomfort.
B. Inquire into the patient's history of previous ear infections.
C. Determine whether the patient notes any degree of hearing loss.
D. Question the patient about recent exposure to immersion in water (swimming).
E. Question the patient as to ear canal cleaning practices and any recent trauma to the canal.

Physical Examination

A. Temperature
B. Inspect
  1. Carefully examine the ear with an otoscope for extreme tenderness.
  2. Observe the ear for erythematous and edematous external canal; look for otorrhea and debris.
  3. Observe the tympanic membrane, which may appear normal.
  4. Inspect nose and throat.
C. Auscultate heart and lungs.
D. Palpate
  1. Apply gentle pressure to tragus and manipulate pinna to assess for tenderness.
  2. Palpate cervical lymph nodes.

Diagnostic Tests

A. Examine ear canal scrapings and drainage under a microscope for hyphae (if fungal infection is suspected from previous history or ineffective topical therapy).
B. Culture vesicular lesions for viruses.

Differential Diagnoses

A. Otitis externa
B. Otitis media
C. Foreign body
D. Mastoiditis
E. Hearing loss
F. Wisdom tooth eruption
G. Herpetic otitis externa (vesicular eruptions in the ear canal are associated with herpetic otitis externa).
H. Necrotizing or malignant otitis externa (life-threatening condition that occurs in diabetic or immunocompromised patients). Cranial nerve palsies (of the seventh, ninth, and twelfth cranial nerves) and periostitis of the skull base have been associated with necrotizing otitis externa.

Plan

A. General interventions
  1. When the patient's ear canal is sufficiently blocked by edema or drainage, preventing passage of ear drops, cautiously irrigate the canal and insert a cotton wick (approximately 1 in. long for adults) to allow passage of drops.
  2. Insert the wick by gently rotating it while inserting it into the ear. The patient then places ear drops on the wick. The drops are absorbed through the wick, which allows medicine to reach the external canal. The provider may need to change the wick daily or several times per week.
B. Patient teaching
  1. *See Section III: Patient Teaching Guide for this chapter, "Otitis Externa."* ◀
  2. The patient should be advised to keep water out of the ear for 4 to 6 weeks. The patient should not swim until symptoms are completely resolved and the wick is removed.
  3. Bathing or showering is permitted with a cotton ball coated with petroleum jelly inserted into the ear to block water passage into the ear canal.
C. Pharmaceutical therapy
  1. For early, mild cases associated with swimming in which the primary symptom is pruritus, homemade preparations of 50% isopropyl alcohol and 50% vinegar can be used as a drying agent and to create an unsatisfactory environment for *Pseudomonas* growth.
  2. Mild infection: Topical therapy—Use of acidifying agent such as Vosol or Vosol HC, which includes a glucocorticoid therapy: Instill five drops in the ear canal three to four times daily. (Vosol and Vosol HC are contraindicated with perforated eardrum; Vosol HC is contraindicated with viral otic infections.)
  3. Moderate infection: Use of an acidifying agent, antibiotic and glucocorticoid therapy (Cipro HC), and Cortisporin is suggested. Other alternatives include Ciprofloxacin (Cipro HC), Ofloxacin (Floxin), Polymyxin B, Neomycin (Cortisporin Otic) suspension or solution. Adults should apply four drops to the canal four times daily for 7 days; children should apply three drops to the canal four times daily for 7 days. The suspension is recommended rather than the solution if the integrity of the tympanic membrane is in question.

a. If fungal infection is suspected, Nystatin 100,000 units/mL or clotrimazole topical solutions may be used for candidal or yeast infections.

4. Severe or resistant infections may require additional management with oral antibiotics and antifungals:

a. Ciprofloxacin for pseudomonal infections; dicloxacillin or cephalexin for staphylococcal infections.

b. Itraconazole (Sporanox) for treatment of otomycosis (fungal otitis externa).

5. For analgesia, use acetaminophen or ibuprofen. Short-term use of opiates may be necessary when acetaminophen and ibuprofen fail to control pain.

Follow-Up

A. Usual follow-up is within 48 hours to assess improvement. Recheck in 1 to 2 weeks.

B. In severe cases requiring antibiotic drops instilled by means of a wick, follow-up may be required daily or several times per week to remove and replace the wick.

Consultation/Referral

A. Parenteral antibiotics are required for necrotizing otitis externa. These patients should be immediately referred to a physician.

B. Consult or refer the patient to a physician if osteomyelitis is suspected.

Individual Considerations

A. Geriatrics

1. Persistent otitis externa in the geriatric patient (especially those who are immunocompromised or diabetic) may evolve into osteomyelitis of the skull base.

2. The external ear is painful and edematous, and a foul, green discharge is usually present.

3. Treatment may require parenteral gentamicin with a beta-lactam agent. Surgery may be necessary.

4. Oral fluoroquinolones may be useful if infection has not progressed to osteomyelitis.

Otitis Media With Effusion

Jill C. Cash and Moya Cook

Definition

A. Otitis media with effusion (OME) is asymptomatic middle-ear fluid without signs of bacterial infection.

Incidence

A. OME is seen in patients of all ages.

B. After the onset of acute otitis media (AOM), approximately 70% of children have fluid present at 2 weeks.

1. 40% have fluid present at 1 month.

2. 20% have fluid present at 2 months.

3. 10% have an effusion at 3 months.

Pathogenesis

A. The effusion may be sterile fluid secondary to upper respiratory infection (URI) and Eustachian tube dysfunction. It may be residual fluid after an episode of AOM.

Predisposing Factors

A. Recent otitis media

B. Concurrent URI

Common Complaints

A. Ear pain

B. Increased pressure sensation in the ears

C. Recent hearing loss

Other Signs and Symptoms

A. The patient has a sense of fullness in the ears.

Subjective Data

A. Elicit the onset and duration of symptoms.

B. Question the patient about recent history of otitis media or URI.

C. Question the patient about hearing loss.

D. Determine if the patient has a past history of frequent otitis media.

Physical Examination

A. Check temperature, pulse, respirations, and blood pressure.

B. Inspect

1. Ears, noting fluid level, serous middle fluid, and a translucent, amber, gray membrane with decreased mobility.

2. Nose, mouth, and throat.

C. Auscultate heart and lungs.

D. Palpate head, neck, and lymph nodes.

E. Neurologic examination

1. Perform the Rinne test. This test is performed by placing the struck tuning fork against the mastoid bone. Begin counting or timing the interval from the start to when the patient can no longer hear. Continue counting or timing the interval to determine the length of time sound is heard by air conduction. Air-conducted sound should be heard twice as long as bone-conducted sound after bone conduction stops.

2. Perform the Weber test.

Diagnostic Tests

A. Pneumatic otoscopy reveals decreased mobility. **Assessment with pneumatic otoscopy is strongly recommended.**

B. Negative pressure on tympanogram.

Differential Diagnoses

A. OME

B. Cerumen impaction

C. AOM

D. Foreign body in the ear

Plan

A. General interventions

1. Patient should be monitored closely for resolution of effusion without treatment within several weeks.

2. Patients who have persistent effusion are at risk for hearing loss, speech, language, and learning disorders.

3. Children with persistent OME should be referred to an otolaryngologist for a hearing evaluation and possible tympanostomy tubes as indicated.

4. Speech and language evaluation or documentation of hearing loss is recommended for children with OME older than 3 months.

B. Patient teaching

1. *See Section III: Patient Teaching Guide for this chapter, "Otitis Media With Effusion."*

2. Educate parents that OME is not treated with antibiotics since no infection is present.

3. If symptoms change, infection should be suspected and the primary care provider should be notified of new symptoms and that reevaluation is needed.

4. Teach the parents/care provider that routine use of antihistamines and decongestants is not recommended.

C. Pharmaceutical therapy

1. The American Academy of Pediatrics, the American Academy of Family Physicians, and the American Academy of Otolaryngology-Head Neck Surgery do not recommend routine use of antibiotic therapy for OME. However, in certain situations, a course of antibiotics (Amoxil) for 10 to 14 days is recommended.

2. Intranasal glucocorticoids are not recommended for routine use for OME in children.

3. Antihistamines and decongestants are not recommended for routine use for OME in children.

Follow-Up

A. Recheck the patient's ears after 4 to 6 weeks to evaluate effectiveness of treatment.

Consultation/Referral

A. Consult or refer the patient to a physician if treatment is not effective or if the patient has a persistent effusion (at least 3 months) along with a hearing loss of 20 dB or more.

B. Consider referring the patient to an otolaryngologist.

Individual Considerations

A. Geriatrics

1. OME may be present in the elderly, usually unilaterally, and usually associated with a URI or allergies due to a blocked Eustachian tube.

2. If there is no accompanying URI, a nasopharyngeal mass must be ruled out.

Tinnitus

Jill C. Cash and Moya Cook

Definition

A. The word *tinnitus* comes from the Latin *tinnire*, which means "to ring." It refers to any sound heard in the ears or head.

Incidence

A. It is estimated that 6.4% of the adult population has experienced tinnitus at some point. More than 7 million people in the United States are thought to experience tinnitus.

Pathogenesis

A. Tinnitus is poorly understood. It is best described as a nonspecific manifestation of pathology of the inner ear, eighth cranial nerve, or the central auditory mechanism.

Predisposing Factors

A. Cerumen impaction

B. Tympanic membrane perforation

C. Fluid in the middle ear

D. Acute otitis media (AOM)

E. Acoustic trauma

F. Ototoxic drugs

1. Sulfas
2. Aminoglycosides
3. Salicylate
4. Indomethacin
5. Propranolol
6. Levodopa
7. Carbamazepine

G. Vascular aneurysm

H. Jugular bulb anomaly. Compression of the ipsilateral jugular vein abolishes the objective tinnitus of a jugular megabulb anomaly

I. Anemia

J. Temporomandibular joint syndrome

K. Hypertension

Common Complaints

A. Ringing

B. Roaring

C. Buzzing

D. Clicking

E. Hissing

F. Hearing loss

Other Signs and Symptoms

A. "Muffled" hearing

B. Change in own voice, lower pitch

Subjective Data

A. Review the onset, duration, course, and type of symptoms; note whether they are bilateral or unilateral.

B. Determine the frequency and quality of sound; is the ringing constant, intermittent, or pulsating?

C. Review all medications, including over-the-counter (OTC) drugs and prescriptions.

D. Determine whether the patient has experienced trauma (domestic violence, motor vehicle accident, and so forth).

E. Rule out a recent sinus, oral, or ear infection.

F. Review any previous occurrences. Ask: How was it treated?

G. Review work, hobbies, and music habits for noise levels (potential damage).

H. Assess the date of last hearing examination and determine whether there was any known hearing loss.

I. Review whether the patient uses cotton-tipped swabs or other small objects for ear cleaning.

Physical Examination

A. Take temperature if infectious cause is suspected.
B. Inspect
1. Observe the external ear for discharge; note color and odor.
2. Conduct otoscopic examination of the auditory canal for cerumen impaction or foreign body.
3. Inspect tympanic membrane for color, landmarks, contour, perforation, and AOM.
a. The landmarks (umbo, handle of malleus, and the light reflex) should be visible on a normal examination.
b. The tympanic membrane should be pearly gray in color and translucent.
c. A bulging tympanic membrane is more conical, usually with a loss of bony landmarks and a distorted light reflex.
d. A retracted tympanic membrane is more concave, usually with accentuated bony landmarks and a distorted light reflex (pathologic conditions in the middle ear may be reflected by characteristics of the tympanic membrane).
C. Auscultation
1. The skull should be auscultated for a bruit if the origin of the problem remains obscure.
D. Palpate
1. Palpate auricle and mastoid area for tenderness, swelling, or nodules.
2. Check lymph nodes if infection is suspected.
E. Visual examination
1. Check for nystagmus if vertigo is reported.
F. Neurologic examination
1. The eighth cranial nerve is tested by evaluating hearing.
2. First evaluate how the patient responds to your questions.
3. Patients who speak in a monotone or with erratic volume may have hearing loss.
4. Check the patient's response to a soft whisper (should respond at least 50% of the time).
5. Perform the Rinne test: The Rinne test is performed by placing the struck tuning fork against the mastoid bone. Begin counting or timing the interval from the start to when the patient can no longer hear. Continue counting or timing the interval to determine the length of time sound is heard by air conduction. Air-conducted sound should be heard twice as long as bone-conducted sound after bone conduction stops.
6. Perform the Weber test.

Diagnostic Tests

A. Audiogram is performed in the primary care setting; other testing is performed by an otolaryngologist. Any association of the sound with respiration, drug use, vertigo, noise trauma, or ear infection should be checked. When the problem is present only at night, it suggests increased awareness of normal head sounds.
B. CT scan or MRI after referral to an otolaryngologist
C. Posterior fossa myelography

Differential Diagnoses

A. Tinnitus
B. Cerumen impaction
C. Foreign body in the ear
D. AOM
E. Otitis externa
F. Acoustic traumas
G. Vascular aneurysm
H. Temporomandibular joint syndrome
I. Otosclerosis
J. Ototoxicity
K. Ménière's syndrome
L. Presbycusis
M. Central nervous system lesion

Plan

A. General interventions
1. Stress the importance of not placing small objects in the ear and using cotton-tipped applicators to clean external ear only.
2. Suggest to the patient that keeping a radio on for background noise often facilitates sleep or work.
3. Address underlying conditions if present (depression, insomnia, hearing loss, drug toxicity).
4. Consider behavioral therapy, such as biofeedback or cognitive behavioral therapy, to teach patient coping strategies.
B. Patient teaching
1. Educate the patient regarding techniques/therapies to improve symptoms of tinnitus.
2. Encourage the patient to attend therapy sessions as indicated.
C. Pharmaceutical therapy
1. No medication "cures" tinnitus.
2. Vasodilators, tranquilizers, antidepressants, and seizure medications have been shown to reduce symptoms.
3. Placebos are also of therapeutic value.

Follow-Up

A. No specific follow-up is required for tinnitus unless a treatable problem is identified.

Consultation/Referral

A. Consult with an otolaryngologist as indicated.
B. Referral of an anxious patient to the otolaryngologist may be necessary to satisfy the patient that everything has been explored and that there is no serious or correctable underlying condition.
C. Any patient with a history of head trauma should be referred to a physician because tinnitus may be associated with an arteriovenous fistula or an aneurysm of the intrapetrous portion of the internal carotid artery.

Bibliography

Bhattacharyya, N., & Meyers, A. D. (2015). Auditory brainstem response auditometry. *Medscape*. Retrieved from http://emedicine.medscape.com/article/836277-overview#a6

Bird, S. (2008). Ear syringing: Minimizing the risks. *Australian Family Physician, 37*(4), 359–360. Retrieved from www.racgp.org.au/afp/backissues/2008

Centers for Disease Control and Prevention, National Institute for Occupational Safety and Health. (2013). *Noise and hearing loss prevention.* DHHS (NIOSH) Pub. No. 2001-103. Retrieved from www.cdc.gov

Dinces, E. (2015). Cerumen. In D. Deschler (Ed.), *UpToDate.* Retrieved from https://www.uptodate.com/contents/cerumen?source=machineLearning&search=ear+lavage&selectedTitle=1%7E150§ionRank=1&anchor=H9#H9

Klein, J. O, & Pelton, S. (2015). Acute otitis media in children: Treatment. In M. Edwards & G. Isaacson (Eds.), *UptoDate.* Retrieved from http://www.uptodate.com/contents/acute-otitis-media-in-children-treatment

Klein, J. O., & Pelton, S. (2016). Management of otitis media with effusion (serous otitis media) in children. In S. Kaplan & G. Isaacson (Eds.), *UpToDate.* Retrieved from http://www.uptodate.com/contents/management-of-otitis-media-with-effusion-serous-otitis-media-in-children?source=search_result&search=otitis+meda+with+effusion&selectedTitle=1~48

Lustig, L. R., Limb, C. J., Baden, R., & LaSalvia, M. T. (2015). Chronic otitis media, cholesteatoma, and mastoiditis in adults. In D. Deschler (Ed.), *UpToDate.* Retrieved from http://www.uptodate.com/contents/chronic-otitis-media-cholesteatoma-and-mastoiditis-in-adults?source=search_result&search=otitis+media+adult&selectedTitle=2%7E150

Mener, D. J., Betz, J., Genther, D. J., Chen, D., & Lin, F. R. (2013). Hearing loss and depression in older adults. *Journal of the American Geriatrics Society, 61*(9), 1627–1629.

National Institute on Deafness and Other Communication Disorders (2016, March). *NIDCD Fact Sheet: Hearing and Balance: Hearing loss and older adults.* NIH Pub. No. 01-4913. Washington, DC: U.S. Department of Health and Human Services. Retrieved from https://www.nidcd.nih.gov/health/hearing-loss-older-adults

National Institutes of Health, National Institute on Deafness and Other Communication Disorders (2015a). *NIDCD Fact Sheet: Hearing and Balance: Pendred Syndrome* (NIH Publication No. 06-5875). November 2012, Reprinted December 2014. Washington, DC: U.S. Department of Health and Human Services. Retrieved from https://www.nidcd.nih.gov/health/pendred-syndrome

National Institutes of Health, National Institute on Deafness and Other Communication Disorders (2015b). Quick statistics about hearing. Retrieved from https://www.nidcd.nih.gov/health/statistics/quick-statistics-hearing

Poe, D., & Bassem, M. (2016). Eustachian tube dysfunction. In D. Deschler (Ed.), *UpToDate.* Retrieved from http://www.uptodate.com/contents/eustachian-tube-dysfunction?source=search_result&search=eustachian+tube+dysfunction&selectedTitle=1%7E39

Roland, P. S. (2015). Presbycusis. *Medscape.* Retrieved from www.medscape.comarticle/855989-overview

Schaefer, P., & Baugh, R. (2012). Acute otitis externa: An update. *American Family Physician, 86*(11), 1055–1061.

Tunkel, D. E., Bauer, C. A., Sun, G. H., Rosenfeld R. M., Chandrasekhar, S. S., Cunningham, E. R., . . . Whamond, E. J. (2014). Clinical guidelines: Tinnitus. *Otolaryngology Head Neck Surgery, 151*(2 Suppl.), S1–40. Retrieved from https://www.guideline.gov/content.aspx?id=48751&search=tinnitus

7 Nasal Guidelines

Allergic Rhinitis

Jill C. Cash and Moya Cook

Definition

A. Allergic rhinitis is a chronic or recurrent condition characterized by nasal congestion, clear nasal discharge, sneezing, nasal itching, conjunctival itching, and periorbital edema. It usually occurs seasonally after exposure to allergens (same time every year, associated with pollen count), or it may be perennial (year-round, related to indoor inhalants, animal dander, and mold). "Allergic" suggests that a specific immunoglobulin E (IgE) antibody mediates the condition.

Incidence

A. Prevalence varies according to geographic region; 20% to 25% of adults have allergic rhinitis.

Pathogenesis

A. This is an immunoglobulin E (IgE) mediated inflammatory disease involving nasal mucosa; IgE antibodies bind to mast cells in the respiratory epithelium, and histamine is released. This results in immediate local vasodilatation, mucosal edema, and increased mucus production.

Predisposing Factors

A. Genetic predisposition to allergy
B. Exposure to allergic stimuli: Pollens, molds, animal dander, dust mites, and indoor inhalants

Common Complaints

A. Nasal congestion
B. Sneezing
C. Clear rhinorrhea
D. Coughing from postnasal drip
E. Sore throat
F. Itchy, puffy eyes with tearing

Other Signs and Symptoms

A. Dry mouth from mouth breathing, snoring
B. Itchy nose
C. Loss of smell and taste
D. Eczema rash
E. Shortness of breath, difficulty breathing, and wheezing
F. Headache
G. Halitosis

Subjective Data

A. Ask about onset, course, and duration of symptoms.
B. Inquire about characteristics of nasal discharge.
C. Inquire about exposure to people with similar symptoms.
D. Ask about seasonal impact on symptoms.
E. Inquire about other diseases caused by allergens, such as asthma, eczema, and urticaria.
F. Rule out pregnancy.
G. Ask female patients about their birth control method, specifically birth control pills.
H. Review exposure to irritants.
I. Ask about any past or recent nasal trauma.

Physical Examination

A. Vital signs: Temperature, blood pressure, pulse, and respirations
B. Inspect
- **1.** Examine face. Note Dennie's lines (skin folds under eyes) and allergic salute (transverse crease on nose from chronic rubbing of nose).
- **2.** Examine eyes and conjunctivae.
  - **a.** Tearing; red, swollen eyelids; and allergic shiners (dark circles under eyes from venous congestion in maxillary sinuses) are seen with allergies.
  - **b.** Palpebral conjunctiva pale and swollen, bulbar conjunctiva is injected.
- **3.** Examine ears, nose, and throat.
  - **a.** Red, dull, bulging, perforated tympanic membrane is seen with otitis media.
  - **b.** Nasal redness, swelling, polyps, and enlarged turbinates are seen with upper respiratory infection (URI). Mucosa appears pale blue, and boggy with clear discharge in chronic allergy.
  - **c.** Cobblestone appearance in pharynx, tonsils, and adenoids seen in chronic allergies.
  - **d.** Use otoscope light to transilluminate under superior orbital ridge of frontal sinus cavity and also maxillary sinus cavity to assess for fluid in sinus cavity. Healthy sinuses contain air and light up symmetrically.

C. Palpate
- **1.** Palpate face and frontal maxillary sinuses for tenderness.

2. Examine the head and neck for enlarged lymph nodes.

D. Percuss

1. Sinus cavities and mastoid bone
2. Chest for consolidation

E. Auscultate heart and lungs.

Diagnostic Tests

Diagnosis may be made from history and physical. Other diagnostic tests include:

A. Wright's stain of nasal secretions; eosinophils present confirm allergy
B. Skin testing for allergies
C. Radioallergosorbent test (RAST)
D. Complete blood count (CBC) with increased eosinophils (confirm allergy)

Differential Diagnoses

A. Allergic rhinitis
B. URI
C. Medication-induced rhinitis
D. Sinusitis
E. Otitis media
F. Deviated septum
G. Nasal polyps
H. Endocrine conditions such as hypothyroidism
I. Influenza

Plan

A. General interventions

1. Avoid allergens (most effective treatment).
2. Keep bedroom as allergen free as possible.

▶ B. Patient teaching: *See Section III: Patient Teaching Guide for this chapter, "Allergic Rhinitis."*

C. Pharmaceutical therapy

1. Antihistamines (H_1 receptor antagonists) are drugs of choice. Several may need to be tried before an effective one is found. Drugs may also need to be switched occasionally to prevent tolerance.

a. Azelastine hydrochloride (HCl; Astelin) metered nasal spray, 137 mcg per metered dose

i. Children younger than 5 years: Not recommended
ii. Children 5 to 11 years: One spray in each nostril twice daily
iii. Adults: Two sprays per nostril twice daily

b. Loratadine (Claritin) 10 mg by mouth daily (adults)

i. Children younger than 2 years: Not recommended
ii. Children 2 to 5 years: 5 mg daily
iii. Children 6 years and older: 10 mg daily

c. Fexofenadine HCl (Allegra) 60 mg capsules orally twice daily (adults) or 180 mg daily

i. Children younger than 6 years: Not recommended
ii. Children 6 to 11years: 30 mg twice daily

d. Cetirizine HCl (Zyrtec)

i. Adults and children 12 years and older: 5 to 10 mg by mouth daily depending on symptom severity
ii. Zyrtec 5 mg daily for patients with renal or hepatic impairment
iii. Children 2 to 6 years: 2.5 mg daily
iv. Children 6 to 11 years: 5 to 10 mg (1–2 teaspoons) by mouth daily depending on symptom severity

e. Montelukast (Singulair): Not recommended for children younger than 6 months

i. Children 6 to 23 months: One 4-mg granule packet
ii. Children 2 to 5 years: One 4-mg chewable tablet or granule packet
iii. Children 6 to 14 years: One 5-mg tablet
iv. Children older than 15 years and adults: One 10-mg tablet daily

f. Levocetirizine dihydrochloride (Xyzal)

i. Children younger than 6 years: Not recommended
ii. Children 6 to 11 years: Maximum 2.5 mg once daily in p.m.
iii. Adults: 2.5 to 5 mg daily in p.m. Precautions for renal impairment

2. Topical decongestants for significant congestion of the mucous membranes. These drugs may also stimulate the sympathetic nervous system and cause insomnia, nervousness, and palpitations. **Use no longer than 3 to 5 days. Discontinuing these drugs after 5 days may result in a rebound effect.**

a. Oxymetazoline hydrochloride (Afrin) spray or drops

i. Adults and children 6 years and older: 2 to 3 drops or sprays of 0.05% solution in each nostril twice daily
ii. Children 2 to 6 years: 2 to 3 drops of 0.025% solution in each nostril twice daily

b. Phenylephrine (Neo-Synephrine) spray or drops

i. Adults and children 12 years and older: 2 to 3 drops or one to two sprays in each nostril, or small amount of jelly applied to nasal mucosa, every 4 hours as needed. Do not use for more than 3 to 5 days.
ii. Children 6 to 12 years: 2 to 3 drops or one to two sprays of 0.25% solution in each nostril every 4 hours as needed. Do not use for more than 3 to 5 days.
iii. Children younger than 6 years: 2 to 3 drops of 0.125% solution every 4 hours in each nostril as needed. Contact physician if symptoms persist beyond 3 days.

3. Steroid sprays may be used to decrease nasal inflammation. Steroid sprays are not recommended in children younger than 6 years old unless there is an

allergic component. Sprays do not cause significant systemic absorption in usual doses, but occasionally they may cause pharyngeal fungal infections.

a. Beclomethasone dipropionate (Beconase AQ, Vancenase): Adults and children older than 6 years: One to two sprays in each nostril twice daily

b. Fluticasone propionate (Flonase): Adults: Two sprays daily or one spray twice daily. Maintenance dosing: One spray in each nostril daily. Children younger than 4 years: Not recommended. Children 4 years and older: One spray in each nostril daily, may increase to two sprays each nostril once daily. Maintenance: One spray daily

c. Triamcinolone acetonide (Nasacort AQ): Adults: Two sprays daily. Children 2 to 5 years: One spray in each nostril once daily. Children 6 to 12 years: One spray in each nostril once daily, maximum one spray in each nostril once daily. Reduce dose as condition improves.

d. Mometasone furoate (Nasonex): Adults: Two sprays in each nostril once daily. Children 2 to 11 years: One spray in each nostril daily

e. Fluticasone furoate (Veramyst)

i. Adults: Two sprays each nostril daily

1) Maintenance: One spray in each nostril daily

ii. Children 2 to 11 years: One spray in each nostril daily; may increase to two sprays daily if needed

1) Maintenance dose: One spray in each nostril daily

f. Budesonide (Rhinocort Aqua): Children younger than 6 years: Not recommended. Adults and children 6 years and older: Two sprays twice daily

g. Qnasl (beclomethasone dipropionate): Children: Not established. Adults: Two sprays in each nostril once daily; maximum four sprays per day

4. Saline spray

a. Saline spray is effective in liquefying thick secretions and helps keep mucosa moist.

b. Use Neti pot to cleanse inside of nasal mucosa; daily use suggested.

5. Petroleum jelly applied with Q-tip to inside mucosa of nares three to four times a day helps to provide lubrication and hold in moisture to prevent nasal dryness and bleeding.

Follow-Up

A. Patient should return for follow-up visit in 2 to 3 weeks if necessary; earlier if symptoms worsen after 3 days of treatment.

Consultation/Referral

A. Refer the patient to an allergist if symptoms continue and interfere with daily activities.

B. Allergist may prescribe immunotherapy following identification of offending allergens.

Individual Considerations

A. Pregnancy

1. Over-the-counter (OTC) antihistamines, such as diphenhydramine HCl (Benadryl), may be used for up to 5 days.

2. OTC decongestants, such as oxymetazoline HCl (Afrin), may be used up to 3 days.

Epistaxis

Jill C. Cash and Moya Cook

Definition

A. Epistaxis is a nosebleed or hemorrhage from the nose.

Incidence

A. About 11% of Americans have had at least one nosebleed.

Pathogenesis

A. Epistaxis is caused by disruption of the nasal mucosa. More than 90% of nosebleeds are related to local irritation rather than underlying anatomic lesions and are self-limiting. Most start in the anterior nasal cavity (Kisselbach's plexus).

B. Posterior nasal bleeding usually originates from the turbinates or lateral nasal wall.

Predisposing Factors

A. Local trauma, usually from nose picking

B. Acute inflammation from an upper respiratory infection (URI; e.g., common cold, acute sinusitis, and allergic rhinitis)

C. Vigorous nose blowing

D. Inhalation of chemical irritants

E. Drying and crusting of nasal septum

F. Trauma

G. Cocaine use

H. Pregnancy

I. Neoplasm

J. Systemic causes

1. Bleeding disorders (most common)

2. Hypertension

3. Arteriosclerosis

4. Renal disease

Common Complaints

A. Common complaint is unusually severe or frequent nosebleeds.

Other Signs and Symptoms

A. Anterior epistaxis

1. Unilateral

2. Continuous, moderate bleeding from septum of nose

B. Posterior epistaxis

1. Brisk (arterial) bleeding
2. Blood flowing into pharynx (indicates a more serious problem)

Subjective Data

A. Inquire about amount, duration, and frequency of bleeding.
B. Ask about use of oral anticoagulants, aspirin, or aspirin-containing compounds (e.g., Pepto-Bismol, aspirin, Excedrin).
C. Ask about recent or current URIs, family history of abnormal bleeding, recent surgery, or trauma.
D. Ask about the first day of female patient's last menstrual period (if appropriate). Determine if the patient is pregnant.
E. Ask about a possible foreign body in the nose.
F. Ask about cocaine use or occupational exposure to irritants or chemicals.
G. If the patient has a history of nosebleeds, how did the patient treat previous nosebleeds?
H. Has the patient ever been evaluated for a blood clotting abnormality, such as thrombocytopenia or platelet dysfunction?
I. Does the patient complain of bruising easily, melena, or heavy menstrual periods?
J. Ask about family history of bleeding disorders, such as hemophilia or von Willebrand's disease.

Physical Examination

A. Check temperature, blood pressure (check for orthostatic hypertension), pulse, and respirations. **If nasal packing is required, take precaution and monitor patient closely for vasovagal episode during insertion of nasal packing.**
B. Inspect
1. Check airway patency with patient sitting and leaning forward.
2. Observe skin, mucous membranes, and conjunctiva for rash, pallor, purpura, petechiae, and telangiectasias.
3. Perform full eye examination, noting pupillary response.
4. Examine nose for septal perforation and ulcerations, which indicate cocaine use. Collagen diseases (such as lupus) are occasionally responsible for ulceration. Epistaxis is rare in hemophiliacs without trauma but is characteristic of von Willebrand's disease.
5. Examine nasal discharge: A unilateral foul discharge with blood indicates a foreign body in the nose.
6. After bleeding has stopped:
   a. Inspect nasal mucosa for color, discharge, masses, lesions, and swelling of turbinates.
   b. Inspect nasal septum for alignment, septal perforation, and crusting.

C. Auscultate heart and lungs.
D. Palpate: Check for enlarged lymph nodes in the neck to rule out sarcoidosis, tuberculosis, or malignancy.
E. Percuss sinuses.

Diagnostic Tests

A. None is required unless the patient has recurrent or severe blood loss.
B. Perform drug screen, if indicated.
C. Hematocrit and hemoglobin if bleeding is severe.
D. Complete blood count (CBC) with differential.
E. Platelets, prothrombin time (PT), and partial thromboplastin time (PTT) if bleeding disorder is suspected.
F. Sinus films if recurrent sinus pain, tenderness, and bleeding.

Differential Diagnoses

A. Epistaxis
B. Foreign body
C. Septal deformity
D. Perforated nasal septum
E. Coagulation disorder (von Willebrand's disease)
F. Nasal tumors
G. Drug-induced coagulopathy
H. Hypertension
I. Pregnancy

Plan

A. General interventions: Main goal is to control episodes of bleeding.
B. Patient teaching: *See Section III: Patient Teaching Guide for this chapter, "Nosebleeds."* ◀
C. Pharmaceutical therapy/medical/surgical management
1. To control *anterior septal bleeding:*
   a. Have patient sit and lean forward, apply pressure to reduce venous pressure, and prevent swallowing of blood.
   b. Soak a cotton pledget in phenylephrine (Neo-Synephrine), oxymetazoline HCl (Afrin), or epinephrine 1:1,000, and apply with pressure against bleeding site for 5 to 10 minutes.
   c. Remove and check for bleeding after 10 minutes.
   d. If this fails, anesthetize mucous membrane by applying cotton soaked with a vasoconstrictor, such as 4% lidocaine (Xylocaine) plus topical epinephrine (1:10,000), cocaine 4%, or phenylephrine 0.25% for 10 to 15 minutes.
   e. Then apply a silver nitrate stick to the bleeding site and any prominent vessels, until gray eschar appears. Warn the patient that this is painful.
   f. If bleeding still does not stop (rare), repeat last two steps. Then place a small amount of oxidized regenerated cellulose (Surgicel) against the bleeding artery, or pack a small petroleum gauze strip in the nasal vestibule for 24 hours. Monitor the patient for vasovagal episode during the insertion of packing.
2. To control *posterior* septal bleeding:
   a. Have the patient sit and lean forward.
   b. Control bleeding: Spray nose with topical anesthetic and vasoconstrictor, and apply pressure to the bleeding site.

c. Consult a physician. The patient needs emergency department care immediately because of rapid blood loss.
d. Take blood pressure and pulse; order hematocrit; blood type and cross-match may be needed.

Follow-Up

A. Anterior septal bleeding: Referral to otolaryngologist is recommended for unsuccessful cessation of hemorrhage.
B. For posterior nosebleeds, admission to hospital and referral to otolaryngologist is recommended.

Consultation/Referral

A. Posterior epistaxis: Refer to a physician and/or otolaryngologist immediately.

Individual Considerations

A. Pregnancy
- **1.** Nosebleeds are common.
- **2.** Suggest use of saline spray to keep mucous membranes moist and use humidifier at bedtime.
- **3.** Follow use of saline spray with Vaseline applied with Q-tip daily to prevent recurrent nosebleeds.

B. Pediatrics
- **1.** The most common cause of nosebleeds is trauma from nose picking or rubbing.
- **2.** Advise parents to keep fingernails short.
- **3.** Applying water-based lubricant on rims of nostrils to maintain mucosal moisture may cause lipoid pneumonia in infants and children.

C. Geriatrics
- **1.** Spontaneous posterior hemorrhage is more common in elderly patients.
- **2.** Epistaxis is classically associated with hypertension or arteriosclerosis.
- **3.** Airway obstruction from posterior packing is especially risky in the elderly.
- **4.** Applying water-based lubricant on rims of nostrils to maintain mucosal moisture may cause lipoid pneumonia in the elderly.

Nonallergic Rhinitis

Jill C. Cash and Moya Cook

Definition

A. Nonallergic rhinitis is an inflammation of nasal mucous membranes, usually accompanied by a nasal discharge and mucosal edema. Nonallergic rhinitis disorder has no correlation to specific allergen exposures. It is classified in several ways: Vasomotor, perennial, atrophic, geriatric, drug induced, or rhinitis of pregnancy.

Incidence

A. Chronic or recurrent nasal congestion occurs in about 15% to 20% of the population.

Pathogenesis

A. Vasomotor and perennial nonallergic rhinitis results from hyperreactive nasal mucosa.
B. Atrophic and geriatric rhinitis results from progressive degeneration and atrophy of the mucous membranes and bones of the nose.
C. Overuse of topical nasal decongestants can worsen symptoms and cause severe rebound congestion.
D. Cocaine abuse causes nasal congestion and discharge.
E. Rhinitis in pregnancy results from hormonal increase; congestion abates with delivery.

Predisposing Factors

A. Adulthood
B. Abrupt changes in temperature, odors, and emotional stress
C. Other predisposing factors depend on type

Common Complaints

A. Nasal congestion
B. Sneezing
C. Clear rhinorrhea
D. Coughing
E. Sore throat
F. Itchy, puffy eyes

Subjective Data

A. Ask about the onset, duration, and course of symptoms.
B. Inquire about the color and other characteristics of nasal discharge.
C. Ask about other discomforts and exposure to people with similar symptoms.
D. Inquire about seasonal impact on symptoms, previous treatments, and results.
E. Rule out pregnancy. Ask female patients about birth control method, specifically contraceptives.
F. Ask about use of prescription drugs, over-the-counter (OTC) drugs (especially aspirin), and illicit drugs (cocaine).
G. Review medical history for other respiratory problems, such as asthma, emphysema, or chronic bronchitis.
H. With children, investigate possibility of a foreign object in nostrils.

Physical Examination

A. Check temperature and blood pressure.
B. Inspect
- **1.** Observe general appearance.
- **2.** Inspect conjunctivae for "allergic shiners" (dark circles under eyes), tearing, and eyelid swelling.
- **3.** Examine ears for signs of otitis media (red, bulging, perforated tympanic membrane, and purulent drainage).
- **4.** Examine nose for redness, swelling, polyps (soft, pedunculated, nontender, pale-gray smooth structures), enlarged turbinates, foreign objects, septal deviation, septal perforation (sign of cocaine abuse), ischemia, mucosal injury, atrophy, and "cobblestoned" pharyngeal mucosa (sign of allergy).

C. Auscultate heart and lungs.
D. Percuss
- **1.** Sinus cavities and mastoid process
- **2.** Chest for consolidation

E. Palpate
1. Face for sinus tenderness
2. Head and neck for enlarged lymph nodes

Diagnostic Test

A. Skin testing for allergies may be done.

Differential Diagnoses

A. Nonallergic rhinitis
B. Allergic rhinitis
C. Upper respiratory infection (URI)
D. Foreign body
E. Sinusitis
F. Otitis media
G. Deviated septum
H. Nasal polyps
I. Endocrine conditions, such as hypothyroidism and pregnancy
J. Drug use: Oral contraceptives, aspirin, alpha-adrenergic blockers, cocaine, and nasal decongestant overuse

Plan

A. General interventions
1. Avoid changes in temperature, odors, and emotional stress.
2. Identify triggers for condition and address alleviating triggers.

B. Patient teaching
1. Teach the patient the significance of individual triggers for nonallergic rhinitis. Encourage use of a journal to learn personal triggers.
2. Avoid triggers, such as smoking, smoke-filled rooms, wood-burning stoves/fireplaces, sprays, and perfumes.
3. Other triggers may include weather changes, hormonal changes, and medications.
4. Teach methods of treatment and identify treatments that work best for the patient.
5. Encourage use of Neti pot daily to cleanse sinus cavity. Cleansing sinus cavity daily will help to remove foreign materials inhaled and will also help with tissue edema. Clean pot after each use and allow to air dry.

C. Pharmaceutical therapy
1. Vasomotor rhinitis: Physiological saline solution as nasal spray, thorough cleansing of nares, topical ipratropium bromide, or inhaled ipratropium bromide (Atrovent) 3 to 6 puffs every 4 hours, not to exceed 12 inhalations per day
2. Atrophic rhinitis: Guaifenesin (Guiatuss) 200 mg/5 mL, 10 mL orally every 4 hours
3. Physiological saline nasal spray to nares three times a day
4. Nasal antihistamines: Azelastine (Astelin): Adults: Two sprays in each nostril daily. Children younger than 5 years: Not recommended. Children 5 to 11 years: One spray in each nostril daily. Olopatadine (Patanase): Adults: Two sprays twice daily. Children younger than 6 years: Not recommended. Children 6 to 11 years: One spray in each nostril twice daily
5. Nasal glucocorticoids: Fluticasone (Flonase): Adults: Two sprays daily or one spray twice daily. Maintenance dosing: One spray in each nostril daily. Children younger than 4 years: Not recommended. Children 4 years and older: One spray in each nostril daily, may increase to two sprays in each nostril once daily. Maintenance: One spray daily. Mometasone (Nasonex): Adults: Two sprays in each nostril once daily. Children younger than 2 years: Not recommended. Children 2 to 11 years: One spray in each nostril daily.
6. Decongestants: Oral and nasal decongestants are not recommended unless the use of antihistamines and glucocorticoids failed. Examples may include: Oral pseudoephedrine or nasal oxymetazoline (Afrin) and phenylephrine (Neo-Synephrine). These should not be used longer than 2 to 3 days at a time for congestion due to the effects of rebound congestion with long-term use.

Follow-Up

A. Have the patient return in 2 to 3 weeks and for biannual examinations and/or as needed.

Consultation/Referral

A. Consult with a physician if symptoms continue despite treatment.
B. If treatment fails, refer the patient to the allergist for testing.

Individual Consideration

A. Pregnancy: Reassure pregnant patients that rhinitis is a common hormonal response. Nonallergic rhinitis is not contagious and cannot cross the placenta.

Sinusitis

Jill C. Cash and Moya Cook

Definition

Sinusitis is the inflammation of mucous membranes lining paranasal sinuses. Sinusitis is often referred to as rhinosinusitis due to the inflammation of the nasal mucosa that almost always accompanies the inflammation of the sinus cavity. It may be acute, subacute, or chronic.

A. Acute sinusitis: Abrupt onset of infection with symptom resolution after therapy. Acute sinusitis lasts less than 4 weeks.
B. Subacute sinusitis: Persistent purulent nasal discharge despite therapy
C. Chronic sinusitis: Episodes of prolonged (greater than 3 months) inflammation and/or repeated or inadequately treated acute infections

Incidence

A. Sinusitis is very prevalent. However, true incidence is unknown because people with frontal headaches or congestion self-medicate with over-the-counter (OTC) decongestants and then request antibiotics if symptoms persist. Most cases of acute sinusitis are viral and last less than 10 days. Incidence increases in spring and fall (allergy seasons) and in winter (cold season).

Pathogenesis

A. One cause is obstruction of mucus flow due to edema of nasal mucosa from allergies and upper respiratory infections (URIs).
B. Another cause is anatomical abnormalities that interfere with the normal mucocilliary clearance mechanism.
C. Exposure to pathogens following URI also causes sinusitis. Pathogens include *Staphylococcus aureus*, *Haemophilus influenzae*, pneumococci, streptococci, and bacteroides. Incubation period depends on the pathogen.
D. Dental abscess is a cause in 10% of cases.
E. Fungi such as *Mucor*, *Rhizopus*, and *Aspergillus* can produce invasive sinusitis in poorly controlled diabetics or people with leukemia.
F. Common cold is a cause in 0.5% to 5.0% of cases.

Predisposing Factors

A. Recent URI
B. Allergens (pollens; molds; smoking; occupational exposure, such as coal mining; and animal dander)
C. Nicotine/smoke exposure (first- or secondhand smoke)
D. Air pollutants
E. Deviated septum
F. Adenoidal hypertrophy
G. Dental abscess
H. Diving and swimming
I. Neoplasms
J. Cystic fibrosis
K. Trauma
L. Medical disorders (diabetes, immune disorders, inflammatory disorders, mucosal disorders, cystic fibrosis, and asthma)
M. Flying or rapid changes in altitude

Common Complaints

A. Yellow or green nasal discharge
B. Fever
C. Sore throat
D. Facial pain, frontal pain, or pressure that worsens when patient bends forward
E. Headache
F. Toothache

Other Signs and Symptoms

A. Anosmia (loss of sense of smell)
B. Nasal congestion
C. Cough (worse when lying down); may be chronic
D. Periorbital edema (especially early morning)
E. Malaise or fatigue
F. Halitosis
G. Snoring, mouth breathing
H. Nasal-sounding speech

Potential Complications to Consider: Immediate Ear, Nose, and Throat Referral

A. Meningitis (symptoms are increased fever, stiff neck)
B. Subdural and epidural purulent drainage
C. Brain abscess
D. Cavernous sinus thrombosis (acute thrombophlebitis due to infection in the area where veins drain into cavernous sinus)
E. Tender periorbital edema (orbital cellulitis)

Subjective Data

A. Elicit the onset, duration, and course of symptoms.
B. Inquire whether seasons affect symptoms.
C. Ask the patient about recent URI and how it was treated.
   1. Did the patient receive antibiotics?
   2. Did the patient finish the full course of antibiotics?
D. Ask about allergies.
E. Inquire about recent dental problems, especially dental abscesses.
F. Find out what home therapies and OTC medications the patient tried before the office visit.
G. Ask if the patient took a trip recently, especially by airplane.
H. With a child, look for a foreign object up the nose.
I. Inquire whether the patient was swimming or diving recently.
J. Review the patient's medical history for cystic fibrosis, asthma, nasal abnormalities (e.g., deviated septum), and other respiratory problems.

Physical Examination

A. Check temperature, blood pressure, pulse, and respirations.
B. Inspect
   1. Observe eyes for periorbital swelling, "allergic shiners" (dark circles under eyes), tearing, and signs of orbital cellulitis (conjunctival edema, drooping lid, decreased extraocular motion, and vision loss).
   2. Examine ears.
   3. Inspect the nose for erythema, edema, discharge, lack of nostril patency, septal deviation and polyps, and presence of a foreign body.
   4. Transilluminate maxillary and frontal sinuses in a darkened room. Absence of light reflection is not definitive.
   5. Examine the mouth and pharynx for erythema and tonsillar enlargement, check teeth for uneven surfaces (sign of grinding), and check retropharynx for evidence of postnasal drip.
C. Auscultate heart and lungs.
D. Palpate
   1. Neck for lymphadenopathy
   2. Sinuses but do not press on eyes
      a. Frontal sinusitis: Pain and tenderness over lower forehead (worse when bending forward) and purulent drainage from middle meatus of nasal turbinates
      b. Maxillary sinusitis: Pain and tenderness over cheeks from inner canthus to teeth (referred pain), edematous hard palate (severe cases), and purulent drainage in middle meatus

c. Ethmoid sinusitis: Frontal or orbital headache, tenderness and erythema over upper lateral aspect of nose, drainage from anterior ethmoid cells through middle meatus, drainage of posterior cells through superior meatus

d. Sphenoid sinusitis (uncommon): Frontal or orbital headache or facial pain (headache referred to top of head and deep into eyes), purulent drainage from superior meatus

E. Percuss

1. Tap maxillary teeth to rule out dental cause.

2. Percussion maxillary and frontal sinuses and do chest percussion, if indicated.

3. Percussion over affected area exacerbates pain.

F. Neurologic examination

1. Evaluate for signs of meningeal irritation, assessing for Brudzinski's sign, Kernig's sign, and nuchal rigidity.

Diagnostic Tests

A. **Diagnosis is usually made through history and physical.**

B. Consider sinus x-ray films, which show air-fluid level and thickening of sinus mucous membranes with sinusitis for chronic or recurrent sinusitis or complicated cases.

C. CT of sinuses if indications include chronic sinusitis, recurrent sinusitis, allergic fungal sinusitis, or osteomeatal complex occusion.

Differential Diagnoses

A. Sinusitis

B. Headache (cluster, migraine)

C. Rhinitis (allergic or vasomotor)

D. Nasal polyps

E. Tumor

F. URI

G. Trigeminal neuralgia

Plan

A. General interventions

1. Preventive techniques suggested to avoid sinus infections.

2. Patients with frequent sinus infections should be encouraged to keep a log of triggers, if present. Avoiding these triggers helps to prevent the onset of infection. Avoid smoking and secondhand smoke; use of nasal saline, Neti pot, and increased fluids also help prevent the onset of infection.

3. Recurrent frequent sinus infections should be further investigated for other causes, such as autoimmune diseases.

B. Patient teaching

1. Teach patient to avoid smoking and secondhand smoke.

2. Drinking extra fluids helps to loosen secretions and hydrate the body.

3. Encourage the patient to use medications as prescribed. OTC medications, such as antihistamines and decongestants, should be used with caution.

4. Application of warm, moist compresses to the face several times a day will help with discomfort.

5. Humidifiers should be used daily.

6. Nasal saline to the nares three times a day will help to keep nasal passages moist.

7. *See Section III: Patient Teaching Guide for this chapter, "Sinusitis."* ◀

C. Pharmaceutical therapy

1. Antibiotics for infection

a. Drugs of choice for acute sinusitis:

i. Children

1) First-line treatment: Augmentin 45 mg/kg/d in twice-daily dosing for 10 to 14 days. Second-line treatment: Augmentin 90 mg/kg/d in twice-daily dosing for 10 to 14 days

2) Beta-lactam allergy: Type I hypersensitivity: Levofloxacin 10 to 20 mg/kg/d orally every 12 to 24 hours for 10 days. Non-type I hypersensitivity:

a) Cefpodoxime 10 mg/kg/d (for a maximum of 400 mg/d) in divided doses every 12 hours or

b) Cefdinir 14 mg/kg/d (for a maximum of 600 mg/d) in divided doses every 12 to 24 hours or

c) Levofloxacin 10 to 20 mg/kg in divided doses every 12 to 24 hours

3) Risk for antibiotic resistance or failed initial therapy:

a) Augmentin 90 mg/kg/d orally twice daily for 10 to 14 days

b) Ceftriaxone 50 mg/kg intramuscular for 3 days followed by Augmentin 90 mg/kg for 10 to 14 days

c) Cefpodoxime 10 mg/kg/d in divided doses every 12 hours

d) Cefdinir 14 mg/kg/d in divided doses every 12 to 24 hours or

e) Levofloxacin 10 to 20 mg/kg/d orally every 12 to 24 hours

ii. Adults

1) First-line treatment: Augmentin 500 mg orally three times a day or 875 mg orally twice daily for 10 to 14 days. Second-line treatment: Augmentin 2,000 mg (two extended-release tablets) by mouth every 12 hours for 10 days or doxycycline 100 mg orally twice daily for 10 to 14 days

2) Beta-lactam allergy: Doxycycline 100 mg orally twice daily or 200 mg orally daily for 10 days, levofloxacin 500 mg orally daily for 10 days, or moxifloxacin 400 mg orally daily for 10 days.

3) Risk for antibiotic resistance or failed initial therapy: Augmentin 2,000 mg orally twice daily for 10 days, levofloxacin 500 mg orally daily for 10 days, or

moxifloxacin (Avelox) 400 mg orally daily for 10 days.

b. The same antibiotics can be used for chronic sinusitis, but treatment should last 3 to 4 weeks. Fluroquinolones should be reserved for those who do not benefit from other medication treatment as the risks associated with these antibiotics outweigh the benefits.

D. Oral and topical decongestants to correct the underlying edematous mucosa (use cautiously with hypertension)

1. Adults and children older than 6 years: Pseudoephedrine sulfate (Afrin) 0.05% spray or drops, 2 to 3 drops or sprays per nostril twice daily; maximum for 3 to 5 days.
2. Adults and children older than 12 years: Phenylephrine (Neo-Synephrine) spray or drops, 2 to 3 drops or one to two sprays of 0.25% solution per nostril, or small amount of jelly to nasal mucosa, every 4 hours as needed. Do not use for more than 3 to 5 days.
3. Pseudoephedrin HCl 30 to 60 mg every 4 to 6 hours as needed for congestion for adults.
4. Nasal saline to nares three times daily as needed for hydrating nasal mucosa: 0.25% solution spray or drops, 2 to 3 drops or one to two sprays per nostril every 4 hours as needed. Do not use for more than 3 to 5 days.

E. Steroid sprays may be used to decrease nasal inflammation. Steroid nasal sprays should only be used on children younger than 6 years of age if there is an allergic component:

1. Beclomethasone dipropionate (Beconase AQ, Vancenase AQ); fluticasone (Flonase):
   - **a.** Adults: Two sprays daily
   - **b.** Children 4 to 12 years: One spray daily
2. Mometasone furoate monohydrate (Nasonex):
   - **a.** Adults: Two sprays daily
   - **b.** Children 6 to 12 years: One spray daily

F. Antihistamines are recommended to block histamine production in response to the allergy triggers and prevent allergy symptoms.

1. Loratadine (Claritin) 10 mg daily for children older than 6 years
2. Fexofenadine (Allegra) 180 mg daily in adults
3. Levocetirizine HCl (Xyzal) 5 mg daily for adults
4. Cetirizine HCl (Zyrtec) 10 mg oral or dissolve tab daily for adults and children older than 6 years; for less severe symptoms, 5 mg daily
5. Leukotriene inhibitors (Singulair, Accolate) for severe allergies and/or asthma

G. Pediatric doses are available for all products.

Follow-Up

A. Recheck the patient in 3 to 4 days if signs and symptoms are not improving with the use of treatment prescribed.

B. Recommend treatment for 10 to 14 days. Patients not improving may be resistant to antibiotics and may be switched to a different antibiotic for 14 days.

Consultation/Referral

A. Admission to hospital is needed if the patient has fever with facial cellulitis and mental changes.

B. Refer chronic sinusitis patients to an otolaryngologist if they do not improve in 4 weeks.

C. Refer patients to a physician or ear, nose, and throat (ENT) specialist for suspected neoplasm, abscess, osteomyelitis, meningitis, or sinus thrombosis.

Individual Considerations

A. Pediatrics: Sinusitis may be considered for children who present with normal to low-grade temperature and green mucus from nose for longer than 2 weeks.

B. Geriatrics

1. Precautionary measures should be used for patients with long-term nasogastric tubes. These patients are at higher risk for the development of occult sinusitis.
2. Precautions should be used with patients currently prescribed warfarin (Coumadin).
3. Avoid use of Bactrim DS (TMP-SMX) with warfarin because the medication can cause a significant increase in prothrombin time/international normalized ratio (PT/INR).

Bibliography

Adelson, R. T., & Adappa, N. D. (2013). What is the proper role of oral antibiotics in the treatment of patients with chronic sinusitis? *Current Opinion in Otolaryngology & Head and Neck Surgery, 21*(1), 61–68.

Center for Disease Control and Prevention. (n.d.). Pediatric treatment recommendations. Retrieved from https://www.cdc.gov/getsmart/community/for-hcp/outpatient-hcp/pediatric-treatment-rec.pdf

DeMuri, G. P., & Wald, E. R. (2012). Clinical practice. Acute bacterial sinusitis in children. *New England Journal of Medicine, 367*(12), 1128–1134.

deShazo, R., & Kemp, S. (2016). Pharmacotherapy of allergic rhinitis. In J. Corren (Ed.), *UpToDate.* Retrieved from http://www.uptodate.com/contents/pharmacotherapy-of-allergic-rhinitis?source=search_result&search=Pharmacotherapy+of+allergic+rhinitis&selectedTitle=1%7E150

Messner, M. D. (2014). Management of epistaxis in children. In A. Stack & G. Isaacson (Eds.), *UpToDate.* Retrieved from http://www.uptodate.com/contents/management-of-epistaxis-in-children?source=search_result&search=epistaxis&selectedTitle=2%7E150

Patel, Z., & Hwang, P. (2016). Acute sinusitis and rhinosinusitis in adults: Treatment. In D. Deschler & S. Calderwood (Eds.), *UpToDate.* Retrieved from http://www.uptodate.com/contents/uncomplicated-acute-sinusitis-and-rhinosinusitis-in-adults-treatment?source=search_result&search=sinusitis&selectedTitle=1%7E150

Ramavaram, S., & Jones, S. M. (2012). Natural course and comorbidities of allergic and nonallergic rhinitis in children. *Pediatrics, 130*(Suppl. 1), S23–S24.

Rosenfeld, R. M., Piccirillo, J. F., Chandrasekhar, S. S., Brook, I., Kumar, K. A., Kramper, M., . . . Corrigan, M. D. (2015). Clinical Practice Guideline (Update): Adult sinusitis executive summary. *Otolaryngology—Head and Neck Surgery, 152*(4), 598–609. Retrieved from https://www.guideline.gov/content.aspx?id=49207&search=acute+rhinitis

Wald, E. (2016). Acute bacterial rhinosinusitis in children: Microbiology and treatment. In S. Kaplan, G. Isaacson, & R. Wood (Eds.), *UpToDate.* Retrieved from http://www.uptodate.com/contents/acute-bacterialrhinosinusitis-in-children-microbiology-and-treatment?source=search_result&search=sinusitis+children+treatment&selectedTitle=3%7E150

8 Throat and Mouth Guidelines

Avulsed Tooth

Jill C. Cash and Moya Cook

Definition

A. A tooth that has been completely displaced from its alveolar socket.

Incidence

A. Avulsion accounts for 0.5% to 16% of all dental injuries to the permanent teeth. It occurs predominantly in children between ages 7 and 10 years. The upper central incisor is the most frequent tooth that is avulsed.

Pathogenesis

A. Trauma causes a tooth to be completely displaced from its alveolar socket.

Predisposing Factor

A. Erupting teeth are most susceptible to avulsion due to immature periodontal ligaments.

Common Complaints

A. Tooth displaced
B. Pain
C. Bleeding

Subjective Data

A. Ascertain the patient's age, and note if the avulsed tooth is primary or permanent.
B. Determine the time span for which the tooth has been avulsed (minutes or hours).
C. Ask the patient about the underlying cause or trauma. Are there any other injuries that need assessment, such as lacerations or concussion?
D. Did the tooth fall out of the mouth or remain in the mouth?

Physical Examination

A. Check temperature, pulse, respirations, and blood pressure.
B. Inspect
  1. Observe general appearance.
    a. Check for signs that are secondary to traumatic etiology, such as lacerations, concussion, facial injury, and eye injury.
    b. Keep the patient calm. Check to be sure that the patient is not in respiratory distress or has not aspirated the tooth.
  2. Inspect gums and avulsed tooth, noting poor dental hygiene. **Do not touch the root surface.**
  3. If the tooth is not in the mouth, rinse off briefly under cold running water (less than 10 seconds) and attempt to reposition the tooth into the socket if there is no concern of the child swallowing the tooth or dropping it.

Diagnostic Tests

A. Dental x-ray should be considered to assess for fracture. Immediate referral to dental specialist for emergency dental evaluation.

Differential Diagnoses

A. Avulsed tooth
B. Luxation injuries: Concussion and subluxation

Plan

A. General interventions
  1. Refer immediately for emergency dental evaluation and treatment.
B. Patient teaching
  1. Tell the patient not to let the tooth air dry; it may cause permanent destruction of periodontal cells.
  2. Instruct the patient to transport the tooth in the tooth socket and bite on gauze or a small handkerchief to help hold the tooth in position.
  3. If unable to transport inside the tooth socket, use another medium to transport the tooth that may include saline, Hanks balanced storage medium, or milk.
C. Pharmaceutical therapy
  1. Consider administering oral antibiotics prophylactically. Consider tetracycline or doxycycline for adults. Amoxicillin may be used for children.
  2. If the tooth had contact with soil, determine tetanus status and administer tetanus booster if necessary.

Follow-Up

A. Follow-up is done with the dentist until stabilization is complete.

Consultation/Referral

A. Immediately refer the patient to a dentist or an emergency department. Teeth replanted within 30 minutes have the best prognosis. Teeth avulsed longer than 2 hours have a poor prognosis. The American Academy of Pediatric Dentistry provides a free algorithm for the treatment of permanent tooth avulsion: www.aapd.org/media/policies_guidelines/rs_traumaflowsheet.pdf

Individual Consideration

A. Pediatrics: Primary teeth do not need to be replaced.

Dental Abscess

Jill C. Cash and Moya Cook

Definition

A. A dental abscess is a space infection of the gingival or periodontal tissues.

Incidence

A. Incidence is unknown.

Pathogenesis

A. An abscess occurs when bacteria gain access into the gingiva or periodontal tissues.

Predisposing Factors

A. Poor dental hygiene
B. Dental caries

Common Complaints

A. Constant, severe jaw pain
B. Swelling
C. Difficulty in chewing with tooth due to pain

Other Signs and Symptoms

A. Fever
B. Warmth, redness
C. Loss of appetite
D. Heat and cold sensitivity
E. Halitosis

Potential Complications

Risk of complications increases with valvular disease. The following are complications:
A. Sepsis
B. Leukocytosis associated with facial cellulitis

Subjective Data

A. Elicit information from the patient regarding the onset, duration, location, and quality of pain.
B. Note the radiation of pain as well as alleviating or aggravating factors.
C. Note if pain is brought on by contact with hot, cold, or sweet substances; this may indicate periapical abscess or dental caries.
D. Ask if the patient has a fever. If so, how high and for how long?
E. Inquire about the history of mitral valve prolapse or rheumatic fever.

Physical Examination

A. Check temperature, pulse, respirations, and blood pressure.
B. Inspect
  1. Inspect teeth for caries, mobility of teeth, or protrusion from sockets, and gum disease.
  2. Examine the teeth for erosion, enamel decalcification, diminished tooth size, discoloration, and sensitivity to temperature changes.
C. Palpate neck and submental area for enlarged, tender lymph nodes.
D. Percuss all teeth. Tenderness is diagnostic of an abscess.
E. Auscultate heart, if indicated.

Diagnostic Tests

A. None usually required.
B. White blood cell count (WBC), if cellulitis is suspected.

Differential Diagnoses

A. Dental abscess
B. Periodontal disease
C. Cellulitis

Plan

A. General interventions
  1. Treat immediate infection.
  2. Refer to the dentist for immediate evaluation and treatment.
B. Patient teaching
  1. Advise the patient to apply a heating pad to the painful facial area for comfort.
  2. Advise soft diet until pain resolves.
  3. Review daily dental care and hygiene with the patient.
C. Pharmaceutical therapy
  1. Drug of choice: Penicillin V potassium (Pen-Vee-K) 250 to 500 mg orally every 6 hours while the patient awaits dental consultation
  2. Other medications
    a. Cephalexin (Keflex) 500 mg every 6 hours until dental consultation
    b. Clindamycin (Cleocin) 300 mg orally every 6 hours until dental consultation
  3. For discomfort and fever: Ibuprofen (Advil) 400 to 600 mg orally every 6 to 8 hours, not to exceed 1,200 mg/d

Follow-Up

A. Follow up 2 to 3 days after dental examination to evaluate results.

Consultation/Referral

A. Advise the patient to see a dentist promptly, even if pain resolves.

Individual Considerations

A. Pregnancy
  1. It is safe for patients to have dental procedures during pregnancy.
  2. X-ray films may be taken with a lead shield over patient's abdomen.
  3. Epinephrine and nitrous oxide should not be used during dental procedures.
  4. Tetracycline should not be used; it causes staining of fetal bones and teeth.

Epiglottitis

Jill C. Cash and Moya Cook

Definition

A. Epiglottitis is the inflammation and swelling of the epiglottis and is a medical emergency.

Incidence

A. Epiglottitis usually occurs in children between ages 2 and 8 years, but it may also occur in adults. Incidence has decreased dramatically since the *Haemophilus influenzae* vaccine was introduced.

Pathogenesis

A. Epiglottitis is almost always caused by *H. influenzae,* although *Streptococcus pneumoniae* and *Streptococcus pyogenes* have also been implicated.

Predisposing Factor

A. Upper respiratory infection

Common Complaints

A. Sudden onset of fever
B. Sudden onset of dysphagia
C. Sudden onset of drooling
D. Sudden onset of muffled voice

Other Signs and Symptoms

A. Respiratory distress
B. Stridor
C. Very ill appearance

Subjective Data

A. Determine the onset, duration, and course of illness.
B. Is the child's breathing labored?
C. Are the child's breathing problems affecting his or her ability to eat or drink?
D. Has he or she had a fever?
E. Has he or she had trouble swallowing or talking?

Physical Examination

A. Check temperature, pulse, respirations, and blood pressure.
B. Inspect
  1. Observe overall appearance.
  2. Check nail beds and lips for cyanosis.
  3. Note drooling or difficulty in swallowing.
  4. Note breathing pattern and rhythm.
  5. Note cough if present.
  6. Do not examine the throat—airway occlusion may result.
C. Auscultate heart and lungs.

Diagnostic Test

A. Lateral neck radiograph confirms diagnosis. However, this test may delay the establishment of an airway.

Differential Diagnoses

A. Epiglottitis
B. Bacterial tracheitis (a pediatric emergency)
C. Viral croup
D. Foreign-body aspiration
E. Retropharyngeal abscess

Plan

A. General interventions
  1. Immediate admission to hospital.
  2. While awaiting transport to hospital, establish patent airway, start oxygen, and assemble airway equipment. Move the child as little as possible.
  3. Insert IV access for fluids and antibiotic administration.
  4. If a respiratory arrest occurs, you may not be able to see the airway to intubate. An Ambu bag and mask may work temporarily, but nasogastric (NG) tube insertion may be necessary to prevent gastric distension.
  5. Prompt recognition and appropriate treatment usually result in rapid resolution of swelling and inflammation.
B. Patient teaching
  1. Educate the patient and the family that epiglottitis is a medical emergency.
  2. If patient has drooling and no cough, diagnosis is most likely epiglottitis. If the child has cough and no drooling, then diagnosis is most likely croup.
C. Pharmaceutical therapy
In-hospital treatment:
1. IV fluids
2. Antibiotics; IV antibiotics after physician consultation
3. Blood and epiglottis cultures obtained before starting antibiotics
4. Drug of choice
  a. Cefotaxime (Claforan) 100 to 200 mg/kg/d every 8 hours IV
  b. Ceftriaxone (Rocephin) 50 to 100 mg/kg/d every 12 hours IV
  c. Ampicillin-sulbactam (Unasyn) 150 mg/kg/d every 6 hours IV
  d. Amoxicillin-clavulanic acid 100 mg/kg/d every 8 hours IV
5. May give Tylenol as needed

Follow-Up

A. Follow-up care occurs in the hospital.
B. An airway specialist should evaluate the patient in the operating room.

Consultation/Referral

A. If you suspect epiglottitis, refer the patient to a physician immediately.

Individual Considerations

A. Pediatrics
  1. Never place a child in supine position because respiratory arrest has been reported.
  2. All close contacts (including children and adults) exposed to a child diagnosed with epiglottitis should be treated with prophylactic antibiotics, such as rifampin, 20 mg/kg, not to exceed 600 mg/day for 4 days

Oral Cancer

Jill C. Cash and Moya Cook

Definition

A. Oral cancer is the cancer of the buccal mucosa, tongue, gingiva, hard palate, soft palate, or lips. White patches, known as *leukoplakia,* or red, velvety patches, known as *erythroplakia,* on the buccal mucosa may indicate premalignant lesions.

Incidence

A. Oral cancer is primarily seen in the elderly. Male-to-female predominance is 2 to 1; oral cancer is equal in African Americans and Caucasian adults. The death rate is fairly high for oral cancer secondary to the cancer being diagnosed in the late stages of development.
B. There are 42,000 Americans diagnosed with new cases of oral cancer, and 8,000 deaths occur each year.
C. Oral cancer represents 3% of all newly diagnosed cancers and 2% of all cancer-related deaths.
D. Frequency of oral cancer of cheek and gum rises 50-fold among long-term users of smokeless tobacco.
E. Patients diagnosed with oral cancer are at greater risk of developing cancer in another part of the body, such as the lung, larynx, esophagus, or other site. Therefore, follow-up examinations are recommended for the remainder of the patient's life.

Pathogenesis

Pathogenesis is unknown; 50% of oral cancers have already been metastasized by the time of diagnosis. The following factors are involved.
A. Use of tobacco in all its forms is highly correlated with the risk of oral cancer.
B. Risk of oral cancer also is high with heavy alcohol consumption. Whether this is due to a direct effect of alcohol on the oral mucosa or associated smoking or vitamin deficiency remains unclear.
C. Chronic iron deficiency leading to Plummer–Vinson syndrome is known to alter mucosal tissues, and this change may be related to increased oral cancer. Research has shown that a diet low in fruits and vegetables contributes to oral cancer.
D. Epstein–Barr virus and papillomavirus have been found in the cells of the tongue manifesting in oral hairy leukoplakia, a hyperplastic change found in AIDS patients. Human papillomavirus (HPV) is found in approximately 20% to 30% of cases of oral cancer.
E. Occupational hazards also exist from sun exposure. It is estimated that 30% of those with oral cancer worked outdoors.

Predisposing Factors

A. Male gender
B. Age greater than 40 years for men, greater than 50 years for women
C. African American ancestry
D. Smoking or use of other tobacco products, including smokeless products such as snuff and dip
E. Alcohol consumption
F. Sun exposure
G. Poor diet, deficient in vitamins A, C, and E, and high in salted or smoked meats, fats, and oils
H. Previous cancer

Common Complaints

A. Oral sores that do not heal, which is the primary reason patients seek medical care
B. Poorly fitting dentures
C. Bleeding mucosa or gingiva without apparent cause
D. Difficulty swallowing, usually indicating more advanced disease
E. Altered sensations: Burning or numbness, usually indicating more advanced disease
F. Leukoplakia or erythroplakia

Other Signs and Symptoms

A. No symptoms, possibly
B. Decreased appetite related to altered taste
C. Increased salivation
D. Sore throat
E. Foul breath odor
F. Neck mass

Subjective Data

A. Review the onset, course, and duration of symptoms. Question the patient regarding altered taste, sensations, difficulty swallowing, and foul breath.
B. Evaluate for risk factors. See Predisposing Factors.
C. Ask the patient about previous history of cancer and treatments.
D. Review the patient's use of tobacco products, including age of onset, amount of daily use, and quit dates.
E. Evaluate amount of alcohol intake, including age of onset, amount of daily use, and quit dates.
F. Review the patient's general health history for other chronic conditions.
G. Review medication history, including prescription and over-the-counter drug use, especially aspirin.
H. Take dental history, including previous gum surgery, how long ago dentures were fitted, and if they always fit well.
I. Establish usual weight. Is there any weight loss related to altered taste, and, if so, how much and during what length of time?

Physical Examination

A. Check temperature, pulse, respirations, blood pressure, and weight.
B. Inspect
  1. Observe general appearance.
  2. Note quality of voice patterns.
  3. Note odor of breath.
  4. Inspect lips, gums, tongue, and buccal mucosa for swelling, discoloration, bleeding, asymmetry, texture, limited movement of tongue, abnormal ulcerations, leukoplakia, and erythroplasia. Take out dentures first.
  5. Assess for tenderness or pain in mouth/tongue.
    a. Leukoplakia ranges from slightly raised, white, translucent areas to dense, white, opaque plaques,

with or without adjacent ulceration. Normal intraoral mucosa is pinkish or salmon colored.

b. Mucosal erythroplasia is red, inflammatory, or shows erythroplastic mucosal changes. It appears smooth, granular, and minimally elevated, with or without leukoplakia, and it persists more than 14 days.

c. Erythroplakia may mimic inflammatory lesions, but it can be differentiated by failure of the affected area to blanch with light pressure. Erythroplakia is a malignant change seen as a red, velvety, plaque-like lesion on the mucous membrane.

d. Other oral lesions appear black, blue, or brown.

e. Approximately 90% of cancers are squamous cell carcinomas, and most occur in sites accessible by clinical examination: Tongue, oropharynx (soft palate, lingual aspect of retromolar trigone, anterior tonsillar pillar), and floor of mouth.

f. Cancer of the lip is a lesion that fails to heal.

g. Signs and symptoms of cancer of the tongue are swelling, ulceration, areas of tenderness or bleeding, abnormal texture, and limited movement.

C. Palpate

1. Palpate mouth for masses. Try to remove or scrape patches.

2. Palpate lymph nodes: Cervical (anterior/posterior chain), submandibular, sublingual, and submental, pre-/postauricular; check nodes for size, firmness, and tenderness.

D. Auscultate lungs and heart. The lungs are the most frequently involved extranodal metastatic site.

Diagnostic Tests

A. Check for HIV, if indicated.

B. Staining of oral lesion with toluidine blue: Lesion stains dark blue after rinsing with acetic acid. Normal tissue does not absorb the stain.

C. Biopsy for persistent lesions (more than 2 weeks): It is essential to differentiate from blue-black lesion of malignant melanoma.

D. Perform chest radiography to rule out metastasis.

E. Consider CT, MRI, or bone scan to rule out metastasis.

Differential Diagnoses

A. Oral leukoplakia

B. Pulpitis

C. Periapical abscess

D. Gingivitis

E. Periodontitis

F. Lichen planus

G. Oral candidiasis

H. Discoid lupus

I. Pemphigus vulgaris

Plan

A. General interventions

1. If oral cancer is suspected, refer to a physician or an otolaryngologist/dentist for evaluation.

2. Suspicious lesions should be biopsied.

B. Patient teaching

1. Advise the patient to stop smoking and stop using oral tobacco products.

2. Advise the patient to decrease/eliminate alcohol consumption.

3. Encourage routine dental care and examinations.

4. Review dietary intake and educate the patient regarding benefits of increasing dietary intake of vitamins A, C, and E. Encourage the patient to decrease dietary intake of foods that are high in salt, smoked meats, fats, and oils.

5. Recommend wearing sunscreen/lip balm with sun protection factor (SPF) of 15 or greater.

6. Avoid contracting the HPV infection. Recommend Gardasil vaccination for girls and boys 9 to 26 years of age.

C. Pharmaceutical therapy

1. Erythroplakia does not respond to antifungal therapy.

2. Treatment is based on diagnosis.

Follow-Up

A. If immediate biopsy is not indicated, ask the patient to return for reevaluation in 2 weeks, after eliminating irritants and noxious agents.

Consultation/Referral

A. Refer the patient to an otolaryngologist and/or a dentist for immediate biopsy for deeply ulcerative or fungating lesions. Follow-up treatment may include one or more of the following: Wide excision, radical neck dissection, radiation, and chemotherapy.

Individual Considerations

A. Pediatrics

1. Currently, the highest rate is in smokeless tobacco use.

2. Oral screening should be considered annually in adolescents who use tobacco and/or alcohol.

B. Adults: The American Cancer Society recommends that people between ages 20 and 40 years undergo an oral cancer screening every 3 years, and that those older than 40 years be screened every year. Oral screening should be considered annually in adults who use tobacco and/or alcohol.

Resources

American Academy of Family Physicians: www.aafp.org

American Cancer Society: www.cancer.org

National Cancer Institute: www.cancer.gov

Oral Cancer Foundation: www.oralcancerfoundation.org

Pharyngitis

Jill C. Cash and Moya Cook

Definition

A. Pharyngitis is the inflammation of the pharynx and the surrounding lymph tissue.

Incidence

A. Pharyngitis is the fourth most common condition seen in medical practice.

Pathogenesis

Pharyngitis may be due to viral, bacterial, and fungal agents, as well as other atypical agents.

A. Viral agents include coxsackievirus, enteric cytopathic human orphan (ECHO) viruses, and Epstein–Barr virus.

B. Bacterial agents include Group A beta-hemolytic *Streptococcus, Neisseria gonorrhoeae*, and *Corynebacterium diphtheriae*.

C. The fungal source is *Candida albicans*.

D. Atypical agents include *Mycoplasma pneumoniae* and *Chlamydia trachomatis* (rare).

E. Noninfectious causes include allergic rhinitis, postnasal drip, mouth breathing, and trauma.

Predisposing Factors

A. Cigarette smoking

B. Allergies

C. Upper respiratory infections

D. Oral sex

E. Drugs (antibiotics and immunosuppressants)

F. Debilitating illnesses (such as cancer) that can cause *C. albicans* to proliferate

Common Complaints

A. Sore and/or scratchy throat

B. Fever

C. Headache

D. Malaise

Other Signs and Symptoms

A. Oral vesicles

B. Exudate on throat or "beefy" red throat without exudate

C. Lymphadenopathy

D. Fatigue

E. Dysphasia

F. Abdominal pain

G. Vomiting

Potential Complications

Without proper antimicrobial treatment, streptococcal pharyngitis can lead to serious complications such as the following:

A. Suppurative adenitis with tender, enlarged lymph nodes

B. Scarlet fever

C. Peritonsillar abscess

D. Glomerulonephritis

E. Rheumatic fever

Subjective Data

A. Ask the patient about the onset, course, and duration of symptoms. Ask about dyspnea or dysphagia.

B. Inquire about mouth lesions, rhinorrhea, cough, drooling, and fever.

C. Ask about malaise, headache, fatigue, and fever; these are symptoms of mononucleosis.

D. Take a sexual history, if indicated. Ask if family members or sexual partners have the same signs and symptoms. Pharyngeal gonorrhea has no symptoms, so high-risk patients should be tested.

E. Ask whether symptoms have caused decreased intake of food and fluid.

F. Determine history of heart disease; previous strep pharyngitis; rheumatic fever; and other respiratory diseases, such as asthma, emphysema, and chronic allergies.

G. If rash is present, find out when it first occurred and if it has spread.

H. Ask about signs and symptoms of urinary tract infection and pyelonephritis.

I. Ask about a history of herpes, immunosuppressive disorders, and steroid use.

J. Review immunization history.

Physical Examination

A. Temperature and blood pressure, if indicated

B. Inspect

  1. Observe general appearance.

  2. Examine the mouth, pharynx, tonsils, and hard and soft palate for vesicles and ulcers, candidal patches, erythema, hypertrophy, exudate, and stomatitis. Check gum and palate for petechiae and tongue for color and inflammation.

  3. Examine the ears, nose, and throat. Assess patency of airway if tonsils are enlarged.

  4. Inspect skin for rashes.

    a. Pastia's lines are petechiae present in a linear pattern along major skin folds in axillae and antecubital fossa that are seen with Group A *Streptococcus*.

    b. Erythema marginatum, caused by Group A *Streptococcus*, is an evanescent, nonpruritic, pink rash mainly on the trunk and extremities. It may be brought out by heat application.

C. Auscultate heart and lungs.

D. Percuss

  1. Abdomen, especially spleen area

  2. Chest

E. Palpate

  1. Palpate lymph nodes, especially of the anterior and posterior cervical chains, axilla, and groin.

  2. Palpate abdomen for organomegaly and suprapubic tenderness.

  3. Palpate back for costovertebral angle (CVA) tenderness.

F. Neurologic examination: Check for nuchal rigidity and meningeal irritation.

Diagnostic Tests

A. Rapid strep test; if negative, then perform throat culture and sensitivity. **Throat culture and sensitivity are the gold standard for diagnosis.**

B. Monospot test

C. Complete blood count with differential

D. Gonorrhea culture

E. Blood cultures if sepsis is suspected

F. Radiograph of neck if possible trauma

Differential Diagnoses

A. Pharyngitis
B. Stomatitis
C. Rhinitis
D. Sinusitis with postnasal drip
E. Epiglottis
F. Peritonsillar abscess
G. Mononucleosis
H. Herpes simplex
I. Coxsackie A virus
J. *C. diphtheriae*
K. Trench mouth
L. Vincent's angina
M. *C. albicans*
N. HIV

Plan

A. General interventions

1. Patients with a history of rheumatic fever and those who have a household member with a documented Group A streptococcal infection need immediate treatment without prior testing.
2. Herpangina are small oral vesicles on the fauces and soft palate caused by the coxsackievirus.
3. Herpes causes vesicles and small ulcers (stomatitis) of the buccal mucosa, tongue, and pharynx.
4. Trench mouth (gingivitis) and necrotic tonsillar ulcers (Vincent's angina) cause foul breath, pain, pharyngeal exudate, and a gray membranous inflammation that bleeds easily.
5. *C. albicans* (thrush) may be painful and causes cheesy, white exudate.
6. Oral candidiasis may be the first symptom of HIV.
7. Peritonsillar cellulitis causes inflamed, edematous tonsils; grayish-white exudate; high fever; rigors; and leukocytosis. Peritonsillar abscess (palpable mass) may also develop.
8. Mononucleosis causes tonsillar exudates in 50% of patients; 33% develop petechiae at junction of the hard and soft palate.
9. *C. diphtheriae* causes a whitish-blue pharyngeal exudate "pseudomembrane" that covers the pharynx and bleeds if removal is attempted.
10. Do not put instruments in the airway if you suspect epiglottitis.

▶ B. Patient teaching: *See Section III: Patient Teaching Guide for this chapter, "Pharyngitis."*

C. Pharmaceutical therapy

1. Drug of choice: Prescribe one of the following penicillins for bacterial pharyngitis.
   a. Penicillin V potassium (Pen-Vee-K)
      i. Children: 250 mg orally two to three times daily for 10 days. Adolescents and adults: 250 mg four times daily or 500 mg twice daily for 10 days
      ii. Children: Amoxicillin 50 mg/kg/d once daily for 10 days (maximum 1,000 mg); alternative, 25 mg/kg (max = 500 mg) twice daily for 10 days
   b. Penicillin G benzathine: Less than 27 kg: 600,000 U × 1 dose intramuscular (IM); greater than or equal to 27 kg: 1,200,000 U × 1 dose IM
2. If the patient is allergic to penicillin:
   a. Cephalexin, oral: 20 mg/kg/dose twice daily (max 500 mg/dose) for 10 days
   b. Cefadroxil, oral: 30 mg/kg once daily (max 1 g) for 10 days
   c. Clindamycin, oral: 7 mg/kg/dose three times daily (max 300 mg/dose) for 10 days
   d. Azithromycin, oral: 12 mg/kg once daily (max 500 mg) daily for 5 days
   e. Clarithromycin, oral: 7.5 mg/kg/dose twice daily (max 250 mg/dose) for 10 days
3. Recurrent bacterial pharyngitis
   a. Clindamycin: 20 to 30 mg/kg/d in three doses (max 300 mg/dose) for 10 days
   b. Penicillin and rifampin: Penicillin V: 50 mg/ kg/d in four doses for 10 days (max 2,000 mg/d); rifampin: 20 mg/kg/d in one dose for last 4 days of treatment (max 600 mg/d)
   c. Amoxicillin-clavulanic acid: 40 mg amoxicillin/kg/d in three doses (max 2,000 mg amoxicillin/d) for 10 days
   d. Benzathine penicillin G (IM) plus rifampin (oral): Benzathine penicillin G: 600,000 U for less than 27 kg and 1,200,000 U for greater than or equal to 27 kg × 1 dose; rifampin: 20 mg/kg/d in two doses (max 600 mg/d) for 4 days
4. For pharyngeal gonorrhea
   a. Adults: Ceftriaxone (Rocephin) 500 mg to 1 g by IM injection
   b. Children: Ceftriaxone (Rocephin) 50 to 75 mg/kg in one dose by IM injection
5. For *M. pneumoniae* and *C. trachomatis*: Erythromycin (E-Mycin) 250 mg orally three to four times daily for 10 days
6. For pharyngeal candidiasis in the immunocompromised patient:
   a. Oral nystatin suspension (100,000 U/mL) 15 mL by swish-and-swallow method four times a day
   b. Clotrimazole troche 10 mg held in mouth 15 to 30 minutes three times daily

Follow-Up

A. If symptoms do not improve in 3 to 4 days, recheck patient.
B. Treat sexual partners of patients with pharyngeal gonorrhea.

Consultation/Referral

A. Consult physician if patient has severe dysphagia or dyspnea, signaling possible airway obstruction.
B. Refer the patient to an otolaryngologist if peritonsillar abscess is noted.

Individual Considerations

A. Pediatrics

1. Rheumatic fever follows between 0.5% and 3% of ineffectively treated cases of Group A streptococcal upper respiratory infections.

2. Approximately 20% of children aged 5 to 15 years who are diagnosed with rheumatic fever had pharyngitis in the preceding 3 months.

Stomatitis, Minor Recurrent Aphthous Stomatitis

Jill C. Cash and Moya Cook

Definition

A. Stomatitis is tender, round, discrete, oval, shallow, 1- to 5-mm ulcers in the oral cavity. The ulcers are gray white or yellow, on nonkeratinized skin, and surrounded by erythematous halos. They typically involve the labial and buccal mucosa and tongue, and adjacent tissue appears healthy.
B. Major recurrent aphthous stomatitis (RAS) has larger, deeper ulcers; lasts a longer period of time; usually recurs up to four times a year; and frequently leaves scars. It can cause significant dysphagia.

Incidence

A. Stomatitis affects 20% to 50% of the population. It is very common in North America.

Pathogenesis

A. Cause is poorly understood. Genetic, immunologic, viral, or nutritional causes are possible.

Predisposing Factors

A. Minor trauma
B. History of RAS
C. Possible nutritional deficiency of iron, folic acid, or zinc
D. Hormonal changes

Common Complaint

A. Painful sore in mouth

Other Signs and Symptoms

A. Burning sensation in mouth for 24 to 48 hours before lesions appear

Subjective Data

A. Elicit history of aphthous stomatitis.
B. Ask the patient about prodrome of burning or stinging in the mouth.
C. Elicit information regarding previous illness and trauma.

Physical Examination

A. Check temperature, pulse, respirations, and blood pressure.
B. Inspect
  1. Mouth for ulcers
  2. Ears, nose, and throat
  3. Skin, especially palms and soles, for lesions; indicates hand, foot, and mouth disease
C. Auscultate heart and lungs.

Diagnostic Tests

A. Specific diagnostic testing for stomatitis is not needed.
B. Consider HSV culture if herpes simplex virus is considered for diagnosis.
C. If syphilis is of concern, order serum rapid plasma reagin (RPR).

Differential Diagnoses

A. Aphthous stomatitis
B. Herpetic stomatitis
C. Behçet's disease
D. Crohn's disease
E. HIV
F. Kawasaki syndrome
G. Hand, foot, and mouth disease

Plan

A. General interventions
  1. Avoid spicy, salty, or hot foods.
  2. Encourage cold foods, such as fluids, ice pops, and so on, to help with pain.
  3. Avoid hard, sharp food that is difficult to chew.
  4. Recommend using a soft-bristle toothbrush when brushing teeth.
B. Patient teaching: *See Section III: Patient Teaching Guide for this chapter, "Aphthous Stomatitis."* ◀
C. Pharmaceutical therapy
  1. Mouthwash made of diphenhydramine (Benadryl), with Kaopectate, or Maalox or sucralfate, and viscous lidocaine three to four times a day. Leave out lidocaine when using in children. Tell the patient not to swallow medication.
  2. Sucralfate (Carafate) suspension 1 teaspoon four times a day may be used to swish in mouth and spit out for oral comfort.
  3. Glucocorticoid gel, such as fluocinonide gel (Lidex), 0.05% two to four times a day, one of which is always at bedtime.
  4. Orabase with or without triamcinolone acetonide (Kenalog).

Follow-Up

A. Follow up as needed for treatment of recurrences.

Consultation/Referral

A. Refer the patient to or consult with a physician if ulcers are deeper or larger than 1 to 5 mm, if Kawasaki disease is suspected, or if no improvement is seen with adequate treatment.
B. Any lesion lasting longer than 3 weeks should be evaluated by a dentist or oral surgeon to rule out cancer.

Individual Considerations

A. Pregnancy: Avoid use of fluocinonide and triamcinolone acetonide (Kenalog) in pregnant or nursing women.
B. Pediatrics
  1. Avoid use of fluocinonide and triamcinolone acetonide (Kenalog).
  2. Do not use viscous lidocaine.

Thrush

Jill C. Cash and Moya Cook

Definition

A. Thrush is a fungal infection of the oral cavity and/or the pharynx caused by *Candida.*

Incidence

A. It is estimated that 5% to 7% of babies younger than 1 month, both bottle-fed and breastfed infants, will develop oral candidiasis. Approximately 9% to 31% of AIDS patients and 20% of patients diagnosed with cancer will have thrush.

Pathogenesis

A. Thrush is an overgrowth of yeast cells, *Candida albicans,* on the oral mucosa, which leads to desquamation of the epithelial cells, creating a psuedomembrane over the normal oral mucosa.

Predisposing Factors

A. Use of broad-spectrum antibiotics
B. Adults
  1. HIV
  2. Prolonged steroid use (systemic or inhaled corticosteroids)
  3. Cancer treatments (radiation/chemotherapy)
  4. Dentures
  5. Malnutrition
C. Children
  1. Endocrine disorders (thyroid disease, diabetes mellitus, and Addison's disease)
  2. HIV
  3. Cancer

Common Complaint

A. Soreness, pain of the mouth

Other Signs and Symptoms

A. Irritability in infants
B. Refusal to eat in infants
C. White plaques coating buccal mucosa

Subjective Data

A. Determine the onset, duration, and course of illness.
B. Ask if the child refuses to eat.
C. Has the patient used antibiotics or other medications in the previous weeks?
D. Does the patient use inhaled or systemic steroids on a daily basis?

Physical Examination

A. Check temperature, pulse, respirations, and blood pressure.
B. Inspect
  1. Oral cavity for white, curd-like plaques that cannot be removed
  2. Ears, nose, and throat
  3. Genital area for red rash and satellite papular lesions

Diagnostic Tests

A. If diagnosis is certain, no testing recommended.
B. If uncertain of diagnosis, swab lesion for KOH testing.
C. If treatment prescribed is not working, fungal culture should be sent for diagnosis.

Differential Diagnoses

A. Thrush
B. Milk deposits on tongue or buccal mucosa
C. Stomatitis
D. Aphthous ulcer
E. Hairy leukoplakia

Plan

A. General interventions
  1. If the infant is breastfeeding, instruct the mother to clean breasts and nipples well with warm water between feedings to prevent contamination. Consider prescribing antifungal cream to be applied to breasts; this should be washed off before feedings.
  2. If bottle feeding, boil all bottles, nipples, and pacifiers to kill the organism.
  3. Instruct caregiver to attempt removal of large plaques with a moistened cotton-tipped applicator and/or small, moist gauze pad before inserting medication in mouth.
  4. If thrush is recurrent or resistant, consider checking the mother for candidal vaginitis.
  5. For adults, instruct the patient/family on proper use and cleaning/rinsing of inhalers/dentures to prevent reoccurrence of thrush.
B. Patient teaching: *See Section III: Patient Teaching Guide for this chapter, "Oral Thrush in Children."* ◀
C. Pharmaceutical therapy
  1. Oral candidiasis: Nystatin (Mycostatin) oral suspension 1 mL four times a day for 1 week. Place medication in front of mouth on each side. Rub directly on plaques with a cotton swab. Adults: Pastilles: 200,000-unit lozenge four times a day for 14 days, or swish-and-swallow 500,000 units four times a day for 14 days or two 500,000-unit tablets three times daily for 14 days.
  2. Clotrimazole troche (Mycelex): 10 mg five times daily for 14 days; monitor for side effects.
  3. Fluconazole: Adults: 200 mg × 1, then 100 mg daily for 5 to 7 days. Children: 5 mg/kg by mouth every day for 5 days or 6 to 12 mg/kg on first day, then 3 to 6 mg/kg for 10 days.
  4. Genital candidal dermatitis: Nystatin cream three to four times a day for 7 to 10 days. Have caregiver discontinue use of all baby wipes, lotions, powders, and creams.

Follow-Up

A. Instruct caregiver to telephone the office if the child refuses to eat, if there is no improvement, if thrush lasts more than 10 days, or if there is unexplained fever.

Consultation/Referral

A. Consult a physician if thrush does not resolve with adequate antifungal treatment.

Bibliography

American Academy of Pediatric Denistry. (n.d.). Decision trees for management of avulsed permanent tooth. Retrievedfrom http://www.aapd.org/media/policies_guidelines/rs_traumaflowsheet.pdf

American Cancer Society. (2013). Oral cavity and pharyngeal cancer. Retrieved from http://www.cancer.org/cancer/oralcavityandoropharyngealcancer/detailedguide/index

Aronson, M., & Auwaerter, P. (2014). Infectious mononucleosis in adults and adolescents. In M. Hirsch & S. Kaplan, (Eds.), *UpToDate.* Retrieved from http://www.uptodate.com/contents/infectious-mononucleosis-in-adults-and-adolescents?source=search_result&search=infectious+mononucleosis&selectedTitle=1%7E150

Doshi, D. (2009). Bet 3. Avulsed tooth brought in milk for replantation. *Emergency Medicine Journal, 26*(10), 736–737.

Goldstein, B., & Goldstein, A. (2015). Oral lesions. In R. Dellavalle & D. Deschler (Eds.), *UpToDate.* Retrieved from http://www.uptodate.com/contents/oral-lesions?source=search_result&search=aphthous+ulcers&selectedTitle=1%7E150

Haddad, R. (2016). Human papillomavirus associated head and neck cancer. In B. Brockstein, D. Brizel, & M. Fried (Eds.), *UpToDate.* Retrieved from http://www.uptodate.com/contents/human-papillomavirus-associated-head-and-neck-cancer?source=search_result&search=oral+cancer+and+hpv&selectedTitle=1%7E150

Kauffman, C. (2016). Treatment of oropharygneal and esophageal candidiasis. In K. Marr (Eds.), *UpToDate.* Retrieved from http://www.uptodate.com/contents/treatment-of-oropharyngeal-and-esophageal-candidiasis?source=search_result&search=oral+candidiasis&selectedTitle=1%7E150

Pichichero, M. (2016). Treatment and prevention of streptococcal tonsillopharyngitis. In D. Sexton & M. Edwards (Eds.), *UpToDate.* Retrieved from https://www.uptodate.com/contents/treatment-and-prevention-of-streptococcal-tonsillopharyngitis?source=see_link§ionName=TREATMENT&anchor=H9#H9

Udeani, J. (2016). Pediatric epiglottitis treatment & management. *Medscape.* Retrieved from http://emedicine.medscape.com/article/963773-treatment#d13

Wald, E. (2016). Approach to diagnosis of acute infectious pharyngitis in children and adolescents. In M. Edwards (Ed.), *UpToDate.* Retrieved from http://www.uptodate.com/contents/approach-to-diagnosis-of-acute-infectious-pharyngitis-in-children-and-adolescents?source=search_result&search=bacterial+pharyngitis+children&selectedTitle=1%7E150

Woods, C. (2015). Epiglottitis (supraglottitis): Clinical features and diagnosis. In M. Edward, G. Isaacson, & G. Fleischner (Eds.), *UpToDate.* Retrieved from http://www.uptodate.com/contents/epiglottitis-supraglottitis-clinical-features-and-diagnosis?source=search_result&search=epiglottitis&selectedTitle=1%7E44

9 Respiratory Guidelines

Asthma

Cheryl A. Glass and Melissa A. Hall

Definition

Pathophysiologically, asthma is defined by airway inflammation, intermittent airflow obstruction secondary to increased smooth muscle tone and bronchial hyperresponsiveness. Episodes are associated with widespread, variable, often reversible airflow obstruction and bronchial hyperresponsiveness when airways are exposed to various stimuli or triggers. Asthma is responsible for lost school days, lost productivity, and presenteeism.

Asthma is classified into four categories:

A. *Step 1—Mild intermittent*: Symptoms less than or equal to two per week; asymptomatic with normal peak expiratory flow rate (PEFR) between attacks; nighttime symptoms less than or equal to two per month; PEFR greater than 80% is predicted with a variability of less than 20%.

B. *Step 2—Mild persistent*: Symptoms greater than two per week but less than one per day; exacerbations may affect activity; nighttime symptoms greater than two per month; PEFR greater than or equal to 80% is predicted with variability of 20% to 30%.

C. *Step 3—Moderate persistent*: Daily symptoms require beta 2 agonist use; attacks affect activity; exacerbations greater than or equal to two per week; nighttime symptoms greater than one per week; PEFRs between 60% and 80% with a variability greater than 30%.

D. *Step 4—Severe persistent*: Continuous symptoms with limited physical activity; frequent exacerbations; frequent nighttime symptoms; PEFR less than or equal to 60% is predicted with greater than 30% variability.

Incidence

A. Asthma affects 25 million people in the United States, or 300 million worldwide.

B. Asthma is the most common chronic disease of childhood, affecting 15% of children.

C. Up to 95% of patients with asthma also suffer from persistent rhinitis.

D. Asthma is often associated with other comorbid conditions, including gastroesophageal reflux disease (GERD) and obesity.

E. Although asthma can present at any age, the peak age of diagnosis is before age 5 years.

Pathogenesis

A. Asthma arises from a complex cycle of processes initiated by airway inflammation resulting from physical, chemical, and pharmacological agents (such as environmental irritants, allergens, furry animals, cockroaches, dust mites, pollen and mold, cold air, viral respiratory infections, and exercise). It progresses to airway hyperresponsiveness, bronchoconstriction, airway wall edema, chronic mucus plug formation, and chronic airway remodeling.

Predisposing Factors

A. In children
   1. Allergy or family history of allergy
   2. Atopy
   3. Ethnicity (Puerto Rican descent, non-Hispanic Black)
   4. Gender: Male during childhood

B. In adults
   1. Family history
   2. Coexisting sinusitis, nasal polyps, and sensitivity to aspirin or other nonsteroidal anti-inflammatory drugs (NSAIDs)
   3. Exposure in workplace to wood dust, metals, and animal products
   4. Premenstrual asthma (PMA)
   5. Gender: Female in adulthood
   6. Ethnicity: Non-Hispanic Black for persistent asthma
   7. Occupational exposures
   8. Comorbidities in older adults

C. In all ages
   1. Inhalation of irritants such as tobacco smoke
   2. Viral respiratory infections
   3. Gastroesophageal reflux
   4. Obesity
   5. Lower socioeconomic level

D. Triggers
   1. Allergen exposure
   2. Viral infections of the upper airways
   3. Medication (potential risk with beta-blockers, angiotensin-converting enzyme [ACE] inhibitors, aspirin, cyclooxygenase [COX] inhibitors)
   4. Exercise

5. Situational factors: Cold air, laughter, strong odors, air pollution, smoke exposure, pregnancy
6. Foods
7. Hormones
8. Gastrointestinal (GI) reflux
9. Stress

Common Complaints

A. Recurrent cough (worse at night and early morning)
B. Recurrent wheezing
C. Recurrent shortness of breath (SOB)
D. Dyspnea (less likely to be reported in the elderly)
E. Recurrent chest tightness (may worsen with moderate activity)

Other Signs and Symptoms

A. Nocturnal awakening from symptoms
B. Variation of symptoms with seasons or environment
C. Chest discomfort, tightness with moderate activity

Subjective Data

A. Ask about the onset, duration, and course of symptoms.
B. Inquire about sudden severe episodes of coughing, wheezing, and SOB and whether precipitating factors can be identified.
C. Ask whether the patient has chest colds that take more than 10 days to resolve.
D. Ask if the patient is a smoker, how much, and for how long he or she has smoked.
E. Ask whether symptoms seem to occur during certain seasons or during exposure to the following environmental irritants:
1. Tobacco smoke
2. Perfume
3. Household pets
4. Fireplaces
5. Woodburning stoves
6. Mold
7. Dust mites
8. Cockroaches

F. Find out how often coughing, wheezing, or SOB awaken the patient.
G. Ask if symptoms are caused or exacerbated by moderate exercise or physical activity.
H. Determine the family history of asthma, allergies, and eczema.
I. Determine whether the patient is pregnant or has medical problems. If so, do not prescribe long term beta 2 adrenergics or NSAIDs. The safest medications are short-acting beta agonists (SABA), cromolyn sodium, and anticholinergic drugs.
J. Administer the asthma control test for adults or the childhood asthma control test for children aged 4 to 11 years. This test is for self-report (or parent-report) to determine whether asthma symptoms are under control. Both tests are available online from www.asthmacontrol.com. A score greater than 20 points indicates that the patient's asthma is well controlled. Scores of 5 to 19 points indicate that the patient is not well controlled.
K. Evaluate whether the patient has ever been tested for allergies.
L. Ask whether the patient has ever needed to go to the emergency room or had to be hospitalized for an asthma attack.
M. Review all medications, including over-the-counter (OTC) and herbal supplements.

Physical Examination

A. Check temperature (if indicated), blood pressure, pulse, respirations, and pulse oximetry. Measure the patient's height and weight to calculate body mass index (BMI) because obesity is associated with asthma, and evaluate failure to thrive if suspected.
B. Inspect
1. Especially in children, observe for hyperexpansion of thorax and signs that accessory muscles are being used (retractions, nasal flaring) or stridor.
2. Note appearance of hunched shoulders and/or chest deformity.
3. In children, inspect the nose for a foreign body.
4. In all patients, inspect ears, nose, and throat. Evaluate the presence of enlarged tonsils and adenoids, and nasal polyps.
5. Inspect skin for eczema, dermatitis, or other irritation that might signal allergy.
6. Observe for allergic shiners and pebbled conjunctiva.
7. Observe for digital clubbing.

C. Auscultate
1. Auscultate lung sounds. Note wheezing during normal expiration and prolonged expiration, which is seen with asthma.
2. Listen to all lung fields for an asymmetric wheeze.
3. Auscultate heart.

D. Percuss lung fields.

Diagnostic Tests

A. **Spirometry is the gold standard.** Peak flow meter measurements are not a substitute for spirometry. Evaluate the forced vital capacity (FVC) and forced expiratory volume in 1 second (FEV_1) before and after the patient inhales a short-acting bronchodilator.
B. Evaluate chest radiograph (CXR) and complete blood count (CBC) to exclude other diagnoses and infection.
C. Allergy testing is recommended for children with persistent asthma.
D. Check PEFR after inhalation of SABA. Diagnosis is confirmed if:
1. There is a 15% increase in PEFR after 15 to 20 minutes.
2. PEFR varies more than 20% between arising and 12 hours later in patients taking bronchodilators (or 10% without bronchodilators).
3. There is a greater than 15% decrease in PEFR after 6 minutes of running or exercise.

E. Consider a bronchial provocation test with histamine or methacholine for nondiagnostic spirometry.

Differential Diagnoses

A. In infants and children

1. Asthma
2. Pulmonary infections:
   - **a.** Pneumonia
   - **b.** Respiratory syncytial virus (RSV)
   - **c.** Viral bronchiolitis
   - **d.** Tuberculosis (TB)
3. Allergic rhinitis and sinusitis
4. Foreign body in the nose, trachea, or bronchus
5. GERD
6. Cystic fibrosis (CF)
7. Bronchopulmonary dysplasia
8. Vocal cord dysfunction
9. Enlarged lymph nodes or tumors

B. In adults

1. Asthma
2. Chronic obstructive pulmonary disease (COPD)
3. GERD
4. Congestive heart failure (CHF)
5. Cough secondary to medications such as ACE inhibitors or beta-blockers
6. Pneumonia, including aspiration pneumonia in elderly or post-cerebrovascular accident (CVA)
7. Pulmonary embolism
8. Laryngeal dysfunction
9. Benign and malignant tumors
10. Vocal cord dysfunction

Plan

A. General interventions

1. Review proper medication dosages. Short- and long-term agents come in several formulations, such as nebulizer, metered-dose inhaler (MDI), and a dry powder inhaler (DPI). Young children should have medication via a nebulizer using an appropriate-size face mask. The "blow-by" technique is not an appropriate means of administering medication.

2. Demonstrate correct use of inhalers, spacers, and nebulizers. If the patient does not use correct technique when using these devices, medication does not get delivered to the bronchioles, and therefore the patient may believe that the medication does not work. Most often, the medication works well when delivered to the bronchioles correctly. ▶ *See Section III: Patient Teaching Guide for this chapter, "Asthma: How to Use a Metered-Dose Inhaler"*

3. Stress the importance of using a peak flow monitor at home to monitor progress of the disease. ▶ See *Section III: Patient Teaching Guide for this chapter, "Asthma: Action Plan and Peak Flow Monitoring."*

4. SABAs are used for rescue from acute symptoms.

5. Use of a SABA more than twice a week for symptom relief indicates that the patient has inadequate asthma control and needs an inhaled corticosteroid (ICS) as controller therapy.

6. Stress the need for an asthma action plan. *See Section III: Patient Teaching Guide for this chapter, "Asthma: Action Plan and Peak Flow Monitoring."* ◀

B. Patient teaching: *See Section III: Patient Teaching Guide for this chapter, "Asthma."* ◀

C. Pharmaceutical therapy: Drugs are prescribed in a stepwise fashion for the type of asthma. The amount of medication used depends on the severity of the asthma (Steps 1–6 in the following list). **Before any medication/dosage changes, monitor the patient's compliance** (see Table 9.1). The following treatments are recommended for children aged 5 years and older and for adults:

1. Step 1: Mild
   - **a.** No long-term preventive medications are needed.
   - **b.** Use SABAs as rescue medication. May be used up to four times a day to treat exacerbations.
   - **c.** Alternative medications include cromolyn, nedocromil, leukotriene modifier, or theophylline.
2. Step 2: Mild to moderate
   - **a.** Low-dose ICSs are used daily as a long-term preventive medication.
   - **b.** Only budesonide inhalation suspension is approved by the Food and Drug Administration (FDA) for use in infants and children younger than 4 years.
   - **c.** Alternative medications include an ICS plus either a leukotriene modifier or theophylline.
3. Step 3: Moderate
   - **a.** Consider referral to asthma specialist at Step 3.
   - **b.** Use low-dose ICS plus a long-acting beta 2 agonist (LABA) *or* a medium-dose ICS.
   - **c.** Use ICS plus either a leukotriene modifier or theophylline or zileuton.
4. Step 4: Moderate to severe
   - **a.** Medium- to high-dose ICS plus either a LABA or Montelukast
   - **b.** Medium-dose ICS plus either a leukotriene modifier or theophylline
   - **c.** Second alternative: Medium-dose ICS plus either leukotriene modifier, theophylline, or zileuton
5. Step 5: Severe
   - **a.** High-dose ICS plus LABA and consider omalizumab for patients with allergies
6. Step 6: Severe
   - **a.** High-dose ICS plus LABA plus oral CS and consider omalizumab for patients who have allergies
7. Acute exacerbations in pediatrics: 0.3 or 0.6 mg/kg orally once daily for 1 or 2 days, up to a max of 16 mg/dose
8. Exercise-induced bronchospasm
   - **a.** Short-acting inhaled beta 2 agonist: Two inhalations shortly before exercise are effective for 2 to 3 hours.
   - **b.** LABA, two inhalations are effective for 10 to 12 hours.

TABLE 9.1 Medications for Asthma and COPD (By Class/Alphabetical Order)

Brand	Generic	Drug Classification	Availability
Short-Acting Beta 2 Agonist (SABA), for Rescue/Fast-Acting Rescue			
Accuneb	albuterol	Beta 2 agonist	Nebulizer
Albuterol	albuterol sulfate	Beta 2 agonist	Inhaler, solution
			Nebulizer
			Syrup
Combivent	ipratropium + albuterol	Combination anticholinergic + beta 2 agonist	MDI
Fenoterol	ipratropium + fenoterol	Beta 2 agonist	Inhaler, MDI, and oral syrup
Maxair Autohaler	pirbuterol acetate	Beta 2 agonist	MDI
ProAir HFA inhaler	albuterol	Beta 2 agonist	MDI
Proventil HFA inhaler	albuterol	Beta 2 agonist	MDI
Terbutaline sulfate	brethine	Beta 2 agonist	Tablet
Ventolin HFA	albuterol sustained release	Beta 2 agonist	MDI
Vospire ER	albuterol	Beta 2 agonist	Extended release tablet
Xopenex	levalbuterol tartrate	Beta 2 agonist	HFA inhaler
			Concentrate solution for nebulizer
Long-Acting Beta 2 Agonist (LABA), for Maintenance/Long-Acting Control			
Advair Diskus	fluticasone + salmeterol	Combination-steroid + LABA	Dry powder diskus
			MD–HFA inhaler
Arcapta	indacaterol	Long-acting beta 1 agonist	Nebulizer
Brovana	arformoterol	Beta 2 agonist	Nebulizer
Foradil Aerolizer	formoterol fumarate	LABA	Nebulizer
			Dry powder diskus
Perforomist	formoterol solution	Beta 2 agonist	Nebulizer
Serevent Diskus	salmeterol	Long-acting beta 2 agonist	Dry powder diskus
Inhaled Corticosteroid Anti-Inflammatory (ICS), for Maintenance or Long-Term Control			
Aerobid and Aerobid M	flunisolide	Inhaled corticosteroid	MDI
			MDI with menthol
Alvesco	ciclesonide	Inhaled corticosteroid	MDI
Asmanex	mometasone	Inhaled corticosteroid	Twisthaler dry powder
Beclovent	beclomethasone dipropionate	Inhaled corticosteroid	Dipro powder inhaler
Dulera	mometasone furoate +	Combination corticosteroid + long-acting	MDI
Flovent HFA	formoterol fluticasone	Beta 2 agonist Inhaled corticosteroid	MDI (also available as a dry powder inhaler as Flovent diskus)
Pulmicort	budesonide	Inhaled corticosteroid	Flexhaler and respules
QVAR	beclomethasone	Inhaled corticosteroid	MDI
Symbicort	budesonide + formoterol	Combination corticosteroid + long-acting beta 2 agonist	MDI
Leukotriene Modifiers—Nonsteroidal Anti-Inflammatory			
Accolate	zafirluklast	Leukotriene modifier	Tablet
Singulair	montelukast	Leukotriene modifier	Chew tablet
			Tablet granules
Zyflo	zileuton	Leukotriene modifier	Filmtab

(*continued*)

TABLE 9.1 Medications for Asthma and COPD (By Class/Alphabetical Order) (*continued*)

Brand	Generic	Drug Classification	Availability
Interleukin-5 agonist			
Cinqair	reslizumab	Interleukin-5 agonist	Intravenous infusion
Nucala	mepolizumab	Interleukin-5 agonist	Subcutaneous injection
Anticholinergics			
Atrovent HFA	ipratropium	Antimuscarinic/antispasmodic	MDI and nebulized
DuoNeb	ipratropium + albuterol	Combination antimuscarinic/ antispasmodic + beta 2 agonist	Nebulizer
Spiriva with HandiHaler	tiotropium	Antimuscarinic/antispasmodic	Dry powder diskus
Mast Cell Stabilizer			
Intal	cromolyn sodium	Mast cell stabilizer	MDI
Tilade	nedocromil	Mast cell stabilizer	MDI
Methylxanthine			
Aminophylline	theophylline	Methylxanthines respiratory smooth muscle relaxant	Tablet
Theo-24	theophylline sustained-release	Methylxanthines respiratory smooth muscle relaxant	Tablet
Anti-IgE (Immunoglobulin E Blocker) Monoclonal Antibody			
Xolair	omalizumab	IgE blocker-immunomodulator	Subcutaneous injection
Systemic Corticosteroids—Used as a Short-Term "Burst" for Control			
Deltasone	prednisone	Systemic corticosteroid	Tablet
Medrol	methylprednisolone	Systemic corticosteroid	Tablet
Prelone	prednisolone	Systemic corticosteroid	Tablet
Phosphodiesterase-4 Inhibitors (PDE4)			
Ariflo	cilomilast	Selective PDE4	Tablet
Daliresp	roflumilast	Selective PDE4	Tablet

HFA, hydrofluoroalkanes; MDI, metered-dose inhaler.

9. Hypertension and asthma: Drug of choice is a calcium channel blocker. Asthmatics also tolerate diuretics well.

10. Theophylline can cause cardiac arrhythmias; therefore, use it with caution and always follow up with theophylline levels.

11. Vaccinations

a. Inhaled flu vaccine is not used in children with asthma. Inactivated influenza vaccine is safe, including for children with severe asthma.

b. Pneumococcal vaccine is recommended for children with asthma.

D. Goal of asthma therapy

1. Minimal to no chronic symptoms, including night-time symptoms

2. Minimal exacerbations

3. No emergency department visits

4. Minimal use of SABA

5. No limitations of activities

6. Peak expiratory flow maintained in normal range

7. Minimal adverse effects of medications

Follow-Up

A. After acute episodes, follow up within 1 to 2 hours or next day to monitor improvement until patient is stable.

B. For patients with mild intermittent or mild persistent asthma under control for at least 3 months, assess and follow up at least every 6 months to provide education and reinforce positive behaviors. Gradually reduce medication dosage. If control is not achieved, consider increasing the dosage after reviewing medication technique, compliance, and environmental control.

Consultation/Referral

A. Consider hospitalization for patients with acute episodes who do not completely respond to treatment within 1 to 2 hours.

B. If all therapies fail—including a short burst of prednisone—refer the patient to an asthma specialist.

C. Consult with a physician when the patient is pregnant or has other medical problems, or when standard treatment is ineffective.

D. Refer if the patient presents with atypical symptoms.

Individual Considerations

Inhaled budesonide is the preferred ICS for treatment of asthma in pregnancy. Cromolyn is generally considered less effective than ICS and is therefore second line in pregnancy (http://acaai.org/asthma/whohasasthma/pregnancy).

A. Pregnancy
  1. Risks of uncontrolled asthma far outweigh risks to mother or fetus from drugs used to control the disease.
  2. Most drugs used to treat asthma and rhinitis, with the exception of brompheniramine and epinephrine, pose little increased risk to the fetus.
  3. Classes of drugs that do cause risk include decongestants, antibiotics (tetracycline, sulfonamides, and ciprofloxacin), live virus vaccines, immunotherapy (if doses are increased), and iodides. Always weigh benefits against risks, because adequate fetal oxygen supply is essential.
  4. If corticosteroids are necessary, recommend aerosolized forms due to their lower systemic effects. Prednisone or methylprednisolone are preferred and should be prescribed at minimum effective doses.
  5. Do not prescribe inhaled triamcinolone because it is teratogenic.
  6. Drugs recommended during pregnancy
    a. A beta 2 agonist, such as terbutaline, is preferred; two inhalations every 4 hours as needed up to eight inhalations per day. Regular daily use suggests a need for additional medications.
    b. Cromolyn; two inhalations four times daily as initial therapy for patients needing regular medication.
    c. Regular inhaled beclomethasone if cromolyn is not effective.
    d. Regular oral theophylline if beclomethasone is not effective.
    e. Oral prednisone if all other therapies fail; 1 week of 40 mg per day, followed by 1 to 2 weeks of tapering. Recommend obstetric consult before prescribing.
  7. Leukotrine inhibitors should be prescribed in pregnancy only if clearly needed.
    a. Accolate is excreted in breast milk and should not be prescribed to mothers who are breastfeeding.
    b. Fetal anomalies have been reported with Zyflo.

B. Geriatrics
  1. Asthma in the elderly is often associated with other comorbidities such as cardiac conditions or dementia.
  2. Half of elderly patients with asthma have the first onset after age 65. Respiratory viruses are a common trigger.
  3. Recurrent episodes of SOB may be primary symptom.
  4. Treatment is the same as with younger patients, with inhaled steroids the mainstay and oral steroids reserved for severe episodes. The elderly have more adverse effects from inhaled ICS.
  5. If steroids are prescribed, carefully monitor the patient for complications, including cataracts, increased intraocular pressure, hyperglycemia, and accelerated loss of bone mass.
  6. Inhaled anticholinergics and beta 2 agonists are second-line treatments.
  7. The elderly may have difficulty with inhaling medications and may require a nebulizer.
  8. Theophylline is rarely effective in the elderly. Asthma medications may have increased adverse effects in the elderly or may aggravate coexisting medical conditions, requiring medication adjustments. Also consider drug interactions and drug-and-disease interactions.

C. Pediatrics
  1. Spacing chambers are recommended to assist in proper delivery of medication.

Resources

Adult and Children Asthma Control tests: www.asthmacontrol.com
American Lung Association: www.lungusa.org
Asthma & Allergy Foundation of America: www.aafa.org
Global Initiative for Asthma (GINA) Instructions for Inhaler and Spacer Use: www.ginasthma.com
National Heart Lung and Blood Institute (NHLBI): www.nhlbi.nih.gov

Bronchiolitis: Child

Cheryl A. Glass and Melissa A. Hall

Definition

A. Bronchiolitis is a narrowing and inflammation of the bronchioles, causing wheezing and mild to severe respiratory distress. Infants are affected most often because of their small airways and insufficient collateral ventilation. It is one of the most common causes of acute hospitalizations in infants, especially in the fall and winter. A small decrease in a broncioles already small airway will have a fourfold increase in airway resistance and accounts for this pathologic manifestation in this age group.

B. The average length of illness with bronchiolitis is 12 days.

Incidence

A. Respiratory infection is seen in one third of children younger than 12 months, with 1 in 10 requiring hospitalization.

B. Bronchiolitis occurs most often in infants and children aged 1 to 2 years. Approximately 2% to 4% of adults with respiratory illnesses, comorbidity of immunosuppression, and the elderly will also be diagnosed with bronchiolitis.

Pathogenesis

The pathology results in obstruction of bronchioles from inflammation, edema, and debris, leading to hyperinflation of the lungs, increased airway resistance, atelectasis, and ventilation–perfusion mismatching.

A. Respiratory syncytial virus (RSV) is the most common cause (50%–80%) of bronchiolitis.

B. Human metapneumovirus (HMPV) is the second most common cause (3%–19%).

C. Other causes include parainfluenza virus, adenovirus, influenza *Chlamydia pneumoniae, Mycoplasma pneumoniae,* and human bocavirus (HBoV).

Predisposing Factors

A. Low birth weight, particularly in premature infants
B. Chronic lung disease (CLD; formerly bronchopulmonary dysplasia)
C. Parental smoking
D. Congenital heart disease
E. Immunodeficiency
F. Lower socioeconomic group
G. Crowded living conditions and day care
H. Gender: Bronchiolitis occurs in males 1.25 times more frequently than in females.

Common Complaints

Clinical manifestations are initially subtle.

A. Infants who become increasingly fussy
B. Difficulty feeding during the 2- to 5-day incubation period. This is because infants prefer to breathe through their nose (obligate nasal breathing) as opposed to their mouths and significant nasal edema and/or rhinorrhea may force mouth breathing and disturb feedings.
C. Low-grade fever (usually less than 101.5°F)
D. Cough
E. Tachypnea
F. Wheezing
G. Retractions
H. Nasal flairing and grunting

Other Signs and Symptoms

A. Coryza
B. Irritability
C. Lethargy
D. Respiratory distress
E. Nasal flaring and grunting
F. Hypothermia (infants younger than 1 month)

Subjective Data

A. Determine the onset, course, and duration of illness.
B. Are breathing problems affecting the ability to eat and drink? Is the baby able to be breastfed?
C. Evaluate a history of fever, nausea, vomiting, or diarrhea.
D. Does the patient or any family members have asthma?
E. Are there any other family members who are ill?
F. Are there smokers in the family environment?

Physical Examination

A. Check temperature, blood pressure, and respirations. **Count respirations for 1 full minute. Respirations greater than 70 breaths per minute in an infant may be associated with risk for severe disease and warrant further evaluation for pneumonia. Tachypnea at any age is a concern for severe lower respiratory illness.**
B. Inspect
  1. Observe overall appearance.
  2. Note respiratory pattern and nasal flaring.
  3. Note the use of accessory muscles for breathing.
  4. Check for tachypnea, which differentiates bronchiolitis from upper respiratory infections and bronchitis.
  5. Examine eyes, ears, and throat, noting other potential infections.
  6. Inspect nose for nasal flaring.
C. Auscultate
  1. Heart
  2. **Lungs. On examination there are fine inspiratory crackles and/or high-pitched expiratory wheezes. A prolonged expiration phase is seen with bronchiolitis.**
D. Palpate liver and spleen.
E. Percuss chest/lungs for hyperresonance.
F. Neurologic examination: Assess for irritability and lethargy.

Diagnostic Tests

A. **Diagnosis is made based on age and seasonal occurrence, tachypnea, and the presence of profuse coryza and fine rales, wheezes, or both on auscultation.**
B. Viral isolation from nasopharyngeal secretions or rapid antigen detection (enzyme-linked immunosorbent assay [ELISA], immunofluorescence) for RSV can confirm diagnosis.
C. Consider pulse oximetry.
D. Routine use of a chest radiograph (CXR) is not recommended by the American Academy of Pediatrics (AAP).

Differential Diagnoses

A. Viral bronchiolitis
B. Asthma
C. Viral or bacterial pneumonia
D. Aspiration syndromes
E. Pertussis
F. Cystic fibrosis (CF)
G. Cardiac disease
H. Reflux
I. Aspiration
J. Tracheoesophageal fistula

Plan

A. General interventions
  1. Use a humidifier in the patient's bedroom.
  2. Clear stuffy nose with saline solution drops and suction out nares with bulb syringe.
  3. Infants should not be exposed to secondhand smoking.
  4. Monitor respiratory pattern.
  5. Use good hygiene practices—handwashing.
B. Patient teaching: *See Section III: Patient Teaching Guide for this chapter, "Bronchiolitis: Child."* ◀
C. Dietary management
  1. Encourage fluids, such as juice and water. Dilute juice for younger infants.
  2. Offer small, frequent feedings.
  3. Breastfeeding should continue.
D. Medical/surgical management
  1. Patients may only require supportive care. Patients with respiratory distress require hospitalization.
  2. Hypoxemic patients need oxygen therapy and possibly mechanical ventilation.
  3. Chest physiotherapy is not recommended.
E. Pharmaceutical therapy
  1. Bronchodilators should not be routinely used. They do not improve the duration of illness or lessen hospitalization.

2. Corticosteroids should not be routinely used. They do not improve the duration of illness or lessen hospitalization.
3. Antibacterials should be used only with proven coexistence of a bacterial infection.
4. There is no vaccine against bronchiolitis. A vaccine against human metapneumovirus (HMPV) is currently in the early stages of development. HMPV has been in existence in humans for more than 60 years, but is only newly categorized. HMPV is most closely related to avian metapneumovirus. The virus most frequently infects young children and the elderly. HMPV is most common in late winter and early spring, and is associated with up to 25% of respiratory infections. Palivizumab (Synagis) prophylaxis should be administered to selective children following the AAP guidelines. HMPV is responsible for the majority of viral upper respiratory infections in children and adults. The virus has a world-wide distribution and is most prevalent in late winter and early spring.
5. Use of the montelukast (Singulair) has not proven beneficial in resolution of symptoms.

Follow-Up

A. Contact the patient within 12 to 24 hours for evaluation.

Consultation/Referral

A. Notify a doctor if the patient's breathing becomes labored, his or her wheezing becomes worse, and/or respiratory distress is suspected.
B. Refer patients with RSV to the emergency room if moderate respiratory distress, dehydration, or hypoxemia occurs.
C. Younger patients in moderate to severe respiratory distress require hospitalization.
D. Infants less than 3 months of age require hospitalization.
E. Patients with pulmonary hypertension, chronic lung disease (CLD; formerly bronchopulmonary dysplasia), or CF need hospitalization if their respiratory rate is greater than 60, their pulse oximetry is less than 92%, or they eat poorly.

Individual Considerations

A. Patients with pulmonary hypertension, bronchopulmonary dysplasia, or CF may have prolonged courses with high morbidity and mortality. Some may have reactive airway diseases in the future.
B. Young children and the elderly are most susceptible to HMPV infection. The majority of children are seropositive for HMPV infection by age 5. History of prematurity and asthma increase risk for hospitalization in children.
C. Human pneumavirus was identified in 8% of adults requiring hospitalization for lower respiratory infections.

Bronchitis, Acute

Cheryl A. Glass and Melissa A. Hall

Definition

A. Acute bronchitis is inflammation of the tracheobronchial tree. Bronchitis is nearly always self-limited in the otherwise healthy individual. Generally, the clinical course of acute bronchitis lasts 10 to 14 days. The cause is usually infectious, but allergens and irritants may also produce a similar clinical profile. Asthma can be mistaken as acute bronchitis if the patient has no prior history of asthma.

Incidence

A. Bronchitis is more common in fall and winter in relation to the common cold or other respiratory illness. It occurs in both children (younger than 5 years of age) and adults and is diagnosed in men more frequently than in women. Fewer than 5% of patients with bronchitis develop pneumonia.

Pathogenesis

A. Most attacks are caused by viral agents, such as adenovirus, influenza, parainfluenza viruses, and respiratory syncytial virus (RSV).
B. Bacterial causes include *Bordetella pertussis, Mycobacterium tuberculosis, Corynebacterium diphtheriae,* and *Mycoplasma pneumoniae. B. pertussis* should be considered in children who are incompletely vaccinated.

Predisposing Factors

A. Viral infection
B. Upper respiratory infection
C. Smoking
D. Exposure to cigarette smoke
E. Exposure to other irritants
F. Allergens
G. Chronic aspiration/gastroesophageal reflux disease (GERD)

Common Complaint

A. The most common symptom initially is a dry, hacking, or raspy-sounding cough. The cough then loosens and becomes productive.

Other Signs and Symptoms

A. Sore throat
B. Rhinorrhea or nasal congestion
C. Rhonchi during respiration
D. Low-grade fever
E. Malaise
F. Retrosternal pain during deep breathing and coughing
G. Decreased/lack of appetite

Subjective Data

A. Ask about the onset, duration, and course of symptoms.
B. Is the cough productive?
C. Is there substernal discomfort?
D. Is there malaise or fatigue?
E. Has the patient had a fever?
F. Does the patient smoke? (Smoking aggravates bronchitis.)
G. A review of occupational history may be important in determining whether irritants play a role in symptoms.
H. Assess for symptoms of gastroesophageal reflux.

Physical Examination

Examinations of children may best be completed with the child sitting on the parent's lap.
A. Check temperature, pulse, and blood pressure (BP). Always check a pulse oximeter.

B. Inspect
1. Observe overall appearance.
2. Inspect eyes, ears, nose, and throat (pharynx may be injected).
3. Transilluminate sinuses.
C. Palpate lymph nodes, maxillary, and frontal sinuses.
D. Auscultate all lung fields for crackles, wheezing, and rhonchi.

Diagnostic Test

A. Consider chest x-ray to exclude pneumonia.

Differential Diagnoses

A. Pneumonia
B. Upper respiratory infection
C. Asthma
D. Sinusitis
E. Cystic fibrosis (CF)
F. Aspiration
G. Respiratory tract anomalies
H. Foreign-body aspiration
I. Pneumonia
J. Chronic obstructive pulmonary disease (COPD) and emphysema
K. Pediatrics: Pertussis

Plan

A. General interventions are primarily supportive and should ensure the patient is adequately oxygenating.
1. Tell the patient to increase fluid intake.
2. Suggest humidity and mist therapy.
3. Avoid irritants, such as smoke.
▶ **B.** Patient teaching: *See Section III: Patient Teaching Guide for this chapter, "Bronchitis, Acute."*
C. Pharmaceutical therapy
1. Acetaminophen (Tylenol) for fever and malaise.
a. Adults: 625 to 1,000 mg orally every 4 hours; not to exceed 4 g/d
b. Pediatrics: For those younger than 12 years: 10 to 15 mg/kg/dose by mouth every 4 to 6 hours; not to exceed 2.6 g/d; for children older than 12 years: 325 to 650 mg by mouth every 4 hours; not to exceed five doses in 24 hours
2. Expectorants, such as guaifenesin with dextromethorphan (Robitussin DM, Humibid DM, Mytussin), can be used to treat minor cough from bronchial/throat irritation.
a. Adults and children older than 12 years: 10 mL by mouth every 4 hours
b. Children younger than 4 to 6 years: Not recommended; for children 6 to 12 years: 5 mL by mouth every 4 hours as needed

In response to child safety concerns, the American Academy of Pediatrics states that cough and cold medications should not be used for children younger than 6 years.

3. Among otherwise healthy individuals, antibiotics have **not demonstrated** benefit for acute bronchitis as the etiology is usually viral. However, oral antibiotics should be considered if symptoms persist for 2 weeks with treatment (indicates bacterial infection).
a. Erythromycin (EES, E-Mycin, Ery-Tab)
i. Adults: 250 to 500 mg by mouth four times a day or 333 mg by mouth three times daily
ii. Pediatrics: 30 to 50 mg/kg/d by mouth divided four times a day
b. Clarithromycin (Biaxin)
i. Adults: 250 to 500 mg by mouth twice a day
ii. Pediatrics: 7.5 mg/kg by mouth twice a day
c. Azithromycin (Zithromax)
i. Adults: Day 1: 500 mg by mouth, then 250 mg by mouth on days 2 to 5.
ii. Pediatrics: 12 mg/kg by mouth every day; do not exceed 500 mg/dose
4. Albuterol (Ventolin) for patients with wheezes or rhonchi, or for patients with a history of bronchoconstriction.
a. Adults: 2 puffs every 4 to 6 hours *or* 2 to 4 mg by mouth for three to four times a day
b. Pediatrics: 0.1 to 2 mg/kg by mouth for three times daily

Follow-Up

A. Follow up if patient does not improve in 48 hours.
B. Recommend yearly influenza vaccinations.

Consultation/Referral

A. In uncomplicated cases, mucus production decreases and cough disappears in 7 to 10 days. If symptoms persist, refer the patient to a physician.
B. Refer the patient if you note respiratory distress or if he or she appears ill and you suspect pneumonia.

Individual Considerations

A. Pediatrics
1. Children who have repeated episodes of bronchitis should be evaluated for congenital defects of the respiratory system.
2. Instruct patients regarding the need for immunization against pertussis, diphtheria, and influenza, which reduces the risk of bronchitis.
3. Children may attend school or day care without restrictions except during acute bronchitis with fever.
B. Geriatrics: Monitor elderly patients for complications such as pneumonia. The elderly have a greater morbidity and mortality rate.

Bronchitis, Chronic

Cheryl A. Glass and Melissa A. Hall

Definition

A. Chronic bronchitis is excessive mucus secretion with chronic or recurrent productive cough occurring three successive months a year for 2 consecutive years.

B. Others limit the definition to a productive cough that lasts more than 2 weeks despite therapy.
C. Patients with chronic bronchitis have more mucus than normal because of either increased production or decreased clearance. Coughing is the mechanism for clearing excess secretion.

Incidence

A. The incidence of chronic bronchitis is uncertain. There is a lack of definitive diagnostic criteria, and there is considerable overlap with asthma. Visits for bronchitis are second only to visits for otitis media and are slightly more common than for asthma.

Pathogenesis

A. Mucociliary clearance is delayed because of excess mucus production and loss of ciliated cells, leading to a productive cough. This is usually secondary to the number of years of cigarette smoke-induced damage. In children, chronic bronchitis follows either an endogenous response to an acute airway injury or continuous exposure to noxious environmental agents such as allergens or irritants.
B. Bacteria most often implicated are *Streptococcus pneumoniae, Haemophilus influenzae, Mycoplasma pneumoniae,* and *Moraxella catarrhalis.* The most common causes of chronic bronchitis in the pediatric population include viral infections such as adenovirus, respiratory syncytial virus (RSV), rhinovirus, and human bocavirus (HBoV).
C. Specific occupational exposures are associated with symptoms of chronic bronchitis, including coal, cement, welding fumes, organic dusts, engine exhausts, fire smoke, and secondhand smoke.

Predisposing Factors

A. Cigarette smoking
B. Cold weather
C. Acute viral infection
D. Chronic obstructive pulmonary disease (COPD)/ emphysema
E. Occupational exposure to other airborne irritants
F. Chronic, recurrent aspiration or gastroesophageal reflux
G. Allergies

Common Complaints

A. Worsening cough: Hacking, harsh, or raspy sounding
B. Changes in color (yellow, white, or greenish), amount, and viscosity of sputum
C. Children younger than 5 years rarely expectorate, and sputum is usually seen in vomitus
D. "Rattling" sound in chest
E. Dyspnea/breathlessness
F. Wheezing

Other Signs and Symptoms

A. Difficulty breathing, retrosternal pain during a deep breath or cough
B. Rapid respirations
C. Fatigue
D. Headache
E. Loss of appetite
F. Fever
G. Myalgias
H. Arthralgias

Subjective Data

A. Determine the onset, course, and duration of illness.
B. Is the patient having trouble breathing?
C. Has there been a fever?
D. How is the patient's appetite? Is the patient drinking enough fluids?
E. Does the patient smoke, or is the patient exposed to secondhand smoke?
F. Review occupational history to evaluate exposure to irritants.
G. Does the patient have a history of asthma?
H. How often is the patient currently using his or her short-acting beta 2 agonist inhaler?

> *Chronic bronchitis has a long history of a productive cough and late-onset wheezing. Patients with asthma with a chronic obstruction have a long history of wheezing with a late-onset of productive cough.*

Physical Examination

Examinations of children may best be started with the child sitting on the parent's lap.
A. Check temperature, pulse, blood pressure, and pulse oximetry.
B. Inspect
  1. Observe overall appearance/mentation.
  2. Inspect eyes, ears, nose, and throat.
    a. Pharynx may be injected.
    b. Conjunctivitis suggests adenovirus.
  3. Transilluminate sinuses.

C. Auscultate
  1. Lungs in all fields; lung sounds may sound normal to scattered, rhonchi, or large airway wheezing
  2. Heart

D. Percuss chest.
E. Palpate
  1. Lymph nodes
  2. Maxillary and frontal sinuses

Diagnostic Tests

A. Patients with uncomplicated respiratory illness need little, if any, laboratory evaluation.
B. Pulse oximetry can help diagnose the issue.
C. Sputum culture is used to identify bacteria.
D. Chest radiograph (CXR) may help exclude other diseases or complications.
E. Pulmonary function studies may be indicated.
F. EKG and pulmonary function tests (PFTs) may be required for COPD patients.
G. Sweat test may be necessary to rule out cystic fibrosis (CF).

Differential Diagnoses

A. Acute bronchitis
B. Pneumonia
C. Asthma

D. Sinusitis
E. CF
F. Bronchiectasis
G. Central airway obstruction
H. Lung cancer
I. Aspiration syndrome
J. Gastroesophageal reflux
K. Tuberculosis (TB)
L. Foreign body

Plan

A. General interventions
  1. Rest during early phase of illness.
  2. Encourage smoking cessation and staying away from secondhand smoke.
  3. Suggest exercise for patients with COPD.
  4. The patient's goal is to improve symptoms and to decrease cough and production of sputum.
  5. Inform patients that increased sputum production may occur after smoking cessation and the patient may have airway reactivity (wheezing), which is especially seen in asthmatics.

▶ B. Patient teaching: *See Section III: Patient Teaching Guide for this chapter, "Bronchitis, Chronic."*

C. Dietary management
  1. Increase fluids.
  2. Eat nutritious food.

D. Pharmaceutical therapy
  1. Bronchodilators should be considered for bronchospasm.
    a. Albuterol sulfate (Proventil, Ventolin, ProAir)
      i. Adults: Metered-dose inhaler (MDI)-2 actuations (90 mcg/actuation) inhaled every 4 to 6 hours
      ii. Pediatrics: MDI or nebulizer
        1) Younger than 1 year: 0.05 to 0.15 mg/kg dose every 4 to 6 hours
        2) 1 to 5 years old: 1.25 to 2.5 mg/dose every 4 to 6 hours
        3) 5 to 12 years old: 2.5 mg/dose every 4 to 6 hours
        4) Older than 12 years: 2.5 to 5 mg/dose every 6 hours
  2. Analgesics and antipyretics are used to control fever, myalgias, and arthralgias.
  3. Consider oral steroids to decrease inflammation.
    a. Adults: 5 to 60 mg/d by mouth
    b. Pediatrics: 1 to 2 mg/kg by mouth daily or in twice a day divided dosing; do not exceed 80 mg/d.
    c. Tapering steroids is not necessary with steroid courses of 10 days' duration or less.
  4. Inhaled corticosteroid (ICS) may be effective.
    a. Beclomethasone (QVAR) is available as an MDI that delivers 40 or 80 mcg/actuation.
      i. Adults MDI: 40 to 80 mcg inhaled by mouth twice a day, not to exceed 320 mcg twice a day
      ii. Pediatrics MDI: 40 mcg inhaled by mouth twice a day, not to exceed 80 mcg twice a day
    b. Fluticasone (Flovent HFA, Flovent Diskus). Available as MDI (44-mcg, 110-mcg, or 220-mcg per actuation) and diskus powder for inhalation (50 mcg, 100 mcg, or 250 mcg per actuation).
      i. Adults
        1) MDI: 88 mcg inhaled by mouth twice a day, dosage not to exceed 440 mcg twice a day.
        2) Diskus: 100 mcg inhaled by mouth twice a day, dosage not to exceed 500 mcg twice a day.
      ii. Pediatrics
        1) MDI: Ages 4 to 11 years: 88 mcg inhaled by mouth twice a day; older than 11 years administer as adults.
        2) Diskus: Ages 4 to 11 years: 50 mcg inhaled by mouth twice a day; older than 11 years administer as adults.
  5. Antibiotics for bacterial infection
    a. Erythromycin (EES, E-Mycin, Ery-Tab)
      i. Adults: 250 to 500 mg by mouth four times a day or 333 mg by mouth three times daily
      ii. Pediatrics: 30 to 50 mg/kg/d by mouth divided four times a day; do not exceed 2 g/d.
    b. Clarithromycin (Biaxin)
      i. Adults: 250 to 500 mg by mouth twice a day
      ii. Pediatrics: 7.5 mg/kg by mouth twice a day
    c. Azithromycin (Zithromax)
      i. Adults: 500 mg by mouth on day 1, then 250 mg by mouth on days 2 to 5
      ii. Pediatrics: 10 mg/kg/d by mouth on day 1, then 5 mg/kg on days 2 to 5; do not exceed adult dose
    d. Amoxicillin-clavuanic acid (Augmentin)
      i. Adult: 250 to 500 mg by mouth every 8 hours
      ii. Pediatrics
        1) Younger than 3 months: 30 mg/kg/d by mouth divided to every 12 hours
        2) 3 months or older: 40 to 80 mg/kg/d by mouth divided to every 12 hours
  6. Over-the-counter cold and cough products: The American Academy of Pediatrics do not recommend use of cold and cough products for use in children 6 years of age or younger. These products have been associated with serious adverse effects.

Follow-Up

A. Follow up if there is no improvement in 3 to 4 days after starting therapy.
B. Recommend yearly influenza vaccinations.

Consultation/Referral

A. Refer patients with respiratory distress to a physician. If respiratory failure occurs (rare), hospitalization may be needed.
B. Refer patients with COPD to a physician or pulmonary specialist.

C. Referral to a pediatric pulmonologist should be considered when symptoms persist and do not respond to initial therapy.

Individual Considerations

A. Pediatrics
  1. Recurrent acute or chronic bronchitis should alert the clinician to the diagnosis of asthma.
  2. Recurrent episodes of acute or chronic bronchitis may also be associated with immunodeficiencies.
  3. Discuss the need for immunization against pertussis, diphtheria, and influenza, which reduces the risk of bronchitis.
  4. Children may attend school or day care without restrictions except during fever.
  5. In children, a foreign body needs to be ruled out either radiographically or by bronchoscopy.

B. Geriatrics
  1. Age-specific changes in elderly include changes in airway size due to connective tissue changes, including shallow alveolar sacs.
  2. Chest wall compliance is reduced, with diaphragmatic strength reduction of 25%.
  3. Older adults may adjust their lifestyle to compensate due to declining lung function.
  4. Dyspnea should be addressed and not associated only with deconditioning with age.

Chronic Obstructive Pulmonary Disease

Cheryl A. Glass and Melissa A. Hall

Definition

Chronic obstructive pulmonary disease (COPD) is progressive, chronic, expiratory airway obstruction due to chronic bronchitis or emphysema. The relief of bronchoconstriction due to inflammation has some reversibility. Chronic bronchitis is a chronic productive cough lasting 3 months during 2 consecutive years, after all causes of chronic cough have been excluded. Emphysema is an abnormal, permanent enlargement (hyperinflation) and destruction of the alveoli air sacs, as well as the destruction of the elastic recoil. Many patients have both types of air-restriction symptoms of chronic bronchitis and emphysematous destruction leading to COPD. Patients with asthma whose airflow obstruction is completely reversible are not considered to have COPD. When asthmatic patients do not have complete reversible airflow obstruction, they are considered to have COPD.

Irreversible airflow obstruction is a key factor in the patient's disability. The goal of COPD management is to improve daily quality of life (QOL) and the recurrence of exacerbations. Smoking cessation continues to be the most important therapeutic intervention.

The Global Initiative for Chronic Obstructive Lung Disease (GOLD) staging criteria are:

A. Stage I—Mild obstruction: Forced expiratory volume in 1 second (FEV_1) greater than 80% of predicted value, some sputum, and chronic cough

B. Stage II—Moderate obstruction: FEV_1 between 50% and 80% of predicted value, shortness of breath (SOB) on exertion, and chronic symptoms

C. Stage III—Severe obstruction: FEV_1 between 30% and 50% of predicted value, dyspnea, reduced exercise tolerance, and exacerbations affecting QOL

D. Stage IV—Very severe obstruction chronic respiratory failure: FEV_1 less than 30% of predicted value or moderate obstruction FEV_1 less than 50% of the predicted value and chronic respiratory failure. Fourteen percent of patients admitted for COPD exacerbation die within 3 months of admission.

E. Comorbidities commonly seen with COPD include hypertension; cardiac disorders, including atrial fibrillation and heart failure; diabetes/metabolic syndrome; gastrointestinal (GI) disorders; lung cancer; depression; and osteoporosis.

Incidence

A. Approximately 6% of the population in the United States has been diagnosed with COPD. It is still an underrecognized diagnosis although it is the third leading cause of death in the United States. COPD is is more commonly seen in males than females, but gender differences are lessening as more females are smoking. The exact worldwide prevalence is unknown.

Pathogenesis

A. Chronic bronchitis leads to the narrowing of the airway caliber and increase in airway resistance. Mucous gland enlargement is the histologic hallmark of chronic bronchitis.

B. In emphysema, loss of the air sac's elastic recoil and alveoli destruction causes air limitation. Emphysema caused by smoking is the most severe in the upper lobes. Most patients with COPD have smoked one pack of cigarettes a day for 20 or more years before the symptomatic dyspnea, cough, and sputum appear.

Predisposing Factors

A. Cigarette smoking

B. Occupational, environmental, or atmospheric pollutants
  1. Dust
  2. Chemical fumes
  3. Secondhand smoke
  4. Air pollution

C. Genetic factor: Alpha 1-antitrypsin (AAT) deficiency

D. Recurrent or chronic lower respiratory infections or disease

E. Age (most common in fifth decade of life)

Common Complaints

A. Chronic cough and colorless sputum, usually worse in morning

B. Dyspnea with exertion, progressing to dyspnea at rest

C. Wheezing

D. Difficulty speaking or performing tasks
E. Weight loss (decrease in fat-free mass)

Other Signs and Symptoms

A. Pursed-lip breathing: induces auto peeping and hence helps keep alveoli open.
B. Use of accessory muscles
C. Tripod position
D. Barrel chest
E. Cyanosis (fingertips, tip of nose, around lips)
F. Tachypnea
G. Tachycardia
H. Difficulty speaking or performing tasks
I. Distended neck veins
J. Abnormal, diminished, or absent lung sounds
K. Mental status changes
L. Anxiety and depression
M. Pulmonary hypertension
N. Cor pulmonale
O. Left-sided heart failure

Subjective Data

A. Ask the patient about past respiratory problems and infections. Does he or she currently have fever, chills, or other signs of infection?
B. Ask about the onset of cough and characteristics of sputum (amount, color, and presence of blood).
C. Determine cigar use and cigarette pack-year history (pack/day × number of years smoked).
D. Inquire about exposure to occupational or environmental irritants.
E. How far can the patient walk before becoming breathless? Is there more breathlessness when the patient walks on a slight incline?
F. Does the patient become breathless or tired when performing activities of daily living (ADLs)?
G. Ask about insomnia, anxiety, restlessness, edema, and weight change.
H. How many pillows does the patient sleep on? Does he or she have to sleep in a recliner or sitting up?
I. Assess the patient's ability to perform ADLs and instrumental activities of daily living (IADLs), including grooming and personal hygiene, performing chores around the house, shopping, cooking, and driving.
J. Ask about alcohol use.
K. Review all medications, including over-the-counter (OTC) and herbal products.
L. Review further assessment questions based on existing comorbidities.

Physical Examination

A. Record temperature (if indicated), blood pressure, pulse, respirations, and pulse oximetry. The respiratory rate increases proportionally to disease severity. Take height and weight to calculate the body mass index (BMI). **The patient may have a fairly normal examination early in the disease.**

B. Inspect
1. Observe general appearance: Skin color, affect, posture, gait, amount of respiratory effort when walking; note increased anterior–posterior chest diameter.
2. Examine sputum: Frothy pink signals pulmonary edema. Hemoptysis as seen in tuberculosis (TB).
3. Examine lips, fingertips, and nose for cyanosis. (Finger clubbing is not characteristic of COPD.)
4. Observe the neck for distended veins and peripheral edema (advanced disease).
5. Check for pursed-lip breathing and use of accessory muscles.

C. Auscultate
1. Auscultate the heart.
2. Auscultate the lungs for wheezes, crackles, decreased breath sounds, and prolonged forced expiratory rate.
3. Assess for vocal fremitus (vibration) and egophony (increased resonance and high-pitched bleating quality). Air trapping causes air pockets that don't transmit sound well. Absent ventricular lung sounds are a distinctive characteristic of COPD.
4. Auscultate the carotids arteries.

D. Percuss the chest for the presence of hyperresonance and for signs of consolidation.
E. Palpation
1. Palpate the neck for lymphadenopathy.
2. Palpate the chest.
3. Evaluate the abdomen for organomegaly.
4. Evaluate pedal edema.

F. Mental status: Assess for decreased level of consciousness.
G. Six-minute walking distance (6MWD) test to evaluate desaturation.
H. Further physical examinations are dependent on comorbidities.

Diagnostic Tests

A. Spirometry is the gold standard for diagnosing COPD. Pulmonary function tests (PFTs) are used to diagnose, determine severity, and follow the disease progression of COPD. Spirometry before and after using a bronchodilator.

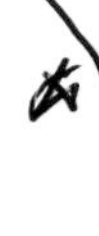

1. FEV_1 is used as an index to airflow obstruction and evaluates the prognosis in emphysema.
2. Forced vital capacity (FVC)
3. FEV_1/FVC ratio less than 0.70

B. Chest radiograph (CXR; not required to diagnose COPD but rules out other diagnoses)
C. Complete blood count (CBC)—evaluate polycythemia due to chronic hypoxia
D. Sputum specimen for culture
E. If the patient is younger than age 40 years or has a family history of early onset of emphysema, measure AAT levels. Patients with a family history of AAT deficiencies are at risk of lung damage early in life as AAT serves to protect lower lung tissue from damage by proteolytic enzymes.
F. Arterial blood gas (ABG)
G. EKG: Note sinus tachycardia, atrial arrhythmias
H. Two-dimensional echocardiogram is used to evaluate secondary pulmonary hypertension.

I. Chest CT is an alternative imaging study for emphysema; however, it is not required as a diagnostic tool.
J. Perform a purified protein derivative (PPD) test if TB is suspected.
K. Brain natriuretic peptide (BNP)
L. Theophylline level (if applicable)

Differential Diagnoses

A. Asthma
B. Heart failure
C. Bronchiectasis
D. Pulmonary edema
E. TB
F. AAT deficiency
G. Pneumonia
H. Pulmonary embolism
I. CF
J. Cancer

Plan

A. General interventions

1. Educate and encourage active participation in the plan of care, including medication adherence.
2. A smoking-cessation plan is an essential part of a comprehensive treatment plan. Develop a smoking-cessation plan; assess readiness to quit. Set a quit date; encourage a group smoking-cessation program. **Discuss smoking at every subsequent visit.** (*See Section III: Patient Teaching Guide for this chapter, "Nicotine Dependence."*)
3. Advise to stay away from secondhand smoke and limit exposure to other pulmonary irritants, including extreme temperature changes.
4. Advise exercise with physician approval.
5. Educate and counsel patients regarding advance directives.
6. Consider pulmonary rehabilitation for all stages of COPD.
7. The selection of inhalers is dependent on the patient's age and ability to use the inhaler. Patients should be evaluated as to their coordination and inspiration abilities necessary to use inhalers; otherwise, aerosol medication via nebulizer is the best delivery method.
8. Have patients bring in their medication/spacers to demonstrate correct use.
9. Consider group visits for teaching sessions.

B. Patient teaching: *See Section III: Patient Teaching Guide for this chapter, "Chronic Obstructive Pulmonary Disease."*

C. Dietary management

1. About 25% of COPD patients are malnourished because of coexisting medical conditions, depression, and inability to shop for or prepare food.
2. Suggest a low-carbohydrate diet. High-carbohydrate intake may increase respiratory work by increasing CO_2 production.

D. Pharmaceutical therapy: Treatment guidelines are based on spirometry.

> *Peak flow meters should not be used to diagnose or monitor COPD.*

1. Stage I (mild FEV_1 80% or greater)—The patient may be unaware that he or she has COPD. Give influenza vaccine and use short-acting beta 2 agonist bronchodilators as needed.
2. Stage II (moderate FEV_1 between 50% and 79%)—Give influenza vaccine, plus short-acting beta 2 agonist bronchodilators, as needed, plus long-acting bronchodilator(s) plus cardiopulmonary rehabilitation.
3. Stage III (severe FEV_1 between 30% and 49%)—Give influenza vaccine, plus short-acting beta 2 agonist bronchodilators as needed, plus long-acting bronchodilator(s), plus cardiopulmonary rehabilitation, plus inhaled glucocorticoid steroids if patient has repeated exacerbations.
4. Stage IV (very severe FEV_1 less than 30%)—Give influenza vaccine, plus short-acting beta 2 agonist bronchodilator, as needed, plus long-acting bronchodilator(s), plus cardiopulmonary rehabilitation, plus inhaled glucocorticoid steroids if repeated exacerbations plus long-term oxygen therapy (if the patient meets criteria for O_2). Medicare guidelines require a patient's PaO_2 (partial pressure of oxygen) to be less than 55 mmHg or his or her resting oxygen saturation to be below 88% on room air.
5. Utilization of a spacer/holding chamber for inhalers should be encouraged.
6. Administer pneumonia vaccines for patients 65 years and older. Prevnar 13 or Pneumovax 23 should be administered according to Centers for Disease Control and Prevention (CDC) recommendations and based on the individual patient's vaccine history. See the CDC website for current recommendations.

> *Administer yearly flu vaccine. Trivalent influenza vaccine is essential for all COPD patients. Give the vaccine each year as soon as it is available.*
>
> *Prescribe pharmacological agents/nicotine replacement therapy for smoking cessation.*

   a. Nicotine chewing gum produces better quit rates than counseling alone.
   b. Transdermal nicotine patches have a long-term success rate of 22% to 42%.
   c. Use of an antidepressant such as Zyban (150 mg twice a day) has been shown to be effective for smoking cessation and may be used in combination with nicotine replacement therapy.
   d. Chantix is a partial agonist selective for alpha 4, beta 2-nicotinic acetylcholine receptors.

7. Antibiotics are not recommended in COPD patients except with acute exacerbation, with symptoms of increased dyspnea, increased sputum volume, and increased sputum purulence, changes in cough, fever, or other evidence of an infection such as an infiltrate on CXR. Antibiotics are prescribed for COPD patients on mechanical ventilation.

8. Consider phosphodiesterase-4 (PDE-4) inhibitors (Roflumilast or Cilomilast) as needed when necessary.
9. Mucolytic agents have small benefits and are not usually recommended.
10. Antitussives are not recommended.
11. Long-term oxygen has been shown to increase survival in patients with severe resting hypoxemia. Target oxygen saturation is 88% to 92% (Long-Term Oxygen Treatment Trial Research Group, 2016).
12. Cardioselective beta-blockers are not contraindicated in COPD. Cardioselective beta-blockers at low dosages do not cause bronchospasm. A noncardioselective beta-blocker or a cardioselective beta-blocker (B1 blocker) at higher dosages may contribute to bronchospasms.

Follow-Up

A. For acute exacerbations, follow up same day or following day.
B. Follow up stable, chronic COPD every 1 to 2 months, depending on the patient's needs.
C. Serial PFTs may help guide therapy and offer prognostic information.
D. Monitor serum theophylline levels. Theophylline has a narrow therapeutic window and the potential for toxicity. Adverse effects, including nausea and nervousness, are the most common. Other adverse effects include abdominal pain with cramps, anorexia, tremors, insomnia, cardiac arrhythmia, and seizures.
E. Reevaluate patients on oxygen therapy 1 to 3 months after starting oxygen.
F. Evaluate for osteoporosis; bone mineral density is lower in COPD patients, and they are at risk for vertebral fractures.
G. Monitor the patient's body weight.

Consultation/Referral

A. Consult with a physician if the patient has acute respiratory decompensation, or severe cor pulmonale (distended neck veins, hepatomegaly, dependent peripheral edema, ascites, and pleural effusion).
B. Refer the patient to a pulmonary specialist for rehabilitation, if available.
 1. Outpatient education for the patient and family
 2. Exercise training
 3. Breathing retraining, that is, pursed-lip breathing, huff coughing
 4. Correct administration of medications
C. Refer to a registered dietitian (RD) to provide medical nutrition therapy (MNT). RDs focus on the prevention and treatment of weight loss associated with COPD and other comorbidities.
D. Send to a pulmonologist for evaluation for continuous positive airway pressure (CPAP) or bi-level positive airway pressure (BiPAP).
E. Send to a pulmonologist to evaluate for surgical intervention such as bullectomy, lung volume reduction surgery, or lung transplantation.

Individual Considerations

A. Pregnancy
 1. COPD is rare except in AAT deficiency.
 2. Monitor drug treatment for potential teratogenic effects.
B. Adults: Sexual dysfunction is common in patients with COPD; encourage other ways to display affection.
C. Geriatrics
 1. Presentation may be atypical.
 2. Patients should have annual flu vaccinations and pneumococcal vaccination every 5 years.
 3. Patients may not have the ability to use inhaler devices because of tremors, muscle weakness, poor hand–eye coordination, and/or poor memory.
 4. Theophylline is on the Beers list of drugs to use with caution in the geriatric population related to cardiovascular, renal, and hepatic concerns; insomnia; and peptic ulcers.
 5. Discuss the course of disease, living wills, advanced directives, and resuscitation status early, before a crisis occurs.

Resources

The Global Initiative for Chronic Obstructive Lung Disease (GOLD) guidelines: www.goldcopd.org

Common Cold/Upper Respiratory Infection

Cheryl A. Glass and Melissa A. Hall

Definition

A. The common cold is a self-limiting acute respiratory tract infection (ARTI) resulting from viral infection of the upper respiratory tract. It is also called *acute nasopharyngitis.* ARTI is characterized by mild coryzal symptoms, rhinorrhea, nasal obstruction, and sneezing.

Incidence

A. Upper respiratory tract infections are among the most frequent reasons for office visits. However, the true incidence is not known because patients treat themselves with over-the-counter (OTC) and home remedies, as well as seasonal and locational variability. Most children have six to eight colds a year; most adults have two to four.

Pathogenesis

A. Over 25% to 80% of ARTIs are caused by a rhinovirus (greater than 100 antigenic serotypes). Other viral agents include coronavirus (10%–20%), RSV, adenoviruses (5%), influenza viruses (10%–15%), and parainfluenza viruses. Incubation period is 1 to 5 days with viral shedding lasting up to 2 weeks.
B. Rhinoviral infections are chiefly limited to the upper respiratory tract but may cause otitis media and sinusitis.

Predisposing Factors

A. Exposure to airborne droplets
B. Direct contact with virus by touching hands or skin of infected people, or by touching surfaces they touched, and then touching eyes or nose

C. Very young or old ages
D. Smoking, which increases risk by 50%
E. Crowded conditions such as day-care centers and schools

Common Complaints

A. Low-grade fever
B. Generalized malaise
C. Nasal congestion and discharge (initially clear, then yellow and thick)
D. Sneezing
E. Sore throat or hoarseness
F. Watery and/or inflamed eyes

Other Signs and Symptoms

A. Headache
B. Cough

Subjective Data

A. Elicit the onset, course, and duration of symptoms.
B. Inquire about color and other characteristics of nasal discharge and sputum. **Purulent nasal discharge after 14 days signals bacterial sinusitis.**
C. Inquire about other discomforts and exposure to people with similar symptoms.
D. Review allergens, seasonal problems, and exposure to irritants and smoke.
E. Review history for other respiratory problems, such as asthma, chronic bronchitis, and emphysema.

Physical Examination

A. Check temperature, pulse, respirations, and blood pressure. Carry out pulse oximetry if difficult respiratory symptoms are noted.
B. Inspect
   1. Observe general appearance.
   2. Inspect eyes. **Note "allergic shiners," tearing, and eyelid swelling.**
   3. Observe ears, throat, and mouth. **Otitis media is indicated by redness and bulging of tympanic membrane, or by membrane perforation with drainage.**
   4. Inspect nose for nasal redness, swelling, polyps, enlarged turbinates, septal deviation, and foreign bodies.
   5. Transilluminate sinuses.
      a. Group A *Streptococcus*: Tonsilar enlargement, exudate, petechiae
      b. Allergies: "Cobblestoned" pharyngeal mucosa
      c. Mononucleosis: About half of patients with mononucleosis develop tonsillar exudates, and about one third develop petechiae at the junction of the hard and soft palates, which is highly suggestive of the disease.
C. Auscultate
   1. All lung fields
   2. Heart
D. Percuss
   1. Sinus cavities and mastoid process of temporal bone to rule out otitis media
   2. Chest for consolidation
E. Palpate
   1. Palpate face for sinus tenderness.
   2. Examine head and neck for enlarged, tender lymph nodes.

Diagnostic Tests

A. Diagnosis may be made from history and physical. Because common cold manifestations are so prevalent, an aggressive workup is rarely necessary.
B. Consider rapid strep test if the patient has symptoms or was exposed to Group A *Streptococcus*.
C. Consider throat culture if negative rapid strep test and symptomatic.

Differential Diagnoses

A. Upper respiratory infection
B. Allergic rhinitis
C. Foreign body
D. Sinusitis
E. Influenza
F. Group A strep pharyngitis
G. Otitis media
H. Pneumonia

Plan

A. General interventions
   1. Controlled trials reveal minimal therapeutic benefits of vitamin C for the treatment and prevention of colds. Zinc has no proven benefit. Echinacea has not shown any differences in rates of infection or severity of symptoms when compared with placebo. Validation and standardization of herbal products have not been completed.
B. Patient teaching: *See Section III: Patient Teaching Guide for this chapter, "Common Cold."* ◀
C. Pharmaceutical therapy
   1. **In 2016, the American College of Chest Physicians released clinical practice guidelines (Gibson et al., 2016) for the management of cough. Health care providers should refrain from recommending cough suppressants and OTC cough medicines for young children because of associated morbidity and mortality. The American Academy of Pediatrics reminds consumers to avoid the use of OTC cough and cold products in children younger than 4 years.**
   2. **Antibiotics are ineffective in treating viral infection.**
   3. Corticosteroids may actually increase viral replication and have no impact on cold symptoms.
   4. Topical decongestants for rhinorrhea and nasal congestion
      a. Adults and children older than 6 years, pseudoephedrine (Afrin) nasal spray 0.05% two to three sprays per nostril twice daily, or phenylephrine (Neo-Synephrine) nasal spray 0.25% to 1% two to three sprays per nostril every 4 hours as needed. Using decongestant-type nasal sprays longer than 2 to 3 days can result in rebound congestion and abuse of the drug.
      b. Children younger than 6 years, saline nasal drops 2 to 3 drops per nostril two to three times daily.

c. As an alternative to pseudoephedrine and other nasal decongestants, consider clearing nasal congestion in infants with a rubber suction bulb; secretions can be softened with saline nose drops or a cool-mist humidifier.

5. Oral decongestants are available such as pseudoephedrine (Sudafed).

a. Adults: Pseudoephedrine (Sudafed) 60 mg every 4 to 6 hours or 120 mg every 12 hours

b. Children 2 to 6 years: Pseudoephedrine (Sudafed) liquid 2.5 mL every 4 to 6 hours

c. Children older than 6 years: Pseudoephedrine (Sudafed) liquid 5 mL every 4 to 6 hours, or pseudoephedrine (Sudafed) 30 mg every 4 to 6 hours

6. Analgesics, such as acetaminophen (Tylenol) and ibuprofen (Advil), may be used for headache relief.

a. Ibuprofen: Adults: 200 to 400 mg by mouth while symptoms persist; not to exceed 3.2 g/d

b. Ibuprofen: Pediatrics

i. Younger than 6 months: Not established

ii. 6 months to 12 years: 4 to 10 mg/kg/dose by mouth three to four times a day

iii. Children older than 12 years: Administered as adults

7. Cough suppressants, if necessary: Dextromethorphan (Benylin DM, Robitussin, Vicks Formula 44 pediatric formula).

a. Adults and children older than 12 years: 10 to 20 mg orally every 4 hours, or 30 mg every 6 to 8 hours, or 60 mg extended-release liquid twice daily, to a maximum of 120 mg/d

b. Children 6 to 12 years: 5 to 10 mg orally every 4 hours

c. Children 2 to 6 years: 2.5 to 5 mg orally every 4 to 6 hours

d. Children younger than 2 years: Few data exist regarding the therapeutic or toxic levels of cough and cold medications in children younger than 2 years.

e. Elderly: Anticholinergic effects from antihistamines may be associated with side effects, including confusion, cognitive impairment, delirium, dry mouth, constipation, urinary retention, and sedation. Diphenhydramine may be appropriate in acute treatment of severe allergic reactions.

8. Colds have no allergic mechanism, so antihistamines are ineffective. The atropine-like drying effect from antihistamines may exacerbate congestion and obstruct the upper airway by impairing mucus flow.

Follow-Up

A. None is recommended unless symptoms persist longer than 7 days from onset.

B. Parents should return to the doctor's office if their child's fever exceeds 102°F, if respiratory symptoms increase, or if symptoms do not resolve in 10 to 14 days.

Consultation/Referral

A. Consult a physician if the patient has been reevaluated and given a new treatment plan but still has symptoms.

B. Refer the patient to an otolaryngologist if tonsillary abscess is suspected.

Individual Considerations

A. Pediatrics

1. Oral decongestants are not recommended for children younger than 24 months of age.

2. The most common reported calls reported to poison control centers that involve OTC medications concern the ingestion of acetaminophen and cough and cold preparations.

a. Accidental pediatric toxic ingestion is reported in children younger than 6 years, and intentional toxic ingestion is more common in adolescents aged 13 to 19 years.

b. Adolescents have used dextromethorphan as a recreational drug.

B. Geriatrics

1. Use of antihistamines with anticholinergic properties may cause side effects of confusion and delirium as listed earlier, along with increased rates of hospitalization.

Cough

Cheryl A. Glass and Melissa A. Hall

Definition

A. Coughing is a mechanism that clears the airway of secretions and inhaled particles. The act of coughing has the potential to traumatize the upper airway (e.g., vocal cords). A chronic cough is one that lasts longer than 8 weeks.

B. Because coughing can be an affective behavior, psychological issues must be considered as a cause or effect of coughing.

Incidence

A. Data on the incidence of coughing are not available. However, most healthy people do not cough, and the main reason for coughing is airway clearance. A chronic cough is the most common presenting symptom in adults who seek medical treatment in an ambulatory setting.

B. Pertussis affects infants and young children; however, the incidence is increasing in adults secondary to the lack of booster vaccination.

Pathogenesis

A. Stimulation of mucosal neural receptors in the nasopharynx, ears, larynx, trachea, and bronchi can produce a cough, as can acute inflammation and/or irritation of the respiratory tract. Cough is a reflex response that is mediated by the medulla but is subject to voluntary control. There is clear evidence that vagal afferent nerves regulate involuntary coughing.

B. Pertussis (whooping cough) is caused by the bacterium *Bordetella pertussis.*

C. The **pathogenic triad of chronic cough** responsible for 92% to 100% of chronic cough is as follows:

1. Upper airway cough syndrome (UACS), previously referred to as postnasal drip syndrome

2. Asthma

3. Gastroesophageal reflux disease (GERD)

Predisposing Factors

A. Pharyngeal irritants
B. Foreign-body aspiration
C. Tuberculosis (TB; persons in prisons and nursing homes and immigrants from areas where TB is endemic)
D. Psychogenic factors (more common in children and those with emotional stress)
E. Mediastinal or pulmonary masses
F. Congestive heart failure (CHF)
G. Cystic fibrosis (CF)
H. Congenital malformations
I. Viral bronchitis
J. Asthma (sole symptom in 28%)
K. Mycoplasma infection
L. UACS, previously referred to as postnasal drip
M. Chronic sinusitis
N. Allergic rhinitis
O. Environmental irritants
P. GERD
Q. Chronic bronchitis
R. Pulmonary edema
S. Medications, including angiotensin-converting enzyme (ACE) inhibitors
T. Impacted cerumen and external otitis
U. Nonasthmatic eosinohilic bronchitis (NAEB; 13%–33%)

Common Complaints

A. Common complaint is a cough that interferes with activities of daily living (ADLs) and sleeping, leading to a decrease in a patient's quality of life (QOL).
B. The pertussis cough is uncontrollable and violent. Following coughing, a "whooping" sound follows with a deep breath.

Other Signs and Symptoms

A. Fatigue
B. Rhinitis
C. Epistaxis
D. Tickle in throat
E. Pharyngitis
F. Night sweats
G. Dyspnea
H. Fever
I. Sputum production
J. Hoarseness
K. Postnasal drip

Subjective Data

A. Elicit information about the onset, duration, and course of the cough. Was the onset recent or gradual? Does the cough occur at night? **Nocturnal cough may be caused by chronic interstitial pulmonary edema and may signal left-sided heart failure. Cough caused by asthma is also worse at night. Morning cough with sputum suggests bronchitis.**
B. Inquire about the cough's characteristics. For example, is it productive, dry, bronchospastic, brassy, wheezy, strong, or weak? If it is productive, is it bloody or mucoid? Note the color, consistency, odor, and amount of sputum or mucus. Dry, irritative cough suggests viral respiratory infection. Severe or changing cough should be evaluated for bronchogenic carcinoma. Rusty-colored sputum suggests bacterial pneumonia. Green or very purulent sputum is due to degeneration of white cells. HIV cough produces purulent sputum.
C. Inquire whether the cough is associated with eating and choking episodes. Wheezing or stridor with coughing may indicate a foreign body or aspiration.
D. Ask whether the cough is associated with postnasal drip, which produces a chronic cough, clear sputum, edematous nasal mucosa, and a "cobblestoned" pharyngeal mucosa.
E. Find out whether if the cough is associated with heartburn or a sour taste in the mouth, indicating GERD.
F. Ask about precipitating factors, such as exercise, cold air, or laughing. Also ask about alleviating factors. **Cough from asthma can be triggered or exacerbated by exposure to environmental irritants, allergens, cold, or exercise.**
G. Ask about current and previous work. Is the patient exposed to occupational and environmental irritants, such as dust, fumes, or gases? If so, what are the type, level, and duration of exposures?
H. Ask about family history of respiratory illness, such as CF or asthma.
I. Is the patient a smoker? If so, how much does he or she smoke, and how long has he or she smoked? Is he or she exposed to secondhand smoke? How much of the day? **Smoking is the main cause of chronic cough.**
J. Find out the date of the patient's last tuberculin skin test. Note recent exposure to TB.
K. Inquire about any exposure to the flu.
L. Does the patient have a history of heart problems?
M. Does the patient have a history of respiratory problems or other medical problems? Chronic bronchitis is a major cause of chronic cough and sputum production. Cough may also be an early sign of lung cancer; in late stages, cough occurs along with weight loss, anorexia, and dyspnea.
N. Review medications such as ACE inhibitors. Cough related to ACE inhibitors usually subsides within 2 weeks, but the median time is up to 26 days.
O. Common causes of chronic cough in the elderly include postnasal drip, asthma, and gastroesophageal reflux.

Physical Examination

A. Record temperature and blood pressure, if indicated.
B. Inspect
   1. Observe general appearance for cyanosis, difficulty breathing, use of axillary muscles, and finger clubbing.
   2. Examine ears, nose, and throat.
C. Auscultate heart and lungs.
D. Percuss
   1. Sinus cavities and mastoid process
   2. Chest and lungs for consolidation
E. Palpate
   1. Palpate face for sinus tenderness.
   2. Examine head and neck for lymph nodes, masses, and jugular vein distension (JVD).

Diagnostic Tests

Testing can be held to a minimum by careful review of history and physical examination. Children with chronic cough should undergo, at a minimum, a chest x-ray and spirometry (if age appropriate).

A. White blood cell (WBC) if infection suspected
B. HIV test if suspected
C. Sputum for eosinophils, Gram stain, and/or culture
D. Mantoux test if indicated
E. Chest radiograph (CXR)
F. Sweat chloride test to rule out CF
G. Pulmonary function testing/spirometry
H. Methacholine challenge to rule out asthma
I. Esophageal pH monitoring to rule out GERD
J. CT scan if necessary

Differential Diagnoses

A. Environmental irritants
  1. Cigarette, cigar, or pipe smoking
  2. Pollutants (wood smoke, smog, burning leaves, etc.)
  3. Dust
  4. Lack of humidity
B. Lower respiratory tract problems
  1. Lung cancer
  2. Asthma
  3. Chronic obstructive lung disease (includes bronchitis)
  4. Interstitial lung disease
  5. CHF
  6. Pneumonitis
  7. Bronchiectasis
C. Upper respiratory tract problems
  1. Chronic rhinitis
  2. Chronic sinusitis
  3. Disease of external auditory canal
  4. Pharyngitis
D. Medication-induced cough from ACE inhibitors
E. Extrinsic compression lesions
  1. Adenopathy
  2. Malignancy
  3. Aortic aneurysm
F. Psychogenic factors, more common in children and those with emotional stress
G. Gastrointestinal (GI) problems such as reflux esophagitis
H. Genetic problems such as CF

Plan

A. General intervention
  1. If sputum is purulent, obtain a sample for examination.
  2. Patients with chronic obstructive pulmonary disease (COPD) and CF should be taught huffing as an adjunct to other methods of sputum clearance.
▶ **B.** Patient teaching: *See Section III: Patient Teaching Guide for this chapter, "Cough."*
C. Pharmaceutical therapy
  1. The American College of Chest Physicians released clinical practice guidelines in 2006 for the management of cough. Health care providers should refrain from recommending cough suppressants and over-the-counter (OTC) cough medicines for young children because of associated morbidity and mortality. The Centers for Disease Control and Prevention (CDC) noted in 2009 that, in response to safety concerns, manufacturers of cough and cold medications for children voluntarily changed labels to include warnings for use in young children.
  2. Antibiotics should not be prescribed for coughs unless a bacterial infection is suspected.
  3. Therapy depends on various acute inflammatory and chronic irritating processes and on the cause of the cough. Refer to applicable sections of this chapter, such as "Asthma," "Tuberculosis," and see Chapter 11, "Gastrointestinal Guidelines."

Follow-Up

A. The patient with a normal CXR and no risk factors for lung cancer (e.g., smoking or occupational exposure) can be followed expectantly without further testing.
B. In patients whose cough resolves after the cessation of ACE inhibitors, and for whom there is a compelling reason to treat with these agents, a repeat trial of ACE inhibitors may be attempted.
C. See applicable sections for specific diagnoses.
D. Pertussis vaccination is available for infants, children, preteens, adults, and the elderly. Pertussis cases should be reported to the local health department.

Consultation/Referral

A. Consult a physician if symptoms persist after treatment. Reevaluate the patient in 2 weeks if he or she is no better.
B. When a cough lasts more than 2 weeks without another apparent cause and it is accompanied by paroxysms of coughing, post-tussive vomiting, and/or an inspiratory whooping sound, the diagnosis of a *Bordetella pertussis* infection should be made unless another diagnosis is proven.
C. Patients whose condition remains undiagnosed after a workup and therapy may need referral to a cough specialist.

Individual Considerations

A. Pregnancy: Cough may be an early symptom of pulmonary edema. Watch intrapartum patients for signs of edema.
B. Pediatrics
  1. The most common reported calls to poison control centers involve the ingestion of acetaminophen and cough and cold preparations. Accidental pediatric toxic ingestion is reported in children younger than 6 years, and intentional toxic ingestion is more common in adolescents aged 13 to 19 years. Adolescents have used dextromethorphan as a recreational drug.
  2. Children with chronic productive purulent cough should always be investigated to document the presence or absence of bronchiectasis and to identify underlying and treatable causes such as CF and immune deficiency.

C. Geriatrics
1. Aspiration should be considered in the elderly with chronic cough, as well as heart failure, laryngeal dysfunction, bronchiectasis, or tumors of the central airway.

Croup, Viral

Cheryl A. Glass and Melissa A. Hall

Definition

A. Viral croup is an acute inflammatory disease of the larynx, also called *laryngotracheobronchitis.* Croup is the most common cause of stridor in febrile children. The uncomplicated disease usually wanes in 3 to 5 days but may persist up to 10 days. Croup is most often self-limited, but occasionally is severe and rarely fatal. Lethargy, cyanosis, and decreasing retractions are indications of impending respiratory failure.
B. Inspiratory stridor suggests a laryngeal obstruction.
C. Poiseuille's equation states that flow (air, fluid) is proportional to the radius of the chamber to the fourth power and inversely to the length. Realizing that pediatric airways are relatively small compared to adult counterparts, a twofold decrease in airway radius decreases the airflow by 16-fold. Therefore, airway resistance is exquisitely sensitive to changes in radius in the pediatric population.
D. Expiratory stridor suggests tracheobronchial obstruction.
E. Spasmodic croup may be a noninfectious variant with symptoms always occurring at night and has the hallmark of reoccurring in children. Although viral illness may trigger this variant, the reaction may be allergic.

Incidence

A. The most common form of acute upper airway obstruction, croup generally affects children aged 3 months to 6 years. Croup has a peak incidence during the second year of life. It is most prevalent in younger children in fall and early winter.

Pathogenesis

A. Parainfluenza viruses types 1, 2, and 3 cause about 80% of croup. The initial port of entry is the nose and nasopharynx. Other viral causes include enterovirus and rhinovirus. Influenza A and B, respiratory syncytial virus (RSV), adenovirus, coronavirus, herpes simplex virus (HSV), and measles are less common causes. In a small number of cases, croup may be caused by *Mycoplasma pneumoniae.* Inflammation usually occurs in the entire airway, and edema formation in the subglottic space accounts for the predominant signs of upper airway obstruction.

Predisposing Factors

A. Upper respiratory tract infection
B. Male-to-female ratio of 1.4:1
C. Ages 6 months to 3 years (mean onset: 18 months)
D. Hyperactive airway
E. Anatomic narrowing of the airway
F. Acquired airway narrowing [from intubation, gastroesophageal reflux disease (GERD) scarring, or human papillomavirus [HPV] papillomas]

Common Complaints

A. Hoarseness
B. Cough progressing to a seal-like barking cough
C. Stridor, especially during sleep
D. Fever, usually absent or low grade, but may be high
E. Runny nose

Subjective Data

A. Determine the onset, duration, and course of illness.
B. Has the child been exposed to respiratory illness?
C. Is the child coughing? Having trouble breathing?
D. Has the child had fever, nausea, vomiting, or diarrhea?
E. Are immunizations up to date?

Physical Examination

Have the child sit upright in a parent's lap to perform the physical examination. Persistent crying increases oxygen demand and respiratory muscle fatigue.
A. Record temperature, pulse, respirations, and blood pressure.
B. Inspect
1. Observe overall appearance, noting respiratory pattern, retractions, nasal flaring, and air hunger. Children often sound terrible but do not look very ill.
2. Check nail beds and lips for cyanosis (ominous sign).
3. Assess skin and mucous membranes for signs of dehydration.
4. Observe for drooling or difficulty swallowing.
5. Inspect throat for foreign body.
6. Inspect eyes, ears, nose, and throat for infection.
C. Auscultate
1. Auscultate heart. Tachycardia is out of proportion to fever.
2. Auscultate lungs for unequal breath sounds (signals foreign-body aspiration). **Stridor is an audible harsh, high-pitched musical sound that may be noted on inspiration or heard during both inspiration and expiration.** Stridor is audible without a stethoscope
3. The Westley score is a way to quantify the severity of respiratory compromise. The severity of croup is evaluated by assessing inspiratory stridor, air entry, retractions, cyanosis, and level of consciousness (see Table 9.2).
D. Percuss chest.
E. Palpate neck to evaluate lymph nodes.
F. Neurologic examination: Assess level of alertness.

Diagnostic Tests

The diagnosis of croup is largely clinical, based on the presenting history and physical examination findings.
A. Pulse oximetry assesses respiratory status.
B. Laboratory testing is usually not needed for croup in a well-hydrated patient. However, a complete blood count (CBC) may be indicated.
C. Imaging is not required in mild cases with a typical history that responds appropriately to treatment.
D. Chest radiograph (CXR) may show the "steeple or pencil sign."
E. Anteroposterior (AP) soft tissue neck radiography may show subglottic narrowing.

TABLE 9.2 Westley Scoring for Croup

Symptom	Scoring
Inspiratory stridor	No inspiratory stridor = 0 points
	Stridor upon agitation = 1 point
	Stridor at rest = 2 points
Retractions	Mild = 1 point
	Moderate = 2 points
	Severe = 3 points
Air entry	Normal = 1 point
	Mild decrease = 1 point
	Marked decrease = 2 points
Cyanosis	None = 0 points
	Cyanosis upon agitation = 4 points
	Cyanosis at rest = 5 points
Level of consciousness	Normal = 0 points
	Disoriented = 5 points

Mild disease = A score of less than 2 points. Occasional barking coughs, no stridor at rest, and mild to no suprasternal or subcostal retraction.
Moderate disease = A score of 3 to 7 points. Frequent cough, audible stridor at rest, visible retractions, but little distress or agitation.
Severe disease = A score of 8 or greater. Frequent cough, prominent inspiratory (occasional expiratory) stridor, obvious retraction, decreased air entry on auscultation, and significant distress and agitation.

Source: Adapted from Woods (2015b).

F. Bronchoscopy or laryngoscopy may be required in unusual circumstances.
G. Arterial blood gases (ABGs) are unnecessary as they do not indicate hypoxia or hypercarbia unless respiratory fatigue is present.

Differential Diagnoses

A. Bacterial croup
B. Epiglottitis
C. Spasmodic croup
D. Membranous croup
E. Bacterial tracheitis
F. Retropharyngeal abscess
G. Diphtheria
H. Foreign bodies (gastrointestinal [GI] or trachea)
I. Respiratory syncytial virus (RSV)
J. Measles
K. Varicella
L. Influenza A or B
M. Mechanical trauma or lesions

Plan

A. General interventions
- **1.** Treatment is supportive for patients without stridor at rest.
- **2.** Stress rest and minimal activity.
- **3.** Cool-mist therapy has not been shown to be clinically effective.
- **4.** Hot steam should be avoided due to the potential of scalding.

B. Patient teaching: *See Section III: Patient Teaching Guide for this chapter, "Croup, Viral."*
C. Dietary management: Give plenty of fluids.
D. Medical/surgical management: If pulse oximetry shows desaturation, administer oxygen and monitor carefully.
E. Pharmaceutical therapy
- **1. Antibiotics are not indicated for the treatment of croup.**
- **2.** Acetaminophen (Tylenol) 5 to 15 mg/kg/dose for fever.
- **3.** In moderate to severe cases requiring hospitalization: Nebulized racemic epinephrine (asthmanefrin solution) 0.5 mL of 2.25% solution in 2.5 mL sterile water may relieve airway obstruction up to 2 hours. Treatment may be repeated three times.
- **4.** Steroid use is controversial but may be considered if the preceding therapy is ineffective. Steroids are used to decrease subglottic edema by suppressing the local inflammatory process. Corticosteroids should not be given to children with untreated tuberculosis (TB).
  - **a.** Decadron (dexamethasone) is the drug of choice. Pediatric dosing is 0.6 mg/kg in single dose orally or intramuscularly.
  - **b.** Budesonide (Pulmicort Respules inhalation suspension) has been shown to be equivalent to oral dexamethasone. Pediatric dosing is 2 mg (2 mL of suspension) nebulized.
  - **c.** Prednisone (deltasone) pediatric dosing is 1 to 2 mg/kg/d orally daily or in a divided dose twice a day for 5 days.
  - **d.** Observation for 3 to 4 hours is recommended following the initial treatment.

Follow-Up

A. Call the parent in 12 to 24 hours to evaluate patient status.

Consultation/Referral

A. Consultation with an otolaryngologist and anesthetist before rapid sequence induction may be necessary if the patient is exhibiting rapid deterioration.
B. Refer the patient to a physician if he or she is a child who is severely ill with respiratory distress or dehydration.
C. Refer the patient to a physician if there is no improvement in 12 to 24 hours.
D. Patients with stridor at rest should be admitted to the hospital.

Individual Considerations

A. Pediatrics
- **1.** Most children improve within a few days.
- **2.** Virus is most contagious during the first few days of fever.

3. Children may return to day care or school when temperature is normal and they feel better, even if cough lingers.

4. Children older than 5 years of age with recurrent croup should be referred to an otolaryngologist for evaluation.

Emphysema

Cheryl A. Glass and Melissa A. Hall

Definition

A. Emphysema is an abnormal dilation and destruction of alveolar ducts and air spaces distal to the terminal bronchioles. Lung function slowly deteriorates over many years before the illness develops. Emphysema is one of the chronic obstructive pulmonary diseases (COPDs)—a term that refers to conditions characterized by continued increased resistance to expiratory airflow. Chronic bronchitis, emphysema, and asthma comprise COPD. Chronic bronchitis and emphysema with airflow obstruction commonly occur together, and as such are usually discussed together in terms of treatment.

B. There are three morphological types of emphysema.

1. Centriacinar emphysema, is associated with long-term smoking and primarily involves the upper half of the lungs.
2. Panacinar emphysema is predominant in the lower half of the lungs. Panacinar emphysema is observed in patients with alpha 1-antitrypsin (AAT) deficiency.
3. Paraseptal emphysema involves the distal airway.

Incidence

A. Emphysema typically occurs in people older than age 50 years, with peak occurrence between ages 65 and 75 years.

B. The prevalence of emphysema is 18 cases per 1,000.

Pathogenesis

A. Decreased gas exchange occurs due to focal destruction limited to the air spaces distal to the respiratory bronchioles causing airway obstruction, hyperinflation, loss of lung recoil, and destruction of alveolar–capillary interface.

Predisposing Factors

A. Long-term cigarette smoking

B. Occupational and environmental exposure to toxic agents

1. Dust
2. Chemical fumes
3. Secondhand smoke
4. Air pollution
5. Gases
6. Respiratory infection

C. Alpha 1-protease inhibitor deficiency

D. Intravenous drug use secondary to pulmonary vascular damage from the insoluble fillers (e.g., cornstarch, cotton fibers, cellulose, talc)

E. Connective tissue disorders (e.g., Marfan syndrome and Ehlers-Danlos)

F. HIV

Common Complaints

A. Gradually progressing exertional dyspnea

B. Chronic cough

C. Wheezing

D. Fatigue

E. Weight loss

Other Signs and Symptoms

A. Cough with mild to moderate sputum production and clear to mucoid sputum

B. Early-morning cough

C. Shortness of breath

D. Tachypnea

E. Use of accessory muscles for breathing; pursed-lip breathing; *prolonged* expiration

F. Barrel chest (increased anterior-to-posterior chest diameter)

G. Flushed skin

H. Clubbed fingers

I. Decreased libido

J. Thin, wasted appearance

K. Wheezing, particularly during exertion and exacerbations of emphysema

Subjective Data

A. Elicit information about the onset, duration, and course of symptoms.

B. Determine whether the patient is a smoker. If so, how much and for how long? Evaluate exposure to secondhand smoke. How much of the day?

C. Ask about current and previous work. Is the patient exposed to occupational and environmental irritants, such as dust, fumes, or gases? If so, what are the type, level, and duration of exposures?

D. Inquire about the cough's characteristics. Is it productive, dry, bronchospastic, brassy, wheezy, strong, or weak?

E. Question the patient about episodes of tachypnea, frequency of respiratory infections, and incidence of angina during exertion.

F. Does the patient have a hereditary disease (e.g., cystic fibrosis [CF] or AAT deficiency), asthma, nasal abnormalities (e.g., deviated septum), or other respiratory problems?

G. When was his or her last tuberculin skin test done?

H. Find out the patient's usual weight, and assess how much weight loss has occurred and over what time period.

I. Evaluate current vaccination status for pneumonia and influenza.

J. Review all medications, including over-the-counter (OTC) and herbal products.

K. Assess the patient's ability to perform activities of daily living (ADLs) and instrumental activities of daily living (IADLs), including grooming and personal hygiene, performing chores around the home, shopping, cooking, and driving.

L. Ask about alcohol use.

Physical Examination

A. Temperature (if indicated), pulse, respirations, blood pressure, and weight. Consider pulse oximetry.

B. Inspect

1. Observe general appearance; note flushed skin color, use of accessory muscles, pallor around lips, pursed-lip breathing, barrel chest (lung hyperinflation), and thinness.

2. Assess for peripheral edema.

3. Dermal examination: Note finger clubbing and cyanosis.

C. Auscultate

1. Auscultate heart.

2. Auscultate lungs for wheezes, crackles, decreased breath sounds (generally diffuse decreased breath sound).

3. Assess for vocal fremitus (vibration) and egophony (increased resonance and high-pitch bleating quality). Air trapping causes air pockets that do not transmit sound well.

D. Percuss chest for presence of hyperresonance and signs of consolidation.

E. Palpate

1. Palpate abdomen.

2. Evaluate pedal edema.

3. Evaluate the abdomen for organomegaly.

F. Further physical examinations are dependent on comorbidities.

Diagnostic Tests

A. Pulse oximetry: Blood gases if indicated

B. AAT deficiency to rule out hereditary deficiency

C. Tuberculin skin test

D. Pulmonary function tests **(PFTs) reveal increased total lung capacity with poor respiratory expulsion and increased respiratory volume.**

E. EKG reveals sinus or supraventricular tachycardia.

F. Chest radiograph (CXR) reveals hyperinflation, flat diaphragm, and enlarged heart.

G. Sputum evaluation and/or culture

Differential Diagnoses

A. Emphysema

B. Chronic bronchitis

C. Chronic asthma

D. Bronchiectasis

E. CF

F. Chronic asthmatic bronchitis

G. Tuberculosis (TB)

H. AAT deficiency

I. Congestive heart failure (CHF)

Plan

A. General interventions

1. Medical management: Supplemental oxygen therapy is indicated if the patient has a resting PaO_2 less than 55 mmHg or a PaO_2 less than 60 mmHg, along with right-heart failure or secondary polycythemia. Goals are to achieve a PaO_2 of greater than 55 mmHg (usually 1–3 L/min).

2. Develop a smoking-cessation plan: Assess readiness to quit. Set a quit date and encourage a group smoking-cessation program. A smoking-cessation plan is an essential part of a comprehensive treatment plan.

a. Nicotine chewing gum produces better quit rates than counseling alone.

b. Transdermal nicotine patches have a long-term success rate of 22% to 42%.

c. The use of an antidepressant, such as Zyban (150 mg twice a day), has been shown to be effective for smoking cessation and may be used in combination with nicotine replacement therapy.

d. Chantix is a partial agonist selective for alpha 4, beta 2 nicotinic acetylcholine receptors.

B. Patient teaching: *See Section III: Patient Teaching Guide for this chapter, "Emphysema."* ◀

C. Pharmaceutical therapy

1. Drugs of choice are inhaled beta 2 agonists. Beta 2 agonists are used primarily for relief of symptoms and, in stable patients, have an additive effect when used with an anticholinergic agent (e.g., ipratropium bromide). A spacer/chamber device should be used to improve delivery and reduce adverse effects. The following inhaled preparations have rapid action and fewer cardiac side effects:

a. Ipratropium bromide (Atrovent) has bronchodilatory activity with minimum side effects.

i. Metered-dose inhaler (MDI): Two to four puffs every 4 to 6 hours

ii. Nebulizer: 250 mcg diluted with 2.5 mL normal saline every 4 to 6 hours

b. Tiotropium (Spiriva) is a bronchodilator similar to ipratropium. Available in a capsule form containing a dry powder or oral inhalation via a HandiHaler inhalation device. Adults: 1 capsule (18 mcg) inhaled every day via the inhaler device

c. Metaproterenol sulfate (Alupent) is available as a liquid for nebulizer and MDI.

i. MDI: Two puffs every 3 to 4 hours

ii. Nebulizer: 0.2 to 0.3 mL of 5% solution diluted to 2.5 mL with normal saline three to four times a day

d. Albuterol (Proventil, Ventolin) is available as a liquid for nebulizer, MDI, and dry powder inhaler (DPI).

i. MDI: One to four puffs every 3 to 4 hours

ii. Nebulizer: 0.2 to 0.3 mL of 5% solution diluted to 2.5 mL with normal saline three to four times a day

2. If improvement is not satisfactory or tachyphylaxis occurs, give theophylline. Theophylline improves respiratory muscle function and stimulates the respiratory center as well as bronchodilates.

a. Initial dose: 10 mg/kg/daily divided in oral doses every 8 to 12 hours

b. Maintenance: 10 mg/kg/daily divided in oral doses every day or twice a day; adjust doses in 25% increments to maintain serum theophylline level of 5 to 15 mcg/mL—not to exceed 800 mg/d

3. Oral steroids should be used to treat outpatients with acute exacerbations. Corticosteroids reduce mucosal edema, inhibit prostaglandins that cause bronchoconstriction, and increase responsiveness to bronchodilators. Taper the dose as soon as bronchospasm is controlled. A minority of patients who respond to oral steroids can be maintained on long-term inhaled steroids.

4. In patients with COPD, chronic infection or colonization of the lower airways is common. The goal of antibiotic therapy is not to eliminate organisms, but to treat acute exacerbations. If infection is present, give one of the following:

a. Doxycycline 100 mg twice daily

b. Trimethoprim-sulfamethoxazole 160/800 mg twice daily

c. Clarithromycin 250 to 500 mg orally twice daily

d. Cefaclor (Ceclor) 250 to 500 mg orally every 8 hours; this drug is active against *Pneumococcus* and *H. influenzae*

5. Mucolytic agents in clinical practice are not recommended currently because of a lack of evidence for their benefit.

6. Trivalent influenza vaccine is essential for all COPD patients. Give the patient the vaccine each October, at least 6 weeks before onset of flu season.

7. Pneumococcal vaccine is essential for COPD patients. Give as a single intramuscular injection of 0.5 mL.

8. AAT is needed for significant antitrypsin deficiency (less than 80 mg/dL). Patients get weekly or monthly infusions. Consult with a physician before therapy. A history of smoking rules out candidacy.

Follow-Up

A. If the patient is acutely ill, contact him or her by phone in 24 to 48 hours and consider immediate referral.

B. Monitor the patient's body weight.

C. Serial PFTs may help guide therapy and offer prognostic information.

D. Monitor theophylline levels because of the drug's potential for toxicity. Adverse effects, including nausea and nervousness, are the most common. Other adverse effects include abdominal pain with cramps, anorexia, tremors, insomnia, cardiac arrhythmia, and seizures. Theophylline doses: 100 to 200 mg every 6 to 8 hours.

Consultation/Referral

A. If the patient's condition remains acute after 48 hours of treatment, consider immediate referral to a physician.

B. Refer the patient to a social worker for help in getting "Meals on Wheels," handicapped parking, and finding other community resources.

C. A consultation with a pulmonary specialist is recommended.

Individual Considerations

A. Adults

1. Sexual dysfunction is common in patients with COPD; encourage other ways to display affection.

B. Geriatrics

1. Discuss course of disease, living wills, advanced directives, and resuscitation status early, before a crisis occurs.

2. Theophylline is on the Beers list of drugs to use with caution in the geriatric population related to cardiovascular, renal, and hepatic effects; insomnia; and peptic ulcers.

Resources

A Patient's Guide to Aerosol Drug Delivery: Retrieved from www.aarc.org/resources/clinical-resources/aerosol-resources

A Guide to Aerosol Delivery Devices for Respiratory Therapists. Retrieved from www.aarc.org/app/uploads/2015/04/aerosol_guide_rt.pdf

National Emphysema Foundation: www.emphysemafoundation.org

The Global Initiative for Chronic Obstructive Lung Disease (GOLD) Guidelines: Retrieved from www.goldcopd.org

Obstructive Sleep Apnea

Cheryl A. Glass and Melissa A. Hall

Definition

Obstructive sleep apnea (OSA) is the periodic reduction (hypopnea) or cessation (apnea) of breathing due to a narrowing or occlusion of the upper airway during sleep. OSA has been linked to traffic accidents, cardiac diseases, stroke, diabetes, and visceral obesity. OSA is also associated with nocturnal cardiac arrhythmias and chronic and acute cardiac events, and is a risk factor for strokes. OSA worsens in the supine sleeping position. The following are diagnostic criteria for OSA if either of these two conditions exists:

A. The presence of 15 or more apneas, hypopneas, or respiratory effort-related arousals per hour of sleep in an asymptomatic patient. More than 75% of the apneas and hypopneas must be obstructive.

B. Five or more obstructive apneas, obstructive hypopneas, or respiratory effort-related arousals per hour of sleep in a patient with symptoms or signs of disturbed sleep. More than 75% of the apneas or hypopneas must be obstructive.

Incidence

A. The incidence of OSA in the morbidly obese population is between 38% and 88%. Otherwise, incidence in males is between 20% and 30% and females between 10% and 15%.

B. In nonobese and otherwise healthy children younger than 8 years, incidence is between 1% and 3%. Obesity adds a fourfold added risk for disordered breathing.

C. Most children with OSA are aged 2 to 10 years, coinciding with adenotonsillar lymphatic tissue growth. (Surgical removal of enlarged tonsils and adenoids usually results in a complete cure.)

D. Most cases in adults are undiagnosed.

Pathogenesis

A. Increased tissue thickness of the structures of the tongue and soft tissues in the pharyngeal cavity, which decreases the passageway for air to the trachea, is thought to be the mechanism of OSA. During the night, the muscles of the oropharynx relax, which result in the relative obstruction of the airway. Obesity and hypertrophy of tonsils and/or adenoids account for most cases of OSA in children. OSA is associated with poor neurocognitive performance and increased risk for mortality, including cardiovascular disease.

Predisposing Factors

A. Obesity
B. Increased neck circumference
C. Age: Increases in older persons (older than 65 years)
D. Gender: Males
E. Postmenopause
F. Hypothyroidism
G. Tonsillar hypertrophy
H. Alcohol
I. Craniofacial abnormalities
J. Medications
  1. Benzodiazepines
  2. Antipsychotics
  3. Opioid analgesics
  4. Beta-blockers
  5. Barbiturates
  6. Antihistamines
  7. Sedative antidepressants

K. Allergic rhinitis
L. Genetic conditions (e.g., Down syndrome, Pierre Robin anomalies, Marfan syndrome, etc.)
M. Ethnicity (e.g., Black, Asian, Hispanic)
N. Acromegaly
O. Family history
P. Diabetes
Q. Hypertension

Common Complaints

A. Daytime sleepiness
B. Loud snoring, gasping, or snorting during sleep
C. Fatigue

Other Signs and Symptoms

A. Adults
  1. Asymptomatic: Patients may not recognize they have OSA because they are able to go to sleep anytime.
  2. Restless sleep
  3. Dry mouth or sore throat
  4. Lack of physical or mental energy
  5. Falling asleep when watching TV, reading, driving/riding in a car
  6. Morning headaches
  7. Decreased libido and impotence
  8. Cognitive deficits

B. Children
  1. Short attention span
  2. Emotional lability
  3. Behavioral problems
  4. Enuresis

Subjective Data

A. Does the patient feel sleepy during the day? Is daytime sleepiness a problem?
B. Does the patient struggle to stay awake during the day?
C. Does the patient take naps? How often and how long does the patient sleep?
D. Does the patient feel physically and mentally exhausted?
E. Does the patient's bed partner complain about snoring, gasping, or snorting?
F. Ask the Epworth Sleepiness Scale questions related to how often the patient dozes off or falls asleep (in contrast to just feeling tired). Each situation is scored from 0 = would never doze, to 1 = a slight change of dozing, 2 = moderate chance of dozing, and 3 = a high chance of dozing. There are eight situations to which the patient should respond:
  1. Sitting and reading
  2. Watching TV
  3. Sitting inactive in a public place (e.g., a theater or meeting)
  4. As a passenger in a car for an hour without a break
  5. Lying down to rest during the day when circumstances permit
  6. Sitting and talking to someone
  7. Sitting quietly after lunch without alcohol
  8. In a car, while stopped for a few minutes in traffic

G. Ask the patient to list all medications currently being taken, particularly substances not prescribed, including over-the-counter (OTC) and herbal products.
H. Review alcohol use.
I. Men who present with sleep disorders should also be questioned about the presence of erectile dysfunction.

Physical Examination

A. Blood pressure, pulse, respirations, height and weight to calculate BMI, and waist measurement
B. Inspect
  1. Oropharynx examination for:
    a. Peritonsillar narrowing or hypertrophy
    b. Tongue (evaluate for macroglossia)
    c. Elongated or enlarged uvula
    d. Palate (high arch or narrow palate)
  2. Nasal examination; look for septal deviation and nasal polyps.
  3. Inspect for signs of pulmonary hypertension or cor pulmonale.
    a. Jugular venous distension
    b. Peripheral edema

C. Palpate thyroid gland.
D. Auscultate heart and lungs.
E. Mental status: Assess for confusion.

Diagnostic Tests

A. Polysomnography (PSG) is the standard method of diagnosis. The apnea hypopnea index (AHI) or the respiratory disturbance index (RDI) is used to quantify hypopneas and classify the degree of sleep disturbance.
  1. Full-night PSG
  2. Split-night PSG
  3. Home testing with portable monitors

B. Routine laboratory work is not helpful in the confirmation or exclusion of OSA.

Differential Diagnoses

A. OSA
B. Primary snoring
C. Narcolepsy

D. Restless leg syndrome
E. Swallowing disorder
F. Nocturnal seizures
G. Gastroesophageal reflux disease (GERD)
H. Obesity hypoventilation syndrome
I. Sleep deprivation
J. Neurodegenerative disease (e.g., Parkinson's, dementia, Alzheimer's)
K. Substance abuse
L. Tonsillar hypertrophy

Plan

A. General interventions

1. Continuous positive airway pressure (CPAP) or bi-level positive airway pressure (BiPAP) is the mainstay of treatment for moderate to severe OSA.

▶ **B.** Patient teaching: *See Section III: Patient Teaching Guide for this chapter, "Sleep Apnea."*

1. Educate the patient about modifying controllable risk factors such as keeping diabetes and hypertension under control, healthy diet, exercise, and stopping smoking.

2. Treatment with CPAP and BiPAP is required at all times during the night and during naps.

3. Behavioral strategies include sleeping in a non-supine position using a positioning device (e.g., alarm, pillow, backpack, tennis ball are used for positional therapy).

4. Give the patient a teaching sheet on sleep apnea.

C. Dietary management

1. Even a modest weight loss of 10% to 20% has been associated with an improvement.

D. Nonsurgical treatment

1. Oral appliances (OAs): Require a thorough dental examination

a. Custom-made OAs may improve airway patency during sleep by enlarging the upper airway and/or by decreasing the upper airway collapse.

b. Mandibular repositioning appliances (MRAs) cover the upper and lower teeth and hold the mandible in an advance position.

c. Tongue retaining devices (TRDs) hold the tongue in a forward position without mandibular repositioning.

E. Surgical treatment

1. Tracheostomy can eliminate OSA but not central hypoventilation syndromes. This procedure should be considered only when other options have failed or when it is considered necessary by clinical urgency.

2. Maxillomandibular advancement (MMA) is indicated when the patient cannot tolerate/refuses CPAP and an OA is not appropriate/effective.

3. Surgical treatment should be considered after using an oral appliance or positive airway pressure for 3 months. Surgical treatment has been shown to benefit patients with tonsillar or adenoid hypertrophy, or craniofacial deformaties (www.uptodate.com/contents/management-of-obstructive-sleep-apnea-in-adults?source=search_result&search=treatment%20obstructive%20sleep%20apnea&selectedTitle=1~150#H15)

4. Weight loss resulting from bariatric surgery has been effective in improving sleep efficiency and increasing amounts of rapid eye movement (REM) sleep. The severity of presurgical OSA determines the degree to which OSA improves postbariatric surgery.

5. Radiofrequency ablation (RFA) is for treatment of mild to moderate OSA when the patient cannot tolerate/refuses CPAP and an OA is not appropriate/effective.

6. Laser-assisted uvulopalatoplasty is not recommended for OSA.

Follow-Up

A. There is no standard for recommending repeat PSG testing or a CPAP titration study after significant weight loss.

Consultation/Referral

A. Refer to a dentist for an OA.
B. Refer to a pulmonologist for management of therapy and/or surgical treatment.
C. Refer the patient to a cardiologist as needed.

Pneumonia (Bacterial)

Cheryl A. Glass and Melissa A. Hall

Definition

A. Pneumonia is inflammation and consolidation of lung tissue caused by a bacterial pathogen. The causative agent and the anatomic location classify pneumonia. It is not uncommon to have acute viral and bacterial pneumonia concurrently.

B. Other types of pneumonia and pulmonary inflammation occur secondary to smoking, exposure to chemicals, fungi, near-drowning, and from recurrent aspiration with gastroesophageal reflux.

C. The CURB acronym represents the assessments for confusion, urea, respiratory rate, and blood pressure. The CURB-65 severity score for community-acquired pneumonia (CAP) is a tool to estimate pneumonia mortality and assist in determining whether the patient should best be treated in the inpatient or outpatient setting. Each parameter is given a score = 1 if present. There are five parameters: Confusion, blood urea nitrogen (BUN) greater than 19 mg/dL, respiratory rate greater than 30/min, systolic blood pressure less than 91 mmHg or diastolic blood pressure less than 60 mmHg, and age greater than 65 years. (http://www.mdcalc.com/curb-65-score-pneumoniaseverity)

Incidence

Pneumonia is the leading cause of death of children worldwide. Approximately 4 million children younger than 5 years worldwide die per year secondary to pneumonia. Pneumonia is also a leading cause of death for patients older than 65 years.

A. Bacterial pneumonia is more prevalent in the very old and very young.
B. A higher mortality rate occurs in young infants, persons with immunodeficiency, and in adults with abnormal vital signs and certain pathogens.
C. The incidence rate also varies by pathogens.

Pathogenesis

Pneumonia results from inflammation of the alveolar space and anatomically can be thought of as an alveolitis. Lobar penumonia has four stages:
A. Vascular congestion and alveolar edema within the first 24 hours of infection
B. Red hepatization (2–3 days), characterized by erythrocytes, neutrophils, and fibrin within the alveoli
C. Gray hepatization (2–3 days), characterized by a gray-brown to yellow color secondary to exudate
D. Resorption and restoration of the pulmonary architecture; a rub may still be ascultated due to the fibrinous inflammation

Bacterial causes include *Streptococcus pneumoniae* (the most common pathogen), *Haemophilus influenzae* type b (Hib; the second most common pathogen), *Staphylococcus aureus, Legionella, Chlamydia trachomatis, Chlamydia pneumoniae, Mycoplasma pneumoniae* (most common pathogen in school-age children and adolescents), and *Pneumocystis jiroveci* pneumonia previously known as *Pneumocystis carinii* pneumonia [PCP] in patients with HIV.

Predisposing Factors

A. Age extremes
B. Chronic obstructive pulmonary disease (COPD)
C. Alcoholism
D. Cigarette smoking
E. Aspiration
F. Heart failure
G. Diabetes
H. Heart failure/heart disease
I. Crowded conditions (day care, dormitories)
J. Immunodeficiency
K. Congenital anomalies
L. Abnormal mucus clearance
M. Lack of immunization
N. Measles
O. Indoor air pollutants from cooking or heating with wood
P. Prematurity

Common Complaints

Acute onset of these symptoms
A. Fever
B. Shaking chills
C. Dyspnea; rapid, labored breathing
D. Cough
E. Rust-colored sputum

Other Signs and Symptoms

A. Increased respiratory rate (tachypnea)
B. Chest pain
C. Upper respiratory tract infection (URI) symptoms such as pharyngitis
D. Headache
E. Nausea
F. Vomiting
G. Vague abdominal pain
H. Diarrhea
I. Myalgia
J. Arthralgias
K. Poor feeding
L. Lethargy in infants

Subjective Data

A. Determine the onset, duration, and course of illness.
B. Has the patient had fever or shaking chills?
C. Has there been breathing trouble? Are the breathing problems interfering with eating and drinking?
D. If a child, review the presence of acute onset of fever, cough, tachypnea, dyspnea, and grunting.
E. Is there a cough? Is the cough productive? What color is the sputum?
F. Are any other family members ill?
G. If a child, has he or she been hospitalized for pneumonia or respiratory distress before?
H. Review the history for any chronic diseases.
I. Has the patient been immunized for pneumonia?
J. Review all medications, including over-the-counter (OTC) and herbal products. Specifically review whether the patient has been on any antibiotics in the past 3 months. **Recent exposure to an antibiotic is a risk factor for antibiotic resistance. Continued or repeated use of that class of antibiotics is not recommended.**

Physical Examination

A. Temperature, blood pressure, pulse, and weight. Count respirations for a full minute.
  1. **Tachypnea is the single best predictor of pneumonia in children and the elderly.**
  2. **In the elderly the blood pressure is usually low.**

B. Inspect
  1. Observe overall appearance. Does the patient appear ill? Consider the clinical presentation, age of the person, and history.
  2. Observe breathing pattern and the use of accessory muscles, grunting, retractions, and tachypnea.
  3. Obtain a pulse oximetry to assess oxygen saturation. **An oxygen saturation less than 92% is an indicator of severity and the need for oxygen therapy.**
  4. Check nail beds and lips for cyanosis.
  5. Examine the eyes, nose, ears, and throat.

C. Auscultate
  1. Heart
  2. Lungs for the following (auscultate bases first in geriatric patients):
    a. Crackles represent fluid in the alveolar sacs (present in 80% of patients), wheezes, and decreased breath sounds
    b. Whispered pectoriloquy (increased loudness of whisper during auscultation)

 c. Egophony (patient's "e" sounds like "a" during auscultation)
 d. Bronchophony (voice sounds louder than usual)
 3. Abdomen (usually hypoactive bowel sounds)

D. Percuss chest to identify areas of consolidation.

E. Palpate
 1. Chest for tactile fremitus (increased conduction when patient says "99")
 2. Lymph nodes for adenopathy
 3. Sinuses for tenderness; sinusitis is a sign of *Mycoplasma* infection

Diagnostic Tests

A. The British Thoracic Society in their 2011 guideline update for CAP in children notes that no diagnostic tests are necessary in the community, but emphasizes the importance of education on management, signs of deterioration, and the need for reassessment.

B. The WHO defines pneumonia solely on the basis of clinical finding observed by inspection and timing of respirations.

C. Chest radiograph (CXR)
 1. Infiltrates confirm diagnosis. False negatives result from dehydration, evaluation in first 24 hours, and infection.
 2. Ordering a posterior, anterior, and lateral CXR ensures adequate visualization for diagnosis.

D. Complete blood count (CBC) with differential.

E. BUN is needed to calculate the CURB-65 score.

F. Cultures
 1. Blood cultures if critically ill, immunocompromised, or for persistent symptoms
 2. Sputum cultures are reserved for very ill patients with unusual presentations.

G. Consider rapid viral testing.

H. Consider skin testing for TB for high-risk exposure.

Differential Diagnoses

A. Pneumonia
 1. Viral pneumonia
 2. Aspiration pneumonia
 3. Chemically induced pneumonia

B. Asthma

C. Bronchitis/bronchiolitis

D. Pertussis

E. Heart failure

F. Pulmonary embolus

G. Empyema and abscess

H. Aspiration of foreign body

Plan

A. General interventions
 1. Encourage rest during acute phase.
 2. Encourage patients to avoid smoking/secondhand smoke.
 3. A vaporizer may be used to increase humidity.
 4. Encourage good handwashing or use of hand sanitizer.
 5. Chest physiotherapy is not prescribed for pneumonia.

B. Patient teaching: *See Section III: Patient Teaching Guides for this chapter, "Bacterial Pneumonia: Adult" and "Bacterial Pneumonia: Child."*

C. Dietary management: Encourage a nutritious diet with increased fluid intake.

D. Pharmaceutical therapy
 1. Treatment with antibiotics is empirical. Oral therapy should continue for 7 to 10 days (see Table 9.3).
  a. Amoxicillin is considered a first-line therapy in pediatrics.
  b. Macrolide antibiotics should not be the first-line therapy, but can be added if there is no response to first-line empirical therapy.
  c. Macrolides are the first choice in otherwise healthy adults.
 2. Administer acetaminophen (Tylenol) for fever.
 3. Avoid cough suppressants. Suppression of a cough may interfere with airway clearance.
 4. Vaccines
  a. Children: Heptavalent pneumococcal vaccine is recommended for all children in the United States.
  b. Geriatrics: Pneumoccocal 13 and 23 vaccines are recommended for the elderly.

Follow-Up

A. Patients/parents should know the signs of increasing respiratory distress and seek immediate medical attention.

B. Follow up with a telephone call in 24 hours.

C. If there is no improvement after 48 hours on antibiotics, the patient is advised to return to the office.

D. Schedule a return visit in 2 weeks for evaluation.

E. Follow up CXR in 4 to 6 weeks for patients older than 60 years and for those who smoke. However, if the patient is younger than 60 years, a nonsmoker, and feels well at 6-week follow-up, there is no need to follow up with a CXR.

Consultation/Referral

A. Patients who are immunocompromised or have signs of toxicity or hypoxia may need hospitalization. Refer them to a physician.

B. If the child is in moderate respiratory distress, dehydrated, or hypoxemic, consult with or refer the patient to a physician/hospital.

C. Poor prognostic signs that require referral are age greater than 65 years, respiration rate greater than or equal to 30 breaths per minute, systolic BP less than 90 mmHg or diastolic BP less than 60 mmHg, temperature greater than 101°F, altered mental status, extrapulmonary infection, and white blood cells (WBC) less than 4,000 or greater than 30,000.

D. Physician consultation is needed for suspected PCP.

Individual Considerations

A. Pregnancy
 1. The annual U.S. rate of antepartum CAP is 0.5 to 1.5 per 1,000 pregnancies.
 2. Perinatal mortality may increase slightly due to an associated increase in prematurity. Pneumonia puts older mothers at high risk of maternal death.

TABLE 9.3 Antibiotic Therapies for Pneumonia

Antibiotic	Adult Dosages	Pediatrics Dosages
Amoxicillin: Oral	250 mg–500 mg TID	90 mg/kg/d divided TID (5 years and older) not to exceed 4,000 mg/d
Amoxil, Trimox	Not to exceed 1,500 mg/d	
Clarithromycin: Oral (Biaxin)	250 mg–500 mg BID	15 mg/kg/d divided every 12 hours
		Not recommended for children <6 months
Cefotaxime: Intramuscular (Claforan)	>50 kg: 1–2 g IM every 6–8 hours. Not to exceed 12 g/d	<50 kg: 100 mg–200 mg/dg/d IM divided doses every 6–8 hours
Doxycycline: Oral (Doryx)	200-mg loading dose then 100 mg BID	>8 years and <100 lb
		2 mg/lb divided in 2 doses for 2 days; then 1–2 mg/lb daily in 2 divided doses
Not recommended for children <9 years		>100 lb: 100 mg orally every 12 hours
Azithromycin: Oral (Zithromax)	500 mg loading dose then 250 mg daily on days 2–5	10 mg/kg initial dose (not to exceed 500 mg/d) then 5 mg/kg daily on days 2–5 (not to exceed 250 mg/d)
Moxifloxacin: Oral (Avelox)	400 mg once a day	Not recommended for children <18 years
Levofloxacin (Levaquin) Adults >18 years of age	500 mg once a day for 7–14 days OR 750 mg once a day for 5 days *Other regimens depend on the pathogen*	Not recommended for children <18 years

Renal dosing should be considered in elders.

3. The symptoms of bacterial pneumonia are the same in pregnancy.
4. CXRs are acceptable in pregnancy to diagnose pneumonia.

B. Pediatrics

1. **Hospitalization is recommended in infants aged 6 months and younger and also in very severe cases of pneumonia.**
2. **Immunization against *Haemophilus influenzae* type B (Hib), pneumococcus, measles, and whooping cough (pertussis) is the most effective way to prevent pneumonia.**

C. Geriatrics

1. Depending on the frailty status of the patient, hospitalization may be required. A calculation to objectively determine patient risk has been developed (CURB-65 Severity Score) and is available at: www.mdcalc.com/curb-65-severity-score-community-acquired-pneumonia/

Pneumonia (Viral)

Cheryl A. Glass and Melissa A. Hall

Definition

A. Viral pneumonia is inflammation and consolidation of lung tissue due to a viral pathogen.

Incidence

A. Viral pneumonia is the most common pediatric pulmonary infection. Viral agents account for only 2% to 15% of pneumonia cases in adults. Viruses were documented in up to 45% of pneumonia cases in children. It is not uncommon to have concurrent viral and bacterial infections.

B. Children younger than 5 years and elderly persons have the highest rate of influenza-associated hospitalizations.

C. Pneumonia is the leading cause of death in children worldwide.

Pathogenesis

A. Pneumonia results from inflammation of the alveolar space and may compromise air at the alveoli–pulmonary capillary interface. Viral pneumonia is caused by influenza viruses, parainfluenza virus, and adenovirus and respiratory syncytial virus (RSV).

B. RSV is the most common viral cause of pneumonia.

C. Viruses and bacteria are spread from a cough or sneeze.

D. Pneumonia can also be spread via blood, especially during and shortly after birth.

Predisposing Factors

A. Age extremes

B. Prematurity

C. Exposure to viral illness
D. Lack of immunization

Common Complaints

A. Fever
B. Cough
C. Dyspnea
D. Tachypnea
E. Wheezing (more common in viral pneumonia)

Other Signs and Symptoms

A. Upper respiratory prodrome
B. Poor appetite
C. Malaise/lethargy in pediatrics
D. Myalgia
E. Muscle aches
F. Headache
G. Fatigue
H. Chest pain/tightness

Subjective Data

A. Determine the onset, duration, and course of illness.
B. Has the patient had fever, cough, and upper respiratory infection?
C. Have there been any flulike symptoms?
D. Has there been any labored breathing?
E. Has there been a cough? Is it a productive cough? What color is the sputum?
F. Are the breathing problems affecting the ability to eat or drink?
G. Has the child had nausea, vomiting, or diarrhea?
H. Review if the patient is up to date on immunizations.
I. Review all medications, including over-the-counter (OTC) and herbal products.

Physical Examination

A. Temperature, blood pressure, pulse, and respirations. Count respirations for a full minute. **Tachypnea is the single best predictor of pneumonia in children.**
B. Inspect
  1. Observe overall appearance. Does the patient appear ill? Consider the clinical presentation, age of person, and history.
  2. Observe respiratory pattern, grunting, nasal flaring, retractions, and use of accessory muscles.
  3. Check pulse oximetry. **An oxygen saturation less than 92% is an indicator of severity and the need for oxygen therapy.**
  4. Check nail beds and lips for cyanosis.
  5. Examine eyes, ears, nose, and throat.
C. Auscultate
  1. Heart
  2. Lungs for the following (auscultate bases first in geriatric patients):
    a. Crackles, decreased breath sounds
    b. Whispered pectoriloquy (Patient's whispered sounds are louder than normal.)
    c. Egophony (patient's "e" sounds like "a")
    d. Bronchophony (Voice sounds louder than usual.)
D. Percuss chest for dull sound (consolidation).
E. Palpate
  1. Lymph nodes for swelling
  2. Chest for tactile fremitus (increased conduction when patient says "99")
  3. Sinuses

Diagnostic Tests

A. Chest radiograph (CXR), which reveals interstitial, perihilar, or diffuse infiltrates
B. Complete blood count (CBC) with differential
C. Rapid viral tests per nasal swab
D. Sputum Gram stain if indicated

Differential Diagnoses

A. Bacterial pneumonia
B. Varicella pneumonia
C. Herpes pneumonia
D. Cytomegalovirus pneumonia
E. Pertussis
F. Asthma
G. Bronchitis/bronchiolitis
H. Sinusitis
I. Foreign body obstruction (usually in small children and the mentally handicapped)
J. Aspiration

Plan

A. General interventions
  1. Recommend to the patient to rest during acute phase.
  2. Avoid smoking or secondhand smoke.
  3. Respiratory isolation; may use facial masks.
  4. Encourage good handwashing or use of hand sanitizer.
  5. Chest physiotherapy is not recommended for pneumonia.
B. Patient teaching: *See Section III: Patient Teaching Guides for this chapter, "Pneumonia, Viral: Adult" and "Pneumonia, Viral: Child."*
C. Dietary management: Encourage fluids and a nutritious diet.
D. Pharmaceutical therapy: Antiviral agents should be considered in immunocompromised patients, those at highrisk for complications, or those requiring hospitalization. High risk includes: Age greater than 65 years; pregnancy or up to 2 weeks postpartum; long-term care residents; pulmonary disease, including asthma; diabetes; cardiovascular disease, excluding hypertension; chronic kidney disease; hepatic dysfunction; and active malignancy.
  1. Zanamivir (Relenza) is the recommended initial choice when influenza A infection or exposure is suspected. Zanamivir is administered by a metered-dose inhaler (MDI). Zanamivir is only effective if it is started within 24 to 48 hours of onset of fever and symptoms.
  2. The combination of Oseltamivir (Tamiflu) and rimantadine, an adamantane, is considered a second-line alternative. Tamiflu resistance should be considered before antiviral selection.

3. Amantadine or rimantadine started within 24 hours of the onset of viral symptoms decreases fever and other symptoms by 1 day in uncomplicated cases.
4. Acyclovir (Zovirax) for herpes viruses is administered as an IV infusion.
5. Ribavirin (Virazole) for RSV is administered as an aerosol. Synagis has also been used in conjunction with ribavirin for high-risk patients.

E. Patients with viral pneumonia who are superinfected with bacterial organisms require antibiotic therapy.
F. Avoid cough suppressants. The suppression of a cough may interfere with airway clearance.
G. Acetaminophen (Tylenol) for fever
H. Immunizations
1. Recommend the influenza vaccine for prevention.
2. Consider RSV vaccine prophylaxis for pediatrics following the current American Academy of Pediatrics (AAP) recommendations.
3. The measles vaccine is recommended except during pregnancy and in immunocompromised patients.

Follow-Up

Signs and symptoms may vary greatly according to the viral pathogen, severity of disease, and patient's age.
A. Recommend to the patient to return to the clinic if no improvement is seen after 48 hours on antiviral agents.
B. Follow up with a phone call in 24 hours.
C. Consider follow-up at 2 weeks if bronchoconstriction is noted on examination.

Consultation/Referral

A. Consult a physician if viral pneumonia is suspected.
B. Consult a physician if the patient is pregnant.
C. Consult a physician or transfer to the hospital if the patient is in respiratory distress, dehydrated, or hypoxemic.
D. Hospitalization should be considered for infants younger than 2 months of age or premature infants with RSV, due to the risk of apnea.
E. Consider consultation with a pulmonologist.

Individual Considerations

A. Pregnancy
1. Ribavirin is contraindicated in pregnancy; it is a class X drug.
2. Acyclovir is given in the third trimester at 10 mg/kg IV every 8 hours for 5 days in cases in which herpes pneumonia is suspected, which carries a high mortality rate.
3. The varicella-zoster immune globulin (VZIG) may be considered in pregnancy. Consultation with a physician is recommended.
4. The measles virus is a live-attenuated virus and should not be given during pregnancy.

B. Pediatrics
1. Hospitalization is recommended in infants aged 2 months and younger and also in very severe cases of pneumonia.

Respiratory Syncytial Virus Bronchiolitis

Cheryl A. Glass and Melissa A. Hall

Definition

A. Respiratory syncytial virus (RSV) is the most frequent cause of viral respiratory tract infection in infants. Most infants develop upper respiratory tract symptoms; 20% to 30% develop lower respiratory tract disease with their first infection. Infection with RSV may produce minimal respiratory symptoms. Most previously healthy infants who develop RSV bronchiolitis do not require hospitalization. Preterm infants with respiratory symptoms with lethargy, irritability, and poor feeding may require admission for treatment. There is no specific treatment for RSV infection.

Incidence

A. RSV is prevalent worldwide and affects all age groups. Infants, the elderly, and adults with chronic heart or lung disease or weakened immune systems are at high risk. Annual epidemics occur in winter and early spring, usually in temperate climates. The peak season in North America is between November and March. Most infants are infected during the first year of life. Peak incidence of occurrence of severe RSV disease is observed at ages of 2 to 8 months. Virtually all children have been infected at least once by their third birthday. Reinfection with RSV throughout life is common.
B. The period of viral shedding usually is 3 to 8 days, but shedding may continue up to 4 weeks. The incubation period ranges from 2 to 8 days.
C. Full recovery from RSV illness occurs in about 1 to 2 weeks.

Pathogenesis

A. RSV is an enveloped, nonsegmented, negative strand RNA virus of the *Paramyxoviridae* family. Two major strains (Groups A and B) have been identified, and strains of both often circulate concurrently.
B. Humans are the only source of infection. Transmission is by direct or close contact with contaminated secretions. RSV can persist on environmental surfaces for several hours and for a half hour or more on hands.

Predisposing Factors

A. Prematurity
B. Congenital heart disease
C. Chronic lung disease (CLD)
D. Immunodeficiency
E. Child-care centers
F. Two or more siblings younger than 5 years
G. Hospitalization

Common Complaints

A. Pediatrics
1. Fever (less than 101°F); 20% of patients have higher temperatures
2. Decreased appetite
3. Irritability
4. Lethargy
5. Rapid respirations
6. Cough

7. Coryza
8. Decreased activity
9. Wheezing

B. Adults
1. Rhinorrhea
2. Pharyngitis
3. Cough
4. Headache
5. Fatigue
6. Fever

Other Signs and Symptoms

A. Tachypnea or apnea
B. Nasal flaring
C. Retractions
D. Crackles
E. Wheezes

Subjective Data

A. Ask about the onset, duration, and course of illness.
B. Inquire whether the child is having trouble eating or drinking because of breathing problems.
C. Review other symptoms, including fever, nausea, vomiting, or diarrhea.
D. Are there any labored breathing patterns?
E. Calculate the child's age—how old the baby is and birth date—if palivizumab (Synagis) is prescribed.
F. Was the baby born preterm and at what gestational age?
G. Has the patient ever been diagnosed with any cardiac or lung problems, including cystic fibrosis (CF)?
H. Do the patient's siblings attend day care?

Physical Examination

A. Record temperature, pulse, respirations, blood pressure, and pulse oximetry.
B. Inspect
1. Observe general appearance.
2. Note respiratory pattern, retractions, nasal flaring, grunting, and circumoral cyanosis.
3. Inspect eyes, ears, nose, and throat. As many as 40% have an associated viral and/or bacterial otitis media.
4. Assess hydration status: Skin turgor, capillary refill, mucous membranes.

C. Auscultate
1. Heart
2. Lungs for crackles and mild to moderate respiratory distress with scattered wheezes

D. Percuss chest.
E. Palpate
1. Lymph nodes for adenopathy
2. Head and fontanelles (if applicable)

Diagnostic Tests

A. Rapid diagnostic assay of nasopharyngeal secretions is reliable in infants and young children.
B. Laboratory studies are frequently not indicated in the infant who is comfortable in room air, is well hydrated, and is feeding adequately. Nonspecific laboratory tests may include complete blood count (CBC), serum electrolytes, and urinalysis.
C. Chest radiograph (CXR) may show hyperexpansion, atelectasis, and/or infiltrates in a specific nonlobar (bacterial) viral pattern.
D. Arterial blood gases (ABGs) or pulse oximetry may show hypoxemia.

Differential Diagnoses

A. Viral or bacterial pneumonia
B. Asthma
C. Croup
D. Influenza
E. Neonatal sepsis
F. Foreign body aspiration

Plan

A. General interventions
1. Most infants require only supportive care, such as nasal suctioning.
2. Infants should never be exposed to cigarette smoke.
3. Hydration is important.
4. Contact precautions are recommended for the duration of RSV-associated illness among infants and young children. Adhere to appropriate hand-hygiene practices.
5. Prevention includes limiting, when feasible, exposure to contagious settings (e.g., child-care centers).

B. Patient teaching: *See Section III: Patient Teaching Guide for this chapter, "Respiratory Syncytial Virus."* ◀
C. Dietary management
1. Tell caregiver to offer juice, water, and other fluids frequently and to dilute juice for younger infants.
2. Suggest offering small, frequent feedings.

D. Pharmacological therapy
1. Ribavirin is an antiviral drug that may be delivered by means of aerosol, but it is reserved for severely ill children or those at high risk.
2. The use of bronchodilators and corticosteroids is controversial, but they may be indicated for hospitalized patients.
3. Antibiotics are not indicated for RSV bronchiolitis or pneumonia unless there is a secondary bacterial infection.
4. Palivizumab (Synagis) immunoprophylaxis is extremely costly and should be limited to infants at risk of hospitalization related to RSV. Dosing: Palivizumab 15 mg/kg intramuscularly every 30 days. Immunizations are given from 3 to 5 months depending on the gestational age, risk factors, and month that prophylaxis is started. The 2012 AAP eligibility criteria for palivizumab prophylaxis criteria includes:
a. Infants with CLD younger than 24 months who receive supplemental oxygen and bronchodilator, diuretic, or chronic corticosteroids. A maximum of five doses is recommended for this category.
b. Infants born before 32 weeks gestation (31 weeks + 6 days or less). A maximum of five monthly doses is recommended depending on gestational age and chronological age at the start of RSV season.

c. Infants born at 32 to younger than 35 weeks gestation (32 weeks + 0 days through 34 weeks + 6 days): Palivizumab prophylaxis should be limited to infants at greatest risk, younger than 3 months of age at the start of RSV season.

d. Infants with congenital abnormalities of the airway or neuromuscular disease may be considered for immunoprophylaxis. A maximum of five doses of palivizumab during the first year of life is recommended.

e. Infants and children with congenital heart disease who are 24 months of age or younger with hemodynamically significant acyanotic congenital heart disease may benefit from immunoprophylaxis. The decision to treat should be based on the degree of physiological cardiovascular compromise.

f. Immunocompromised children with severe immunodeficiency or advanced AIDS may benefit from prophylaxis.

g. There is insufficient data to determine the efficacy of palivizumab with patients with CF.

Follow-Up

A. Call the patient's caregiver in 12 to 24 hours to assess feeding and respiratory status.

Consultation/Referral

A. Refer the patient to a physician or emergency room if the infant is in moderate respiratory distress, is dehydrated, is hypoxemic, or is less than 6 months of age.

B. Admit hypoxemic infants to the hospital for hydration, oxygen therapy, and, possibly, mechanical ventilation.

C. Age is a significant factor in the severity of infection: The younger the patient is, the more severe the infection/hypoxemia tends to be. Infants younger than 6 months are most severely affected secondary to their smaller, more easily obstructed airways and their decreased ability to clear secretions.

Individual Considerations

A. Adults: Palivizumab (Synagis) is not approved for adults.

B. Pediatrics

1. All high-risk infants 6 months of age and older and their contacts should be administered the influenza vaccine as well as other recommended age-appropriate immunizations.

2. Palivizumab does not interfere with response to vaccines.

C. Pregnancy: Ribavirin is contraindicated during pregnancy. A negative pregnancy test and assurance of contraception should be obtained before prescribing.

Shortness of Breath

Mellisa A. Hall

Definition

A. Shortness of breath (SOB; dyspnea) is derived from the Greek terms for *difficult* and *breath*. Dyspnea may be experienced by patients with or without respiratory disorders. SOB/dyspnea is clinically significant when it interferes with normal functioning. Dyspnea is considered chronic when it persists longer than 4 to 8 weeks. SOB is a subjective symptom, reported by the patient. As self-reported, SOB may cause greater distress than pain.

Incidence

A. Dyspnea affects millions of people and is commonly associated with pulmonary disease, cardiovascular disease, anemia, obesity, and deconditioning. Dyspnea is reported in more than one fourth of the elderly. An estimated 25 million people with asthma or chronic obstructive pulmonary disease (COPD) experience SOB during the course of their illness. SOB is reported in more than 95% of patients in terminal stages of lung cancer, COPD, and heart failure.

Pathogenesis

A. The sensation of SOB can involve psychological, physical, social, and environmental factors. A sensation of SOB is stimulated by chemoreceptors that respond to changes in pH and carbon dioxide. Mechanoreceptors are located in upper airways, lungs, and the chest wall.

B. A sensation of SOB occurs with ventilation–perfusion mismatch, metabolic acidosis, increase in respiratory dead space, or stimulation of chest wall or pulmonary respiratory receptors.

C. SOB is perceived more by patients with existing lung disease.

D. Anemia and cardiovascular disease compromise the amount of oxygen delivered to tissues, worsening the sensation of dyspnea.

E. Interstitial lung disease associated with autoimmunity increases dyspnea/SOB, and with disease progression tissue oxygenation is reduced.

Predisposing Factors

A. Exertion
B. Asthma
C. COPD
D. Congestive heart failure (CHF)
E. Cardiac valve disorders
F. Cardiac anomalies
G. Pulmonary embolism
H. High altitudes
I. Environmental air pollution
J. Respiratory muscle weakness or paralysis, including neuromuscular disorders
K. Metabolic acidosis (renal failure)
L. Hemoglobinopathies
M. Hyperventilation syndrome, anxiety disorder, panic episodes
N. Reduced vital capacity and thoracic expansion with aging
O. Severe kyphoscoliosis
P. Obesity
Q. Pregnancy
R. Pleural effusions
S. Pulmonary hypertension
T. Foreign body aspiration

U. Obstructive sleep apnea
V. End-stage terminal illness (lung cancer, COPD, CHF)

Common Complaint

A. Discomfort with breathing or air hunger, worsening with positioning or activity

Subjective Data

A. How long have the symptoms been present?
B. How do they interfere with functioning?
C. What worsens and what improves the SOB?
D. Associated with syncope?
E. Associated with palpitations?
F. Increased anxiety before episodes?
G. History of similar symptoms?
H. Associated with odors (including household cleaners)?
I. Associated with certain social environments?
J. Weight changes since symptoms began?
K. History of lung or cardiac disease?
L. Treatments used to relieve the SOB?
M. Family history of similar issues?
N. If using a short-acting beta 2 agonist, how often, and has it helped?
O. Is cough associated?
P. Is it hemoptysis?
Q. Is the patient smoking now or ever? Pack years?
R. Did the patient use illicit substances? What type? In what amount? When was the most recent use?
S. Has the patient taken any new medications, foods, or been stung by an insect?
T. Has the patient been injured in the chest or neck?
U. Does the patient's chest hurt anywhere?
V. What is the patient's history of sickle cell disease?
W. What does the patient feel is causing the SOB?

Physical Examination

A. Record temperature, pulse, respirations, blood pressure, and pulse oximetry.
B. Inspect
   1. Observe general appearance, including morbid obesity, gravid uterus, skin tones, and use of accessory muscles of breathing, and facial appearance for fear or reduced level of consciousness, as well as tobacco or other chemical odors.
   2. Position in the tripod position for ability to speak in complete sentences.
   3. Assess hydration status: Skin turgor, capillary refill, and mucous membranes. Note distal fingers for clubbing.
   4. Pharynx and tonsils for erythema or hypertrophy
   5. Trachea for deviation
   6. Chest for barrel appearance or obvious trauma
   7. Spine for scoliosis or kyphosis
   8. Abdomen for distension
   9. Infants: Note respiratory pattern, retractions, nasal flaring, grunting, and circumoral cyanosis.
C. Auscultate
   1. Heart for murmur, rate, irregular rhythm, S3 or S4
   2. Lungs for crackles and mild to moderate respiratory distress with wheezing
D. Percuss chest.
E. Palpate
   1. Palpate lymph nodes for adenopathy.
   2. Perform strength testing against resistance of upper and lower extremities to assess for lethargy/atonia.
F. Neurologic examination
   1. Assess mentation.

Diagnostic Tests

A. Labs: CBC, blood urea nitrogen (BUN), creatinine, electrolytes, cardiac troponin, brain natriuretic peptide (BNP), D-dimer, carbon monoxide levels
B. EKG
C. Chest x-ray
D. Pulmonary function tests
E. Echocardiogram if heart failure is suspected
F. Anxiety and depression scales as indicated

Differential Diagnoses

A. Cardiovascular anomalies, dysfunction, or acute ischemia
B. Pulmonary disease, including autoimmune disorders affecting lung tissue
C. Anxiety
D. Foreign body or other aspiration syndromes
E. Anaphylaxis
F. Airway trauma
G. Infection of upper or lower airways
H. Pulmonary hypertension

Plan

A. General interventions
   1. The underlying etiology of the SOB should be considered and treated.
   2. Severe airway compromise should be considered in patients with stridor or change in level of consciousness. Emergency medical services (EMS) should be activated immediately with airway support, including supplemental oxygen.
B. Patient teaching: *See Section III: Patient Teaching Guide for this chapter, "Shortness of Breath."* ◀
   1. Discuss the underlying etiology of SOB with the patient and family and establish strategies to prevent further episodes of SOB.
C. Dietary management
   1. Foods associated with worsening SOB should be avoided.
   2. Swallowing studies should be considered for patients at risk for aspiration.
D. Pharmaceutical therapy
   1. Medications should be prescribed according to the underlying etiology. Products specific for dyspnea relief in terminal illness in patients under hospice care are outlined in the following. Medication adjustments should follow dyspnea assessment scales.
   2. Weak opioids: Codeine (30 mg q 4 hours)
   3. Strong opioids: Morphine 5–10 mg q 3 hours
   4. Anxiolytics: Lorazepam 0.5–2 mg PO/SL/IV q hour
   5. Anxiolytics: Clonazepam 0.25–2 mg q 12 hours

Follow-Up

A. Follow-up should occur frequently until symptoms of SOB have been controlled and the underlying etiology treated.

Consultation/Referral

A. Activate EMS in acute respiratory distress.
B. Provide supplemental oxygen for all ages until EMS has transported the patient.
C. Refer to appropriate specialty care depending on underlying cause of SOB.
D. Consultation to palliative care or hospice services should be considered to relieve dyspnea based on patients' advance care planning.

Individual Considerations

A. Pediatrics
  1. Acute respiratory distress should be immediately ruled out in infants and children in an emergency department setting.
B. Pregnancy
  1. Dyspnea occurs in up to two thirds of patients beginning in the first or second trimester of pregnancy. Underlying pathology during pregnancy should be considered as with all ages.
C. Geriatrics
  1. Avoid sedating medications that would increase the risk for hypoventilation or aspiration.
  2. Physical changes associated with aging increase the risk for hypoxia.
  3. Elderly patients may report SOB less frequently and assume it is an expectation of aging.

Tuberculosis

Cheryl A. Glass and Melissa A. Hall

Definition

A. Tuberculosis (TB) is an infectious disease. TB is a granulomatous disease caused by *Mycobacterium tuberculosis*, *Mycobacterium bovis*, and other mycobacteria. Humans are the only reservoirs for *M. tuberculosis*. TB may involve multiple organs, including the lungs, liver, spleen, lymph nodes, kidney, brain, eyes, and bone. The WHO estimates that one third of all people in the world are infected with *M. tuberculosis*.
B. In most immunocompetent individuals, macrophages are successful in containing the bacilli, and the infection is self-limited and often subclinical. As many as 60% of children and 5% of adults with primary TB are asymptomatic. When the pulmonary macrophages are unable to contain the bacilli, this leads to clinically apparent infection-progressive primary TB.
C. Postprimary (reactivation) TB occurs when the initial infection was successfully contained by the pulmonary macrophages, with bacilli remaining viable within the macrophages. Infection results when the host's immune status (T cells) is compromised.
D. Patients with fever of unknown origin, failure to thrive, significant weight loss, or unexplained lymphadenopathy should be evaluated for TB.
E. The lungs are the most common site for the development of TB; 85% of patients present with pulmonary complaints.

Incidence

A. TB is a worldwide infection and is considered a global public health emergency by the World Health Organization (WHO).
  1. The WHO reports more than 9 million new cases of TB every year.
  2. TB can affect any age group. More than 60% of cases are in those 25 to 40 years old. TB is uncommon in children between ages 5 and 15 years.
  3. Child-to-child transmission is not common because children rarely develop a cough and the sputum is scant.
  4. The incidence of TB in the United States is 3.4 cases per 100,000 population.
  5. Due to the high risk among immigrants, California, New York, Texas, and Florida accounted for half of the TB cases reported in the United States.
B. Postprimary TB is a significant cause of worldwide morbidity and mortality. Pulmonary morbidity results from a chronic cough, hemoptysis, fibrosis, superinfection, bronchial stenosis, repeated pulmonary infections, or empyema. Morbidity also arises from chronic TB osteomyelitis, chronic renal insufficiency, and central nervous system (CNS) TB.

Pathogenesis

A. Mycobacteria are non-spore-forming, slow-growing bacilli. TB infection occurs by means of inhalation of airborne bacillus droplets from an infected host. The development of an infection depends on prolonged exposure (weeks) to an individual with active pulmonary TB. Bacilli travel through the pulmonary lymphatics or enter the vascular system and are disseminated to the brain, meninges, eyes, bones, joints, lymph nodes, kidneys, intestines, larynx, pericardium, genitourinary system, and skin. The incubation period from infection to positive skin test reaction is 2 to 10 weeks, although disease may not occur for many years or may never occur. The risk of disease is greatest within 2 years following infection.

Predisposing Factors

A. Exposure to someone with active disease
B. High-risk groups: Minorities, young children (before age 5 years) and the elderly, foreign-born people, prisoners, nursing home residents, teachers, indigents, migrant workers, and health care providers
C. HIV infection is one of the most significant risk factors for TB.
D. Steroid therapy, cancer chemotherapy, and hematologic malignancies increase the risk of TB.
E. Tumor necrosis factor-alpha (TNF-alpha) antagonist is used for rheumatoid arthritis, psoriasis, and other autoimmune disease is associated with a significant risk for TB. Before beginning any TNF-alpha treatment, a TB skin test should be given.

F. Non-TB infections, such as measles, varicella, and pertussis, may activate quiescent TB.
G. Smoking
H. Malnutrition
I. Alcoholism
J. Intravenous (IV) drug abuse
K. Congenital TB (rare)

Common Complaints

A. Fever (usually low grade at onset but becoming marked with progression of disease)
B. Malaise
C. Weight loss/difficulty gaining weight
D. Cough
E. Night sweats
F. Chills
G. Occasional hemoptysis
H. Fatigue
I. Pediatric symptoms
  1. Nonproductive cough
  2. Failure to thrive
  3. Difficulty gaining weight
  4. Fever
  5. Night sweats
  6. Anorexia

Other Signs and Symptoms

A. Pulmonary TB: Fatigue, irritability, undernutrition, with or without fever and cough
B. Glandular TB: Chronic cervical adenitis
C. Meningeal TB: Fever and meningeal signs, positive cerebrospinal fluid
D. Failure to thrive
E. Anorexia

Subjective Data

A. Determine the onset, duration, and course of illness.
B. Review symptom history: Fever, night sweats, chills, or cough
C. Review history of weight loss.
D. Review exposure history to someone who has TB.
E. What is the patient's living situation (including past history of homelessness)?
F. Review travel history to endemic areas with TB, including China, Pakistan, the Philippines, Thailand, Indonesia, Bangladesh, and the Democratic Republic of Congo.
G. Review HIV status or need for testing.

Physical Examination

A complete physical examination is mandatory. Physical findings of pulmonary TB are not specific and usually are absent in mild or moderate disease.

A. Record temperature, respirations, pulse, blood pressure, and weight.
B. Inspect
  1. Observe overall appearance.
  2. Check skin for pallor.
  3. Inspect eyes, ears, nose, and throat.
C. Auscultate
  1. Heart
  2. Lungs and chest for the following:
    a. Rales in upper posterior chest
    b. Bronchophony: Voice sounds louder than usual.
    c. Whispered pectoriloquy: Patient's whispered sounds are louder than normal.
D. Percuss chest.
E. Palpate
  1. For lymphadenopathy, usually anterior or posterior cervical and supraclavicular nodes. Less commonly involved lymph nodes include submandibular, axillary, and inguinal lymph nodes.
  2. To evaluate hepatosplenomegaly
F. Neurologic examination
  1. Evaluate the presence of nuchal rigidity.
  2. Assess deep tendon reflexes.

Diagnostic Tests

Diagnosis is based on a combination of tuberculin skin testing, purified protein derivative (PPD) testing, and sputum cultures. Bronchoscopy may be required to obtain specimens. Patients with primary TB may not undergo imaging; however, conventional CXR may be performed, and 15% of patients with primary TB have normal chest radiograph (CXR) findings.

Patients with progressive primary or postprimary TB may need a CT to evaluate parenchymal involvement, satellite lesions, bronchogenic spread, and miliary disease. MRI may be ordered to evaluate complications, such as the extent of thoracic wall involvement with empyema.

A. Tuberculin skin test using the Mantoux test is the recommended method. The dosage of 0.1 mL or 5 tuberculin units (TU) of PPD should be injected intradermally into the volar aspect of the forearm using a 27-gauge needle. A wheal should be raised and should measure approximately 6 to 10 mm in diameter. Skilled personnel should read the test in 48 to 72 hours after administration. Measure the amount of induration and note the erythema. Measure transverse to the long axis of the forearm (see Table 9.4).
B. The Food and Drug Administration (FDA) has approved QuantiFERON-TB Gold as an alternative TB test for detecting both TB and latent TB infection.
C. Annual Mantoux tests are given for those at high risk. There is no need to repeat PPD once the patient has reacted and had a positive PPD.
D. AP and lateral CXR films: "Snowstorm" appearance indicates miliary TB; segmental consolidation and hilar adenopathy are common; pleural effusion may be present.
E. CBC with differential may be performed.
F. Sputum culture with acid-fast smear
  1. Nasopharyngeal secretions and saliva are not acceptable.
  2. Gastric aspirate specimens for children younger than 6 years old. (Young children do not have a cough deep enough for a sputum specimen.)

TABLE 9.4 Interpretation of Mantoux Tuberculin Skin Test

Positive Reaction—Induration Size	Risk Factors
5 mm or more	Close contact with a known or suspected tuberculosis; immunosuppressive conditions (e.g., HIV); on immunosuppressive medications; or an abnormal chest x-ray—consistent with active TB, previously active TB, or clinical evidence of the disease, children, organ transplant recipients, other immunosuppressive illnesses or high-risk medical conditions (silicosis and end-stage renal disease on dialysis).
10 mm or more	High-risk categories (i.e., homeless, HIV infected, users of illicit drugs, residents in nursing homes, incarcerated, or institutionalized); travel histories or recent immigration to high-prevalence areas of world; mycobacteriology lab personnel, employees of high-risk settings).
15 mm or more	Low-risk persons

TB, tuberculosis.

G. Interferon-gamma release assay (IGRAs) test
H. HIV testing as indicated by risk factors to guide management
I. Pregnancy test (if indicated) to guide management

Differential Diagnoses

A. TB
B. Bronchiectasis
C. Asthma
D. Histoplasmosis
E. Coccidioidomycosis
F. Blastomycosis
G. Malignancies
H. Other pulmonary infections
I. Aspiration pneumonia

Plan

A. General interventions
  1. Report all suspected and confirmed cases of TB to the local health department.
  2. Directly observed therapy (DOT) is mandatory for the treatment of patients with coexistent HIV disease, those with multidrug-resistant (MDR) TB, and those who may be noncompliant.
B. Patient teaching
  1. Educate patients regarding compliance to therapy, adverse effect of medications, and follow-up care.
C. Pharmaceutical therapy: The American Thoracic Society (ATS) and the CDC provide the standard guidelines for therapy.
  1. Contact public health authorities for up-to-date recommendations on medications. Medication protocols vary and include the following first-line agents: Isoniazid (INH), rifampin (Rifadin), pyrazinamide (Tebrazid), and ethambutol (Etibi); (see Table 9.5).
    a. Isoniazid (Laniazid, Nydrazid) dosing
      i. Adults: 5 mg/kg by mouth (not to exceed 300 mg/d)
      ii. Pediatrics: 10 to 20 mg/kg by mouth every day; not to exceed 300 mg/d
    b. Rifampin (Rifadin) dosing
      i. Adults: 10 mg/kg, max 600 mg/d
      ii. Pediatrics: 10 to 20 mg/kg by mouth every day; not to exceed 600 mg/d
    c. Pyrazinamide (Tebrazid) dosing
      i. Adults: 25 mg/kg by mouth every day; not to exceed 2 g/d
      ii. Pediatrics: Not routinely recommended in children receiving INH. Public health authorities should be contacted for current guidelines.
    d. Ethambutol (Myambutol) dosing
      i. Adults with no previous anti-TB therapy: 15 mg/kg by mouth every day
      ii. Pediatrics: For those older than 13 years administer as in adults; not recommended for those younger than 13 years
  2. Compliance with drug regimen is most important.
  3. Drug resistance averages 5% to 10% nationally and is increasing.
  4. The bacilli Calmettend–Guerin (BCG) vaccine is available for the prevention of disseminated TB. BCG is a live vaccine. BCG does not prevent infection with *M. tuberculosis.*

Follow-Up

A. Regular follow-up every 4 to 8 weeks to ensure compliance and to monitor the adverse effects and response of the medications.
B. Repeat CXR may be performed after 2 to 3 months of therapy to observe the response to treatment for patients with pulmonary TB.
C. Consider monitoring liver enzymes monthly in the following patients:
  1. Severe or disseminated TB
  2. Concurrent or recent hepatic disease or hepatobiliary tract disease from other causes
  3. Those receiving high doses of INH (10 mg/kg/d) in combination with rifampin, pyrazinamide, or both drugs
  4. Women who are pregnant or within the first 6 weeks postpartum
  5. Clinical evidence of hepatotoxic effects

TABLE 9.5 Treatment of Tuberculosis

Tuberculosis	Regimen	Duration
Pulmonary and cervical lymphadenopathy	Isoniazid (INH) + rifampin	6 months
	Supplement with pyrazinamide	First 2 months only
Hilar adenopathy	Isoniazid + rifampin daily or INH + rifampin daily then INH + rifampin twice a week	9 months 1 month 8 months
Bone and joint disease and miliary disease	INH + rifampin + pyrazinamide and streptomycin once a day then INH + rifampin once a day	2 months 7–10 months
Tuberculosis in patients with HIV	Consult with a specialist	

Current guidelines should be in accordance with the Centers for Disease Control and Prevention (CDC).

Consultation/Referral

A. An infectious diseases consultation for the management of affected patients

Individual Considerations

A. Pregnancy

1. Manage TB on a case-by-case basis with a physician.

2. Chemotherapy must be started immediately after the first trimester to protect both mother and fetus.

a. First-line agents recommended by the American Academy of Pediatrics (AAP) include INH, rifampin, and ethambutol.

b. Streptomycin is contraindicated in pregnancy.

3. All pregnant women on INH therapy should receive pyridoxine.

4. The mother who has current disease but is noncontagious at delivery does not require separation of the infant and mother. The mothers can also breastfeed.

a. Evaluation of the infant includes CXR and Mantoux test at age 4 to 6 weeks.

b. If the Mantoux test is negative, a repeat test is warranted at age 3 to 4 months and at age 6 months.

c. INH should be administered even if the Mantoux results and CXR do not suggest TB because sufficient cell-mediated immunity to prevent progressive disease may not develop until age 6 months.

5. The mother who has current disease and is contagious at delivery requires separation of the mother and infant until the mother is noncontagious. The management is the same as noted earlier.

B. Pediatrics

1. Most children and adolescents with positive skin tests are asymptomatic.

2. Mantoux tests are given at ages 1 year, between 4 and 6 years, between 11 and 16 years, and annually to children at risk.

3. Neonatal symptoms of TB typically develop in the second or third week of life and include poor feeding, poor weight gain, cough, lethargy, and irritability.

4. The AAP recommends administration of 9 months of therapy for latent TB. The drug of choice is INH.

5. INH tablets can be crushed and added to food. Isoniazid liquid without sorbitol should be used to avoid osmotic diarrhea.

6. Rifampin capsules can be opened and the powder added to food.

7. Young children are at high risk of disseminated TB and permanent sequela. Timely treatment is essential.

8. TB is commonly diagnosed clinically and should be considered in children presenting with superficial lymph adenopathy and central nervous system dysfunction.

C. Geriatrics

1. The majority of cases of TB in older adults are due to reactivation of previous TB exposure.

2. Most cases of TB in older adults have pulmonary involvement (75%).

3. For long-term care, use a two-step TB PPD test for initial screening of newly admitted residents.

4. Treatment of active TB is the same as in younger adults. Renal and hepatic labs should be monitored according to the manufacturer's recommendations.

5. Adult patients who have recently converted to positive TB status should receive prophylaxis with INH for 9 months.

Bibliography

Adams, L. V., & Starke, J. R. (2015, October). Tuberculosis disease in children. Retrieved from http://www.uptodate.comcontents/tuberculosis-disease-in-children

American Academy of Pediatrics. (2015). Respiratory syncytial virus. In D. Kimberlin, M. T. Brady, M. A. Jackson, & S. S. Long (Ed.), *Red book: 2015 Report of the Committee on Infectious Diseases* (30th ed., pp. 667–676). Elk Grove Village, IL: Author. Retrieved from http://redbook.solutions.aap.org/chapter.aspx?sectionId=88187226&bookId=1484.

American Academy of Pediatrics. (2016). Cough and cold medicine—Not for children. Retrieved from https://www.aap.org/en-us/about-the-aap/aap-press-room/aap-press-room-media-center/Pages/Cough-and-Cold-Medicine-Not-for-Children.aspx?nfstatus=401&nftoken=00000000-0000-0000-0000-000000000000&nfstatusdescription=ERROR:+No+local+token

American Lung Association. (n.d). Tuberculosis. Retrieved from http://www.lung.org/lung-health-and-diseases/lung-disease-lookup/tuberculosis

Barnes, P. J. (2015). Asthma. In D. L. Kasper, A. S. Fauci, S. L. Hauser, D. L. Longo, J. L. Jameson, (Eds.), *Harrison's principles of internal medicine* (19th ed.). New York, NY: McGraw-Hill.

Barr, R. G., & Graham, B. S. (2015, July). Respiratory syncytial virus: Treatment. Retrieved from http://www.uptodate.com/contents/respiratory-syncytial-virus-infection-treatment?source=search_result&search=Respiratory+syncytial+virus%3A+Treatment&selectedTitle=1~147

Barr, R. G., & Graham, B. S. (2016, March). Respiratory syncytial virus: Prevention. Retrieved from http://www.uptodate.com/contents/respiratory-syncytial-virus-infection-prevention?source=search_result&search=Respiratory+syncytial+virus%3A+Treatment&selectedTitle=2~147

Bartlett, J. G., & Sethi, S. (2016, March). Management of infection in exacerbations of chronic obstructive pulmonary disease. Retrieved from http://www.uptodate.com/contents/management-of-infection-in-exacerbations-of-chronic-obstructive-pulmonary-disease?source=search_result&search=Management+of+infection+in+exacerbations+of+chronic+obstructive+pulmonary+disease&selectedTitle=1~150

Center for Medicare & Medicaid Services. (n.d.). Medicare coverage of durable medical equipment and other coverage. Retrieved from https://www.medicare.gov/Pubs/pdf/11045.pdf

Centers for Disease Control and Prevention. (n.d.). Bronchitis (chest cold). Retrieved from https://www.cdc.gov/getsmart/antibiotic-use/url/bronchitis.html

Centers for Disease Control and Prevention. (2010). Infant deaths associated with cough and cold medications: Two states, 2005. *Morbidity and Mortality Weekly Report, 56*(1), 1–4. Retrieved from https://www.cdc.gov/mmwr/preview/mmwrhtml/mm5601a1.htm

Centers for Disease Control and Prevention. (2009, September 11). For parents: Young children and adverse drug events. Retrieved from https://www.cdc.gov/MedicationSafety/parents_childrenAdverseDrugEvents .html

Centers for Disease Control and Prevention. (2015a, April 20). Respiratory syncytial virus infection (RSV). Retrieved from www.cdc.gov/rsv

Centers for Disease Control and Prevention. (2015b, August 7). Prevention and control of influenza with vaccines: Recommendations of the Advisory Committee on Immunization Practices, United States, 2015–16 Influenza Season. Retrieved from https://www.cdc.gov/mmwr/preview/mmwrhtml/mm6430a3.htm

Centers for Disease Control and Prevention. (2015c, August 31). Pertussis (whooping cough) surveillance & reporting. Retrieved from www.cdc.gov/pertussis/surv-reporting.html

Centers for Disease Control and Prevention. (2016a, February 10). FastStats chronic obstructive pulmonary disease (COPD) includes: Chronic bronchitis and emphysema. Retrieved from www.cdc.gov/nchs/fastats/copd.htm

Centers for Disease Control and Prevention. (2016b, February 16). FastStats asthma. Retrieved from www.cdc.gov/nchs/fastats/asthma.htm

Centers for Disease Control and Prevention. (2016c). Recommended adult immunization schedule. U.S.–2016. Retrieved from http://www.cdc.gov/vaccines/schedules/downloads/adult/adult-schedule.pdf

CNBC News. (2016, March 17). Cold remedies and kids: Study finds some parents ignoring warnings against use. Retrieved from http://www.cbc.ca/news/health/cold-medicines-children-1.3496164

Crow, J. E. (2015, November). Human metapneumovirus infections. Retrieved from http://www.uptodate.com/contents/human-metapneumovirus-infections

Dolin, R. (2015). Common viral respiratory infections. In D. L. Kasper, S. L. Hauser, J. L. Jameson, A. S. Fauci, D. L. Longo, & J. Loscalzo (Eds.), *Harrison's principles of internal medicine* (19th ed.). New York, NY: McGraw-Hill.

Emanuel, E. J. (2015). Palliative and end-of-life care. In D. L. Kasper, A. S. Fauci, S. L. Hauser, D. L. Longo, J. L. Jameson, (Eds.), *Harrison's principles of internal medicine* (19th ed.). New York, NY: McGraw-Hill.

Fanta, H. (2014, July). Diagnosis of asthma in adolescents and adults. Retrieved from http://www.uptodate.com/contents/diagnosis-of-asthma-in-adolescents-and-adults

Ferguson, E., & Make, B. (2016, January 21). Management of stable chronic obstructive pulmonary disease. Retrieved from http://www.uptodate.com/contents/management-of-stable-chronic-obstructive-pulmonary-disease

File, T. M. (2016, February 24). Acute bronchitis in adults. Retrieved from http://www.uptodate.com/contents/acute-bronchitis-in-adults

Flaherty, E., & Resnick, R. (Eds.). (2014). *Geriatric nursing review syllabus: A core curriculum in advanced practice geriatric nursing* (4th ed.). New York, NY: American Geriatrics Society.

Gibson, P., Wang, G., McGarvey, L., Vertigan, A. E., Altman, K. W., & Birring, S. S.; CHEST Expert Cough Panel. (2016). Treatment of unexplained chronic cough: CHEST guideline and Expert Panel report. Online supplement. *Chest.*

Global Initiative for Chronic Obstructive Lung Disease. (2016). Global strategy for the diagnosis, management, and prevention of COPD. Retrieved from http://goldcopd.org/global-strategy-diagnosis-management-prevention-copd-2016

Goldblatt, D., & O'Brien, K. L. (2015). Pneumococcal infections. In D. L. Kasper, A. S. Fauci, S. L. Hauser, D. L. Longo, J. L. Jameson, (Eds.), *Harrison's principles of internal medicine* (19th ed.). New York: McGraw-Hill.

Han, M. K., Dransfield, M. T.. & Martinez, F. J. (2015, September 29). Chronic obstructive pulmonary disease: Definition, clinical manifestations, diagnosis, and staging. Retrieved from http://www.uptodate.com/contents/chronic-obstructive-pulmonary-disease-definition-clinical-manifestations-diagnosis-and-staging

Harding, S. M. (2015, August 11). Gastroesophageal reflux and asthma. Retrieved from http://www.uptodate.com/online/contents/gastroesophageal-reflux-and-asthma

Hopewell, P. C., Kato-Maeda, M., & Ernst, J. D. (2016). Tuberculosis. In V. C. Broaddus, R. J. Mason, J. D. Ernst, T. E. King, , S. C. Lazarus, J. F. Murray, . . . M. B. Gotway (Eds.), *Murray & Nadel's textbook of respiratory medicine* (6th ed., Vol. 1, pp. 593–628). Philadelphia, PA: Elsevier Saunders.

Horsburgh, C. R., Jr. (2016). Treatment of latent tuberculosis infection in HIV-uninfected adults. Retrieved from https://www.uptodate.com/contents/treatment-of-latent-tuberculosis-infection-in-hiv-uninfected-adults

King-Han, M., Dransfield, M. T., & Martinez, F. J. (2015, September 29). Chronic obstructive pulmonary disease: Definition, clinical manifestations, diagnosis, and staging. Retrieved from http://www.uptodate.com/contents/chronic-obstructive-pulmonary-disease-definition-clinical-manifestations-diagnosis-and-staging

Kline, L. R. (2016, March 23). Clinical presentation and diagnosis of obstructive sleep apnea in adults. Retrieved from http://www.uptodate.com/contents/clinical-presentation-and-diagnosis-of-obstructive-sleep-apnea-in-adults

Krawczyk, J., Gharahbaghian, L., & Rutkowski, A. (2006, July 14). Toxicity, cough and cold preparation. *emedicine*. Retrieved from http://emedicine.medscape.com/article/1010513-print

Kritek, P. A., & Fanta, C. H. (2015). Cough and hemoptysis. In D. L. Kasper, A. S. Fauci, S. L. Hauser, D. L. Longo, J. L. Jameson, & J. Loscalzo (Eds.), *Harrison's principles of internal medicine* (19th ed.). New York, NY: McGraw-Hill.

Long-Term Oxygen Treatment Trial Research Group. A randomized trial of long-term oxygen for COPD with moderate desaturation. *New England Journal of Medicine, 375*(17), 1617–1627.

Medscape Drug Reference. (n.d.). Theophylline oral. *Medscape.* Retrieved from http://www.medscape.com/druginfo/dosage?drugid=3591&drugname=Theophylline+Oral&monotype=default

MPR: Nurse Practitioner's Edition. (2016, Spring). New York, NY: Haymarket Media.

Munoz, F. M., & Flomenberg, P. (2015, June). Diagnosis, treatment, and prevention of adenovirus infection. Retrieved from http://www.uptodate .com

National Guideline Clearinghouse. (2013 October). Guideline summary: Management of obstructive sleep apnea in adults: A clinical practice guideline from the American College of Physicians. Rockville, MD: Agency for Healthcare Research and Quality. Retrieved from https://www.guideline.gov/summaries/summary/47136/management-of-obstructive-sleep-apnea-in-adults-a-clinical-practice-guideline-from-the-american-college-of-physicians

Pappas, D. E. (2015, August 4). Patient information: The common cold in children (Beyond the Basics). Retrieved from http://www.uptodate.com/contents/the-common-cold-in-children-beyond-the-basics

Piedra, P. A. (2016, February 23). Bronchiolitis in infants and children: Clinical features and diagnosis. Retrieved from http://www.uptodate.com/contents/bronchiolitis-in-infants-and-children-clinical-features-and-diagnosis

Pozniak, A. (2016, January 16). Clinical manifestations and complications of pulmonary tuberculosis. Retrieved from http://www.uptodate.com/contents/clinical-manifestations-and-complications-of-pulmonary-tuberculosis

Prescriber's Letter. (2013, May, Vol. 29). Appropriate med use. Retrieved from http://prescribersletter.therapeuticresearch.com/pl/ArticleDD.aspx?cs=&s=PRL&pt=6&fpt=31&dd=290501&pb=PRL&searchid=55980185

Prescriber's Letter. (2015a, January, Vol. 3). Pediatrics. Retrieved from http://prescribersletter.therapeuticresearch.com/pl/ArticleDD.aspx?cs=&s=PRL&pt=6&fpt=31&dd=310118&pb=PRL&searchid=55978611

Prescriber's Letter. (2015b, September, Vol. 22). Infectious disease. Retrieved from http://prescribersletter.therapeuticresearch.com/pl/ArticleDD.aspx?cs=&s=PRL&pt=6&fpt=31&dd=310922&pb=PRL&searchid=55978639

Prescriber's Letter. (2016a, January Vol. 23). Asthma. Retrieved from prescribersletter.therapeuticresearch.com

Prescriber's Letter. (2016b, March, Vol. 30). Poison prevention. Retrieved from http://prescribersletter.therapeuticresearch.com/pl/ArticleDD.aspx?nidchk=1&cs=&s=PRL&pt=6&fpt=31&dd=300305&pb=PRL&searchid=55978305

Rains, S. G. (2013). Fifteen-to-eighteen-month visit. In B. Richardson (Ed.), *Pediatric primary care: Practice guidelines for nurses* (2nd ed., pp. 113–124). Burlington, MA: Jones & Bartlett.

Raviblione, M. C. (2015). Tuberculosis. In D. L. Kasper, A. S. Fauci, S. L. Hauser, D. L. Longo, J. L. Jameson, (Eds.), *Harrison's principles of internal medicine* (19th ed.). New York, NY: McGraw-Hill.

Reilly, J. J., Silverman, E. K., & Shapiro, S. D. (2015). Chronic obstructive pulmonary disease. In D. L. Kasper, A. S. Fauci, S. L. Hauser, D. L. Longo, J. L. Jameson, (Eds.), *Harrison's principles of internal medicine* (19th ed.). New York, NY: McGraw-Hill.

Sawicki, G., & Haver, K. (2015, December 9). Acute asthma exacerbations in children: Outpatient management. Retrieved from http://www.uptodate.com/contents/acute-asthma-exacerbations-in-children-home-office-management-and-severity-assessment?source=search_result&search=acute+asthma+exacerbations+in+children&selectedTitle=3%7E150

Schatz, M., & Weinberger, S. E. (2015, December). Management of asthma during pregnancy. Retrieved from http://www.uptodate.com/contents/management-of-asthma-during-pregnancy

Schwartzstein, R. M. (2013, July). Physiology of dyspnea. Retrieved from http://www.uptodate.com/contents/physiology-of-dyspnea

Schwartzstein, R. M. (2015, November). Approach to the patient with dyspnea. Retrieved from http://www.uptodate.com/contents/approach-to-the-patient-with-dyspnea

Schwartzstein, R. M., & Adams, L. (2016). In *Murray & Nadel's textbook of respiratory medicine* (6th ed.). Philadelphia, PA: Elsevier-Saunders.

Sterling, T. R. (2016, January). Treatment of pulmonary tuberculosis in HIV-uninfected adults. Retrieved from http://www.uptodate.com/contents/treatment-of-pulmonary-tuberculosis-in-hiv-uninfected-adults

Strohl, K. P. (2016, March). An overview of sleep apnea in adults. Retrieved from http://www.uptodate.com/contents/overview-of-obstructive-sleep-apnea-in-adults?source=search_result&search=sleep+apnea&selectedTitle=1%7E150

Terry, E. G. (2017). Seven-to-ten-year visit (school age). In B. Richardson (Ed.), *Pediatric primary care: Practice guidelines for nurses* (3rd ed., pp. 143–158). Burlington, MA: Jones & Bartlett.

Valentine, N. (2017). Respiratory disorders. In B. Richardson (Ed.), *Pediatric primary care: Practice guidelines for nurses* (3rd ed., pp. 143–158). Burlington, MA: Jones & Bartlett.

Vaz Fragoso, C. (2016). Diagnosis and managment of asthma in older adults. Retrieved from UpToDate: http://www.uptodate.com/contents/diagnosis-and-management-of-asthma-in-older-adults?source=search_result&search=diagnosis+and+management+in+older+adults&selectedTitle=1%7E150

Weinburger, S. E. (2015, June). Dyspnea during pregnancy. Retrieved from http://www.uptodate.com/contents/dyspnea-during-pregnancy

Weiner, D. L. (2014, November). Causes of acute respiratory distress in children. Retrieved from http://www.uptodate.com/contents/causes-of-acute-respiratory-distress-in-children

Weiss, S. T. (2016, March 17). Chronic obstructive pulmonary disease: Risk factors and risk reduction. Retrieved from http://www.uptodate.com/contents/chronic-obstructive-pulmonary-disease-risk-factors-and-risk-reduction

Wellman, A., & Redline, S. (2015). Sleep apnea. In D. L. Kasper, A. S. Fauci, S. L. Hauser, D. L. Longo, J. L. Jameson, (Eds.), *Harrison's principles of internal medicine* (19th ed.). New York, NY: McGraw -Hill.

Woods, C. R. (2015a, April). Croup: Approach to management. Retrieved from http://www.uptodate.com/contents/croup-approach-to-management

Woods, C. R. (2015b, December). Croup: Clinical features, evaluation, and diagnosis. Retrieved from http://www.uptodate.com/contents/croup-clinical-features-evaluation-and-diagnosis

World Health Organization. (2015, November). Pneumonia fact sheet N331. Retrieved from http://www.who.int/mediacentre/factsheets/fs331/en

Zachary, K. C. (2015, December). Treatment of seasonal influenza in adults. Retrieved from http://www.uptodate.com/contents/treatment-of-seasonal-influenza-in-adults

10 Cardiovascular Guidelines

Acute Myocardial Infarction

Jill C. Cash and Debbie Gunter

Definition

A. Acute myocardial infarction (MI) is a prolonged lack of myocardial oxygenation leading to necrosis of a portion of the heart muscle. It is caused by atherosclerotic coronary artery disease (CAD), which alone or in association with other factors causes complete blockage of one of the coronary arteries.

Incidence

A. According to the CDC in 2015, approximately 735,000 Americans suffer an acute MI annually in the United States (Mozaffarian, Benjamin, & Go, 2015). Of these, 525,000 are the first event and for 210,000, it is a subsequent MI. Despite a marked decrease in incidence and mortality during the past three decades, MI continues to be the leading cause of death in this country, accounting for one fourth of all fatalities. More women die from heart disease than men.

Pathogenesis

A. Abrupt coronary artery occlusion is the primary cause of most MIs. Occlusions can result from atherosclerotic plaque, intracoronary thrombus formation, or arterial spasm.

Predisposing Factors

A. Hypercholesterolemia: Increased low-density lipoprotein (LDL), decreased high-density lipoprotein (HDL)
B. Hypertriglyceridemia
C. Premature familial onset of coronary heart disease (CHD), formerly called CAD, before age 55 years
D. Smoking
E. Hypertension (HTN)
F. Obesity
G. Sedentary lifestyle
H. Diabetes mellitus
I. Aging
J. Stress

Common Complaints

A. Primary complaint: Pain somewhere in chest, described as worst pain ever experienced
B. Nausea
C. Vomiting
D. Diaphoresis
E. Indigestion

Other Signs and Symptoms

A. Pain in abdomen, arm, back, jaw, and neck
B. Chest heaviness or tightness
C. Anxiety
D. Cough
E. Dyspnea
F. HTN or hypotension
G. Weakness, light-headedness, syncope
H. Pallor
I. Orthopnea
J. Fatigue
K. Malaise

Potential Complications

A. Arrhythmias
B. Heart failure (HF)
C. Cardiogenic shock
D. Rupture of left ventricular (LV) papillary muscle
E. Ventricular septal rupture
F. Pericarditis or Dressler's syndrome
G. Ventricular aneurysm
H. Thromboembolism
I. Death

Subjective Data

A. Ask the patient what activity brought about or preceded the episode of chest pain.
B. Ask the patient to describe the duration of pain and what time of day symptoms began.
C. Ask the patient to describe the pain; for example, crushing, stabbing, or burning.
D. Ask the patient where sensation began and in what direction it radiates.
E. Identify the degree of pain by using a pain scale of 1 to 10, with 1 being the least painful.
F. Ask the patient to list all medications currently being taken, particularly substances not prescribed and illicit drugs such as cocaine.

Physical Examination

Patients presenting with acute chest pain should be quickly assessed for the need to callV emergency services/ 911 for immediate transport to the hospital.

A. Check pulse, respirations, blood pressure (BP), and pulse oxygenation.

B. Inspect
 1. General appearance, noting dyspnea and weakness
 2. Skin for pallor and diaphoresis
 3. Legs for edema
 4. Chest wall for visible pulsations
 5. Neck for jugular vein distension
 6. Nail beds for signs of cyanosis and note capillary filling time
C. Palpate
 1. Abdomen for organomegaly
 2. Peripheral pulses in legs
 3. Femoral pulses
D. Auscultate
 1. Auscultate carotid arteries.
 2. Auscultate abdomen.
 3. Conduct a complete heart examination, checking for dysrhythmias.
 4. Conduct a complete lung examination.
E. Mental status: Assess for confusion and anxiety.

Diagnostic Tests

A. EKG: Shows inverted T waves and ST segment elevation; depending on the timing, Q waves may also be present. One normal EKG initially does not always rule out MI; perform serial EKGs if MI is suspected.
B. Laboratory testing
 1. Cardiac biomarkers/enzymes
 2. Troponins: Troponins increase within 3 to 4 hours of injury and may remain elevated for 1 to 2 weeks.
 3. Creatine kinase (CK): CK-MB levels increase 3 to 12 hours after the chest pain begins, peak at 24 hours, and return to normal in 48 to 72 hours.
 4. Myoglobin: Urine myoglobin levels rise 1 to 4 hours after the chest pain begins.
 5. Complete blood count (CBC)
 6. Chemistry profile
 7. Lipid profile
 8. C-reactive protein (CRP) and inflammatory markers
C. Cardiac imaging: Coronary angiogram

Differential Diagnoses

A. Acute MI
B. Unstable angina pectoris
C. Aortic dissection
D. Pulmonary embolism (PE)
E. Pericarditis
F. Esophageal spasm
G. Pancreatitis
H. Biliary tract disease

Plan

A. General interventions
 1. Educate the patient and family regarding the signs and symptoms of an acute MI.
 2. Long-term care and treatment should be reinforced at each patient visit.
B. Patient teaching
 1. Educate the patient about modifying controllable risk factors, such as keeping diabetes and HTN under control, diet, exercise, and smoking cessation.
 2. If known CHD is present
  a. Instruct the patient on signs and symptoms of an acute MI.
  b. Advise the patient to have a plan for seeking medical attention or dialing 911 if signs and symptoms occur.
  c. Advise the patient to carry nitroglycerin at all times and to take the nitroglycerin at the first sign of chest pain. If there is no relief after 5 minutes, 911 should be called. Nitroglycerin may be repeated every 5 minutes up to a total of three doses.
  d. Encourage cardiopulmonary resuscitation (CPR) training for family members and close friends.
  e. Exercise regimen: Encourage routine exercise for the patient most days of the week, such as walking, treadmill use, and so on, once released by the cardiologist.
  f. Advise smoking cessation as indicated. Encourage support groups, classes, and smoking-cessation aids as indicated (*see Section III: Patient Teaching Guide for Chapter 9, "Nicotine Dependence"*). ◀
C. Dietary management: Counsel the patient on nutrition and low-fat, low-cholesterol, low-sodium diet. Recommend the Dietary Approaches to Stop Hypertension (DASH) diet and lifestyle changes. Provide dietary handouts on the DASH diet, a low-fat/low-cholesterol/low-sodium diet. See Appendix B for the DASH diet.
D. Pharmaceutical therapy
 1. When MI is suspected: Aspirin 160 to 325 mg (four 81-mg baby aspirin) chewed or swallowed as soon as possible. Enteric-coated aspirin delays absorption and therefore is not recommended.
 2. Instruct the patient on how to take sublingual nitroglycerin tablets and other medications.
 3. Nitrates: Nitroglycerin sublingual 0.2 to 0.6 mg every 5 minutes for ischemic chest pain in the absence of hypotension up to three doses. Monitor side effects: headache, hypotension.
 4. If pain persists after three doses of nitroglycerin:
  a. Morphine sulfate IV: 2 to 4 mg IV, repeating every 5 minutes until pain resolves. Dose may be increased at 2 to 8 mg per dose as tolerated. Monitor side effects: Nausea/vomiting, dizziness, hypotension.
 5. Oxygen therapy: 2 to 4 L per nasal cannula
 6. If there are no contraindications (bradycardia, HF, second- or third-degree heart block, asthma, shock), beta-blockers may be started IV during the acute phase and changed to oral therapy during the course of the treatment.
 7. Fibrinolytic therapy may be used for patients with suspected MI with ST-elevation myocardial infarction

(STEMI) or non-ST-elevation myocardial infarction (NSTEMI) with left bundle branch block.

8. After an MI, if the patient is not currently on a statin, a statin should be started.

Follow-Up

A. Follow-up is determined by the patient's needs, severity of acute MI, and whether complications are present.

Consultation/Referral

A. If MI is suspected, call 911 and refer the patient for immediate hospitalization.

B. According to the 2013 American College of Cardiology/American Heart Association (ACC/AHA) guidelines, a patient who is a candidate for reperfusion who is seen at a percutaneous coronary intervention (PCI)-capable hospital should be sent to the catheterization lab for primary PCI in 90 minutes or less. If the patient is at a facility that is non-PCI capable, then a transfer should be made to a PCI facility as soon as possible in 120 minutes or less than or equal to 120. If time lapse will be more than 120 minutes, then it is recommended to administer fibrinolytic therapy within 30 minutes of arrival.

C. Follow up with cardiologist as scheduled when discharged from the hospital.

Individual Considerations

A. Adults

1. Women do not always complain of typical chest pain. Suspect MI in patients who complain of shortness of breath, back pain, jaw pain, nausea, just not feeling right. Men may also exhibit these symptoms.

B. Geriatrics

1. Consider MI in patients complaining of atypical chest pain. Symptoms may include dyspnea, fatigue, dizziness, confusion, altered mental state.

2. Older adults may not perceive chest pain as being severe and may not consider that symptoms may be related to a heart attack because of an altered pain perception. Educate older adults that pain perception may be diminished as one ages.

Arrhythmias

Jill C. Cash and Debbie Gunter

Definition

Arrhythmias are abnormal heart rhythms. Common types are the following:

A. Bradycardia: Heart rate less than 60 beats per minute (bpm); impulse originates in sinoatrial (SA) node.

B. Tachycardia: Heart rate greater than 100 to 160 bpm; impulse originates in SA node.

C. Supraventricular tachydysrhythmias (SVTs): Heart rate greater than 100 bpm; the origin of impulse is listed as follows:

1. Atrioventricular (AV) nodal reentrant tachycardia (NRT) is intranodal reentry by means of fast and slow conduction pathways within the AV junction.

2. Orthodromic atrioventricular reentrant tachycardia (AVRT) is tachycardia across accessory pathways associated with preexcitation.

D. Atrial fibrillation (AF): Chaotic electrical activity caused by rapid discharges from numerous ectopic foci in atria. Atrial rate is difficult to count. There are three types of AF:

1. Paroxysmal AF occurs in patients who usually have normal sinus rhythm (NSR), but then have an episode of faulty electrical signals and rapid heart rate. This usually starts suddenly and stops on its own. Symptoms can be mild or severe and usually stop in less than 24 hours, but may last for several days.

2. Persistent AF is a condition in which the abnormal heart rhythm continues for more than a week. It may stop on its own, or it can be stopped with treatment.

3. Permanent AF is a condition in which a normal heart rhythm cannot be restored with treatment. Both paroxysmal and persistent AF may become more frequent and, over time, result in permanent AF.

E. Premature ventricular contractions (PVCs) are impulses that form within the Purkinje network.

Incidence

A. SVTs are the most common cardiac arrhythmias presenting to health care providers.

B. Atrioventricular nodal reentrant tachycardia (AVNRT) accounts for 60% to 70% of all SVTs.

C. AVRTs account for 30% to 40% of all SVTs. Greater than 90% of younger children who present with SVTs are likely to have an AVRT, but once they reach adolescence, AVNRT is the primary cause of SVT in about one third of these patients.

D. AF is the most common cardiac tachydysrhythmia, affecting approximately 2% of the general population. Prevalence increases with age to 5% of those older than 69 years. The presence of AF is associated with a fivefold increase in the risk of morbidity, a twofold increase in mortality, and an increased incidence of embolic stroke.

E. PVCs are common, and their frequency increases with age.

Pathogenesis

A. Bradycardia: Dominance of the parasympathetic nervous system, with excessive vagal stimulation to the heart, causes a decreased heart rate of sinus node discharge.

B. Tachycardia: Dominant sympathetic nervous system stimulation of the heart or vagal inhibition results in positive chronotropic, dromotropic, and inotropic effects.

C. AVRT: The most classic form of this SVT is Wolff–Parkinson–White (WPW) syndrome. Reentry occurs in a loop using atrial myocardium, AV node–His–Purkinje system, ventricular myocardium, and an accessory AV connection. During sinus rhythm, antegrade conduction through the accessory connection depolarizes the myocardium earlier than would occur by conduction through the AV node–His–Purkinje system, preexcitation is present, and a delta wave (slurring of initial deflection of the QRS complex) is usually seen on the surface 12-lead EKG.

D. AVNRT: The most common form is antegrade conduction, which occurs through a pathway with a short effective refractory period (ERP) and a longer conduction time. This pathway is often referred to as the *slow pathway*.

E. AF: Multiple, rapid impulses from many foci depolarize the atria in a totally disorganized manner. In the chaos, no P waves, no atrial contraction, no atrial kick, and a totally irregular ventricular response occur. The atria quiver, which leads to formation of mural thrombi and potential embolic events.

F. PVCs: These originate in the ventricles as a result of increased irritability in those cells.

Predisposing Factors

A. Bradycardia
  1. Increased vagal tone
  2. Decreased sympathetic drive
  3. Ischemia to SA node
  4. Drugs: Digitalis, propranolol, sedatives, propylthiouracil (PTU) or Tapazole, aminophylline, caffeine, alcohol, nicotine, and sympathomimetics
  5. Normal variant in athletes
  6. Normal body response to insult
  7. Atrial enlargement
  8. Acute myocardial infarction (MI)
  9. Congestive heart failure (CHF)
  10. Rheumatic heart disease
  11. Hypertensive heart disease
  12. Hypothyroidism
  13. Hypothermia
  14. Electrolyte abnormality
  15. Acidosis
  16. Infection

B. Tachycardia
  1. Decreased vagal tone
  2. Increased sympathetic tone
  3. MI
  4. Hyperthyroidism

C. SVT
  1. Digitalis toxicity
  2. Catecholamine surge

D. AF
  1. Myocardial ischemia
  2. Thyrotoxicosis

E. PVC: Stress

Common Complaints

A. Symptoms may not be present; however, patient may note irregular heartbeat.
B. Palpitations
C. Chest discomfort
D. Shortness of breath (SOB)
E. Dizziness
F. Diaphoresis
G. Weakness
H. Syncope
I. Nausea

Subjective Data

A. Obtain an accurate health and medical history.
B. Explore precipitating factors such as emotional stress, alcohol or drug use, or hot tub or bath use.
C. Inquire about the onset and duration of symptoms, also noting the patient's age when symptoms began.
D. Explore whether the patient has had concomitant weight loss, mood changes, and tremor, which are often associated with hyperthyroidism.
E. Carefully determine the number of previous episodes of palpitations or symptoms and what treatment, if any, was initiated.
F. Review all medications, including prescription, over-the-counter (OTC), and herbal products.

Physical Examination

A. Check pulse, respirations, blood pressure (BP), and weight.
  1. Sinus bradycardia: Pulse rate decreased below 60 bpm
  2. EKG: Normal
  3. Sinus tachycardia: Pulse rate increased above 100 bpm
    a. Pulse regular
    b. Systolic BP (SBP) constant
  4. AF
    a. Pulse irregular
    b. SBP changing
  5. AVNRT
    a. Pulse regular; AV block usual
    b. SBP constant; electrical alternans rare
  6. AVRT
    a. Pulse regular; AV block not present
    b. SBP constant; electrical alternans common, especially at high heart rates
  7. PVC: Pulse diminished or absent during the PVC

B. Inspect
  1. General appearance
    a. Is the patient in respiratory distress? Note SOB, chest pain, dyspnea.
    b. Does the patient look apathetic? This is a sign of a thyroid problem.
  2. Inspect the skin for flushing or pallor.
  3. Examine the eyes, noting lid lag.
  4. Assess the neck for jugular vein distension or thyromegaly.
    a. With sinus tachycardia, neck vein pulsation is normal.
    b. With AF, neck vein pulsation is irregular; assess for thyromegaly.
    c. AVNRT: Assess the neck veins for "frog sign," in which the atria contract against closed AV valves, producing rapid, regular, expansive venous pulsation in the neck, resembling the rhythmic puffing motion of a frog.
    d. AVRT: Assess for frog sign.

C. Auscultate the neck for carotid artery bruits and the heart for abnormal heart sounds. Heart rhythm may be regular or irregular, depending on type of dysrhythmia. Have the patient perform vagal maneuver (Valsalva's maneuver). If the rapid heart rate responds to the vagal maneuver and the cycle is broken, it is likely the patient has AVRT. If it does not respond, it is possible the patient has AVNRT.

1. Sinus bradycardia
   a. Rate less than 60 bpm
   b. Rhythm regular
2. Sinus tachycardia
   a. Rate greater than 100 bpm
   b. Rhythm regular; gradual onset and cessation
   c. Constant loudness of first heart sound
3. AF
   a. Rate: Atrial rate is nonmeasurable, ventricular rate is variable, usually rapid at onset.
   b. Rhythm: Atrial and ventricular rhythms are irregular.
   c. Loudness of first heart sound changes.
4. AVNRT
   a. AV block is usually present.
   b. Loudness of first heart sound is constant.
5. AVRT
   a. AV block is not present.
   b. Constant loudness of first heart sound
6. PVC
   a. Rate depends on underlying rhythm.
   b. Rhythm: Prematurity interrupts regularity of rhythm.

Diagnostic Tests

A. EKG
B. Drug screen
   1. Digitalis
   2. Aminophylline
   3. Illicit drugs
C. Electrolytes
D. Arterial blood gases (ABGs) if indicated

Differential Diagnoses

A. Multifocal atrial tachycardia
B. Sinus tachycardia with multiple premature atrial contractions
C. Atrial flutter
D. Ventricular tachycardia
E. AV blocks

Plan

A. General interventions
   1. Remove as many predisposing factors as possible.
   2. Stop smoking.
   3. Decrease or stop caffeine use.
B. Patient teaching
   1. Teach relaxation techniques.
   2. Teach the patient and his or her family signs of hemodynamic compromise, including rapid heart rate, unexplained weight gain or loss, worsening dyspnea on exertion, and decreased exercise tolerance.
   3. Teach and reassure the patient about long-term medication therapy and its side effects.
   4. Educate the patient and family regarding safety, dietary restrictions, and complications that may occur (bleeding) with the use of anticoagulant therapy.
   5. Discuss the need for a pacemaker/defibrillator or surgical ablation.
C. Pharmaceutical therapy
   1. Initial treatment usually is prescribed by a physician.
   2. Selection of treatment modality should be based on underlying pathophysiology.
   3. For reentrant cases (AVNRT, AVRT), agents that block the reentrant circuit are more effective.
      a. Calcium channel blockers (CCBs)
      b. Beta-blockers—long acting
      c. Digitalis
   4. Episodes caused by increased automaticity are treated with antiarrhythmic therapy.
   5. Chronic AF is treated with anticoagulants such as warfarin sodium (Coumadin).
      a. Start therapy as soon as possible if a history of underlying heart disease is present.
      b. Evaluate prothrombin time/international normalized ratio (PT/INR) on a regular basis to monitor for therapeutic response to warfarin sodium treatment.

Follow-Up

A. Patients who have their first episode of AF should return to the clinic within 24 to 48 hours for reevaluation.
B. Patients on antiarrhythmic agents should have liver enzymes measured during the first 4 to 8 weeks of therapy.
C. Patients with risk factors for developing cardiac complications to therapy, like QT prolongation, should have EKG during the first weeks of therapy and every 3 to 6 months thereafter.
D. Monitor patients on digoxin carefully for digitalis toxicity.
E. Patients on digitalis should be carefully monitored for signs of toxicity. Caution the patient regarding interactions of medication with digitalis.

Consultation/Referral

A. Patients with hemodynamic instability should be referred to a hospital or 911 immediately.
B. Patients unable to tolerate their dysrhythmia should be hospitalized immediately.
C. Consult a physician if the patient has an abnormal EKG pattern, refractory AF, suspicion of WPW syndrome, or sick sinus syndrome.
D. Consult a physician when questions arise about the difference between a narrow and wide QRS complex.

Individual Considerations

A. Pregnancy: Digitalis is safe during pregnancy.
B. Pediatrics
   1. Paroxysmal supraventricular tachycardia (PSVT) is probably the most common pediatric arrhythmia.

2. Instruct young adult patients without underlying heart disease to quit/avoid smoking, avoid sleep deprivation, and limit use of alcohol and stimulants.

Atherosclerosis and Hyperlipidemia

Jill C. Cash and Debbie Gunter

Definition

A. Atherosclerosis is a systemic disease characterized by lipid deposition and smooth muscle cell migration and proliferation in the intima of the larger arteries. Atheromatous changes lead to thrombotic stroke, peripheral vascular disease (PVD), atherosclerotic cardiovascular disease (ASCVD), and myocardial infarction (MI).

B. Hyperlipidemia is an elevation in serum lipoproteins and a major risk factor in the development of cardiovascular disease (CVD). The two main lipids in blood are cholesterol and triglyceride. Cholesterol is a relatively insoluble lipid that is necessary for cell membrane formation, steroid and bile salt production, and the development of nerve sheaths. Cholesterol is composed of three clinically significant components: High-density lipoprotein cholesterol (HDL-C), low-density lipoprotein cholesterol (LDL-C), and very-low-density lipoprotein (VLDL). Triglyceride is found in VLDL particles, but its role in atherosclerosis is not clear.

C. The atherosclerotic buildup of lipids, cholesterol, calcium, and cellular debris within the intima of the blood vessels causes plaque formation, vascular remodeling, and acute and chronic obstruction of the lumen of the blood vessels, which in turn decreases blood flow causing myocardial ischemia and decreased oxygen to other vital organs.

D. In 2013, the American College of Cardiology (ACC) and the American Heart Association (AHA) published guidelines on the assessment of cardiovascular risk, lifestyle management, and treatment of cholesterol to reduce ASCVD risks. A downloadable spreadsheet enabling estimation of 10-year and lifetime risk for ASCVD and a web-based calculator are available (see www.my.americanheart.org/cvriskcalculator and www.cardiosource.org/science-and-quality/practice-guidelines-andquality-standards/2013-prevention-guideline-tools.aspx). These risk tools are used to drive conversations on patient risk factors for ASCVD, potential benefits, negative aspects of risk, and patient preferences regarding initiation of relevant therapies. The assessment of ASCVD risk factors is recommended every 4 to 6 years in adults 20 to 79 years of age who are free from ASCVD and estimate 10-year ASCVD risk every 4 to 6 years in adults aged 40 to 79 years who are free from ASCVD. Long-term and lifetime risk information may be used to motivate therapeutic lifestyle changes (TLCs), and encourage adherence to these changes and pharmacological therapies.

Incidence

A. Atherosclerosis begins in childhood with the development of fatty streaks. The incidence of atherosclerotic diseases increases with age. CVD causes one in three deaths reported each year in the United States. The annual direct cost of CVD is estimated at $273 billion and the overall cost of CVD is estimated at $444 billion annually.

B. The leading risk factors for CVD are hypertension (HTN), high cholesterol, and smoking.

1. HTN can increase arterial wall tension, potentially leading to disturbed repair processes and aneurysm formation.
2. Cigarette smoking is associated with an increase in multiple inflammatory markers, including C-reactive protein (CRP), interleukin-6, and tumor necrosis factor.

Pathogenesis

A. Atherosclerosis is in part attributed to the deposition of cholesterol and lipoproteins in arterial smooth muscle cells. Dietary factors, obesity, drugs, and genetic defects in lipoprotein particle metabolism influence lipid and lipoprotein concentrations in blood.

B. Primary hyperlipoproteinemias are either caused by single-gene disorders transmitted by simple dominant or recessive mechanisms, or to multifactorial disorders with complicated inheritance patterns.

C. Secondary hyperlipoproteinemias (such as in thyroid disease and diabetes mellitus) occur as part of a constellation of abnormalities in certain metabolic pathways. The association among atherosclerosis, CVD, and hypercholesterolemia is well documented. HDL-C comprises about one fourth of the total serum cholesterol and acts as a scavenger, removing cholesterol from peripheral tissues and returning it to the liver, which produces a favorable cardioprotective effect. Elevated HDL-C levels are desirable. HDL-C levels greater than 60 mg/dL are a negative risk factor for CVD; those below 35 mg/dL are a major risk factor for CVD.

D. LDL-C constitutes 70% of the total serum cholesterol. It is the most atherogenic cholesterol subgroup. LDL-C particles interact with platelets, damaged arterial endothelium, and smooth muscle cells in the process of plaque formation. LDL-C levels of 160 mg/dL or greater are associated with an increased number of cardiac events.

E. VLDL accounts for a small amount of total serum cholesterol and is responsible for carrying triglycerides from the liver. Its role in atherogenesis is uncertain, but an inverse relationship has been observed between VLDL and HDL-C.

Predisposing Factors

A. High-risk factors for coronary vascular disease (CVD) events (CVD risk equivalent)

1. Clinical CVD
2. Symptomatic carotid artery disease
3. Peripheral arterial disease (PAD)
4. Abdominal aortic aneurysm

B. Presence of major risk factors (other than LDL-C)

1. **Age is the strongest risk factor for the development of CVD:**
   a. Age greater than 45 years for men and greater than 55 years for women
   b. Elderly persons experience a higher morbidity and mortality.
2. Cigarette smoking
3. Low HDL-C level, less than 40 mg/dL
4. Family history of early CVD: MI or sudden cardiac death younger than 55 years in father or other male first-degree relative, or before age 65 years in mother or other female first-degree relative
5. HTN (blood pressure [BP] > 140/90 mmHg or on antihypertensive medication)
6. Sedentary lifestyle
7. Obesity
8. Metabolic syndrome
9. Diabetes
10. Chronic inflammation

HDL-C greater than 60 mg/dL is equal to a "negative" risk factor and removes one risk factor from the total count.

Common Complaints

A. There are no complaints or symptoms associated with atherosclerosis and hyperlipidemia. Most lipid abnormalities are detected by routine laboratory testing or as part of a cardiovascular evaluation.

Subjective Data

A. Ask the patient if there is a history of CVD.
B. Discuss his or her past medical history, including predisposing factors for CVD.
C. Have the patient list current medications, including over-the-counter (OTC) and herbal products.
D. Have the patient discuss his or her current diet and exercise routine.
E. Explore the patient's social habits, including use of alcohol and tobacco.

Physical Examination

A. Check pulse, respirations, BP, height, and weight. Calculate body mass index (BMI) at each subsequent visit. An adult BMI calculator and a child and teen BMI calculator are located at www.cdc.gov/healthyweight/assessing/bmi

B. Inspect
1. Funduscopic examination: Examine eyes for premature arcus cornealis, which is a gray opaque line around the cornea caused by lipoid degeneration, and for lipemia retinalis, or a pale retina with white blood vessels caused by excess serum lipids because of VLDL of more than 2,000 mg/dL or alcoholism.
2. Inspect skin for xanthomas, which appear as red-brown or yellow papules, nodules, or plaque, caused by lipid deposits from high VLDL. Tendinous xanthomas are found on Achilles tendons, patellae, and hands.
3. Inspect joints for Achilles tendonitis and arthritis.

C. Palpate
1. Palpate abdomen for hepatomegaly or splenomegaly.
2. Palpate neck and thyroid.

D. Auscultate
1. Perform a complete heart examination.
2. Perform a complete vascular examination.

Diagnostic Tests

A. Laboratory testing
1. Lipid profile and lipoprotein analysis (see Table 10.1)
2. Complete blood count (CBC)
3. Complete metabolic panel (CMP)
4. Thyroid function studies to exclude disorders of the thyroid
5. C-reactive protein (CRP)
6. Hemoglobin A1C (if appropriate)

B. Tests/imaging
1. Treadmill stress test
2. Nuclear stress test
3. Echocardiogram
4. Ultrasound
5. CT
6. Coronary angioplasty

Differential Diagnoses

Assess the patient for the following secondary causes of ASCVD and hyperlipidemia:

A. Atherosclerosis
B. Hyperlipidemia
C. Diabetes mellitus
D. Hypothyroidism
E. Nephrotic syndrome

TABLE 10.1 ATP III Classification of LDL-C, Total Cholesterol, and HDL-C (mg/dL)

Determine lipoprotein levels. Obtain complete lipoprotein profile after 9- to 12-hour fast	
LDL-C—primary target of therapy	
<100	Optimal
100–129	Near optimal/above optimal
130–159	Borderline high
160–189	High
≥190	Very high
Total cholesterol	
<200	Desirable
200–239	Borderline high
≥240	High
HDL-C	
<40	Low
≥60	High

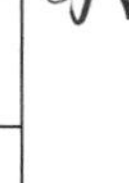

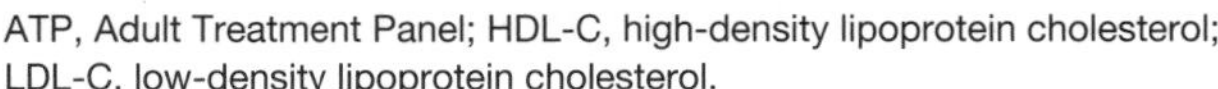

ATP, Adult Treatment Panel; HDL-C, high-density lipoprotein cholesterol; LDL-C, low-density lipoprotein cholesterol.

F. Porphyria
G. Obesity
H. Obstructive liver disease
I. Diuretic use

Plan

A. General interventions

1. TLCs, including exercise, diet, and weight management, are recommended for all patients.

2. Increased physical activity. The 2013 ACC/AHA guidelines on lifestyle management outline the newest physical activity recommendations advising adults to engage in 40 minutes of aerobic physical activity three to four times a week. The aerobic exercise should involve moderate to vigorous intensity to reduce BP, LDL-C, and non-HDL-C.

B. Dietary management

1. Advise the patient that diet modification is the first line of therapy for hyperlipidemia.

2. Explain cholesterol-lowering diet. Give dietary recommendation sheets. See Appendix B for low-fat/low-cholesterol and DASH dietary approaches to stop HTN.

C. Patient teaching

1. Weight reduction

a. Explain that weight reduction in patients greater than 20% over ideal body weight can lower LDL-C and triglyceride levels.

2. Other key dietary recommendations include:

a. Reduce intake of saturated fats and trans fats. Aim for 5% to 6% of calories from saturated fat.

b. Increase intake of poly- and monounsaturated fats.

c. Increase intake of soluble fiber (psyllium supplement).

d. Limit intake of alcohol: One drink per day for women and two drinks per day for men.

e. Increase intake of plant stanols and sterols (1 oz of Promise Activ or Benecol spread per day).

f. Increase intake of omega-3 fatty acids from marine sources (salmon or tuna twice a week or supplements).

g. Follow the Dietary Approaches to Stop Hypertension (DASH), Mediterranean, or AHA diet.

h. Lower sodium intake. Consume no more than 2,400 mg/d of sodium. Further reductions to 1,500 mg/d of sodium are associated with greater reduction in BP.

▶ **3.** Discuss smoking cessation (*see Section III: Patient Teaching Guide for Chapter 9, "Nicotine Dependence"*).

D. Pharmaceutical therapy: **Use clinical judgment when deciding potential benefits, possible side effects, and costs of drug treatment.**

1. Drug of choice: HMG-CoA reductase inhibitors (statins)

a. Statins suppress the activity of the key enzyme in cholesterol synthesis in the liver; they are

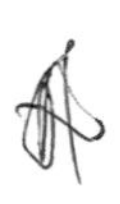
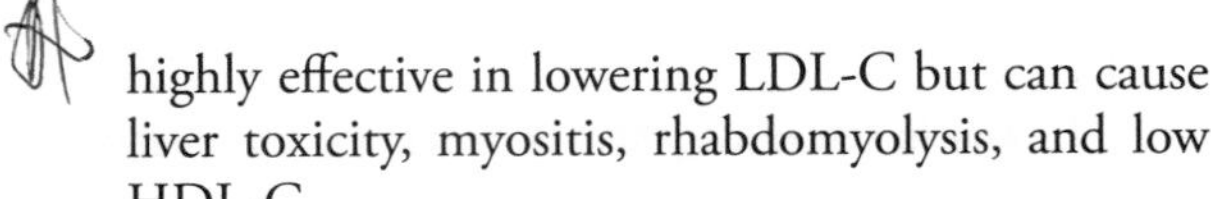

highly effective in lowering LDL-C but can cause liver toxicity, myositis, rhabdomyolysis, and low HDL-C.

b. There are four major statin benefit groups:

i. Individuals with the presence of clinical ASCVD, including acute coronary syndromes, a history of MI, stable or unstable angina, coronary or other arterial revascularization, stroke, transient ischemic attack (TIA), or PAD

ii. Individuals with primary elevations of LDL-C ≥ 190 mg/dL

iii. Individuals 40 to 75 years of age with diabetes and LDL-C 70 to 189 mg/dL and without clinical ASCVD (refer to Chapter 20, "Endocrine Guidelines")

iv. Individuals without clinical ASCVD or diabetes who are 40 to 75 years of age with an LDL-C 70 to 189 mg/dL and an estimated 10-year ASCVD risk of 7.5% or higher

c. ASCVD events are reduced by using the maximum tolerated statin intensity in those groups shown to benefit. The expert panel defines intensity of statin therapy on the basis of the average expected LDL-C response to a specific statin and dose. The intensity levels are "high-intensity," "moderate-intensity," and "low-intensity" statin therapy. Full statin treatment recommendations for primary and secondary prevention as well as the high-, moderate-, and low-intensity statin therapy from the 2013 ACC/AHA guidelines on the treatment of cholesterol are available at content.onlinejacc.org/article.aspx?articleid=1770217

d. Monitor liver function tests (LFTs) before therapy begins, then 4 to 6 weeks after starting drug therapy. Check at 6- to 12-month intervals or more frequently, if necessary.

e. Discontinue medications if abnormal laboratory values or adverse symptoms appear.

f. Use caution with the use of statins and other medications. Avoid concomitant drugs such as erythromycin, nicotine, azole antifungals, clofibrate, and gemfibrozil.

2. Category X drugs

a. Statins are category X drugs and are contraindicated in pregnancy.

3. Nonstatin drug therapy (see Table 10.2 for the nonstatin drugs that affect cholesterol)

a. Bile acid sequestrants bind bile acids in the gastrointestinal (GI) tract; lower moderately elevated LDL-C by 20%; and may cause constipation, bloating, and poor absorption of other drugs. Bile acid sequestrant therapy is not recommended if triglycerides are greater than 300 mg/dL.

b. Nicotinic acid or niacin: Broad-spectrum lipid-regulating agent. Niacin has been documented to exhibit anti-inflammatory properties (reduction of lipoprotein-associated phospholipase A_2 and CRP). Discuss possibilities of flushing. Contraindicated with chronic liver disease

TABLE 10.2 **Non-Statin Drugs Affecting Lipoprotein Metabolism**

Drug Class	Agents and Daily Doses	Lipid/Lipoprotein Effects	Side Effects	Contraindications
Bile acid sequestrants	Cholestyramine (4–16 g), Colestipol (5–30 g), Colesevelam (1,875–3,750 mg)	LDL-C ↓ 15%–30% HDL-C ↑ 3%–5% TG No change or increase	Gastrointestinal distress Constipation Decreased absorption of other drugs	Absolute: • Dysbeta-lipoproteinemia • TG >400 mg/dL Relative: • TG >200 mg/dL
Nicotinic acid	Immediate release (crystalline) nicotinic acid (1.5–3 g), extended release nicotinic acid (Niaspan®; 500–2,000 mg), sustained release nicotinic acid (1–2 g)	LDL-C ↓ 5%–25% HDL-C ↑ 15%–35% TG ↓ 20%–50%	Flushing Hyperglycemia Hyperuricemia (or gout) Upper GI distress Hepatotoxicity	Absolute: • Chronic liver disease • Severe gout Relative: • Diabetes • Hyperuricemia • Peptic ulcer disease
Fibric acids	Gemfibrozil (600 mg BID); Fenofibrate (145–200 mg) Clofibrate (500–2,000 mg)	LDL-C ↓ 5%–20% (may be increased in patients with high TG) HDL-C ↑ 10%–20% TG ↓ 20%–50%	Dyspepsia Gallstones Myopathy	Absolute: • Severe renal disease • Severe hepatic disease

GI, gastrointestinal; HDL-C, high-density lipoprotein cholesterol; LDL-C, low-density lipoprotein cholesterol; TG, triglyceride.

and severe gout. The niacin-treated subjects in the Atherothrombosis Intervention in Metabolic Syndrome with Low HDL/High Triglycerides: Impact on Global Health (AIM-HIGH) clinical trial had a trend toward increased stroke incidence.

c. Fibric acid derivatives: Highly effective in lowering triglycerides; it lowers VLDL-C, causes modest reduction in LDL-C, and raises HDL-C.

i. The combination of niacin with other lipid-lowering drugs has been shown to reduce progression and promote regression of coronary and carotid atherosclerosis and improve clinical outcomes.

ii. Fibrates may cause GI distress, rash, pain, blurred vision, anemia, and gallstones.

iii. Fibrates may inhibit insulin and oral hypoglycemic absorption, and potentiates oral anticoagulants.

Follow-Up

A. Measure patient's total cholesterol 4 weeks after initiation of diet and then at 3- to 4-month intervals.

B. If initiating medication therapy, obtain baseline blood work, including fasting lipid profile with LFTs and a CBC. Recheck tests 4 to 6 weeks after starting drug therapy. Then check at 6- to 12-month intervals or more frequently, if necessary.

Consultation/Referral

A. Refer to dietitian for nutritional counseling for dietary modifications.

Individual Considerations

A. Adults

1. Patients with high cholesterol who are otherwise at low risk for ASCVD (particularly men older than age 35 years and premenopausal women) are candidates for primary prevention emphasizing diet modification and increased physical activity. It is recommended that drug therapy be used sparingly in these patients.

2. Lowering serum cholesterol reduces morbidity and mortality in patients with ASCVD, and it also reduces the number of new cardiac events in those without known ASCVD.

3. Elevated triglycerides increase the risk of pancreatitis and diabetes.

B. Children

1. It is uncommon for children to have events secondary to atherosclerosis during childhood; however, the build-up of plaque begins during childhood and progressive changes can lead to heart events during early adulthood. Risk factors for children for this to occur include obesity, high BP, family history of heart disease, depression/bipolar disorder, exposure to cigarette smoking, and underlying chronic conditions.

2. Educate and lifestyle changes during childhood are imperative to prevent these events in children and early adulthood. Education should include healthy diet, exercise, and avoiding exposures (cigarette smoke) that increase risk factors.

3. Guidelines for screening children have been developed according to risk factors. The U.S. Preventive Services Task Force (USPSTF) is currently updating the guidelines for screening in children. Please refer to the USPTF for current guidelines.

Atrial Fibrillation

Laura A. Petty

Definition

A. Atrial fibrillation (AF) is the irregular and rapid heart rhythm caused by abnormal electrical impulse formation and/or propagation. These impulses make the heart's upper chambers (the atria) beat chaotically and out of sync with the heart's lower chambers (the ventricles), resulting in poor circulation of blood throughout the body.
B. Classification of AF
  1. Paroxysmal AF
    a. Also called *intermittent AF*
    b. Two or more episodes of AF that end spontaneously within 7 days or less and usually last less than 24 hours
  2. Persistent AF
    a. AF that does not end spontaneously within 7 days
    b. Usually requires pharmacological interventions and/or cardioversion to restore sinus rhythm
  3. Permanent AF
    a. Persistent AF in which rhythm control strategies are no longer effective (Such strategies are not utilized to restore sinus rhythm.)
  4. "Lone" AF
    a. The term used to reference patients with paroxysmal, persistent, or permanent AF who do not have structural heart disease

Incidence

A. The Centers for Disease Control and Prevention (CDC) notes that as of 2005, AF is the most frequently managed cardiac arrhythmia in the United States with an estimated 2.7 to 6.1 million patients.
B. AF is more common in women than in men. Men of any age are more likely than women to develop AF. However, because AF occurs much more often in older adults, and because there are more women than men over age 75, the total number of women and men with AF in this age group is essentially the same.
C. AF is more common in Caucasians.

Pathogenesis

A. Multiple impulses travel throughout the atria, yielding continuous electrical activity and an atrial rate in excess of 300 beats per minute (bpm). The impulses enter the atrioventricular (AV) node in a completely random manner. A small percentage of the impulses are conducted to the ventricle, which results in a lower ventricular rate, usually 100 to 180 bpm, and an irregularly irregular rhythm. This leads to ineffective atrial contractions, a decrease in cardiac output, and an increased risk of thrombus formation.

Predisposing Factors

A. Age, increased occurrence after age 65 years
B. Coronary artery disease (CAD)
C. Hypertension (HTN)
D. Diabetes
E. Rheumatic heart disease
F. Valvular heart disease
  1. Mitral valve stenosis
  2. Mitral regurgitation
  3. Tricuspid regurgitation
G. Fibrosis or calcification in the vicinity of the AV node
H. Left ventricular hypertrophy (LVH)
I. Heart failure (HF)
J. Myocardial infarction (MI)
K. Sick sinus syndrome
L. Hyperthyroidism
M. Infection
N. Pericarditis
O. Obstructive sleep apnea (OSA)
P. Obesity
Q. Recent cardiac surgery, including heart transplantation
R. Pulmonary diseases (related to hypoxia)
  1. Chronic obstructive pulmonary disease (COPD)
  2. Bronchitis, acute or chronic
  3. Asthma
  4. Emphysema
S. Electrolyte imbalances
  1. Hyperkalemia and hypokalemia
  2. Hypercalcemia and hypocalcemia
  3. Hypermagnesemia and hypomagnesemia
T. Factors that can trigger episodes of AF
  1. Physical or emotional stress
  2. Nicotine
  3. Caffeine
  4. Alcohol
  5. Exercise

Common Complaints

A. Palpitations
B. Angina
C. Fatigue
D. Dyspnea at rest or on exertion
E. Vertigo or dizziness
F. Disorientation
G. Confusion
H. Syncope
I. Headache
J. Urinary frequency or urgency
K. Anxiety
L. Asymptomatic presentation, most often seen in the elderly and in patients with permanent AF

Potential Complications

A. Stroke
  1. The risk for stroke increases five times during an episode of AF.
B. Pulmonary embolism (PE)
C. Peripheral emboli
  1. May present as an ischemic extremity or ischemic bowel

Subjective Data

A. Ask the patient what activity brought about or preceded the episode.

B. Have the patient describe the duration of pain, if any, and what time of day the symptoms began.
C. Ask the patient to describe his or her symptoms.
D. Ask the patient whether any previous episodes have occurred.
E. Ask the patient to list all medications, over-the-counter (OTC), and herbal products currently being taken or recently stopped.
  1. Medications with links to AF
    a. Common complication with AF
      i. Theophylline (theophylline anhydrous, Theo-24, Elixophyllin)
      ii. Digoxin (Lanoxin)
      iii. Quinidine (quinidine gluconate, Nuedexta)
      iv. Tricyclic antidepressants (TCAs)
    b. Rare complication with AF
      i. Aricept (donepezil hydrochloride)
    c. Questionable complication with AF
      i. Bisphosphonates (alendronate, risedronate, etidronate)
F. Ask the patient to quantify his or her smoking history, alcohol history, and caffeine intake.

Physical Examination

A. Patients presenting with an acute cardiovascular episode should be quickly assessed for the need to call emergency services/911 for immediate transport to the hospital.
B. Vital signs: Check BP, pulse, and respirations. Count heart rate for 1 full minute.
  1. Check orthostatic BP: Sitting, standing, and lying down.
C. Inspect
  1. Inspect overall physical appearance, noting any distress.
  2. Inspect the neck: Check jugular vein distension and pulsations.
    a. Provoking maneuvers (i.e., carotid massage) should only be performed by a cardiologist.
  3. Inspect extremities: Note edema, pallor, and cyanosis.
  4. Perform a funduscopic examination: Note hemorrhage, exudates, and papilledema to determine the presence of malignant HTN.
D. Palpate
  1. Palpate extremities for peripheral pulses in arm and groin; determine rate and regularity.
  2. Assess capillary refill.
  3. Palpate carotid arteries for thrills and heaves.
E. Auscultate
  1. Heart: While the patient is sitting, standing, and in left lateral recumbent positions, note normal and extra heart sounds (S3 and S4)
    a. S4 is not present during AF
  2. Neck for carotid bruits
  3. Lungs: Note the presence of wheezing and crackles
F. Additional areas for physical examination
  1. Assess for focal neurologic deficits (orientation, unilateral weakness, dysarthria).

Diagnostic Tests

A. CBC, basic metabolic panel (BMP; including electrolytes, blood glucose, blood urea nitrogen [BUN], creatinine), magnesium, and liver function tests (LFTs)
B. Thyroid profile and lipid profile
C. Brain natriuretic peptide (BNP) and N-terminal pro b-type natriuretic peptide (NT-proBNP)
D. Cardiac profile (including troponin, creatine phosphokinase test [CPK], creatine kinase, muscle and brain [CK-MB])
E. Serum drug levels, digoxin, amiodarone, quinidine (if applicable)
F. International normalized ratio (INR), if applicable
G. Creatinine clearance (CrCl)
H. EKG
I. 2-D echocardiogram
J. Chest x-ray
K. Exercise stress test or thallium stress test, if exercise-induced arrhythmia or CAD is suspected
L. Holter monitoring
M. Evaluation of sleep apnea

Differential Diagnoses

A. AF
B. MI
C. CAD
D. HF
E. Mitral stenosis
F. HTN
G. Hyperthyroidism
H. Digitalis intoxication
I. Acute infections

Plan

A. General interventions
  1. The goal of therapy is to improve the patient's quality of life by reducing morbidity and prolonging survival.
B. Patient teaching
  1. Encourage weight loss, smoking cessation, and stress management. *See Section III: Patient Teaching Guide for this chapter, "Atrial Fibrillation."* ◀
  2. Educate patients about the adverse effects of their anticoagulant and antiarrhythmic medications.
  3. Instruct patients taking Coumadin (warfarin) to take steps to lessen their risk of falls.
  4. Educate patients with implanted defibrillators and pacemakers about their susceptibility for external electrical fields and avoidance of exposure.
C. Prevention
  1. Control other chronic medical conditions, that is, HTN, diabetes, HF, pulmonary diseases, and hyperlipidemia.
D. Dietary management
  1. Counsel patient on proper nutrition, specifically a low-fat, low-cholesterol, low-sodium diet. Give diet handouts.
  2. Patients taking Coumadin should be educated regarding foods that are high in vitamin K. Some

foods will interfere with clotting factors. Please see Appendix B, "Foods to Avoid While Taking Warfarin (Coumadin, Jantoven)," for common foods that interfere with clotting factors.

E. Pharmaceutical therapy

1. Anticoagulant therapy

a. Goal of therapy: Prevention of thromboembolism

i. Coumadin (warfarin sodium, Jantoven)

1) Doses: 1 mg, 2 mg, 2.5 mg, 3 mg, 4 mg, 5 mg, 6 mg, 7.5 mg, and 10 mg tablets

2) Warfarin Dose Calculator is located at www.globalrph.com/warf-maint.htm

3) Review all medications that may affect the anticoagulant effects of warfarin. Globalrph is a resource with a list of medications that both increase and decrease the INR (www.globalrph.com/warfarin_calc.htm).

ii. Pradaxa (dabigatran etexilate mesylate)

1) 75 mg and 150 mg tablets

a) Dosage indications based on CrCl

i) CrCl greater than 30 mL/min: 150 mg, taken twice a day

ii) CrCl of 15 to 30 mL/min: 75 mg, taken twice a day

iii. Xarelto (rivaroxaban)

1) 10 mg, 15 mg, and 20 mg tablets

a) Dosage indications based on CrCl

i) CrCl greater than 50 mL/min: 20 mg with evening meal

ii) CrCl of 15 to 50 mL/min: 15 mg with evening meal

iv. Eliquis (apixaban)

1) 2.5 mg and 5 mg tablets

a) Dosage indications

i) Recommended dose is 2.5 mg, taken twice a day in patients who fit any of the following criteria:

- 80 years of age or older
- Weight greater than or equal to 60 kg (132 lb)
- Serum creatinine greater than or equal to 1.5 mg/dL

v. Savaysa (edoxaban)

1) 15 mg, 30 mg, and 60 mg tablets

a) Dosage indications

i) CrCl between 15 and 50 mL/min: 30 mg, once daily

ii) CrCl >95 mL/min: Do not prescribe

2. Antiplatelet therapy

a. Goal of therapy: Prevention of thromboembolism; modest preventative effect

i. Aspirin: 81 mg and 325 mg tablets

ii. Plavix (clopidogrel bisulfate): 75 mg and 300 mg

3. Combined anticoagulant and antiplatelet therapies

a. Prescription of both antiplatelet medications (Plavix and aspirin) in addition to an anticoagulant is referred to as *triple therapy*. Triple therapy is commonly used to prevent complications when two or more of the following conditions are present:

i. AF

ii. Mechanical valve prosthesis

iii. Drug-eluting coronary stent

b. Triple therapy is linked with an increase in bleeding complications ranging from mild to life-threatening.

4. Heart rate control therapy

a. Goal of therapy: Varies based on patient age, but typically involves achieving a ventricular rate between 60 and 80 beats per minute (bpm) at rest and 90 and 115 bpm during moderate exercise.

b. Beta-blockers

i. Acebutolol (Sectral, acebutolol hydrochloride)

1) 200 mg and 400 mg capsules

ii. Atenolol (Tenormin)

1) 25 mg, 50 mg (scored), and 100 mg tablets

iii. Betaxolol (Betoptic, Betoptic S, betaxolol hydrochloride)

1) 10 mg and 20 mg tablets, all scored

iv. Bisoprolol (Zebeta, bisoprolol fumarate)

1) 5 mg (scored) and 10 mg tablets

v. Metoprolol (Lopressor, Toprol-XL, metoprolol tartrate)

1) 50 mg and 100 mg tablets, all scored

vi. Nadolol (Corgard)

1) 20 mg, 40 mg, and 80 mg tablets, all scored

vii. Nebivolol (Bystolic)

1) 2.5 mg, 5 mg, 10 mg, and 20 mg tablets

viii. Propranolol (propranolol hydrochloride)

1) 10 mg, 20 mg, 40 mg, 60 mg, and 80 mg tablets, all scored

ix. Sotalol (Betapace, sotalol hydrochloride)

1) 80 mg, 120 mg, and 160 mg tablets, all scored

x. Timolol (timolol maleate)

1) 5 mg, 10 mg (scored), and 20 mg (scored) tablets

c. Calcium channel blockers (CCBs)

i. Diltiazem (Cardizem, diltiazem hydrochloride)

1) 30 mg, 60 mg (scored), 90 mg (scored), 120 mg (scored) tablets

ii. Verapamil (Calan, verapamil hydrochloride, Tarka)

1) 40 mg, 80 mg (scored), and 120 mg (scored) tablets

d. 4th generation calcium channel blockers

i. Cilnidipine (Cilacar)

1) 5 mg, 10 mg, and 20 mg tablets

ii. Digoxin
1) Digoxin (Lanoxin)
a) 0.125 mg and 0.25 mg tablets, all scored
5. Heart rhythm control therapy
a. Goal of therapy: The maintenance of a normal rhythm and suppression of AF
i. Sodium channel blockers
1) Disopyramide (Norpace): 100 mg and 150 mg capsules
2) Quinidine (quinidine gluconate): 200 mg and 300 mg tablets, all scored
ii. Potassium channel blockers
1) Amiodarone (Cordarone, Pacerone, Nexterone, amiodarone hydrochloride): 200 mg tablet, scored
2) Dofetilide (Tikosyn): 125 mcg, 250 mcg, and 500 mcg capsules
3) Dronedarone (Multaq): 400 mg tablet
4) Sotalol (Betapace, sotalol hydrochloride): 80 mg, 120 mg, and 160 mg tablets, all scored
F. Surgical therapies
1. Ablation therapy
a. Goal of therapy: Prevention of recurrent AF
b. Preferred clinical characteristics include the following:
i. Symptomatic paroxysmal AF
ii. Failure of one or more antiarrhythmic medications
iii. Normal to mildly dilated atria
iv. Normal to mildly reduced ventricular function
v. Absence of severe pulmonary disease
c. The long-term efficacy of ablation therapy requires further study, especially with regard to patients with HF and structural heart disease.

Follow-Up

A. AF patients should be comanaged with a physician.
B. AF that is resistant to routine therapy should always be followed by a cardiologist.
C. Laboratory monitoring as indicated by the patient's anticoagulant and antiarrhythmic medications
1. CrCl for patients taking Pradaxa and Xarelto
2. INR for patients taking Coumadin. Multiple medications affect the anticoagulant property of Coumadin.
a. The INR labs are located on Globalrph at www.globalrph.com/warfarin_drug_interactions.htm
D. Follow-up is determined by the patient's needs, frequency of AF reoccurrence, and the presence of other medical conditions.
E. After defibrillator or pacemaker placement, monitor the patient using regular follow-up appointments and EKGs to identify failure of the implanted device, thromboembolism, lead dislodgement, infection, and complicating arrhythmias.

Consultation/Referral

A. If you suspect an acute cardiovascular episode, refer the patient for immediate hospitalization in order to initiate thrombolytic therapy, cardioversion, hypertensive management, and additional diagnostic testing.
B. Refer to cardiology as indicated by the patient's clinical situation, specifically the frequency of AF reoccurrence and the presence of other complex medical conditions.
C. AF that is resistant to routine therapy should always be followed by a cardiologist.

Individual Considerations

A. Pediatrics: AF is uncommon in the pediatric population; however, when present AF occurs secondary to structural heart disease.

Chest Pain

Cheryl A. Glass and Debbie Gunter

Definition

A. Chest pain is a localized sensation of distress or discomfort that may or may not be associated with actual tissue damage.

Incidence

A. Chest pain is one of the most common complaints of adult patients. Causes can range from minor disorders to life-threatening diseases; every patient must be assessed carefully.

Pathogenesis

A. Cardiac etiology: Ischemia, atherosclerosis, inflammation, or valvular problems caused by angina, myocardial infarction (MI), pericarditis, endocarditis, dissecting aortic aneurysm, or mitral valve prolapse (MVP; see Table 10.3)
B. Musculoskeletal etiology: Muscle strain and inflammation caused by costochondritis, chest wall syndrome, cervicodorsal arthritis, or intercostal myositis
C. Neurologic etiology: Nerve inflammation and/or compression caused by herpes zoster and nerve root compression
D. Gastrointestinal (GI) etiology: Structural defects, inflammation, or infection caused by gastroesophageal reflux disease (GERD), hiatal hernia, esophageal spasm, pancreatitis, cholecystitis, or peptic ulcer disease (PUD)
E. Pleural etiology: Inflammation, distension, or compression of pleural membranes caused by pneumonia, pulmonary embolus, pulmonary hypertension (HTN), spontaneous pneumothorax, and lung and mediastinal tumors
F. Psychogenic etiology: Stress caused by anxiety, depression, or panic disorders

Predisposing Factors

A. These vary depending on the etiology of pain.

TABLE 10.3 Comparison of Common Chest Pain Etiologies

Condition	Pain Findings	Associated Symptoms	Precipitating Factors	Relieving Factors	Physical Findings	Diagnostic Tests	Treatment Modalities
Cardiac-stable angina	Substernal, tight, dull pressure, usually lasts longer than 15 minutes		Exertion, cold, emotional stress	Rest, nitroglycerin, Valsalva's maneuver	Sinus tachycardia, bradycardia, xanthomas, signs of HF	Resting EKG, stress EKG, cardiac enzymes, echocardiogram, angiogram	ASA, BB, nitrate, CCB
Prinzmetal's angina (variant)	Substernal, achy, tight, dull pressure		Often occurs at rest; may awaken from sleep	Nitroglycerin	Same as stable angina	Resting EKG, angiogram	ASA, nitrate, CCB
MI	Precordial, substernal, severe, crushing, squeezing, lasts >15 minutes	Dyspnea, sweating, dizzy, pain radiates to neck/arm/jaw, N&V, cough, fever, unstable V/S	Oxygen	Not relieved by nitroglycerin	S3 or S4 murmur, tachycardia, bradycardia, pericardia, friction rub, hyper/hypotension	EKG, serial CK enzymes, echo, radionuclide studies	Analgesia, reperfusion, prevention and treatment complications limit infarcts Thrombolytic therapy for acute MI
MVP	Usually not substernal, often knifelike, may last 1 to 3 hours	Palpitations, fatigue, lightheaded, arrhythmia, syncope		Recumbent position, BB, nitroglycerine	Midsystolic click and/or murmur, thin body status, SOB	Echo, EKG	Usually none, BB if palpitations or ventricular ectopy becomes disabling
Hypertrophic cardiomegaly	Similar to angina	Dyspnea with exertion, arrhythmias, light-headed syncope	May be increased by nitroglycerin, exertion	BB, squatting	Systolic murmur, increased upright position, Valsalva's maneuver, more forceful PMI	EKG, CXR, echo, Doppler, cardiac catheterization	BB, CCB, possible pacing and myomectomy, exercise restriction
Pericarditis	Retrosternal, sharp or dull; sudden onset; long duration; radiates to one side of the trapezius	Fever, myalgia, anorexia, anxiety, recent viral infection		Sitting up, leaning forward	Friction rub, SVT1, tachypnea, crackles, signs of cardiac tamponade	EKG, echo, CBC, ESR	Hospitalize; rule out purulent process Analgesics

Endocarditis	Usually dull, retrosternal, may radiate to back	Fever, night sweats, joint pain, back pain, weight loss, headache, murmur			Systolic–diastolic murmur, petechiae, Osler's modes, Roth spots, neck vein distension, pleural or pericardia rub, pain in extremities, splenomegaly, hematuria	CBC, ESR blood cultures, echo	Hospitalize, for antibiotic therapy
GI-esophageal spasm	May be identical to angina		Alcohol or cold liquids	May be relieved by nitroglycerin		Esophageal manometry	Nitroglycerin anticholinergics, esophageal dilation
Esophagitis	Burning, tightness	Heartburn, water brash	Overeating, alcohol, recumbent position	Antacids	May have slight to moderate epigastric tenderness	Esophagoscopy	Lifestyle modification, antacid, H2 blocker, PPI, promotility agent
Musculoskeletal costochondritis	Sharp, sometimes pleuritic, parasternal costochondral pain		Sneezing, cough on deep inspiration, or twisting motions, reaching overhead		Erythema at sites of tenderness; positive pinpoint tenderness at costochondral junctions	CXR to rule out other causes	NSAIDs, ASA, ibuprofen, naproxen, heat application

ASA, acetylsalicylic acid; BB, beta-blocker; CBC, complete blood count; CCB, calcium channel blockers; CK, creatine kinase; CXR, chest x-ray; ESR, eosinophilic sedimentation rate; GI, gastrointestinal; HF, heart failure; MI, myocardial infarction; MVP, mitral valve prolapse; NSAIDs, nonsteroidal anti-inflammatory drugs; N&V, nausea and vomiting; PMI, point of maximal impulse; PPI, proton pump inhibitor; SOB, shortness of breath; SVT, supraventricular tachydysrhythmias; VS, vital signs.

Common Complaints

A. Primary complaint: Pain somewhere in the chest
B. "Levine's sign": Placing the fist on the center of the chest to demonstrate pain
C. Fatigue
D. Cough
E. Indigestion
F. Dyspnea
G. Syncope
H. Palpitations
I. Profound fatigue

Other Signs and Symptoms

A. Pain may be typical of angina and MI.
B. Musculoskeletal pain may be relieved by position change, aggravated by body movement, reproducible, or caused by injury or trauma.
C. Neurologic pain is associated with skin lesion if herpes zoster is the causative agent.
D. GI pain may be associated with meals, certain positions, belching, or an acid "brash" taste in mouth, or it may be referred to other sites.
E. Pleural pain is accompanied by cough, upper respiratory infection (URI) symptoms, or shortness of breath (SOB).
F. Psychogenic pain or pressure along with SOB and dizziness may be associated with a specific event or time.

Subjective Data

A. How long has the patient had chest pain?
B. Has the patient ever been treated for chest pain? What treatment, tests, and medications (such as nitroglycerin) were used?
C. What precipitates and relieves the patient's chest pain?
  1. Precipitates pain: Exertion, taking a deep breath, eating, cold, stress, and sexual intercourse
  2. Relieves pain: Resting, eating, taking an antacid, taking nitroglycerin, and positional change
D. Inquire about character of pain:
  1. Location: Neck, throat, chest, epigastric area, and shoulder
  2. Radiation: Neck, throat, shoulder, lower jaw, and upper extremity
    a. Radiation to both arms is a predictor of acute MI.
    b. Chest pain that radiates between the scapulae may be because of thoracic aortic dissection.
  3. Quality: Squeezing, pressure, strangling, fullness, heavy weight, tightening, constriction, and ripping/tearing (acute aortic dissection)
  4. Intensity: Abrupt onset, gradually getting worse, dull, or insidious
  5. How long has the pain been occurring? Seconds, minutes, hours, or years?
  6. Frequency: Intermittent, occurs every morning/evening
E. Are other associated symptoms present?
F. Discuss any risk factors the patient may have for cardiac disease: Smoking, hyperlipidemia, HTN, sedentary lifestyle, diabetes, and family history
G. Review medical history as noted earlier.
H. Review all medications including prescription (such as sildenafil), over-the-counter (OTC), and herbal products.
I. Review recreational/illicit drug use.
J. Inquire about any new physical labor if musculoskeletal etiology is suspected.
K. Has the patient had any trauma (including domestic violence)?
L. Has the patient had a recent infection?

Physical Examination

A. Check temperature (if infection is suspected), pulse, respirations, blood pressure (BP), and pulse oximetry.
B. Inspect
  1. Inspect general appearance.
    a. Appearance of discomfort/distress
    b. Any appearance of respiratory distress
    c. Evaluate jugular venous distension (JVD).
    d. Note patient position: Sitting, lying, squatting. Relief of chest pain with recumbency suggests MVP; relief with squatting suggests hypertrophic cardiomyopathy. Noncardiac chest pain may be present along with cardiac chest pain.
  2. Inspect skin for diaphoresis, jaundice, pallor, herpes zoster lesions, rash, or cyanosis.
  3. Inspect chest wall for herpes zoster lesions or signs of trauma.
  4. Inspect eyes by performing funduscopic examination.
  5. Inspect legs for signs of phlebitis: Unilateral swelling, cyanosis, venous stasis, and diminished pulses.
  6. Inspect neck for enlarged thyroid and lymph nodes, midline trachea, and JVD.
C. Palpate
  1. Palpate chest wall for tenderness and swelling. Chest pain present in only one body position is usually not cardiac in origin.
  2. Palpate abdomen for masses, tenderness, bounding pulses, organomegaly, and ascites.
  3. Palpate femoral and distal pulses.
D. Auscultate
  1. Auscultate carotid arteries for bruits.
  2. Auscultate lungs for crackles, wheezes, equal breath sounds, and pleural rub.
  3. Auscultate abdomen for bruits and bowel sounds.
  4. Auscultate heart for murmurs, rubs, clicks, irregularities, or extra sounds.
E. Neurologic examination: Perform this examination if neurologic etiology is suspected.

Diagnostic Tests

A. Testing depends on information collected in the examination. A normal physical examination, EKG, and/or laboratory test results in a patient with chest pain does not rule out coronary heart disease (CHD). Typical tests include the following:
  1. EKG
  2. Chest radiography, whenever diagnosis of chest pain is not clear

3. Echocardiogram
4. Stress test
5. Cardiac catheterization
6. Barium tests
7. Endoscopy to rule out GI etiology
8. Esophageal pH, low
9. Laboratory tests
   a. Troponin I or T
   b. Myoglobin
   c. Creatine kinase (CK)
   d. Creatine kinase—muscle and brain (CK-MB)
   e. C-reactive protein (CRP)
   f. Brain natriuretic peptide (BNP) for clinical findings/risk of heart failure (HF)
   g. D-dimer for suspected venous thrombotic event (deep vein thrombosis [DVT] or pulmonary embolism [PE])

Differential Diagnoses

A. Cardiac causes
   1. CHD
      a. Acute MI: Chest pain lasting more than 15 minutes
      b. Unstable angina pectoris
      c. Stable angina pectoris
      d. Prinzmetal's or variant angina
   2. Valvular heart disease
      a. MVP
      b. Aortic stenosis
   3. Hypertrophic cardiomyopathy
   4. Pericarditis
   5. Endocarditis
   6. Aortic dissection
B. Noncardiac causes
   1. Pulmonary causes
      a. Pneumonia
      b. Pleurisy
      c. PE
      d. Pulmonary HTN
      e. Pneumothorax
      f. Tracheobronchitis
      g. Lung cancer
   2. GI causes
      a. GERD
      b. Esophageal spasm
      c. PUD
      d. Pancreatitis
      e. Cholecystitis
      f. Flatulence
   3. Rheumatology causes
      a. Fibromyalgia
      b. Costochondritis
      c. Arthritis
   4. Chest wall causes
      a. Rib fracture
      b. Muscle strain
      c. Cervical or thoracic spine disease
      d. Metastatic bone disease
      e. Breast conditions
   5. Neurologic causes
      a. Herpes zoster
      b. Postherpetic pain syndrome
      c. Nerve root compression
   6. Psychogenic causes
      a. Panic disorder
      b. Generalized anxiety
      c. Depression
      d. Somatoform disorders

Plan

A. General interventions: Direct management toward primary disorder causing the symptom.
B. Patient teaching
   1. Teach the patient about medications.
   2. Encourage cardiopulmonary resuscitation (CPR) training for the patient's family and/or close friends if chest pain is cardiac in origin.
   3. Explain to the patient and family when and how to call 911 and the importance of going to the ER immediately so that thrombolytic therapy can be considered. A positive response to nitroglycerin does not confirm the presence of coronary artery disease (CAD).
C. Pharmaceutical therapy
   1. Cardiac pain: Nitroglycerin
   2. GI pain: H2 blocker, proton pump inhibitor (PPI)
   3. Musculoskeletal pain: Nonsteroidal anti-inflammatory drugs (NSAIDs)
   4. Psychogenic pain
      a. Selective serotonin reuptake inhibitors (SSRIs)
      b. Tricyclic antidepressants (TCAs)
      c. Benzodiazepines

Follow-Up

A. Follow-up of patients with CAD to be carried out for an indefinite period of time to detect the recurrence or progression of disease.
B. Other follow-up depends on the etiology of chest pain.

Consultation/Referral

A. Consult a physician when chest pain is cardiac in origin. If a cardiac origin is found in a pregnant patient, schedule a cardiology consultation as soon as possible for comanagement.

Individual Considerations

A. Pregnancy
   1. Evaluate chest pain in the same manner as in non-pregnant patients.
   2. Rule out pregnancy-induced hypertension (PIH) and hemolysis, elevated liver enzymes, low platelets (HELLP) syndrome when a third-trimester patient presents with upper epigastric/chest pain.
B. Pediatrics
   1. Chest pain usually does not represent serious cardiovascular disease (CVD).
   2. Pericarditis is one of the most frequent causes of chest pain associated with a febrile illness.

3. Exercise-induced chest pain may be indicative of asthma.
4. A chest wall syndrome, such as costochondritis, is another frequent etiology.

C. Geriatrics
1. Frail elderly patients usually do not present with the "typical" symptom complex of chest pain. Often, the only symptoms of acute MI are lethargy, decreased level of consciousness (LOC), crackles, congestive heart failure (CHF), persistent cough, or hypotension.
2. Prescribe medications for frail elderly patients in half the usual dosage and then slowly taper upward to the desired effect.

Chronic Venous Insufficiency and Varicose Veins

Laura A. Petty

Definition

Peripheral vascular disease (PVD) is a general term that encompasses all occlusive or inflammatory diseases that occur within the peripheral arteries, veins, and lymphatics. These conditions include peripheral arterial disease (PAD), deep vein thrombosis (DVT), superficial thrombophlebitis, lymphedema, and chronic venous diseases. Chronic venous diseases include chronic venous insufficiency (CVI) and varicose veins.

A. CVI
1. It is estimated that 20% of adults in the United States have CVI. CVI is twice as common in females than in males.
2. Peak incidence is seen in women older than 50 years.

B. Varicose veins
1. This is the most common circulatory condition of the lower extremities, affecting more than 20 million Americans. Varicose veins are usually thought to be more common in females; however, in certain populations the rate is higher in males.

Pathogenesis

A. CVI: Venous insufficiency is caused by incompetent valves that allow valvular reflux and subsequently venous hypertension (HTN). In CVI, venous HTN leads to obstruction of venous flow, which produces local tissue anoxia, inflammation, and at times even tissue necrosis. This process eventually causes subcutaneous fibrosing panniculitis and additional venous and lymphatic outlet obstruction.

B. Varicose veins: Varicose veins are a form of CVI. The same incompetent valves that cause valvular reflux and subsequently venous HTN in CVI also cause varicose veins. This influx of volume and pressure causes the vessels to dilate, twist, and bulge.

Predisposing Factors

A. CVI
1. Age
2. Female gender
3. Prolonged standing or sitting
4. Prior history of DVT
5. Stature, more common in tall persons
6. Obesity
7. Sedentary lifestyle

B. Varicose veins
1. Genetics
a. Risk increases to 90% if both parents have varicose veins.
b. If one parent is affected, the risk increases by 25% for men and 62% for women.
2. Age
3. Pregnancy
4. Prolonged standing
5. Restrictive clothing
6. Obesity
7. Ligamentous laxity
a. A history of hernia(s) or flat feet
8. Smoking

Common Complaints

A. CVI
1. Extremity edema
2. Pain worse when standing, usually dull, aching, or cramping
3. Pain improved with elevation
4. Itching sensation
5. Feeling of heaviness in extremity
6. Hyperpigmentation
7. Thickening and hardening of the skin
8. Ulcerations

B. Varicose veins
1. Pain, usually burning, aching, or itching
2. Blue veins that protrude above the surface of the skin
3. Leg fatigue
4. Edema
5. Symptoms worsened toward the end of the day
6. Leg heaviness

Potential Complications

A. CVI
1. Cellulitis
2. Peripheral neuropathy
3. Varicose veins
4. Abscess
5. Ulceration
6. Stasis dermatitis
7. DVT

B. Varicose veins
1. Stasis dermatitis
2. Stasis ulceration
3. Petechial hemorrhage
4. Chronic edema
5. Superficial thrombophlebitis
6. Hyperpigmentation
7. Eczema

Subjective Data

A. Ask the patient when the symptom(s) were first noticed.

B. Have the patient describe the duration of symptoms.

C. Ask the patient to describe pain, for example, crushing, stabbing, or burning.
D. Ask the patient what makes the symptoms better and what makes them worse.
E. Have the patient rate pain on a scale of 1 to 10, with 1 being the least painful.
F. Ask the patient to list all medications currently being taken, particularly substances not prescribed and illicit drugs such as cocaine.
G. Review recent history of invasive procedures or surgery.

Physical Examination

A. CVI
  1. Vital signs
    a. Check blood pressure (BP) and document resting heart rate, respirations, temperature, height, and weight.
  2. Inspect
    a. Inspect extremity for edema, hyperpigmentation, erythema, and difference in temperature.
    b. Inspect and document any varicosities.
  3. Palpate
    a. Palpate distended veins noting tenderness.
    b. Perform the cough impulse test to determine turbulent retrograde flow.
    c. Perform the tap test to determine if the great saphenous vein is distended with blood.
  4. Auscultate
    a. Heart: Rate rhythm, heart sounds, murmur, and gallops.
    b. Lungs: Assess lung sounds in all fields
B. Varicose veins
  1. Patient presenting with any of the following should be quickly assessed for the need to call emergency services/911 for immediate transport to the hospital:
    a. A bleeding varicosity with eroded surrounding skin
    b. A varicosity that has bled and is at risk of bleeding again
    c. An ulceration that is worsening and/or painful despite treatment
  2. Vital signs
    a. Check BP and document resting heart rate, respirations, temperature, height, and weight.
  3. Inspect
    a. Inspect skin for superficial veins that are raised above the skin's surface; patient should be standing.
    b. Inspect extremity for edema, hyperpigmentation, and eczema.
  4. Palpate
    a. Palpate distended veins, noting tenderness.
  5. Auscultate
    a. Auscultate heart: Rate rhythm, heart sounds, murmur, and gallops.
    b. Auscultate lungs: Assess lung sounds.

Diagnostic Tests

A. CVI
  1. Trendelenburg test
  2. Perthes test
  3. Doppler ankle/brachial index (ABI)
  4. Duplex ultrasound
  5. Venography, not utilized often because of expense and risk of phlebitis
B. Varicose veins
  1. Trendelenburg test
  2. Perthes test
  3. Duplex ultrasound

Differential Diagnoses

A. CVI
  1. DVT
  2. Ulceration
  3. Infection
  4. PAD
  5. Varicose veins with risk of hemorrhage
B. Varicose veins
  1. Arthritis
  2. Peripheral neuritis
  3. Nerve root compression
  4. Telangiectasia
  5. DVT
  6. Inflammatory liposclerosis

Plan

A. Prevention: General
  1. Avoid prolonged standing or sitting.
  2. Exercise on a regular basis.
  3. Encourage smoking cessation, weight loss, and exercise, if applicable.
  4. Encourage strategies to better manage other chronic medical conditions that directly affect the progression of PAD, that is, diabetes, dyslipidemia, obesity, and HTN.
B. CVI
  1. Nonpharmaceutical therapy
    a. Extremity elevation
    b. Compression stockings
    c. Exercise
    d. Venous ulcerations treated with wound care and compression therapy
  2. Pharmaceutical therapy
    a. Diuretics: Management of edema, short-term administration
      i. Hydrochlorothiazide
      ii. Antiplatelet: May increase the speed of healing to ulcerations
        1) Aspirin: 325 mg tablet
        2) Systemic antibiotics: Management of infection in persons demonstrating an increase in pain, erythema, or size of ulceration.
  3. Surgery
    a. Venous ablation for patients who continue to be symptomatic after 6 months of nonpharmacological, therapies. Types of ablation: Chemical, thermal, and mechanical
C. Varicose veins
  1. Patient teaching: *See Section III: Patient Teaching Guides for this chapter, "Chronic Venous Insufficiency" and "Varicose Veins."* ◀

a. If prolonged standing is required, shift weight from one leg to the other.
b. Do not sit with legs dependent.
2. Nonpharmaceutical therapy
a. Extremity elevation
b. Compression stockings
c. Exercise
3. Surgery
a. Radiofrequency ablation
b. Endovenous laser therapy
c. Phlebectomy
d. Foam sclerotherapy
e. Vein litigation

Follow-Up

A. Follow-up is determined by patient's needs, frequency and intensity of symptoms, and the presence of other medical conditions.
B. PVD manifesting persistent symptoms should always be followed by a cardiologist.

Consultation/Referral

A. If you suspect acute limb ischemia, refer patient for immediate hospitalization in order to obtain diagnostic testing to determine the presence of a thrombus and restore circulation to the affected extremity.
B. If chronic limb ischemia has led to ulceration and/or superimposed infection, hospitalization is indicated to initiate a wound care consultation and diagnostic testing to determine the degree of arterial occlusion.
C. Referral to a cardiologist is indicated in the presence of persistent PVD symptoms.
D. Referral to a podiatrist becomes necessary to trim toenails and assess patient for proper-fitting shoes.
E. Referral to pain management is indicated if pain is resistant to treatment.

Individual Considerations

A. Nonambulatory patients
1. Using rocking chairs is a possible substitute for persons unable to participate in a walking program.
B. Geriatrics
1. Be alert to signs and symptoms of depression related to immobility and pain.

Deep Vein Thrombosis

Laura A. Petty

Definition

A. Peripheral vascular disease (PVD) is a general term that encompasses all occlusive or inflammatory diseases that occur within the peripheral arteries, veins, and lymphatics. PVD includes deep vein thrombosis (DVT). DVT is a condition in which a thrombus forms in one or more veins. DVT greatly increases the risk of pulmonary embolism (PE).

Incidence

A. The Centers for Disease Control and Prevention (CDC) estimates that as many as 900,000 Americans are affected by DVT or PE annually. Of those, between 60,000 and 100,000 persons die from complications from DVT.

Pathogenesis

A. Changes within the venous system precipitate the formation of a DVT. These changes are formally called Virchow's triad. This triad includes hypercoagulability, venous stasis, and injury to the vessel wall. At least two of the three must be present for a DVT to form. Essentially, an injury to the vessel wall causes inflammation that attracts platelets, especially in a state of altered coagulation. The thrombus that forms spreads in the direction of blood flow and additional layers of platelets are added to the thrombus as time progresses. As it grows, the vessel becomes more occluded and symptoms worsen.

Predisposing Factors

A. Age, 60 years and older
B. Hip or femur fracture
C. Recent surgery, especially cardiac or extremity surgery
D. Prolonged inactivity/immobility
E. Pregnancy
F. Medication
1. Hormone replacement therapy (HRT)
2. Oral contraceptives
3. Tamoxifen
G. Smoking
H. Obesity
I. Cancer
J. Inherited hypercoagulable conditions

Common Complaints

Symptoms of a DVT are usually unilateral and have a sudden onset.
A. Extremity edema
B. Extremity pain
C. Increased temperature of extremity
D. Change in color or extremity
E. Asymptomatic, depending on the size and location of the thrombus

Potential Complications

A. PE
B. Arterial embolism with atrioventricular (AV) shunting
C. Myocardial infarction (MI)
D. Chronic venous insufficiency (CVI)
E. Postphlebitic syndrome
F. Phlegmasia cerulea dolens

Subjective Data

A. Ask the patient when the symptom(s) were first noticed.
B. Have the patient describe the duration of the symptoms.
C. Ask the patient to describe pain, for example, crushing, stabbing, or burning.
D. Ask the patient what makes the symptoms better and what makes them worse.
E. Have the patient rate pain on a scale of 1 to 10, with 1 being the least painful.

F. Ask the patient to list all medications currently being taken, particularly substances not prescribed and illicit drugs such as cocaine.
G. Review recent history of invasive procedures or surgery.

Physical Examination

Patients presenting with acute shortness of breath (SOB) and/or chest pain should be quickly assessed for the need to call emergency services/911 for immediate transport to the hospital. Patients presenting with symptoms of DVT that include cyanosis of the distal extremity should be quickly assessed for the need to call emergency services/911 for immediate transport to the hospital.

A. Vital signs
  1. Check blood pressure (BP) and document resting heart rate, respirations, height, and weight.
B. Inspect
  1. Assess for signs of erythema, increased temperature, and edema.
  2. Assess for a Homans' sign (i.e., calf pain with forced plantar flexion).
  3. Assess for Moses' or Bancroft's sign (i.e., pain when calf muscle is compressed forward against the tibia).
  4. Assess the Lisker sign (i.e., pain upon tibial percussion).
C. Palpate
  1. Pulses distal to affected area, noting symmetry
  2. Capillary refill
  3. Extremity for tenderness. Do not perform deep palpation.
D. Auscultate
  1. Heart: Rate, rhythm, heart sounds, murmur, and gallops
  2. Lungs: Assess lung sounds in all fields.

Diagnostic Tests

A. DVT
  1. Serum laboratory testing
    a. D-dimer
    b. Complete blood count (CBC) with differential
    c. Coagulation panel (prothrombin time [PT], partial thromboplastin time [PTT], international normalized ratio [INR]
    d. Testing for idiopathic DVT: Add Factor V Leiden, homocysteine, G20210A prothrombin, Factor VIII, lupus anticoagulant antibody, protein C and protein S levels anticardiolipin antibodies, and antithrombin
  2. Compression ultrasound
  3. MRI, if thrombus is suspected in the pelvic veins or vena cava
  4. Venography, not utilized often because of expense and risk of phlebitis

Differential Diagnoses

A. DVT
B. Cellulitis
C. Fracture
D. Lymphedema
E. Congestive heart failure (CHF)
F. Vein compression (caused by enlarged lymph nodes or mass)
G. Filariasis (parasitic disease)
H. Allergic reaction, localized
I. Compartment syndrome

Plan

A. Patient teaching: *See Section III: Patient Teaching Guide for this chapter, "Deep Vein Thrombosis."*
  1. Patients taking Coumadin should be educated regarding foods that are high in vitamin K. Some foods will interfere with clotting factors. Please see Appendix B, "Diet Recommendations" for common-foods that interfere with clotting factors.
  2. Avoid prolonged standing or sitting.
  3. Avoid crossing the legs.
  4. Gradually resume normal activity.
  5. Avoid immobility.
  6. Exercise on a regular basis.
  7. Stop smoking.
  8. Encourage strategies to better manage other chronic medical conditions that directly affect the progression of peripheral arterial disease (PAD), that is, diabetes, dyslipidemia, obesity, and hypertension (HTN).
B. Nonpharmaceutical therapy
  1. Compression stockings
C. Pharmaceutical therapy
  1. Thrombolytics: Administered in the inpatient setting
  2. Anticoagulants
    a. Heparin, intravenous, administered in the inpatient setting
    b. Coumadin (warfarin sodium, Jantoven)
      i. Doses: 1 mg, 2 mg, 2.5 mg, 3 mg, 4 mg, 5 mg, 6 mg, 7.5 mg, and 10 mg tablets
      ii. See "Atrial Fibrillation" section in this chapter for specifics on Coumadin therapy
  3. Low-molecular-weight heparin (LMWH)
    a. Lovenox (enoxaparin sodium)
      i. Doses: 300 mg/3 mL multidose vial
      ii. Doses: 30 mg/0.3 mL, 40 mg/0.4 mL, 60 mg/0.6 mL, 80 mg/0.8 mL, 100 mg/mL, 120 mg/0.8 mL, and 150 mg/mL prefilled syringes
    b. Fragmin (dalteparin sodium)
      i. Doses: 95,000 IU/9.5 mL multidose vial
      ii. Doses: 2,500 IU/0.2 mL, 5,000 IU/0.2 mL, 7,500 IU/0.3 mL, 10,000 IU/0.4 mL, 10,000 IU/mL, 12,500 IU/0.5 mL, 15,000 IU/0.6 mL, 18,000 IU/0.72 mL by injection
  4. Specific factor Xa inhibitor
    a. Arixtra (fondaparinux sodium): 2.5 mg/0.5 mL, 5 mg/0.4 mL, 7.5 mg/0.6 mL, and 10 mg/0.8 mL by injection
    b. Savaysa (edoxaban): 15 mg, 30 mg, and 60 mg
    c. Eliquis (apixaban): 2.5 mg and 5 mg
    d. Xarelto (rivaroxaban): 10 mg, 15 mg, and 20 mg
    e. Pradaxa: 75 mg and 150 mg

D. Surgery
   1. Insertion of vena cava filter to prevent PE
   2. Venous thrombectomy

Follow-Up

A. Follow-up is determined by patient's needs, frequency and intensity of symptoms, and presence of other medical conditions.
B. DVT manifesting persistent symptoms should always be followed by a cardiologist.
C. Patients taking anticoagulants are best followed by an anticoagulant clinic and/or cardiologist.

Consultation/Referral

A. If you suspect acute limb ischemia, refer patient for immediate hospitalization in order to obtain diagnostic testing to determine the presence of a thrombus and restore circulation to the affected extremity.
B. If chronic limb ischemia has led to ulceration and/or superimposed infection, hospitalization is indicated to initiate a wound care consultation and diagnostic testing to determine the degree of arterial occlusion.
C. Referral to a cardiologist is indicated in the presence of persistent PVD symptoms.
D. Refer to pain management if pain is resistant to treatment.
E. Refer to a registered dietitian as indicated by the patient's understanding of dietary modification necessary to improve status of risk factors.

Individual Considerations

A. Nonambulatory patients
   1. Using rocking chairs is a possible substitute for persons unable to participate in a walking program.
B. Geriatrics
   1. Be alert to signs and symptoms of depression related to immobility and pain.

Heart Failure

Cheryl A. Glass and Debbie Gunter

Definition

Heart failure (HF) is failure of the heart to pump sufficient blood to meet the metabolic demands of the tissues. The previous guidelines, published in 1999, defined HF according to primary dysfunction and clinical manifestations. However, the 2013 guidelines from the American College of Cardiology/American Heart Association (ACC/AHA) address management of HF with reduced ejection fraction (HFrEF) and preserved ejection fraction (HFpEF).

The 2013 ACC/AHA guidelines for HF are available at http://circ.ahajournals.org/content/early/2013/06/03/CIR.0b013e31829e8776. These guidelines include:

A. HFrEF
   1. Ejection fraction (EF) less than 40% because of weak, inefficient systolic contractions. The left ventricular ejection fraction (LVEF) is a measurement of systolic failure.
   2. An S3 ventricular gallop rhythm commonly occurs.
   3. Systolic failure is often the result of coronary heart disease (CHD) and/or myocardial infarction (MI).
   4. It can result from right- or left-sided failure, or both.
B. HFpEF
   1. EF is greater than 50%, but with poor compliance of the ventricle, which impedes ventricular diastolic filling (the ventricle is unable to relax).
   2. There are two subgroups.
      a. HFpEF borderline (or intermediate): Patients with an EF of 41% to 49%
      b. HFpEF with EF greater than 40% who previously had HFrEF (EF < 40%) but improvement or recovery was noted in EF
   3. The patient may be asymptomatic for years. HFpEF presents with the same symptoms of systolic failure, pulmonary congestion, and peripheral edema.
   4. An S4 atrial gallop rhythm commonly occurs.

Incidence

A. HFrEF incidence is higher in older women, chronic hypertension (HTN), obesity, left ventricular hypertrophy (LVH), cardiomyopathy, excessive alcohol use, end-stage chronic obstructive pulmonary disease (COPD), valvular disorders, anemia, renal failure, atrial fibrillation (AF), coronary artery disease (CAD), or diabetes.
B. Approximately 5.7 million people in the United States have HF. By the year 2030, the AHA estimates that there will be over 8 million people affected with HF.
C. It is also estimated that the costs of direct patient care (health care services, hospitalization, medications, etc.) for these patients with chronic disease will increase to approximately $53 billion by the year 2030.

Pathogenesis

A. Injuries to the myocardium may cause loss of functioning muscle. Compensatory mechanisms, including cardiac hypertrophy and neurohumoral processes, lead to adverse long-term effects. An inotropic insult results in incomplete emptying (systolic failure), and a compliance abnormality results in incomplete filling (diastolic failure). Most HF has some degree of both abnormalities.

Predisposing Factors

A. Atherosclerotic heart disease
B. Myocardial infarction
C. Rheumatic heart disease involving mitral and aortic valves
D. Cardiomyopathies
E. Hypertensive heart disease
F. Aortic stenosis or regurgitation
G. Thyrotoxicosis

H. Pregnancy-related disorders such as multiple births with preexisting heart disease
I. Volume overload
J. Beta-blockers or other cardiac depressants
K. Pulmonary embolism (PE)
L. Systemic infection
M. Arrhythmias
N. Renal disease

Common Complaints

Patients are assigned the New York Heart Association classifications by their tolerance of physical activity and shortness of breath (SOB). This classification may change according to the progression or regression of their cardiovascular disease (CVD; see Table 10.4).

A. Dyspnea on exertion
B. Hemoptysis
C. Fatigue
D. Cough
E. Orthopnea
F. Edema/weight gain
G. Paroxysmal nocturnal dyspnea
H. Nausea
I. Right upper abdominal pain or fullness
J. Chest pain
K. Palpitations

TABLE 10.4 New York Heart Association Functional Classification for Heart Failure

Functional Class	Activities	Objective Assessment
AHA Class I ACCF Stage A	No limitation. Ordinary activity does not cause undue fatigue, palpitation, dyspnea, or angina.	No objective evidence of CVD
AHA Class II ACCF Stage B	Slight limitations. Fatigue, palpitation, SOB, angina with ordinary physical activity.	Objective evidence—minimal CVD
AHA Class III ACCF Stage C	Marked limitations. No discomfort at rest. Fatigue, palpitation, SOB, and angina with less than usual activities.	Objective evidence—moderately severe CVD
AHA Class IV ACCF Stage D	Inability to do physical activity without discomfort. Symptoms are present at rest and become worse with activity.	Objective evidence—severe CVD

ACCF, American College of Cardiology Foundation; AHA, American Heart Association; CVD, cardivascular disease; SOB, shortness of breath.
Source: Modified from the American Heart Association and includes staging by the American College of Cardiology Foundation.

Other Signs and Symptoms

A. Hemoptysis
B. Bibasilar crackles
C. S3 gallop
D. Murmurs
E. Exercise intolerance
F. Weakness
G. Cough
H. Orthopnea
I. Nocturnal dyspnea
J. Tachycardia
K. Pallor
L. Cyanosis
M. Anorexia
N. Constipation
O. Jugular venous distension (JVD)
P. Hepatomegaly
Q. Hepatojugular reflux (HJR)
R. Murmurs
S. Exercise intolerance

Subjective Data

A. Ask the patient if he or she has difficulty breathing.
B. Ask how many pillows he or she sleeps on. Does the patient need to sit up in a recliner to sleep?
C. Inquire about how often he or she wakes up at night with SOB.
D. Inquire about how far the patient can walk without getting SOB. Have the patient describe his or her routine activities of daily living (ADLs) and how well the patient tolerates each activity.
E. Discuss the patient's history of heart disease, heart attack, HTN, or hyperlipidemia.
F. Ask the patient about current medications, prescription, over-the-counter (OTC), and herbal products.
G. Question the patient regarding all symptoms found in the "Common Complaints" section.
H. Discuss drug and alcohol history.
I. Has the patient ever been treated for cancer/chemotherapy, and how long ago?
J. What is the patient's usual weight; has he or she experienced more symptoms if he or she has pedal edema?
K. Does the patient have a cough (consider angiotensin-converting enzyme inhibitors [ACEI] as the cause)?

Physical Examination

A. Check pulse, respirations, blood pressure (BP), height, and weight.

1. Check BP while patient is sitting, standing, and lying down.
2. Be alert for abnormal vital signs: Hypotension, narrow or wide pulse pressure, tachycardia, bradycardia, and tachypnea.
3. Calculate body mass index (BMI).
4. On all subsequent visits, note weight gain of more than 1 pound per day over 3 consecutive days or 3 lb in 1 day.

B. Inspect
1. Overall physical appearance. Is the patient in distress?
2. Skin: Note pallor, cyanosis, and temperature.
3. Neck: Check jugular veins for distension.
4. Extremities: Note edema, cyanosis, pallor, and ulcers.

C. Auscultate
1. Heart for murmurs; tachycardia; S1, S3, or S4 gallops; and other abnormalities
2. Lungs: Note moderate to severe crackles/rales and other abnormal sounds
3. Neck and carotid arteries

D. Palpate
1. Abdomen for hepatomegaly and HJR
2. Extremities for peripheral pulses
3. Chest wall for displaced point of maximal impulse (PMI), lifts, heaves, and thrills

E. Mental status: Check mental status because confusion may occur, especially in the elderly.

Diagnostic Tests

A. Two-dimensional echocardiography with Doppler to evaluate LVEF
B. Radionuclide ventriculography may be used to measure LVEF and LV volumes
C. Coronary angiography
D. Anterior/posterior chest x-ray
E. EKG for patients with suspected arrhythmia, ischemia, or cardiac disease. Identify acute and old EKG changes to rule out pathologic Q wave, ST segment elevation, and LV hypertrophy.
F. Natriuretic peptides (brain natriuretic peptide [BNP] or N-terminal pro brain natriuretic peptide [NT-proBNP])

Differential Diagnoses

A. HF
1. HFrEF
2. HFpEF
a. HFpEF borderline patients with an EF of 41% to 49%
b. HFpEF patients with an EF greater than 40% who previously had HFrEF (EF, 40%) with improvement noted in EF

B. Renal disease or nephrotic syndrome
C. Liver disease
D. Asthma
E. COPD: To distinguish between progressing HF and a COPD exacerbation when both conditions are present, the presence of weight gain and an S3 gallop indicates HF, not COPD.

Plan

A. General interventions
1. Determine the etiology of the failure state and treat appropriately.
2. Treat HF stages:
a. Stage A: Treat/manage the patient's underlying conditions (HTN, AF, hyperlipidemia, diabetes, tobacco cessation, obesity, substance abuse [alcohol, cocaine, etc.]).
b. Stage B: Begin ACEI with beta-blockers for patients with HFrEF. Add statin therapy if patient has a history of MI.
c. Stage C: HFrEF: Implantable cardioverter defibrillators and consider cardiac resynchronization therapy
i. Digoxin may be used to manage symptoms. Hydralazine and isosorbide dinitrate are indicated for African American patients with HFrEF, patients with kidney dysfunction, or patients who cannot take ACEI or angiotensin receptor blocker (ARB) therapy. A diuretic agent is also recommended.
d. Stage D: Provide advanced treatment such as cardiac transplant, mechanical support, and/or palliative care.
3. The goals of therapy are to improve the patient's quality of life by reducing symptoms, decreasing morbidity, and prolonging survival.

B. Patient teaching
1. Teach the patient to weigh daily at the same time, on the same scale, and in the same clothing. Instruct the patient should call if there are gains of more than 3 lb in 1 day or more than 1 lb a day over a 3-day period.
a. Develop a plan of care for the increase of diuretic dosing for edema/weight gain in order to decrease dyspnea and prevent hospitalization.
2. Encourage weight loss.
3. Recommend regular, moderate exercise as long as dyspnea is not induced. Encourage exercise to increase endurance and strengthen muscles even though the patient may only tolerate a few minutes of walking.
4. Encourage smoking cessation.
5. Encourage medication adherence. Instruct the patient about all medications and possible side effects. Do not use OTC medicines without consulting the provider. Nonsteroidal anti-inflammatory drugs (NSAIDs) are contraindicated in HF.
6. Use continuous positive airway pressure (CPAP) or bilevel positive airway pressure (BiPAP) for nighttime sleep and naps for treatment of obstructive sleep apnea (OSA).

C. Dietary management
1. Read food labels for sodium content.
2. Teach dietary modifications, especially salt restriction of 2,000 to 3,000 mg/d for HFrEF and

HFpEF. Less than 2,000 mg sodium per day is recommended in patients with moderate to severe HF symptoms.

3. Fluid restriction is not recommended unless the patient is classified as Stage D or is diagnosed with hyponatremia with sodium levels less than 130 mEq/L. Restrict fluid intake to 2,000 mL/d or less for patients with chronic fluid retention despite use of diuretics and sodium restrictions.

4. Alcohol consumption should be limited to one glass of beer or wine per day. This amount should be counted in the daily fluid restriction.

5. See Appendix B for the DASH diet (Tables B.3 and B.4).

6. Other diet changes include low-fat/low cholesterol foods and the use of

   a. Monounsaturated fats, which decrease cholesterol
      i. Canola oil
      ii. Olive oil
   b. Polyunsaturated fats, which decrease cholesterol but not as well as monounsaturated fats
      i. Vegetable and fish oils
      ii. Corn, safflower, peanut, and soybean oils
   c. Avoid saturated fats.
      i. Animal fats and some plant fats
      ii. Butter and lard
      iii. Coconut oil and palm oil

D. Pharmaceutical therapy

1. Therapy is based on the extent of cardiac impairment and severity of symptoms. Medication regimens include a combination of the following classes: Diuretics, ACEI (ARB if unable to tolerate ACEI), cardioselective beta-blockers, inotropic agents such as digoxin, vasodilators, nitrates, and anticoagulants if there is an increased risk of thrombus formation. In general, calcium channel blockers (CCBs) are not used in HF management.

2. Drug classifications for antihypertensive and cardiac medication are noted in Table 10.5.

E. Drugs that should be avoided and/or used with caution in HF because they cause exacerbations or are at high risk of adverse reactions include:

1. NSAIDs: Increased renal dysfunction, edema, impaired response to ACEI
2. Cyclooxygenase (COX-2) inhibitors: Increased rate of HF and increased mortality
3. Aspirin: Interaction between ASA and ACEI and interference with benefits of beta-blockers on LVEF
4. Metformin: Increased risk of lethal lactic acidosis
5. Thiazolidinediones: Causes fluid retention that may precipitate HF.
6. CCBs: Some data exist on possible effects on systolic dysfunction.
7. Antidepressants (tricyclic antidepressants [TCAs]) and selective serotonin reuptake inhibitors (SSRIs): Major adverse cardiovascular events, including HF, MI, stroke, and cardiovascular death
8. Phosphodiesterase inhibitors (PDE-3, PDE-4, and PDE-5): Increased mortality
9. Antiarrhythmic: Negative inotropic activity and further reduction in LV function can impair the elimination and result in toxicity of the antiarrhythmic.
10. Chemotherapy: Many are cardiotoxic.
11. Androgen-testosterone patch: Edema may increase the rate of HF.
12. Theophylline-serum levels may increase and cause toxicity because of acute decompensation of HF.
13. Sodium bicarbonate and Fleet Phospho-Soda contain significant quantities of sodium.
14. Herbal/supplements may also affect HF.

F. Biventricular pacing or an implantable defibrillator may be necessary for advanced HF.

G. Discuss the need for palliative/hospice care when HF does not respond despite maximal therapy.

H. Discuss the patient's desire for advanced therapies that might include an evaluation for heart transplant or ventricular assist device.

I. The pneumonia vaccination as well as yearly influenza immunization should be encouraged.

Follow-Up

A. HF patients should be comanaged with a physician.

B. Close follow-up is essential if the patient is to be maintained as an outpatient.

C. Appointments every 1 to 2 weeks may be necessary, with additional appointments depending on the patient's symptoms such as increasing SOB, inability to lie flat to sleep, nocturnal moist cough, and increase in daily weight.

D. Laboratory monitoring is required for electrolytes, blood urea nitrogen (BUN), creatinine, proteinuria, and digoxin level.

Consultation/Referral

A. Consult a physician when the patient requires the next level up in pharmacological management.

B. Consult a cardiologist for staging and hospital management.

Individual Considerations

A. Pregnancy

1. HF is uncommon in healthy women without coexisting heart disease.
2. Pregnancy in a patient with heart disease is considered high risk.
3. Refer to a high-risk obstetrician.

B. Pediatrics: HF is usually associated with congenital heart defects.

C. Adults

1. The 5-year survival rate is 25% for men and 38% for women.
2. Predictors of poor outcome include an EF of less than 25%, ischemic etiology, ventricular arrhythmias, serum sodium less than 130 mEq/L, poor functional class, low cardiac index, and high-filling pressures.

TABLE 10.5 **Antihypertensive and Cardiac Medications (Sorted Alphabetically)**

Brand Name	Generic Name	Drug Class
Accupril	quinapril	ACEI
Aceon	perindopril erbumine	ACEI
Adalat CC	dihydropyridine/nifedipine	CCB
Aldactazide	spironolactone + HCTZ	Combination—K + sparing + thiazide
Aldactone	spironolactone	Diuretic—K + sparing
Altace	ramipril	ACEI
Amiloride/HCTZ	amiloride/HCTZ	Combination + diuretic
Atacand	candesartan cilexetil	Angiotensin II receptor blocker
Atacand HCT	candesartan + HCTZ	Combination—ARB + diuretic
Avalide	irbesartan + HCTZ	Combination—ARB + diuretic
Avalide Avapro	irbesartan + HCTZ irbesartan	Combination—ARB + diuretic angiotensin II receptor blocker
Azor	amlodipine + olmesartan	CCB + ARB
Benicar	olmesartan medoxomil	Angiotensin II receptor blocker
Benicar HCT	olmesartan + HCTZ	Combination—ARB + diuretic
Betapace	sotalol	Beta-blocker/class II and III antiarrhythmic
Betapace AF	sotalol	Class II and III antiarrhythmics
Betaxolol Bidil	betaxolol HCl isosorbide dinitrate + hydralazine	Beta-blocker-cardioselective nitrate + diuretic
Bumex	bumetanide	Loop diuretic
Bystolic	nebivolol	Beta-blocker-cardioselective
Caduet	amlodipine + atorvastatin	CCB/amlodipine/atorvastatin
Calan	verapamil	CCB/antianginal
Calan SR	verapamil	CCB
Capoten	captopril	ACEI/CHF
Capozide	captopril + HCTZ	Combination—ACE + diuretic
Cardizem LA	diltiazem	CCB
Cardura	doxazosin	Alpha 2 blocker AAB
Catapres	clonidine	Central alpha agonist
Chlorothiazide	various	Thiazide diuretic
Chlorthalidone	various	Monosulfamyl diuretic
Cleviprex	clevidipine	CCB
Cordarone	amiodarone	Class II and III antiarrhythmics
Coreg CR	carvedilol	Beta-blocker-noncardioselective/CHF
Corgard	nadolol	Beta-blocker-noncardioselective/antianginal
Corzide	nadolol + HCTZ	Combination beta-blocker (noncardioselective) + diuretic
Covera-HS	verapamil	CCB/antianginal
Cozaar	losartan	Angiotensin II receptor blocker (ARB)
Demadex	torsemide	Loop diuretic
Lanoxin	digoxin	Cardiac glycoside/antiarrhythmic
Dilacor XR	diltiazem	Calcium channel blocker/antianginal
Dilatrate SR	isosorbide dinitrate	Nitrate
Diovan	valsartan	Angiotensin II receptor blocker/CHF class II-IV
Diovan HCT	valsartan + HCTZ	Combination—ARB + diuretic

(*continued*)

TABLE 10.5 Antihypertensive and Cardiac Medications (Sorted Alphabetically) (*continued*)

Brand Name	Generic Name	Drug Class
Diuril	chlorothiazide	Thiazide diuretic
Dutoprol Dyazide	metoprolol ext. release + HCTZ triamterene + HCTZ	Beta-blocker (cardioselective) + thiazide combination—K + sparing + thiazide
Dynacirc CR	isradipine controlled release	CCB
Edarbi	azilsartan	Angiotensin II receptor blocker
Edarbyclor	azilsartan + chlorthalidone	Angiotensin II receptor blocker + diuretic
Edecrin	ethacrynic acid	Loop diuretic
Exforge	amlodipine + valsartan	CCB + ARB
Fosinopril HCTZ	various hydrochlorothiazide	ACEI thiazide diuretic
Hytrin	terazosin	Alpha 1 blocker
Hyzaar	losartan potassium + HCTZ	Combination ARB + diuretic
Imdur	isosorbide dinitrate	Nitrate
Inderal	propranolol	Beta-blocker-noncardioselective/antianginal/antiarrhythmic
Inderide	propranolol + HCTZ	Combination-beta-blocker (noncardioselective) + diuretic
Innopran XL	propranolol HCL ext. release	Beta-blocker-noncardioselective
Inspra	eplerenone	Aldosterone receptor blocker—mineralocorticoid selective/CHF
ISMO	isosorbide mononitrate	Nitrate
Isoptin SR	verapamil	CCB
Isordil	various	Nitrate
Kerlone	betaxolol	Beta-blocker-cardioselective
Lanoxin	digoxin	Cardiac glycoside/antiarrhythmic
Lasix	furosemide	Loop diuretic
Levatol	penbutolol sulfate	Beta-blocker-noncardioselective
Lopressor	metoprolol tartrate	Beta-blocker-cardioselective/antianginal
Lopressor HCT	metoprolol + HCTZ	Combination-beta-blocker (cardioselective) + diuretic
Lotensin	benazepril	ACEI
Lotensin HCT	benazepril + HCTZ	Combination—ACE + diuretic
Lotrel	amlodipine + benazepril	Combination—CCB + ACEI
Mavik	trandolapril	ACE inhibitor/CHF
Maxide	triamterene + HCTZ	Combination—K + sparing + thiazide
Micardis	telmisartan	Angiotensin II receptor blocker
Micardis HCT	telmisartan + HCTZ	Combination—ARB + diuretic
Microzide	hydrochlorothiazide (HCTZ)	Diuretic
Minitran	nitroglycerin	Nitrate
Monoket	isosorbide dinitrate	Nitrate
Monopril	fosinopril	ACEI/CHF
Multaq	dronedarone	Antiarrhythmic
Nicardipine	various	Calcium channel blocker
Nitro-BID	nitroglycerin	Nitrate
Nitro-Dur	nitroglycerin	Nitrate
Nitrolingual	nitroglycerin	Nitrate
Nitrostat	nitroglycerin	Nitrate
Normodyne	labetalol	Beta-blocker

(*continued*)

TABLE 10.5 Antihypertensive and Cardiac Medications (Sorted Alphabetically) (*continued*)

Brand Name	Generic Name	Drug Class
Norpace	disopyramide	Antiarrhythmics-class 1 ventricular
Norvasc	amlodipine	CCB/antianginal
Pindolol	pindolol	Beta-blocker-noncardioselective
Plendil	felodipine	CCB
Prinivil	lisinopril	ACEI/CHF
Prinzide	lisinopril + HCTZ	Combination-ACE inhibitor + thiazide diuretic
Procanbid	procainamide	Antiarrhythmics-class 1a ventricular
Procardia XL	nifedipine	CCB/antianginal
Quinidine gluconate	various	Antiarrhythmics-class 1 atrial and ventricular
Quinidine sulfate	various	Antiarrhythmics-class 1 atrial and ventricular
Ranexa	ranolazine	Antianginal
Rythmol	propafenone	Antiarrhythmics-class 1c ventricular
Sectral	acebutolol	Beta-blocker-cardioselective
Sular	nisoldipine	CCB
Tambocor	flecainide	Antiarrhythmics-class 1c-ventricular
Tarka	trandolapril + verapamil	Combination—ACE + CCB
Tekamlo	aliskiren + amlodipine	Direct renin inhibitor + DHP CCB
Tekturna	aliskiren	Direct renin inhibitor
Tekturna HCT	aliskiren + HCTZ	Direct renin inhibitor + thiazide diuretic
Tenex	guanfacine	Central alpha agonist
Tenoretic	atenolol + chlorthalidone	Combination-beta-blocker (cardioselective) + diuretic
Tenormin	atenolol	Beta-blocker-cardioselective/antianginal
Teveten	eprosartan	Angiotensin II receptor blocker
Teveten HCT	eprosartan + HCTZ	Combination—ARB + diuretic
Thalitone	chlorthalidone	Antihypertensive/diuretic
Tiazac	diltiazem	CCB/antianginal
Timolide	timolol maleate + HCTZ	Combination-beta-blocker (noncardioselective) + diuretic
Toprol-XL	metoprolol	Beta-blocker-cardioselective/antianginal/CHF class II or III
Trandate	labetalol	Beta-blocker-noncardioselective
Tribenzor	olmesartan + amlodipine + HCTZ	ARB + calcium channel blocker + thiazide diuretic
Twynsta	telmisartan + amlodipine	ARB + calcium channel blocker
Uniretic	moexipril + HCTZ	Combination—ACE + diuretic
Univasc	moexipril	ACEI
Valturna	aliskiren + valsartan	Direct renin inhibitor + ARB
Vaseretic	enalapril + HCTZ	Combination—ACE + diuretic
Vasotec	enalapril	ACEI/CHF with digitalis and diuretics
Verelan PM	verapamil	CCB
Zaroxolyn	metolazone	Diuretic—Quinazoline
Zebeta	bisoprolol	Beta-blocker—cardioselective
Zestoretic	lisinopril + HCTZ	Combination—ACE + diuretic
Zestril	lisinopril	ACEI/CHF with digitalis and diuretics
Ziac	bisoprolol + HCTZ	Combination-beta-blocker (cardioselective) + diuretic

AAB, alpha adrenergic blocker; ACEI, angiotensin-converting enzyme inhibitor; ARB, angiotensin receptor blocker; CCB, calcium channel blocker; CHF, congestive heart failure; DHP, dihydropyridine; HCTZ, hydrochlorothiazide.

D. Geriatrics

1. In very frail elderly patients or those in long-term care settings, the only sign may be increased agitation or acute change in level of consciousness (LOC).

Hypertension

Jill C. Cash, Cheryl A. Glass, and Debbie Gunter

Definition

A. Hypertension (HTN) is considered to be a systolic blood pressure (SBP) of 140 mmHg or more, a diastolic blood pressure (DBP) of 90 mmHg or more, or describes a condition in which a person is taking antihypertensive medications. The Eighth Joint National Committee (JNC) defines HTN in adults as follows (see Table 10.6).

B. Resistant HTN is defined as:

1. BP that is not at target despite a three-drug regimen, with one of the agents being a diuretic appropriate for the patient's glomerular filtration rate (GFR).
2. BP that is controlled while taking four or more medications is also considered resistant HTN.

C. Standing and supine BPs should be measured before the initiation of combination antihypertensive therapy. Orthostatic (postural) hypotension is diagnosed when, within 2 to 5 minutes of quiet standing, one or more of the following is present:

1. At least a 20 mmHg fall in systolic pressure
2. At least a 10 mmHg fall in diastolic pressure
3. Symptoms of cerebral hypoperfusion, such as dizziness

D. The average nocturnal BP is approximately 15% lower than daytime values. Failure of the BP to fall by at least 10% during sleep is called "nondipping" and is a stronger predictor of adverse cardiovascular outcomes than daytime BP.

E. *Isolated systolic HTN (ISH)* is when the SBP is greater than or equal to 140 with DBP normal or below normal (<90 mmHg). ISH usually affects the elderly, increasing their risk of stroke or myocardial infarction (MI).

F. *Isolated diastolic hypertension (IDH)* is defined as a diastolic pressure greater than or equal to 90 mmHg with a systolic pressure less than 140 mmHg. IDH is more common in younger men who are overweight/obese and in individuals younger than 40 years.

TABLE 10.6 JNC 8 Classification of Blood Pressure in Adults 18 Years or Older

Blood Pressure Classification	Systolic Blood Pressure (mmHg)	Diastolic Blood Pressure (mmHg)
Normal	<120	and <80
PreHTN	120–139	or 80–89
Stage 1 HTN	140–159	or 90–99
Stage 2 HTN	≥160	or ≥100

HTN, hypertension; JNC, Joint National Committee.
Source: U.S. Department of Health and Human Services, National Institutes of Health, & National Heart, Lung, and Blood Institute (2004).

G. Malignant HTN is marked HTN with retinal hemorrhages, exudates, or papilledema. Malignant HTN is usually associated with diastolic pressures above 120 mmHg.

Incidence

A. Worldwide, HTN affects about 975 million people.

B. Approximately 77.9 million or one in three adults in the United States has HTN.

C. The incidence of resistant HTN is being studied more closely and the current average rate is about 12% of all patients with hypertension.

D. The 2009 overall death rate from high BP was 18.5 per 100,000. Death rates were:

- 17.0 for White males
- 14.4 for White females
- 51.6 for Black males
- 38.3 for Black females

Pathogenesis

More than 90% of cases have no identifiable cause, thus constituting the category of primary or essential HTN. The remaining 10% of cases have the following secondary causes:

A. Renal causes

1. Glomerulonephritis
2. Pyelonephritis
3. Polycystic kidney disease

B. Endocrine causes

1. Primary hyperaldosteronism
2. Pheochromocytoma
3. Hyperthyroidism
4. Cushing's syndrome

C. Vascular causes

1. Coarctation of aorta
2. Renal artery stenosis

D. Chemical/medication induced

1. Oral contraceptives
2. Nonsteroidal anti-inflammatory drugs (NSAIDs)
3. Decongestants
4. Antidepressants
5. Sympathomimetics
6. Corticosteroids
7. Lithium
8. Ergotamine alkaloids
9. Cyclosporine
10. Monoamine oxidase inhibitors (MAOIs), in combination with certain drugs or foods
11. Appetite suppressants, in combination with certain drugs or foods
12. Cocaine
13. Amphetamines

E. Obstructive sleep apnea (OSA)

Predisposing Factors

When making a diagnosis, consider not only the absolute BP reading, but also the presence or absence of other cardiovascular risk factors. Factors include the following:

A. Family history of HTN

B. Obesity

C. Alcohol consumption
D. Stress
E. Sedentary lifestyle
F. African American ancestry
G. Male gender
H. Age greater than 30 years
I. Excessive salt intake
J. Medications
K. Drug use

Common Complaint

A. HTN is asymptomatic in the majority of patients.

Other Signs and Symptoms

A. Headaches
B. Advanced disease: Organ-specific complaints with end-organ damage
C. Retinopathy

Potential Complications

A. Cerebral vascular accident (CVA)
B. MI
C. Renal failure
D. Heart failure (HF)
E. Peripheral arterial disease (PAD)

Subjective Data

A. Ask the patient about any family history of HTN or cardiac or renal disease.
B. Ask if the patient has ever been diagnosed with HTN or cardiac or renal disease.
C. Ask if the patient ever had any high BP readings.
D. Ask if the patient has ever been treated for any of the aforementioned problems.
E. Ask the patient about other risk factors such as smoking, drinking, high-fat intake, obesity, and/or diabetes.
F. Inquire about the patient's lifestyle, exercise regimen, work environment, and stress level.
G. Ask the patient about symptoms that suggest secondary etiology.
 1. Palpitations, headache, diaphoresis (pheochromocytoma)
 2. Anxiety, weight gain or loss (thyroid abnormality)
 3. Muscle weakness, polyuria (primary hyperaldosteronism)
H. Find out if the patient is taking drugs that elevate BP (noted under "Pathogenesis").
I. Ask whether the patient feels nervous when having his or her BP taken in the office ("white coat HTN").
J. Review current medications, including prescription, over-the-counter (OTC), and herbal products.
K. Review current recreational/illicit drug use.

Physical Examination

A. Check pulse, BP, height, weight, waist circumference, and distribution of body fat. Calculate body mass index (BMI).
 1. The diagnosis of HTN is made after averaging two or more properly measured readings at each of two or more visits after an initial screen.
 2. When the patient's SBP and DBP fall into two different categories, use the higher category to classify his or her BP.
 3. For accurate measurement, use the correct size cuff for the patient (adult, large adult, or thigh cuff).
B. Inspect
 1. Observe overall appearance.
 2. Conduct funduscopic examination; look for papilledema, exudates, atrioventricular (AV) nicking, anterior nicking.
 3. Inspect the neck for jugular vein distension.
 4. Observe for pedal edema.
C. Auscultate
 1. Heart; note the point of maximal impulse (PMI).
 2. Lungs; check for bronchospasm and rales.
 3. Neck; assess carotid arteries for bruits.
D. Palpate
 1. Palpate the neck; check thyroid for enlargement.
 2. Palpate the abdomen for masses or organomegaly.
 3. Palpate the extremities; assess peripheral pulses and note edema.
 4. Assess deep tendon reflexes (DTRs).

Diagnostic Tests

A. Hematocrit
B. Liver function tests (LFTs; lactate dehydrogenase [LDH], uric acid)
C. Chemistry profile
D. Lipid profile (total and HDL cholesterol and triglycerides)
E. Urinalysis for proteinuria
F. Estimated GFR
G. EKG
H. If history, physical examination, or laboratory tests indicate the need, obtain the following:
 1. Intravenous pyelography (IVP)
 2. Renal arteriogram
 3. Plasma renin
 4. Catecholamines
 5. Chest radiography
 6. Aortogram
 7. Ultrasonography
 8. Sleep study
I. Monitor potassium levels if on angiotensin-converting enzyme inhibitor/angiotensin receptor blocker (ACEI/ARBs) or spironolactone.

Differential Diagnoses

A. Primary HTN
B. Secondary HTN
C. Drug-induced HTN
D. White coat syndrome

Plan

A. General interventions (see Table 10.7)
 1. Advise overweight patients to lose weight. Loss of as little as 10 pounds reduces BP in many patients.

TABLE 10.7 Modifiable and Nonmodifiable Risk for Control of HTN

Modifiable	Nonmodifiable
Sedentary lifestyle	Age
Smoking	Gender
Diet	Ethnicity
Lipid control	Diabetes
Sodium intake	Postmenopausal
Alcohol intake	Family history
Obesity	

HTN, hypertension.

2. Advise the patient to limit or discontinue alcohol intake.
3. Encourage the patient to stop smoking.
4. Encourage increased physical activity. The 2013 American College of Cardiology/American Heart Association (ACC/AHA) guidelines on lifestyle management outline the newest physical activity recommendation, which advises adults to engage in 40 minutes of aerobic physical activity three to four times a week. The aerobic exercise should involve moderate to vigorous intensity.
5. Encourage some form of relaxation technique.

B. Patient teaching
1. Stress asymptomatic nature of disease.
2. Stress importance of ongoing monitoring and treatment under the direction of a health care provider.
3. Review risk factors for cardiac, renal, and cerebrovascular disease and possible preventive measures.
4. The ACC maintains the CardioSmart Patient Education Portal for an online BP management tool to educate and motivate patients. ACC's CardioSmart is a free resource located at www.cardiosmart.org CardioSmartTXT PREVENT is a 6-month program of health tips and reminders sent via two text messages a week. CardioSmartTXT QUIT is a 2-month program to assist patients in smoking cessation. Four text messages are sent a day with information and assistance with smoking cessation. Patients can sign up at http://author.cardiosmart.org/Tools/CardioSmartTXT-Prevent

C. Dietary management: Review specific dietary measures. Give dietary recommendation sheets. See Appendix B for low-fat/low-cholesterol and DASH dietary approaches to stop HTN.
1. Diet alone will make only the lowest incremental change in BP; therefore, it should be combined with lifestyle modification and lower sodium intake; smoking cessation; weight loss and exercise are essential.
2. It is essential for the patient/family to read labels for sodium, fat content, and serving sizes.
3. Other dietary changes include low-fat/low-cholesterol diets and limiting fats.
   a. Use monounsaturated fats to decrease cholesterol.
      i. Canola oil
      ii. Olive oil
   b. Use in limited quantities: Polyunsaturated fats decrease cholesterol, but not as well as monounsaturated.
      i. Vegetable and fish oils
      ii. Corn, safflower, peanut, and soybean oils
   c. Limit saturated fats.
      i. Animal fats and some plant fats
      ii. Butter and lard
      iii. Coconut oil and palm oil

D. Pharmaceutical therapy
1. If lifestyle changes alone are not adequate to control HTN, consider drug therapy. Medication doses are dependent on age, ethnicity, and comorbid conditions. Most patients will require two or more medications to control their BP. Consider starting antihypertensives and/or diuretics (see Table 10.5 for drugs and classifications). The Eighth Joint National Committee (JNC 8) recommendations were released in 2014 for the initiation of BP goals (see Table 10.8). The JNC 8 published an extensive algorithm for the treatment of hypertension. The algorithm is available at www.nmhs.net/documents/27JNC8HTNGuidelinesBookBooklet.pdf
2. The 2013 Science Advisory recommendations from the AHA, the ACC, and the Centers for Disease Control and Prevention (CDC) provide medication classifications for the treatment of HTN in the presence of medical conditions (see Table 10.9).
3. Antihypertensives/diuretics should be started low and increased if there is inadequate response to initial therapy and nonadherence is ruled out. Consider the following:
   a. Increasing drug dose
   b. Substituting another drug
   c. Adding a second drug from another class; a diuretic is recommended if one is not already being used.
   d. Beta-blockers are no longer first-line antihypertensive agents. Atenolol may increase central aortic pressure.
   e. ACEIs and ARBs are critical medications to prescribe and titrate to maximum dose as a first-line medication in people with renal disease, diabetes, and proteinuria.
4. If response is still inadequate, add a second or third drug or diuretic if one has not already been tried.
5. Evaluate the patient for secondary causes if severe HTN is resistant to therapy.
6. Resistant HTN; rule out all inadequate responses to the three-drug therapy (ACEI or ARB or CCB + diuretic):
   a. "White coat" HTN: Have the patient begin to take and record his or her BP at home and report the values.

TABLE 10.8 **Eighth Joint National Committee (JNC 8) Recommendations for the Management of Hypertension**

Ethnicity/ Population	Age (Years)	Begin Initiation of Pharmacological Treatment to Lower BP	BP Goals for Treatment	Other Comments
General population	≥60	Initiate therapy for SBP ≥150 mmHg OR DBP ≥90 mmHg	Treat to goal of SBP <150 mmHg *and* DBP <90 mmHg	If pharmacological treatment results in a lower achieved SBP and treatment is well tolerated, treatment does not need to be adjusted.
	<60	Initiate therapy to lower BP at SBP ≥140 mmHg	Treat to goal of SBP <140 mmHg	
		Initiate therapy to lower BP at DBP ≥90 mmHg	Treat to goal of DBP <90 mmHg	
Patients with chronic kidney disease	≥18	Initiate therapy to lower the SBP ≥140 mmHg OR DBP ≥90 mmHg	Treat to goal of SBP <140 mmHg *and* DBP <90 mmHg	
Patients with chronic kidney disease (regardless of race or diabetes status)	≥18			Initial or add-on antihypertensive therapy should include an ACEI or ARB to improve kidney outcomes.
Patients with diabetes	≥18	Initiate therapy to lower BP at SBP ≥140 mmHg *or* DBP ≥90 mmHg	Treat to goal of SBP <140 mmHg *and* DBP <90 mmHg	The American Diabetes Association recommends diabetics with hypertension should be treated to an SBP goal of <140 mmHg and to a DBP of <80 mmHg.
General non-Black population, including those with diabetes				Initial antihypertensive therapy should include a thiazide-type diuretic, CCB, ACEI, or ARB.
General Black population, including those with diabetes				Initial antihypertensive therapy should include a thiazide-type diuretic *or* CCB.

ACEI, angiotensin-converting enzyme inhibitor; ARB, angiotensin receptor blocker; BP, blood pressure; CCB, calcium channel blocker; DBP, diastolic blood pressure; SBP, systolic blood pressure.

TABLE 10.9 **AHA, ACC, and CDC 2013 Suggested Hypertensive Medications by Medical Condition**

Medical Condition	BB	ACEI or ARB	ALDO ANTAG	Thiazide	CCB
Coronary artery disease/post MI	X	X			
Systolic heart failure	X	X	X	X	
Diastolic heart failure	X	X		X	
Diabetes	X	X		X	X
Kidney disease		X			
Stroke or TIA		ACEI		X	

ACC, American College of Cardiology; ACEI, angiotensin-converting-enzyme inhibitor; AHA, American Heart Association; ALDO ANTAG, aldosterone antagonist; ARB, angiotensin II blocker; BB, beta-blocker; CCB, calcium channel blocker; CDC, Centers for Disease Control and Prevention; MI, myocardial infarction; TIA, transient ischemic attack.

b. Use size-appropriate BP cuffs on obese patients.
c. Nonadherence to therapy, including side effects, medication regimen too complex, and/or cost/affordability
d. Volume overload because of excessive salt intake, progressive renal damage, fluid retention from BP reduction, and inadequate diuretic therapy
e. Drug problems: Dose too low, wrong type of diuretic, inappropriate combinations, rapid inactivation, drug actions, and interactions
f. Associated conditions: Smoking, obesity, sleep apnea, insulin resistance, ethanol intake more than 30 mL (1 oz) per day, panic attacks, chronic pain, and organic brain syndrome
g. Adding spironolactones can decrease SBP by 25 mmHg on average and DBP by an average of 12 mmHg in resistant hypertensives.

7. Treat with decongestants very cautiously. Pseudoephedrine HCl (Sudafed) has the least cardiovascular effect.
8. Diuretics may worsen gout and diabetes.
9. Beta-blockers are contraindicated in asthma, HF, and heart block.
10. Use diltiazem HCl (Cardizem) and verapamil HCl (Calan) cautiously in HF or block.
11. ACEI may cause coughing.
12. Abrupt cessation of therapy with a short-acting beta-blocker, such as propranolol, or the short-acting alpha-2-agonist clonidine, can lead to a potentially fatal withdrawal syndrome. Gradual discontinuation of these agents over a period of weeks should prevent this syndrome.

Follow-Up

A. If drug therapy is initiated, see the patient again in 2 to 4 weeks for follow-up.
B. Once the patient is stable, see him or her every 3 to 6 months.
C. Evaluate the patient yearly, including uric acid, creatinine, and potassium.
D. Review and discuss drug therapy compliance, effectiveness, and adverse reactions (including effect on sexual activity) at each visit.
E. Home and ambulatory blood pressure monitoring (ABPM) is an adjunctive tool for the management of HTN.

1. BP tracking apps are available on iTunes for the iPhone, iPod touch, and iPad.
2. BP tracking apps for Androids are available on Google Play and Amazon Appstore.
3. The AHA/American Stroke Association has BP tracker instructions located at https://www.heart.org/idc/groups/heart-public/@wcm/@hcm/documents/downloadable/ucm_305157.pdf
4. A printable BP tracker log is located at www.organizedhome.com/sites/default/files/image/pdf/health_blood_pressure_tracker.pdf

F. Consider a sleep study for diagnosis of OSA (see Chapter 9, section on "Obstructive Sleep Apnea").
G. Patients with pre-HTN without diabetes, chronic kidney disease (CKD), or cardiovascular disease (CVD) should be treated with nonpharmacological therapy (i.e., diet, sodium reduction, weight loss, exercise, smoking cessation) and should be evaluated annually.

Consultation/Referral

A. If the patient is pregnant, consult a physician before prescribing medications. Many antihypertensive drugs are harmful to the fetus.
B. Consult a physician if the patient is having an acute hypertensive emergency: DBP greater than 130 mmHg.
C. Consult/comanage with a physician if the patient needs more than three drugs for therapy.

Individual Considerations

A. Pregnancy. Refer to Chapter 13, "Obstetrics Guidelines."

1. HTN may be either chronic or pregnancy induced.
2. HTN is considered chronic if it is present before pregnancy or diagnosed before the 20th week of gestation.
3. Pregnancy-induced hypertension (PIH) is diagnosed if SBP increases 30 mmHg or more, or if DBP increases 15 mmHg or more, compared with BP readings before the 20th week of gestation. When BP readings are not known, a reading of 140/90 or higher is considered abnormal.
4. Maternal as well as fetal mortality and morbidity improve with treatment.

B. Pediatrics

1. Evaluate BP at every visit starting at the age of 3 years.
2. HTN can occur in many acute illnesses, or it may be a chronic problem.
3. Determine high BP by correlating height indexes with BP readings.

C. Geriatrics

1. The optimal BP treatment goal in the elderly has not been determined as there is not a concensus among various national and international organizations. In the most recent JNC 8 guideline, treatment goals for individuals older than 65 years were changed to a goal of less than 150/90 mmHg. HTN in the elderly places the patient at risk of coronary events, stroke, HF, and PAD.
2. Elderly persons with HTN are more likely to develop orthostatic and postprandial hypotension, which may result in falls or syncope.
    a. Evaluate side effects, including dizziness and sedation. Beta-blockers may cause depression or confusion in the elderly.
3. The general approach to drug therapy in the geriatric population is to start low and go slow.
4. Check the Beers list for harmful drugs in the geriatric population. The 2015 American Geriatrics Society's,

Updated Beers Criteria for Potentially Inappropriate Medication Use in Older Adults is available at http://geriatricscareonline.org/ProductAbstract/american-geriatrics-society-updated-beers-criteria-for-potentially-inappropriate-medication-use-in-older-adults/CL001. A printable pocketcard is available for download at www.americangeriatrics.org/files/documents/beers/PrintableBeersPocketCard.pdf

5. To avoid hyperkalemia in the elderly, potassium-sparing diuretics should not be given with ACEI or ARBs.

Resource

The National Kidney Foundation provides online calculators: www.kidney.org/professionals/KDOQI/gfr_calculator

Lymphedema

Laura A. Petty

Definition

A. Peripheral vascular disease (PVD) is a general term that encompasses all occlusive or inflammatory diseases that occur within the peripheral arteries, veins, and lymphatic. Lymphedema is a chronic condition caused by the accumulation of lymphatic fluid in the interstitial tissue.

Incidence

A. The Vascular Disease Foundation reports that almost 1 million Americans have lymphedema. The incidence worldwide is projected to approach 100 million.

Pathogenesis

A. Lymphedema occurs when lymph fluid is unable to flow in a normal manner and accumulates in an extremity. The propensity for lymphedema can be inherited or caused by another condition such as lymphangitis, malignancy, filariasis, or removal of lymph nodes.

Predisposing Factors

A. Cancer
B. Radiation therapy
C. Surgical removal of lymph nodes
D. Parasitic infection (Filariasis)
E. Congenital disorders involving the structure of the lymph system
  1. Milroy's disease
  2. Meige's disease
F. Obesity
G. Surgical implantation of pacemaker or arteriovenous shunt
H. Systemic diseases (hyperthyroidism, hypertension, renal or cardiac disease)
I. Vascular disease (chronic venous insufficiency or post-thrombotic syndrome)

Common Complaints

A. Severe edem, that is consistent to the distal aspect of the extremity
B. Hard skin over edematous area
C. Loss of range of motion

Potential Complications

A. Infection, including lymphangitis and cellulitis
B. Lymphangiosarcoma

Subjective Data

A. Ask the patient when the symptom(s) were first noticed.
B. Have the patient describe the duration of symptoms.
C. Review any history of cancer, radiation, and chemotherapy.
D. Review recent history of invasive procedures or surgery.
E. Ask the patient to list all medications currently being taken, particularly substances not prescribed and illicit drugs.
F. Ask the patient to describe any pain.
G. Ask the patient what makes the symptoms better and vwhat makes them worse.
H. Have the patient rate discomfort on a scale of 1 to 10, with 1 being the least uncomfortable.

Physical Examination

A. Vital signs
  1. Check blood pressure (BP) and document resting heart rate, respirations, temperature, height, and weight.
B. Inspect
  1. Assess for signs of erythema, increased temperature, and edema.
C. Palpate
  1. Lymph nodes distal and proximal to the site
  2. Pulses distal and proximal in all extremities
  3. Extremity for tenderness
D. Auscultate
  1. Heart: Rate, rhythm, heart sounds, murmur, and gallops.
  2. Lungs: Assess lung sounds in all fields.

Diagnostic Tests

A. Serum laboratory tests (complete blood count [CBC] with differential and brain natriuretic peptide [BNP])
B. CT scan of the affected extremity
C. Doppler ultrasound of the affected extremity
D. Testing to assess the extent of the lymphedema or to rule in/out an etiology
  1. CT scan, MRI, and/or Doppler
E. Lymphoscintigraphy
F. Additional tests to monitor coexisting systemic and/or vascular disease

Differential Diagnoses

A. Unilateral limb edema
  1. Lymphedema
  2. Venous insufficiency
  3. Deep vein thrombosis or post-thrombotic syndrome
  4. Arthritis
  5. Baker's cyst
  6. Presence or reoccurrence of cancer
B. Symmetrical limb edema
  1. Congestive heart failure (CHF)

2. Chronic venous insufficiency
3. Renal dysfunction
4. Hepatic dysfunction
5. Hypothyroidism (Myxoedema)
6. Medication-induced edema
7. Lipoedema

Plan

A. Patient teaching: *See Section III: Patient Teaching Guide for this chapter, "Lymphedema."*
   1. Protect the arm or leg while recovering from cancer treatment.
   2. Avoid heavy lifting, if an arm is affected.
   3. Avoid strenuous exercise.
   4. Avoid heat on the arm or leg.
   5. Avoid tight clothing.
   6. Inspect the affected limb daily, noting any cracks or cuts.
   7. Apply lotion daily to protect and prevent dry skin.

B. Nonpharmaceutical therapy
   1. Extremity elevation
   2. Compression stockings or wrapping of affected limb
   3. Pneumatic compression boot
   4. Therapeutic massage, specifically manual lymph drainage
   5. Referral to a lymphedema therapist
   6. Referral to physical therapy for home exercise program

C. Surgery
   1. Lymphaticovenular bypass
   2. Lymphovenous bypass

Follow-Up

A. Follow-up is determined by patient's needs, frequency and intensity of symptoms, and presence of other medical conditions.
B. PVD manifesting persistent symptoms should always be followed by a cardiologist.

Consultation/Referral

A. If you suspect acute limb ischemia, refer the patient for immediate hospitalization in order to obtain diagnostic testing to determine the presence of a thrombus and restore circulation to the affected extremity.
B. If chronic limb ischemia has led to ulceration and/or superimposed infection, hospitalization is indicated to initiate a wound care consultation and for diagnostic testing to determine the degree of arterial occlusion.
C. Referral to a cardiologist is indicated in the presence of persistent PVD symptoms.
D. Referral to a lymphedema therapist and physical therapist is indicated to best manage chronic lymphedema.

Murmurs

Jill C. Cash and Debbie Gunter

Definition

A murmur is turbulent blood flow through the heart as a result of one or more of the following etiologies:

A. Narrow valve opening, stenosis
B. Incomplete valve closure, regurgitant or insufficient blood flow
C. Abnormal opening through chambers, atrial or ventricular septal defect
D. Rapid blood flow through normal valve structures; occurs during pregnancy, with increased physiological demand states, and in children
E. No abnormality; occurs in patients with thin chest walls and in children

Incidence

A. Approximately 80% of children have a physiological murmur at one time or another. Four percent of women studied in the Framingham study had a murmur related to mitral valve prolapse (MVP).

Pathogenesis

A. Pathogenesis depends on specific etiology, but rheumatic disease, calcific changes, ischemic insults, congenital abnormalities, and degenerative diseases all contribute to the development of a murmur.

Common Complaints

A. Often no symptoms are present, and murmur is found on routine examination.
B. Complaints with advanced valvular disease:
   1. Chest pain
   2. Dyspnea
   3. Palpitations
   4. Shortness of breath (SOB)
   5. Exercise intolerance
   6. Postural light-headedness

Subjective Data

A. Has the patient ever been diagnosed with a murmur?
B. Did the patient have frequent strep infections as a child?
C. Ask the patient about any recent viral infections.
D. Question the patient about chest pain; SOB; palpitations; diaphoresis; light-headedness; or syncope, especially with exertion.
E. Ask the patient whether any family members had sudden cardiac death before the age of 55 years.

Physical Examination

A. Check temperature, if indicated, pulse, respirations, and BP.
B. Inspect
   1. Chest for lifts and heaves.
C. Palpate
   1. Chest for lifts, heaves, and thrills.
D. Auscultate
   1. Heart for splitting of heart sounds, clicks, rubs, and murmurs; use the bell and diaphragm of the stethoscope to auscultate the patient in the left lateral, supine, standing, sitting (and leaning forward), and squatting positions and after having patient run in place or do jumping jacks for 2 to 3 minutes.

a. A new, systolic, regurgitant murmur in the setting of an acute myocardial infarction (MI) may indicate a ruptured papillary muscle and possible cardiogenic shock.
b. When a new murmur is audible, differentiate location, timing, quality, intensity, and duration. Note if radiation to the neck, axilla, or back is present.
c. Note location of murmur.
i. Aortic: Second right intercostal space (ICS) next to sternum
ii. Pulmonic: Second left ICS next to sternum
iii. Tricuspid: Fifth left ICS next to sternum
iv. Mitral: Fifth left ICS at midclavicular line
d. If murmur is heard, have the patient squat, stand, and/or perform the Valsalva maneuver. Squatting will increase the blood to the heart and increase the left ventricle blood volume and stroke volume, which will increase the sound of the murmur. Standing and the Valsalva maneuver will provide the opposite, in which the venous return will drop and decrease the ventricle size and stroke volume and soften the sound of the murmur.
e. If the sound of the murmur occurs during the opposite action, softer when squatting and louder when standing or during the Valsalva maneuver, consider hypertrophic cardiomyopathy or MVP as the diagnosis.
2. Assess the neck and axilla for radiation

Diagnostic Tests

A. EKG
B. Echocardiogram
C. Chest radiography

Differential Diagnoses

Major differentiation should be in the description of murmur, as this aids in identification of the murmur.
A. Timing
1. Identify when the murmur occurs in the cardiac cycle.
2. Systolic murmurs may or may not be normal.
a. Occurs between the S1 "lub" and the S2 "dub."
3. Diastolic murmurs are always abnormal and need further evaluation.
a. Occurs between the S2 "dub" and the S1 "lub."
B. Quality: Is the sound harsh, blowing, musical, rumbling, vibratory, or soft?
C. Intensity: Murmurs are usually graded on a six-point scale:
- Grade I. Barely audible
- Grade II. Audible but soft
- Grade III. Easily audible without thrill
- Grade IV. Easily audible, thrill usually palpable
- Grade V. Audible with only the rim of the stethoscope on the chest wall; thrill present
- Grade VI. Audible with the stethoscope barely off the chest wall; thrill present

D. Duration: Identify location and timing in the specific phase of the cardiac cycle:
1. Holosystolic: Throughout systole
2. Holodiastolic: Throughout diastole
3. Midsystolic: Midway between S1 and S3
4. Mid-diastolic: Midway between S2 and S1
5. Decrescendo: Starts loud at the beginning, then tapers off
6. Crescendo: Starts soft at the beginning, then gets louder
E. Radiation: Murmur can be heard in another place, such as the neck, back, left axilla, or across precordium. Sound usually radiates in the direction of blood flow.
F. Location: Identify location on chest wall where murmur is heard the best. Identify site: Apex, pulmonary area, tricuspid, and aortic areas. Radiation murmur may also include axilla, left fourth ICS, or base of heart.
G. Configuration: The intensity of the murmur over time: Does it plateau, crescendo, decrescendo, or crescendo-decrescendo?
H. Systolic murmurs: Systolic murmurs are benign or pathologic.
1. Early systolic murmurs
a. Mitral regurgitation: Holosystolic, blowing may be loud. Located at fifth ICS and radiates to left axilla/back. Heard best in left lateral position and with sudden squatting; intensity decreases with the Valsalva maneuver and standing.
b. Tricuspid regurgitation: Holosystolic, heard in left lower sternal border or apex when right ventricle is enlarged. Intensity increases with inspiration and decreases with expiration. Straight leg raises may increase intensity. May also see hepatojugular reflux (HJR).
c. Physiological: Early to midsystolic, low-pitch normal S1–S2, located at left lower sternal edge at third to fourth ICS. Heard best with bell and supine and disappears when sitting up or holding breath. Commonly seen in children, pregnancy, and infection.
2. Midsystolic to late systolic murmurs
a. Aortic stenosis: Loud, hard crescendo–decrescendo at second right ICS that radiates to the neck. Heard best when patient is leaning forward, increases with leg raise and lying flat. Decreases with Valsalva and handgrip standing.
b. Pulmonic stenosis: Prolonged, loud S2 or crescendo-decrescendo, usually greater than 3/6 at second ICS and radiates to neck; increases with inspiration.
c. Hypertrophic cardiomyopathy (aortic outflow obstruction): Peaks at midsystole; loud, harsh tone at left, lower sternal border that may radiate to neck. Increases with Valsalva maneuver and standing, decreases with sudden squatting. Note brisk carotid upstroke.

3. Late systolic murmurs

a. MVP: Midsystolic click heard before late systolic murmur, heard best at fifth left ICS. Heard best with diaphragm; sitting or squatting may increase intensity.

b. Tricuspid valve prolapse: Heard over the left lower sternal border, delayed onset of murmur with inspiration secondary to an increase in the right ventricular volume.

I. Diastolic murmurs: Murmurs are always pathologic.

1. Early diastolic murmur

a. Aortic regurgitation: High-pitch faint, decrescendo may start with S2, at third left ICS and radiate down sternal edge. Heard best when patient is leaning forward, holding breath. Increases with sudden squatting or handgrip. May hear displaced PMI, S3, bounding pulse.

b. Pulmonary regurgitation: Valvular, dilation of valve annulus, congenital defect (tetralogy of Fallot ventricular septal defect [VSD]), pulmonic stenosis. Best heard over left second/third ICS. May sound high pitched with "blowing" sound in patients with hypertension (HTN). May be pansystolic, having decrescendo configuration.

2. Middiastolic murmur

a. Mitral stenosis: Rumbling extends beyond mid-diastole at fifth ICS, heard best using the bell of the stethoscope. Increases with left lateral position. May hear snap after S2.

b. Tricuspid stenosis: Increased flow across the tricuspid valve, heard best at the left sternal border. Identified by its increase in intensity of the murmur with inspiration (Carvallo's sign). Commonly seen with mitral stenosis.

Plan

A. General interventions

1. Major therapeutic goals are to preserve quality of life, increase life expectancy and exercise capacity, and reduce risk of complications.

2. Activity restriction is not necessary in patients with asymptomatic valvular disease.

B. Patient teaching

1. Reassure the patient regarding specific diagnosis.

2. Counsel the patient regarding his or her specific condition. Teach the patient signs and symptoms to report to the health provider, including chest pain, SOB, difficulty breathing, and so forth.

C. Medical and surgical management: Patients who need progressive increases in medications to control symptoms may be candidates for valve replacement surgery.

D. Pharmaceutical therapy

1. The 2007 American Heart Association (AHA) guidelines (these remain the most up to date) do not recommend endocarditis antimicrobial prophylaxis treatment for common valvular lesions that include bicuspid aortic valve, acquired aortic or mitral valve disease (including MVP with regurgitation), and hypertrophic cardiomyopathy with latent or resting obstruction.

2. The European Society of Cardiology (ESC) published a recent guideline in 2015, which continued to support the recommendations from the AHA 2007 guideline.

E. Endocarditis prophylaxis treatment: Cardiac conditions

1. It is recommended for high-risk cardiac condition abnormalities to have prophylactic treatment. Specific cardiac conditions are as follows:

a. Prosthetic cardiac valve or prosthetic material used for cardiac valve repair

b. Previous infective endocarditis

c. Certain congenital heart diseases, such as cyanotic congenital heart disease that has not been repaired; a congenital heart disease that has been repaired with an artificial material or device for 6 months after repair; and repaired congenital heart defects with continued problems, such as leaks or insufficient flow at the prosthetic device or adjacent to the repair endocarditis prophylaxis treatment

d. Postcardiac transplant valvulopathy

2. Procedures for high-risk patients mentioned earlier that require prophylaxis treatment:

a. All dental procedures with manipulation of gingival tissue or periapical region of teeth or perforation of oral mucosa

b. Incision or biopsy of respiratory mucosa or any invasive procedure of the respiratory tract system

c. Procedures that include infected skin or musculoskeletal tissue

d. Preventative treatment with antibiotics is not recommended for procedures that include the reproductive tract, urinary tract, or gastrointestinal (GI) tract.

3. Antibiotic prophylactic regimens include a single dose 30 to 60 minutes before procedure:

a. Amoxicillin single dose: 2 g by mouth, intramuscular (IM), or intravenous (IV) for adults or 50 mg/kg for children

b. Ampicillin 2 g IM or IV or 50 mg/kg IM or IV

c. Allergy to penicillin (PCN): Cephalexin 2 g by mouth for adults or 50 mg/kg for children

d. Azithromycin or clarithromycin 500 g for adults or 15 mg/kg for children

e. Allergic to aforementioned: Consider cefazolin or ceftriaxone 1 g IM or IV for adults or 50 mg/kg IM or IV for children, or clindamycin 600 mg IM or IV for adults or 20 mg/kg IM or IV children.

4. Other pharmaceutical treatments depend on the specific valvular abnormality.

a. Mitral stenosis: The mitral valve has a narrowing that does not allow adequate blood to the left ventricle during diastole, usually because of rheumatic heart disease. Mitral heart disease is the most commonly seen valve effect with rheumatic heart disease.

b. Diuretics, such as furosemide (Lasix) or hydrochlorothiazide (HydroDiuril), are used to control edema.

c. Digoxin (Lanoxin) or beta-blockers are used to control atrial fibrillation (AF) and irregular heart rate.

d. Warfarin (Coumadin) and the antiplatelet agent aspirin (Bayer) are used to prevent clotting.

e. MVP: The echocardiogram is the recommended test for diagnosis of MVP. Usually no medications are recommended except when symptomatic and required.

i. Beta-blockers (such as Atenolol) may be used for palpitations.

ii. Diuretics should be avoided in patients who are volume reserved.

iii. Oral contraceptives should be avoided in women who exhibit neurologic symptoms.

f. Mitral regurgitation: Diuretics, digitalis, and afterload-reducing agents for congestive heart failure (CHF):

i. Aortic stenosis

ii. Diuretics are used for CHF.

iii. Avoid vasodilators; they may result in profound, irreversible hypotension.

iv. Echocardiograms should be performed every 6 to 12 months to follow the progression of narrowing of the left ventricle across the aortic valve.

g. Aortic regurgitation: Afterload-reducing agents, digitalis, and diuretics are recommended.

Follow-Up

A. Most patients with valvular disease should be evaluated at least once a year.

B. Patients on oral anticoagulation drugs need monthly follow-up or as needed prothrombin time/international normalized ratios (PT/INRs).

Consultation/Referral

A. Consult a physician if the patient is diagnosed with a new murmur or exercise-induced symptoms during a sports physical.

B. Refer patients with newly diagnosed murmurs to a cardiologist after obtaining echocardiogram results. Drug therapy should be initiated according to diagnosis and symptoms.

C. Onset of AF with rapid ventricular response is an indication for immediate hospitalization.

D. Refer patients with systemic embolization to a physician for emergent anticoagulation therapy and chronic oral anticoagulant therapy. Discuss the possibility of valve replacement with a cardiologist.

E. If a new murmur is diagnosed in a pregnant patient with a history of cardiac disease, refer her to a physician immediately.

F. All diastolic murmurs in pediatric patients indicate pathology and need to be evaluated by a physician.

Individual Considerations

A. Pregnancy

1. The development of a new, "high-flow" murmur in a healthy woman is not uncommon because of physiological changes occurring during pregnancy.

B. Pediatrics

1. Perform a thorough cardiac examination on patients from the time they are newborns through adolescence, so that if a murmur is detected, it can be compared.

C. Geriatrics

1. A systolic murmur heard best in the aortic area may indicate aortic sclerosis because of aging of the aortic valve rather than true aortic stenosis.

Palpitations

Jill C. Cash and Debbie Gunter

Definition

A. Palpitations are a feeling or an unpleasant awareness of the heartbeat in the chest. It may be described as feeling a sensation of the heart "flip-flopping" or feeling a "rapid flutter" of the heart.

Incidence

A. The incidence of palpitations may range from 1% to 8% of patients in a general practice setting.

Pathogenesis

Palpitations may be caused by the following:

A. Increase in stroke volume or contractility

B. Sudden change in heart rate or rhythm

C. Unusual cardiac movement within thorax

D. Hyperkinetic states, which cause constant pounding; hyperthyroidism, late-stage pregnancy

E. Valvular heart disease that produces large stroke volumes

F. Catecholamine release during anxiety or panic attacks

Predisposing Factors

A. Cardiac defects

B. Severe anemia

C. Hyperthyroidism

D. Pregnancy

E. Fever

F. Anxiety

G. Stimulants such as caffeine and certain drugs

H. Emotions such as fear

I. Exertion

J. Diabetes mellitus and insulin reaction

Common Complaints

A. Palpitations are often described as a turning over or flopping sensation in the chest, but symptoms vary enormously.

B. Most patients are free of palpitations at the time of the examination.

Other Signs and Symptoms

A. Fluttering in the chest

B. Shortness of breath (SOB)

C. Pounding in the chest and neck

D. Diaphoresis
E. Lightheadedness
F. Anxiety or fear

Subjective Data

A. Ask the patient when symptoms first presented, including age, and how they have changed.
B. Have the patient describe the characteristics of the palpitations such as rapid, regular, irregular, or slow.
C. Ask the patient what precipitates the palpitations. Does anything terminate them, or do they go away on their own?
D. Inquire whether symptoms occur or change with position (standing, bending over, lying down, left lateral decubitus position) and/or exercise.
E. Ask the patient about other associated symptoms with the palpitations such as dizziness or syncope.
F. Ask how often the episodes occur and how long each lasts.
G. Discuss any previous treatments for this condition and the results.
H. Ask the patient about risk factors for coronary heart disease (CHD) and prior cardiac history.
I. Question the patient's use of over-the-counter (OTC) decongestants and diet pills. Are there any new medications or change in routine medications? Obtain a complete list of medications the patient is currently taking.

Physical Examination

A. Check pulse (count the pulse for 1 full minute), respirations, and blood pressure (BP).
B. Inspect
  1. Overall appearance
  2. The skin for diaphoresis and pallor
  3. The neck for thyromegaly or jugular vein distension
  4. The legs for edema
C. Palpate
  1. The skin for temperature and dryness
  2. The lower extremities for edema and calf tenderness
  3. The neck for thyroid enlargement
D. Auscultate
  1. The heart for abnormal rhythms. Auscultate heart with the patient in the sitting, standing, and left lateral decubitus positions. Ask the patient to walk quickly down the hallway and back and then auscultate the heart in all positions again.
  2. The lungs
  3. The neck and carotid arteries for bruits
E. Mental status: Does the patient appear lightheaded, anxious, or fearful?

Diagnostic Tests

Diagnostic testing is highly recommended for patients with an arrhythmia, who at risk of an arrhythmia, and patients who are anxious and want to explore causes for their symptoms.

Testing recommended:

A. Hemoglobin (Hgb) to rule out anemia, if suggestive on examination
B. Thyroid-stimulating hormone (TSH) to rule out hyperthyroidism, if suggestive on examination
C. EKG during episode, if possible
D. Ambulatory monitoring if symptoms continue, either 24-hour Holter monitor or patient-activated transtelephonic monitoring
E. Treadmill test if palpitations are provoked by exercise

Differential Diagnoses

A. Palpitations are secondary to the underlying problem such as anxiety, medications, or cardiac or pulmonary origin.

Plan

A. General interventions:
  1. Provide reassurance if the palpitations result from a neurotic concern.
B. Patient teaching
  1. Caution the patient to avoid any factors that trigger episodes. Factors may include stress, exercise, foods, and medications.
  2. Teach the patient a vagal maneuver, which is effective in halting palpitations.
C. Medical and surgical management: Correct any underlying problem (e.g., cardiac or pulmonary). Treat medical conditions accordingly. Management of arrhythmias should be monitored by a cardiologist.
D. Pharmaceutical therapy: Discontinue all nonessential medications that could cause palpitations.

Follow-Up

A. Depending on the etiology of palpitations and the existence of comorbid conditions, the prognosis in patients with no underlying cardiac disease is generally favorable.

Consultation/Referral

A. Consult a physician if the patient has a history of palpitations leading to syncope or near syncope, angina-like chest pain, or dyspnea. These patients are candidates for referral to a cardiologist and/or inpatient evaluation. Refer any patient with an arrhythmia to a cardiologist.
B. Hemodynamically compromised patients need prompt hospital admission.

Peripheral Arterial Disease

Laura A. Petty

Definition

A. Peripheral arterial disease (PAD) is a circulatory disorder generally characterized by the build-up of plaque on the interior surface of arteries. These plaques harden and narrow the diameter of the arteries, which reduces the volume of blood circulating to internal organs and extremities. The arteries affected by PAD include all arteries in the body with the exception of the cerebral and coronary arteries. The decreased circulation seen in PAD can also be caused by nonatherosclerotic conditions. Some of these conditions are arteritis, trauma, radiation damage, and fibromuscular dysplasia. Symptoms of PAD can occur in upper or lower extremities.
B. Classification of PAD
  1. Asymptomatic PAD

a. No symptoms but the presence of risk factors or a new diagnosis of a common coexisting disease (coronary artery disease [CAD] or cerebrovascular disease) should prompt further evaluation.

2. Intermittent claudication (IC)

a. Discomfort with physical exertion that remits a few minutes after activity ceases.

3. Chronic limb ischemia

a. Pain at rest and/or skin ulceration

4. Acute limb ischemia

a. Pain at rest with a pulseless extremity

C. Other conditions contained within PAD

1. Buerger's disease (thromboangiitis obliterans): A disease manifested by inflammation, peripheral edema, and micro thrombi leading to gangrene of the hands and feet. Usually caused by tobacco abuse; patients are thought to have a genetic predisposition to develop this condition.

2. Raynaud's disease/phenomenon: A vasospastic disorder manifested by a response in the extremities to cold temperatures or stress during which pallor, cyanosis, numbness, and/or pain are experienced

3. Leriche syndrome: Involves the triad of claudication, absent or diminished femoral pulses, and erectile dysfunction

Incidence

A. Approximately 8 million adults in the United States have PAD. This correlates to between 12% and 20% of Americans older than 60 years of age.

B. PAD is more common in men than in women.

C. PAD is more common in patients of African and Hispanic descent.

Pathogenesis

A. PAD is most commonly precipitated by atherosclerosis. An atherosclerotic plaque develops in response to turbulent blood flow on the endothelial cells of the vessel wall. The plaque contains inflammatory cells and a thrombogenic lipid core that is covered by a fibrous cap. When the fibrous cap is disturbed, the lipid core can precipitate to development of a thrombus and lead to occlusion of the vessel.

Predisposing Factors

A. Smoking

B. Diabetes

C. Dyslipidemia

D. Hypertension (HTN)

E. Obesity

F. Age, increased occurrence after the age of 60 years

Common Complaints

A. Pain with activity is commonly characterized as cramping and/or aching

1. Upper extremity pain in the forearm, hand, and digits.

2. Lower extremity pain in the foot, calf, hip, thigh, and/or buttocks

a. Foot pain is most common in tibial or peroneal artery stenosis.

b. Calf pain is most common with superficial femoral or popliteal artery stenosis.

c. Thigh pain is most common in aortoiliac and common femoral artery stenosis.

d. Hip and buttock pain are most common with aortoiliac arterial stenosis.

B. Pain at rest

C. Calf weakness or fatigue

D. Numbness or tingling

E. Dizziness with upper extremity exertion

F. Syncope with upper extremity exertion

G. Extremity ulceration

Other Signs and Symptoms

A. Decreased peripheral pulses

B. Blanching of the affected limb with elevation

C. Ulcerations or infection on distal aspects of extremities

D. Erectile dysfunction

Potential Complications

A. Nonhealing lower extremity ulcerations

B. Infection

C. Amputation

D. Common coexisting diseases:

1. Coronary Artery Disease (CAD); also known as Coronary Heart Disease (CHD)

2. Cerebrovascular disease

Subjective Data

A. Ask the patient what activity brought about or preceded the episode or whether it occurs at rest. If ambulation was the precipitating factor, how far was the patient able to walk?

B. Have the patient describe the duration of pain and what time of day symptoms began.

C. Ask the patient what alleviates his or her pain.

D. Ask the patient whether any previous episodes have occurred.

E. Ask the patient to list all medications, including over-the-counter (OTC) and herbal products, currently being taken or recently stopped.

F. Ask the patient to quantify his or her smoking history.

G. Ask the patient if he or she has a past medical history of an MI or cerebrovascular accident.

H. If the patient is male, ask if he has any history of impotence or erectile dysfunction.

Physical Examination

A. Patients presenting with acute limb ischemia should be quickly assessed for the need to call emergency services/911 for immediate transport to the hospital.

1. Symptoms of acute limb ischemia as evidenced by the six Ps—pain, pallor, paresthesia, paralysis, pulselessness, and poikilothermia (the inability to maintain a constant core temperature).

B. Vital signs

1. Check blood pressure (BP) in both upper extremities.

a. A difference in SBP of 10 mmHg or greater in the upper extremities is associated with the upper extremity PAD and cerebrovascular disease.
b. A difference in systolic BP (SBP) of 15 mmHg or greater in the upper extremities is associated with lower extremity PAD.
2. Check BP in both lower extremities.
3. Document resting heart rate, respirations, height, and weight.

C. Inspect
1. Perform a funduscopic examination: Check for retinal vascular changes that indicate a retinal vascular occlusion such as macular edema and neovascularization.
a. Macular edema is the swelling of the central part of the retina.
b. Neovascularization is the growth of abnormal vessels secondary to decreased perfusion of the retina.
2. Inspect abdomen for a pulsating abdominal mass.
3. Inspect extremities. Note edema, pallor, and cyanosis. Note color of extremities in dependent and elevated positions.
4. Inspect distal skin, hair, and nails. Note any temperature discrepancies or trophic changes that are indicative of ischemia.
5. Assess lower extremities for any ulcerations or diffuse erythema.
6. Assess for a Homans' sign (i.e., calf pain with forced dorsiflexion).
7. Assess whether pain occurs when affected limb is elevated.

D. Palpate
1. Palpate pulses, noting symmetry.
a. Bilateral upper extremities (brachial and radial)
b. Abdominal (aorta)
c. Bilateral groin (femoral)
d. Bilateral lower extremity pulses (popliteal, dorsalis pedis, and posterior tibialis)
2. Palpate capillary refill.
3. Perform an Allen test: Occlude the radial and ulnar arteries with the fist closed. Open the hand and then release one of the occluded arteries. Repeat but release the other artery. Each time, prompt capillary refill should occur.
4. Palpate neck for carotid bruits.
5. Palpate the abdominal aorta noting any lateral pulsation, indicative of an aortic aneurysm.

E. Auscultate
1. Heart: Assess the rate, rhythm, heart sounds, murmur, and gallops.
2. Carotids, abdomen, and bilateral groin for bruits
3. Lungs: Assess lung sounds, noting any sign of heart failure (HF).

Diagnostic Tests

A. Doppler ankle/brachial index (ABI)
1. Interpretation of ABI ratios
a. 1.00 to 1.29: Normal
b. 0.91 to 0.99: Borderline PAD
c. 0.41 to 0.90: Mild to moderate PAD
d. 0.00 to 0.40: Severe PAD

B. Basic metabolic panel (BMP; including blood urea nitrogen [BUN], creatinine, sodium, and potassium)
C. Lipid profile
D. C-reactive protein (CRP), homocysteine, D-dimer
E. EKG (12 lead)
F. Doppler ultrasound
G. Abdominal ultrasound
H. Treadmill testing
I. Computed tomography angiography (CTA)
J. Magnetic resonance angiography (MRA)
K. Arteriography, ordered and performed by surgeon

Differential Diagnoses

A. PAD
B. Venous stasis
C. Venous obstruction/claudication
D. Spinal stenosis
E. Nerve root compression
F. Arthritis of the hip
G. Peripheral neuropathy
H. Arteritis

Plan

A. General interventions
1. The goal of therapy is to improve the patient's quality of life by reducing morbidity and prolonging survival.

B. Patient teaching: *See Section III: Patient Teaching Guide for this chapter, "Peripheral Arterial Disease."* ◀
1. Encourage smoking cessation, weight loss, and exercise, if applicable.
2. Encourage strategies to better manage other chronic medical conditions that directly affect the progression of PAD, that is, diabetes, dyslipidemia, obesity, and HTN.
3. Proper foot care
a. Instruct the patient to wear proper-fitting shoes that protect the feet.
b. Inspect inside of shoes before donning.
c. Encourage the patient to inspect feet daily for signs of trauma or infection.
d. Instruct the patient to dry feet well, including between toes, after bathing.

C. Prevention
1. Control other chronic medical conditions, that is, diabetes, dyslipidemia, HTN, and obesity.

D. Dietary management
1. To manage dyslipidemia and HTN: Counsel patient on nutrition and low-fat, low-cholesterol, low-sodium diet.
2. To manage diabetes: Counsel patient on diabetic diet and carbohydrate counting.
3. To manage infection related to PAD: Counsel patient on high-calorie, high-protein diet. Consider the addition of vitamins and minerals to promote wound healing, specifically zinc, and vitamins A and C.
4. Give diet handouts and/or refer to a registered dietitian.

E. Pharmaceutical therapy
1. Goal of therapy: Prevention of thromboembolism
a. Trental (pentoxifylline)
i. 400 mg tablet
1) Dosage indications based on creatinine clearance (CrCl)
a) CrCl less than 10 mL/min: 400 mg, taken once a day
b) CrCl = 10 to 50 mL/min: 400 mg, taken twice daily
c) CrCl greater than 50 mg/min: 400 mg, taken three times a day
b. Pletal (cilostazol)
i. 50 mg and 100 mg tablets
1) Warning: Metabolites of Pletal are inhibitors of phosphodiesterase III and are contraindicated in patients with congestive heart failure (CHF) of any severity.
2) Dosage indications
a) 50 mg, taken twice daily if taken in coadministration with ketoconazole, itraconazole, erythromycin, and diltiazem
b) 100 mg, taken twice daily at least half an hour before or 2 hours after breakfast and dinner
c. Aspirin (acetylsalicylic acid, Ecotrin)
i. 81 mg, 325 mg tablets, taken once daily
d. Plavix (clopidogrel bisulfate)
i. 75 mg, taken once daily
2. Risk factor reduction
a. Manage dyslipidemia
i. Low-density lipoprotein (LDL) cholesterol goal: Less than 100 mg/dL and less than 70 mg/dL for patients at high risk of CAD
b. Manage HTN
i. BP goal in patients without diabetes: Less than 140/90 mmHg
ii. BP goal in patients with diabetes or chronic kidney disease (CKD): Less than 130/80 mmHg
c. Manage diabetes
i. Hemoglobin A1C goal: Less than 7.0%

F. Surgical therapies: Considered in patients with pain at rest, tissue loss, or significant physical limitations that prevent exercise
1. Bypass
2. Stenting
3. Angioplasty/percutaneous transluminal angioplasty

G. Nonsurgical therapies
1. Smoking-cessation program
2. Daily walking program
a. Instruct patient to walk to the point of pain, then stop and resume walking when pain remits.
b. May need to obtain medical clearance for the patient to exercise.

Follow-Up

A. PAD manifesting persistent symptoms should always be followed by a cardiologist visit.

B. Follow-up is determined by the patient's needs, frequency and intensity of symptoms, and the presence of other medical conditions.

Consultation/Referral

A. If you suspect acute limb ischemia, refer the patient for immediate hospitalization in order to obtain diagnostic testing to determine the presence of a thrombus and restore circulation to the affected extremity.

B. If chronic limb ischemia has led to ulceration and/or superimposed infection, hospitalization is indicated to initiate a wound care consultation and diagnostic testing to determine the degree of arterial occlusion.

C. Referral to a cardiologist in the presence of persistent PAD symptoms

D. Referral to a vascular surgeon for further evaluation of angioplasty, stenting, or bypass surgery

E. Referral to a podiatrist to trim toenails and assess patient for proper-fitting shoes

F. Referral to pain management if pain is resistant to treatment

G. Referral to a registered dietitian as indicated by the patient's understanding of dietary modification necessary to improve status of risk factors

Individual Considerations

A. Nonambulatory patients
1. Using rocking chairs is a possible substitute for persons unable to participate in a walking program.

B. Geriatrics
1. Be alert to signs and symptoms of depression related to immobility and pain.

Superficial Thrombophlebitis

Cheryl A. Glass and Laura A. Petty

Definition

A. Superficial thrombophlebitis is inflammation of a vessel wall accompanied by blood stasis in varicose veins, which may also have clot formation in a vein close to the surface.
1. Most superficial thrombophlebitis occurs in the lower extremity, but may also occur in the breast and in the penis (Mondor disease).
2. Superficial thrombophlebitis may also occur in the upper extremities and in the neck after invasive intravenous catheters are used in medical procedures.
3. Generally superficial thrombophlebitis is self-limiting but may persist for a period of time (3–4 weeks or longer) before resolution.

B. Superficial phlebitis with an infection is referred to as a *septic thrombophlebitis*.

Incidence

A. Pregnancy carries an increased risk of phlebitis. Eighty percent of thromboembolic events in pregnancy are venous. The incidence of PE in pregnancy accounts for 1.1 deaths per 100,000 deliveries.

B. The prevalence of superficial thrombophlebitis ranges from 4% to 8% of patients with an indwelling intravenous catheter.
C. Superficial phlebitis after a vein radiofrequency or laser ablation is common.

Pathogenesis

A. Superficial thrombosis is caused by infection, abuse of intravenous (IV) drugs, chemical irritation from overuse of IV route for diagnostic tests and drugs, and/or trauma. Several episodes can signal an underlying problem such as carcinoma of the pancreas.
B. A common cause of varicose veins is blood-flow stasis, basically caused by valvular incompetence and/or dilation of the vessel lumen.
C. Thrombi in the upper extremities commonly have iatrogenic causes such as IV catheters.
D. Thrombophlebitis during pregnancy through the first 6 weeks postpartum is linked to a reduced fibrinolytic state.

Predisposing Factors

A. Previous thrombophlebitis is the highest risk factor for recurrence.
B. Hypercoagulability such as pregnancy (50% of events) through 6 weeks postpartum (50% of events)
C. Hemoglobinopathies
  1. Factor V Leiden mutation
  2. Protein C deficiency
  3. Protein S deficiency
  4. Prothrombin gene mutation
  5. Antithrombin III deficiency
  6. Factor XII deficiency
D. Estrogen therapy
  1. Oral contraceptives
  2. High-dose hormone replacement therapy (HRT)
E. Malignancy (especially in the tail of the pancreas)
F. Lupus, positive anticardiolipin antibody
G. Sepsis
H. Surgery
I. Long bone trauma
J. Recent IV catheter access
K. Prolonged immobilization
L. Obesity
M. Varicose veins
N. Age older than 60 years
O. Stroke
P. Myocardial infarction (MI)
Q. Family history of deep vein thrombosis (DVT)
R. Smoking
S. Hypertension (HTN)
T. Infection

Common Complaints

A. Warm, tender, inflamed vessel with palpable cord
B. Redness along the course of the superficial vein
C. Tenderness or pain localized to the affected vein

Other Signs and Symptoms

A. Fever/no fever
B. Localized edema

Potential Complications

A. Superficial thrombophlebitis extending into the deep venous system
B. DVT
C. Conversion to suppurative thrombophlebitis
  1. Metastatic abscess formation
  2. Septicemia
  3. Septic emboli

Subjective Data

A. Query the patient regarding the onset, duration, and intensity of symptoms.
B. Ask the patient about fever or other related symptoms.
C. Obtain a thorough medical history and account of recent physical activity.
D. Ask the patient about any recent experience of any type of injury.
E. Inquire whether the patient has ever had similar symptoms or history of previous thrombophlebitis. If so, discuss previous treatment and therapy used and the results.
F. Review current medications: Prescription, over-the-counter (OTC), and herbal products.
  1. Ask specifically about oral contraceptives and hormone therapy.
G. Review the patient's occupation for sedentary lifestyle.
H. Review any recent plane travel.
I. Review history for recent invasive procedures.

Physical Examination

A. Check temperature (if indicated with inflammation), pulse, respirations, and blood pressure (BP).
B. Inspect
  1. Assess overall appearance. Evaluate for the presence of respiratory distress.
  2. Inspect extremities, noting erythema and edema.
  3. Assess for increased warmth over the affected vein.
C. Auscultate
  1. Heart, noting rate, rhythm, heart sounds, murmurs, and gallops
  2. Lungs for lung sounds in all fields
D. Palpate
  1. Palpate extremities; check all pulses, including femoral, posttibial, pedal, and radial.
  2. Palpate extremities for tenderness and palpable cord.
  3. Palpate lymph nodes distal and proximal to the site.
  4. Test for Homans' sign in lower extremities bilaterally if DVT is suspected.

Diagnostic Tests

A. Duplex ultrasound identifies the presence, location, and extent of venous thrombosis.
B. Doppler ultrasound
C. Laboratory tests are ordered dependent on the clinical situation.
  1. Complete blood count (CBC) with differential

2. Screening for hypercoagulability should not be considered for one episode of superficial thrombophlebitis.
3. Screening for hypercoagulability should be considered for recurrent superficial thrombophlebitis.
4. Blood cultures

Differential Diagnoses

A. Thrombophlebitis
B. Varicose veins
C. Cellulitis
D. Strained muscle
E. Insect bites
F. Erythema nodosum
G. Cutaneous polyarteritis nodosa
H. Kaposi's sarcoma
I. Hyperalgesic pseudothrombophlebitis

Plan

A. General interventions
   1. Advise all patients to stop smoking.
   2. Tell the patient to avoid prolonged sitting or standing and not to cross or massage legs. *See Section III: Patient Teaching Guides for this chapter, "Superficial Thrombophlebitis" and "Varicose Veins."*
   3. Advise the patient to avoid constrictive clothing such as knee-high hosiery.
   4. Prescribe supportive hose/compression stockings.
   5. Have the patient apply heat and elevate extremity for varicose veins or superficial thrombophlebitis.
   6. Prescribe bed rest for superficial thrombophlebitis.
   7. DVT: Hospitalization is required.
   8. Tell patients with thrombophlebitis to discontinue oral contraceptives and hormone replacement.
   9. Alternative forms of birth control recommended by the American College of Obstetricians and Gynecologists (ACOG) include
      a. Intrauterine device, including intrauterine devices (IUDs) that contain progestin
      b. Progestin-only oral contraceptives
      c. Progestin-only implants
      d. Barrier methods
      e. Surgical procedures: Vasectomy and tubal ligation

B. Patient teaching: See *Section III: Patient Teaching Guide for this chapter, "Superficial Thrombophlebitis."*

C. Pharmaceutical therapy for superficial thrombophlebitis
   1. Nonsteroidal anti-inflammatory drugs (NSAIDs) are used for treatment of pain. No NSAID has been identified as superior for treatment.
   2. The use of anticoagulation therapy for the treatment of lower extremity superficial thrombophlebitis is controversial. Unfractionated heparin and low-molecular-weight heparin (LMWH) are both used for treatment to reduce risk of DVT and/or recurrent phlebitis.
   3. The American College of Chest Physicians recommends anticoagulation for patients with lower extremity superficial thrombophlebitis at increased risk of thromboembolism. This is defined as the affected venous segment greater than or equal to 5 cm in proximity (less than or equal to 5 cm) to deep venous system and positive medical risk factors. The American College of Chest Physicians' full evidence-based clinical practice guidelines on antithrombotic therapy are available at http://journal.publications.chestnet.org/article.aspx?articleID=2479255
   4. Antibiotics, if infection is suspected

D. Surgery
   1. Biopsy
   2. Vein ablation, only if symptoms are significant and persistent
   3. Vein ligation, only if symptoms are significant and persistent

Follow-Up

A. Schedule a return appointment for patients with superficial thrombophlebitis to return in 7 to 10 days or earlier as needed. Repeat physical examination as needed to evaluate resolution or progression of the thrombophlebitis.
B. Periodic follow-up is needed to monitor patients on anticoagulation therapy.
C. After an acute problem is resolved, consider laboratory evaluation for hypercoagulation syndrome (protein C, protein S, and antithrombin III).
D. Monitor bone loss with dual-energy x-ray absorptiometry (DEXA) scan with prolonged use of heparin.
E. Screening all women for thrombophilias before starting oral contraceptives is not recommended by the ACOG.
F. Women with a history of thrombosis who have not had a complete evaluation should be tested for both antiphospholipid antibodies and inherited thrombophilias.

Consultation/Referral

A. If septic thrombophlebitis or DVT is diagnosed, refer the patient to a physician.
B. Hospitalization is required to initiate heparin therapy.
C. Comanage pregnancy with an obstetrician.

Individual Considerations

A. Pregnancy
   1. Routine anticoagulation therapy for all pregnant women is not recommended. Therapeutic anticoagulation is recommended for women with acute thromboembolism during the current pregnancy or those at high risk of thrombosis such as women with mechanical heart valves.
   2. Warfarin and NSAIDs are contraindicated.
   3. Heparin is the preferred anticoagulant in pregnancy. Neither unfractionated heparin nor LMWH crosses the placenta.
   4. Warfarin, LMWH, and unfractionated heparin do not accumulate in breast milk and do not induce an anticoagulant effect in the infant and therefore are considered compatible with breastfeeding.

B. Geriatrics
   1. Prognosis is poor for patients with septic thrombophlebitis.

2. Using a rocking chair is a possible substitute for persons unable to participate in a walking program.
3. Be alert to signs and symptoms of depression related to immobility and pain.

Syncope

Jill C. Cash and Debbie Gunter

Definition

A. Syncope is a brief, sudden loss of consciousness and muscle tone secondary to cerebral ischemia, or inadequate oxygen or glucose delivery to brain tissue. Recovery is spontaneous.

Incidence

A. Syncope is a common problem in all age groups. An estimated 15% of children experience an episode by adulthood. Between 12% and 48% of healthy young adults have lost consciousness (one third following trauma), but most do not seek medical attention. Adults older than age 75 years in long-term care facilities have a 6% annual incidence of syncope, and 23% have had previous episodes. Syncopal episodes account for approximately 1% to 6% of hospital admissions and 3% of emergency room visits.

Pathogenesis

The most common cause of syncope is inadequate cerebral perfusion caused by one of the following:

A. Vasomotor instability associated with a decrease in systemic vascular resistance and/or venous return. The following may cause syncope:
1. Vasovagal episodes
2. Situational syncope, from coughing, micturition, and defecation
3. Medications
a. Vasodilators
b. Antiarrhythmics
c. Diuretics
d. Neurologic agents
e. Glucose-regulating drugs
f. Impotence therapy

B. Decrease in cardiac output caused by blood-flow obstruction within the heart or pulmonary circulation or by arrhythmias. This may be caused by the following:
1. Aortic, pulmonic, and mitral stenosis
2. Idiopathic hypertrophic subaortic stenosis (IHSS)
3. Pump failure
4. Subclavian steal syndrome
5. Seizures

C. Focal or generalized decrease in cerebral perfusion leading to transient ischemia because of cerebrovascular disease.

D. Metabolic abnormalities
1. Hypoglycemia
2. Hypocarbia and hypoxia usually do not result in syncope unless they are profound, although consciousness may be altered.

E. Psychiatric illnesses associated with syncope include:
1. Generalized anxiety
2. Panic attacks
3. Major depressive disorders

F. Unexplained cause

Predisposing Factors

A. Advanced age, caused by altered regulation of cerebral blood flow and/or systemic arterial pressure because of aging process and increased medication use
B. Other factors, depending on etiology
C. Medication use (noted earlier)

Common Complaints

A. Dizziness
B. Light-headedness
C. Fainting with no memory of events

Other Signs and Symptoms

A. Neuroautonomic regulations
1. Event triggered by changing position, turning head, wearing tight collars
2. Nausea, warmth, diaphoresis, weakness 1 hour after eating

B. Cardiac causes: Exercise-induced palpitations, chest pain, shortness of breath (SOB) with no warning before episode

C. Neurologic causes
1. Vertigo
2. Diplopia
3. Facial paresthesias
4. Ataxia
5. Auditory, visual, or vestibular disturbances

D. Metabolic or endocrine causes
1. Restlessness
2. Anxiety
3. Confusion
4. No recent food intake, low glucose level

E. Psychiatric: Graceful fainting in presence of an audience

Subjective Data

A. Inquire if the patient ever experienced similar symptoms or episodes before. If so, when and at what age did it begin?

B. Ask the patient or witness of the episode to give a detailed description of the loss of consciousness. Was loss of consciousness complete, and, if so, for how long? What was the posture of the patient before, during, and after the event? Did it occur abruptly, or were there symptoms leading up to the event?

C. Question the patient regarding events leading up to the episode, noting prodromal symptoms such as headache, aura, nausea/vomiting, light-headedness, diaphoresis, feeling of warmth.

D. Obtain a detailed account of symptoms during and after the episode, noting mental status. Did the patient recover on his or her own, or did the patient require assistance? Were there any associated symptoms that occurred during the event—SOB, chest pain, loss of bowel or bladder control?

E. If syncope has occurred in the past, are there any events that precipitate an episode? Exertion, exercise, coughing, standing quickly?
F. Obtain a detailed medication history, addressing prescribed and OTC drugs, alcohol, and illicit preparations.
G. Review the patient's past medical history.

Physical Examination

A. Check temperature, if indicated, pulse, respirations, and blood pressure (BP).
  1. Measure BP and pulse in both arms and legs. Note BP differences between the arms.
  2. Measure BP several times during a 2-minute period with the patient standing.
  3. Check for orthostatic hypotension, which is defined as a drop of 20 mmHg or more in systolic BP (SBP) on standing:
    a. First, measure BP after the patient lies supine for 5 to 10 minutes.
    b. Then have the patient stand, and measure BP several times during a 2-minute period.
B. Inspect
  1. Assess overall appearance of the patient, skin color.
  2. Note the range of motion in the neck.
C. Auscultate
  1. The heart with position changes. Note murmurs or extra heart sounds to rule out structural disease.
  2. The carotid arteries
  3. The abdomen for bruits
D. Palpate
  1. The abdomen, noting pulsatile expansion.
E. Neurologic examination
  1. Perform a complete examination, if indicated, including assessing 2nd to 12th cranial nerves, Babinski's reflex, and gait.
F. Mental status
  1. Assess mental health, if indicated.

Diagnostic Tests

The following tests are performed depending on history and physical examination results. The 2009 ESC guidelines recommend the following testing: The ESC guidelines are current.
A. Carotid sinus massage in patient older than 40 years of age. Avoid if patient has a history of transient ischemic attack (TIA) or stroke in the past 3 months and in patients with carotid bruits. Recommend physician or cardiology specialist assistance when performing carotid massage. Use caution when performing carotid sinus massage. Please consider contraindications, complications, and protocol for performing procedure.
B. Echocardiogram for patients with a history of heart disease, structural heart disease, or syncope secondary to cardiovascular cause (known heart disease, family history of unexplained sudden death, syncope with exertion or supine, abnormal EKG, sudden onset of palpitation before syncope, or arrhythmia on EKG [UpToDate, 2016]).
C. EKG for patients with suspected arrhythmia or cardiac disease. Identify acute and old EKG changes to rule out pathologic Q wave, ST segment elevation, and left ventricular hypertrophy (LVH).
D. Orthostatic challenge test if syncope is related to position change or suspect reflex mechanism
E. Neurologic/serum laboratory testing for other concerns of nonsyncopal loss of consciousness. Laboratory testing includes chemistry profile, thyroid-stimulating hormone (TSH), and free T4. Consider a glucose tolerance test if diabetes is suspected. Brain natriuretic peptide (BNP) may be useful to evaluate cardiac versus noncardiac cause for syncope.
F. Chest radiography, for essential baseline data. Wide mediastinum signals aortic dissection.
G. In-hospital monitoring recommended for unstable, life-threatened patients.
H. Holter monitor for 24 to 48 hours
I. External event monitor
J. Exercise testing recommended for patients with syncope that occurs during, or quickly after, cessation of exercise. Echocardiogram is recommended before this testing.
K. Cardiac catheterization
L. Lung scan
M. Treadmill test
N. Electrophysiological studies recommended for patients with unexplained syncope.

Differential Diagnoses

A. Irregular neuroautonomic regulations
  1. Neurocardiogenic causes
  2. Situational causes, such as coughing, defecation, diving, micturition, sneezing, swallowing, trumpet playing, vagal stimulation, weight lifting, postprandial state
  3. Orthostatic causes
    a. Hyperadrenergic state
    b. Hypoadrenergic state, primary or secondary autonomic insufficiency
    c. Carotid sinus syncope
    d. Cardioinhibitory state
    e. Vasodepressor stimulation
    f. Mixed
B. Cardiac causes
  1. Mechanical causes such as aortic dissection, aortic stenosis, atrial myxoma, cardiac tamponade, global myocardial ischemia, hypertrophic cardiomyopathy, mitral stenosis, myocardial infarction (MI), prosthetic valve dysfunction, pulmonary embolism (PE), pulmonary HTN, pulmonary stenosis, and Takayasu's arteritis
  2. Electrical causes, such as atrioventricular (AV) block, long QT syndrome, pacemaker, sick sinus syndrome, supraventricular tachyarrhythmias, and ventricular tachyarrhythmias
C. Neurologic causes
  1. Neuralgias: Glossopharyngeal, trigeminal
  2. Normal pressure hydrocephalus

3. Subclavian steal
4. Vertebrobasilar artery disease: Compression, migraine, TIA

D. Metabolic or endocrine causes: Hypoadrenalism, hypoglycemia, hyponatremia, hypothyroidism, and hypoxia

E. Psychiatric causes: Anxiety, hysteria, major depression, panic disorder, somatization, and hyperventilation syndrome

Plan

A. General interventions
1. Management is directed at primary cause for the episode.

B. Patient teaching
1. If the patient has orthostatic hypotension, suggest that he or she wear elastic stockings, change positions slowly, sleep with the head of the bed elevated, and exercise legs before standing.
2. If syncope is induced by situations, warn the patient to avoid or alter his or her approach to such precipitating events.
3. If the patient has prodromal symptoms, such as nausea, light-headedness, pallor, sweating, or palpitations, advise him or her to lie down when they occur.
4. If the patient has hypersensitive carotid sinus reflex, recommend that he or she loosen his or her collar.
5. Tell patients to avoid prolonged standing. If they cannot avoid it, they should contract their calf muscles to increase venous blood flow.
6. Some driving restrictions exist for patients at risk of recurrent syncope. Driving restrictions are enforced by the state law. Review restrictions with the patient and family as indicated by diagnosis.

C. Dietary management: If not contraindicated, instruct patients with orthostatic hypotension to use salt liberally.

D. Pharmaceutical therapy will depend on the etiology of the syncope. Therapy for neurocardiogenic syncope includes the following:
1. Nonpharmacological methods suggested: Avoid volume depletion. Maintain adequate sodium levels by increasing salt intake in the diet. Wear thigh-high elastic support hose with 30- to 40-mmHg pressure. Orthostatic training is also recommended two times a day.
2. Drugs of choice: Beta-blockers (Inderal 80–160 mg/d, metoprolol 50–100 mg/d)
3. Fludrocortisone acetate (Florinef Acetate), a corticosteroid, may be used alone or with beta-blockers. Initial dosage is 0.1 to 0.4 mg/d; this may be increased gradually to 1.0 to 2.0 mg/d.
4. Other drugs include anticholinergic agents (Disopyramide 100–200 mg twice daily sustained release) and SSRIs (Zoloft 50 mg/d, Prozac 20 mg/d, Paxil 20 mg/d).

Follow-Up

A. Scheduling of return visits depends on etiology and severity of syncope and whether the patient has been placed on medications.

Consultation/Referral

A. Consult with or refer the patient to a physician when cardiac or neurologic involvement is suspected.

B. Consult with or refer the patient to a physician if medication therapy is required.

Individual Considerations

A. Adults
1. In young adult athletes, be aware of symptoms of Marfan syndrome.
2. In older adults, coronary atherosclerosis may present along with syncope.

B. Geriatrics
1. Elderly patients may have multiple comorbid conditions such as decreased cerebral blood flow and acute viral illness.

Bibliography

Abid, S., & Shuaib, W. (2015). Chest pain assessment and imaging practices for nurse practitioners in the emergency department. *Advanced Emergency Nursing Journal, 37*, 12–22.

Alguire, P. C., & Mathes, B. M. (2015, September). Diagnostic evaluation of chronic venous insufficiency. *UpToDate*. Retrieved from http://www.uptodate.com/contents/diagnostic-evaluation-of-chronic-venous-insufficiency

Alguire, P. C., & Scovell, S. (2015, March). Overview and management of lower extremity chronic venous disease. *UpToDate*. Retrieved from www.uptodate.com/contents/overview-and-management-of-lower-extremity-chronic-venous-disease

Al Shammeri, O., AlHamdan, N., Al-Hothaly, B., Midhet, F., Hussain, M., & Al-Mohaimeed, A. (2014). Chronic venous insufficiency: Prevalence and effect of compression stockings. *International Journal of Health Sciences, 8*(3), 231–236.

American Diabetes Association. (2013). Executive summary: Standards of medical care in diabetes—2013. *Diabetes Care, 36*(Suppl. 1), S4–S10.

American Geriatrics Society. (2015). Updated Beers criteria for potentially inappropriate medication use in older adults. *Journal of the American Geriatrics Society, 63*, 2227–2246.

American Heart Association. (2013). Infective endocarditis. Retrieved from http://www.heart.org/HEARTORG/Conditions/CongenitalHeartDefects/TheImpactofCongenitalHeartDefects/Infective-Endocarditis_UCM_307108_Article.jsp#.WGFOlLnT8rM

Amsterdam, E. A., Wenger, N. K., Brindis, R. G., Casey, D. E., Ganiats, T. G., Holmes, D. R., . . . Zieman, S. J. (2014). AHA/ACC guideline for the management of patients with non-ST-elevation acute coronary syndromes: A Report of the American College of Cardiology/American Heart Association Task Force on Practice Guidelines and the Heart Rhythm Society. *Circulation, 130*(25), e344–e426.

Anderson, J. L., Halperin, J. L., Albert, N. M., Bozkurt, B., Brindis, R. G., Curtis, L. H., . . . Shen, W. K. (2013). Management of patients with peripheral artery disease (compilation of 2005 and 2011 ACCF/AHA guideline recommendations): A report of the American College of Cardiology Foundation/American Heart Association Task Force on Practice Guidelines. *Circulation, 127*(13), 1425–1443.

Aschenbrenner, D. (2013). Drug watch: New labeled indications for an anticoagulant. *American Journal of Nursing, 113*(3), 22–23.

Batra, G., Svennblad, B., Held, C., Jernberg, T., Johanson, P., Wallentin, L., & Oldgren, J. (2016). All types of atrial fibrillation in the setting of myocardial infarction are associated with impaired outcome. *Heart (British Cardiac Society), 102*(12), 926–933.

Bernas, M. (2013). Assessment and risk reduction in lymphedema. *Seminars in Oncology Nursing, 29*(1), 12–19.

Boudi, F. B. (2016, April 25). Coronary artery atherosclerosis. *Medscape*. Retrieved from emedicine.medscape.com/article/153647-overview

Bowers, M. T. (2013, November). Managing patients with heart failure. *Journal for Nurse Practitioners, 9*, 621–628.

Brazziel, T., Cox, L., Drury, C., & Guerra, M. (2011). Stopping the wave of PAD. *Nurse Practitioner, 36*(11), 28–33; quiz 33–34.

Centers for Disease Control and Prevention. (2012, June 8). Deep vein thrombosis (DVT)/pulmonary embolism (PE)—Blood clot forming in a vein. Retrieved from www.cdc.gov/ncbddd/dvt/data.html

Centers for Disease Control and Prevention. (2012, October 17). Heart failure fact sheet. Retrieved from https://www.cdc.gov/dhdsp/data_statistics/fact_sheets/fs_heart_failure.htm

Centers for Disease Control and Prevention. (2014, March 7). CDC grand rounds: Preventing hospital-associated venous thromboembolism. Retrieved from https://www.cdc.gov/mmwr/preview/mmwrhtml/mm6309a3.htm

Centers for Disease Control and Prevention. (2015, June). Venous thromboembolism (blood clots). Retrieved from www.cdc.gov/ncbddd/dvt/data.html

Centers for Disease Control and Prevention. (2015, August). Atrial fibrillation fact sheet. Retrieved from https://www.cdc.gov/dhdsp/data_statistics/fact_sheets/fs_atrial_fibrillation.htm

Chao, T.-F., Liu, C.-J., Tuan, T.-C., Chen, S.-J., Wang, K.-L., Lin, Y.-J., . . . Chen, S.-A. (2015). Rate-control treatment and mortality in atrial fibrillation. *Circulation, 132*,1604–1612. Retrieved from http://circ.ahajournals.org/content/early/2015/09/17/CIRCULATIONAHA.114.013709.abstract

Cheng, A., & Kumar, K. (2016, February). Overview of atrial fibrillation. *UpToDate*. Retrieved from www.uptodate.com/contents/overview-of-atrial-fibrillation

Davis, L. L. (2013, November). Using the latest evidence to manage hypertension. *Journal for Nurse Practitioners, 9*, 621–628.

Di Nisio, M., & Middeldorp, S. (2014). Treatment of lower extremity superficial thrombophlebitis. *The Journal of the American Medical Association, 311*(7), 729–730.

Dumitru, I. (2013, May 6). Heart failure medication. *Medscape*. Retrieved from emedicine.medscape.com/article/163062-medication

Eckel, R. H., Jakicic, J. M., Ard, J. D., de Jesus, J. M., Houston Miller, N., Hubbard, V. S., . . . Yanovsk, S. Z. (2014). 2013 AHA/ACC guideline on lifestyle management to reduce cardiovascular risk: A report of the American College of Cardiology/American Heart Association Task Force on practice guidelines. *Circulation, 129*(25 Suppl. 2), S76–S99. Retrieved from http://circ.ahajournals.org/content/129/25_suppl_2/S76

Faiz, A. S., Khan, I., Beckman, M. G., Bockenstedt, P., Heit, J. A., Kulkarni, R., . . . Philipp, C. S. (2015). Characteristics and risk factors of cancer associated venous thromboembolism. *Thrombosis Research, 136*(3), 535–541.

Fernandez, L., & Scovell, S. (2016, Apr). Superficial thrombophlebitis of the lower extremity. *UpToDate*. Retrieved from http://www.uptodate.com/contents/superficial-thrombophlebitis-of-the-lower-extremity

Ganz, L. (2015, October). Epidemiology of and risk factors for atrial fibrillation. *UpToDate*. Retrieved from http://www.uptodate.com/contents/epidemiology-of-and-risk-factors-for-atrial-fibrillation

Go, A. S., Bauman, M., King. S. M. C., Fonarow, G. C., Lawrence, W., Williams, K. A., & Sanchez, E. (2013, November 15). An effective approach to high blood pressure control: A science advisory from the American Heart Association, the American College of Cardiology, and the Centers for Disease Control and Prevention. *Hypertension*. Epub ahead of print. Retrieved from http://hyper.ahajournals.org/content/early/2013/11/14/HYP.0000000000000003.reprint

Go, A. S., Mozaffarian, D., Roger, V. L., Benjamin, E. J., Berry, J. D., Borden, W. B., . . . Turner, M. B.; American Heart Association Statistics Committee and Stroke Statistics Subcommittee. (2013). Heart disease and stroke statistics—2013 update: A report from the American Heart Association. *Circulation, 127*(1), e6–e245.

Goff, D. C., Lloyd-Jones, D. M., Bennett, G., Coady, S., D'Agostino, Sr., R. B., Gibbons, R., . . . Wilson, P. W. F. (2014). 2013 ACC/AHA guideline on the assessment of cardiovascular risk: A report of the American College of Cardiology/American Heart Association Task Force on practice guidelines. *Circulation, 129*(25 Suppl. 2), S49–S73. Retrieved from http://circ .ahajournals.org/content/129/25_suppl_2/S49

Gonsalves, W. I., Pruthi, R. K., & Patnaik, M. M. (2013). The new oral anticoagulants in clinical practice. *Mayo Clinic Proceedings, 88*(5), 495–511.

Guyatt, G. H., Akl, E. A., Crowther, M., Gutterman, D. D., & Schuünemann, H. J. (2012). Executive summary: Antithrombotic therapy and prevention of thrombosis, 9th ed: American College of Chest Physicians evidence-based clinical practice guidelines. *Chest, 141*(2 Suppl.), 7S–47S.

Harris, L., & Dryjski, M. (2015, Nov). Epidemiology, risk factors, and natural history of peripheral artery disease. *UpToDate*. Retrieved from http://www.uptodate.com/contents/epidemiology-risk-factors-and-natural-history-of-peripheral-artery-disease

Heidbuchel, H., Verhamme, P., Alings, M., Antz, M., Hacke, W., Oldgren, J., . . . Kirchhof, P. (2013). EHRA practical guide on the use of new oral anticoagulants in patients with non-valvular atrial fibrillation: Executive summary. *European Heart Journal, 34*(27), 2094–2106.

Isl, I. (2013). The diagnosis and treatment of peripheral lymphedema: 2013 consensus document of the International Society of Lymphology. *Lymphology, 46*(1), 1–11.

Jackson, S. M. (2013). Diastolic heart failure. *Advance for NPs & PAs, 4*(2), 23–25, 34.

James, P. A., Oparil, S., Carter, B. L., Cushman, W. C., Dennison-Himmelfarb, C., Handler, J., . . . Ortiz, E. (2014). 2014 evidence-based guideline for the management of high blood pressure in adults: Report from the panel members appointed to the Eighth Joint National Committee (JNC 8). *The Journal of the American Medical Association, 311*(5), 507–520. doi: 10.1001/jama.2013.284427.

January, C. T., Wann, L. S., Alpert, J. S., Calkins, H., Cigarroa, J. E., Cleveland, J. C., . . . Yancy, C. W. (2014). 2014 AHA/ACC/HRS guideline for the management of patients with atrial fibrillation: A report of the American College of Cardiology/American Heart Association Task Force on Practice Guidelines and the Heart Rhythm Society. *Journal of the American College of Cardiology, 64*(21), e1–e76.

Judd, E., & Calhoun, D. A. (2014). Apparent and true resistant hypertension: Definition, prevalence and outcomes. *Journal of Human Hypertension, 28*(8), 463–468.

Kearon, C., Akl, E. A., Ornelas, J., Blaivas, A., Jimenez, D., Bounameaux, H., . . . Moores, L. (2016). Antithrombotic therapy for VTE disease: CHEST Guideline and Expert Panel Report. *Chest, 149*(2), 315–352.

Klever, R. G. (2015, June). Superficial thrombophlebitis. *Medscape*. Retrieved from emedicine.medscape.com/article/463256-overview

Lavigne, P. M., & Karas, R. H. (2013). The current state of niacin in cardiovascular disease prevention: A systematic review and meta-regression. *Journal of the American College of Cardiology, 61*(4), 440–446.

Lip, G., & Hull, R. (2016, May). Overview of the treatment of lower extremity deep vein thrombosis (DVT). *UpToDate*. Retrieved from http://www.uptodate.com/contents/overview-of-the-treatment-of-lower-extremity-deep-vein-thrombosis-dvt

Madhur, M. S. (2013, December 3). Hypertension. *Medscape*. Retrieved from emedicine.medscape.com/article/241381-overview

Mann, J. F. E. (2013, May 25). Choice of therapy in primary (essential) hypertension: Recommendations. *UpToDate*. Retrieved from www.uptodate.com

Mann, J. F. E., & Hilgers, K. F. (2015, January 20). Hypertension: Who should be treated? *UpToDate*. Retrieved from http://www.uptodate.com/contents/hypertension-who-should-betreated?topicKey-NEPH

McLafferty, R. B., Lohr, J. M., Caprini, J. A., Passman, M. A., Padberg, F. T., Rooke, T. W., . . . Wakefield, T. W. (2007). Results of the national pilot screening program for venous disease by the American Venous Forum. *Journal of Vascular Surgery, 45*(1), 142–148.

Mohler III, E. (2014, June). Clinical features and diagnosis of lower extremity peripheral artery disease. *UpToDate*. Retrieved from http://www.uptodate.com/contents/clinical-features-and-diagnosis-of-lower-extremity-peripheral-artery-disease

Mohler III, E. (2015, October). Overview of upper extremity peripheral artery disease. *UpToDate*. Retrieved from http://www.uptodate.com/contents/overview-of-upper-extremity-peripheral-artery-disease

Moss, J. D., & Cifu, A. S.; ACC/AHA Task Force on Practice Guidelines. (2015). Management of anticoagulation in patients with atrial fibrillation. *The Journal of the American Medical Association, 314*(3), 291–292.

Mozaffarian, D., Benjamin, E. J., & Go, A. S. (2015). Heart disease and stroke statistics—2015 update: A report from the American Heart Association. *Circulation, 131*(4), e29–322.

Nasr, H., & Scriven, J. M. (2015). Superficial thrombophlebitis (superficial venous thrombosis). *The BMJ, 350*, h2039. Retrieved from http://www.bmj.com/content/350/bmj.h2039

National Institute for Health and Care Excellence. (2016, July). Prophylaxis against infective endocarditis: Clinical guideline 64.1: Methods, evidence and recommendations. Retrieved from https://www.nice.org.uk/guidance/cg64

O'Gara. P. T., Kushner, F. G., Ascheim, D. D., Casey, D. E., Chung, M. K., de Lemos, J. A., . . . Zhao, D. X. (2013). 2013 ACCF/AHA guideline for the management of ST-elevation myocardial infarction: A report of the American College of Cardiology Foundation/American Heart Association Task Force on Practice Guidelines. *Circulation, 127*(4), e362–e425.

O'Gara, P. T., Kushner, F. G., Ascheim, D. D., Casey, D. E., Chung, M. K., de Lemos, J. A., . . . Zhao, D. X. (2013, January). 2013 ACCF/AHA guideline for the management of ST-elevation myocardial infarction: A report of the American College of Cardiology Foundation/American Heart Association Task Force on Practice Guidelines. *Journal of the American College of Cardiology, 61*(4), e78–140. Retrieved from http://content.onlinejacc.org/article.aspx?articleid=1486115

Palmer, S. (2015). Atrial fibrillation. *British Journal of Cardiac Nursing, 10*(11), 567.

Patel, M. R., Conte, M. S., Cutlip, D. E., Dib, N., Geraghty, P., Gray, W., . . . Krucoff, M. W. (2015). Evaluation and treatment of patients with lower extremity peripheral artery disease: Consensus definitions from Peripheral Academic Research Consortium (PARC). *Journal of the American College of Cardiology, 65*(9), 931–941. Retrieved from http://content.onlinejacc.org/article.aspx?articleid=2174621#tab1

Payne, A. B., Miller, C. H., Hooper, W. C., Lally, C., & Austin, H. D. (2014). High factor VIII, von Willebrand factor, and fibrinogen levels and risk of venous thromboembolism in Blacks and Whites. *Ethnicity & Disease, 24*(2), 169–174.

Physicians' Desk Reference. Drug information. (2016). Retrieved from www.pdr.net

Piller, N., Partsch, H., Hays, S., & Woodman, R. (2014). What's best for our lymphedema patients? *Journal of Lymphoedema, 9*(2), 6–10.

Robert, L. (2013, May 15). Hypertension meeting has primary care track [Web blog]. Retrieved from www.consultantlive.com/print/article/10162/2142634

Rooke, T. W., & Felty, C. L. (2014). A different way to look at varicose veins. *Journal of Vascular Surgery. Venous and Lymphatic Disorders, 2*(2), 207–211.

Ruff, C. T., Giugliano, R. P., Braunwald, E., Hoffman, E. B., Deenadayalu, N., Ezekowitz, M. D., . . . Antman, E. M. (2014). Comparison of the efficacy and safety of new oral anticoagulants with warfarin in patients with atrial fibrillation: A meta-analysis of randomised trials. *Lancet, 383*(9921), 955–962.

Rutecki, G. W. (2013, May 16). Some do's and don'ts for tough-to-treat hypertensives [Web blog]. Retrieved from http://www.consultantlive.com/print/article/10162/2142822?printable=true

Rutecki, G. W. (2013, May 22). Reflections on ASH 2013: Lessons in quality improvement [Web blog]. Retrieved from www.consultantlive.com/conference-reports/ash2013/content/article/10162/2143452

Saklani, P., Krahn, A., & Klein, G. (2013). Syncope. *Circulation, 127*(12), 1330–1339.

Spencer, A., Jablonski, R., & Loeb, S. J. (2012). Hypertensive African American women and the DASH diet. *Nurse Practitioner, 37*(2), 41–46.

Stone, N. J., Robinson, J., Lichtenstein, A. H., BaireyMerz, C. N., Lloyd-Jones, D. M., Blum, C. B., . . . Wilson, P. W. (2013, November 7). 2013 ACC/AHA guidelines on the treatment of blood cholesterol to reduce atherosclerotic cardiovascular risk in adults: A report of the American College of Cardiology/American Heart Association Task Force on practice guidelines. *Journal of the American College of Cardiology, 53*(25), 2889–2934.

Summary of the Second Report of the National Cholesterol Education Program Expert Panel on Detection, Evaluation, and Treatment of High Blood Cholesterol in Adults (Adult Treatment Panel II). (1993). *The Journal of the American Medical Association, 269*, 3015–3023.

Trayes, K. P., Studdiford, J. S., Pickle, S., & Tully, A. S. (2013). Edema: Diagnosis and management. *American Family Physician, 88*(2), 102–110.

Tsai, J.-R., Liu, P.-L., Chen, Y.-H., Chou, S.-H., Cheng, Y.-J., Hwang, J.-J., & Chong, I.-W. (2015). Curcumin inhibits non-small cell lung cancer cells metastasis through the adiponectin/NF-κb/MMPs signaling pathway. *PLOS ONE, 10*(12), e0144462.

U.S. Department of Health and Human Services, National Institutes of Health, & National Heart, Lung, and Blood Institute. (2006). Your guide to lowering your blood pressure with DASH (NIH Publications No. 06-4082). Washington, DC: U.S. Government Printing Office Retrieved from http://www.nhlbi.nih.gov/health/public/heart/hbp/dash/new_dash.pdf

U.S. Department of Health and Human Services, National Institutes of Health, National Heart, Lung, and Blood Institute, & National High Blood Pressure Education Program. (2004). Seventh report of the Joint National Committee on prevention, detection, evaluation, and treatment of high blood pressure (2003). Retrieved from https://www.nhlbi.nih.gov/files/docs/public/heart/new_dash.pdf

Vascular Cures. (2016a). Chronic venous insufficiency. Retrieved from http://www.vascularcures.org/about-vascular-disease/2011-05-05-02-02-59/chronic-venous-insufficiency

Vascular Cures. (2016b). Lymphedema. Retrieved from http://vasculardisease.org/images/VDF-Diseases-Flyers/lymphedema-flyer%20Vascular%20Cures.pdf

Verma, A., Cairns, J. A., Mitchell, L. B., Macle, L., Stiell, I. G., Gladstone, D., . . . Healey, J. S. (2014). 2014 focused update of the Canadian Cardiovascular Society guidelines for the management of atrial fibrillation. *Canadian Journal of Cardiology, 30*(10), 1114–1130.

Vongpatanasin, W. (2014). Resistant hypertension: A review of diagnosis and management. *The Journal of the American Medical Association, 311*(21), 2216–2224.

Walsh, K., Hoffmayer, K., & Hamdan, M. H. (2015). Syncope: Diagnosis and management. *Current Problems in Cardiology, 40*(2), 51–86.

Wigle, P., Hein, B., Bloomfield, H. E., Tubb, M., & Doherty, M. (2013). Updated guidelines on outpatient anticoagulation. *American Family Physician, 87*(8), 556–566.

Wittens, C., Davies, A. H., Bækgaard, N., Broholm, R., Cavezzi, A., Chastanet, S., . . . Rosales, A.; European Society for Vascular Surgery. (2015). Editor's choice—Management of chronic venous disease: Clinical Practice Guidelines of the European Society for Vascular Surgery (ESVS). *European Journal of Vascular and Endovascular Surgery: The Official Journal of the European Society for Vascular Surgery, 49*(6), 678–737.

Wright, B. M., Rutecki, G. W., & Bellone, J. (2013, January). Resistant hypertension: An approach to diagnosis and treatment. *Consultant, 53*(1), 9–16. Retrieved from www.Consultant360.com

Yancy, C. W., Jessup, M., Bozkurt, B., Butler, J., Casey, D. E., Drazner, M. H., . . . Wilkoff, B. L. (2013). 2013 ACCF/AHA guideline for the management of heart failure: A report of the American College of Cardiology Foundation/American Heart Association Task Force on Practice Guidelines. *Journal of the American College of Cardiology, 62*(16), e147–e239.

Yancy, C. W., Jessup, M., Bozkurt, B., Butler, J., Casey, D. E., Drazner, M. H., . . . Wilkoff, B. L. (2013). 2013 ACCF/AHA guideline for the management of heart failure: A Report of the American College of Cardiology/American Heart Association Task Force on Practice Guidelines and the Heart Rhythm Society. *Circulation, 128*(16), e240–e327.

Yao, S., & Tong, L. (2012). Comparison of anticoagulants used for stroke prevention in patients with atrial fibrillation. *American Journal for Nurse Practitioners, 16*, 29–34.

Zhang, S., & Melander, S. (2014). Varicose veins: Diagnosis, management, and treatment. *Journal for Nurse Practitioners, 10*(6), 417–424.

11 Gastrointestinal Guidelines

Abdominal Pain

Cheryl A. Glass and Audra Malone

Definition

A. Abdominal pain is a common nonspecific complaint. The responsibility is for clinicians to determine that patients can be safely observed and treated symptomatically and that require further investigation or a specialist referral. Pain in the abdomen is secondary to problems relating to abdominal organs, and it is categorized as follows:

  1. Acute pain: Pain of less than a few days that has worsened progressively until presentation.
  2. Chronic pain: Interval of 12 weeks can be used to separate acute from chronic pain, that is, pain has remained unchanged for months or years.
  3. Emergent: Pain that lasts 3 hours or longer, accompanied by fever or vomiting.

B. Pain may be categorized by description:

  1. Visceral pain is usually dull and aching in character.
  2. Parietal pain is sharp and well localized.
  3. Referred pain is aching and perceived to be near the surface of the body.

Incidence

Abdominal pain is very common. On questioning, abdominal pain is present in 75% of adolescents and in about 50% of all adults. Gastroenteritis and irritable bowel syndrome (IBS) are the most common cause of acute pain, and chronic stool retention is the most common cause of chronic pain. Other causes of abdominal pain include the following:

A. Acute appendicitis: Occurs 10:100,000.
B. Acute cholecystitis: Varies according to age and ethnic origin.
C. Intestinal obstruction, usually small intestines: Accounts for 20% of acute abdominal conditions.
D. Abdominal pain associated with pregnancy: Ectopic pregnancy (1:200 pregnancies), miscarriage, and abruptio placenta.

Pathogenesis

A. Pathogenesis depends on the origin of pain. Pain may result from inflammation, ischemia, distension, altered motility, obstruction, or ulceration.

Predisposing Factors

A. Abdominal trauma
B. Motor vehicle accidents
C. Lactose intolerance
D. Pregnancy
E. Torsion
F. Psychogenic pain
G. Sickle cell disease
H. Infection

Common Complaints

Clinical presentation of abdominal pain is determined in part by the site of the involvement.

A. Acute or chronic onset of pain
B. Vomiting
C. Diarrhea

Other Signs and Symptoms

A. Bleeding
B. Referred shoulder pain
C. Fever
D. Nausea and/or projectile vomiting
E. Rigid abdomen
F. Changes in vital signs
G. Abdominal distension
H. Constipation
I. Guarding
J. Rebound tenderness
K. Biliary pain and right subcostal tenderness
L. Anorexia
M. Periumbilical discomfort; consider appendicitis if within 2 to 12 hours, pain localizes in right lower quadrant (RLQ) at McBurney's point.
N. Dysuria
O. Abdominal mass: Do not overlook the possibility of pregnancy as the cause of a mass.
P. Melena (most common in peptic ulcer disease [PUD])

Subjective Data

Evaluate for a "surgical abdomen," defined as a rapidly worsening prognosis in the absence of surgical intervention. Patients should not eat or drink while a diagnosis of a surgical abdomen remains under consideration. Once a surgical abdomen has been excluded, the remainder of the evaluation will be guided by the chronicity of symptoms along with the location of pain.

A. Review the onset, duration, course, and quality of pain.

  1. When did the pain start?

2. What were you doing when the pain started?
3. Has this ever occurred before?
4. What was the primary diagnosis?
5. What was the previous treatment, and was it effective?
6. Is there anyone else in your home having the same symptoms?
7. Review the progression of pain.

B. Determine the pain rating on a 10-point scale, with 0 being no pain and 10 being equivalent to the worst pain the patient has ever felt.
C. Qualify the duration of pain in minutes, hours, days, weeks, or months. Does the pain interfere with sleep?
D. Review the pattern of pain.
1. Review aggravating factors.
2. Review alleviating factors
3. Does the pain radiate?
4. Does the pain have any relationship to food intake?

E. Questions specific to females:
1. Determine the patient's last menstrual period (LMP).
2. Has she had a hysterectomy or tubal ligation?
3. Does she have a recent history of dyspareunia or dysmenorrhea that suggests pelvic pathology?
4. Is there any history of physical abuse?
5. **What type of contraception is used? (Specifically evaluate for an intrauterine device (IUD).**

F. Review the patient's current medications and drug history, especially antibiotic, laxative, acetaminophen, aspirin, and nonsteroidal anti-inflammatory drug (NSAID) use. Pain may be significantly masked in patients taking corticosteroids.
G. Rule out abdominal trauma from domestic violence, motor vehicle accidents, falls, or assaults.
H. Review bowel habits and note changes: Constipation, diarrhea, anorexia, food intolerance, nausea, vomiting, or bloating
I. Review the patient's history for sickle cell disease. Any individual of African American or Mediterranean descent presenting with leg or abdominal pain should be questioned regarding sickle cell disease or trait.
J. Review urinary function. Is there any urinary frequency, urgency, dysuria, flank pain, or back pain? If the patient is male, does he have any hesitancy, difficulty starting the urine stream, nocturia, low urinary volume, or any lower abdominal distension indicating urinary retention?
K. Review alcohol intake/history.
L. Has the patient had any unexplained weight loss?
M. Evaluate sexual activity to rule out potential sexually transmitted infection (STI).
1. Evaluate whether the patient has new partners.
2. Are the partners experiencing any symptoms?

Physical Examination

A. Check temperature, pulse, respirations, and blood pressure; include orthostatic blood pressure.

> *Tachycardia or hypotension may be signs of a ruptured aortic aneurysm, septic shock, gastrointestinal (GI) hemorrhage, or volume depletion. Absence of a fever in the elderly or immunosuppressed does not exclude a serious illness.*

B. Inspect
1. Observe general appearance: Facial expressions, walk, skin turgor, refusal to move/writhing; note grimace during examination.
2. Perform eye and mouth examination to rule out iritis and aphthous ulcers of the mouth (extraintestinal manifestations of inflammatory bowel disease [IBD]). Examine eyes for jaundice.
3. Examine the abdomen for the presence of hernia at the umbilicus, groin, or near the site of prior surgical incisions.
4. Examine the abdomen for overt masses or pulsations.
5. Examine skin for jaundice. Observe for any bruising or other signs of domestic violence in the "bathing suit" areas: Breasts, abdomen, and the back that would be easily covered with clothes.

C. Auscultate
1. Auscultate for bowel sounds in all four quadrants of the abdomen.
2. Evaluate heart and lungs.
3. Check for aortic, iliac, and renal bruits.

D. Percuss the abdomen for tympany and dullness.
E. Palpate
1. Abdomen for masses, rebound tenderness, and peritoneal signs
   a. Before palpating the abdomen, ask the patient to bend the knees to help with relaxation of the wall musculature.
   b. Elderly patients may lack classical peritoneal signs of rebound and guarding.
2. Check the abdomen for tender pulsatile mass at midline; it may indicate abdominal aortic aneurysm (AAA).
3. Palpate back; check for costovertebral angle (CVA) tenderness.
4. Perform a bimanual examination in women regardless of whether the patient has had a hysterectomy or is postmenopausal.
   a. Evaluate the size and symmetry of the uterus.
   b. Evaluate the adnexal areas for presence of appropriately sized mobile ovaries. A fixed, painful adnexal mass is suggestive of an endometrioma or tubo-ovarian abscess.
   c. Endometriosis is suggested by localized tenderness in the cul-de-sac or uterosacral ligaments, palpable tender nodules, pain with uterine movement, and tenderness fixation of adnexal mass or uterus in a retroverted position.
5. Check for obturator sign, which is abdominal pain in response to passive internal rotation of the right hip from the 90° angle knee–hip flexion position; perform this when an inflamed appendix is suspected.
6. Check for iliopsoas sign; perform this when an inflamed appendix is suspected. Positive psoas sign is the presence of lower quadrant pain noted as the supine patient raises his or her right leg from the hip while the examiner pushes downward against his or her lower thigh.

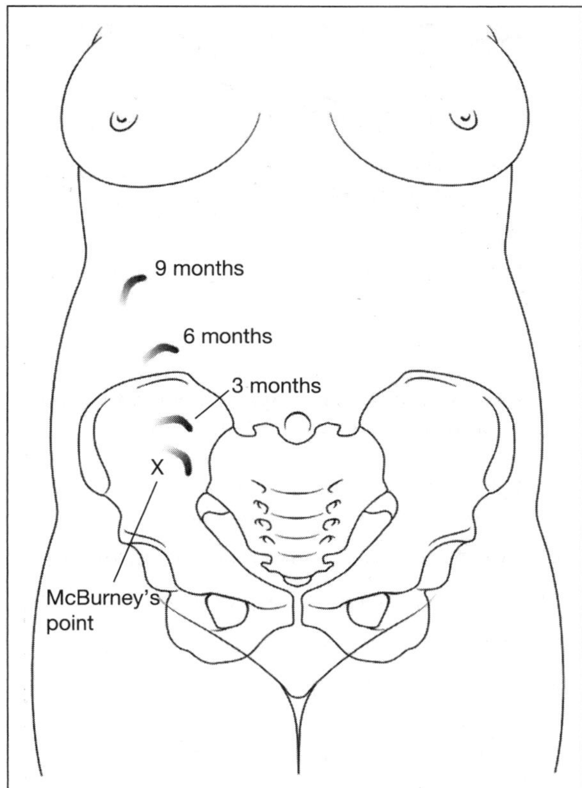

FIGURE 11.1 The position of the appendix alters during pregnancy and so must the site of incision to gain access.

3. Check for rebound tenderness.
4. Check for jar tenderness.

Diagnostic Tests

A. **Serum human chorionic gonadotropin (HCG): Pregnancy should be excluded in all women of childbearing age. Assume that the woman is pregnant until proven otherwise.**
B. Complete blood count (CBC) with differential
C. C-reactive protein (CRP)
D. Urinalysis, to rule out urinary disorders
E. Abdominal ultrasonography; any person with trauma to the abdomen should have an abdominal ultrasound.
F. CT scan with or without contrast
G. MRI may be used as an alternative diagnostic test in pregnancy to avoid exposure to ionizing radiation.
H. Stool guaiac test for occult blood

Differential Diagnoses

The appendix has no fixed position. Duration of pain can significantly help in narrowing differential diagnosis. Nonspecific dysfunctional abdominal pain and psychogenic abdominal pain are diagnoses of exclusion.

A. Appendicitis
B. Regional enteritis
C. Leaking aneurysm
D. Ruptured ectopic pregnancy
E. Ovarian cyst
F. Ovarian torsion
G. Pelvic inflammatory disease (PID)
H. Mittelschmerz, or ovulatory bleeding or pain
I. Endometriosis
J. Ureteral calculi
K. Incarcerated, strangulated groin hernia
L. Meckel's diverticulitis
M. Abdominal wall hematoma
N. Bowel obstruction
O. Intestinal malrotation
P. Intussusception
Q. Testicular torsion
R. Inflammatory bowel disease (IBD)/Crohn's
S. Parasites
T. Intrauterine device (IUD)
U. Constipation

Plan

A. Patient teaching: *See Section III: Patient Teaching Guides for this chapter, "Abdominal Pain: Adults" and "Abdominal Pain: Children."*
B. Medical and surgical management: Appendectomy may need to be performed.
C. Pharmaceutical therapy
   1. Antibiotics are currently used to treat uncomplicated, nonsurgical appendicitis; however, there is a 5% to 15% rate of complications and a 15% to 30% recurrence rate. More studies are needed to determine the efficacy of antibiotic therapy alone.
   2. Do not give antipyretics to mask fever.
   3. Do not administer cathartics because they may cause rupture.

Follow-Up

A. Postoperative follow-up is with the surgeon.

Consultation/Referral

A. Physician consultation and possible emergency transport and hospitalization are often required.

Individual Considerations

A. Pregnancy
   1. Any abdominal pain or bleeding in the first 8 weeks after a missed menstrual period must be considered a symptom of possible *ectopic pregnancy.*
   2. The identification of intra-abdominal masses may be compromised by the enlarged uterus, but this problem may be partially obviated by examining the woman in the lateral position.
   3. The intestinal tract is progressively displaced upward, outward, and backward during pregnancy; bowel sounds are best heard lateral or superior to the uterus.
B. Pediatrics
   1. The caregiver's lap makes the best examining surface; it is much better than having the child lie fixed and supine on a table.
   2. If possible, examine the infant's abdomen during a time of relaxation and quiet. It is often best to do this at the start of the overall examination, especially before initiating any procedure that might cause distress. Allowing the infant to suck on a bottle or pacifier may help relax him or her.
   3. Tenderness or pain on palpation may be difficult to detect in the infant. However, pain and tenderness are assessed by such behaviors as change in the pitch of

crying, facial grimacing, rejection of the opportunity to suck, and drawing knees to the abdomen with palpation.

4. Intestinal malrotation must be considered when a healthy infant suddenly refuses to eat, vomits, becomes inconsolable, and develops abdominal distension.

5. Young children have inaccurate body perceptions and are inaccurate historians, so rely on caregivers and examination for data, and consider psychosocial aspects such as child care and child abuse.

6. Intussusception presents as paroxysmal, colicky pain, and the infant often has currant-jelly stools, a palpable right upper quadrant (RUQ), abdominal mass, and ultimately distension.

C. Adults

1. Obesity distorts abdominal examination, making organ palpation or pelvic examination difficult.

2. Immunocompromised patients are susceptive to infection. They may not exhibit the typical signs and symptoms of appendicitis; only mild tenderness on examination.

3. CT examination is useful for diagnosis in the immunocompromised.

D. Geriatrics

1. The elderly tend to have a diminished inflammatory response, resulting in a less remarkable history and physical examination. Be aware of vague symptoms, such as milder pain, less pronounced fever, and leukocytosis with shift to left on differential.

2. Confusion is a common presenting symptom.

3. A redundant sigmoid colon may also cause right-sided pain from sigmoid disease.

4. Prompt CT scanning is used for diagnosis and differential.

Celiac Disease

Cheryl A. Glass and Audra Malone

Definition

A. Celiac disease, previously known as *celiac sprue*, is an autoimmune disorder triggered by a well-defined environmental factor, gluten. Celiac disease is a permanent sensitivity to gluten, specifically; the people are unable to tolerate gliadin, the alcohol-soluble fraction of gluten. Three cereals contain gluten and are considered toxic for patients with celiac disease: Wheat, rye, and barley. The disease primarily affects the small intestine. Onset of symptoms depends on the amount of gluten in the diet. Dietary nonadherence is the chief cause of persistent or recurrent symptoms (see Appendix B, Table B.5).

B. Celiac disease is one of the most common causes of chronic malabsorption as a result of injury to the small intestine with loss of absorptive surface area, reduction of digestive enzymes, and consequential impaired absorption of micronutrients such as fat soluble vitamins, iron, and potentially vitamin B_{12} and folic acid.

C. Celiac disease is strongly associated with autoimmune conditions, including type 1 diabetes, Addison disease, and thyroiditis, as well as genetic syndromes, including Down syndrome, Williams syndrome, and Turner syndrome. The complications from celiac disease include osteopenia, osteoporosis, infertility, short stature, delayed puberty, anemia, gastrointestinal (GI) malignancies, and non-Hodgkin's lymphoma (NHL).

D. After GI symptoms, the second most common manifestation of celiac disease in patients with type 1 diabetes is diminished or impaired bone mineralization.

E. Celiac disease is the most common cause of steatorrhea in people older than 50 years and the second most common cause in people older than 65 years.

F. A substantial number of patients are misdiagnosed as having irritable bowel syndrome (IBS) for years before the diagnosis of celiac disease.

Incidence

A. Celiac disease can occur at any stage of life. The prevalence of celiac disease in children is unknown. Its prevalence is approximately 1% of the general population in North America. The highest incidence (5%) is noted in the Sub-Saharan African population. The true incidence is undetermined due to asymptomatic disease and underdiagnosis. It is estimated that 75% of those affected by celiac disease remain underdiagnosed or misdiagnosed.

B. Screening of the general population is not recommended.

C. Newly diagnosed patients with celiac disease should inform their first-degree family members of their increased risk of celiac disease and the American College of Gastroenterology (ACG) recommendation for testing.

Pathogenesis

A. Interactions between gluten and immune and genetic factors result in celiac disease. Gluten is poorly digested. The enzyme tissue transglutaminase (tTG) is the autoantigen against which abnormal immune response is directed. The immune responses promote an inflammatory reaction. Celiac disease primarily affects the mucosal layer of the small intestine. The classic celiac lesion is noted in the proximal small intestine.

B. A hallmark on histology is the presence of villous atrophy. The Marsh Classification is used to describe the progressive histologic stages of celiac disease. Marsh 1 and Marsh 2 may be seen in sow and cow's milk allergies.

- Marsh 0: Preinfiltrative stage (normal)
- Marsh 1: Infiltrative lesion (increased intraepithelial lymphocytes)
- Marsh 2: Hyperplastic lesion (type 1 plus hyperplastic crypts)
- Marsh 3: Destructive lesion (type 2 plus villous atrophy of progressively more severe degrees [termed 3a, 3b, and 3c])
- Marsh 4: (atrophic-hypoplastic) Total villous atrophy, crypt hypoplasia

Predisposing Factors

A. Female gender

B. May be precipitated by an infectious diarrheal episode or other intestinal disease (e.g., rotavirus)

C. Genetic disorders

1. Down syndrome (8%–12%)

2. Type 1 diabetes (10%)
3. Turner syndrome (2%–10%)
4. Williams syndrome (8.2%)

D. Strong hereditary component (10% in first-degree relatives)
E. The introduction of gluten before 4 months of age is associated with increased disease development.
F. Autoimmune thyroiditis
G. Selective immunoglobulin A (IgA) deficiency

Common Complaints

A. Asymptomatic
B. Chronic diarrhea or explosive watery diarrhea
C. Foul-smelling voluminous stools
D. Anorexia
E. Abdominal distension
F. Abdominal pain
G. Poor weight gain or weight loss
H. Vomiting
I. Steatorrhea (malabsorption of ingested fat)
J. Refusal to eat (children)

Other Signs and Symptoms

A. Behavioral changes, including irritability
B. Dehydration
C. Lethargy
D. Constipation
E. Failure to thrive (FTT)
F. Short stature and delayed puberty
G. Dermatitis herpetiformis
H. Arthritis
I. Seizures
J. Weakness and fatigue
K. Dental enamel hypoplasia of permanent teeth
L. Iron-deficiency anemia unresponsive to treatment
M. Bruising/bleeding tendency
N. Osteopenia/osteoporosis
O. Hair loss
P. Lactose intolerance
Q. Aphthous stomatitis
R. Ataxia
S. Neuropathy

Subjective Data

A. Review the onset, duration, course, and type of symptoms.
B. Review the patient's weight history.
C. Evaluate family history for celiac disease or members with similar histories.
D. Review current medications and drug history, especially antibiotic, laxative, and herbal products.
E. Review bowel habits and note changes: Constipation, diarrhea, anorexia, and/or food intolerance
F. Review the patient's tolerance to lactose products.

Physical Examination

A. Check vital signs, including height and weight. Follow serial weights and plot serial height/weight on growth charts.
B. Inspect
   1. Observe general overall appearance.
   2. Oral examination to evaluate glossitis, dry mucosal membranes (dehydration), and the presence of oral aphthae
   3. Examine the skin for the presence of dermatitis herpetiformis: A blistering rash involving the scalp, neck, elbows, knees, and buttocks.
   4. Evaluate the abdomen for the presence of bloating and protuberant "potbelly."
   5. Evaluate the patient's weight loss, including muscle wasting.

C. Auscultate
   1. For bowel sounds in all four quadrants of the abdomen

D. Percuss abdomen.
E. Palpate
   1. Palpate the abdomen for masses, rebound tenderness, and peritoneal signs.
      a. Before palpating the abdomen, ask the patient to bend his or her knees to help with relaxation of the wall musculature.
   2. Perform a rectal examination, including testing stool for occult blood.

Diagnostic Tests

The confirmation of a diagnosis of celiac disease is based on the combination of findings from the medical history, physical examination, serology, and upper endoscopy, with histologic analysis of multiple biopsies of the duodenum. **All testing should be performed while patients are following a gluten-rich diet.**

A. **Endoscopy for duodenal biopsies is the standard and a critical component for diagnosing celiac disease.**
B. Screening and monitoring tests for celiac disease (see Table 11.1 for celiac disease tests and possible results):
   1. tTG antibody, IgA class
      a. Primary test ordered to screen for celiac disease
      b. Used for monitoring and evaluating the effectiveness of treatment
      c. Antibody levels should fall when gluten is removed from the diet
   2. Anti-tTG antibodies, immunoglobulin G (IgG)
   3. Anti-tTG, IgG class
   4. Deamidated gliadin peptide antibodies (anti-DGP, IgA)
   5. Anti-gliadin antibodies (AGAs) IgG (gliadin is a component of wheat storage protein gluten)
   6. AGA IgA
   7. IgA endomysial antibody (EMA)—less frequently ordered, measures same as the anti-tTG
   8. Antireticulin antibody (ARA)—rarely ordered
   9. Anti-F-actin—is ordered if the disease has been diagnosed; evaluates the severity of intestinal damage. May be used for monitoring.

C. Complete blood count (CBC) and electrolytes
D. Aspartate transaminase (AST) and alanine transaminase (ALT; liver enzymes normalize on a gluten-free diet)
E. Prothrombin time (PT) may be prolonged with malabsorption of vitamin K.
F. C-reactive protein (CRP)
G. Erythrocyte sedimentation rate (ESR)

TABLE 11.1 What Does the Test Result Mean? Some Celiac Disease Tests and Positive Results

Anti-TTG Antibodies, IgA	Total IgA	Anti-TTG Antibodies, IgG	Anti-DGP, IgA	AGAs, IgG	Diagnosis
Positive	Normal	Not performed	Not performed	Not performed	Presumptive celiac disease
Negative	Normal	Negative	Negative	Negative	Symptoms not likely due to celiac disease
Negative	Low	Positive	Negative	Positive	Possible celiac disease (false negative anti-tTG, IgA, and anti-DGP, IgA are due to total IgA deficiency)
Negative	Normal	Negative	Positive	Positive (or not performed)	Possible celiac disease (may be seen in children younger than 3 years old)

AGA, anti-gliadin antibodies; DGP, deamidated gliadin peptide; IgA, immunoglobulin A; IgG, immunoglobulin G; TTG, tissue transglutaminase.
Source: © 2015 American Association for Clinical Chemistry. Reprinted with permission from Lab Tests Online.

H. Total protein
I. Albumin
J. Calcium
K. Iron, transferrin, and ferritin
L. Vitamin B_{12} and folate levels
M. Thyroid screen (autoimmune thyroid disorders and hypothyroidism common in the elderly)
N. Stool culture, ova, and parasites
O. Fecal fat
P. Bone density (bone mineral density improves on gluten-free diet)
Q. Human leukocyte antigen (HLA) haplotypes
R. Colonoscopy if bloody stools or symptoms of colitis
S. Sweat test to exclude cystic fibrosis (CF)
T. Other testing specific to nutritional deficiencies as needed (vitamin D, B_{12}, folate)
U. Radiograph, including barium swallow study with a small-bowel follow-through, is usually nonspecific and is not indicated.

Differential Diagnoses

A. Celiac disease
B. FTT
C. Food allergies
D. Inflammatory bowel disease (IBD)
  1. Crohn's disease (CD)
  2. Ulcerative colitis (UC)
E. Immunodeficiency disorders
F. Gastroenteritis (viral or bacterial)
G. Parasites
H. Fungal infection
I. Irritable bowel syndrome (IBS)
J. Malabsorption
K. Lymphomas of the small intestine

Plan

A. Nutrition therapy is the only accepted treatment for celiac disease.
  1. Gluten-free dietary instructions should be given and reinforced.
  2. Reinforce the need to read all food labels.
  3. Stress that wheat-free is not the same as gluten-free.
  4. The gluten-free diet must continue throughout the patient's life.

B. The ACG recommends a referral to a registered dietitian in order to receive a thorough nutritional assessment and education on a gluten-free diet. A gluten-free diet should be maintained for life. Nutriguides "nutrition guides" apps are available from the iTunes Store for iPhone and iPad and from the Google Store for Android products.
C. Genetic testing does not diagnose celiac disease.
D. Monitor for iron and vitamin deficiencies because substitute flours are not fortified with B vitamins. Supplement with iron, folate, and vitamin B_{12} as needed.
E. Screen for osteoporosis. Up to 70% of adult and elderly patients with celiac disease have osteopenia.
F. Keep a food/symptom diary in order to eliminate trigger foods. See Appendix B, Table B.5.
G. Gluten has been identified in dietary supplements, over-the-counter (OTC) medications, and nonfood items such as lipstick and envelope adhesive, and in food items with gluten additives such as condiments.
H. Gluten rechallenge is not generally recommended unless the diagnosis remains uncertain.
  1. The rechallenge is not mandatory for patients with good improvement of symptoms.
  2. HLA-DQ2/DQ8 gentoyping for genetic risk factors should be used to try to exclude celiac disease prior to a formal gluten challenge.
I. Pharmacology: Corticosteroids may be prescribed for rapid control of symptoms: Prednisone (Deltasone, Orasone, Sterapred)
  1. Adults: 30 to 40 mg/d; taper off completely in 6 to 8 weeks.
  2. Pediatrics: 1 mg/kg/d; not to exceed 30 mg/d. Taper off completely in 6 to 8 weeks. Children with celiac disease are rarely given steroids.
  3. Bisphosphonates for osteoporosis

Follow-Up

A. After the diagnosis of celiac disease and a strict diet has been started, follow up in 4 to 8 weeks or earlier if the patient has other comorbidities.

F. Perform a rectal examination, including testing of stool for occult blood. **Failure to perform a rectal examination in patients with abdominal pain may be associated with an increased rate of misdiagnosis and should be considered a medicolegal pitfall.**

Diagnostic Tests

Diagnostic testing is ordered based on the following differential diagnoses.

A. In all women of childbearing age, assume the woman is pregnant until proven otherwise. Vaginal bleeding with or without abdominal pain should prompt a transvaginal ultrasound and a serum human chorionic gonadotropin (HCG) test. HCG should be tested before performing the transvaginal ultrasound.

B. Complete blood count (CBC) with differential
C. Electrolytes
D. Complete metabolic panel
E. Blood urea nitrogen (BUN)
F. Amylase
G. Aminotransferases, alkaline phosphatase (ALP), and bilirubin
H. Lipase
I. Urinalysis; save sample for culture.
J. Coproporphyrin, if lead poisoning is suspected
K. Plain x-ray films of abdomen to rule out obstruction
L. CT of abdomen with or without contrast
M. Abdominal ultrasonography
N. GI series radiography
O. Endoscopy; consider *Helicobacter pylori* testing.
P. Sigmoidoscopy
Q. Barium enema (BE): Avoid with suspected obstruction.
R. Stool guaiac test for occult blood
S. Consider endoscopic retrograde cholangiopancreatography (ERCP) to visualize the distal common bile duct.
T. EKG to rule out cardiac pain.
U. Consider blood cultures for elderly who present with abdominal pain associated with either fever or hypothermia or when sepsis is suspected.
V. Chest radiography

Differential Diagnoses

Location and duration of abdominal pain can often significantly help in narrowing the differential diagnosis.

A. Right upper quadrant (RUQ) pain
  1. Acute cholecystitis and biliary colic
    a. Biliary tract: Increased serum amylase
    b. Ascending cholangitis presents with fever and jaundice in a patient with RUQ pain.
    c. In acute cholecystitis, the typical pain is maximal in the RUQ or epigastrium, radiating to the scapular region, and is accompanied by nausea, vomiting, and fever without jaundice. Murphy's sign, or inspiratory arrest in response to upper quadrant palpation, may be seen with acute cholecystitis. RUQ tenderness to percussion or pressure of the gallbladder is also a suggestive finding.
    d. Ketoacidosis has been found to present with severe abdominal pain in 8% of instances and may be accompanied by emesis and an elevated white cell count. Acute intra-abdominal events, such as cholecystitis, may be the precipitant of ketoacidosis.
  2. Acute hepatitis
  3. Hepatic abscess
  4. Hepatomegaly due to congestive heart failure (CHF)
  5. Perforated duodenal ulcer (DU)

A perforated ulcer is accompanied by an increased serum amylase.

  6. Acute pancreatitis: bilateral pain-right and left upper quadrant pain.

Pancreatitis is accompanied by an increased serum amylase.

  7. Herpes zoster
  8. Myocardial ischemia
  9. Pleural or pulmonary pathology (e.g., pneumonia, pulmonary embolism, or empyema)

B. Right lower quadrant (RLQ) pain
  1. Appendicitis often begins with symptoms of dull, steady, periumbilical pain and anorexia before localizing to the RLQ at McBurney's point.
  2. Regional enteritis
  3. Leaking aneurysm
  4. Ruptured ectopic pregnancy
  5. Ovarian cyst
  6. Ovarian torsion
  7. Pelvic inflammatory disease (PID)
  8. Ureteral calculi
  9. Incarcerated, strangulated inguinal hernia
  10. Endometriosis
  11. Meckel's diverticulitis
  12. Abdominal wall hematoma

C. Left upper quadrant (LUQ) pain
  1. Gastritis
  2. Acute pancreatitis: Epigastric pain that is relatively sudden, bores in to the back, and is associated with nausea, vomiting, and anorexia.
  3. Splenic enlargement, rupture, infarction, aneurysm
  4. Myocardial ischemia
  5. Left lower lobe pneumonia
  6. Renal colic: Radiates to the groin

D. Left lower quadrant (LLQ) pain
  1. Sigmoid and/or descending diverticulitis
  2. Regional enteritis
  3. Leaking aneurysm

AAA may present with a tender pulsatile mass at the abdominal midline. Vascular disorders such as acute arterial insufficiency due to atherosclerosis or embolus, may present with severe abdominal pain, although mild, constant pain may be the only symptom for several days. Dissection or rupture of an AAA produces severe acute abdominal pain and often radiates to the back or genitalia.

4. Ruptured ectopic pregnancy

Rupture of the fallopian tube generally causes sudden, acute, and localized abdominal pain. Internal hemorrhage causes syncope and referred shoulder pain, caused by phrenic nerve irritation. Diagnosis before tubal rupture may be difficult because symptoms and physical findings mimic other conditions such as appendicitis.

5. Ovarian cyst
6. Ovarian torsion
7. PID
8. Ureteral calculi
9. Incarcerated, strangulated inguinal hernia

E. Generalized abdominal pain
1. Trauma
a. **Any person with a possible blow to the abdomen should have orthostatic blood pressure taken, careful palpation of the abdomen, serial abdominal circumferences measured, and be considered for abdominal imaging. Serial hemoglobin and hematocrit (Hct) measurements should be obtained, if necessary.**
b. In abdominal trauma, the spleen is the most commonly injured organ, especially in blunt abdominal trauma; the onset can be immediate or delayed.
c. Nontraumatic splenic rupture is often associated with acute infectious mononucleosis.
2. Intestinal obstruction: Obstruction that develops slowly over weeks to months may be relatively subtle in presentation.

Acute obstruction presents with severe "colicky" pain or pain that is wavelike in nature; it makes the pain relentless.

3. Peritoneal irritation: Severe pain due to the rich innervation of the parietal peritoneum. Focal injury results in well-localized discomfort that is described as a sharp aching or burning sensation.
4. Metabolic disturbances may mimic intra-abdominal etiologies.

Porphyria and lead poisoning sometimes simulate bowel obstruction because they can cause cramping, abdominal pain, and hyperperistalsis.

5. Nonspecific dysfunctional abdominal pain and psychogenic abdominal pain are diagnoses of exclusion.

Plan

A. General interventions
1. If necessary, prepare the patient for emergency transport and hospitalization.
2. Management and follow-up of other causes of abdominal pain are variable and depend on diagnosis.

B. Patient teaching
1. *See Section III: Patient Teaching Guides for this chapter, "Abdominal Pain: Adults" and "Abdominal Pain: Children."*
2. Counsel the patient to keep a pain diary to include activity, foods, and other pain triggers; duration of pain; and what provides relief of symptoms.

C. Pharmaceutical therapy: Treatment depends on the findings from the history, physical, and testing and clinical diagnosis.

Follow-Up

A. Variable, depending on diagnosis
B. Review pain diary

Consultation/Referral

A. Consult the physician for the patient with acute abdominal pain and pain related to abdominal trauma.
B. For the obstetric patient, consult a physician for any bleeding or abdominal pain.

Individual Considerations

A. Pregnancy: There is no evidence that acute intra-abdominal surgical emergencies are more common during pregnancy if ectopic pregnancy is excluded.
1. The presence of peritoneal signs, rebound tenderness, and abdominal guarding is never normal in pregnancy.
2. Bleeding complications include the following:
a. First trimester: Miscarriage and ectopic pregnancy
b. Second and third trimester: Abruptio placenta
3. Physiological changes of pregnancy may affect the presentation and evaluation of abdominal pain. The enlargement of the uterus can impede physical examination, affect the normal location of pelvic and abdominal organs, and mask or delay peritoneal signs.
4. Severe preeclampsia: The clinical manifestations of liver involvement include RUQ or midepigastric pain, elevated transaminases, and, in severe cases, subcapsular hemorrhage or hepatic rupture.

B. Pediatrics
1. The caregiver's lap makes the best examining surface; it is much better than having the child lie fixed and supine on a table.
2. Observe the child's interaction and gait prior to examination. If able to stand, ask the child to hop as an assessment of peritoneal irritation. If the child is unwilling to stand, shaking the examination table or pelvis can also evaluate for peritoneal signs.
3. An infant's abdomen should be examined during a time of relaxation and quiet, if possible. It is often best to do this at the start of the overall examination, especially before initiating any procedure that may cause distress.
4. Allowing an infant to suck on a pacifier may help relax him or her.
5. Tenderness or pain on palpation may be difficult to detect in an infant. However, pain and tenderness are assessed by such behaviors as change in the pitch of crying, facial grimacing, rejection of opportunity to suck, and drawing the knees to the abdomen with palpation.

6. Urinary tract infections (UTIs) can cause abdominal pain, and often the child with a UTI does not complain of dysuria and frequency as adults typically do.
7. Young children have inaccurate body perceptions and are inaccurate historians. The practitioner must rely on the caregiver and the examination for data. Consider psychosocial aspects of child care and possible abuse.
8. Appendicitis is the most common pediatric surgical emergency. The diagnosis can be difficult, because the classic symptoms are often not present.
9. Intestinal malrotation must be considered when a healthy infant suddenly refuses to eat, vomits, becomes inconsolable, and develops abdominal distension.
10. Intussusception presents as paroxysmal, colicky pain, and the infant often has currant-jelly stools; a palpable right upper quadrant (RUQ) abdominal mass; and, ultimately, distension.
11. Young male patients may hesitate to report testicular pain.

C. Adults
1. Obesity distorts the abdominal examination, making organ palpation or pelvic examination difficult.
2. With men older than age 40 and women older than age 50, suspect cardiac origin when presenting with epigastric pain. Consider obtaining EKG for patients in this age group.

Although myocardial infarction "classically" presents with anterior chest pressure or pain, the patient may also have a gastritis or heartburn sensation, coupled with nausea and diaphoresis.

D. Geriatrics
1. Elderly patients may have a vague or atypical presentation of pain, varying in location, severity, and presence of a fever or nonspecific findings on examination.
a. Classic findings of acute peritonitis, rebound tenderness, and local rigidity occur less in the elderly.
2. Elderly patients have a diminished sensorium, allowing pathology to advance to a dangerous point prior to symptom development.
a. The level of pain is much less severe at presentation and continues to be at a lower level of pain.
b. The elderly may present with altered mental status.
3. In an older patient, a similar presentation to IBD with abdominal pain and a change in bowel habits can be the first sign of colon cancer.
4. AAA is observed almost exclusively in elderly patients. Maintain a high index of suspicion in patients who present with a clinical picture suggestive of renal colic or musculoskeletal back pain.
a. Approximately 5% of men 65 years and older have AAA.
b. Maintain a high index of suspicion in patients who present with a clinical picture suggestive of renal colic or musculoskeletal back pain.
5. Elderly patients with UTI are less likely to have dysuria, frequency, or urgency.
6. Patients older than 65 years have a 30% to 50% risk of gallstones and may not present with significant pain; less than half have fever, vomiting, or leukocytosis.
7. Fever and an elevated white blood cell (WBC) count, occur in less than half of the elderly patients with diverticulitis. Only about 25% of the elderly with diverticulitis present with a guaiac positive stool.
8. The incidence of peptic ulcer disease (PUD) is more common in the elderly due to the availability and use of nonsteroidal anti-inflammatory drugs (NSAIDs). The most common presenting symptom with PUD in the elderly is melena.

Resource

Rome Foundation: http://romecriteria.org/criteria

Appendicitis

Cheryl A. Glass and Audra Malone

Definition

A. Appendicitis is acute inflammation of the appendix caused by the obstruction of the appendiceal lumen. There is no single sign, symptom, or diagnostic test that accurately confirms the diagnosis of inflammation. Perforation is rare in the first 12 hours, but the rate of possible perforation increases after 72 hours. Prompt, early diagnosis and intervention are the goal of treatment. The differential diagnoses for appendicitis include all abdominal sources of pain.

Incidence

A. Acute appendicitis occurs at a rate of 10:100,000. It is the most common condition in children (1%–8%) and during pregnancy (0.06%–0.1%) that requires emergency abdominal surgery. One in every 2,000 adults older than age 65 years will develop appendicitis.

Pathogenesis

A. Foreign bodies, fecal material, tissue hypertrophy, strictures, or a bend or twist on the organ may cause obstruction of the appendix. The obstruction causes colicky pain. Bacterial invasion causes inflammation and leads to gangrene and perforation. The most common bacteria are *Escherichia coli*, pseudomonas, *Bacteroides fragilis*, and *Peptostreptococcus* species.

Predisposing Factors

A. Pregnancy
B. Torsion
C. Abdominal trauma
D. Male gender, age: 10 to 30 years

Common Complaints

The classic history of anorexia and periumbilical pain followed by nausea, right lower quadrant (RLQ) pain, and vomiting occurs in only 50% of cases.

A. Adults
1. Generalized or localized abdominal pain in the epigastric or periumbilical areas. Within 2 to 12 hours, pain localizes in RLQ at McBurney's point, and intensity increases.
2. The location of the appendix is altered in pregnancy and with anatomical variations.
3. Pain typically develops before vomiting.
4. Nausea and/or vomiting (may be projectile).
5. Anorexia signals organic cause of abdominal pain.
6. Elderly may present with confusion.

B. Pediatrics
1. Children younger than 2 years
a. Abdominal distension
b. Irritability
c. Lethargy
d. Fever
2. Children older than 2 years
a. Vomiting is often the first symptom
b. Abdominal pain in RLQ
c. Fever

Other Signs and Symptoms

A. Rigid abdomen
B. Changes in pulse (tachycardia), breathing (tachypnea), or skin temperature
C. Involuntary guarding
D. Rebound tenderness

Subjective Data

Evaluate for a "surgical abdomen," defined as a rapidly worsening prognosis in the absence of surgical intervention. Patients should not eat or drink while a diagnosis of a surgical abdomen remains under consideration. Once a surgical abdomen has been excluded, the remainder of the evaluation will be guided by the chronicity of symptoms along with the location of pain.

A. Review the onset, duration, course, and quality of pain. Has pain ever occurred before? If so, what was the primary diagnosis? What was the previous treatment, and was it effective?
B. Qualify the duration of pain in minutes, hours, days, weeks, or months. Does it interfere with sleep? Is there a pattern to the pain?
C. Have the patient rate the pain on a 10-point pain scale, with 0 being no pain and 10 being the worst pain the patient has ever felt.
D. Review the pattern of pain.
1. Review aggravating factors.
2. Review alleviating factors.
3. Does the pain radiate?
4. Does the pain have any relationship to food?
E. Questions specific to females:
1. Determine the patient's last menstrual period (LMP) to rule out pregnancy.
2. What type of contraception is used (specifically evaluate for an intrauterine device [IUD])?
3. Has she had a hysterectomy or tubal ligation?
4. Does she have a recent history of dyspareunia or dysmenorrhea that suggests pelvic pathology?
F. Review current medications and drug history, especially antibiotic and laxative use. Patients taking corticosteroids may have a significant masking of pain.
G. Rule out abdominal trauma, motor vehicle accidents, falls, and assault.
H. Discuss bowel habits, including any changes, such as constipation or diarrhea, anorexia, food intolerance, nausea and vomiting, and bloating.
I. Ask the patient about urinary frequency, urgency, dysuria, flank pain, and back pain. In males, ask about hesitancy, difficulty starting the urine stream, nocturia, low urinary volume, or lower abdominal distension (urinary retention).

Physical Examination

A. Check temperature, pulse, respirations, and blood pressure (BP), including orthostatic BP.
B. Inspect
1. Observe general appearance: Facial expressions (grimace during examination), walk, skin color and turgor, level of consciousness, and acuity level of pain.
2. Inspect abdomen for surgical scars.
3. Observe for any bruising or other signs of domestic violence in the "bathing suit" area: breasts, abdomen, or the back—that would be easily covered by clothes.
C. Auscultate
1. Abdomen for bowel sounds in all quadrants
2. Heart and lungs
D. Palpate: Note guarding with examination.
1. Palpate back; note costovertebral angle (CVA) tenderness.
2. Check for obturator sign, or abdominal pain in response to passive internal rotation of right hip from 90° angle hip–knee flexion position. A positive sign indicates pain secondary to irritation of obturator muscle with inflamed appendix.
3. Assess psoas sign or increased abdominal pain occurring when the patient attempts to raise his or her right thigh against the pressure of your hand placed over his or her right knee. Pain is caused by inflammation of the psoas muscle in acute appendicitis.
4. Check for the Apley rule; the farther the pain from the navel, the more likely it is organic in origin.
5. Check for Rovsing's sign, or pain in the right lower quadrant (RLQ) on palpation of the left side.
6. Anatomical variations of the appendix may lead to differences in the location of the pain. For example, the location of the appendix changes with pregnancy (see Figure 11.1), retrocecal appendix may lead to right loin pain.
E. Percuss abdomen.
F. Perform rectal or pelvic examination if needed. May have right side pain with subcecal or pelvic appendix.
G. Palpate abdomen. Palpate at the end of the examination because positive response produces pain and muscle spasm that can interfere with subsequent examination.
1. Ask the patient to bend his or her knees to help relax abdominal wall musculature.
2. Check for Murphy's sign, which is inspiratory arrest in response to right upper quadrant (RUQ) palpation, seen in acute cholecystitis.

B. The Celiac Disease Guideline Committee recommends the measurement of tTGA after 6 months of a gluten-free diet.
C. Newly diagnosed patients with celiac disease should undergo testing and treatment for micronutrient deficiencies. Deficiency testing should include, but not be limited to, iron, folic acid, vitamin D, and vitamin B_{12}.
D. Refer for dietary consultation with a nutritionist with experience in gluten-free diets.
E. Consider allergy testing.

Consultation/Referral

A. If the gluten-free diet fails or the patient experiences new symptoms, a systematic evaluation is required.
B. Endocrine consultation for patients with Hashimoto thyroiditis and celiac disease
C. Consultation with a pediatric gastroenterologist

Individual Considerations

A. Pregnancy: Women with untreated celiac disease are at risk for preterm birth, low-birth-weight babies, recurrent loss, and reduced fertility.
B. Pediatrics
  1. Children may appear to have a "potbelly" with muscle wasting from malnutrition.
  2. Monitor growth and development. Utilize a growth chart to plot growth rates. As many as 10% of children with idiopathic short stature may have celiac disease.
  3. Breastfeeding has a protective role even if gluten is introduced while breastfeeding.
  4. Biliary sludge and/or gallstones are likely to form in one in five children with hemolytic anemia before their adolescent years.
C. Geriatrics
  1. The elderly may present with nonspecific GI symptoms, abdominal discomfort, bloating, constipation, or dyspepsia.
  2. Diarrhea may be mild or intermittent in the elderly.
  3. Iron-deficiency anemia may also be a presenting symptom. Anemia is present in 60% to 80% of elderly patients with celiac disease.
  4. The elderly are at increased risk for falls related to osteopenia, ataxia, neuropathy.
  5. Autoimmune thyroid disorders are common with elderly celiac patients. The majority present with hypothyroidism.
  6. The risk for non-Hodgkin's lymphoma (NHL) is increased in people with celiac disease aged 50 years and older.

Resources

www.celiac.com
http://www.celiac.com/categories/Gluten-Free--Recipes-c-3400.html
www.celiac.org
www.glutenfreedrugs.com

Reference

Rubio-Tapia, A., Hill, I. D., Kelly, C. P., Calderwood, A. H., & Murray, J. A. (2013). Diagnosis and mangement of celiac disease. *The American Journal of Gastroenterology, 108,* 656–676 Retrieved from http://gi.org/guideline/diagnosis-and-management-of-celiac-disease

Cholecystitis

Cheryl A. Glass and Audra Malone

Definition

A. Cholecystitis is the acute or chronic inflammation of the gallbladder. Acute cholecystitis has associated stone formation (cholelithiasis) in 90% of all cases, causing obstruction and inflammation. Biliary sludge is a feature of chronic cholecystitis.

Incidence

A. Gallbladder disease afflicts 10% to 20% of Americans. The incidence in children is not known. Most patients with an acute attack of cholecystitis have complete remission in 1 to 5 days; however, approximately 20% require surgical intervention. Mortality related to acute cholecystitis is 5% to 10%, with the highest risk for patients older than 60 years. The most common complication is the development of gallbladder gangrene with the potential for subsequent perforation (2%). Gangrenous cholecystitis is most common in older patients, diabetics, or patients who delay treatment.
B. Cholecystectomy for recurrent biliary colic or acute cholecystitis is the most common major surgical procedure performed by general surgeons.

Pathogenesis

A. Cholecystitis occurs subsequent to bile stasis, bacterial infection, ischemia, or obstruction by a gallstone. Acute cholecystitis is related to the impaction of a calculus in the neck of the gallbladder in approximately 90% of cases. Spontaneous resolution may occur after the reestablishment of cystic duct patency.
B. *Escherichia coli* is the primary microorganism in 80% of cholecystitis infections.
C. Estrogen-induced alteration in bile salts may favor stone formation. Stones occur when cholesterol supersaturates the bile in the gallbladder and precipitates out of the bile. Cholesterol stones are the most common type of gallstones in the United States.
D. Pigment stones occur when free bilirubin combines with calcium. Pigment stones are found in patients with cirrhosis, hemolysis, and infections in the biliary tree.
E. Acalculous cholecystitis is associated with infection and local inflammation. Formation of gallstones is not necessary for the obstruction of the bile duct.

Predisposing Factors

A. Female gender
B. Sudden starvation/prolonged fasting
C. Medications
  1. Cholesterol-lowering drugs: Stone formation increases in users of cholesterol-lowering drugs, which are known to increase biliary cholesterol saturation.
  2. Estrogen usage (oral contraceptives [OCPs] and hormone replacement therapy [HRT]): Stone

formation increases in users of contraceptives and estrogens, which are known to increase biliary cholesterol saturation.

3. Furosemide
4. Ceftriaxone
5. Cyclosporine
6. Opiate narcotic analgesics
7. Octreotide

D. Bile acid malabsorption
E. Genetic predisposition: Native Americans and those of Chinese or Japanese descent have a high incidence.
F. Total parenteral nutrition (TPN)
G. Obesity
H. Status post-bariatric surgery
I. Pregnancy secondary to elevated progesterone
J. Increasing age
K. Hemolytic anemia
L. Diabetes
M. High serum triglyceride and low high-density lipoprotein (HDL) levels
N. High-caloric and refined carbohydrate diet
O. Cirrhosis, Crohn's disease, and gallbladder stasis

Common Complaints

A. Abrupt, severe abdominal pain lasting 24 hours
B. Constant aching pain in the right upper quadrant (RUQ), right subcostal region, with radiation to the back and right shoulder
C. Nausea and vomiting
D. Acalculous cholecystitis may present with fever and sepsis alone

Other Signs and Symptoms

A. Anorexia
B. Heartburn
C. Upper abdominal fullness
D. Biliary colic: Sudden onset of severe pain in the epigastrium or right hypochondrium that subsides relatively slowly. Tenderness may remain for days.
E. Fat intolerance
F. Fever (low grade)
G. Mild jaundice (20%)
H. Complicated disease such as an abscess or perforation; symptoms include more severe localized persistent pain, tenderness, fever, chills, and leukocytosis.
I. Chronic diarrhea (4–10 bowel movements every day for at least 3 months)

Subjective Data

A. Review the onset, location, duration, course, and quality of pain.
B. Use a pain-rating scale, such as a 10-point pain scale, with 0 being no pain and 10 being equivalent to the worst pain the patient has ever felt. Determine the progression of the pain as well.
C. Review any alleviating factors, such as antacids, and any worsening factors, such as deep inspiration.
D. Review any pain radiating to the jaw, neck, shoulder, or arm.
E. Review the onset of pain in relation to last meal and foods ingested.
F. Ask the patient about recurrent history of epigastric pain.
G. Obtain history and demographic data that may indicate the risk factors for biliary disease.
H. Review the date of the patient's last menstrual period (LMP), and, if she is pregnant, establish gestational age.

Physical Examination

The absence of physical findings does not rule out the diagnosis of cholecystitis.

A. Check temperature, pulse (tachycardia), respirations, and blood pressure.
B. Inspect: Observe general appearance, facial expressions, walk, skin color (15% have jaundice) and turgor, and grimace during examination. Overall appearance is generally unremarkable between attacks; ill appearance occurs during acute attack.
C. Auscultate

1. Heart
2. Lung fields
3. Abdomen for bowel sounds in all four quadrants

D. Percuss the abdomen
E. Palpate

1. Palpate the abdomen; check for tenderness in the right upper quadrant (RUQ), especially with inspiration; assess for guarding and rebound tenderness.
2. Check Murphy's sign. Positive Murphy's sign is inspiratory arrest secondary to extreme tenderness when the subhepatic area is palpated during deep inspiration.

F. Perform rectal examination, if indicated.

Diagnostic Tests

A. Laboratory tests

1. Amylase (will be normal in classic cholecystitis)
2. Complete blood count (CBC) with differential (leukocytosis)
3. Alkaline phosphate (normal in classic cholecystitis)
4. Bilirubin (normal to mildly elevated in classic cholecystitis)
5. Aspartate transaminase (AST; slightly elevated to normal)
6. Alanine transaminase (ALT; slightly elevated to normal)
7. Urinalysis to rule out pyelonephritis and renal calculi
8. Pregnancy test if childbearing age
9. Stool guaiac test for occult blood to rule out bleeding

B. Radiography

1. **Ultrasonography: Study of choice and can often establish the diagnosis. Positive findings include presence of stones, gallbladder wall thickening, or enlargement and fluid.**
2. Cholescintigraphy (hepatobiliary [HIDA]) scan is indicated if the diagnosis is uncertain after an ultrasound.
3. MR cholangiography
4. CT scan (can identify extrabiliary disorders and complications of acute cholecystitis)
5. Chest radiography to rule out pneumonia

C. EKG to rule out myocardial infarction (MI)

Differential Diagnoses

A. Acute cholecystitis
B. Biliary colic
C. Acute pancreatitis
D. Appendicitis
E. Peptic ulcer disease (PUD)/perforation
F. Acute hepatitis
G. Pneumonia or pleurisy
H. MI
I. Renal calculi
J. Gastroesophageal reflux disease (GERD)
K. Pregnancy: Urolithiasis, pyelonephritis

Plan

A. General interventions: Patients with a single episode of biliary colic are reasonable candidates for expectant management, as long as they continue to be free of recurrent pain.

B. Patient teaching
- **1.** No activity restriction is required.
- **2.** Treatment depends on acuteness of attack. Heat may be used as needed for pain. If pain continues to worsen, have the patient contact his or her health care provider. Hospitalization and/or surgery may be required depending on the severity of the attack.

C. Dietary management
- **1.** Counsel the patient to avoid fatty foods.
- **2.** Encourage the patient to avoid fasting and starvation diets, which make the bile even more lithogenic.

D. Surgical management
- **1.** Cholecystectomy may be recommended for symptomatic patients. **The standard of care is the laparoscopic cholecystectomy.** Conversion from a laparoscopic procedure to an open surgical procedure is approximately 5%.

E. Pharmaceutical therapy
- **1.** Acetaminophen (Tylenol) may be used as needed for pain.
- **2.** Anticholinergics are not helpful.
- **3.** Oral bile acid therapy decreases the amount of cholesterol produced by the liver and absorbed by the intestines.
  - **a.** Actigall (Ursodiol)
    - **i.** Dissolution of stones: 8 to 10 mg/kg/d in two or three divided doses.
    - **ii.** Urso (Ursodiol) 250 mg tablets also available as Urso Forte 500 mg tablets
    - **iii.** 13 to 15 mg/kg/d in two or four divided doses
- **4.** Antibiotics, such as ampicillin or cefazolin (Ancef), Flagyl, may be used for mild attacks.
- **5.** Antiemetics for nausea and vomiting.
- **6.** Drug dissolution therapy with ursodeoxycholic acid and extracorporeal shock wave lithotripsy have lower cure rates.

Follow-Up

A. See the patient at next pain attack to reevaluate.
B. Surgical follow-up in 2 weeks

Consultation/Referral

A. For acute attack, consult a physician for possible surgical consultation referral.

B. Refer the patient for elective cholecystectomy when he or she has documented gallstones and recurrent biliary colic or a history of complication of gallstone disease such as pancreatitis.

C. Refer to a gastroenterologist for consideration of endoscopic retrograde cholangiopancreatography (ERCP).

Individual Considerations

A. Pregnancy
- **1.** Right upper quadrant (RUQ) pain in pregnancy differential includes preeclampsia, pancreatitis, and appendicitis.
- **2.** In the absence of pancreatitis, maternal mortality should be rare, and fetal loss is generally estimated to be no more than 5%. However, if secondary pancreatitis is present, maternal mortality is 15%, and fetal loss is reported as high as 60%.

B. Pediatrics
- **1.** Patients with sickle cell disease are at higher risk for developing cholecystitis.
- **2.** Infants with cholecystitis may present with irritability, jaundice, and acholic (pale white) stools.
- **3.** The most common complication of gallstones in children is pancreatitis.

C. Geriatrics
- **1.** Signs and symptoms may be nonspecific and vague.
- **2.** Localized tenderness may be the only presenting sign.
- **3.** The response of Murphy's sign may be diminished in the elderly.
- **4.** Early cholecystectomy is advocated for elderly patients with gallstone disease. The most important risk factor for postoperative morbidity and mortality is advanced age.
- **5.** Biliary sludge and/or gallstones are likely to form in one in five children with hemolytic anemia before their adolescent years.

Colic

Cheryl A. Glass

Definition

A. Colic is a benign disorder characterized by abdominal spasms and rigidity that results in abdominal pain. Infants with colic exhibit persistent, unexplained, and inconsolable crying lasting more than 3 hours a day, occurring more than 3 days in a week for 3 weeks in an otherwise healthy infant aged 2 weeks to 4 months. The infant is in good health, eats well, and gains weight appropriately, despite the daily crying episodes. Colic is self-limited.

Incidence

A. Between 8% and 30% of all infants exhibit colic, regardless of ethnicity, gender, gestational age, breast-versus bottle-fed, or socioeconomic status.

Pathogenesis

A. Research has never conclusively identified a cause for colic, and many interventions are based on hypothesized causes, such as immature gastrointestinal (GI) function, milk allergy to casein or whey, and maternal anxiety.

Exposure to cigarette smoke may be linked to colic. There has been a causal relationship between colic and family stress.

Predisposing Factors

A. Age: 2 weeks to 4 months; usually resolves by 6 months of age
B. Male gender: Occurs more in males than females
C. First in birth order
D. Fruit juice intolerance (sorbitol-containing fruit juices)

Common Complaints

Crying characteristics:
A. Intense crying: Louder, higher, and more variable in pitch
B. The cry may sound like the baby is in pain or is screaming rather than crying.
C. Inconsolable

Other Signs and Symptoms

A. Hands clenched
B. Abdominal distension
C. Legs flexed over abdomen
D. Short sleep cycles
E. Flatus
F. Fussiness
G. No disease process found on examination
H. Red flags include distended abdomen, fever, and lethargy.

Subjective Data

A. Review when the crying occurs and how long it lasts. What techniques help?
B. Review basic infant needs with caregivers, such as determining whether the infant is hungry or wet, has air bubbles, or is in an uncomfortable position.
C. Review feeding methods, technique, and burping. Crying that occurs directly after feeding may be associated with swallowing too much air or gastroesophageal reflux.
D. If the infant is breastfed, review maternal diet for offending foods, including chocolate, pizza, spicy foods, cabbage, and so forth.
E. If the infant is breastfed, review prescribed maternal drugs and any over-the-counter (OTC) medications that she is taking, such as laxatives.
F. If the infant is bottle-fed, review preparation of formula and type of formula.
G. Review intake of fruit juices for possible carbohydrate intolerance to sorbitol.
H. Rule out the early introduction of solid foods.
I. Review any history of fever and high-pitched or shrill cry.
J. Have caregiver describe color, frequency, and softness of stools.
K. Review secondhand smoke exposure: There is an association between maternal smoking and colic.

Physical Examination

A. Check temperature, pulse, respirations, blood pressure, and weight.
B. Plot growth parameters: Length, head circumference, and weight. **Note signs of failure to thrive (FTT). Failure to gain approximately 1 ounce per day may indicate FTT.**
C. Inspect
 1. Evaluate the skin for signs of abuse.
 2. Check fontanelles.
 3. Conduct ear, nose, and throat examination.
 4. Evaluate the skin and mucosa for signs of dehydration.
D. Auscultate abdomen, heart, and lungs.
E. Percuss the abdomen.
F. Palpate
 1. Palpate the abdomen for tenderness, masses, and distension.
 2. Feel anterior and posterior fontanelles.
 3. Perform testicular examination to evaluate torsion.

Diagnostic Tests

A. Colic is a diagnosis of exclusion and must be differentiated from identifiable causes of prolonged crying.
B. Laboratory tests and radiographic examination are not required if the infant is gaining weight and has a normal physical examination.
C. Consider urinalysis.
D. Check stool for occult blood to rule out cow's milk allergy.

Differential Diagnoses

A. Colic
B. Infection
C. Obstruction
D. Injury
E. Abuse
F. FTT
G. GERD
H. Intussusception
I. Meningitis
J. Otitis media
K. Protein intolerance
L. Testicular torsion
M. Strangulated inguinal hernia

Plan

A. Patient teaching
 1. Encourage parents and caregivers to keep a diary on crying and fussing spells for review.
 2. Review feeding and burping techniques, making sure the baby is not over- or underfed.
 3. Reassure the family that the baby has no evidence of infant developmental problems and the problem is not related to poor parenting skills.
 4. Reassure families that colic does resolve over time.
 5. Encourage parents to take time away from the infant to rest and recoup the energy needed to deal with the demands of a crying baby.
 6. Empathize with parental frustration and provide coping techniques.

Physical abuse of the infant with colic may occur when crying is prolonged and parents have inadequate resources to cope.

7. Consider a hypoallergenic diet (e.g., protein hydrolysate formula such as Alimentum, Nutramigen, or Pregestimil). The literature does not support the use of fiber-enriched formulas.

8. *See Section III: Patient Teaching Guide for this chapter, "Colic: Ways to Soothe a Fussy Baby."*

9. Teach caregivers to assess the child for signs of emergent abdominal problems such as fever, pallor, sweating, vomiting, diarrhea, a rigid and tender abdomen.

B. Dietary management

1. Dietary changes such as eliminating cow's milk proteins is indicated only in cases of suspected intolerance to protein (e.g., positive family history, eczema, onset after the first month, association with other GI symptoms such as vomiting or diarrhea).

2. Use of soy-based formula is not recommended because many infants allergic to cow's milk protein may also develop an intolerance to soy protein.

3. For breastfeeding mothers, suggest a period of elimination of allergic foods (e.g., dairy, nuts, soy, citrus) in order to evaluate the baby's response.

4. For formula-fed infants, consider hydrolyzed formula.

5. Educate caregivers to avoid the use of homegrown mint teas for fussy babies. Fatalities have been reported secondary to ingestion of the pennyroyal form of mint, which produces toxic oil.

C. Pharmaceutical therapy

1. Simethicone has little therapeutic benefit versus a placebo for treating colic by randomized controlled trials.

2. Antispasmodics have adverse effects, including apnea, seizures, and coma. Dicyclomine is contraindicated in infants younger than 6 months of age and is not considered for the indication of colic by the manufacturer.

3. Lactase is not a therapeutic option for colic.

4. For breastfed infants, consider 5 drops of *Lactobacillus reuteri* DSM 17938 per day. Evidence does not support other forms of probiotics or prebiotics.

5. Sedatives should not be used for the treatment of colic.

6. Herbal remedies are common in many cultures, but few herbal products have been evaluated for colic.

Follow-Up

A. Reevaluate the child periodically to provide support and assess for other problems.

B. Review signs of emergent abdominal problems such as fever, pallor, sweating, vomiting, diarrhea, and rigid and tender abdomen.

Consultation/Referral

A. Consult a physician as necessary.

B. Consider a home-based nursing consultation.

C. Refer the breastfeeding mother for an observational feeding.

Colorectal Cancer Screening

Cheryl A. Glass

Definition

Screening for colorectal cancer has increased early detection and the ability for early intervention of premalignant localized cancer. There are multiple screening guidelines; the U.S. Preventive Services Task Force (USPSTF) recommendations are presented in this review. Screening is done for men and women between the ages of 50 and 75 years. There are two categories of screening:

A. Stool-based testing

B. Endoscopic and radiologic testing

Incidence

A. In the United States, colorectal cancer is the second leading cause of cancer-related death in both men and women.

B. Americans have a 5% lifetime risk of colorectal cancer.

C. Colorectal cancer is rare before age 40 years. Colorectal cancer is most frequently diagnosed among adults aged 65 to 74 years. You would consider screening in older patients if symptoms are present and life expectancy is >10 years.

D. 90% of the cases of colorectal cancer occur after 50 years.

E. Up to 20% of colorectal cancer in the United States is associated with smoking.

F. Obesity is associated with colon cancer but not an increase in rectal cancer. Abdominal obesity is a stronger risk factor than truncal obesity or body mass index (BMI).

Pathogenesis

A. The usual pathogenesis is an adenomatous polyp that grows slowly, followed by dysplasia and final cancerous cells.

Predisposing Factors

A. Age: 50 years and older

B. African American (screening is recommended at age 40 years)

C. Inflammatory bowel diseases (IBDs; Crohn's disease [CD], and ulcerative colitis [UC])

D. Family history/genetic

1. Familial adenomatous polyposis (FAP)
2. Nonpolyposis colorectal cancer (Lynch syndrome)

E. Smoking

F. Obesity

G. Diet high in red meat and fats

Common Complaint

A. Asymptomatic screening

Subjective Data

A. Review the patient's age and risk factors to discuss screening for colorectal cancer.

B. Review family history of colorectal cancer.

C. Review smoking history.

D. Review the patient's diet evaluating red meat; processed meats; and lack of grains, fruits, and vegetables.

E. Review all medications currently being taken, including over-the-counter (OTC) medications and herbal products.

Physical Examination

A. Examinations are not required for discussion on colorectal screening testing.

B. A physical examination and vital signs should be taken as indicated for other presenting complaints.

Diagnostic Tests

See Table 11.2 for frequency of tests.

A. Stool-based testing
  1. Guaiac-based fecal occult blood test (FOBT)
  2. Fecal immunochemical test (FIT) is replacing the FOBT as the preferred cancer detection test.
  3. FIT DNA panel

B. Endoscopic and radiological
  1. Flexible sigmoidoscopy
  2. Colonoscopy: The American College of Gastroenterology (ACG) recommends colonoscopy as the preferred strategy for screening.
  3. Double-contrast barium enema (DCBE): The ACG recommends the DCBE as a screening test; however, it has limited effectiveness for polyp detection.
  4. Computed tomography colonography (CTC)

Differential Diagnosis

A. None related to screening

TABLE 11.2 Screening Tests At-a-Glance Based on U.S. Preventive Services Task Force (USPSTF) Colorectal Cancer Screening

Name	Preparation	What Happens?	Frequency
High-sensitivity FOBT or stool test; or FIT Note: There are two types of FOBT: One uses the chemical guaiac to detect blood. The other—an FIT—uses antibodies to detect blood in the stool. Ask your doctor for a *high-sensitivity* FOBT or FIT.	Your doctor may recommend that you follow a special diet before taking the FOBT.	You receive a test kit from your health care provider. At home, you use a stick or brush to obtain a small amount of stool. You may be asked to do this for several bowel movements in a row. You return the test kit to the doctor or a lab, where stool samples are checked for blood.	This test should be done every year. (If anything unusual is found, your doctor will recommend a follow-up colonoscopy.)
The one-time FOBT done by the doctor in the doctor's office is *not* appropriate as a screening test for colorectal cancer. FIT-DNA is an emerging screening strategy. This is a multitargeted stool DNA test combined with FIT testing.			The FIT-DNA test should be done every year or once in 3 years (suggested by the manufacturer).
Flexible sigmoidoscopy (flex sig) *Note*: This is sometimes done in combination with *high-sensitivity* FOBT.	Your doctor will tell you what foods you can and cannot eat before the test. The evening before the test, you use a strong laxative and/or enema to clean out the colon.	During the test, the doctor puts a short, thin, flexible, lighted tube into the rectum. This tube allows the doctor to check for polyps or cancer inside the rectum and lower third of the colon.	This test should be done every 10 years. When it is done in combination with high-sensitivity FIT, the FIT should be done every year. (If anything unusual is found, your doctor will recommend a follow-up colonoscopy.)
Colonoscopy *Note*: Colonoscopy also is used as a follow-up test if anything unusual is found during one of the other screening tests.	Before this test, your doctor will tell you what foods you can and cannot eat. You use a strong laxative to clean out the colon. Some doctors recommend that you also use an enema. Make sure you arrange for a ride back home, as you will not be allowed to drive.	You will receive medication during this test to make you more comfortable. This test is similar to flex sig, except the doctor uses a longer, thin, flexible, lighted tube to check for polyps or cancer inside the rectum and the entire colon. During the test, the doctor can find and remove most polyps and some cancers.	This test should be done every 10 years. If polyps or cancers are found during the test, you will need more frequent colonoscopies in the future.

FIT, fecal immunochemical test; FOBT, fecal occult blood test.

Plan

A. Patient teaching

1. Educate the patient about modifying controllable risk factors with diet, exercise, and smoking cessation.

2. Discuss the procedures and the preparation needed for each test.

B. Pharmaceutical therapy

1. Bowel prep depends on the test, patient's age, and other comorbidities.

Follow-Up

A. Follow-up and consultations are determined by patient's needs, severity, and whether complications are present.

B. Patients with classic FAP (greater than 100 adenomas) should be advised to have genetic counseling.

C. Nonsteroidal anti-inflammatory drugs **(NSAIDs) have been associated with a decrease in the risk of developing colorectal cancer. There is insufficient evidence to recommend the use of NSAIDs as a prevention strategy.**

D. The USPSTF has made a recommendation on aspirin use for primary prevention of cardiovascular disease and colorectal cancer in average-risk adults (www.uspreventiveservicestaskforce.org).

Consultation/Referral

A. Referral to a gastroenterologist and/or surgeon as indicated.

Individual Considerations

A. Geriatrics

1. The benefit of early detection of and intervention for colorectal cancer declines after age 75 years. Screening for adults aged 76 to 85 years should be made on an individual basis, taking into account the patient's overall health and prior screening history.

2. Medicare Part B covers several colorectal screening tests.

a. Medicare covers a screening barium enema (BE) when used instead of a flexible sigmoidoscopy or colonoscopy once every 48 months for 50 years or older and once every 24 months if at high risk.

b. Screening colonoscopy is covered every 24 months if at high risk for colorectal cancer. If not at high risk, Medicare covers the colonoscopy once every 120 months, or 48 months after a previous flexible sigmoidoscopy.

3. FOBT is covered by Medicare once every 12 months for ages 50 years or older.

4. Flexible sigmoidoscopy is covered by Medicare every 48 months for most people older than 50 years. If not at high risk, Medicare covers the flexible sigmoidoscopy every 120 months after a previous screening colonoscopy.

5. Multitarget stool DNA at-home test is covered once every 3 years for people who meet *all* of the following criteria:

a. Between ages 50 and 85 years

b. No signs or symptoms of colorectal disease, including, but not limited to, lower gastrointestinal pain, blood in stool, positive guaiac fecal occult blood test, or FIT.

c. Average risk for developing colorectal cancer, meaning:

i. No personal history of adenomatous polyps, colorectal cancer, or inflammatory bowel disease, including Crohn's disease and ulcerative colitis

ii. No family history of colorectal cancers or adenomatous polyps, FAP, or hereditary nonpolyposis colorectal cancer

Resources

CDC website—Screening Tests at-a-Glance includes the 2008 Screening for Colorectal Cancer from the USPTF website: www.cdc.gov/cancer/colorectal/pdf/SFL_inserts_screening.pdf

Medicare.gov Your Medicare Coverage Colorectal cancer screenings: www.medicare.gov/coverage/colorectal-cancer-screenings.html

National Cancer Institutes at the National Institutes of Health Colon and Rectal Cancer: www.cancer.gov/cancertopics/types/colon-and-rectal

National Cancer Institutes at the National Institutes of Health Tests to Detect Colorectal Cancer and Polyps. www.cancer.gov/cancertopics/factsheet/detection/colorectal-screening

National Comprehensive Cancer Network website: www.nccn.org

Professional National Cancer Institute at the National Institutes of Health Rectal Cancer Treatment (PDQ®): www.cancer.gov

Constipation

Cheryl A. Glass and Audra Malone

Definition

Constipation is infrequent and difficult defecation of hard stools and a sensation of incomplete evacuation or straining. Constipation may also refer to a decrease in the volume or weight of stool, and the need for enemas, suppositories, or laxatives to maintain bowel regularity. Constipation is a symptom, not a disease. The lower limit of normal stool frequency is three bowel movements (BMs) a week. The Rome consensus criterion defines constipation as two or fewer stools weekly, lumpy/hard stools, straining, sensation of incomplete evacuation/obstruction or blockage, and/or the need for digital removal of stool.

Classification of constipation includes:

A. Normal-transit constipation (most common)

B. Functional constipation (slow transit)

C. Irritable bowel syndrome (IBS; constipation dominant)

D. Outlet obstruction (sudden onset)

Incidence

A. The incidence of constipation is unknown due to frequent self-treatment. Constipation is commonly self-reported. Constipation occurs in more than 50% of patients with colorectal cancers; it may be an early symptom of rectal cancer or an symptom of advanced disease in colon cancer.

Pathogenesis

A. Constipation can be caused by an alteration of the filling of the rectum by colonic transportation and/or reflex defecation of stool.

B. Lack of exercise decreases propulsion of bowel contents.
C. During pregnancy, progesterone has a relaxing effect on the muscles of the gastrointestinal (GI) tract and causes a decrease in peristalsis. The compression of the intestines by the enlarging uterus causes constipation during pregnancy.
D. Habitual use of laxatives is associated with impaired motor activity and has the potential of producing hypokalemia.
E. Hypokalemia can produce a generalized ileus and is most often seen in patients who take diuretics.
F. Psychiatric disease and psychosocial distress have important roles. The exact mechanisms by which emotional difficulties lead to constipation remain unclear, but their contribution is widely recognized.
G. Drugs (see Table 11.3).

Predisposing Factors

A. Insufficient nutrition
  1. Low-fiber diet
  2. Low-fluid intake
B. Neurologic causes
  1. Spinal cord injury
  2. Parkinson's disease
  3. Multiple sclerosis
  4. Aganglionosis (Hirschsprung's disease [HD])
  5. Sacral nerve trauma/tumor
C. Sedentary lifestyle
D. Laxative abuse
E. Travel
F. Ignoring urge to defecate
G. Drug use (individual medications and polypharmacy)
H. Pregnancy, especially third trimester
I. Psychosocial problems
  1. Depression
  2. Sexual abuse
  3. Unusual attitudes to food and bowel function
J. Extremes of ages: Infants and geriatrics
K. Hypothyroidism
L. Colorectal cancer
M. Irritable bowel syndrome (IBS)
N. Pelvic floor disorders
  1. Impaired function of the pelvic floor and/or external sphincter
  2. Pelvic floor obstruction
  3. Rectal prolapse
  4. Enterocele and/or rectocele
  5. Rectal intussusception

Common Complaints

A. Hard, infrequent stools
B. Straining
C. Inability to defecate when desired
D. Need for digital manipulation to facilitate evacuation

Other Signs and Symptoms

A. Hard, pebbly, rocklike stools
B. Painful defecation
C. Abdominal pain
D. Weight loss
E. Blood in stools

Potential Complications

A. A rectal prolapse of the mucosa is pink and looks like a doughnut or rosette. Complete prolapse involving the muscular wall is larger and red, and it has circular folds.

Subjective Data

A. Review the onset, duration, and course of symptoms.
  1. Is constipation a chronic or acute problem?
  2. If there has been a change in bowel habits, was it gradual or sudden?
  3. What feature does the patient rate most distressing?
B. Review bowel habits.
  1. Does the patient have a regular time for defecation?
  2. Review size, color, consistency, and frequency of stools. Has there been a change in the caliber of stools?
  3. Is there any blood?
  4. Are there any periods of diarrhea?
  5. How often are laxatives being used, and at what doses?
  6. Are suppositories and enemas also required?
  7. Does the patient have the urge to defecate?
  8. Does the patient have a sensation of incomplete evacuation?
  9. Does the patient need to digitally remove stool?
  10. Does the patient have fecal incontinence?
C. Review the patient's daily diet and fluid intake. Has there been any dietary change?

TABLE 11.3 Drugs/Drug Classifications That Cause and Increase Constipation

Anticholinergics (atropine, antidepressants, neuroleptics, antiparkinsonian drugs)	Opiates
Antipsychotics	Cholestyramine (binds bile salts)
Anticonvulsants	Antacids (aluminum hydroxide and calcium carbonate)
Antihistamines	Iron supplements
Antihypertensives (calcium channel blockers, clonidine, hydralazine, MAOI, methyldopa)	NSAIDs
Diuretics	Ganglionic blockers

MAOI, monoamine oxidase inhibitor; NSAIDs, nonsteroidal anti-inflammatory drugs.

D. Review the patient's medication history: Prescription and over-the-counter (OTC; refer to Table 11.3).
E. Review the patient's daily physical activity.
F. Review the patient's psychosocial history of stress, depression, anxiety, and coping mechanisms.
G. Review the patient's other health problems such as diabetes, depression, hypothyroidism, and hypercalcemia.
H. Review family history of constipation and colorectal cancer.
I. Review surgical history.

Physical Examination

A. Check pulse, respirations, blood pressure, and weight. Check temperature if indicated.
B. Inspect
- **1.** General overall assessment of nutritional status.
- **2.** Examine the skin, especially the rectum, for pallor and signs of dehydration and hypothyroidism.
- **3.** Evaluate for the presence of hernias.
- **4.** Inspect the anus, including the position, anal wink, prolapse, presence of excoriation, presence of perianal erythema, hemorrhoids, fissures, and skin tags.
- **5.** Examine the lower back to rule out spinal lesions—hairy or hyperpigmented patches, gluteal fold asymmetry, cutaneous dimples, sinus tracts, and lipomas.

C. Auscultate all four abdominal quadrants for bowel sounds. Bowel sounds may be high pitched or absent.
D. Percuss the abdomen.
E. Palpate
- **1.** The abdomen for masses, tenderness, distension, and fecal mass
- **2.** The liver and spleen

F. Digital rectal examination
- **1.** Examine the rectum for an anorectal mass, stricture, hemorrhoids, fissures, fistula, prolapse, inflammation, and anal warts.
- **2.** Evaluate for impaction, hard stool in ampulla.
- **3.** Perform an anal reflex test by a light pinprick or scratch.
- **4.** Evaluate sphincter tone.
  - **a.** Disordered innervation of the anus is indicated by finding that the anal canal opens wide when the puborectalis muscle is pulled posteriorly.
  - **b.** Evaluate the resting tone of the sphincter and squeezing effort.
  - **c.** Instruct the patient to "expel the examination finger" to evaluate the force of expulsion.
  - **d.** Have the patient do a Valsalva maneuver to diagnose a rectocele, prolapse, pelvic floor descent, or puborectalis dysfunction.
  - **e.** In women, the vagina should also be evaluated for rectocele and cystocele.

G. Perform a neurologic examination for tone, strength, and reflexes to search for focal deficits and the delayed relaxation phase of the ankle jerks, suggestive of hypothyroidism.
H. Perform pelvic examination to evaluate a prolapse or rectocele. Evaluate when the patient is at rest and with straining.
I. Perform mental status examination for signs of depression and somatization.

Diagnostic Tests

A. No tests are required for *common* constipation.
B. Tests to rule out differential diagnoses
- **1.** Complete blood count (CBC) with differential
- **2.** Thyroid studies
- **3.** Potassium and calcium: Patients taking diuretics should have serum potassium checked. Hypokalemia may reduce bowel contractility and produce an ileus.
- **4.** Urinalysis
- **5.** Serum glucose to rule out diabetes
- **6.** Barium enema (BE) to evaluate megacolon and redundant sigmoid colon.
- **7.** Flexible sigmoid or colonoscopy is recommended if the patient meets the guidelines for general screening or weight loss greater than 10 pounds, anemia, or blood in the stool.
- **8.** Stool for occult blood
- **9.** Anorectal function tests
  - **a.** Manometry
  - **b.** Electromyography

Differential Diagnoses

A. Constipation
B. Intestinal obstruction: Acute onset of constipation requires ruling out an ileus, especially when accompanied by abdominal discomfort.
C. Hypothyroidism
D. Psychosocial dysfunction
E. Fecal impaction
F. Neurologic disorders
G. Multiple sclerosis
H. Spinal cord injury
I. Cancer
J. Drug use
K. Crohn's disease (CD): Constipation is often the presenting complaint in CD.
L. Diabetes (chronic dysmotility)

Plan

A. Patient teaching:
- **1.** *See Section III: Patient Teaching Guide for this chapter, "Constipation Relief."* ◀
- **2.** Encourage the patient to exercise. Both exercise and dietary fiber stimulate the natural wavelike contraction of the colon that triggers the urge to defecate.
- **3.** Reassure the patient that recommended dietary changes and exercise help with constipation.
- **4.** Warn chronic laxative users that it may take 4 to 6 weeks before spontaneous BMs return.
- **5.** Teach the patient about potential complications of long-term constipation.
- **6.** Ask the patient to keep a stool diary to bring to the next appointment.

B. Dietary management: See Appendix B.
C. Surgical and medical management
- **1.** Treatment of constipation is symptomatic and should begin with lifestyle and dietary changes.
- **2.** Evaluate and stop medications, if possible, that cause constipation.

3. Glycerin suppositories may be needed for rectal disimpaction in infants. Enemas are to be avoided.

4. Fecal impaction may require enemas or manual removal to relieve the situation. Enemas should not be given routinely to treat constipation because they disrupt normal defecation reflexes and the patient becomes dependent. Disimpaction by enema treatments includes three enemas per day:

a. The first enema of the day includes the use of a phosphate-based enema.

i. Patients older than 12 years—one adult phosphate-based enema, plus 1 L of saline solution.

ii. Patients aged 4 to 12 years—one pediatric phosphate-based enema, plus 1 L of saline solution.

iii. Patients younger than 4 years—one half of a pediatric phosphate-based enema, plus 500 mL of saline solution.

b. The second and third enema of the day includes only the saline solution and no phosphate-based enema.

c. Patients should never receive more than one phosphate enema per day because of the risk of phosphate intoxication, hypoglycemia, and hyponatremia.

d. Soap suds, tap water, and magnesium enemas in children are not recommended because of potential toxicity.

5. Pelvic floor physiotherapy may be offered.

6. Biofeedback has been effective for short-term treatment of intractable constipation.

7. Manual removal of fecal impaction can stimulate the vagus nerve and cause syncope and tachycardia. It is contraindicated in the following conditions:

a. Pregnancy

b. After genitourinary, rectal, perineal, abdominal, or gynecologic surgery

c. Myocardial infarction, coronary insufficiency, pulmonary embolus, congestive heart failure (CHF), or heart block

d. GI or vaginal bleeding

e. Blood dyscrasias or bleeding disorders

f. Hemorrhoids, fissures, and rectal polyps

D. Pharmaceutical therapy

1. Bulk-forming agents decrease abdominal pain and improve stool consistency. They should be used if an increase in dietary fiber does not work. They act by causing retention of fluid and increasing fecal mass. They must be taken with plenty of fluids to prevent formation of an obstructing bolus. Flatulence and abdominal distension may occur, but long-term use is safe.

2. Stimulant laxatives act by directly stimulating the colonic nerves. Suppositories are faster (20–60 minutes) versus oral laxatives (8–12 hours).

3. Osmotic laxatives act by retaining fluid in the bowel by osmosis, changing the water distribution in the feces. Good hydration is important. (Table 11.4).

TABLE 11.4 Laxatives

Bulk laxatives	Psyllium (Konsyl, Metamucil) Polycarbophil Methylcellulose (Citrucel)
Lubricating agents	Mineral oil[a]
Stimulant laxatives	Docusate Bile acids Bisacodyl[b] Castor oil Senna[a] Cascara Aloes Rhubarb
Osmotic agents	Magnesium and phosphate salts Lactulose (Kristalose)[a] Sorbitol[a] Polyethylene glycol (Colyte, Glycolax, Miralax)[b] Glycerin suppositories[a]
Selective 5-HT_4 receptor agonists	Prucalopride
Type-2 chloride channel	Tegaserod (Zelnorm, HTF-919)[c]
Activator	Lubiprostone (Amitiza)
Guanylate cyclase C agonist	Linaclotide (Linzess)[d]

[a]Considered safe and effective in children.
[b]After a thorough evaluation, use in low doses for selected children when constipation is hard to manage.
[c]Tegaserod is prescribed under limited restrictive authority.
[d]The safety and efficacy of Linzess has not been established in pediatric patients younger than 18 years. Contraindicated in pediatric patients up to 6 years of age.

4. Lubiprostone (Amitiza) 24 mcg orally twice a day is approved for treatment of chronic idiopathic constipation in adults, opioid-induced constipation in adults with chronic noncancer pain, and IBS–constipation predominant in women 18 years or older in age.

5. Methylnaltrexone bromide (Relistor) 450 mg tablet once per day is currently approved by the Food and Drug Administration (FDA) for treatment of opioid-induced constipation in adult patients with chronic noncancer pain.

6. When severe depression requires the use of antidepressants, the least constipating agent should be selected (i.e., one with minimal anticholinergic activity).

7. Treat other identified causes, for example, hypothyroidism.

Follow-Up

A. Repeat assessment in 4 to 6 weeks. Ask the patient to keep a stool diary and bring it for subsequent appointments.

B. If there is no evidence of obstruction, anemia, or occult blood loss, follow the patient expectantly for a few weeks on a conservative program that includes increased dietary fiber and increased exercise, and follow stool guaiac.

C. Failure to improve may indicate a serious underlying cause and need for referral.

Consultation/Referral

A. Consider consultations with a gastroenterologist (adult or pediatric), pediatrician, gynecologist, surgeon, or psychologist/psychiatrist as indicated.

Individual Considerations

A. Pregnancy

1. Constipation is very common in pregnancy secondary to progesterone and the enlarging uterus (see "Pathogenesis" section).

2. Constipation that results from iron supplementation can be avoided by increasing the intake of fluid and high-fiber foods, and increasing physical activity such as walking.

3. Bulking agents and lactulose will not enter breast milk. Senna, in large doses, will enter breast milk and may cause diarrhea and colic in infants.

B. Pediatrics

1. In infancy and childhood, most constipation is functional. Constipation can be associated with coercive toilet training, sexual abuse, excessive parental interventions, and toilet phobia.

2. An empty contracted anal canal in a constipated child may suggest HD.

a. Bloody mucoid diarrhea in an infant with a history of constipation could be an indication of enterocolitis complicating HD.

b. If HD is suspected, the patient should be evaluated by a pediatric gastroenterologist and a pediatric surgeon.

3. Reinforce the idea that each infant has individual stool patterns. Formula-fed infants generally pass at least one stool each day, whereas breastfed infants may pass a stool after every feeding or, occasionally, only one every 2 to 3 days.

4. Educate the parent that constipation really is dry, hard, and marblelike stools.

5. Infants may get red in the face and appear to be straining when having a BM, but it is normal behavior and does not indicate constipation.

6. Rectal prolapse in children has been associated with cystic fibrosis (CF).

7. Use a high-fiber diet and fluids first before other therapies. Prune, pear, and apple juices may decrease constipation.

8. Common times when constipation is likely to occur in the pediatric population are

a. Upon introduction of solid foods or cow's milk

i. Recommended fiber intake is 20 g/d.

ii. Minimum fluid intake depends on the child's age.

iii. Consumption of cow's whole milk should be limited to 24 oz/d.

b. During toilet training: A potty seat that provides appropriate foot support and leverage for elimination should be used.

c. On school entry

C. Adults

1. The most common cause of chronic constipation in adults is failure to initiate defecation.

2. Diabetics should avoid stimulant laxatives such as lactulose and sorbitol. Their metabolites may influence blood glucose levels.

D. Geriatrics

1. Constipation in old people is not a result of aging; it is usually related to an increase in constipating factors such as chronic illnesses, immobility, dietary factors, medications, neurologic factors, and psychiatric conditions. **Acute onset of constipation is considered a red flag in the geriatric population.**

2. An important diagnostic concern in the elderly is the possibility of constipation due to a colonic neoplasm. More than 25% of patients with colorectal carcinomas present with constipation.

3. Check for a fecal impaction, especially in elderly patients with a history of chronic constipation. Fecal impaction ranks as one of the major sources of anorectal discomfort among the elderly and bedridden. Chronic, incomplete evacuation leads to formation of an obstructing bolus of desiccated hard stool in the rectum. Fecal incontinence may be a sign of fecal impaction.

4. Diarrhea, rather than constipation, is sometimes the only complaint because of the collection of liquid stool distending the proximal colon and passing around the obstructing bolus.

5. Dietary fiber supplementation has been shown to allow discontinuation of laxatives in 59% to 80% of elderly patients with chronic idiopathic constipation.

Resource

Rome Foundation: http://romecriteria.org/criteria

Crohn's Disease

Cheryl A. Glass and Audra Malone

Definition

A. Crohn's disease (CD) is a chronic inflammatory bowel disease (IBD) of the gastrointestinal (GI) tract that produces ulceration, fibrosis, and malabsorption. CD can involve any segment of the GI tract from the mouth to the anus; the terminal ileum and colon are the most common sites. Pediatric patients are more likely to present with the disease limited to the small intestine.

1. In 2003, CD was subclassified based on age, location (ileal, colonic, ileocolonic, or upper GI), and clinical presentation (nonstricturing/nonpenetrating to penetrating) using the Montreal classification.

2. Elderly patients with IBD can be subdivided into two groups:

a. Elderly patients with onset of IBD at a late age (late-onset IBD)

b. Elderly patients with long-standing IBD; first diagnosed as having IBD at a younger age (long-standing IBD)

B. The disease is chronic, relapsing, and incurable. CD is characterized by episodes of remission and exacerbation.

The most frequent cause of death in persons with IBD is the primary disease, followed by malignancy and thromboembolic disease. In most cases, symptoms do correspond well with the degree of inflammation present. The diagnosis is usually established with endoscopic finding in a patient with a compatible clinical history. Objective evidence for disease activity should be sought before administering medication with significant adverse effects.

C. More than 70% of patients with CD undergo surgery within 20 years of the diagnosis. Indications for surgery include stricture, intractable or fulminant disease, anorectal disease, and intra-abdominal abscess. Approximately 30% of patients who have surgery for CD have a recurrence within 3 years, and up to 60% will have a recurrence within 10 years.

D. The lifetime risk of fistulaw development is 20% to 40%.

E. The incidence of small bowel and colorectal adenocarcinoma in CD is higher than in the general population. Lymphoma is also increased, especially for patients with IBD treated with azathioprine (AZA; 6-mercaptopurine [6-MP]).

Incidence

A. The incidence rate ranges from 3.1 cases per 100,000 to 20.2 cases per 100,000. An estimated 1 to 2 million people in the United States have ulcerative colitis (UC) or CD. The incidence of IBD has been reported to be highest in Jewish populations. IBD is very prevalent among the American Jewish population—four to five times that of the general population.

B. The peak incidence of CD is most common in late adolescence to the third decade of life: Children younger than 5 years and elderly persons aged 70 to 80 years. CD may involve the entire GI tract; note the incidence according to the location.

- **1.** About 80% have small-bowel involvement, usually in the distal ileum. In severe cases of ileitis, complications may include fistulas or an abscess in the right lower quadrant (RLQ) of the abdomen.
- **2.** About 50% have ileocolitis (involving both the ileum and colon). This type is associated with significant weight loss.
- **3.** About 20% have disease limited to the colon, with roughly one half having sparing of the rectum.
- **4.** A small percentage has predominant involvement of the mouth (aphthous ulcers) or gastroduodenal area; fewer have involvement of the esophagus (odynophagia and dysphagia) and proximal small bowel.
- **5.** One third have perianal disease (perianal pain, drainage from large skin tags, anal fissures, perirectal abscesses, and anorectal fistulae).
- **6.** 15% to 20% have arthralgias. Arthritis is the most common complication.

Pathogenesis

Pathogenesis is unknown. The common end pathway is inflammation of the mucosal lining of the intestinal tract, causing ulceration, edema, bleeding, and fluid and electrolyte loss. Speculation for the pathogenesis includes:

A. Pathogenic organism (remains unidentified)

B. Immunologic response

C. Autoimmune process

D. Potential genes linked to IBD

- **1.** Chromosome 16 (*IBD1* gene).
- **2.** *CARD15* gene, which is noted to be a susceptibility gene for CD
- **3.** Susceptibility genes on chromosomes 5 (5q31) and 6 (6p21 and 19p)

Predisposing Factors

A. Age between 15 and 35 years

B. Genetic predisposition/family history of CD

- **1.** First-degree relatives 5- to 20-fold increased risk
- **2.** Children of a parent with IBD have 5% risk
- **3.** About 70% incidence in identical twins versus 5% to 10% in nonidentical twins
- **4.** Jewish populations

C. Smoking (increased risk for CD, but reduces risk in UC)

Common Complaints

The following cardinal symptoms occur in about 80% of patients.

A. Chronic or nocturnal diarrhea

B. Abdominal pain, the classic location being in the right lower quadrant (RLQ; appendicitis like)

C. Fatigue, commonly related to pain, inflammation, and anemia

Other Signs and Symptoms

Symptoms vary, depending on the location of the intestinal tract and extent of disease:

A. Constipation: Early sign

B. Weight loss

C. Abdominal mass

D. Cramping with bowel movement (BM)

E. Urgent need to move bowels

F. Rectal bleeding or blood in stools

G. Perianal discomfort or soft or semiliquid irritating rectal discharge

H. Vomiting

I. Low-grade fever

J. Folate deficiency

K. Anorexia

L. Fissures and fistulas, abscesses sometimes extending to skin

M. Weight loss, diarrhea, and growth retardation may be presenting signs in children.

N. Extraintestinal symptoms

- **1.** Erythema nodosum (correlates well with the activity of disease)
- **2.** Inflammation of the eyes
- **3.** Inflammation of the skin

O. Pediatric

- **1.** Failure to grow
- **2.** Delayed development of secondary sex characteristics

P. Loss of normal menstrual cycle

Subjective Data

A. Ask about the onset, duration, and course of symptoms. Have any of the presenting symptoms occurred at any time in the past (flares of CD may have gone undiagnosed in the past)?

B. Review the patient's history and extent of diarrhea, including frequency, consistency, color, quantity, and odor of stools. Evaluate if there is blood, mucus, pus, or food particles in the stools.
C. Inquire about recent travel to foreign countries.
D. Ask the patient if diarrhea represents a change in bowel habits. Is there nocturnal diarrhea?
E. Ask the patient what makes the diarrhea worse or better.
F. Inquire about previous GI surgery.
G. Review the patient's usual weight and any history of weight loss. If weight loss has occurred, how many pounds? How is patient's appetite?
H. Review family history of CD, colon cancer, UC, and malabsorption syndrome.
I. How has the duration of current complaints affected the patient's work or usual social activities?
J. Review for duration and extraintestinal symptoms, including:
1. Urinary complications: Renal calculi
2. Sclerosing cholangitis: Fatigue and jaundice
3. Skin diseases
a. Erythema nodosum: Painful, tender, raised, purple lesion on the tibia
b. Pyoderma gangrenosum: Inflamed patch of skin that has progressed to ulceration
c. Herpetic lesions related to immune suppression
4. Arthritic symptoms
5. Occular inflammation
6. Hypercoagulabilty
K. Review medications, especially antibiotics and nonsteroidal anti-inflammatory drugs (NSAIDs).
L. Review the patient's current tobacco/cigarette use.

Physical Examination

A. Check temperature, pulse, respirations, blood pressure, and weight. Pediatrics: Plot height/weight on growth curves to follow growth failure.
B. Inspect
1. Observe general appearance, noting pallor, wasting, apathetic appearance, ecchymosis, skin ulcerations, jaundice, and signs of Kaposi's sarcoma.
2. Inspect the head and neck for aphthous ulcers, glossitis, stomatitis, and poor dentition.
3. Inspect the abdomen for surgical scars.
4. Order eye examination for uveitis.
5. Inspect joints for warmth and redness.
C. Auscultate the abdomen in all quadrants for altered bowel sounds (obstruction).
D. Palpate
1. Palpate the neck for goiter and lymphadenopathy.
2. Palpate the abdomen for distension, ascites, tenderness rebound, guarding, and masses.
3. Palpate for hepatomegaly in right lower quadrant (RLQ).
4. Palpate the joints for tenderness.
E. Rectal examination
1. Check anal sphincter for tags, control, and discharge.
2. Palpate for masses, fissures, fistulas, tags, and inflammation.
3. Perform digital rectal examination to assess for anal strictures and rectal mass.
F. Neurologic examination: Assess for signs of vitamin B_{12} deficiency, including tingling sensation and numbness in the hands or feet.

Diagnostic Tests

A. Laboratory tests
1. Complete blood count (CBC) with differential
2. Electrolytes and albumin
3. Erythrocyte sedimentation rate (ESR)
4. Serum cobalamin (vitamin B_{12})
5. Serum iron studies
6. Folate
7. Liver enzymes and functioning tests (international normalized ratio [INR]) and bilirubin
8. HIV
9. Celiac antibody testing should be considered.
10. Thiopurine methyltransferase (TPMT) activity should be assessed before AZA or MP.
B. Stool studies
1. Guaiac
2. Stool culture
3. *Clostridium difficile* toxin assay
4. Ova and parasites
C. Imaging
1. Abdominal flat plate
2. Barium enema (BE)
a. Classic "string sign": Narrow band of barium flowing through an inflamed or scarred area in terminal ileum; differentiates CD from UC
b. "Rectal sparing": Suggests CD in the presence of inflammatory changes in other parts of the colon
c. "Thumbprinting": Indicates mucosal inflammation (may be seen on flat plate of abdomen)
d. "Skip lesions": Areas of inflammation with normal-appearing areas
3. Small-bowel follow-through GI series
4. Fistulogram: Used to guide the surgical correction
5. CT scan of the abdomen and pelvis (limited use in IBD but may detect fistulae)
D. Procedures with/without biopsy
1. Colonoscopy: Mucosa has a characteristic cobblestone appearance.
2. Flexible sigmoidoscopy with biopsy: Reveals "skip areas" in colon, significant small-bowel involvement, fistulas, and granulomas.
3. Upper endoscopy: Aphthous ulcerations occur in the stomach and duodenum in 5% to 10%.
4. Capsule enteroscopy: The major risk is the potential for the camera to become lodged at the point of stricture and require operative intervention.
5. Skin biopsy
E. Tuberculin purified protein derivative (PPD) skin test

Differential Diagnoses

A. CD
B. UC
C. Appendicitis
D. Colon cancer

E. Irritable bowel syndrome (IBS)
F. Anorexia nervosa
G. Perianal abscess
H. Intestinal protozoan and bacterial etiologies
I. Food poisoning
J. Cytomegalovirus (CMV)
K. Intestinal tuberculosis (TB)
L. Other forms of colitis (ischemic, medication induced)

Plan

A. CD should be managed jointly with a gastroenterologist, colorectal surgeon, and specialists such as a rheumatologist and a nutritionist.

▶ **B.** *Patient teaching: See Section III: Patient Teaching Guide for this chapter, "Crohn's Disease."*

C. Dietary management

1. Adequate nutrition is critical to promote healing. Sufficient protein and calories limit the stress on an inflamed and often strictured bowel.

2. Patients with cramps and diarrhea should alter the fiber content of their diets. Diet should include high fiber, low fat (see Appendix B).

3. Those with steatorrhea benefit from decrease in fat intake to less than 80 g/d. Give the patient a copy of the low-fat/low-cholesterol diet (see Appendix B).

4. An empiric trial of restricting milk products may terminate diarrhea due to lactase deficiency.

5. Patients with severe diarrhea may require partial bowel rest, which removes the stimulus that food has on bowel motility and secretion.

6. Elemental diet preparations, such as Ensure, Sustacal, or Isocal, have been found to induce remission, improve symptoms, and decrease disease activity in patients with acute disease.

7. Total parenteral nutrition (TPN) is used when the patient's oral intake is not adequate or when surgery is indicated.

8. Pretreatment screening for TB, using Mantoux (a PPD) skin testing, is needed prior to initiation of immunomodulators and thiopurines.

9. Immunization status

a. Immunizations with inactivated vaccines should be brought up to date and rigorously maintained during treatment, including influenza, meningococcus, and pneumococcus.

b. Check varicella titers prior to treatment with immunomodulators and reimmunize if titers are low.

c. The risk of administering live vaccines (polio, rubella, and yellow fever) to patients on immunomodulators has not been established; however, most experts avoid live vaccines during treatment.

D. Medical and surgical management

1. Consider hospitalization for fulminate disease, cachexia, fever, vomiting, and evidence of obstruction and/or abscess.

a. Surgery does not cure the patient and is reserved for intractable disease, perforation, obstruction, or severe bleeding.

b. The objective of surgery is to remove grossly involved bowel and to spare as much normal-appearing bowel as possible.

c. Postoperative recurrence rates are estimated at 30% to 50% per decade and are inversely related to preoperative disease duration.

E. Pharmaceutical therapy: The medical management of CD can be divided into treatment of an acute exacerbation and maintenance of remission. In acute exacerbation, triggers, such as underlying infection, fistula, perforation, and other pathology, must be ruled out prior to the intravenous (IV) administration of glucocorticoids. The goal of chronic therapy is the remission of bowel inflammation. Therapies include the following:

1. Vitamin, mineral, and folic acid supplements are necessary for proper healing and avoidance of secondary complications, such as bone disease and anemia.

a. Patient should take a multiple vitamin supplement containing about five times the normal daily vitamin requirements.

b. Folic acid supplementation is required for patients on sulfasalazine because it impairs folic acid absorption.

c. Vitamin B_{12} replacement is required for patients who have ileal surgery.

d. Vitamin D, 4,000 international units (IU), is required for patients with steatorrhea.

2. Opiates provide symptomatic relief of diarrhea during acute phases of illness and chronic active colitis. Diphenoxylate and atropine (Lomotil), codeine, tincture of opium (Paregoric), and loperamide (Imodium A-D) all limit the number of BMs. Tincture of belladonna and other anticholinergics help control cramping.

3. Stepwise medication approach (see Table 11.5 for adult dosing)

a. Aminosalicylates (5-ASA) are a mainstay of therapy because of their anti-inflammatory activities and rapid absorption throughout the small intestines. Several formulations are available for targeting a specific region of the bowel. The 5-ASA drugs are not specifically approved by the Food and Drug Administration (FDA) for use in CD.

i. Sulfasalazine and balsalazide are primarily released in the colon.

1) Pediatrics: 50 to 75 mg/kg/d is given in three or four divided doses of with a maximum dose of 1 g/dose.

2) Reduced absorption of folic acid and digoxin have been reported when administered with sulfasalazine.

ii. Mesalamine (Pentasa) can be released in the duodenum to the distal colon.

1) Pediatrics: 50 to 75 mg/kg/d is given in three or four divided doses with a maximum dose of 1 g/dose.

iii. Asacol is targeted for release in the distal ileum and colon.

1) Pediatrics: For patients 5 years or older, dose is weight based (up to a maximum of

TABLE 11.5 Medications for Crohn's Disease and Ulcerative Colitis—Adult Dosing

		Induction Therapy	Maintenance Therapy
Aminosalicylates (5-ASA) anti-inflammatory activities and rapid absorption throughout the GI tract. The 5-ASA drugs are not specifically approved by the FDA for CD.			
sulfasalazine (Azulifidine)	Treatment of mild to moderate UC, and as adjunctive therapy in severe UC. Converted to mesalamine in the colon	**UC and Crohn's** Initial 1 to 2 g per day in divided doses. Gradual increase to 3 to 4 g per day in divided doses	**UC** For the prolongation of the remission period between acute attacks: 2 to 4 g per day in divided doses
olsalazine (Dipentum)	Release is delayed in the colon. Converted to mesalamine in the colon	**UC** Maintenance of remission of UC in patients intolerant of sulfasalazine	**UC** Maintenance: 500 mg orally. Take with food in evenly divided doses
balsalazide (Colazal)	Mild to moderately active CD. Release is delayed until the terminal ileum and cecum. Converted to mesalamine in the colon	**UC and Crohn's** 6.75 g per day in divided doses Duration 8 to 12 weeks	**UC and Crohn's** Safety and effectiveness have not been established beyond 12 weeks
mesalamine (Asacol)	Targeted for release in the distal ileum and colon	**UC and Crohn's** 2.4 to 4.8 g per day in divided doses	**UC and Crohn's** Maintenance: 2.4 to 4.8 g per day in divided doses
mesalamine (Pentasa)	Mild to moderate disease. Released in the duodenum to the distal colon	**UC and Crohn's** 4 g/day in divided doses for up to 8 weeks	**UC and Crohn's** 2 to 4 g per day in divided doses
mesalamine (Apriso)	Locally acting aminosalicylates, 24-hour delayed and extended release. Release occurs at a pH $\geq$ 6, then is prolonged throughout the colon	**UC** 1.5 to 3 g per day in divided doses	**Maintenance of remission of UC**. 1.5 g every day
mesalamine suppository	Specific to the rectum and distal colon	**Ulcerative Proctitis** **Rectal Suppository** One 500-mg suppository rectally twice a day **OR** one 1,000-mg rectally at night. Suppositories should be retained 1 to 3 hours to achieve maximal benefit	**Maintaining Remission of ulcerative Proctitis** **Rectal Suppository** One 500-mg suppository rectally twice a day **OR** one 1,000-mg rectally at night. Suppositories should be retained 1 to 3 hours to achieve maximal benefit
mesalamine retention enema (Rowasa)	Specific to the rectum and distal colon	**Retention enema**—60 mL (4 g) at bedtime, retained overnight (8 hours)	**Retention enema**—60 mL (4 g) at bedtime, retained overnight (8 hours)
Corticosteroids nonspecifically suppress the immune system. They are the mainstay of treatment for active flares			
budesonide (Uceris, Entocort EC)	Treatment of mild to moderate CD involving the ileum and/or ascending colon Released in the distal small intestine and right colon **Rectal 5-ASA is the first-line therapy in distal UC**	**UC and Crohn's** 9 mg daily for up to 8 weeks TAPER to 6 mg daily for 2 weeks prior to complete cessation For recurring episodes of active CD, a repeat 8-week course can be given	**UC and Crohn's** Maintenance of clinical remission of mild to moderate CD of ileum and/or ascending colon 6 mg per day up to 3 months. Maintenance treatment beyond 3 months has no proven substantial clinical benefit

(continued)

TABLE 11.5 Medications for Crohn's Disease and Ulcerative Colitis–Adult Dosing (*continued*)

		Induction Therapy	Maintenance Therapy
Prednisone (most common oral steroid used) Methylprednisolone (IV)	Used in acute treatment but is not preventative IV steroids are used in patients in severe disease who require hospitalization	**UC and Crohn's** Dosage and length of treatment vary Steroids should not be stopped abruptly, tapering should begin concomitant with initiating other treatments to maintain remission	**UC and Crohn's** Not for maintenance therapy
Hydrocortisone enemas (Cortenema) Hydrocortisone acetate foam and steroid suppositories (Cortifoam, ProctoFoam-HC)	Colonic disease—proctitis requiring topical/rectal formulations	**UC and Crohn's** **Enema**—One nightly at HS; usual length of treatment 2 to 3 weeks **Suppository**—One twice a day (a.m. and p.m.). Severe proctitis may require using a suppository three times a day or using two suppositories twice a day **Foam**—One applicator once daily or every 12 hours for 2 to 3 weeks, then one applicator every other day if needed	**UC and Crohn's** Dosage and length of treatment are based on medical treatment and response to treatment
Immunomodulatory Agents: Thiopurines—The 2013 AGA recommends against using thiopurine monotherapy to induce remission with patients with moderately severe CD. Because of the delay in the onset of action of 6-thiopurines, concomitant therapy with systemic corticosteroids or an anti-TNF-α drug is required for rapid system relief with moderately severe CD. **AGA suggests against using MTX to induce remission in patients with moderately severe CD.** **AGA suggests using MTX over no immunomodulator therapy to maintain corticosteroid-induced remission in patients with CD.**			
6-Mercaptopurine (6-MP; Purinethol)	Slow onset—The onset of therapy is noted after 3 to 6 months.	**CD** Weight-based dosage and response to therapy 1.5 mg/kg/day	**CD** Weight-based dosage and response to therapy 1.5 mg/kg/day
Azathioprine (Imuran) Used off-label for UC and CD	Converts to its active form 6-MP. Slow acting, can take up to 3 months to work	**UC and Crohn's** Weight-based dosage and response to therapy 2.5 mg/kg/day	**UC and Crohn's** Weight-based dosage and response to therapy 2.5 mg/kg/day
MTX Folic acid antagonist	Improvement generally in 3 to 6 weeks; full benefit may not be seen for 12 weeks	**CD** 15 mg to 25 mg once a week by injection Patients also need to take folic acid: 1 mg per day	**CD** 15 mg per week Patients also need to take folic acid 1 mg per day
Biologics—TNF-alpha blocker **The AGA recommends using anti-TNF-α *monotherapy* to induce remission in patients with moderately severe CD.** **The AGA recommends using anti-TNF-α with thiopurines over *thiopurines monotherapy* to induce remission in patients with moderately severe CD.** **The AGA recommends using anti-TNF-α over no anti-TNF-α to maintain corticosteroid or anti-TNF-α-induced remission in patients with CD.**			
Infliximab Remicade IV infusion	Moderate to severe CD with fistulizing CD or resistance to steroids and conventional therapy	**CD** 5 mg/kg IV over 2 hr at 0, 2, and 6 weeks	**CD** 5 mg/kg every 6 to 8 weeks thereafter. If no response by week 14, consider discontinuing therapy

Infliximab-dyyb (Inflectra)	Approved for adult and pediatric patients with moderate to severe Crohn's disease.	**CD** IV infusion given at 2 to 4 hr at 0, 2, and 6 weeks	**CD** Every 8 weeks thereafter
Certolizumab Pegol (Cimzia) Subcutaneous (subq) in the abdomen or thigh	Moderate to severe CD resistance to steroids and conventional therapy	**CD** 400 mg (two 200 mg) subcutaneous injections on day 1, then at 2 weeks, and at 4 weeks	**CD** 400 mg every 4 weeks
Adalimumab (Humira) Subcutaneous in the abdomen or thigh	Moderate to severe CD resistance to steroids and conventional therapy	**CD** Prefilled syringes: On day 1, four injections are self-administered. On day 15, two injections are self-administered	**CD** One injection every 2 weeks
Golimumab (Simponi)	Moderate to severe UC resistance to steroids and conventional therapy	**UC** 200-mg injections are self-administered at initiation, 100-mg subq at week 2	**UC** 100-mg injection every 4 weeks
Vedolizumab (Entyvio)	Moderate to severe CD and UC resistance to steroids and conventional therapy	**UC and Crohn's** 300 mg IV infused over 30 minutes at initiation, week 2 and week 6	**UC and Crohn's** 300-mg IV every 8 weeks thereafter
Antiadhesion molecule			
Natalizumab (Tysabri)[a] ***Distribution is restricted and infusion is available only through a close monitored infusion center program known as TOUCH***	***Moderate to severe CD for adults who failed anti-TNF therapy.***	***CD*** ***300 mg every 4 weeks. Given by IV infusion over 1 hour.*** ***Discontinue after 12 weeks based on individual response/protocol***	***CD*** ***300-mg IV monthly—Restricted distribution***
Antibiotics—Used for treatment of bacterial infections that cause abscesses and can be helpful with treatment of fistulas			
Ciprofloxacin (Cipro)		**UC and Crohn's** Dosage and length of treatment vary	**UC and Crohn's** Dosage and length of treatment vary
Metronidazole (Flagyl)		**UC and Crohn's** Dosage and length of treatment vary	**UC and Crohn's** Dosage and length of treatment vary

AGA, American Gastroenterology Association; CD, Crohn's disease; FDA, Food ad Drug Administration; 5-ASA, aminosalicylates; GI, gastrointestinal; HS, bedtime; IV, intravenous; MTX, methotrexate; TNF, tumor necrosis factor; TOUCH, TYSABRI Outreach: Unified Commitment to Health; UC, ulcerative colitis.

[a]Natalizumab users carry an increased risk of a severe brain condition called *progressive multifocal leukoencephalopathy (PML)*, resulting from infection with the John Cunningham (JC) virus. It is important to be tested for JC virus prior to starting natalizumab; patients who are negative for JC virus have a much lower risk of developing PML.

Source: Adapted from the American College of Gastroenterology Guidelines (2013): gastro.org/guidelines

2.4 g/d), divided into two daily doses for a duration of 6 weeks.

2) Two Asacol 400 mg tablets are not interchangeable or substitutable with one mesalamine delayed-release 800 mg tablet.

iv. Multi-Matrix System (MMX) marketed as Lialda releases mesalamine in the colon. *Lialda is not recommended for children younger than 18 years.* Dosage is 2.4 to 4.8 mg once a day with meals, taken for 8 weeks.

v. Rowasa is specific for the rectum and distal colon. Mesalamine (Rowasa) 800 mg tablets are given three times daily for a total of 2.4 g/d for 6 weeks. Alternatively, 1 g control-release capsule four times daily for a total of 4 g/d for up to 8 weeks; or 40 g/60 mL as a retention enema or suppository once daily, preferably at bedtime. Rectal form should be retained overnight, for about 8 hours. Usual course of therapy for rectal form is 3 to 6 weeks.

b. Corticosteroids are used if IBD fails to respond to 5-ASA. Corticosteroids should be tapered as rapidly as possible and do not have a role in maintaining remission.

i. Budesonide (Entocort) is designed to be effective only in the treatment of disease involving the ileum and ascending colon. Budesonide is effective in the maintenance of short-term (3 months) but not long-term (1 year) remission.

1) Pediatrics: For children 6 years of age and older: The dose is 0.45 mg/kg/d (maximum of 9 mg/d), tapered by 3-mg increments.

ii. Prednisone or prednisolone

1) Pediatrics: Prednisone or prednisolone 1 to 2 mg/kg per day (maximum 60 mg/d) given orally or IV brings rapid improvement but should serve as a short-term induction therapy due to long-term side effects, including growth failure, osteopenia, hirsutism, diabetes, psychosis, cataracts, and altered body shape and image.As soon as the acute disease subsides, steroid taper for 2 weeks to minimum is necessary to control symptoms.

c. Immunomodulatory agents may be initiated for IBD refractory to corticosteroids or frequent flares that require steroids. These agents require monitoring of blood counts due to hematologic toxicity. A 3% incidence of pancreatitis, allergic reactions, infections, and marrow toxicity is associated with their use. The main drawback to the use of AZA and 6-MP is their slow onset. The effect of therapy is noted after 3 to 6 months of treatment. The FDA recommends that individuals should have TPMT genotype or phenotype assessment before initiation of therapy with AZA or 6-MP to detect individuals who have low-enzyme activity or who are homozygous deficient in TPMT.

i. 6-MP

1) Pediatrics: 1.0 to 2.0 mg/kg per day orally (maximum of 150 mg per day)

2) Patients with inherited little or no TPMT activity are at increased risk for severe Purinethol toxicity and generally require substantial dose reduction.

ii. AZA (Imuran)

1) Monitoring includes: CBC, including platelet counts weekly during the first month, twice monthly for the second and third months of therapy, then monthly or more frequently if dosage alteration is necessary.

2) TPMT testing: Testing is recommended for consideration to either genotype or phenotype patients for TPMT.

3) Pediatrics: 1.5 to 2.5 mg/kg/d orally (maximum 200 mg/d)

4) Doses for adults and pediatrics must be lowered for reduced TPMT activity.

iii. Methotrexate ([MTX] folic acid antagonist) has adverse effects, including leukopenia, GI upset, and hypersensitivity pneumonitis.

1) Pediatrics: Doses typically start at 15 mg/m^2 per week and are advanced as tolerated to a maximum of 25 mg/m^2 per week. Subcutaneous dosing for children is recommended to ensure absorption until the patient enters remission; then switch to oral MTX.

2) Folic acid supplement (1 mg/d) may reduce the likelihood of oral ulcers.

d. Tumor necrosis factor (TNF)-alpha blocker

i. Infliximab (Remicade) is a chimeric monoclonal antibody to TNF alpha. Infliximab is effective for moderate to severe CD and for patients with fistulizing CD or who are resistant to steroids and conventional therapy. Infliximab can close perianal fistulas refractory to therapy with antibiotics and 6-MP. Infliximab has a half-life of approximately 10 days.

1) Pediatrics: Recommended for people age 6 to 17 years with severe active CD whose disease has not responded to conventional therapy, including corticosteroids, immunomodulators, and conventional therapy; 5 mg/kg in a single IV dose.

ii. Certolizumab (Cimzia) is given subcutaneously in the abdomen or thigh.

1) *Pediatrics: Not recommended*

iii. Adalimumab (Humira) is an antibody directed against TNF. It is also administered subcutaneously in the abdomen or thigh.

1) *Pediatrics: Not recommended for those younger than 18 years.*

e. Natalizumab (Tysabri), a monoclonal antibody, is an effective induction agent for CD in adults. It is given in a certified TOUCH center. IV infusion is given over 1 hour and requires a 1-hour observation period postinfusion.

i. *Pediatrics: Not recommended for those younger than 18 years.*

f. Antibiotics are utilized in adults for perianal disease or inflammatory mass. Pediatric doses have not been established in either metronidazole or ciprofloxacin for CD.

g. Thalidomide, an inhibitor of both TNF and angiogenesis, has been used off-label to treat refractory IBD.

Follow-Up

A. Have the patient record his or her weight daily to monitor changes.

B. Assess frequency and consistency of stools to evaluate volume losses and effectiveness of therapy.

C. Instruct patients on self-medication to call the health provider's office if fever develops, diarrhea worsens, bleeding occurs, or abdominal pain becomes marked.

D. Monitoring patients on 5-ASA should include a CBC at least twice a year and urinalysis at least annually.

E. Monitoring patients on 6-MP requires frequent monitoring, including CBC and aminotransferase levels (alanine transaminase [ALT] and aspartate transaminase [AST]) before treatment, and again at 2, 3, 8, and 12 weeks after initiating therapy. When stable, monitor every 3 months thereafter, and 2 to 3 weeks after a change in dosage.

F. Monitoring patients on MTX includes a CBC and aminotransferases as with 6-MP/thiopurine therapies.

G. Periodic bone mineral density assessment is recommended for patients on long-term corticosteroid therapy (longer than 3 months). Osteopenia should be treated aggressively. The primary intervention includes dietary counseling and supplementation to ensure adequate intake of vitamin D and calcium.

H. Annual ophthalmologic examinations are recommended for patients on long-term corticosteroids.

I. Patients who are using corticosteroids should be monitored for glucose intolerance and other metabolic abnormalities.

Consultation/Referral

A. Refer the patient to a gastroenterologist initially for evaluation. Treatment requires multidisciplinary management with the gastroenterologist and other subspecialists, including a nutritionist, surgeon, rheumatologist, ophthalmologist, and social workers.

B. Promptly hospitalize for parenteral management patients who are toxic, bleeding heavily, in severe pain, or too sick to obtain adequate nutrition orally.

C. Consider a referral for genetic testing.

Individual Considerations

A. Pregnancy

1. Active disease at the time of conception is associated with increased incidence of miscarriage and postpartum exacerbation. It may also predispose the patient to other maternal and prenatal risks, such as premature labor, small-for-gestational-age babies, and stillbirth.

2. Oral and topical mesalamine, oral balsalazide, sulfasalazine, corticosteroids, and ciprofloxacin (after the first trimester) are safe and effective during nursing or pregnancy.

3. Women on prednisone should receive supplementary steroids during labor and delivery as well as during other highly stressful times.

4. Counsel women to attempt pregnancy only when the disease has been quiescent for several months.

5. Withholding sulfasalazine for 2 to 3 days before delivery may be advisable to minimize neonatal jaundice due to bilirubin displacement.

6. MTX is a FDA category X drug.

B. Pediatrics

1. Approximately 30% of children with CD are refractory to or dependent on steroids despite concomitant use of 6-MP. These patients may require conversion from thiopurine to MTX maintenance therapy, or treatment with a biologic agent.

2. Sulfasalazine and olsalazine can be compounded into a suspension for young children to drink. It is recommended that other 5-ASA be swallowed whole; however, Pentasa may be opened and administered by sprinkling the granules on soft food.

3. Psychological counseling may be required in children secondary to the chronic relapsing nature of the illness, effects on body appearance and image such as short stature, and pubertal delay.

4. Children with CD should undergo colonoscopy for cancer screening beginning 8 to 10 years after the diagnosis of CD. The frequency of screening should be determined by the findings on the initial colonoscopy (around every 1–3 years).

5. The National Institute for Health and Clinical Excellence (NICE) clinical guideline recommendations include consideration of monitoring for changes in bone mineral density in children and young people with risk factors, such as low body mass index (BMI), low-trauma fracture, or continued or repeated glucocorticosteroid use.

C. Geriatrics

1. **Unexplained diarrhea, weight loss, and perianal disease in the elderly should arouse suspicions regarding CD. Elderly patients have worse outcomes because of delayed presentation and comorbid conditions.**

2. Elderly patients tend to have CD confined to the distal colon, with only 40% having proctitis.

3. With an increase in cancers in elderly patients with CD, it is imperative to evaluate and exclude cancer before beginning immunosuppressant or biologic therapies.

4. Review CD therapies, with comorbid conditions in mind, due to side effects, interactions, need for increased laboratory monitoring (e.g., INR, as well as digoxin levels and phenytoin levels), and risk of infection.

5. Anti-TNF-α agents are contraindicated in patients with New York Heart Association (NYHA) class III and IV heart failure (HF).

Resource

Crohn's and Colitis Foundation of America: www.ccfa.org

Cyclosporiasis

Cheryl A. Glass and Audra Malone

Definition

A. Cyclosporiasis is a one-cell parasite that infects the upper small intestines. Causes of cyclosporiasis include ingesting infected water or produce (fresh fruits, especially raspberries, and vegetables) or exposure to the organism during travel to countries where it is endemic.
B. Cyclosporiasis manifests as protracted and relapsing gastroenteritis. The clinical syndrome consists of explosive watery diarrhea, nausea, anorexia, weight loss, fatigue, and abdominal cramps that may persist for 7 days to several weeks, with a waxing and waning course.
C. In an immunocompromised host, onset is insidious; the condition becomes chronic with symptoms, and the shedding of oocysts continues indefinitely.
D. The oocysts are resistant to most disinfectants used in food and water processing and can remain viable for prolonged periods.

Incidence

A. The incidence of infection is unknown, although it is common around the world.
B. Most outbreaks in the United States and Canada have been associated with consumption of imported fresh produce, including raspberries, basil, snow peas, and mesclun lettuce.

Pathogenesis

A. Infection is caused by an 8- to 10-μm, spore-forming coccidian protozoan called *Cyclospora cayetanensis.* Transmission of oocysts is by the oral–fecal route. The incubation period ranges from 2 days to 2 weeks after excretion, depending on temperature and humidity.

Predisposing Factors

A. Incompetent or compromised immune system (e.g., infection with AIDS)
B. Travel to underdeveloped or tropical countries
C. Ingestion of contaminated food or water
D. Contact with animals that carry the parasite

Common Complaints

A. Abrupt, profuse, malodorous, watery diarrhea
B. Nausea
C. Vomiting
D. Anorexia
E. Substantial weight loss
F. Flu-like symptoms
G. Abdominal cramps and bloating

Other Signs and Symptoms

A. Asymptomatic
B. Low-grade fever
C. Nausea and vomiting
D. Profound fatigue
E. Yellow- to khaki-green stools
F. Flatus
G. Dehydration

Subjective Data

A. Review the onset, duration, and course of symptoms. Is diarrhea acute or chronic?
B. Question the patient about travel to areas known for cyclospora, such as Haiti, Puerto Rico, Pakistan, India, Mexico, Nepal, New Guinea, and Peru. It has also been seen in Chicago, Los Angeles, New York, Florida, and Massachusetts.
C. Review the patient's intake of medications and other substances that can cause diarrhea, especially antibiotics, laxatives, quinidine, magnesium-containing antacids, digitalis, loop diuretics, antihypertensives, alcohol, caffeine, herbal teas, and sorbitol-containing (sugar-free) gum and mints.
D. Ask about the nature of the patient's bowel movements (BMs), including frequency; consistency; volume; and presence of blood, pus, or mucus.
E. Review associated symptoms that need evaluation: Fever, abdominal pain, and anorexia.
F. Ask the patient if other family members or sexual contacts are also ill.
G. Establish the patient's normal weight and any recent weight loss. How much weight was lost and over what period of time?

Physical Examination

A. Check temperature, pulse, respirations, blood pressure, and weight (vital signs are normal in most cases).
B. Inspect
  1. General appearance for signs of illness and dehydration
    a. Inspect mucous membranes.
    b. Inspect infants' fontanelles.
    c. Note for decreased skin turgor.
C. Auscultate the abdomen for bowel sounds in all quadrants.
D. Palpate
  1. The abdomen for masses, rebound tenderness, and guarding; may exhibit right upper quadrant (RUQ) pain (biliary disease)
  2. Lymph nodes for enlargement
E. Perform rectal examination.

Diagnostic Tests

Identification may be made by microscopic examination of stool under ultraviolet light, by modified acid-fast staining, or by review of wet mounts of stool by experienced microscopists. Finding large numbers of white cells suggests an inflammatory or invasive diarrhea. The following tests are done:
A. Acid-fast Ziehl–Neelsen stained slide of stool
B. Stool culture for ova and parasites: Parasites are passed intermittently, so three or more stools on alternating days should be examined.
C. Endoscopy with small-bowel biopsy

Differential Diagnoses

A. Cyclospora infection
B. Giardiasis
C. Malabsorption

D. *Escherichia coli* infection: *E. coli* causes diarrhea within hours of ingesting contaminated food. Confirm by checking if others were affected.
E. IBS: Leukocyte-free mucus is the hallmark of IBS.
F. Viral diarrhea
G. Lactose intolerance
H. Other bacterial infections, for example, *Shigella, Salmonella,* and *Campylobacter*
I. Cholera
J. Inflammatory bowel disease (IBD; Crohn's disease [CD] or ulcerative colitis [UC])

Plan

A. General interventions
- **1.** Avoid food and water that is contaminated with feces.
- **2.** Fresh produce should always be washed thoroughly before it is eaten.

▶ **B.** Patient teaching: *See Section III: Patient Teaching Guide for this chapter, "Diarrhea."*
- **1.** Teach contact precautions to those caring for diapered and/or incontinent children.

C. Dietary management
- **1.** Tell the patient to increase fluids. Fluid replacement is the basic approach to prevent dehydration from diarrhea.
- **2.** Tell the patient to restrict milk products to rule out lactose intolerance.
- **3.** Give the patient a copy of a diet plan to control nausea and vomiting (children and adults).

D. Pharmaceutical therapy
- **1.** Drugs of choice are trimethoprim with sulfamethoxazole (TMP–SMZ). They can reduce shedding, and stop diarrhea within 2 days.
  - **a.** Adults
    - **i.** Immunocompetent host: TMP 160 mg/SMZ 800 mg tablet orally twice a day for 7 to 10 days
    - **ii.** Immunocompromised host: TMP 160 mg/SMZ 800 mg tablet orally four times a day for 10 days, followed by prophylaxis with TMP 160 mg/SMZ 800 mg orally three times per week
  - **b.** Children
    - **i.** For those younger than 2 months, do not prescribe TMP/SMZ.
    - **ii.** For those older than 2 months: TMP 8 mg/kg, SMZ 40 mg/kg orally twice a day for 7 days for acute infections
- **2.** Ciprofloxacin (Cipro) is the alternative treatment for patients with allergies to sulfamethoxazole.
  - **a.** Adults: Cipro 500 mg orally twice a day for 5 to 7 days for acute infection
  - **b.** Adults: Prophylaxis in HIV: Cipro 500 mg orally three times a week
  - **c.** Pediatrics: Not recommended for those younger than 18 years

Follow-Up

A. See the patient in 1 week to verify continuing clinical improvement.
B. If diarrhea persists 2 weeks or longer, a second evaluation is indicated.
C. Retest stools for blood and leukocytes; do a stool culture for ova and parasites.
D. Report cases of cyclosporiasis to the health department.

Consultation/Referral

A. Consult an infectious disease specialist and/or gastroenterologist if the patient has no symptom relief after completing therapies or has a prolonged or severe case.

Individual Considerations

Pregnancy:
A. TMP–SMZ is a pregnancy category C drug. Use during pregnancy if the potential benefits outweigh the risk to the fetus.
B. TMP–SMZ should be avoided near term because of the potential for hyperbilirubinemia and kernicterus in the newborn.

Diarrhea

Cheryl A. Glass and Audra Malone

Definition

A. Diarrhea is an abnormally high fluid content in the stool. Generally, diarrhea also involves an increase in the frequency of bowel movements (BMs), which can range from four to five to more than 20 times a day. Diarrhea may be an acute onset or chronic/persistent diarrhea.
B. Acute diarrhea is usually self-limited; the most common complication of diarrhea is dehydration.
C. Chronic diarrhea is defined as lasting longer than 14 days.

Incidence

A. The incidence of diarrhea is unknown; however, it is responsible for 20% of pediatric referrals in children younger than 2 years and for 10% in children younger than 3 years. Morbidity has decreased because of the use of oral rehydration solutions; however, the global rate of mortality from acute diarrhea is 18% of children younger than age 5 years.
B. The incidence of *Clostridium difficile* infection is approximately 7%, and 28% of patients who were hospitalized have positive cultures for the organism. *C. difficile*–associated diarrhea has a mortality rate as high as 25% in the frail elderly.
C. 20% to 27% of cases of *C. difficile* are community acquired.

Pathogenesis

A. The increased water content in diarrhea stools is due to an imbalance in the physiology of the small and large intestinal processes. A bacterial infection is usually the cause of acute diarrhea in children. Other causes of diarrhea in children include malabsorption syndrome (see Table 11.6).

TABLE 11.6 Organisms That Cause Diarrhea

Viral organisms	Rotavirus Norovirus Adenovirus Calicivirus Astrovirus
Invasive bacteria	*Escherichia coli* *Klebsiella* *Clostridium difficile* *Clostridium perfringens* *Shigella* *Salmonella* *Campylobacter* *Cholera* *Yersinia* *Plesiomonas* *Aeromonas*
Parasites	*Giardia* *Entamoeba* organisms *Cryptosporidium* *Giardia lamblia*

Predisposing Factors

A. Enteric infections
B. Females have a higher incidence of *Campylobacter* species infections.
C. Young children
D. Institutional: Day care and skilled nursing facilities
E. Food: Raw or contaminated food
F. Contaminated water or inadequate chlorinated water supply
G. Travel
H. Chemotherapy or radiation induced
I. Vitamin deficiencies (niacin and folate)
J. Vitamin toxicity (C, niacin, and vitamin B_3)
K. Ingestion of heavy metals (copper, tin, or zinc) or toxins
L. Ingestion of plants, mistletoe, or mushrooms
M. Antibiotics
N. Antacids containing magnesium

Common Complaints

A. Frequent watery stool
B. Foul-smelling stools (fat malabsorption)
C. Flatulence
D. Abdominal cramping

Other Signs and Symptoms

A. Lethargy
B. Fever
C. Nausea and vomiting
D. Currant jelly stool (blood and mucus)
E. Anorexia
F. Dehydration in adults
   1. Thirst
   2. Less frequent urination
   3. Dark urine
   4. Dry skin
   5. Fatigue
   6. Dizziness
   7. Lightheadedness
G. Dehydration in infants and young children
   1. Dry mouth and tongue
   2. No tears when crying
   3. No wet diapers for 3 hours or more
   4. Sunken eyes, cheeks, or fontanelles
   5. High fever
   6. Listlessness or irritability

Subjective Data

A. Review the onset of diarrheal stools. What is the normal stool pattern?
B. Review the consistency, color, volume, and frequency of the stools.
C. Review dietary intake of raw foods, contaminated food, and nonabsorbable sugars, including lactulose or lactose in lactose malabsorbers.
D. Review any contact with others who may have the same symptoms.
E. Have any of the stools contained blood? Bloody stool may be an indication of bacterial infection.
F. Review travel history, including camping vacations.
G. Review any exposure to turtles or young dogs or cats.
H. Review medication history, including antibiotics, vitamins, herbal production, laxatives, antacids that contain magnesium, opiate withdrawal, Olestra, and methylxanthines (caffeine, theobromine, and theophylline).
I. Review any food allergies and history of lactose intolerance.
J. Evaluate the presence of other symptoms such as fever, nausea, vomiting and abdominal pain, or tenesmus.
K. Evaluate for symptoms of dehydration, including thirst, dizziness, mental status changes, and decreased urine output.

Physical Examination

A. Check temperature, pulse, respirations, blood pressure (standing and sitting), and weight.
B. Inspect
   1. Observe the patient's general overall appearance, the presence of lethargy or depressed consciousness, or grimace during examination.
   2. Evaluate muscle tone, skin turgor, reduced muscle, and fat mass.
   3. Examine mouth, lips, and mucus membranes for signs, symptoms, and severity of dehydration.
   4. Perianal examination for skin breakdown, erythema, and fissures.
C. Auscultation
   1. Assess heart and lungs.
   2. Auscultate the abdomen in all four quadrants.
   3. Assess the presence of borborygmi (significant increase in peristaltic action that may be audible and/or palpable).
D. Percuss abdomen.
E. Palpate
   1. Palpate the abdomen for masses, guarding, rebound tenderness, and peritoneal signs.
   2. For a newborn, palpate fontanelles.
   3. Palpate for lymphadenopathy.

4. Perform a rectal examination, including testing of stool for occult blood.

Diagnostic Tests

A. Stool specimens for the evaluation of
  1. *C. difficile*
  2. Fecal leukocytes
  3. Blood
  4. Culture
  5. Ova and parasites
  6. Fecal alpha-1 antitrypsin levels
  7. Viral antigen testing
B. Specific enzyme immunoassay (EIA) and direct florescence antibody (DFA) assays are becoming the standard for the diagnosis of giardiasis.
C. Complete blood count (CBC): White blood cell (WBC) may be elevated.
D. Albumin
E. Electrolytes
F. A colonoscopy for intestinal biopsy for chronic or protracted diarrhea or patients with AIDS should be done. A sigmoidoscopy alone may not reveal any abnormality.
G. Abdominal ultrasound to identify intussusception
H. Abdominal CT

Differential Diagnoses

A. Diarrhea: Infectious etiology
B. Inflammatory bowel disease (IBD)
  1. Crohn's disease (CD)
  2. Ulcerative colitis (UC)
C. Cystic fibrosis (CF)
D. Giardiasis
E. Protozoan
F. Malabsorption syndromes
G. Intussusception
H. Stool impaction
I. Irritable bowel syndrome (IBS)
J. Meckel's diverticulum
K. Intolerance to lactose, carbohydrates, and protein
L. Medication induced
  1. Antibiotic-associated diarrhea
  2. Antacids containing magnesium
  3. Cancer drugs
M. Pseudomembranous colitis
N. Toxic megacolon
O. Appendicitis

Plan

► **A.** Patient teaching: *See Section III: Patient Teaching Guide for this chapter, "Diarrhea."*
B. Examination of stools for ova and parasites should be done every other day or every 3 days.
C. Rehydrate with oral fluids for each diarrheal stool. Administer small amounts at frequent intervals.
D. Hold foods until hydration is completed. No evidence shows that bananas, rice, applesauce, and toast (BRAT) are useful; these are not currently recommended.
E. Use antibiotics (or the discontinuation of antibiotics in the case of *C. difficile*) or use antiparasitic agents, depending on the etiology.
F. The use of probiotics, *Lactobacillus GG* (I, A) and *S. boulardii* (II, B), has been found to be effective and may reduce the spread of rotavirus.
G. Encourage proper hygiene and food preparation to prevent spread and future infections.
H. Water should be boiled for at least 1 minute if contamination is suspected.

Follow-Up

A. Follow-up depends on the severity of diarrhea and the age of the patient. Neonates require strict follow-up within a few days of illness.
B. Monitor children who require labor-intensive oral hydration. Hospitalization for intravenous (IV) hydration may be required.
C. Rotavirus vaccine is available for the prevention of rotavirus gastroenteritis. RotaTeq is administered in a three-dose series for infants aged 6 to 12 weeks and completed before 32 weeks. *Or* ROTARIX oral vaccine is available in a two-dose administration to patients aged 6 to 24 weeks.

Consultation/Referral

A. Evaluate the need for a surgical consultation (fulminant colitis, peritonitis, and toxic megacolon) or one with an infectious-disease specialist or a gastroenterologist.

Individual Considerations

A. Pediatrics
  1. Stool patterns vary widely. Breastfed children may have up to five to six stools per day. Breastfed infants with acute diarrhea should continue on breast milk.
  2. The younger the child, the higher the risk for severe, life-threatening dehydration and nutrient malabsorption.
B. Geriatrics
  1. Review any hospitalizations within the last 72 hours as a cause of diarrhea.
  2. Advanced age is a risk factor for *C. difficile* infection.
  3. Diarrhea may be related to fecal impaction.
  4. Dehydration is more common in the elderly.
  5. Because of polypharmacy risk in the elderly, review all medications for drug-to-drug interactions.

Resources

Drugs.com Drug Interaction Checker: https://www.drugs.com/drug_interactions.html
Medscape Drug Interaction Checker: http://reference.medscape.com/drug-interactionchecker
RxList Drug Interaction Checker: http://www.rxlist.com/drug-interaction-checker.htm

Diverticulosis and Diverticulitis

Cheryl A. Glass and Audra Malone

Definition

A. Diverticula are saclike protrusions of mucosa through the muscular colonic wall. Protrusions can occur in weakened areas of the bowel wall and blood vessels. Diverticulosis is the presence of diverticula, but it does not imply a pathologic condition. Diverticulitis occurs when the diverticula become plugged and inflamed. Surgery is often the treatment of choice for young symptomatic patients. Diverticular disease is one of the most common causes of lower gastrointestinal (GI) hemorrhage and a leading consideration in patients who present with brisk rectal bleeding.

B. There is no evidence of a relationship between the development of diverticula and smoking, caffeine, and alcohol consumption. However, an increased risk of developing diverticular disease is associated with a diet that is high in red meat and total fat content. This risk can be reduced by a diet high in fiber content, especially with fruits and vegetables (cellulose); see Appendix B, Table B.6).

C. Diverticulosis is often diagnosed as an incidental finding on a BE or sigmoid/colonoscopy.

D. Recurrent attacks of diverticulitis can result in the formation of scar tissue, leading to narrowing and obstruction of the colonic lumen.

E. Complicated diverticulitis includes those episodes associated with free perforation, abscess, fistula, obstruction, or stricture.

Incidence

Diverticulosis is very common and increases with age.

A. Prevalence by age
- **1.** Age 40 years: 5%
- **2.** Age 60 years: 30%
- **3.** Age 80 years: 65% to 80%

B. No significant difference in prevalence by gender

Diverticulosis is symptomatic in 70% of cases. It leads to diverticulitis in 5% to 25%; and is associated with bleeding in 5% to 15%. The sigmoid colon is commonly affected. There are two types of diverticular disease and diverticulitis.
- **1.** Simple, with no complications; responds to treatment such as dietary changes without the need for surgery
- **2.** Complicated, with abscesses, fistula, obstruction, perforation, and peritonitis leading to sepsis; usually requires surgery

Pathogenesis

A. The exact etiology of diverticular disease is not known.

B. The present theory that fiber is a protective agent against the development of diverticula and subsequent diverticulitis holds that insoluble fiber causes the formation of more bulky stool, which leads to decreased effectiveness in colonic segmentation. The overall result is that intracolonic pressure remains close to the normal range during colonic peristalsis. Diverticular sac can become inflamed when undigested food residues and bacteria get trapped in the thin-walled sacs. If this occurs, blood supply is mechanically compromised and bacterial invasion ensues.

Predisposing Factors

A. Advanced age

B. Obesity (84%–96%)

C. Low-residue diet

D. Complicated diverticular disease is exacerbated by
- **1.** Smoking
- **2.** Nonsteroidal anti-inflammatory drugs (NSAIDs)
- **3.** Acetaminophen use (especially paracetamol)
- **4.** Opioids
- **5.** Steroids

E. Indication that genetics is a predisposing factor
- **1.** Left-sided diverticula is predominant in the United States.
- **2.** Right-sided (cecal) diverticula is predominant in Asia.

Common Complaints

A. Diverticulosis is usually asymptomatic.

B. Painless rectal bleeding is the hallmark of diverticular bleeding, with intermittent passage of maroon or bright red blood.

C. Common diverticulitis symptoms
- **1.** Left lower quadrant (LLQ) pain
- **2.** Constipation

Other Signs and Symptoms

A. Back pain

B. Flatulence

C. Periodic abdominal distension

D. Borborygmi, or loud, prolonged gurgles caused by hyperactive intestinal peristalsis

E. Diarrhea

F. Nausea or vomiting

G. Dysuria

H. Tenderness on palpation, possible guarding

I. Fever, low-grade

Subjective Data

A. Review the onset, duration, and course of symptoms, including size, color, consistency, and frequency of stools.

B. Ask the patient if constipation is a chronic or acute problem, and if it alternates with diarrhea. Has the patient ever had a bowel obstruction?

C. Review the patient's daily diet and fluid intake.

D. Ask the patient about medication use, including iron supplements, nonsteroidal anti-inflammatory drugs (NSAIDs), and acetaminophen.

E. Inquire about the color, amount, and frequency of rectal bleeding. Does the patient strain when having a bowel movement (BM)?

F. Review the patient's history of pain with defecation.

G. Review the patient's history of kidney stones as it can mimic diverticulitis.

Physical Examination

The constellation of LLQ tenderness with or without peritoneal findings, fever, and leukocytosis is suggestive of sigmoid diverticulitis.

A. Check temperature, pulse, respirations, blood pressure, and weight.

B. The physical examination may be relatively unremarkable but most commonly reveals abdominal tenderness or a mass.

C. Inspection

1. Observe the general overall appearance for signs of pain.
2. Inspect the abdomen in detail, assessing for distension and guarding.

D. Auscultate all four quadrants of the abdomen. Bowel sounds may be decreased or normal in early diverticulitis.
E. Percuss the abdomen.
F. Palpate
1. Palpate the abdomen for rebound tenderness or masses signaling possible abscess and tenderness.
2. Palpate beneath the right costal arch, checking for Murphy's sign or pain on deep inspiration.
3. Consider a pelvic examination to rule out gynecologic sources of the abdominal pain.

G. Rectal examination: Evaluate for hemorrhoids, masses, fissures, fistulas, inflammation, and stool in the ampulla.

Diagnostic Tests

The diagnosis of acute diverticulitis can often be made following a focused history and physician examination, especially in patients with recurrent diverticulitis whose diagnosis has been previously confirmed.

A. The diagnosis of diverticular colitis is made endoscopically and histologically.
B. CT scan of the abdomen and pelvis is the optimal method of investigation for suspected acute diverticulitis.
C. Complete blood count (CBC) with differential: White blood cell (WBC) may show leukocytosis with a shift to the left; hemoglobin and hematocrit (Hct) may be low with chronic or acute bleeding.
D. C-reactive protein (CRP; greater than 50 in the patient with LLQ pain and no vomiting is highly suggestive of diverticulitis)
E. Radiography: Flat plate and upright films of abdomen to evaluate ileus or obstruction, free air, and perforation.
F. Abdominal ultrasonography to evaluate masses or abscess
G. Proctosigmoidoscopy
H. BE after infection subsides. Caution: A BE during the acute phase may increase intraluminal pressure and cause bowel perforation.
I. Hemoccult: Stool
J. Pregnancy test if there is a possibility of pregnancy.
K. Urinalysis (excludes urinary tract infections)

Differential Diagnoses

A. Diverticulitis
B. Diverticulosis
C. Acute appendicitis
D. Bowel obstruction
E. Ischemic colitis
F. Colon cancer
G. Hemorrhoids
H. Constipation or impaction
I. Inflammatory bowel disease (IBD)
J. Urologic disorder: Pyelonephritis
K. Tubo-ovarian abscess/pelvic inflammatory disease (PID)
L. Torsion (testicular or ovarian)
M. Ectopic pregnancy
N. Cholecystitis
O. Hernia
P. Renal colic
Q. Urinary tract infection

Plan

A. Stress the importance of strict adherence to diet.
B. Dietary management
1. Nothing by mouth (NPO) status for acute treatment
2. Full-liquid diet or low-fiber diet if not on bowel rest
3. Long-term dietary management
a. High-fiber diet, including bran, beans, fruits, and vegetables
b. Bulk agents if unable to tolerate bran
c. Note foods to avoid, such as nuts

C. Medical and surgical management: Acute treatment has not been well defined in diverticular disease.
1. Acute treatment may include the following:
a. Nasogastric (NG) tube placement
b. Intravenous (IV) fluids
2. Surgical intervention is required for abscess, peritonitis, obstruction, fistula, or failure to improve after several days of medical management, or recurrence after successful medical management.

D. Pharmaceutical therapy: Optimal treatment has not been defined.
1. Conservative management of diverticulosis: Psyllium (Metamucil) one to three teaspoons in 8 oz of liquid three times a day
2. Diverticulitis initial attack: Ciprofloxacin (Cipro) 500 mg orally twice daily and metronidazole (Flagyl) 500 mg orally three times a day for 7 to 14 days. Amoxicillin/clavulanic acid or sulfamethoxazole-trimethoprim may also be used with metronidazole.
3. Aminosalicylates (5-ASA) may be added if there is a lack of response.
4. Relapse: May repeat with the same antibiotic regimen for 1 month
5. Chronic disease: Use long-term ciprofloxacin but not metronidazole.
6. Avoid laxatives, enemas, and opiates.
7. Nonsteroidal anti-inflammatory drugs (NSAIDs) should be avoided due to a moderately increased risk of occurrence of diverticulitis.

Follow-Up

A. Follow up in 2 to 3 days. Continue conservative management if the patient has no signs of complications.
B. A colonoscopy should be performed from 6 to 8 weeks after recovery to evaluate the extent of the diverticulosis/rule out other manifestations.

Consultation/Referral

A. Consult a physician if the patient has mild diverticulitis: Temperature less than 101°F; WBC less than 13,000 to 15,000.
B. Arrange for prompt hospitalization and surgical consultation if the patient's temperature rises above 101.0°F, his or her pain worsens, peritoneal signs develop, or WBC continues to rise. Surgery consultation is required

for abscess, peritonitis, obstruction, fistula, or failure to improve after several days of medical management.

Individual Considerations

A. Immunocompromised and elderly patients may have a normal WBC without a left shift and still have a severe infection.

Elevated Liver Enzymes

Cheryl A. Glass and Audra Malone

Definition

Liver function tests (LFTs) used to determine the health of the liver are not direct measures of its function. The liver has excretory, metabolic, protective, detoxification, hematologic, and circulatory functions. LFTs may be abnormal even in patients with a healthy liver. Normal laboratory chemistry values may vary according to age, gender, ethnicity, blood group, and postprandial state, as well as other factors such as exercise and pregnancy. Common rationales for ordering liver chemistry tests (see Table 11.7) include the following:

A. Making differential diagnosis of the different types of jaundice
B. Assessing the severity of hepatocellular injury
C. Following the trend of the disease
D. Diagnosing of the presence of latent liver disease (i.e., differential diagnosis of ascites or hematemesis)
E. Screening the suspected case during outbreaks of infective hepatitis
F. Screening the persons exposed to hepatotoxic drugs
G. Evaluating cholestatic problems

Incidence

A. The incidence of elevated liver enzymes is undetermined. Abnormal elevations of serum liver chemistries may occur in 1% to 4% of the asymptomatic population.

Pathogenesis

A. Pathogenesis varies by diagnosis.

Predisposing Factors

A. Predisposing factors are dependent on the suspected or known medical diagnosis.

Common Complaints

A. Asymptomatic
B. Pruritus
C. Jaundice
D. Ascites
E. Fatigue
F. Weight loss
G. Change in the color of urine (dark) or stools (clay colored)
H. Loss of appetitie

TABLE 11.7 Liver Chemistry Tests and Implications

Liver Chemistry Test	Clinical Implication of Abnormality
ALT	Hepatocellular damage
AST	Hepatocellular damage
ALP	Cholestasis, infiltrative disease, or biliary obstruction
Albumin	Synthetic function
Alpha-fetoprotein	Cancer marker when elevated
Bile acids: Urine bile salts, bile pigments, and urobilinogen	Cholestasis or biliary obstruction, impaired hepatic update or secretion, or portal-systemic shunting
Bilirubin: Serum total, direct, and indirect bilirubin	Cholestasis, impaired conjugation, or biliary obstruction
Cholesterol, serum triglycerides	Lipoprotein production and metabolism, chronic cholestasis
Fibrinogen	Liver damage/cirrhosis, acute liver insufficiency, poisoning
GGT	Cholestasis or biliary obstruction, malignant involvement in hepatocellular disease, more sensitive than other enzymes in alcoholism
Hepatitis surface antigen, IgM, antibody, RNA, genotype, viral load	Differentiation of type of hepatitis
LDH	Hepatocellular damage not specific for hepatic disease
Total proteins, albumin globulin (A/C ratio)	Hepatitis, advanced liver disease
PT	Synthesis function in hepatocellular disease, fulminate hepatitis
Plasma ammonia	Central nervous system dysfunction/toxicity or end-stage liver disease
5NT	Cholestasis or biliary obstruction
Urea	End-stage liver disease

ALP, alkaline phosphatase; ALT, alanine transaminase; AST, aspartate transaminase; CNS, central nervous system; 5NT, 5'-nucleotidase; GGT, gamma-glutamyl transpeptidase; IgM, immunoglobulin M; LDH, lactate dehydrogenase; PT, prothrombin time; RNA, ribonucleic acid.

Subjective Data

A complete medical history is the single most important part of the evaluation of the patient with elevated LFTs.

A. Review medications, including prescription medications, statins, and over-the-counter (OTC) medications, as well as herbal therapies.
B. Determine the duration of LFT abnormalities (if known).
C. Review the presence of accompanying symptoms, including arthralgias, myalgias, rash, abdominal pain, fever, pruritus, and changes in the color of urine or stool.
D. Has the patient experienced any anorexia or weight loss? Over what period did weight loss occur?
E. Review parenteral exposures, including transfusions, IV and intranasal drug use, tattoos, and sexual history.
F. Review the patient's recent travel history and possible exposure to contaminated foods.
G. Review the patient's exposure to people with jaundice.
H. Review the patient's occupational history and exposure to hepatotoxins.
I. Review the patient's history of alcohol consumption, including when started, amount, type of alcohol (beer, liquor, and moonshine), and frequency.
J. Evaluate the gestational age of pregnancy. Hemolysis, elevated liver enzymes, and low platelets (HELLP) syndrome is generally present in the third trimester of pregnancy.

Physical Examination

A. Temperature (if indicated), pulse, respirations, and blood pressure.
B. Observation
   1. Observe for temporal and proximal muscle wasting.
   2. Perform eye and mouth (mucous membranes) examination for icterus.
   3. Perform dermal examination for icterus, spider nevi, palmar erythema, and presence of caput medusae (the presence of dilated veins seen on the abdomen; noted with cirrhosis of the liver and portal hypertension).
   4. Evaluate the presence of gynecomastia.
   5. Observe for the presence of jugular venous distension (JVD), a sign of right-sided heart failure (HF) that suggests hepatic congestion.
C. Auscultate heart and lungs.
D. Percuss the abdomen.
E. Palpate
   1. Abdominal examination
      a. Evaluate the presence of hepatomegaly; focus on the size and consistency of the liver.
      b. Evaluate the presence of splenomegaly; focus on the size of the spleen. An enlarged spleen is most easily appreciated with the patient in the right lateral decubitus position.
      c. Assess for ascites: Note presence of a fluid wave or shifting dullness.
      d. Assess for an abdominal mass.
   2. Lymph nodes: Evaluate lymphadenopathy.
   3. Conduct testicular examination for testicular atrophy (increased estrogen/reduced testosterone).

Diagnostic Tests

A. The particular LFT tests ordered are related to the suspected or identified medical diagnosis. Table 11.8 shows common serologic tests for viral hepatitis.

TABLE 11.8 Serologic Tests for Hepatitis

Virologic Test	Usual Clinical Implication of a Positive Test
Hepatitis A-IgM	Positive in acute hepatitis A
Hepatitis A-IgG	Positive in response to previous hepatitis A infection or vaccination
HBsAg	Positive during active hepatitis B infection
HBsAg	Positive in response to previous hepatitis B infection or vaccination
Hepatitis B core antibody-IgM	Positive during active hepatitis B infection
Hepatitis B core antibody-IgG	Positive in response to current or prior hepatitis B infection
HBV-DNA	Positive during active hepatitis B infection
Hepatitis B e antigen	Positive test indicates replicative state of wild-type hepatitis B infection
Hepatitis B e antibody	Positive after replicative state of wild-type hepatitis B infection
HBV viral load	Assess hepatitis B virology
HCV antibody ELISA	Positive during or after hepatitis C infection
HCV-immunoblot assay (RIBA)	Positive during or after hepatitis C infection
HCV-RNA	Positive during hepatitis C infection
HCV viral load	Assess hepatitis C virology
HCV genotype	Genotyping is used for evaluation of the length of therapy

ELISA, enzyme-linked immunosorbent assay; HBV, hepatitis B virus; HCV, hepatitis C virus; HBsAg, hepatitis B surface antigen; IgG, immunoglobulin G; IgM, immunoglobulin M, RIBA, Recombinant ImmunoBlot Assay; RNA, ribonucleic acid.

Differential Diagnoses

A. Table 11.9 shows differential diagnoses with elevated liver enzymes.

Plan

A. **The clinical significance of any liver chemistry test abnormality must be interpreted in the context of the clinical situation.** The plan of care is dependent on the suspected or identified medical diagnosis. Lifestyle modifications, including discontinuance of medications and alcohol, weight loss, and dietary changes, can be recommended as appropriate.

B. Patients with marked abnormalities of liver tests, or with signs and symptoms of chronic liver disease or hepatic decompensation (i.e., ascites, encephalopathy, coagulopathy, or portal hypertension), should be evaluated and treated in a more expeditious manner than asymptomatic patients.

Follow-Up

A. Follow-up testing for elevated LFTs, including abdominal/liver ultrasonography, CT, MRI, and liver biopsy, is dependent on the risk factors for disease, symptoms and history, and physical finding of the suspected or identified medical diagnosis. A liver chemistry test that is normal does not ensure that the patient is free of liver disease. If a laboratory error is suspected, the laboratory test should be repeated.

Consultation/Referral

A. Consider a consultation or referral to a hepatologist, gastroenterologist, or infectious disease specialist.

Individual Considerations

Pregnancy: HELLP syndrome is a severe form of pregnancy-induced hypertension (PIH or preeclampsia). It may occur anywhere from the mid second trimester to immediately postpartum. The HELLP syndrome occurs in 0.1% to 0.8% of pregnancies. The etiology is unknown. The presence of laboratory abnormalities confirms the diagnosis. Treatment of the HELLP syndrome will not be covered. However, the laboratory abnormalities that are noted include the following:

A. Hemolytic anemia
B. Proteinuria
C. Serum aspartate transaminase (AST) level (greater than 70 IU/L)
D. Low platelet count (less than 10,000 cells/mL)
E. Serum lactate dehydrogenase (LDH) level (greater than 600 IU/L)
F. Total bilirubin level (greater than 1.2 mg/dL)

Gastroenteritis, Bacterial and Viral

Cheryl A. Glass and Audra Malone

Definition

A. Bacterial and viral gastroenteritis is an acute inflammation of the gastrointestinal (GI) mucosa of the middle or lower intestine. It is primarily an acute, self-limiting illness. Immunocompromised patients can develop unremitting or fatal symptoms from gastroenteritis.

Incidence

A. Gastroenteritis is very common, occurring in all age groups. Epidemic outbreaks of bacterial gastroenteritis occur in groups who have ingested contaminated food. Viral excretion can begin before symptoms. Gastroenteritis is responsible for an estimated 8 million health care visits and 250,000 hospitalizations a year.

B. Rotovirus is most common in young children with peak incidence at 3 to 15 months of age.

C. Norovirus most commonly infects older children and adults.

TABLE 11.9 Differential Diagnosis With Elevated Liver Enzymes

Infiltrating Diseases of the Liver	
• Sarcoidosis • TB • Fungal infection • Amyloidosis • Lymphoma • Metastatic malignancy • Hepatocellular carcinoma	
Acute viral hepatitis (A–E, EBV, CMV, herpes)	Wilson's disease (genetic disorder of biliary copper excretion)
Cholestasis disease	Acute bile duct obstruction
Chronic hepatitis B, C	Hemolysis
Steatosis/nonalcoholic steatohepatitis	Myopathy
Hereditary hemochromatosis	Thyroid disorders
Medication/herbal induced	Strenuous exercise–induced changes
Alpha-1-antitrypsin deficiency	Pregnancy—HELLP syndrome
Cirrhosis	Toxin(s) exposure
Celiac disease	Acute Budd–Chiari syndrome
Alcohol-related liver injury	Anorexia nervosa

CMV, cytomegalovirus; EBV, Epstein–Barr virus; HELLP, hemolysis, elevated liver enzymes, and low platelets; TB, tuberculosis.

D. Astrovirus usually infects infants and young children; however, it can infect people of all ages.
E. Adenoviruses primarily affect children younger than 2 years.

Pathogenesis

A. Gastroenteritis is commonly caused by infectious agents—viruses, bacteria, and parasites (see Table 11.10). There are four viral agents: rotavirus, norovirus, enteric adenovirus, and astrovirus (Lee et al., 2013). Rotavirus is the most common cause of severe diarrhea in children. Exotoxins produced by some organisms induce hypersecretion or increased peristalsis resulting in diarrhea or vomiting. Bacteria, such as *Escherichia coli* and *Salmonella*, penetrate and invade the gastric mucosa and lead to diarrhea accompanied by fever and fecal leukocytes. Viruses destroy enterocytes of the upper jejunal villi, often producing secondary lactose intolerance.

Predisposing Factors

A. Travel to areas where cholera or *Giardia* is epidemic
   1. Ingestion of raw or undercooked seafood or drinks containing cholera-contaminated ice or water
   2. Ingestion of *Giardia*-contaminated water supplies
B. Ingestion of food contaminated with *Salmonella* or *Shigella*. Foods that are often implicated are domestic fowl and eggs, custard-filled pastries, processed meats, foods warmed on steam tables, poultry, red meat, raw seafood, raw milk, rice, and bean sprouts due to the following:
   1. Inadequate cooking time and temperatures
   2. Poor hygiene, lack of handwashing
   3. Improper storage of food
   4. Ingestion of fruits and vegetables contaminated by an infected person or by animal products
C. Infection by person-to-person spread
   1. Day-care centers: Rotavirus can be found on toys and hard surfaces.
   2. Overcrowded environments, inadequate health care or education.

TABLE 11.10 Infectious Agents Causing Gastroenteritis

Causative Agent	Incubation Period
Noroviruses	12 hours–2 days
Escherichia coli	24–72 hours
Campylobacter	2–5 days
Staphylococcus	1–6 hours
Shigella	8–24 hours
Botulism	12–36 hours
Giardia lamblia	7–21 days
Salmonella	6–72 hours
Rotaviruses	1–3 days
Astrovirus	1–5 days
Adenoviruses	5–8 days
Clostridium perfringens	10–12 hours
Clostridium difficile	Variable
Listeria species	20 hours

   3. Schools/dormitories
   4. Nursing homes
   5. Banquet halls, cruise ships
D. Contact with *Salmonella*-infected turtles, iguanas, and other reptiles.
E. Seasonal outbreaks
   1. Rotavirus and astrovirus occur from October to April.
   2. Adenovirus occurs throughout the year.
   3. Norovirus occurs throughout the year but tends to increase in cooler months (November to April).
   4. Astrovirus is most common in the winter.

Common Complaints

A. Abrupt onset of nausea and vomiting
B. Abrupt onset of diarrhea (with or without blood and mucus)
C. Fever, sometimes

Other Signs and Symptoms

A. Explosive flatulence
B. Cramping abdominal pain
C. Abdominal tenderness
D. Frequent watery diarrhea
E. Mucoid stools with or without blood
F. Tenesmus
G. Myalgia
H. Headache
I. Weakness
J. Malaise
K. Potential for seizures in children with high fever or electrolyte abnormalities

Subjective Data

A. Review the onset, duration, and course of symptoms, including presence of abdominal pain and frequency of bowel movements (BMs). Ask the patient if anyone else in the family has the same symptoms.
B. Ask the patient about travel history, including travel by cruise ships or travel to foreign countries and camping with ingestion of water from streams, springs, or untreated wells.
C. Ask the patient about crowded or unsanitary living conditions, use of day-care centers, and institutional living.
D. Take a 24-hour diet history, including ingestion of prunes or beans.
E. Review diarrhea history.
   1. How many stools?
   2. How frequent are the diarrheal stools?
   3. What color is the stool?
   4. Does the stool contain mucus?
   5. Has there been blood in the stool?
   6. Does the patient have tenesmus (constant feeling of the need to pass stool)?
F. Inquire about other symptoms, such as fever or respiratory problems.
G. If the patient is an infant, ask the caregiver about activity level, irritability, sleep pattern, fluid intake, and number of wet diapers.
H. If the patient is a child, ask about activity level and dietary and fluid intake.

I. Review drug history intake, including laxatives, antacids, antibiotics, quinine, or anticancer medications.
J. Has the patient been vaccinated with the rotavirus vaccine?

Physical Examination

A. Check temperature, pulse, respirations, blood pressure, and weight.
 1. Bacterial infections: Temperatures between 101°F and 102°F
 2. Viral infections: Temperatures of 103°F and above
 3. Note hypotension and tachycardia.
B. Inspect
 1. Inspect general appearance; note if the patient is very ill.
 2. Assess hydration status. Signs of dehydration:
  a. Mild: Slightly dry buccal mucous membranes, increased thirst, decreased urine output
  b. Moderate: Sunken eyes, sunken fontanelle in infants, loss of skin turgor, dry buccal mucous membranes, decreased urine output
  c. Severe: Signs of moderate dehydration and one or more of the following: Rapid thready pulse, tachypnea, lethargy, and postural hypotension
 3. Assess activity level and behavior in infant or child.
C. Auscultate the abdomen in all quadrants for bowel sounds; note hyperactive bowel sounds, absent or hypoactive bowel sounds (common with botulism), and borborygmi.
D. Palpate the abdomen for diffuse tenderness, slight distension, masses, rebound tenderness, and spasm. Observe for muscle guarding during the examination.
E. Rectal examination: Check for masses, fissures, inflammation, perianal erythema, or stool in ampulla.
F. Neurologic examination
 1. Check for dizziness, difficulty swallowing, and other neurologic signs.
 2. Neurologic signs and symptoms indicate botulism and require emergency intervention.

Diagnostic Tests

A. No immediate labatory tests are required if dehydration is absent or mild and the patient feels well except for frequent diarrhea.
B. Complete blood count (CBC) with differential: Serologic studies can detect viral pathogens.
C. Sedimentation rate: Elevated with infections or inflammation
D. Electrolytes, sodium, chlorides, potassium, and BUN
E. Blood gases to assess acid–base balance, if indicated
F. Blood cultures, if indicated
G. Stool for guaiac, leukocytes, ova, and parasites; test specimens three times, every other day. Stool guaiac is usually negative in viral infections, positive in invasive bacterial infections. Large numbers of white cells in stool suggest inflammatory or invasive diarrhea, such as occurs with *Shigella, Salmonella, Campylobacter,* invasive *E. coli,* or *Entamoeba.* Mononuclear cells in stool are characteristic of salmonellosis.
H. Stool culture if blood or mucus, fever more than 24 hours, or leukocytes are present.
I. Special cultures for *Campylobacter* and cholera are required.
J. Urinalysis: Excludes urinary tract infection (UTI) as cause of nonspecific diarrhea; urine specific gravity to assess dehydration.
K. Sigmoidoscopy: Skip bowel prep with gross blood, large numbers of leukocytes in stool, or severe illness.
L. Culture food from suspected foci for *Salmonella.*
M. Real-time reverse transcriptase-polymerase chain reaction (RT-qPCR) is the most widely used assay for detecting norovirus in stool, vomitus, and environmental specimens. The best detection is in stool specimens.

Differential Diagnoses

A. Gastroenteritis, bacterial and viral
B. Acute viral hepatitis
C. Acute appendicitis
D. Cholecystitis
E. Inflammatory bowel disease (IBD)
F. Pelvic inflammatory disease (PID)
G. Intussusception
H. Bowel obstruction for other causes

Plan

A. General interventions
 1. Meticulous handwashing is the single most important measure to decrease transmission. Hand sanitizers are an option when access to soap or clean water is limited.
 2. Advise the patient to begin bed rest with progression to regular activities.
 3. If the patient is diapered and/or incontinent, tell the patient or caregiver to adhere strictly to contact precautions. Alcohol-based handwashing may decrease the spread.
 4. Diaper changing areas should be separate from food preparation areas.
 5. Chlorine-based disinfectants inactivate rotavirus and may prevent disease transmission from contact with environmental surfaces.
B. Patient teaching: *See Section III: Patient Teaching Guide for this chapter, "Diarrhea."* ◀
C. Dietary management
 1. Patients should comply with nothing by mouth (NPO) and then slowly add clear liquids to maintain hydration.
 2. Hydration is one of the most important factors in the prevention of complications.
 3. Rehydrate with oral fluids for each diarrheal stool.
 4. Administer small amounts at frequent intervals.
 5. Hold foods until hydration is completed. No evidence shows that bananas, rice, applesauce, and toast (BRAT) are useful; these are not currently recommended. See Appendix B for "Nausea and Vomiting Diet Suggestions (Children and Adults)."
D. Pharmaceutical therapy
 1. The primary treatment for viral gastroenteritis is fluid replacement. There are no specific antiviral

pharmaceutical therapies. IV rehydration of fluids and electrolytes may be required in severe dehydration.
2. Antibiotics may or may not be prescribed according to the bacterial source. Antimicrobial therapy is not indicated for uncomplicated (noninvasive) gastroenteritis because therapy does not shorten duration of the disease and can prolong duration of excretion of *Salmonella* organisms.
3. Antidiarrheal therapy delays transit time and can reduce the severity and duration of abdominal cramping; however, it may prolong the course of some bacterial diarrhea such as *Shigella* and *E. coli.* Bismuth subsalicylate (Pepto-Bismol; OTC) is not recommended for young children with gastroenteritis due to the potential toxicity from salicylate absorption.
4. Stop other medications that may be triggering diarrhea.
5. Vaccinate children with rotavirus live vaccine. Both vaccinations are oral.
  a. RotaTeq is given in three doses at 6 to 12 weeks of age with subsequent doses administered at 4- to 10-week intervals. The third dose should not be given after 32 weeks of age.
  b. ROTARIX is given in two doses, the first at 6 weeks of age then the second dose after an interval of at least 4 weeks and before 24 weeks of age.
  c. The rotavirus vaccine can be administered together with diphtheria, tetanus, and pertussis (DTaP) vaccine, *Haemophilus influenzae* type b (Hib) vaccine, inactivated polio vaccine (IPV), hepatitis B vaccine, and the pneumococcal conjugate vaccine.
  d. In March 2010, the Centers for Disease Control and Prevention (CDC) learned that a virus (or parts of a virus), *Porcine circovirus* (PCV), is present in both rotavirus vaccines. There is no evidence that PCV is a safety risk or causes illness in humans. Information related to PCV and rotavirus vaccines is available on the Food and Drug Administration (FDA) and CDC websites.
  e. Some postmarketing studies from outside the United States have detected a low-level increased risk of intussusception following rotavirus vaccination, particularly shortly after the first dose. The CDC continues to recommend both ROTARIX and RotaTeq to prevent severe rotavirus disease in infants and children. The CDC continues to monitor data on intussusception.

Follow-Up

A. Tell the patient to return if the condition worsens or if signs and symptoms have not abated in 48 to 72 hours. However, diarrhea due to *Salmonella* may be expected to persist for up to 2 weeks.
B. Renal function tests and CBC should be done in approximately 1 week after the start of symptoms in patients with *E. coli* O157:H7 to detect early-onset hemolytic-uremic syndrome.
C. If diarrhea persists for 2 weeks or more, the patient should present for a secondary evaluation.
D. Reporting surveillance systems
  1. In 2009, the CDC launched the National Outbreak Reporting System (NORS) to collect information for public health agencies on outbreaks of foodborne, waterborne, and enteric disease that is spread from person to person, animals, environmental surfaces, and other ways.
  2. In 2009, the CDC developed CaliciNet for public health and food regulator laboratories to submit outbreak information to a national database.
  3. New Vaccine Surveillance Network (NVSN)
  4. Foodborne Disease Active Surveillance Network (FoodNet)

Consultation/Referral

A. Refer patients to a physician immediately if they have dehydration, rebound tenderness, severe abdominal pain, neurologic symptoms, and intussusception.
B. Immediately refer infants under age 2 years with paroxysmal, severe abdominal pain and vomiting followed by currant-jelly stool; they need immediate evaluation for intussusception.
C. Refer any patient with diarrhea longer than 7 days who has had no response to usual treatment.
D. Refer an immunocompromised patient.

Individual Considerations

A. Pediatrics
  1. Very young children are at a higher risk of mortality.
  2. Affected children may exhibit chronic diarrhea, or more than five watery or loose stools a day, but they develop normally and show no signs of malnutrition.
  3. Rotavirus is the most common cause of nosocomial diarrhea in children and an important cause of acute gastroenteritis in day-care centers. Children whose stool cannot be contained by diapers or toilet use should be excluded from day care until diarrhea stops.
  4. Breastfeeding can continue during diarrhea.
  5. Children should not attend day-care facilities until 24 hours or more after diarrhea ceases.
  6. In cases of *Shigella*: The health department may not permit return to day-care facilities until there are one or more stool cultures negative for Shigella.
  7. Children should not go to water parks/swimming pools for 1 week after symptoms resolve.
B. Adults: Those with concomitant chronic debilitating disease are at a higher risk of mortality.
C. Geriatrics
  1. Elderly are at a higher risk of mortality secondary to dehydration. Signs of dehydration include:
    a. Confusion
    b. Muscle weakness
    c. Fever
    d. Dizziness
    e. Poor skin turgor
    f. Hypotension
    g. Tachycardia
  2. Diminished thirst mechanism and decreased body water exacerbate dehydration.
  3. New residents to nursing/group homes should be isolated from ill patients.

Resource

Centers for Disease Control and Prevention: www.cdc.gov

Gastroesophageal Reflux Disease

Cheryl A. Glass and Audra Malone

Definition

A. The American College of Gastroenterology (ACG) defines gastroesophageal reflux disease (GERD) as symptoms or complications resulting from the reflux of gastric contents into the esophagus or beyond, into the oral cavity (including larynx) or lung.
B. GER is considered a normal physiological process in healthy infants, children, and adults. Most episodes last less than 3 minutes, and most often occur 30 to 60 minutes after meals and with reclining positions. GERD is present when the symptoms occur more than twice a week.
C. Complications of GERD include erosive esophagitis (ERD), esophageal strictures, and Barrett's esophagus.
D. A very large population of patients will present after self-medicating with antacids, bicarbonate soda, and over-the-counter (OTC) medications. Management of GERD should be tailored to the frequency, severity, and duration of symptoms.

Incidence

A. GERD is very common. Daily heartburn typically occurring postprandially has been estimated to affect 17% to 65% of the normal adult population. Reflux esophagitis affects 30% to 80% of women at some time during pregnancy. It is estimated that 30% to 90% of asthmatics have GERD. Barrett's esophagus, which affects fewer than 1% of adults, is commonly associated with GERD.

Pathogenesis

A. GERD is relaxation or incompetence of the lower esophagus persisting beyond the newborn period. Relaxation of the lower esophageal sphincter (LES) allows reflux of gastric acid and pepsin into the distal esophagus. Heartburn occurs when reverse peristaltic waves cause regurgitation of acidic stomach contents into the esophagus. Anatomical abnormalities, such as a hiatal hernia, predispose persons to GERD. Improper diet and nervous tension are also precipitating factors.
B. GERD has been identified as a trigger for asthma, possibly by the activation of vagal reflexes and/or microaspiration. Asthma may promote GERD, and GERD may provoke asthma. Some asthma medications may reduce LES tone, further complicating the picture. Conversely, a patient with GERD may experience pulmonary disease as a response to the esophageal acid exposure.

Predisposing Factors

A. Obesity
B. Consuming large meals
C. Pregnancy
D. Immature, weak sphincter in newborns
E. Emotional stress
F. Increased abdominal pressure from tight clothes, straining to lift or defecate, or swallowing air
G. Ingesting drugs and foods that promote LES relaxation.
  1. Nonsteroidal anti-inflammatory drugs (NSAIDs)
  2. Benzodiazepines
  3. Calcium channel blockers
  4. Theophylline
  5. Nitrates
  6. Anticholinergics
  7. Alcohol
  8. Chocolate and peppermint
H. Smoking: Increases stomach acid and LES pressure
I. Ingestion of caustic agents such as lye
J. Infection by agents, such as *Candida,* herpes simplex, or cytomegalovirus (CMV), which directly attack the esophageal mucosa
K. Compromised immunity, from AIDS, diabetes, or chemotherapy
L. Asthma

Common Complaints

A. Heartburn
B. Regurgitation of fluid or food
C. Chest pain

Alarm Symptoms

A. Dysphagia (difficulty swallowing)
B. Unintentional weight loss
C. Predominant upper abdominal pain
D. Hematemesis (vomiting blood)
E. Melena (black feces/blood stool)
F. Odynophagia (painful swallowing)
G. Severe symptoms

Other Signs and Symptoms

A. Retrosternal aching or burning
B. Nocturnal aspiration, water or "acid" brash
C. Harsh taste in the mouth upon awakening
D. Chronic cough, especially at bedtime
E. Hoarseness
F. Globus sensation
G. Nausea
H. Dental erosion
I. Infants: FTT, vomiting

Subjective Data

A. Review the onset, duration, and course of heartburn or other symptoms.
B. Review medication history, including OTC medication and herbals.
  1. Has the patient been taking OTC antacids, H_2 blockers, or OTC proton pump inhibitors (PPIs)?
  2. How long has the patient been using these OTCs?
  3. Is the patient taking drugs that induce esophagitis such as
    a. Antibiotics
    b. Alendronate
    c. NSAIDs
    d. Ascorbic acid
    e. Potassium chloride
    f. Quinidine
    g. Iron
C. Ask the patient about alleviating and aggravating factors.

D. Review the patient's habits, including smoking and alcohol intake.
E. Inquire about other symptoms, such as weight loss, dysphagia, blood loss, regurgitation, and diarrhea.
F. Establish the patient's usual weight to determine the extent of the problem.
G. Ask the patient about any history of asthma and Crohn's disease (CD).
H. Rule out ingestion of caustic agents especially in the pediatric population.
I. Review the patient's dietary history for bulimia.

Physical Examination

A. Check pulse, respirations, blood pressure, and weight.
B. General observation of respiratory distress, including stridor
C. Inspect
  1. Examine throat and evaluate mouth for dental erosion.
  2. Assess swallowing ability.
D. Auscultate
  1. Evaluate the presence of wheezing in the lungs.
  2. Auscultate the heart.
  3. Evaluate the abdomen in all four quadrants.
E. Palpate
  1. Palpate the abdomen for the presence of hepatosplenomegaly and masses.
  2. Assess the abdomen for tenderness or distension.
F. Perform rectal examination (if indicated for any history of hematemesis).

Diagnostic Tests

A. Clinical examination and history alone usually confirm the diagnosis in the vast majority of reflux sufferers.
B. Rule out cardiac/noncardiac chest pain before institution of therapy (see Chapter 10, section on chest pain).
C. Endoscopy is not required for the presence of typical GERD symptoms but is recommended for the presence of alarm symptoms or for screening patients at high risk for complications.
D. Endoscopy with biopsy is usually the first diagnostic tool in cases of caustic ingestion or suspected infectious etiology. The ACG does not recommend an endoscopy to establish the diagnosis of GERD-related asthma, chronic cough, or laryngitis.
E. Ambulatory 24-hour pH monitoring: Prolonged monitoring is the best clinical tool for diagnosing GERD in asthmatics. However, it is very expensive and not universally available.
F. Upper GI series or barium contrast radiography is not used to diagnose GERD but rules out anatomic abnormalities of the upper digestive tract.
G. Esophageal manometry is not used for the diagnosis of GERD. It is used to evaluate patients who have failed to respond to an empiric trial of PPIs.
H. Guaiac test for occult blood: Bleeding may accompany reflux esophagitis and be slow and chronic, resulting in iron-deficiency anemia, or brisk, resulting in hematemesis. GERD may not be obvious to the clinician when obtaining a patient history, especially in an asthmatic patient with confounding respiratory symptoms.
I. Consider *H. pylori* testing.

Differential Diagnoses

A. GERD
B. Myocardial infarction (MI)/angina
C. Esophageal spasm
D. Gallbladder disease
E. Cancer—gastric or esophageal
F. Infections: CMV, herpes simplex virus, and *Candida*
G. Peptic ulcer
H. Ingestion of caustic substance
I. Self-induced vomiting/bulimia
J. Pyloric stenosis
K. Food allergy
L. Eosinophilic esophagitis
M. Autoimmune skin disorders affecting the esophagus

Plan

A. General interventions: Management depends on the cause and severity of symptoms.
B. Patient teaching: *See Section III: Patient Teaching Guide for this chapter, "Gastroesophageal Reflux Disease."* ◀
C. Dietary management
  1. Weight loss is advised for overweight or obese patients with GERD symptoms.
  2. At present, there is no supporting data for special dietary precautions; however, a dietary elimination of foods helps to identify triggers.
D. Medical and surgical management
  1. The Nissen fundoplication is a surgical procedure used to treat GERD in asthmatics. It improves the antireflux barrier and provides a lasting solution. Because it is not always successful, it is reserved for severe cases. The Nissen operation is often performed as a laparoscopic procedure. Achalasia or severe hypomotility (scleroderma-like esophagus) are conditions that would be contraindications to Nissen fundoplication.
  2. Surgical therapy is not recommended for patients who do not respond to proton pump inhibitor (PPI) therapy.
  3. The ACG guidelines note that surgical therapy is as effective as medical therapy for carefully selected patients with chronic GERD when performed by an experienced surgeon.
  4. Patients on NSAIDs who experience upper gastric pain, including reflux, need to be referred for endoscopy as soon as possible.
E. Pharmaceutical therapy
  1. The potentially adverse effects of acid suppression include the increased risk of community-acquired pneumonia and GI infections, including, *C. difficile*–associated diarrhea.
  2. Long-term use of acid suppression therapy without a diagnosis is not advised.
  3. The target of pharmaceutical therapy is improvement in quality of life through the reduction/relief of symptoms and healing of erosive esophagitis (EE).

4. On-demand or self-directed therapy has been shown to be effective; however, patient's use and response should be evaluated.

5. Histamine-2 receptor antagonists (H_2 blockers) are effective in managing milder, infrequent GI symptoms. Tolerance occurs with chronic use of H_2 blockers. Several H_2 blockers are currently available by prescription or OTC: Nizatidine (Axid), famotidine (Pepcid), cimetidine (Tagamet), and ranitidine (Zantac).

6. PPIs are used for both GERD and EE and are considered the "gold standard" of treatment.

a. Initiation of a PPI should be prescribed once a day, before the first meal of the day. For maximal pH control, the traditional delayed-release PPI should be administered 30 to 60 minutes before a meal.

b. Avoid the concomitant use of clopidogrel (Plavix) with omeprazole or esomeprazole because of the significant reduction of the antiplatelet activity of copidogrel. This is an FDA safety labeling change.

c. Dosages are age and weight based.

d. Long-term therapy should be titrated down to the lowest effective dose based on symptom control.

e. Patients may experience a relapse in their GERD symptoms after discontinuance, and therefore may need to be tapered off or use a stepdown approach with an antacid or an H_2 blocker.

f. No PPI is approved for use in infants younger than 1 year.

g. PPIs are currently available by prescription and OTC (see Table 11.11).

h. Patients with known osteoporosis can remain on PPI therapy except for long-term use in patients with other risks for hip fracture.

i. PPI therapy can be a risk factor for *Clostridium difficile* infection, and should be used with care for patients at risk.

Follow-Up

A. Noncardiac chest pain due to GERD should have a diagnostic evaluation before institution of therapy.

B. Empiric treatment with a PPI may be attempted for a short period except for patients presenting with any alarm symptoms. Schedule a return visit in 1 to 2 weeks to evaluate the relief of symptoms.

C. Patients have been having frequent relapses; failure to adequately respond or long-term OTC H_2 blockers and PPI use should have an endoscopic evaluation.

D. The need for prescribed long-term PPI treatment or the presence of alarm symptoms requires a gastroenterology consultation.

E. Consider bone density studies for patients with long-term PPI use.

Consultation/Referral

A. GERD diagnosis should not be made without a full evaluation in infants with vomiting or poor weight gain; refer to a pediatric gastroenterologist for evaluation.

B. Referral is necessary if the patient fails to improve after trying two different medications, or if the patient has dysphagia, recent weight loss, or blood loss.

C. PPI nonresponders need to be referred for evaluation.

Individual Considerations

A. Pregnancy

1. The diagnosis of heartburn during pregnancy is usually made by taking a thorough history. Underlying causes of GERD in pregnancy are diminished gastric

TABLE 11.11 Proton Pump Inhibitors

PPI	Available Dosages	Over the Counter
Omeprazole (Prilosec, Losec, Omesec)	Capsules: 10 mg, 20 mg, and 40 mg	Tablet 20 mg
Lansoprazole (Prevacid)	Capsules: 15 mg and 30 mg	Capsules: 15 mg
	Oral suspension and SoluTab: 15 mg and 30 mg	
	IV: 30 mg	
Rabeprazole (Aciphex)	Capsules: 20 mg	Not available
Pantoprazole (Protonix)	Capsules: 20 mg and 40 mg	Not available
	Oral suspension: 30 mg	
	IV: 40 mg	
Esomeprazole (Nexium)	Capsules: 20 mg and 40 mg	Not available
	Oral suspension: 20 mg and 40 mg	
	IV: 20 mg and 40 mg	
Dexlansoprazole (Dexilant)	Capsules: 30 mg and 60 mg	Not available
Omeprazole + sodium bicarbonate (Zegerid)	Capsules: omeprazole 20 mg and 20 mg plus 300 mg Na^+	Capsules: 20 mg
	Oral suspension: omeprazole 20 mg and 40 mg plus 460 mg Na^+	

IV, intravenous; PPI, proton pump inhibitor.

motility and displacement of stomach by enlarging uterus.

2. Sodium bicarbonate-containing antacids should be avoided as they may lead to metabolic alkalosis and fluid overload in both the fetus and mother.

3. To rule out pregnancy-induced hypertension (PIH), evaluate the patient immediately for signs and symptoms of sudden-onset discomfort with no relief from antacids (PIH or hemolysis, elevated liver enzymes, and low platelets [HELLP] syndrome).

B. Pediatrics

1. Some regurgitation is normal in neonates because the cardiac sphincter is immature and weak. However, vomiting is an abnormal sign associated with overfeeding, sepsis, metabolic disorders such as galactosemia, increased intracranial pressure (ICP), and intestinal atresia and stenosis. Regurgitation and vomiting must be differentiated:

a. Regurgitation most frequently occurs within the first hour after feeding in conjunction with burping or spontaneous eructation of air.

b. Infants may exhibit refusal to eat, irritability, or arching of their back during or immediately after feeding.

c. Vomiting, often projectile in nature, can occur at any time and results in the loss of significant amounts of body fluids and electrolytes.

2. Milk protein sensitivity should be ruled out.

3. There is no evidence to eliminate specific foods in children and adolescents to manage GERD.

4. The major agents used in children are gastric acid buffering agents, mucosal surface barriers, and gastric antisecretory agents.

C. Geriatrics

1. GERD prevalence increases with age and may be associated with a hiatal hernia.

2. Prolonged reflux results in esophagitis and may lead to stricture development. Chronic recurrence may develop into Barrett's syndrome.

3. Treatment of GERD is the same as for general adults; however, do diagnostic testing in short-time sequence secondary to stricture and cancer in the elderly.

Resources

American Gastroenterological Association: www.gastro.org

Rome Foundation: http://romecriteria.org/criteria

The 2013 guidelines for the diagnosis and management of gastroesophageal reflux disease: http://gi.org/wp-contents/uploads/2013/03/ACG_Guideline_GERD_March_2013.pdf

Giardiasis intestinalis

Cheryl A. Glass and Audra Malone

Definition

A. *Giardiasis intestinalis* (formerly *Giardia lamblia*) is the leading parasitic cause of diarrhea. Infestation can lead to malabsorption by coating large areas of the small bowel, particularly the lower duodenum and upper jejunum. Most people infected with *G. intestinalis* remain asymptomatic, and most infections are self-limited.

Incidence

A. Giardiasis has a worldwide distribution. It is common in areas where water supplies are contaminated by human sewage. The age-specific prevalence of giardiasis is highest in children 1 to 9 years and adults 35 to 44 years of age. The peak onset occurs annually during early summer through early fall.

Pathogenesis

A. *G. intestinalis* is a flagellated protozoan. The infective form is the cyst. Humans are the principal reservoir of infection, but *Giardia* can infect dogs, cats, beavers, and other animals that can contaminate water with feces containing cysts.

B. People become infected either directly, by hand-to-mouth transfer of cysts from feces of an infected person (e.g., child care), or indirectly, by ingestion of fecal-contaminated water or food. Most community-wide epidemics result from contaminated water supplies.

C. Incubation period is 1 to 3 weeks, with an average of 7 to 10 days. The infective form is the cyst, with infection limited to the small intestine and the biliary tract. Disease is communicable for as long as the infected person excretes cysts.

Predisposing Factors

A. About 50% to 75% of outbreaks occur in child care settings.

B. Travel to endemic areas

C. Subjection to unsanitary food handling

D. Exposure to contaminated water supplies

E. Male homosexuality

F. Cystic fibrosis (CF)

G. Immunocompromised individuals are at high risk.

Common Complaints

Acute complaints

A. Explosive, foul-smelling diarrhea

B. Mucus in stools, bulky stools

C. Upper abdominal pain or discomfort

D. Flatulence

E. Nausea

F. Anorexia

G. Weight loss

Other Signs and Symptoms

Chronic complaints

A. Intermittent loose stools (but not diarrhea)

B. Steatorrhea

C. Increased flatulence or distension

D. Vague abdominal discomfort

E. Fatigue related to anemia

F. Profound weight loss (10%–20% of body weight)

G. Malabsorption

H. Urticaria

I. Dehydration

Subjective Data

A. Review the onset, duration, and course of symptoms. Is diarrhea acute or chronic?

B. Ask the patient about travel to areas known for giardiasis.

C. Review the patient's intake of medications and other substances that can cause diarrhea, especially antibiotics, laxatives, quinidine, magnesium-containing antacids, excess alcohol, caffeine, herbal teas, digitalis, loop diuretics, antihypertensive agents, and sorbitol-containing (sugar-free) gums and mints.

D. Review the nature of the patient's bowel movements (BMs), including frequency; consistency; volume; and presence of blood, pus, or mucus.

E. Does diarrhea have any relationship to meals? Onset of diarrhea within hours of ingesting a potentially contaminated food is suggestive of bacterial infection such as *E. coli*; this is confirmed by checking if others were similarly affected.

F. Ask the patient about associated symptoms that need evaluation, such as fever, abdominal pain, or rash.

G. Ask the patient if other family members or sexual contacts are also ill.

H. Establish the patient's normal weight, and, if any weight has recently been lost, review amount and over what period of time.

Physical Examination

The physical examination may reveal no specific finding.

A. Check temperature (if indicated), pulse, respirations, blood pressure, and weight.

B. Inspect: general appearance for signs of dehydration; include evaluation of mucous membranes and infants' fontanelles.

C. Auscultate: abdomen for bowel sounds in all quadrants

D. Palpate

- **1.** Palpate the abdomen for masses, tenderness, guarding, and rebound. Patients with periumbilical or right lower quadrant (RLQ) pain and copious volumes of watery stool are likely to have a small-bowel etiology.
- **2.** Palpate lymph nodes for enlargement.

E. Perform rectal examination.

Diagnostic Tests

A. EIA and direct fluorescence antibody (DFA) are becoming the standard for diagnosis of giardiasis in the United States.

B. Stool bacteria culture and sensitivity

C. Mucus stool for leukocytes: Mucus free of leukocytes is the hallmark of irritable bowel syndrome (IBS); a large number of white cells suggests inflammatory or invasive diarrhea.

D. Stool for ova and parasites; test three times on alternate days. Parasites are passed intermittently, so examine stools on alternating days.

E. Stool for occult blood

F. Endoscopy to identify cyst in duodenal fluid or small-bowel tissue.

Differential Diagnoses

A. Giardiasis

B. Malabsorption

C. *E. coli* infection

D. IBS

E. Viral diarrhea

F. Lactose intolerance

G. Other bacterial infections, such as *Shigella, Salmonella,* and *Campylobacter*

H. Crohn's disease (CD)

I. Sprue

Plan

A. General interventions

- **1.** Advise children and adult workers with diarrhea to stay away from day-care centers until they become asymptomatic.
- **2.** Advise the patient's household and sexual contacts to seek medical examination and treatment.

B. Patient teaching:

- **1.** *See Section III: Patient Teaching Guide for this chapter, "Diarrhea."* ◀
- **2.** Discuss safe sexual practices. Avoiding oral–anal and oral–genital sex can decrease venereal transmission.
- **3.** Recommend contact precautions for duration of illness for diapered and/or incontinent children.
- **4.** People with diarrhea caused by giardia should not use recreational water venues, including swimming pools and water slides, for 2 weeks after symptoms resolve.

C. Dietary management

- **1.** Tell the patient or caregiver to prevent dehydration from diarrhea by increasing fluids.
- **2.** Advise restricting milk products to rule out lactose intolerance. Post-giardia lactose occurs in 20% to 40% of patients.
- **3.** Tell backpackers, campers, and people likely to be exposed to contaminated water to avoid drinking directly from streams. To make water for safe drinking, boil water, or use chemical disinfection or filtration. Boiling water is the most reliable method to make water safe for drinking.

D. Pharmaceutical therapy

- **1.** Treatment of asymptomatic carriers is not generally recommended.
- **2. Fluid and electrolyte management is critical in patients with large-volume diarrheal losses.**
- **3.** Treat children with acute or chronic diarrhea who manifest failure to thrive (FTT), malabsorption, or other GI tract symptoms when giardia has been identified.
- **4.** Metronidazole, tinidazole, and nitazoxanide are the drugs of choice for treatment.
  - **a.** Metronidazole (Flagyl) is the principal agent used to treat giardiasis in the United States.
    - **i.** Adults: 250 mg orally three times daily for 5 to 7 days
    - **ii.** Pediatric: 5 mg/kg/d orally divided in three times daily dosing for 5 to 7 days; not to exceed 750 mg/d
  - **b.** Tinidazole (Tindamax) is a one-time dose for children 3 years of age and older; it has fewer side effects than metronidazole.
    - **i.** Adults: 2 g single dose
    - **ii.** Pediatrics: 50 mg/kg single dose (maximum 2 g)
  - **c.** Nitazoxanide (Alinia) oral suspension has similar efficacy to metronidazole and has the advantage of treating other intestinal parasites; it has been approved for children 1 year of age and older.
    - **i.** Age 1 to 3 years: 5 mL (100 mg) oral suspension every 12 hours with food for 3 days

ii. Age 4 to 11 years: 10 mL (200 mg) oral suspension every 12 hours with food for 3 days
iii. Age 12 years and older: 500 mg tablet every 12 hours or 25 mL oral suspension every 12 hours with food for 3 days

5. Paromomycin (Humatin), a nonabsorbable aminoglycoside, is recommended for treatment of symptomatic infection in pregnant women in the second and third trimesters.
   a. Adults: 100 mg three times daily for 5 to 7 days
   b. Pediatrics: 20 mg/kg/d three times daily with meals for 5 to 7 days

Follow-Up

A. Relapses after treatment are common, especially in immunocompromised patients.
B. Schedule follow-ups at 6 weeks and 6 months after treatment, as indicated.
C. If diarrhea persists for 2 weeks or more, secondary evaluation is indicated. Stools should be examined again for blood, leukocytes, and parasites.
D. Patients who remain undiagnosed after an extensive evaluation and trial of metronidazole (Flagyl) often turn out to have IBS or surreptitious laxative abuse.

Consultation/Referral

A. Severely dehydrated or malnourished patients should be admitted for further care.
B. Consult a physician if the patient has no relief of symptoms after completion of therapies.
C. Consultations with a pediatric infectious disease specialist and pediatric gastroenterologist are recommended.

Individual Considerations

A. Pregnancy
   1. Treatment of patients during pregnancy is recommended. Giardiasis in pregnancy is associated with dehydration, malabsorption, or severe symptoms.
   2. Malabsorptive symptoms may persist as regeneration of functioning intestinal mucosa requires time.
   3. Breastfeeding appears to protect infants from *G. intestinalis.*
B. Pediatrics
   1. **When an outbreak is suspected in a child-care setting, the local health department should be notified to investigate.**
   2. Children who are carriers do not have to be excluded from child care; however, personal hygiene/universal precautions should be followed.

Hemorrhoids

Cheryl A. Glass and Audra Malone

Definition

A. Hemorrhoids are clusters of vascular tissues, smooth muscle, and connective tissue of the anal canal. Internal hemorrhoids are above the anorectal line, covered by rectal mucosa, and can be found at any position in the rectum. Hemorrhoids can be found at any position of the rectum. Internal hemorrhoids are graded by severity (see Table 11.12).
B. External hemorrhoids are below the anorectal line, covered by anal skin, and appear as painless, flaccid skin tags (see Figure 11.2).
C. When blood within the hemorrhoid becomes clotted due to obstruction, the hemorrhoids are referred to as thrombosed and appear as blue, shiny masses.
D. Although rectal bleeding is commonly associated with hemorrhoids, it may be a symptom of other disease processes, such as colorectal cancer, inflammatory bowel disease (IBD), other colitides, diverticular disease, and angiodysplasia.

Incidence

A. The incidence of hemorrhoids is unknown. Patients tend to present after utilization and failure of over-the-counter (OTC) treatments. Hemorrhoids are common in people more than 20 years of age. They are uncommon in people under age 20 years except secondary to pregnancy.

Pathogenesis

A. Mechanism is unknown. Prolapse may be initiated by shearing force from passage of large firm stool, by increased venous pressure from heart failure (HF) or pregnancy, or by straining that occurs with lifting or defecation.

Predisposing Factors

A. Increased abdominal pressure (constipation, pelvic congestion, pregnancy, portal hypertension, cirrhosis).
B. Altered bowel function (constipation, diarrhea).
C. Poor muscle tone
D. Low-fiber diet
E. Sedentary jobs, such as driving trucks, piloting planes
F. Loss of muscle tone due to advanced age
G. Anal intercourse
H. Obesity
I. Colon malignancy
J. Rectal surgery
K. IBD

Common Complaints

A. Cardinal features
   1. Bleeding: Painless, bright red bleeding with defecation (internal)
   2. Anal pruritus
   3. Prolapse
   4. Pain related to thrombosis

TABLE 11.12 Severity of Hemorrhoids to Guide Treatment Options

Grade	Severity
I	The hemorrhoids bleed but do not prolapse.
II	The hemorrhoids prolapse upon defecation but reduce spontaneously.
III	The hemorrhoids prolapse upon defecation and must be reduced manually.
IV	The hemorrhoids are prolapsed and cannot be reduced manually.

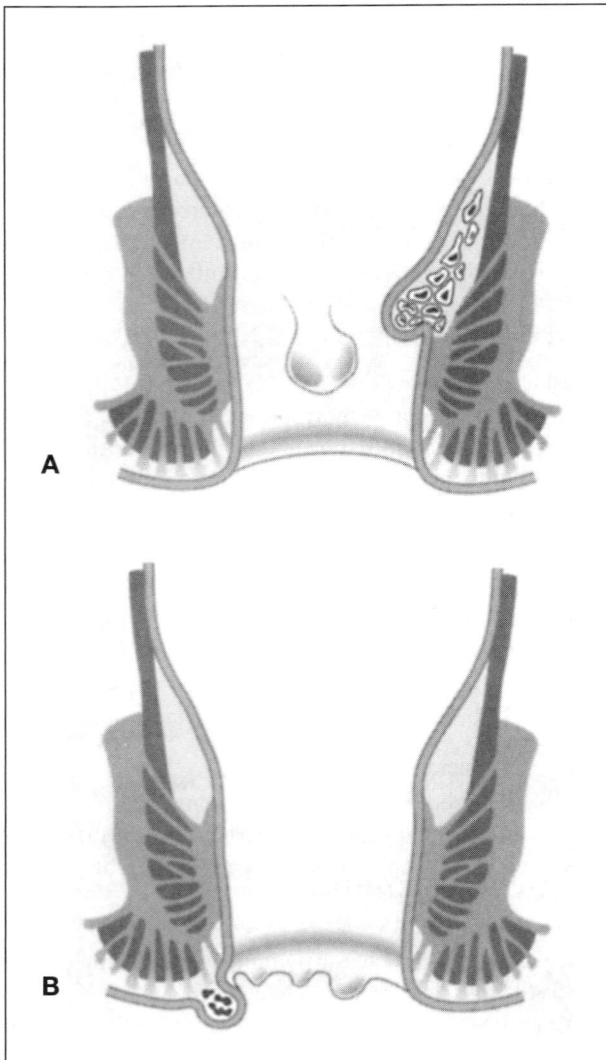

FIGURE 11.2 Internal (A) and external (B) hemorrhoids.
A. Internal hemorrhoid: Covered by a thin sheet of tissue called mucous membrane, an internal hemorrhoid bulges into the rectal opening and may sink a bit during bowel movements.
B. External hemorrhoid: Covered by skin, an external hemorrhoid protrudes from the rectum.

Other Signs and Symptoms

A. Visible prolapsed mass
B. Incomplete defecation
C. Leakage of feces (internal hemorrhoids)
D. Excessive moisture
E. Weakness or fatigue, with anemia
F. External hemorrhoid: Covered by skin, an external hemorrhoid protrudes from the rectum.

Subjective Data

A. Review the onset and duration of symptoms, especially the history of rectal bleeding, prolapse, and issues of hygiene and pain.
B. Review the patient's history of hemorrhoids and treatments, including surgery.
C. Ask the patient about recent pregnancy, liver disease, and constipation.
D. Inquire about the patient's job and level of daily activity.
E. Review the patient's sexual practices for anal intercourse.
F. Review the patient's dietary history for fluid intake and sources/amount of fiber.
G. Ask about bowel habits, including frequency, consistency, and ease of evacuation.
H. Review a detailed family history, with emphasis on intestinal disease.

Physical Examination

A. Check temperature (if indicated), pulse, respirations, blood pressure, and weight.
B. Inspection
- **1.** Observe of rectal area for skin tags, prolapse, irritation, fissures, and condyloma.
  - **a.** Internal hemorrhoids are usually not visible unless prolapsed.
  - **b.** External hemorrhoids protrude with straining or standing.
- **2.** Using anoscopy: Visualize internal rectum for hemorrhoids, fissures, or masses.

C. Palpate
- **1.** Palpate abdomen for masses.
- **2.** Internal hemorrhoids are usually not palpable unless thrombosed.
- **3.** Perform digital rectal examination.

Diagnostic Tests

A. Hematocrit (Hct) and hemoglobin, if bleeding present
B. Anoscopy: Reveals internal hemorrhoids as bright red to purplish bulges. Digital rectal examination alone can neither diagnose nor exclude internal hemorrhoids; anoscopy is required.
C. Sigmoidoscopy or colonoscopy (geriatric population)
D. Stool for guaiac testing
E. Air-contrast barium enema (BE) for atypical bleeding

Differential Diagnoses

A. Hemorrhoids
B. Condyloma acuminata
C. Rectal prolapse
D. Rectal bleeding due to one of the following
- **1.** Colorectal cancer
- **2.** Polyps
- **3.** Anal fissure
- **4.** Fistula
- **5.** Perianal abscess
- **6.** IBD, including ulcerative colitis (UC) and Crohn's disease (CD)
- **7.** Diverticulitis
- **8.** Pelvic tumor

Plan

A. General interventions: No treatment is necessary if the patient is asymptomatic except for maintaining regular bowel habits and performing comfort measures.
B. Patient teaching: *See Section III: Patient Teaching Guide for this chapter, "Hemorrhoids."* ◀
C. Dietary management: High-fiber diet and an adequate fluid intake should be continued indefinitely in order to maintain a soft bulky stool that can be passed without straining (see Appendix B, Table B.6).

D. Medical and surgical management

1. Use warm sitz baths up to three times a day for irritation and pruritus.

2. Conservative treatment for thrombosed hemorrhoid includes lying prone and applying ice pack to the area.

3. Incision and evacuation of thrombosis or clot may be performed under local anesthesia. Other treatments for thrombosed hemorrhoids noted in clinical trials have included the following:

- **a.** Topical nitroglycerin 0.2% topical ointment for temporary analgesia. The most common side effect was headache.
- **b.** Topical nifedipine
- **c.** In a small study, one intrasphincter injection of botulinum toxin relieved pain within 24 hours.

4. Symptomatic Grade I, Grade II, and some Grade III hemorrhoids may be treated by the following:

- **a.** Rubber band ligation is the treatment of choice for Grades I and II hemorrhoids. Rubber band ligation is the most widely used and is associated with fewer complications than surgery.
- **b.** Bipolar, infrared, and laser coagulation (may require more than one treatment)
- **c.** Sclerotherapy
- **d.** Stapled hemorrhoidopexy can be performed in patients with Grade III hemorrhoids.

5. External hemorrhoids usually do not require surgical therapy except in cases of thrombosis. For selective Grade III and Grade IV internal and strangulated hemorrhoids that fail medical and nonoperative therapies, surgical treatment is required. **Stapled hemorrhoidopexy has a faster recovery but has a higher recurrence rate. Hemorrhoidectomy is the treatment of last choice because it requires hospitalization and an extended recovery period, and it risks compromising competence of the anal sphincter.** Hemorrhoidectomy complications include

- **a.** Urinary retention
- **b.** Urinary tract infection (UTI)
- **c.** Fecal impaction
- **d.** Pain
- **e.** Hemorrhage
- **f.** Stricture formation (1%) or sphincter damage (rare)
- **g.** Nonhealing wound
- **h.** Fistula formation
- **i.** Anal leakage

E. Pharmaceutical therapy

1. Drug of choice: Bulk-forming agents such as psyllium seed (Metamucil), methylcellulose (Citrucel), or calcium polycarbophil (Fibercon), 1 to 3 teaspoons in 8 oz of liquid three times a day. Maintenance dose is 1 to 3 teaspoons after dinner.

2. Stool softener: Docusate sodium (Colace) or docusate calcium (Doxidan) 100 mg three times daily.

3. For irritation and pruritus, topical creams and anesthetics are found in OTC products such as Anusol, pramoxine HCl (Tronolane Cream), Preparation H, and topical hydrocortisone preparations.

4. Nonsteroidal anti-inflammatory drugs (NSAIDs) supplemented with narcotics: An oral analgesic such as codeine may be prescribed for thrombosed hemorrhoids. However, codeine causes constipation.

Follow-Up

A. None is necessary if resolution occurs and the patient is asymptomatic.

B. Reevaluate the patient in 2 weeks for further treatment if symptoms persist.

C. Evaluate the patient with an intervention in 7 to 10 days.

Consultation/Referral

A. The onset of urinary retention and fever immediately after an office-based procedure may be the initial sign of perianal sepsis and mandates emergent patient evaluation.

B. Refer the patient with acute thrombosis of external hemorrhoids to a physician.

C. Refer the patient to a surgeon if hemorrhoids bleed repeatedly, prolapse, produce intractable pain, or are thrombosed, and if 3 to 5 consecutive days of treatment do not provide relief.

Individual Considerations

A. Pregnancy

1. Labor, which results in pressure on the pelvic floor by the presenting part of the fetus and the expulsive efforts of the woman, may aggravate hemorrhoids, causing protrusion and inflammation during the puerperium. Hemorrhoids may be pushed back after delivery to prevent them from becoming swollen and painful.

2. Surgical treatment is contraindicated in pregnancy because of the risk of inducing labor.

3. Conservative treatment is recommended with excision of thrombosed external hemorrhoids if necessary.

B. Pediatrics: Rectal prolapse in children is associated with cystic fibrosis (CF).

> *Prolapse looks like a pink doughnut or rosette; complete prolapse involving the muscular wall is larger and red, and it has circular folds.*

C. Geriatrics

1. Prolapse of rectal mucosa is more common in the elderly.

2. Colonoscopy is recommended in the geriatric population to exclude malignancy or other underlying disease.

Hepatitis A

Cheryl A. Glass and Audra Malone

Definition

A. Hepatitis A is an acute self-limited illness with inflammation of the liver caused by a viral infection. Hepatitis A virus (HAV) is spread by viral shedding. All cases of hepatitis A are reportable to the public health department.

B. The highest titers of HAV in the stool of infected patients occur 1 to 2 weeks before the onset of illness (jaundice or elevation of liver enzymes), during which time patients are most likely to transmit infection. Risk subsequently diminishes and is minimal in the week after the onset of jaundice. Few children younger than 6 years have concomitant jaundice, whereas up to 70% of older children and adults will have jaundice. Fulminant hepatitis is rare, and chronic infectious and carrier states do not occur.
C. Duration of HAV infection is typically 8 weeks, but prolonged disease, as long as 6 months, can occur in 10% to 15% of symptomatic patients, especially in neonates and young children.
D. The major methods of prevention include improved sanitation of water sources, improved hygiene practice prior to food preparation and diaper changes, immunization with the hepatitis A vaccine, and administration of immune globulin (IG).

Incidence

A. From 30% to 35% of acute hepatitis cases in the United States are due to HAV. In developing countries, where infection is endemic, most people are infected during the first decade of life. In the United States, the incidence of HAV has declined since 1995 due to the administration of the HAV vaccine.
B. Outbreak in custodial institutions accounts for about 10% to 15% of reported HAV in the United States. No appreciable seasonal variation in incidence has been noted.
C. The incidence of mortality from HAV is 0% to 1%. The single most important determinant of illness severity is age; a direct correlation between increasing age and the likelihood of adverse events is present.

Pathogenesis

A. HAV is a small, RNA enterovirus classified as a member of the picornavirus group. Viral replication depends on hepatocyte uptake and synthesis, and assembly occurs exclusively in liver cells. Transmission of HAV is person-to-person primarily by the fecal–oral route and parenterally. The incubation period is 15 to 50 days, with an average of 25 to 30 days. It does not cause chronic infection.
B. Common-source, food-, and waterborne epidemics have occurred, including several caused by shellfish contaminated with human sewage. Nosocomial outbreaks have occurred as a result of shedding of HAV from infected, asymptomatic neonates, children, or adults.

Predisposing Factors

A. Ingestion of infected water, food, and shellfish
   1. Undercooked HAV-contaminated foods are a source of outbreaks.
   2. Cooked foods also can transmit HAV if the temperature during food preparation is inadequate to kill the virus.
   3. Food contaminated after cooking is associated with infected food handlers.
B. Close personal contact with an HAV-infected person
   1. Contact with a child who attends a child-care center (especially with children in diapers)
   2. Male homosexual activity
   3. Vertical transmission from mother to fetus (limited)
   4. Personal contact with a newly arriving international adoptee
C. Poor sanitation or personal hygiene
D. Crowded living conditions
E. International travel
F. Intravenous (IV) drug abuse
G. Persons with clotting factor disorders
H. Persons working with nonhuman primates

Common Complaints

A. Asymptomatic, particularly in young children
B. Malaise
C. Anorexia
D. Nausea with/without vomiting
E. Low-grade fever
F. Jaundice—icteric phase (70% of older children and adults)
   1. Tea-colored urine
   2. Clay-colored stool
   3. Abdominal pain
   4. Pruritus
   5. Enlarged liver

Other Signs and Symptoms

A. Infants and children: Mild, nonspecific, flu-like symptoms without jaundice
B. Adults: Severe, prolonged course with fatigue, headache, vomiting, and symptoms noted earlier
C. Relapsing hepatitis A is more common in the elderly. There generally has been a protracted course of symptoms then a relapse of symptoms following an apparent resolution.

Subjective Data

A. Review the duration, onset, and severity of symptoms, including specifics about urine or stool color changes.
B. Ask the patient about family members and sexual contacts with similar symptoms.
C. Review the patient's history of blood transfusions, IV drug use, and alcohol abuse.
D. Inquire about occupational exposure.
E. Ask the patient about recent international travel or exposure to newly arrived international adoptees.
F. Review immunization status.
G. Review medications for a possible Tylenol overdose or Ecstasy use as a cause for acute drug-induced liver injury.

Physical Examination

A. Check temperature (acute illness), pulse, respirations, blood pressure, and weight.
B. Inspect
   1. Note general appearance.
   2. Inspect the skin for slight jaundice or rash.
   3. Inspect mucous membranes and nail beds.
   4. Inspect eyes for yellow sclera.
C. Auscultate lung fields, all quadrants of the abdomen, and the heart.
D. Percuss the abdomen.

E. Palpate
 1. Palpate all quadrants of the abdomen for masses, liver tenderness, and hepatosplenomegaly (about 10% of cases).

Diagnostic Tests

A. Viral serology for typing HAV, immunoglobulin G (IgG), and immunoglobulin M (IgM). Serum IgM presents at the onset of illness and disappears within 4 months, generally indicating current or recent infection. However, it may persist for 6 months or longer. Presence of IgG anti-HAV antibodies without virus-specific IgM indicates past infection and lifelong immunity.
B. Liver function studies, including alanine transaminase (ALT), aspartate transaminase (AST), lactate dehydrogenase (LDH), and alkaline phosphatase (ALP)
C. Bilirubin, direct and indirect
D. Complete blood count (CBC)
E. Prothrombin time (PT)
F. Urinalysis: Reveals proteinuria and bilirubinuria
G. Imaging studies are usually not indicated for hepatitis A infection. An ultrasound may be used to exclude other pathology.

Differential Diagnoses

A. Hepatitis A virus (HAV)
B. Mononucleosis
C. Cancer
D. Obstructive jaundice
E. Alcoholic hepatitis or cirrhosis
F. Hepatotoxic drug use
 1. Drug-induced liver injury (e.g., Tylenol, Ecstasy)
 2. Drug-induced hypersensitivity reaction (e.g., sulfasalazine hypersensitivity)
G. Food poisoning
H. Exclusion of other hepatitis types
I. Cytomegalovirus (CMV)
J. Acute HIV infection

Plan

A. General interventions
 1. Contact precautions are recommended for diapered and/or incontinent patients for 1 week after the onset of symptoms.
 2. Children and adults with acute HAV infection should be excluded from school, work, and child-care centers for 1 week after the onset of illness.
 3. Hepatitis is self-limiting and does not require therapy. Treatment is supportive.
  a. Limit activities secondary to malaise.
  b. Oral contraceptives (OCPs) and hormone replacement therapy (HRT) should be stopped to avoid cholestasis.
  c. Alcohol consumption is not advised.
  d. Adults who work as food handlers should not work for 1 week after the onset of the illness.
 4. Encourage strict handwashing.
B. Patient teaching:
 1. *See Section III: Patient Teaching Guide for this chapter, "Jaundice and Hepatitis."*
 2. Teach the patient that major methods for prevention are improved sanitation (e.g., of water sources and in food preparation) and personal hygiene.
 3. Food and travel precautions include the following:
  a. Avoid uncontrolled water resources: Use bottled water, boil water, or add iodine to inactivate the virus.
  b. Avoid raw shellfish.
  c. Avoid uncooked foods.
  d. All fruit should be washed and peeled.
C. Dietary management: Encourage optimum nutrition.
D. Pharmaceutical therapy
 1. IG (Gamastan, Gammar-P): Preexposure administration is 0.02 mL/kg, two doses intramuscularly (IM). HAV vaccine preexposure is preferred in all populations unless contraindicated.
 2. Postexposure IG administration given IM within 2 weeks of HAV exposure is 80% to 90% effective in preventing symptomatic infection.
  a. Time of exposure: 2 weeks or less
   i. Younger than 12 months: 0.02 mL/kg of IG given IM into a large muscle. No more than 3 mL in one site should be given to small children and infants.
   ii. 12 months to 40 years: Hepatitis A vaccine.
   iii. 41 years and older: 0.02 mL/kg IG is given IM into a large muscle. No more than 5 mL should be administered into one site for an adult or large child.
  b. Postexposure prophylaxis with IG is recommended for the following:
   i. Household and sexual contacts of infected persons
   ii. Newborn infants of HAV-infected mothers
   iii. Child-care center staff, children, and their household contacts
   iv. Students when transmission within school is documented
   v. Staff in institutions and hospitals
   vi. People who ingested HAV-contaminated food or water, within 2 weeks of last exposure
 3. Vaccines
  a. Two inactivated HAV vaccines, HAVRIX and VAQTA, are available in the United States.
  b. TWINRIX is a combination of hepatitis A (HAVRIX) and hepatitis B (Engerix-B) vaccine available in the United States for those aged 18 years or older (see Table 11.13).
 4. Hepatitis A vaccine is recommended for the following:
  a. Children 1 year and older in defined and circumscribed communities with high endemic rates and/or periodic outbreaks of HAV infection. Children who have not been vaccinated by age 2 can be vaccinated at subsequent visits.
  b. Children and adolescents ages 2 to 18 years who live in states or communities where routine hepatitis A vaccination has been implemented because of high disease incidence.

TABLE 11.13 Licensed Dosages and Schedules for Hepatitis A Vaccines

A. HAVRIX[a]				
Age	**Dose (ELISA units)[b]**	**Volume (mL)**	**No. of Doses**	**Schedule (mo)[c]**
12 months to 18 years	720	0.5	2	0, 6–12
≥19 years	1,440	1.0	2	0, 6–12
B. VAQTA[d]				
Age	**Dose (U.)[e]**	**Volume (mL)**	**No. of Doses**	**Schedule (mo)[f]**
12 months to 18 years	25	0.5	2	0, 6–18
≥19 years	50	1.0	2	0, 6–18
C. TWINRIX[g, h]				
Age	**Dose (ELISA units)[b]**	**Volume (mL)**	**No. of Doses**	**Schedule[i]**
≥18 years	720	1.0	3	0, 1, 6 mo
≥18 years	720	1.0	4	0, 7, 21–30 d + 12 mo[b]

[a]Hepatitis A vaccine, inactivated, GlaxoSmithKline.
[b]Enzyme-linked immunosorbent assay units.
[c]0 months represents timing of the initial dose; subsequent numbers represent months after the initial dose.
[d]Hepatitis A vaccine, inactivated, Merck & Co., Inc.
[e]Units.
[f]0 months represents timing of the initial dose; subsequent numbers represent months after the initial dose.
[g]Combined hepatitis A and hepatitis B vaccine, inactivated, GlaxoSmithKline.
[h]Not recommended for postexposure prophylaxis.
[i]This four-dose schedule enables patients to receive three doses in 21 days; this schedule is used before planned exposure with short notice and requires a fourth dose at 12 months.
Source: Centers for Disease Control and Prevention: www.cdc.gov/hepatitis/hav/havfaq.htm#B1

  c. Patients with chronic liver disease
  d. Homosexual and bisexual men (both adolescents and adults)
  e. Users of illegal injected and noninjected drugs
  f. Those with occupational risk of exposure, such as handlers of nonhuman primates and persons working with HAV in a laboratory setting
  g. Travelers who need preexposure immunoprophylaxis: The first dose of hepatitis A vaccine should be administered as soon as travel is considered.
  h. Patients with clotting-factor disorders such as hemophilia.

5. Routine HAV vaccination is *not* indicated for the following groups:
  a. Child-care center staff and children
  b. Patients and staff in custodial care institutions
  c. Hospital personnel; if a patient with hepatitis A is admitted to the hospital, routine infection-control precautions will prevent transmission to hospital staff.
  d. Food service workers.
  e. Patients with hemophilia
  f. Sewage workers

6. HAV vaccine may be administered simultaneously with other vaccines, including hepatitis B, diphtheria, polovirus (oral and inactivated), tetanus, oral and IM typhoid, cholera, Japanese encephalitis, rabies, and yellow fever. The HAV vaccine should be given in a separate syringe and at a separate site.

7. The need for an additional hepatitis A booster beyond the two-dose primary immunization has not been established; however, the CDC reports that extra doses of HAV vaccine are not harmful.

8. Immune response in immunocompromised patients, such as those with HIV or on hemodialysis, may be suboptimal. The vaccine is inactivated; therefore, no special precautions are needed when vaccinating immunocompromised patients.

9. Vaccine side effects are generally mild and may include
  a. Local pain at the immunization site
  b. Localized induration at the injection site

10. Tylenol may be administered for fever and arthralgia but is strictly limited to a maximum dose of 3 to 4 g/d in adults.

Follow-Up

A. Dehydration may require hospital admission.
B. Follow up in 2 weeks for reevaluation.
C. Check for hepatitis B immunity and vaccinate.
D. Hepatitis A is reportable to the public health department.

Consultation/Referral

A. Consult a physician if necessary.

Individual Considerations

A. Pregnancy
  1. Pregnant women recently exposed to HAV should receive prophylactic gamma globulin.

2. HAV is an inactivated vaccine and is considered safe during pregnancy.
3. HAV infection during pregnancy is associated with increased risk of premature labor and delivery.

B. Pediatrics
1. In the United States, the highest rates for symptomatic HAV infection occur in children 5 to 14 years of age, and the lowest rates occur in children from birth to 4 years.
2. Children who have received HAV vaccine rarely have detectable anti-HAV IgM titers.
3. Risk of outbreak in child-care centers increases with the number of children under age 2 years who wear diapers.
4. Immunization is recommended routinely for children 12 through 23 months of age (follow the childhood immunization schedule).
5. The hepatitis A vaccine is not currently licensed for children younger than 12 months.

C. Adults: In the United States, the lowest rate of HAV infection is in people older than 40 years.

D. Geriatrics
1. The elderly have greater numbers of HAV antibodies, resulting in fewer cases.
2. Symptoms are usually vague. Fatigue; pruritus; and the classic symptoms of jaundice, hepatomegaly, and liver tenderness are commonly absent in the elderly.
3. Diagnostic test results in the elderly include elevated bilirubin, lower or normal transaminase and ALP, and normal ultrasonography.
4. Treatment is supportive. Corticosteroids may relieve symptoms but prolong the disease state due to prolonged viral replication.

E. Special populations
1. People with chronic liver disease are at risk of fulminant hepatitis and should be immunized.
2. People who are awaiting or have received liver transplants should be immunized.

Hepatitis B

Cheryl A. Glass and Audra Malone

Definition

A. Hepatitis B is inflammation of the liver caused by hepatitis B virus (HBV). Acute HBV infection cannot be distinguished from other forms of acute viral hepatitis on the basis of clinical signs and symptoms or nonspecific laboratory findings. Acutely infected patients may be asymptomatic or symptomatic. The likelihood of developing symptoms of acute hepatitis is age dependent.

B. Chronic HBV infection is defined as the presence of hepatitis B surface antigen (HBsAg) in serum for at least 6 months or by the presence of HBsAg in a person who tests negative for antibody of the immunoglobulin (Ig) M subclass to hepatitis B core antigen (IgM anti-hepatitis B core antigen).

C. HBV is the main cause of cirrhosis and hepatocellular carcinoma (HCC) worldwide. For selected candidates, liver transplantation currently seems to be the only viable treatment for the latest stages of hepatitis B.

D. Antiviral treatment may be effective in approximately one third of the patients who receive it. Eight different genotypes (A through H) have been identified. The progression of the disease seems to be more accelerated, and the response to treatment with antiviral agents is less favorable for patients infected by genotype C compared with those infected by genotype B. Genotypes A or B have a better response to interferon (IFN) treatment compared with patients infected by genotype C or D.

E. Acute HBV is undistinguishable from other forms of hepatitis in the acute viral stage on the basis of clinical symptoms.

F. In 2012, the Centers for Disease Control and Prevention (CDC) recommended testing for the following:
1. All pregnant women
2. Persons born in regions with intermediate or high rates of hepatitis B (HBsAg prevalence greater than or equal to 2%)
3. U.S.-born persons not vaccinated as infants whose parents were born in regions with high rates of hepatitis B (HBsAg prevalence of greater than or equal to 8%)
4. Infants born to HBsAg-positive mothers
5. Household, needle-sharing, or sex contacts of HBsAg-positive persons
6. Men who have sex with men
7. Injection drug users
8. Patients with elevated liver enzymes (alanine transaminase [ALT]/aspartate transaminase [AST]) of unknown etiology
9. Hemodialysis patients
10. Persons needing immunosuppressive or cytotoxic therapy
11. HIV-infected persons
12. Donors of blood, plasma, organs, tissues, or semen.
13. Adults with diabetes mellitus are at an increased risk of acquiring HBV infection if they share diabetes care equipment such as blood glucose meters, finger-stick devices, syringes, and/or insulin pens. Adults with diabetes aged less than 60 years are, therefore, recommended by the CDC to receive hepatitis B vaccination and those aged greater than 60 years are to be considered for vaccination.

Incidence

A. An estimated one third of the global population has been infected with HBV. Approximately 350 million people are lifelong carriers, and only 2% spontaneously seroconvert annually. Of chronically infected patients, 15% to 40% will develop cirrhosis, progressing to liver failure and/or HCC.

B. In 2014, rates were highest for persons aged 30 to 39 years (2.23 cases/100,000 population); the lowest rates were among children and adolescents aged less than 19 years (0.02 cases/100,000 population).

C. Acute hepatitis B occurs in 1 to 2 out of every 1,000 pregnancies in the United States, and chronic infection occurs in 5 to 15 out of every 1,000 pregnancies. The course of maternal HBV infections does not seem to be affected by coexistent pregnancy. However, premature labor and delivery is increased.

D. Chronic HBV infections with persistence of HBsAg occur in as many as 90% of infants infected by perinatal transmission; in 30% of children 1 to 5 years old infected after birth; and in 5% to 10% of older children, adolescents, and adults with HBV infection.

Pathogenesis

A. HBV is a hepadnavirus. HBV-related liver injury is largely caused by immune-mediated mechanisms mediated via cytotoxic T-lymphocyte lysis of infected hepatocytes. The virus is transmitted through blood or body fluids, such as wound exudates, semen, cervical secretions, and saliva that are HBsAg positive. It is not transmitted by the fecal–oral route or by water. Blood and serum contain the highest concentration of virus; saliva contains the lowest.

B. The incubation period is 45 to 160 days (2–5 months), with an average of 120 days. An infected person can infect others 4 to 6 weeks before symptoms appear and for an unpredictable time thereafter.

C. The production of antibodies against HBsAg confers protective immunity and can be detected in patients who have recovered from HBV or in those patients who have been vaccinated. The immunoglobulin M (IgM) subtype indicates an acute infection or reactivation. IgG subtype indicates chronic infection.

Predisposing Factors

A. Higher prevalence in non-Hispanic Blacks and other populations
- **1.** Asian origin
- **2.** American Indian/Alaskan Eskimos
- **3.** Asian Pacific islanders

B. Sexual contact is the major mode of transmission.
- **1.** High number of sexual partners
- **2.** An early age of first intercourse
- **3.** Homosexuality/bisexuality

C. Intravenous (IV) drug use, sharing needles

D. Occupational exposure

E. Household exposure

F. Perinatal exposure, by vertical infection

G. Receiving blood transfusions or blood products for hemophilia and hemodialysis

H. Breastfeeding, by transmission in breast milk

I. Staffing or residing in institutions

J. International travel

K. Incarceration in long-term correctional facilities

L. Percutaneous contact with inanimate objects contaminated with HBV; virus can survive 1 week or longer

M. Diabetics

N. Recipient of dialysis or kidney transplant

Common Complaints

A. The following symptoms occur in the acute phase of HBV.
- **1.** Anicteric hepatitis: Asymptomatic (majority of patients)
- **2.** Icteric hepatitis: Associated with a prodromal period
  - **a.** Anorexia
  - **b.** Nausea and vomiting
  - **c.** Low-grade fever
  - **d.** Headache
  - **e.** Diarrhea
  - **f.** Myalgia
  - **g.** Fatigue
  - **h.** Aversion to food and cigarettes
  - **i.** Intermittent, mild to moderate right upper quadrant (RUQ) and epigastric pain
- **3.** Hyperacute, acute, and subacute hepatitis symptoms
  - **a.** Hepatic encephalopathy
  - **b.** Somnolence
  - **c.** Disturbances in sleep pattern
  - **d.** Mental confusion
  - **e.** Coma

B. The following symptoms occur in the chronic phase of HBV:
- **1.** Asymptomatic: May be healthy carriers without any evidence of active disease
- **2.** During the replicative state common symptoms are:
  - **a.** Fatigue
  - **b.** Anorexia
  - **c.** Nausea
  - **d.** Mild upper quadrant pain or discomfort
  - **e.** Hepatic decompensation

Other Signs and Symptoms

A. In young children
- **1.** Jaundice and other symptoms may not be present.
- **2.** Symptoms may be prolonged and insidious compared with HAV.

B. Icteric phase (10 days after the appearance of constitutional symptoms and lasts for 1–3 months)
- **1.** Jaundice of sclera and skin
- **2.** Tea-colored urine
- **3.** Clay-colored stools, often precede jaundice
- **4.** RUQ tenderness
- **5.** Enlarged liver

Subjective Data

A. Review the onset, duration, course, and severity of symptoms. Ask the patient for specifics about urine and stool color.
- **1.** Ask whether the patient has ever been treated for any type of hepatitis.

B. How long ago was her or she treated?
- **1.** Did the patient complete the therapy? If not, why?
- **2.** What was their response to therapy (i.e., nonresponder, etc.)?

C. Review vaccination status.

D. Review family history for hepatocellular carcinoma (HCC).

E. Ask the patient about other family members and sexual contacts with similar symptoms.

F. Discuss the patient's history of blood transfusions, IV drug use, and alcohol abuse.

G. Review the patient's occupational exposure.

H. Inquire about recent international travel.

I. Review for a history of variceal bleeding.

J. Is the patient coinfected with hepatitis C virus (HCV) or HIV?

Physical Examination

A. Check temperature (if indicated), pulse, respirations, blood pressure, and weight. Establish the patient's usual weight; note amount of any weight lost and over what length of time.
B. Inspect
  1. Observe general appearance, muscle wasting, ascites, and peripheral edema.
  2. Inspect the skin for jaundice, palmar erythema, rash, spider nevi, spider angioma, and dehydration.
  3. Inspect the eyes for yellow sclera.
  4. Inspect the mucous membranes and nail beds.
  5. Evaluate for the presence of gynecomastia.
C. Auscultate
  1. Lung fields and the heart
  2. All quadrants of the abdomen
D. Percuss the abdomen.
E. Palpate
  1. All quadrants of the abdomen for masses, liver enlargement or tenderness, hepatomegaly, and splenomegaly
  2. The lymph nodes for lymphadenopathy
  3. For testicular atrophy

Diagnostic Tests

A. Diagnostic tests for HBV antigens and antibodies (see Table 11.14).
B. Complete blood count (CBC) with differential
C. Complete liver panel
  1. AST/ALT
  2. Total bilirubin
  3. International normalized ratio (INR)
  4. Albumin
  5. Alkaline phosphatase
D. Other viral infection markers: HCV and hepatitis delta virus (HDV)
E. Alkaline phosphatase (ALP)
F. Serum iron levels
G. Gamma-glutamyl transpeptidase (GGT; rule out other causes of chronic liver disease)
H. Alpha-fetoprotein (AFP; rule out other causes of liver disease)
I. HBV genotype
J. HBV DNA viral load quantitation
K. Serum fibrosis panel
  1. APRI = aspartate aminotransferase (AST)-to-platelet ratio index used for estimating hepatic fibrosis. Online calculator can be found at: www.hepatitisc.uw.edu/page/clinical-calculators/apri
  2. Fibrosis-4 (FIB-4) is an index for estimating hepatic fibrosis based on a calculation derived from AST, ALT, platelet concentrations, and age. Online calculator can be found at: www.hepatitisc.uw.edu/page/clinical-calculators/fib-4
  3. FibroTest (FibroSure)—commercial biomarker test that uses the results of six blood markers to estimate hepatic fibrosis
L. Imaging
  1. Abdominal ultrasound
  2. FibroScan—Transient shear wave elastography measures liver stiffness as a surrogate for fibrosis
  3. CT or MRI to help exclude biliary obstruction
M. Liver biopsy to assess the severity of disease
N. Pregnancy testing before antiviral therapy
O. Before oral antiviral therapy is introduced, all patients should be screened for HIV.
P. HCV and HIV testing to rule out co-infection.

Differential Diagnoses

A. Hepatitis B
B. Exclusion of other types of hepatitis (A, C, D, E, viral, or autoimmune hepatitis)
C. Infectious mononucleosis
D. Hepatotoxic drug ingestion, for example, chloramphenicol, acetaminophen, or methyldopa
E. Metastatic cancer to the liver
F. Alcoholic cirrhosis

TABLE 11.14 Diagnostic Tests for HBV Antigens and Antibodies

Factors to Be Tested	HBV Antigen or Antibody	Indication
HBsAg	HBsAg	Detects acutely or chronically infected; antigen used in hepatitis B vaccine
Anti-HBs	Antibody to HBsAg	Identifies resolved HBV infections; determines immunity after immunization
HBeAg	HBeAg	Identifies at risk of transmitting HBV
Anti-HBe	Antibody to HBeAg	Identifies lower risk of transmitting HBV
Anti-HBc	Antibody to hepatitis B core antigen; IgM (HBcAg)	Identifies acute, resolved, or chronic HBV infection. Anti-HBc is not present after immunization
IgM anti-HBc Anti-HAV	IgM antibody to HBcAg	Identifies acute or recent HBV infections (includes HBsAg-negative during the window phase of infection) Determines need for vaccination

HAV, hepatitis A virus; HB, hepatitis B: HBcAg, hepatitis B core antigen; HBeAg, hepatitis B envelope antigen; HBsAg, hepatitis B surface antigen; HBV, hepatitis B virus; IgM, immunoglobulin M.

G. Hemochromatosis
H. Wilson's disease

Plan

A. General interventions
1. No specific therapy for acute HBV infection is available.
2. Before any form of HBV therapy is started, and optimally at the first presentation, the patient needs to be provided with information about the natural history of chronic hepatitis B infection and the fact that most infections remain entirely without symptoms even in those with severe disease, so that there is a need for regular lifelong monitoring.
3. Hepatitis B immune globulin (HBIG) and corticosteroids are not effective treatment.
B. Patient teaching:
▶ **1.** *See Section III: Patient Teaching Guide for this chapter, "Jaundice and Hepatitis."*
2. Tell the patient to avoid sexual activity until he or she is free of HBsAg.
3. History of anaphylactic reaction to common baker's yeast is a contraindication to HBV vaccination.
4. There are no dietary restrictions with acute and chronic hepatitis (without cirrhosis). Decompensated cirrhosis, portal hypertension, or encephalopathy are prescribed.
a. Low-sodium diet (1.5 g/d)
b. High-protein diet (white-meat protein, e.g., pork, turkey, and fish)
c. Fluid restriction of 1.5 L/d in the presence of hyponatremia
C. Pharmaceutical therapy: The goal of treatment is to prevent progression to cirrhosis, hepatic failure, and hepatocellular cancer.
1. Primary prevention includes vaccination of high-risk individuals, including teens. Vaccination is up to 95% effective.
2. HBV vaccine is the recommended preexposure for the following groups:
a. Prevention of perinatal HBV infection through routine screening of all pregnant women for HBV infection and provision of hepatitis B vaccine and immunoprophylaxis to infants born to hepatitis B surface antigen (HBsAg)-positive mothers
b. All infants: All major authorities recommend that all children receive a complete series of HBV immunizations during the first 18 months of life. **Universal immunization of infants begins at birth.**
c. Routine vaccination of previously unvaccinated children and adolescents
d. Children at risk of acquiring HBV by person-to-person (horizontal) transmission
e. All adolescents
f. IV drug users
g. Sexually active individuals with more than one sex partner in the previous 6 months or those who have a sexually transmitted infection (STI), men who have sex with men (MSM), and persons who inject drugs (PWID).
h. Health care workers and others at occupational risk
i. Residents and staff of institutions for developmentally disabled persons
j. Staff of nonresidential child care centers
k. Patients undergoing hemodialysis
l. Patients with bleeding disorders who receive clotting factor concentrates
m. Household contacts and sexual partners of HBV carriers
n. Members of households with adoptees who are HBsAg positive
o. International travelers to areas of high or intermediate endemicity
p. Inmates of long-term correctional facilities
3. Hepatitis B vaccine can be given concurrently with other vaccines.
4. Early prophylaxis is paramount after an HBsAg needle stick. HBIG should be administered immediately, no later than 48 hours, after exposure. Postexposure prophylaxis HBV vaccine is recommended.
5. The length of therapy is dependent on the genotype and previous treatment:
a. Treatment: Naïve—not previously treated for HCV.
b. Relapser: Reappearance of HCV occurs after therapy is discontinued.
c. Partial responder: HCV declines at week 12 of therapy but is still positive at week 24 after completion of treatment.
6. Management of side effects with therapeutic agents is targeted to the symptoms.
7. There are multiple drug–drug interactions; consult with a pharmaceutical reference before instituting of drug therapy.
8. Dose adjustment is required in the presence of renal impairment and dialysis, and is used with caution in patients with a history of pancreatitis.
9. Orthotopic liver transplantation (OLT) is the treatment of choice for patients with fulminant hepatic failure who do not recover and for patients with end-stage liver disease.
10. The guidelines for treatment are rapidly changing. The most current guideline recommendations are available at the American Association for the Study of Liver Diseases at www.aasld.org/publications/practice-guidelines-0. Guidelines include:
a. Acute liver failure, management
b. Ascites due to cirrhosis, management
c. Gastroesophageal varices and variceal hemorrhage in cirrhosis, management
d. Hepatic encephalopathy
e. Hepatitis B, guidance
f. Hepatitis C, guidance
g. Hepatocellular carcinoma, management
h. Liver biopsy
i. Several chapters in the AASLD guideline recommendations are related to liver transplantation.

11. The current World Health Organization (WHO) *Guidelines for the Prevention, Care, and Treatment of Persons With Chronic Hepatitis B Infection* is located at www.who.int/hiv/pub/hepatitis/hepatitis-b-guidelines/en

Follow-Up

A. Laboratory monitoring
  1. Monitor liver function (alanine transaminase [ALT]) every 3 to 6 months for active disease.
  2. Monitor hepatitis B envelope antigen (HBeAg) every 3 to 6 months, depending on ALT levels.
  3. Monitor CBC and creatinine every month (1–2 days before treatment).
  4. Monitor HBV DNA every 3 to 6 months when the patient is on treatment in the reactivation phase.

B. Risk of exposure to HBsAg ceases when antigen disappears from the bloodstream, usually within 6 to 8 weeks of infection. Repeated serum determinations of HBsAg can help define when precautions may be relaxed.

C. Laboratory, physical examination, and psychosocial evaluation are required for antiviral therapy.

D. The American Association for the Study of Liver Disease (AASLD) recommends HCC surveillance using ultrasound in the following types of patients with chronic HBV.
  1. Asian men older than 40 years and Asian women older than 50 years
  2. All patients with cirrhosis, regardless of age
  3. Patients with a family history of HCC; any age
  4. Africans older than the age of 20 years and any carriers older than 40 years with persistent or intermittent ALT evaluation and/or HBV DNA level greater than 2,000 IU/mL should be screened with an ultrasound every 6 to 12 months.
  5. Any individual with HBV/HIV coinfection

E. Routine booster doses of hepatitis B vaccine are not recommended for children or adults with normal immune status.

Consultation/Referral

A. Patients with persistently elevated serum transaminase concentrations (exceeding twice the upper limits of normal), as well as those with elevated serum AFP concentrations or abnormal ultrasounds, should be referred to a gastroenterologist for further management.

Individual Considerations

A. Pregnancy
  1. No adverse effect on the developing fetus has been observed when pregnant women are vaccinated against HBV.
  2. There is insufficient data to recommend delivery by cesarean section.
  3. The AASLD suggests antiviral therapy to reduce the risk of perinatal transmission of hepatitis B in HBsAg-positive pregnant women with an HBV DNA level greater than 200,000 IU/mL.
  4. The only antivirals studied in pregnant women are lamivudine, telbivudine, and tenofovir.
  5. Antiviral therapy was started at 28 to 32 weeks of gestation and discontinued at birth to 3 months postpartum in most studies.
  6. Pregnancy and lactation are not a contraindication to vaccination.
  7. Prenatal HBsAg testing of all pregnant women is recommended to identify newborns who require immediate postexposure prophylaxis.
  8. Breastfeeding by an HBsAg-positive mother poses no additional risk for acquisition of HBV infection by infant.

B. Pediatrics
  1. Infants born to HBsAg-positive mothers need no special precautions for spread of infectious disease other than removal of maternal blood by a gloved attendant and standard universal precautions.
  2. Infants of all HBsAg-positive women should receive immunoprophylaxis (HBV vaccination ± hepatitis B immunoglobulin) per WHO and CDC recommendations.
  3. All infants, including those who are premature, born to HbsAg-positive mothers need HBIG within 12 hours of birth.
  4. More than 90% of infants infected perinatally will develop chronic HBV infection.
  5. Adoptees from countries where HBV infection is endemic should be screened for HBsAg. If a child is HBsAg positive, previously unimmunized family members and other household contacts should be vaccinated, preferably before adoption.
  6. Persons infected as infants or young children are at higher risk of death due to liver disease than those infected as adults. Children with chronic HBV should be screened periodically for hepatic complication using serum liver transaminase tests, alpha-fetoprotein concentration, and abdominal ultrasound.
  7. All children 11 to 12 years should have their immunization records reviewed and should complete the vaccine series if they have not received the vaccine or did not complete the immunization series.
  8. Children who stop antiviral therapy should be monitored every 3 months for at least 1 year for recurrent viremia, ALT flares, and clinical decompensation.

C. Adults
  1. Most HBV infections are acquired in adolescence or adulthood, largely as a result of IV drug use, sexual contact, or occupational or household exposure. HBV infection is associated with other sexually transmitted diseases, including syphilis.
  2. Patients who have received a blood transfusion should refrain from blood donation for 6 months, the incubation period for HBV. Blood should never be donated if the patient is a hepatitis B carrier or was infected with hepatitis C.

D. Geriatrics
  1. The elderly have fewer cases of HBV due to diminished immune response; however, they tend to be asymptomatic HBV carriers.
  2. The disease has a greater tendency to deteriorate into chronic liver failure or chronic hepatitis.

Resources

American Association for the Study of Liver Diseases: www.aasld.org
American Liver Foundation: www.liverfoundation.org
Centers for Disease Control and Prevention: www.cdc.gov/hepatitis
Hepatitis and HIV: www.hivandhepatitis.com
Hepatitis B Foundation: www.hepb.org
Hepatitis Foundation International: www.hepfi.org
Immunization Action Coalition: www.immunize.org
National Institute of Diabetes and Digestive and Kidney Diseases: www2.niddk.nih.gov
United Network for Organ Sharing: www.unos.org
World Health Organization: who.int

Hepatitis C

Cheryl A. Glass

Definition

A. Hepatitis C is an inflammation of the liver caused by the hepatitis C virus (HCV). HCV has signs and symptoms often undistinguishable from those of hepatitis A virus (HAV) or hepatitis B virus (HBV). The disease tends to be asymptomatic to mild and has an insidious onset. Acute fulminate infection is rare. The major feature of HCV is its propensity to become chronic. Persistent infection occurs in at least 75% to 85% of patients, even in the absence of biochemical evidence of liver disease. Approximately 60% to 70% of patients develop chronic hepatitis, and 5% to 20% develop cirrhosis.

B. Multiple (six) HCV genotypes and subtypes exist. The genotype is a major factor in the effectiveness of the patient's response to therapy. Approximately 50% of patients infected with genotype 1 and approximately 80% of patients with genotypes 2 and 3 achieve a sustained virologic response (SVR). SVR is defined as undetectable HCV RNA 12 months or more after treatment cessation.

C. The development of chronic hepatitis and its complications increase with several factors, including older age at acquisition, HIV infection, excessive alcohol consumption, and male gender. Among children, liver disease progression appears to be accelerated with comorbid conditions, including cancer, iron overload, thalassemia, or coinfection with HIV.

D. HCV is the leading cause of nonalcoholic hepatic failure and cirrhosis, and the cause of 90% of post-transfusion hepatitis. Primary hepatic cellular carcinoma (HCC) also occurs in these patients.

Incidence

A. Worldwide, more than 170 million individuals are chronically infected with HCV.

B. The "emerging epidemic" of acute HCV resulted from people who have transitioned from oral prescription opioid abuse to injection of these opioids and heroin.

C. Seroprevalence rates among individuals vary according to their associated risk factors. The highest rates occur in persons with large or repeated direct percutaneous exposure to blood or blood products, such as intravenous (IV) drug users and patients with hemophilia who have received multiple blood transfusions.

D. Seroprevalence among pregnant women in the United States has been estimated at 1% to 2%. Maternal–fetal (vertical) transmission is only 5% from women who are HCV RNA positive at the time of delivery. Maternal coinfection with HIV has been associated with increased risk of perinatal transmission of HCV RNA.

E. Serum anti-HCV antibody and HCV RNA have been detected in colostrum. However, although only a limited number of patients have been studied, the rate of transmission among breastfed infants is the same as among bottle-fed infants.

F. More than 20% of adults with chronic infection progress to cirrhosis an average of 20 years after their initial infection. Patients with cirrhosis have a secondary risk of portal hypertension, liver failure, and other complications. HCV is the leading indication for liver transplantation among adults in the United States.

G. HCC is diagnosed an average of 30 years after initial HCV infection in 1% to 5% of patients, most of whom have underlying cirrhosis.

Pathogenesis

A. HCV is a small, single-stranded RNA virus with a lipid envelope and is a member of the Flavivirus family. Infection is spread primarily by parenteral exposure to blood and blood products from HCV-infected persons. In the United States, the current risk of HCV infection following blood transfusion is estimated at 0.1% or less because of exclusion of high-risk individuals from the pool of blood donors and screening for HCV. Sexual transmission of HCV is uncommon except with high-risk behavior.

B. The incubation period averages 6 to 7 weeks, with a range of 2 weeks to 6 months. The time from exposure to the development of viremia generally is 1 to 2 weeks.

Predisposing Factors

All people with HCV RNA in their blood are considered to be infectious. The following groups are at high risk of HCV infection and should be tested:

A. IV drug users who have shared needles
B. Intranasal cocaine users, presumably resulting from epistaxis and shared equipment
C. Hemophiliacs, hemodialysis patients, and those who received blood transfusions before 1992
D. Recipients of solid organ transplants before 1992
E. Health care workers with percutaneous exposures
F. Individuals with multiple sexual partners
G. Transmission among contacts living with infected persons may occur with percutaneous or mucosal exposure to blood.
H. Infants of infected mothers, by vertical transmission
I. More common in males than females.
J. Tattooing, body piercing, and acupuncture with unsterile equipment
K. HIV

Common Complaints

A. Chronic HCV is asymptomatic unless there is progressive inflammation and complications from cirrhosis.
B. Malaise
C. Anorexia

D. Nausea
E. Myalgia
F. Fever
G. Abdominal pain

Other Signs and Symptoms

A. Jaundice (occurs in fewer than 20% of patients)
B. Hepatomegaly is present in one third of patients with an acute infection.
C. Ascites
D. Spider nevi
E. Dark urine

Subjective Data

A. Review the onset, duration, course, and severity of symptoms. Ask the patient for specifics about urine and stool color.
B. Ask the patient about other family members and sexual contacts with similar symptoms.
C. Review the patient's history of blood transfusions, tattoos, incarnation, IV drug use, and alcohol abuse.
D. Ask the patient about occupational exposure.
E. Ask about high-risk sexual practices.
F. Review family history of HCC.
G. When was HCV diagnosed?
H. Has the patient had a liver biopsy? when?
I. Ask if the patient has ever been treated for any type of hepatitis.
   1. How long ago the patient treated?
   2. Did the patient complete therapy? If not, why?
   3. What was the patient's response to therapy (i.e., nonresponder, relapser, etc.)?
J. Review for a history of variceal bleeding.

Physical Examination

A. Check temperature (acute infection), pulse, respirations, blood pressure, and weight.
B. Inspect
   1. Observe general appearance, muscle wasting, edema, and demeanor. **Administer a depression self-assessment tool at each visit when on HCV therapy.**
   2. Inspect the skin for jaundice, rash, dehydration, palmar erythema, excoriations, spider nevi, and tattoos/piercings.
   3. Inspect the eyes for yellow sclera.
   4. Inspect mucous membranes and nail beds for clubbing and cyanosis.
   5. Inspect for gynecomastia and small testes.
C. Auscultate
   1. Lung fields and heart
   2. All quadrants of the abdomen and evaluate for abdominal bruit
D. Percuss the abdomen.
E. Palpate
   1. All quadrants of the abdomen for masses; liver enlargement or tenderness; characteristics of cirrhosis; and hepatosplenomegaly, which occurs in about 10% of cases.
   2. The lymph nodes for lymphadenopathy and enlarged parotid.

Diagnostic Tests

A. Laboratory tests
   1. Immunoglobulin G (IgG) antibody enzyme immunoassays (EIAs) for HCV and nucleic acid amplification (NAA) tests to detect HCV RNA
   2. HCV genotyping
   3. HCV viral load: Quantitative assay used as a prognostic indicator for patients undergoing antiviral therapy
   4. Alanine transaminase (ALT) and aspartate transaminase (AST)
   5. Hepatitis A IgM and IgG
   6. Hepatitis B surface antigen (HBsAg) and antibody, core antibody
   7. Cytomegalovirus (CMV) immunoglobulin (IgM) and IgG (and/or CMV in urine culture)
   8. Epstein–Barr virus IgM and IgG
   9. HIV IgG enzyme-linked immunoassay (ELISA)
   10. Alpha-fetoprotein
B. Ultrasonography is used for monitoring HCV-related complications. FibroScan—transient shear wave elastography—measures liver stiffness as a surrogate for fibrosis
C. Serum fibrosis panel
   1. APRI = AST-to-platelet ratio index used for estimating hepatic fibrosis. Online calculator can be found at: www.hepatitisc.uw.edu/page/clinical-calculators/apri
   2. FIB-4 is an index for estimating hepatic fibrosis based on a calculation derived from AST, ALT, platelet concentrations, and age. Online calculator can be found at: www.hepatitisc.uw.edu/page/clinical-calculators/fib-4
   3. FibroTest (FibroSure): Commercial biomarker test that uses the results of 6 blood markers to estimate hepatic fibrosis.
D. Liver biopsy is the most accurate method of evaluating the extent of HCV-retlated liver disease. Liver biopsy is the gold standard for determining the histologic grade and stage of fibrosis/cirrhosis. The *absolute* requirement for a liver biopsy prior to the institution of medication therapy is currently under discussion. For patients with genotypes 2 and 3, the likelihood of response to therapy is so high that the benefits of treatment may outweigh the risk of biopsy and histologic considerations.
E. Prior to the institution/during antiviral therapy, perform the following tests:
   1. Complete blood count (CBC) with platelets
   2. Viral load
   3. Liver function (ALT/AST)
   4. Pregnancy test
   5. Thyroid profile
   6. Blood glucose/A1C
   7. Consider a dilated retinal examination.
   8. Consider a stress test.
   9. Screen for alcohol abuse, drug abuse, and/or depression.

Differential Diagnoses

A. Hepatitis C
B. Hepatitis A

C. Hepatitis B
D. Alcoholic liver disease
E. Drug toxicities
F. Opportunistic infections associated with HIV infection

Plan

A. Patient teaching:
1. *See Section III: Patient Teaching Guide for this chapter, "Jaundice and Hepatitis."*
2. Warn the patient of the possibility of transmission to others, and tell the patient to refrain from donating blood, organs, tissues, or semen and from sharing toothbrushes and razors.
3. All patients with chronic HCV should be immunized against hepatitis A and hepatitis B.
4. Counsel the patient to avoid hepatotoxic medications and alcohol.
5. Immunoprophylaxis for postexposure prophylaxis with IG is not recommended.
6. The Centers for Disease Control and Prevention (CDC) recommends anyone born between 1945 and 1965 be tested for HCV.

B. Patients and their spouses should be counseled to not become pregnant while on therapy and for 6 months after the completion of treatment. Pregnancy tests should be done prior to institution of HCV therapy and monthly thereafter.

C. Pharmaceutical therapy is aimed at inhibiting HCV replication, eradicating infection, progression of fibrosis, and prevention of HCC.
1. The length of therapy is dependent on the genotype and previous treatment:
a. Treatment: Naïve—not previously treated for HCV.
b. Relapser: Reappearance of HCV after therapy is discontinued
c. Partial responder: HCV declines at week 12 of therapy but is still positive at week 24 after completion of treatment.
i. Manage side effects with therapeutic agents related to symptoms.
ii. If there are multiple drug–drug interactions, consult with a pharmaceutical reference before instituting of drug therapy.
iii. The guidelines for treatment are rapidly changing. The most current guideline recommendations are available from the American Association for the Study of Liver Diseases (AASLD) and the Infectious Diseases Society of America (IDSA) at www.aasld.org/publications/practice-guidelines-0. Guidelines break down therapy in detail by genotype, length of therapy, and medications. The AASLD guidelines also include:
1) Acute liver failure, management
2) Ascites due to cirrhosis, management
3) Gastroesophageal varices and variceal hemorrhage in cirrhosis management
4) Hepatic encephalopathy
5) Hepatitis B guidance
6) Hepatitis C guidance
7) Hepatocellular carcinoma management
8) Liver biopsy
9) Several chapters in the AASLD guideline recommendations are related to liver transplantation

2. The WHO *Guidelines for the Screening, Care, and Treatment of Persons With Hepatitis C Infection* is available at: apps.who.int/iris/bitstream/10665/111747/1/9789241548755_eng.pdf?ua=1&ua=1

Follow-Up

A. Test the patient within 5 to 6 weeks after the onset of hepatitis; 80% of patients are positive for serum anti-HCV antibody.
B. Persons with chronic HCV infections should be vaccinated against hepatitis A and B, unless they have previously been demonstrated to be nonsusceptible.
C. Children with chronic infection should be screened periodically for chronic hepatitis with serum liver function tests (LFTs) because of their potential long-term risk for chronic liver disease. Definitive recommendations on frequency have not been established.
D. Monitor for mental dysfunction related to interferon (IFN), including depression, psychosis, aggressive behavior, hallucinations, violent behavior, suicidal ideation, suicide attempt, and homicidal ideation (rare), even without previous history of psychiatric illness.

Consultation/Referral

A. Referrals include gastroenterologist, psychiatrist, endocrinologist, neurologist, hematologist, dietitian, and social workers.
B. Patients who are coinfected with HBV or HIV or have end-stage renal disease should be referred for treatment.
C. Children with severe disease or histologically advanced pathology (bridging necrosis or active cirrhosis) should be referred to a specialist in the management of chronic HCV infection.
D. Children with persistently elevated serum transaminase concentrations, or those exceeding twice the upper limits of normal, should be referred to a gastroenterologist for further management.

Individual Considerations

A. Pregnancy
1. No data currently exist to support counseling a woman against pregnancy (unless under active treatment).
2. Routine serologic testing of pregnant women for HCV infection is not recommended. Women with significant risk factors for HCV should be offered antibody screening.
3. According to current guidelines of the U.S. Public Health Service and the American Academy of Pediatrics, maternal HCV infection is not a contraindication to breastfeeding. HCV-positive mothers should consider abstaining from breastfeeding if their nipples are cracked or bleeding.
4. Ribivarin (RBV) is a pregnancy category X drug with abortifacients potential.

5. Interferon (IFN) is a pregnancy category C drug and should be used only if the benefits outweigh the risk to the fetus. **IFN is a pregnancy category X drug when combined with RBV.**
6. The method of delivery has not been shown to increase the risk of vertical transmission of HCV. Cesarean delivery is reserved for obstetric indications.

B. Pediatrics
1. Serologic testing for anti-HCV antibodies in children born to women previously identified to be HCV infected is recommended because approximately 5% acquire the infection. Duration of passive maternal antibody in infants is unknown. Testing for anti-HCV antibodies should not be performed until after 12 months of age.
2. Exclusion of children with HCV infections from out-of-home child-care centers is not indicated.
3. The Food and Drug Administration (FDA) does not approve IFN-alpha or the direct-acting antivirals (DAAs) telaprevir or boceprevir for children younger than 18 years.
4. The need for testing for alpha-fetoprotein concentration and for abdominal ultrasonography in children has not been determined.
5. Routine serologic testing of adoptees, either domestic or international, is not recommended.

C. Adults
1. The CDC recommends anyone born between 1945 and 1965 be tested for HCV.
2. Infected persons with steady partners do not need to change their sexual practices. However, they should be informed of the possible risk of transmission and of what precautions to use to prevent transmission.
3. Persons with multiple partners should be advised to reduce the number of partners and to use condoms to prevent transmission.
4. The best means of limiting transfusion-associated HCV is to rely exclusively on volunteer rather than commercial blood donors and to screen donors for anti-HCV antibodies.

D. Geriatrics: There are fewer cases of HCV in the elderly than in other age groups. However, they tend to develop chronic hepatitis or hepatic failure.

Resources

American Association for the Study of Liver Diseases: www.aasld.org
American Liver Foundation: www.liverfoundation.org
Centers for Disease Control and Prevention: www.cdc.gov/hepatitis
Hepatitis and HIV: www.hivandhepatitis.com
Hepatitis Foundation International: www.hepfi.org
Immunization Action Coalition: www.immunize.org
National Institute of Diabetes and Digestive and Kidney Diseases: www.niddk.nih.gov
United Network for Organ Sharing: www.unos.org
World Health Organization: www.who.int/en

Hernias, Abdominal

Cheryl A. Glass

Definition

A hernia is the protrusion of a peritoneum-lined sac through a defect in the abdominal wall. Abdominal wall hernias are the most common of surgical procedures. Hernias are a leading cause of disability and work loss. Abdominal hernias can be congenital or acquired. Types include the following:

A. Umbilical hernia: Occurs when the intestinal muscles fail to close around the umbilicus, allowing the omentum and/or intestines to protrude into the weaker area
B. Incisional hernia: Caused by a defect in the abdominal musculature that develops after a surgical incision
C. Epigastric hernia: Protrusion of fat or omentum through the linea alba between the umbilicus and the xiphoid. Epigastric hernias are generally less than 2 cm in diameter.
D. Diastasis recti: Acquired hernia most often due to pregnancy and obesity. The right and left rectus muscles separate, but there is no facial defect.
E. Obturator hernia: Follows the path of the obturator nerves and muscles

Incidence

A. Umbilical hernias are more common in African American infants, women, and the elderly. This type of hernia has a higher risk of incarceration and strangulation and, therefore, a greater mortality because the large bowel is frequently entrapped.
B. Epigastric hernias are most common in men 20 to 50 years old.
C. Incisional hernias typically are noted in the early postoperative period; however, there is an increase in incisional hernias during pregnancy. These iatrogenic hernias occur in 2% to 10% of abdominal operations. In addition to hernias, separation of the recti abdominis muscles (diastasis recti) is often caused by pregnancy or obesity.
D. Obturator hernias occur more commonly in females. Females have a larger canal diameter, which is noted predominantly in thin elderly women.

Pathogenesis

A. Incisional hernias are due to failure of fascial tissues to heal and close.
B. Epigastric hernias are defects in the abdominal midline between the umbilicus and the xiphoid process. They are usually related to a congenital weakness, increased intra-abdominal pressure, surrounding muscle weakness, or chronic abdominal wall strain.
C. An umbilical hernia is caused by failure of the umbilical ring to obliterate after birth. In the infant, the umbilical ring often closes spontaneously within the first 1 to 2 years of life. Increased abdominal pressure or congenital defects cause abdominal hernias that allow abdominal contents to protrude through the opening defect. In adults with an umbilical hernia, obesity increases the danger of incarceration.
D. Parastomal hernia is caused by the bowel intrusion into the defect in the abdominal wall when the ileostomy or colostomy was created.

Predisposing Factors

A. Congenital predisposition
B. Gender
C. Obesity
D. Multiparity
E. Cirrhosis and ascites

F. Trauma or straining
G. African American ancestry and infancy
H. Chronic cough; can precipitate or worsen herniation
I. Previous abdominal surgery
J. Straining, coughing, and sneezing in infancy
K. Straining with chronic constipation
L. Incisional hernia factors
  1. Smoking
  2. Connective tissue disorder
  3. Infection
  4. Malnutrition
  5. Immunosuppressive medications
M. Age: Obturator hernias occur predominately in the elderly
N. Maternal smoking is associated with an increased prevalence of omphalocele and gastroschisis

Common Complaints

A. Bulge of abdomen or of a previous scar
B. Symptoms aggravated by cough and straining
C. Small hernias may be asymptomatic, or, as the hernia progresses, varying degrees of discomfort and pain occur
D. The only sign of a hernia may be increased irritability.

Other Signs and Symptoms

A. Incisional: Bulge through incision wall (may be intermittent)
B. Epigastric: Small, usually painless subcutaneous mass
C. Umbilical
  1. Adult: Vague, intermittent pain; palpable mass
  2. Infant: Vomiting and irritability
D. Reducible or irreducible: Signs and symptoms are related to the degree of pressure of their contents rather than to size. Most patients are asymptomatic or complain of only mild pain.
E. Strangulated: Colicky abdominal pain, nausea, vomiting, abdominal distension, hyperperistalsis

Subjective Data

A. Review the onset, duration, and course of symptoms.
B. Ask the patient about previous abdominal surgeries, wound infection, and pregnancies.
C. Review the history of straining, trauma, or physical labor.
D. Determine if the patient has signs and symptoms of strangulation of entrapped bowel: Pain, nausea, vomiting, distension, and fever.
E. Determine if the patient can reduce the hernia.
F. Ask the patient whether the hernia is enlarging and uncomfortable.
G. Review the patient's bowel history, specifically constipation.
H. Review the patient's history for chronic obstructive pulmonary disease (COPD)/chronic cough.
I. Review the patient's history for symptoms of obstructive uropathy.
J. Review how the hernia affects the patient's activities of daily living (ADLs).

Physical Examination

Examination is the same for all types of abdominal hernias. Perform examination while the patient is standing and supine. History and physical examination are the best means of diagnosing hernias.

A. Check temperature (if indicated), pulse, respirations, and blood pressure.
B. Inspect
  1. Inspect contour and symmetry of the abdomen for bulges or masses. The bulge may be asymmetric.
  2. Inspect irreducible hernias for discoloration, edema, and ascites.
  3. Assess
    a. Have the patient perform Valsalva's maneuver while standing.
    b. Have the patient lie supine, lift head from examination table, and then bear down to tense abdomen.
C. Auscultate all quadrants of the abdomen for bowel sounds.
D. Percuss liver, spleen, and abdomen.
E. Palpate
  1. The entire abdomen for masses, hepatomegaly, and ascites. Umbilical hernias may be obscured by subcutaneous fat.
  2. The groin
  3. The hernia, to try to gently reduce it

Diagnostic Tests

A. None is required if the hernia is easily reducible (depending on the type of hernia).
B. Complete blood count (CBC): White blood cell (WBC) increased, hematocrit (Hct) increased
C. Electrolytes: Na^+ increased or decreased
D. Abdominal radiography: Reveals abnormally high levels of gas in bowel
E. Ultrasonography, if strangulation is suspected
F. CT scan of the abdomen and pelvis may be indicated. In obese patients, the CT of the abdomen is the best imaging study.

Differential Diagnoses

A. Abdominal hernia
B. Diastasis recti
C. Ascites
D. Abdominal wall tumor or cyst
E. Bowel obstruction

Plan

A. Patient teaching
  1. Discuss the hernia and available options for treatment.
  2. Teach the patient signs and symptoms of strangulation.
  3. Instruct the patient to refrain from heavy lifting.
  4. Advise the patient to wear a support garment.
B. Medical and surgical management

> *Reduction should not be attempted if there are signs of inflammation or obstruction.*

  1. Try to reduce the hernia unless strangulated. See Section II: Procedure, "Hernia Reduction (Inguinal/Groin)."
    a. Easily reducible: Abdominal contents can be easily returned to their original compartment. Allows symptomatic relief.

b. Incarcerated: Cannot be returned to its original compartment. The incarcerated tissue may be bowel, omentum, or other abdominal contents.

c. Strangulated: Surgical emergency—blood supply to the herniated tissue is compromised.

2. Do not try to reduce strangulated hernias because reduction can cause gangrenous bowel to enter the peritoneal cavity.

3. A truss fits snugly over a hernia to prevent abdominal contents from entering the hernial sac. It does not cure a hernia and is used only when the patient is not a surgical candidate.

4. Umbilical hernia repair is best performed under general anesthesia in children.

5. Surgery may be done laparoscopically or through an open procedure and by sutured or mesh repair, depending on the age of the person, type and size of the hernia, and the presence of strangulation.

Follow-Up

A. Instruct the patient to call the office if fever or severe pain occurs. Otherwise, no follow-up is required unless for postoperative repair. Postoperative follow-up is with the physician who performed the surgery.

Consultation/Referral

Consult a physician if the patient has abdominal tenderness, discoloration, or edema at the site; fever; or signs of bowel obstruction.

A. Pregnancy

1. Incisional hernias are more common during pregnancy because of increased intra-abdominal pressure.

2. Bowel obstruction secondary to previous scarring may also be seen and is most common when the uterus emerges from the pelvis early in the second trimester, when the uterus is maximally distended at term, and in immediate puerperium when the uterus promptly decreases in size.

B. Pediatrics

1. Infants with umbilical hernias require no special treatment because the majority of these hernias close by the fifth year.

2. The infant's abdomen should be soft. Masses may be due to enlargement of tumors or liver. The liver is normally felt 1 to 3 cm below the right costal margin.

3. Tell caregivers that the umbilicus normally everts when a baby cries. However, they should report if the lump becomes large or irreducible, particularly if the baby is vomiting. These signs indicate strangulation and the need for urgent surgery.

4. Genetic testing should be considered in infants with an omphalocele. An omphalocele is associated with chromosomal abnormalities, including trisomy 13, trisomy 18, trisomy 21, or Klinefelter syndrome.

C. Geriatrics

1. Because of the anatomic position of the obturator hernia, the presentation is more common as a bowel obstruction than as a protrusion of bowel contents.

a. The geriatric population is more prone to develop electrolyte and acid–base imbalances from obstruction.

2. The geriatric population has a higher rate of ventral hernias attributed to the loss of muscle strength in the anterior abdominal wall and the prevalence of comorbidities that lead to an increased intra-abdominal pressure.

Hernias, Pelvic

Cheryl A. Glass

Definition

A hernia is the protrusion of a peritoneum-lined sac through some defect from one anatomical space to another. As shown in Figure 11.3, there are three types of pelvic (inguinal) hernias distinguished by presentation:

A. Indirect: Protrudes through internal inguinal ring; can remain in canal, exit external ring, or pass into scrotum; unilateral or bilateral

B. Direct: Protrudes through external inguinal ring; is located in region of Hesselbach's triangle; rarely enters scrotum

C. Femoral: Protrudes through femoral ring, femoral canal, and fossa ovalis

Incidence

A. Indirect inguinal hernias are the most common type of hernia. They affect both sexes, but most often are seen in children and young males (7:1 male-to-female ratio). Incidence increases with age.

B. Direct inguinal hernias are less common than indirect inguinal hernias. They occur more often in males and are more common in those older than age 40. Primary inguinal hernias occur in 1% to 5% of infants and in 9% to 10% of those born prematurely.

C. Femoral hernias are the least common type of hernias. They are rarely seen in children and occur more often in females (1.8:1 female-to-male ratio). Right-side presentation is more common than left.

D. Among inguinal hernias, a sliding component is found in 3%; they are overwhelmingly on the left side (left-to-right ratio, 4.5:1). Sliding hernias are much more common in men than in women, and the predominance increases with age. Female infants have a high incidence of sliding tube, ovary, or broad ligament hernias.

E. Primary perineal hernias occur most often in elderly multiparous women.

Pathogenesis

Pelvic hernias occur because there is a potential space for protrusion—commonly of the bowel but occasionally of the omentum.

A. Indirect and direct hernias arise along the course that the testicle travels as it exits the abdomen and enters the scrotum during intrauterine life. Indirect hernias may be due to a congenital defect in which the processus vaginalis remains patent.

B. Femoral hernias occur at the fossa ovalis, where the femoral artery exits the abdomen.

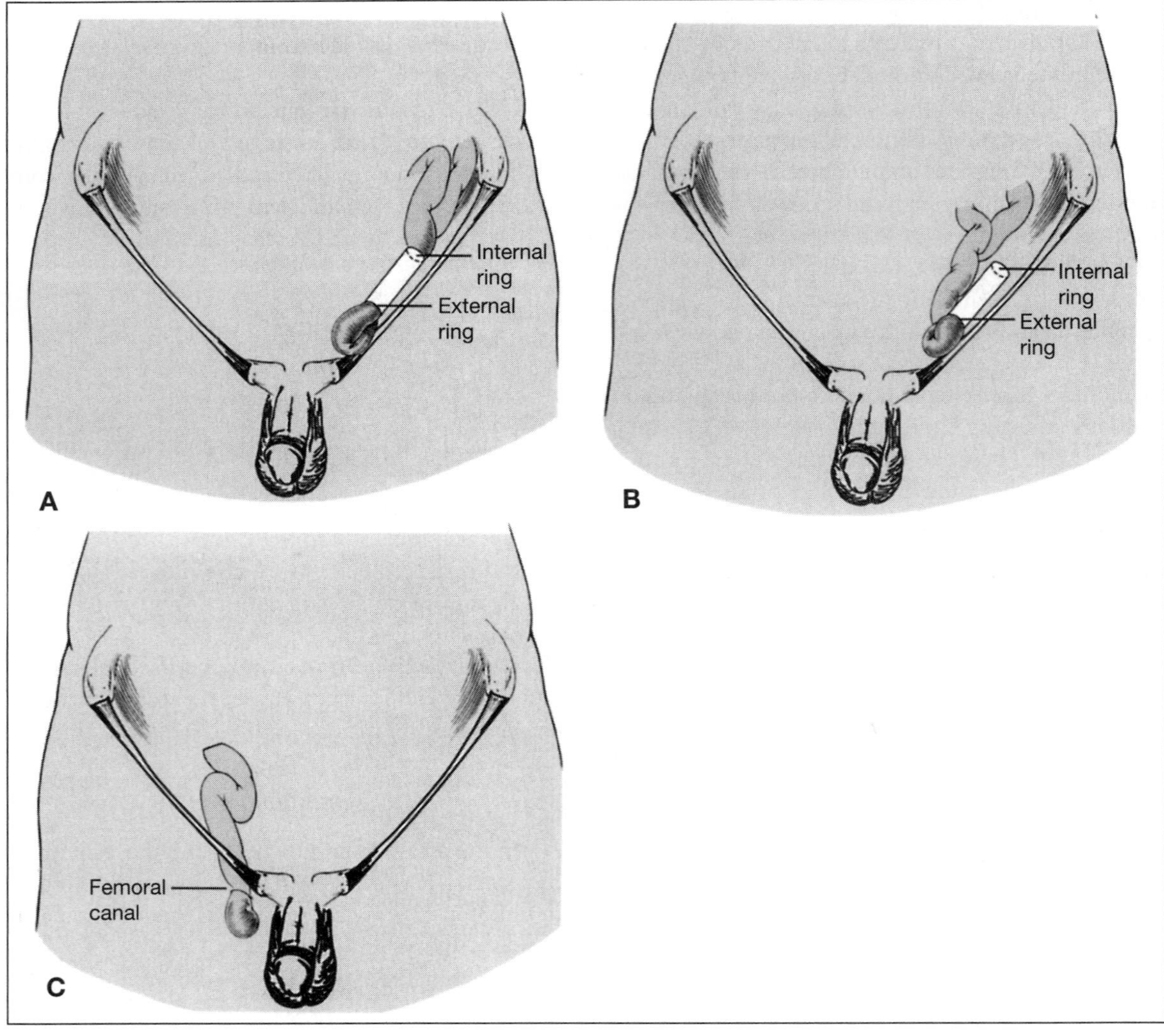

FIGURE 11.3 Pelvic hernias. A. Indirect hernia comes down the canal and touches the fingertip on examination. B. Direct hernia bulges anteriorly and pushes against the side of the finger on examination. C. Femoral hernia protrudes through the femoral ring, femoral canal, and fossa ovalis, so the inguinal canal is empty on examination.

Predisposing Factors

A. Pregnancy
B. Straining
C. Age
D. Obesity
E. Gender
F. Repetitive stress/hard physical labor
G. Congenital defect
H. Premature birth
I. Chronic cough
J. Chronic constipation
K. Family history of hernia
L. History of an abdominal aortic aneurysm (AAA)

Common Complaints

A. Bulging or swelling localized in the groin or scrotum
B. Dull ache in lower abdomen or groin
C. Swelling of labia majora in women
D. Children with inguinal hernias have minimal symptoms and may present with a history of an intermittent mass noted when straining or crying
E. Bowel obstruction

Other Signs and Symptoms

A. Ability to reduce hernia
B. Exacerbation on standing, straining, or coughing
C. Strangulation
  1. Colicky abdominal pain
  2. Nausea or vomiting
  3. Hyperperistalsis
  4. Fever
  5. Edema
  6. Discoloration
  7. Tenderness
D. Infants:
  1. Distress
  2. Vomiting
  3. Poor feeding
  4. Irritable and crying

Subjective Data

A. Review the time of onset, duration, and course of hernia, and swelling.
B. Review any symptoms and quality of pain. Outright pain with hernias is unusual, and its presence should raise the possibility of incarceration or strangulation.

C. Ask the patient about history of straining, trauma, physical labor, and pregnancy.
D. Inquire about symptoms of obstruction or strangulation of entrapped bowel: Pain, nausea, and vomiting. Groin pain and tenderness are generally absent in strangulated femoral hernias.
E. Determine if the patient can reduce the hernia.
F. Review irritating (e.g., exercise, straining, cough) and alleviating factors.
G. Review bowel habits, particularly constipation.
H. Evaluate history of COPD and cough.

Physical Examination

Physical examination is the same for all types of hernias and is directed at determining the type of hernia and whether it is reducible, incarcerated, or strangulated. Perform the examination while the patient is standing or supine. Palpation is best done with the patient standing.

A. Check temperature (if indicated), pulse, respirations, and blood pressure.
B. Inspect
  1. Inspect for discoloration and edema of the herniated area.
  2. Inspect for visible hernia. Instruct the patient to perform Valsalva's maneuver to increase intra-abdominal pressure.
  3. Transillumination of the scrotum is performed to evaluate any bowel contents
  4. Inspect for the presence of ascites.
C. Auscultate abdomen for bowel sounds.
D. Palpate
  1. Palpate the groin for lymphadenopathy, masses, and tenderness. *The right side is more commonly affected in both genders.*
    a. Males: Using the second or third finger, invaginate the scrotal skin, with and without cough and strain. There will be some degree of pressure with this maneuver, but a true hernia can typically be felt as a "silky" impulse tapping against the finger. Palpate the scrotum: Scrotal lump is either soft or unusually firm.
    b. Females: Visually examine for a bulge, and then place two or three fingers across the inguinal canal and ask the patient to bear down or cough to elicit the characteristic bulge or impulse. Palpate the labia for swelling: Either soft or unusually firm.

Diagnostic Tests

A. History and physical examination remain the best means of diagnosing hernias.
B. Ultrasonography for abdominal masses and strangulation
C. MRI appears to be able to differentiate inguinal and femoral hernias with a high sensitivity.
D. Sigmoidoscopy is not recommended as a screening test.
E. Plain abdominal x-rays are of limited value in the evaluation of an incarcerated hernia.
F. Karyotyping should be considered when a testicle is palpable in the inguinal canal or found at herniorrhaphy in phenotypic females
G. Routine laboratory work is not recommended.

Differential Diagnoses

A. Inguinal or pelvic hernia
B. Acute conditions
  1. Testicular torsion causes sudden, excruciating pain in or around the testicle, which may spread to the lower abdomen; the pain may get worse with standing. Other signs and symptoms include swelling, rising of the affected testicle, nausea, vomiting, fever, and fainting or lightheadedness.
  2. Epididymitis
C. Nonacute conditions
  1. Testicular tumor
  2. Muscle strain
  3. Hip arthritis
  4. Undescended testicle
  5. Hydrocele
  6. Varicocele
  7. Spermatocele
D. Bowel obstruction

Plan

A. Patient teaching
  1. Tell the patient to call the office right away if he finds a lump or swelling in the scrotum, even if it is small or painless. Testicular tumors are usually painless.
  2. Discuss the condition and treatment options with the patient.
    a. Surgery is the only effective treatment. Open hernia repair and laparoscopic repair are the two types of herniorrhaphy.
    b. Watchful waiting rather than surgical repair is an option if the patient is asymptomatic as long as he is aware of the risk and understands the need for prompt attention should symptoms of complication occur.
    c. Nonsurgical therapy for groin hernias is the use of a truss. There is insufficient data to determine the efficacy of trusses in controlling symptoms. A truss has the potential risk of bowel constriction; prolonged use of a truss can lead to atrophy of the spermatic cord or fusion to the hernial sac.
  3. Teach the patient signs of strangulation.
  4. Instruct the patient to avoid heavy lifting.
B. Medical and surgical management: Gently reduce a groin hernia while the patient lies supine with hips slightly flexed to relax the abdominal muscles.

Follow-Up

A. Tell the patient to return to the office if fever, severe pain, or strangulation occurs.
B. Postoperative evaluation for hernia recurrences as needed.
  1. Immediately from repair
  2. Greater than 6 months and up to 5 years from repair
  3. Late recurrences beyond 5 years from the repair

Consultation/Referral

A. Refer patients with femoral hernias to a physician. These hernias need to be repaired as soon as possible because of increased risk of incarceration and strangulation.

B. Contemporary practice triages surgical repair versus watchful waiting according to the severity of symptoms, type of hernia, and gender.

1. Females should undergo inguinal herniorrhaphy once a diagnosis is established instead of watchful waiting.

2. Surgical repair is indicated for males with moderate to severe symptoms from an inguinal hernia.

3. Surgical repair is indicated in men with scrotal or recurrent hernias, even though they are asymptomic or may only have minimal symptoms.

4. Strangulated hernias are nonreducible, and blood supply to protruded tissue is compromised. Refer patients for immediate surgical intervention.

Individual Considerations

A. Pregnancy

1. Preexisting groin hernias may become more symptomatic during the first trimester of pregnancy. The symptoms must be differentiated from round ligament pain.

2. Surgical repair of a groin hernia during a pregnancy is generally contraindicated. Generally, elective repair is deferred until 4 weeks postpartum.

B. Pediatrics

1. A high incidence (16%–25%) of inguinal hernias occurs in premature infants. The incidence is inversely related to weight.

2. In infants, the only symptom of a hernia may be increased irritability.

C. Geriatrics

1. Groin hernias are one of the most frequently encountered pathologies occurring in old age, secondary to the presence of constipation, coughing, abdominal fat deposits and loss of strength of the abdominal wall.

2. Signs and symptoms of prostatism are frequently present in men with hernias and may require relief before herniorrhaphy.

3. Excessive waiting time for elective repair increases the risk of strangulation, bowel resection, and mortality, especially with older patients.

Hirschsprung's Disease or Congenital Aganglionic Megacolon

Cheryl A. Glass

Definition

A. Hirschsprung's disease (HD) is the major cause of intestinal obstruction in newborns. HD is congenital or present at birth. HD is a motor disorder of the gut. The aganglionic segment is aperistaltic and remains in a state of contraction, causing a functional obstruction. The majority of HD patients are diagnosed in the neonatal period. Although infants appear normal at birth, more than half do not pass meconium for more than 48 hours. Absence of peristalsis causes feces to accumulate proximal to the defect and leads to intestinal obstruction. Bacterial enterocolitis is the most severe complication of untreated HD, and mortality from the complications may be as great as 25% to 30%.

Incidence

A. HD occurs in 1 in every 5,400 to 7,200 live births. It is uncommon in premature infants.

B. Occurrence is more common in males; however, long-segment disease increases in females. The incidence is roughly three times more common among Asian Americans.

C. About 10% to 50% of cases have familial incidence. Around eight genetic mutations have been identified. One in 100 children with Down syndrome also have HD.

D. HD is associated with other chromosomal abnormalities and syndromes:

1. Trisomy 21 (Down syndrome)

2. Cardiac disease (septal defects)

3. Bardet–Biedl syndrome (BBS)

4. Congenital central hypoventilation syndrome (CCHS)

5. Waardenburg syndrome

6. Smith–Lemli–Opitz syndrome

7. Multiple endocrine neoplasia type 2

8. Shprintzen–Goldberg syndrome

9. Piebaldism

10. Yemenite deaf–blind syndrome

11. Neurocristopathy syndromes

E. Approximately 80% of affected patients have the disorder limited to the rectum or rectosigmoid region.

F. From 3% to 5% of affected patients have aganglionosis of the entire colon.

G. The disease is three times more common in people of European ancestry.

H. Around 25% of HD patients have associated congenital anomalies of the kidney and urinary tract (hydronephrosis and renal hypoplasia).

Pathogenesis

A. The disorder is due to congenital absence of ganglion cells in both Meissner's (submucosal) and Auerbach's (myenteric) plexus. It occurs secondary to the failure of migration of ganglia from the neural crest, which normally occurs before the 12th week of gestation. The disorder starts in the distal rectum and extends proximally to involve a varying amount of the bowel.

Predisposing Factors

A. Full-term infant of normal weight

B. European ancestry

C. Male gender

D. Family history of disorder

E. Down syndrome

Common Complaints

A. Newborns: Failure to pass meconium for more than 48 hours

B. Blast sign: Explosive expulsion of gas and stool after the use of a digital rectal examination

C. Children: Failure to grow

D. Constipation

E. Abdominal distension

Other Signs and Symptoms

A. Newborns

1. Overflow-type diarrhea

2. Bile- or feces-stained vomitus
3. Failure to thrive (FTT)
4. Anorexia due to early satiety, abdominal discomfort, and distension
5. Temporary relief with enema

B. Older infants and children (nearly all children with HD are diagnosed during the first 2 years of life)
1. Constipation since birth; may have a history of requiring a daily enema
2. Older presentation is more common in breastfed infants; constipation will typically develop around the time of weaning.
3. Intestinal obstruction
4. Progressive abdominal distension with visible peristaltic activity
5. Temporary relief with enema
6. Ribbonlike, fluidlike, or pellet stools
7. FTT
8. Anemia

Subjective Data

A. In newborns, review the onset, duration, and course of symptoms, including number of bowel movements (BMs), passage of first stool, and expulsion of flatus.
B. Ask the patient or caregiver about family history of HD.
C. Review the infant's weight and growth parameters.
D. Inquire about other symptoms of bowel obstruction, such as vomiting and diarrhea.
E. Ask about other complications such as blood in stool.
F. Review the history of BMs and feeding habits, including onset of constipation, character of stools (ribbonlike or fluid filled), frequency of BMs, and use of enemas.

Physical Examination

A. Check temperature (if indicated), pulse, respirations, blood pressure, weight, and growth parameters, including length and head circumference.
B. Inspect
1. Note general appearance, level of activity, abdominal distension, and signs of malnutrition.
2. Inspect fontanelles for signs of dehydration.
3. Inspect the lower back for evidence of spinal cord involvement such as a hairy or hyperpigmented patch, gluteal fold asymmetry, cutaneous dimples, sinus tracts, and lipomas.

C. Auscultate the abdomen for bowel sounds in all quadrants.
D. Percuss the abdomen for organomegaly.
E. Palpate the abdomen for distension and masses. Specifically examine the left quadrant for the presence of stool.
F. Neurologic examination to evaluate other systemic disease related to constipation.
G. Rectal examination
1. Check for "tight" anal sphincter and absence of stool in rectal ampulla.
2. Many infants have relief of symptoms and pass large amounts of stool and flatus after examination (Blast sign).
3. Test the perineal sensation and the anocutaneous "wink" reflex by stroking the skin around the anus using a cotton-tipped swab.

Diagnostic Tests

A. Full-thickness rectal biopsy is considered the gold standard for diagnosis of HD. The biopsy is obtained by mucosal suction.
B. Contrast barium enema (BE): 25% of cases appear normal.
C. Anorectal manometry
D. Ultrasonography
E. Plain abdominal x-ray (distended bowel loops and air in the rectum)
F. Chemistry panel to evaluate fluid and electrolyte management

Differential Diagnoses

A. HD
B. Meconium peritonitis
C. Meconium plug syndrome
D. Meconium ileus
E. Intestinal obstruction
F. Enterocolitis
G. Megacolon (acute, chronic, or toxic)
H. Hypothyroidism
I. Constipation
J. Irritable bowel syndrome (IBS)

Plan

A. Patient teaching
1. Prepare caregivers or the patient for referral or consultation.
2. Teach caregivers or the patient about HD and treatment therapy.

B. Medical and surgical management
1. Treatment consists of colostomy performed proximal to aganglionic segment with biopsies taken at the time of surgery to identify level of involvement. Definitive repair can then be performed when the infant is 6 to 12 months old.
   a. There are two types of surgical procedures:
      i. Pull-through procedure involves removal of the affected part of the large intestine and anastomose to the healthy part of the anus.
      ii. Ostomy surgery reroutes the intestine through the abdominal wall, forming a stoma.
2. The mainstay of treatment is surgery; however, in older children when symptoms are chronic, but not severe, treatment may consist of isotonic enemas, stool softeners, and low-residue diet.

Follow-Up

A. Pediatric surgeons and gastroenterologists should generally care for children with HD.

Consultation/Referral

A. Consult or refer the patient to a physician if HD is suspected in an infant.

1. Bloody mucoid diarrhea in an infant with a history of constipation could be an indication of enterocolitis complicating HD.
2. An empty contracted anal canal in a constipated child may suggest HD.

B. Consider genetic testing.

Individual Considerations

A. Pediatrics
1. Recurrence risk is proportional to the length of aganglionic segment of the colon.
2. Infants who have symptom relief after rectal examination and pass large amounts of stool and gas (Blast sign) can have recurrence of symptoms, often fail to grow normally, can have constipation or diarrhea, and may have protein loss in their stool.

Hookworm

Cheryl A. Glass

Definition

A. Hookworm is a chronic, debilitating parasitic disease with vague symptoms that vary in proportion to the degree of iron-deficiency anemia and hypoproteinemia of the host. The adult hookworm attaches to the small intestinal wall and ingests the host's blood and nutrients. Chronic infection in children may lead to physical growth delay, cognitive deficits, and developmental delay. Anemia and hypoproteinemia are produced by the blood-clotting activity of adult nematodes in the intestines.

Incidence

A. Incidence in the United States is unknown. Globally, about 740 million are infected with hookworms.

Pathogenesis

A. Disease is caused by infection with *Ancylostoma duodenale, Ancylostoma ceylonicum,* and *Necator americanus* (soil-transmitted helminthes) intestinal parasites. Mixed infections are common. Humans are the major reservoir. *A. duodenale* may be ingested. Eggs of the nematode hatch into larvae that penetrate the soles of feet and palms of hands from contact with contaminated soil. Contact for 5 to 10 minutes results in skin penetration. Larvae are carried by circulation to lungs and eventually to their final habitat, the small intestines. Eggs are passed in stools of infected persons. Although hookworms are not transmitted from person to person, infected persons can contaminate soil by defecation as long as they are untreated.

B. Incubation period, or the time from exposure to eggs excreted in stool to the development of noncutaneous symptoms, is 4 to 12 weeks. The appearance of parasites in the blood is 4 to 6 weeks. Adult worms or larvae are rarely seen.

Predisposing Factors

A. Living in or traveling to rural, tropic, or subtropic areas where soil contamination with human feces is common

B. Exposure to loose, sandy, moist, shady, well-aerated, warm soil where larvae and eggs thrive

C. Agricultural workers

D. Tourists with bare feet or open footwear that exposes skin to contaminated soil

E. Military troops in endemic areas

F. Children

Common Complaints

A. Intense stinging or burning at penetration site, followed by pruritus and papulovesicular rash that persists for 1 to 2 weeks

B. Fatigue

C. Weight loss

D. Vague abdominal discomfort

E. Loss of appetite

Other Signs and Symptoms

A. **Anemia is the principal manifestation of hookworm infestation; it occurs secondary to blood loss.** *Severe anemia affects children and pregnant women disproportionately due to their preexisting iron stores.* **Severe anemia symptoms include:**
1. Fatigue
2. Syncope
3. Exertional dyspnea
4. Tachycardia
5. Pallor

B. Pharyngeal itching after oral ingestion

C. Hoarseness

D. Nausea or vomiting

E. Cough or wheeze from pulmonary infiltration due to heavy infestation

F. Colicky abdominal pain or diarrhea: Late sign, occurring with marked eosinophilia 29 to 38 days after exposure

G. Edema

H. Mild diarrhea

Subjective Data

A. Review the onset, duration, and course of symptoms, including recent episodes of intense itching of feet, palms of hands, or buttocks.

B. Establish patient's normal weight and amount of any weight lost, over what length of time.

C. Inquire about abdominal symptoms, including onset and intensity.

D. Review other gastrointestinal (GI) symptoms such as diarrhea.

E. Review any transitory chest symptoms, such as cough or wheezing. Is there a history of asthma?

F. Ask the patient if any other family members are exhibiting the same symptoms.

Physical Examination

A. Check temperature (if indicated), pulse, respirations, blood pressure, and weight.

B. Inspect skin on the entire body, especially the soles of both feet. Erythematous, papular vesicular lesions may be excoriated from scratching. Rash persists for 1 to 2 weeks.

C. Palpate the abdomen for masses and tenderness.

D. Auscultate the abdomen and lungs.

Diagnostic Tests

A. Identification of hookworm eggs in feces is diagnostic. Fecal egg excretion does not become detectable until around 2 months after dermal exposure. Repeated stool samples may be needed for diagnosis.
B. Hgb and hematocrit (Hct) for anemia
C. Complete blood count (CBC) with differential: May have mild eosinophilia.
D. Beaver direct smear, Stoll egg-counting, or Kato–Katz techniques quantify infection.
E. Endoscopic examination may reveal the adult worms.

Differential Diagnoses

A. Hookworm
B. Acute or chronic anemia
C. Asthma
D. Poor nutrition
E. Giardiasis
F. Amebiasis
G. Ascariasis
H. Gastroenteritis
I. Growth failure/failure to thrive (FTT)

Plan

A. Patient teaching
 1. Discuss the dangers of going barefoot outdoors with the patient.
 2. Explain that good handwashing is critical, especially after defecation.
 3. There is no direct person-to-person transmission.
 4. Use good sanitary practices to prevent soil contamination.
B. Dietary management: Teach the patient how to correct anemia through good nutrition.
C. Pharmaceutical therapy
The dosage is the same for children as adults.
 1. Mebendazole (Vermox) 100 mg orally twice a day for 3 days *or* a one-time single dose of 500 mg is a drug of choice.
  a. Mebendazole is available in the United States only through compounding pharmacies.
  b. The WHO recommends that 1-year-old children be given half of the dose (50 mg) prescribed for older children and adults.
 2. Albendazole (Albenza) 400 mg, one-time dose, is also a drug of choice.
 3. Pyrantel pamoate (Pyrantel) 11 mg/kg/d for 3 days; do not exceed 1 g/d.
 4. Thiabendazole applied topically
 5. Iron replacement therapy and nutritional supplements (proteins and vitamins including folate) may be needed to correct anemia.
 6. At the present time, there is no hookworm vaccine.
 7. Ivermectin (Stromectol) is ineffective against hookworms.

Follow-Up

A. Stool should be examined again 2 weeks after therapy is completed. If results are positive, repeat therapy is indicated.
B. Reinfection is common.
C. Iron supplement should be continued even after hemoglobin values return to normal.

Consultation/Referral

A. Refer pregnant patients to a physician.
B. Refer children to a physician if hemoglobin is less than 6 g/dL. Cardiac decompensation occasionally develops in children with hemoglobin concentrations of less than 6 g/dL.

Individual Considerations

A. Pregnancy
 1. Anthelmintics are in pregnancy category C; however, the potential risks to the fetus versus benefits should be considered.
 2. The WHO has determined that the benefit of pharmaceutical treatment outweighs its risk.
  a. WHO allows the use of albendazole in the second and third trimesters of pregnancy.
  b. WHO allows the use of pyrantel pamoate in the second and third trimesters of pregnancy.
 3. Adequate protein and iron nutrition should be maintained throughout pregnancy.
 4. Consider delaying treatment until after delivery if necessary.
B. Pediatrics
 1. All medications are advised for children.
  a. WHO guidelines for mass prevention campaigns indicate albendazole can be used in children as young as 1 year old.
  b. Mebendazole and pyrantel pamoate are on the WHO Model List of Essential Medicines for Children intended for the use in children up to 12 years of age.
 2. Severely affected children may require a blood transfusion.
 3. The physical and cognitive growth can be affected.

Irritable Bowel Syndrome

Cheryl A. Glass

Definition

Irritable bowel syndrome (IBS) is the most common of the gastrointestinal (GI) motility disorders. IBS is responsible for significant direct and indirect health care costs. It is a relapsing functional disturbance of intestinal motility marked by a common symptom complex that includes bloating and abdominal pain or discomfort associated with defecation. Bladder dysfunction has been identified in 50% of patients with IBS. Patients commonly transition between subgroups.

IBS is defined by symptom-based diagnostic criteria, in the absence of detectable organic causes. Rome III criteria for IBS are related to stool characteristics.

A. IBS with diarrhea predominant (IBS-D): Loose stools (small volume, pasty/mushy or watery) more than 25% of the time and hard stools less than 25% of the time

B. IBS with constipation (small, hard, pelletlike stools) predominant (IBS-C): Hard stools more than 25% of the time and loose stools less than 25% of the time

C. IBS with alternating bouts of constipation and diarrhea, mixed or cyclic pattern (IBS-M): Both hard and soft stools more than 25% of the time

D. On clinical grounds, other subclassifications are used.

- **1.** Based on symptoms
  - **a.** IBS with predominant bowel dysfunction
  - **b.** IBS with predominant pain
  - **c.** IBS with predominant bloating
- **2.** Based on precipitating factors
  - **a.** Postinfectious (PI-IBS)
  - **b.** Food induced (meal induced)
  - **c.** Stress related

Incidence

A. IBS is common, accounting for about 50% of GI complaints seen by health care professionals, and is a major cause of morbidity in the United States. Studies suggest nearly 20% of all adults suffer from some form of the condition; however, only a fraction seek medical help. IBS is recognized in children; symptoms consistent with IBS are reported in 16% of students aged 11 to 17 years. IBS is not described in preschool-aged children.

B. IBS with diarrhea is more common in men.

C. IBS with constipation is more common in women.

D. The American College of Gastroenterology (ACG) has recognized IBS as a key component of the Gulf War syndrome.

Pathogenesis

A. IBS has an absence of detectable pathology, and laboratory tests are unrevealing. The understanding of IBS has evolved from a disturbance in bowel motor activity to a more integrated understanding of visceral hypersensitivity and brain–gut interaction. It is thought to be both a normal response to severe stress and a learned visceral response to stress:

- **1.** Nonpropulsive colonic contractions lead to IBS-C predominant.
- **2.** Increased contraction in the small bowel and proximal colon with diminished activity in the distal colon lead to IBS-D predominant.

B. Most patients with functional disorders appear to have inappropriate perception of physiological events and altered reflex responses in different gut regions.

C. The brain–gut transmitters act at different sites in the brain and gut and lead to varied effects on GI motility, pain control, emotional behavior, and immunity. Serotonin plays a critical role in the regulation of GI motility, secretion, and sensation. Studies have shown that IBS may be related to an imbalance in mucosal serotonin and 5-hydroxytryptamine (5-HT) availability caused by defects in 5-HT production, serotonin receptors, or serotonin transport.

Predisposing Factors

A. Age

- **1.** IBS mainly occurs between the ages of 15 and 65 years.
  - **a.** About 50% of IBS occurs before age 35 years.
  - **b.** About 40% of IBS occurs between ages 35 and 50 years.

B. Gender

- **1.** Women are two to three times more likely to have IBS.
- **2.** In pediatrics, both sexes are equally affected.

C. Emotional factors and situational stress

D. Prior GI infection-induced IBS

E. Genetics is considered a factor.

F. Carbohydrate intolerance may produce significant symptoms.

Common Complaints

A. Chronic relapsing stool pattern

- **1.** Diarrhea, over three loose stools per day, *or*
- **2.** Alternation of diarrhea with constipation. Diarrhea is typically small in volume, has visible mucus, and may follow a hard movement by a few hours, *or*
- **3.** Constipation: Less than three bowel movements (BMs) per week.

B. Feeling of incomplete evacuation

C. Abdominal distension and bloating

D. Straining with BMs

E. Aching or cramps in periumbilical or lower abdominal region

F. Pain relief with BM

Other Signs and Symptoms

A. Change in bowel function

B. Clear mucus stool

C. Pain may be precipitated by meals

D. Pain radiates to the left chest or arm, from gas in splenic flexure. Nocturnal pain is unusual and is considered a warning sign.

E. Flatulence

F. Nausea

G. Anxiety

H. Depression

I. Preoccupation with bowel symptoms

J. Extraintestinal symptoms

- **1.** Dysmenorrhea
- **2.** Urinary frequency, urgency, and incomplete bladder emptying
- **3.** Impaired sexual function and dyspareunia
- **4.** Fibromyalgia

K. Menses may exacerbate IBS symptoms

L. Red-flag symptoms and differential diagnoses for IBS (see Table 11.15)

Subjective Data

A. Review pattern of main symptoms, including the onset, duration, and usual course.

B. Ask the patient what are the predominant symptoms—abdominal pain, diarrhea, or constipation.

C. Review the patient's history for stress factors, and ask whether recurrent symptoms occur in relation to them.

D. Ask what other symptoms occur with the pain, diarrhea, or constipation, such as bloating, blood in stool, or nighttime BMs. **Bleeding, weight loss, and nocturnal diarrhea are not characteristic of IBS. IBS symptoms disappear during sleep.**

E. Establish patient's normal weight history, and determine amount of weight loss, if any, over what time period.

TABLE 11.15 Common and Red-Flag Differential Diagnoses for IBS

Disorder	Signs and Symptoms	Diagnostic Tests
Ulcerative colitis	Peaks ages 15–35 years	Sigmoidoscopy, colonoscopy, BE
	Bloody diarrhea with mucus, fever, abdominal pain, tenesmus, weight loss	
Crohn's disease	Onset ages 15–35 or 70–80 years Fever, abdominal pain, diarrhea, fatigue, weight loss, anorectal fissures, fistulae, abscesses	Sigmoidoscopy, colonoscopy, BE
Infectious diarrhea	Chronic diarrhea with cramps with or without blood and mucus	Microscopy, stool studies, sigmoidoscopy
Diverticulitis	Lower left abdominal pain, fever, altered bowel habits	CBC, CT, BE
Colorectal malignancy	Age 50 years or older Rectal bleeding, altered bowel habits, abdominal or back pain, anemia, occult blood in stool, weight loss	Colonoscopy
Medication side effects	Antacids, laxatives, SSRIs, thyroid hormones, metformin, narcotics, calcium channel blockers, anticholinergics	History of concordance of symptoms with medication initiation, trial of drug holiday or reducing dosage, rechallenge

BE, barium enema; CBC, complete blood count; IBS, irritable bowel syndrome; SSRIs, selective serotonin reuptake inhibitors.

F. Review the patient's diet, including
 1. Response to milk or lactose products
 2. Artificial sweeteners
 3. Alcohol intake
 4. Irregular or inadequate meals
 5. Insufficient fluid intake
 6. Excessive fiber intake
 7. Obsession with dietary hygiene
 8. Response to gluten (wheat, barley, rye) ingestion

G. Inquire about the patient's prescription, herbal, and over-the-counter (OTC) medications. Ask specifically about the use of laxatives.

H. Review travel and food history for dominant history of diarrhea.

I. Ask the patient if there is a family history of colon cancer, ulcerative colitis (UC), Crohn's disease (CD), or malabsorption.

J. Is there any fever accompanying lower abdominal pain?

K. What is the relation of symptoms to menstruation?

Physical Examination

A. Check temperature (if indicated), pulse, respirations, blood pressure, and weight.

B. Inspect
 1. Observe general appearance. Does the patient appear anxious or depressed?
 2. Inspect abdominal contour for masses and bulges.

C. Auscultate all quadrants of the abdomen for bowel sounds; note whether they are normal or mildly hyperactive.

D. Percuss the abdomen for tympany or dullness.

E. Palpate the abdomen
 1. Evaluate the abdomen for mild tenderness, rigidity, guarding, and masses.
 2. Evaluate for hepatosplenomegaly.
 3. Evaluate for lymphadenopathy.

F. Rectal examination
 1. Check for masses and tenderness.
 2. Obtain stool for diagnostic tests.
 3. Rectal examination is normal with irritable bowel syndrome (IBS).

Diagnostic Tests

A. The AGA Task Force on IBS recommends that patients younger than 50 years who do not have alarm features need not undergo routine colonic imaging. Patients with IBS symptoms who have alarm features, such as anemia or weight loss, or those who are older than 60 years, should undergo colonic imaging to exclude organic disease.

B. Diagnosis of IBS is usually suspected on the basis of the patient's history and physical examination without additional tests (see Table 11.16).

C. Diagnostic tests are performed to exclude organic disease that may masquerade as IBS.
 1. Complete blood count (CBC)
 2. Sedimentation rate or C-reactive protein (CRP)
 3. Serum potassium, if the patient is on diuretics; hypokalemia may reduce bowel contractility and produce an ileus.
 4. Blood glucose, if diarrhea predominates; rule out diabetes mellitus, which may present as diarrhea resulting from diabetic gastroenteropathy.
 5. Thyroid function study
 6. Stool specimen: Culture for leukocytes and fat, ova and parasites, and occult blood; leukocyte-free mucus is a hallmark of IBS.
 7. Stool cultures for *C. difficile* toxin assay, if clinically indicated
 8. BE and/or proctosigmoidoscopy for severe signs and symptoms, after consultation or referral
 9. Celiac serology, if appropriate

TABLE 11.16 Rome III Diagnostic Criteria for IBS

Onset of symptoms at least 6 months before diagnosis
Recurrent abdominal pain or discomfort for more than 3 days per month during the past 3 months
At least two of the following features: A. Improvement with defecation B. Association with a change in frequency of stool C. Association with a change in stool form

IBS, irritable bowel syndrome

10. A mucosal biopsy is appropriate if a colonoscopy or sigmoidoscopy is performed
11. Esophagogastroduodenoscopy (EGD) and distal duodenal biopsy in patients with diarrhea should be considered to rule out celiac disease, tropical sprue, giardiasis, and for patients in whom abdominal pain and discomfort is located more in the upper abdomen
12. Hydrogen breath test to evaluate lactose intolerance and small-intestinal bowel overgrowth (SIBO)

Differential Diagnoses

A. IBS
B. Inflammatory bowel disease (IBD; CD/UC)
C. Viral or bacterial gastroenteritis
D. GI neoplasm
E. Acute diarrhea caused by protozoa or bacteria
F. Lactose insufficiency/deficiency
G. Laxative abuse
H. Drug side effect
I. Diabetes
J. Celiac spruce/gluten etiology
K. Diverticulitis
L. FTT in children
M. Endometriosis/PID
N. Zollinger–Ellison syndrome
O. Diverticulitis

Plan

A. General interventions
   1. Advise the patient to keep a diary of events of BMs and precipitating factors.
   2. Encourage the patient to quit smoking because nicotine may aggravate symptoms.
   3. Recommend daily exercise to reduce stress.
   4. Stress management should be encouraged, including counseling, tapes, meditation, and yoga.

▶ B. Patient teaching: *See Section III: Patient Teaching Guide for this chapter, "Irritable Bowel Syndrome."*

C. Dietary management
   1. Prescribe a high-fiber diet.
   2. Tell the patient to avoid foods that aggravate the bowel, including gas-producing foods, such as broccoli, beans, onions, garlic, and so forth. When diarrhea predominates, dietary review is essential for clues of intolerance to lactose or sorbitol.

D. Pharmaceutical therapy
   1. Tell the patient to stop all nonessential medications that may affect bowel function, especially irritant laxatives. Avoid narcotics, depressants, and other long-term drug use if possible.
   2. Recommend eliminating sorbitol-containing candy and restricting lactose-containing milk products.
   3. Drug of choice: Psyllium hydrophilic mucilloid (Metamucil) 1 tablespoon per day in 8 oz of juice or water, followed with another 8 oz of liquid. This treats both diarrhea and constipation.
   4. Pain relief
      a. Opiates should be avoided due to the risk of dependence and addiction in chronic conditions.
      b. Nonsteroidal anti-inflammatory drugs (NSAIDs) have an undesirable side effect on the GI tract.
      c. Antispasmodics and anticholinergic agents (IBS-D predominant):
         i. Hyoscyamine (Levsin, Levbid)
            1) Levsin 0.125 to 0.25 mg (1–2 tablets) orally or sublingual every 4 hours; not to exceed 12 tablets a day.
            2) Levbid tablets for adults and pediatric patients 12 years or older: Take 2 tablets every 12 hours. Do not crush or chew tablets, not to exceed 4 tablets in 24 hours.
            3) Pediatric doses are dependent on age and weight.
            4) Hyoscyamine is available in immediate-release, extended-release, time capsules, biphasic tablets, elixir, and drop formulations.
         ii. Dicyclomine (Bentyl) 20 to 40 mg four times a day; discontinue if not effective within 2 weeks or if 80 mg daily is associated with adverse effects. Also available in intramuscular formulation.
      d. Tricyclic antidepressants for diarrhea-predominant IBS. Tricyclics should be avoided for constipated patients.
         i. Amitriptyline (Elavil) 10 mg every bedtime initially; titrate up slowly to 75 mg/d at bedtime as needed
         ii. Desipramine (Norpramin) 10 mg every bedtime initially; titrate up slowly up to 75 mg/d
         iii. Imipramine (Tofranil) 10 to 50 mg orally every bedtime
   5. Selective serotonin reuptake inhibitors (SSRIs)
      a. Paroxetine (Paxil) 10 to 60 mg/d
      b. Citalopram (Celexa) 5 to 60 mg/d
   6. Antidiarrheals
      a. Opiate-derived medications are reserved for very severe cases secondary to the potential for abuse.
      b. Loperamide (Imodium)
         i. Adults: 2 to 12 mg orally in divided twice a day/three times daily doses; doses differ greatly among individuals.
         ii. Pediatrics older than 2 years: 0.08 mg to 0.24 mg/kg/d orally divided in twice a day/three times daily doses; not to exceed 2 mg/dose.

c. Alosetron (Lotronex), a 5-HT_3 receptor antagonist, is indicated only for women with severe IBS-D predominant. Starting dose is 0.5 mg twice a day, may increase to 1 mg twice a day (bid) after 4 weeks of starting dose. Discontinue if no relief after 4 weeks of 1 mg dosing.

7. Laxatives and stool softeners (IBS-C predominant) along with dietary measures and fiber supplements.

a. Mineral oil 15 to 45 mL orally daily or in divided three times daily dosing.

b. Stimulant laxatives may be necessary intermittently for short periods, but prolonged use of stimulant laxatives should be avoided.

c. Lactulose is a colonic acidifier that promotes laxation. Transit time through the colon may be slow; 24 to 48 hours may be required to produce a bowel movement. The usual dose is 1 to 2 tablespoons daily. Lactulose contains galactose and lactose and should be used with caution for patients with diabetes. Safety in pediatric patients has not been established.

8. Lubiprostone (Amitiza), a selective C-2 chloride-channel activator, is indicated for women 18 years and over with IBS-C predominant. 8 mcg twice a day with food and water.

9. Probiotics

10. Linaclotide (LINZESS), guanylate cyclase-C (GC-C) agonist is used for both IBS-C and chronic idiopathic constipation (CIC).

11. Eluxadoline (Viberzi), a mu-opioid receptor agonist, is indicated for IBS-D predominant. There are two recommended dosings:

a. Dosing is 100 mg tablet twice a day taken with food.

b. The alternative dosing is 75 mg twice a day taken with food for patients with the following conditions:

i. Do not have a gallbladder

ii. Unable to tolerate 100 mg bid

iii. Are receiving concomitant OATP1B1 inhibitor, such as the lipid-lowering drug gemfibrozil and its metabolite gemfibrozil 1 O β.

iv. Have mild or moderate hepatic impairment

c. If a dose is missed, patients should not compensate by taking two doses at once.

Follow-Up

A. Reevaluate the effectiveness of treatment in 2 weeks. Treatment may be challenging for symptom management and numerous tests that are inconclusive but rule out pathology.

B. If symptoms persist without relief, have the patient return as needed.

C. Return if diarrhea/constipation lasts more than 2 weeks on medication therapy.

Consultation/Referral

A. Refer to a gastroenterologist for red-flag symptoms.

B. Refer to a pediatric gastroenterologist if findings from the patient's history, physical examination, or screening laboratory tests are suggestive of organic disease.

C. Alosetron (Lotronex) is prescribed under a restricted distribution program through a gastroenterologist.

D. Consult a physician if all treatment options fail.

E. Consider a psychiatric consultation, if indicated for anxiety, depression, somatization, and symptom-related fears.

Individual Considerations

A. Pediatrics

1. IBS is recognized in children, and many patients trace the onset of symptoms to childhood.

2. Children who have a history of recurrent abdominal pain are at increased risk of IBS during adolescence and young adulthood.

3. The recommended daily intake of fiber (in grams) for children is estimated by adding four to their age in years.

B. Adults

1. Annual rectal examination and sigmoidoscopy are recommended after age 50 years.

2. When constipation predominates, rule out malignancy, particularly in patients older than age 40 years who have weight loss or a family history of colon cancer.

Resource

Rome Foundation: http://romecriteria.org/criteria

Jaundice

Cheryl A. Glass

Definition

A. Jaundice is a yellow tinge to the skin or mucous membranes. It is a symptom, not a disease. The diagnostic approach begins with gathering a comprehensive history, physical examination, and screening laboratory tests. The differential diagnosis is formulated, and further testing may be warranted. The onset of jaundice usually prompts the patient or family to seek medical attention. Jaundice can reflect a medical emergency secondary to massive hemolysis, ascending cholangitis, unconjugated hyperbilirubinemia in the neonatal period, and fulminant liver failure.

Incidence

A. Incidence is variable according to pathogenesis, age, and population.

Pathogenesis

The mechanism responsible for jaundice includes excess bilirubin production, decreased hepatic uptake, impaired conjugation, intrahepatic cholestasis, extrahepatic obstruction, and hepatocellular injury (see Table 11.17).

However, it is important to recognize that more than one mechanism can be operating in a given case (i.e., sickle cell anemia and HIV).

A. Excess bilirubin production results from accelerated red cell destruction. The excessive amounts of hemoglobin and resultant bilirubin released into the bloodstream overwhelm the liver's normal capacity for uptake, and an unconjugated hyperbilirubinemia ensues.

TABLE 11.17 Classification of Jaundice According to Bile Pigment and by Mechanism

Unconjugated Hyperbilirubinemia	Conjugated Hyperbilirubinemia
Increased/overproduction of bilirubin	Hepatocellular injury/disease
Impaired/decreased hepatic uptake of bilirubin	Intrahepatic cholestasis
Impaired/decreased conjugation	Extrahepatic cholestasis (biliary obstruction)

B. With decreased uptake and conjugation, there is often a concurrent, acquired illness such as infection, cardiac disease, or cancer. Hereditary conditions, such as Gilbert and Crigler–Najjar syndromes, are responsible.
C. Intrahepatic cholestasis may occur at a number of levels: Intracellularly (e.g., hepatitis), at the canalicular level (when estrogen is induced), at the ductule (phenothiazine exposure), at the septal ducts (primary biliary cirrhosis), and at the intralobular ducts (cholangiocarcinoma).
D. Extrahepatic obstruction occurs when a stone, stricture, or tumor blocks the flow of bile within the extrahepatic biliary tree. A history of gallstones, biliary tract surgery, or malignancy may be elicited.

Predisposing Factors

A. Previous blood transfusion
B. Travel to an area endemic for hepatitis
C. Raw shellfish consumption
D. Intravenous (IV) drug abuse
E. High-risk sexual practices
F. Family history of episodic jaundice
G. History of gallstones
H. Biliary obstruction/previous biliary tract surgery
I. Alcoholism
J. Chemical exposure
K. Working in the health care profession
L. Sickle cell disease
M. Pregnancy (intrahepatic cholestasis)
N. Cancer

Common Complaints

A. Pruritus
B. Dark, tea-colored urine, from conjugated bilirubinuria
C. Light, clay-colored stools, from absence of bile
D. Fatigue
E. Right upper quadrant (RUQ) pain

Other Signs and Symptoms

A. Enlarged liver
B. Splenomegaly
C. Fever
D. Chills
E. Gastrointestinal (GI): Appetite loss, weight loss, abdominal pain, nausea, or vomiting
F. Ascites

TABLE 11.18 Drugs and Herbals Associated With Jaundice

ACE inhibitors
Acetaminophen (Tylenol)
Alkylated steroids
Aminobenzoic acid
Antibiotics
Antidiabetic drugs
Arsenic
Chloramphenicol
Chlorpromazine
Ethinyl estradiol/oral contraceptives/hormone replacement
Herbal medications (e.g., Jamaican bush tea)
Isoniazid (INH)
Mercaptopurine (Purinethol)
Methyldopa (Aldomet)
Monoamine oxidase inhibitors Nitrofurantoin
Perphenazine (Trilafon)
Phenothiazine derivatives
Propylthiouracil (PTU) Probenecid
Rifampin
Sulfonamides
Tamoxifen
Total parenteral nutrition (TPN)

G. Shortness of breath
H. Palpitations
I. Ecchymosis
J. Steatorrhea, severe
K. Asterixis (tremor)
L. Myalgias
M. Malaise

Subjective Data

A. Review the onset, duration, and course of symptoms.
B. Review medication history for drugs/herbals that may induce jaundice (see Table 11.18).
C. Inquire about recent blood transfusions. Are there any known blood disorders in the patient's family history?
D. Ask about contact with a person who has an infection, such as infectious hepatitis.
E. Ask about unprotected sexual activity/HIV status.
F. Review ingestion of potentially contaminated food or water, including *Amanita* mushrooms, milk, or shellfish.
G. Ask about the patient's exposure to any toxic chemicals, such as carbon tetrachloride, chloroform, phosphorus, arsenic, ethanol, or halothane (Fluothane).
H. Review the patient's history of nonsterile needle punctures.
I. Review the patient's medical/surgical history for gallstones, hepatitis, tumor, pancreatitis, Wilson's disease,

Budd–Chiari syndrome, liver surgery, or transplantation. Is there a family history of gallstones?

J. Ask how much alcohol the patient has ingested over the years.

K. Ask about dark urine or white or clay-colored stool.

L. Inquire about dyspepsia, anorexia, nausea, vomiting, RUQ or epigastric pain, or pain radiating to back or shoulder blade. Ask about the relationship of pain to eating?

M. Inquire about fever, fatigue, malaise, loss of vigor and strength, easy bruising, and weight loss.

N. Review travel history.

Physical Examination

A. Check temperature (if indicated), pulse, respirations, blood pressure, and weight. Marked weight loss accompanied by jaundice suggests carcinoma of the head of the pancreas or metastatic disease obstructing the common duct. Note breath odor for fetor hepaticus (breath of the dead).

B. Inspect

- **1.** Skin, mouth, palms, and sclera for yellow tinge. Severe jaundice may cause greenish tinge from oxidation of bilirubin to biliverdin.
  - **a.** In fair-skinned people, discoloration is most evident on the face, trunk, and sclera (sclera icterus).
  - **b.** In dark-skinned people, discoloration is most evident in sclera and roof of mouth.
  - **c.** In newborns, jaundice first appears over the face or upper body, then progresses over larger areas; it can also be seen in conjunctivae of the eyes.
  - **d.** Jaundice is most noticeable in natural sunlight. In artificial or poor light, it may be hard to detect.
- **2.** The skin for spider angiomata, rashes or scratches from severe itching due to pruritus, and for bruising or petechiae
- **3.** The palms for erythema or overt bleeding
- **4.** The chest for gynecomastia

C. Palpate the abdomen for tenderness, masses, liver enlargement in RUQ, and ascites.

- **1.** Extrahepatic obstruction and intrahepatic cholestasis may be identical in presentation.
- **2.** Tenderness is minimal unless cholangitis or rapid distension occur.
- **3.** Splenomegaly is unlikely except in primary biliary cirrhosis.
- **4.** Gallbladder may be palpable (Courvoisier sign). Sudden onset of pain results from passage of stone that becomes wedged into a common duct; fever and sepsis shortly thereafter indicates cholangitis.
- **5.** Malignancy usually presents as a rock-hard mass.
- **6.** Absence of abdominal pain does not rule out obstruction, especially when it develops slowly from tumor growth or primary biliary cirrhosis.
- **7.** Advanced hepatocellular disease is indicated by a small liver, signs of portal hypertension (ascites, splenomegaly, prominent abdominal venous pattern), asterixis, peripheral edema (from hypoalbuminemia), spider angiomata, gynecomastia, palmar erythema, and testicular atrophy.

D. Percuss the abdomen.

E. Auscultate the heart, lungs, and abdomen for bowel sounds.

F. Neurologic examination

- **1.** Note level of consciousness.
- **2.** Asterixis test can be used to test for peripheral neuritis caused by impaired liver function. Screen for a flapping tremor occurring with wrist dorsiflexed.

G. Rectal examination: Check for masses and occult blood.

Diagnostic Tests

The diagnostic approach begins with a careful history, physical examination, and screening laboratory studies. A differential is formulated and appropriate further testing is performed to narrow the diagnosis.

A. Initial laboratory tests

- **1.** Serum bilirubin: Direct, indirect (unconjugated), and total; clinically, jaundice becomes noticeable when levels reach 2.0 to 2.5 mg/dL.
  - **a.** Intrahepatic cholestasis and extrahepatic obstruction: Elevated conjugated bilirubin, elevated serum alkaline phosphatase (ALP), mild to moderate rise in transaminase
  - **b.** Gilbert syndrome is the most common cause of decreased uptake and unconjugated hyperbilirubinemia. It is a benign disorder that produces recurrent self-limited episodes of mild jaundice. Typically, the unconjugated fraction rises to no more than 1.5 to 3.0 mg/100 mL. In Gilbert syndrome, fasting and minor illness can precipitate jaundice.
- **2.** ALP
- **3.** Aspartate transaminase (AST)/alanine transaminase (ALT)
  - **a.** Elevation of ALT and AST may indicate liver cell damage or may be caused by opiates and aspirin.
  - **b.** Aspirin may also decrease AST and ALT.
- **4.** Prothrombin time (PT)
  - **a.** PT may be prolonged due to malabsorption, but it is reversible by vitamin K injection.
  - **b.** Prolonged PT unresponsive to parenteral vitamin K strongly suggests hepatocellular failure.
  - **c.** Cholestasis and obstruction may also produce prolongation of PT but can be reversed by vitamin K.
  - **d.** Phenazopyridine (Pyridium) may cause a false-positive bilirubin result.

B. Other laboratory testing as needed

- **1.** Total serum protein
- **2.** Serum albumin and globulin
  - **a.** Albumin decreases with cirrhosis and chronic hepatitis.
  - **b.** Globulin increases with cirrhosis, chronic obstructive jaundice, and viral hepatitis.
  - **c.** To interpret albumin level, consider dietary intake and sources of possible protein loss.
- **3.** Cholesterol
- **4.** Lactate dehydrogenase (LDH)
- **5.** Gamma-glutamyl transpeptidase (GGT)

6. Serum ammonia
7. Bile acid radioimmunoassay: Elevated levels indicate hepatic disease.
8. Serologic tests for viral hepatitis
9. Serum iron, transferrin, and ferritin to evaluate hemochromatosis
10. Serum ceruloplasmin levels to evaluate Wilson's disease
11. Alpha-1 antitrypsin activity to evaluate alpha-1 antitrypsin deficiency
12. Urine for bilirubin-bilirubinuria may be an early sign of liver disease
   a. Collect specimens over a 2-hour period after lunch.
   b. Place specimen in a dark brown container and send to the laboratory immediately to prevent decomposition.

C. Abdominal ultrasound is considered the screening procedure of choice. More selective imaging procedures are ordered based on clinical evaluation.
D. Other imaging procedures
   1. Endoscopic ultrasound
   2. HIDA scan: Uses radioactive isotopes
   3. Oral cholecystography
   4. Endoscopic retrograde cholangiopancreatography (ERCP)
   5. Percutaneous transhepatic cholangiography (PTC)
   6. Helical CT
   7. Magnetic resonance cholangiopancreatography (MRCP) is an alternative to ERCP.
   8. Liver biopsy may be indicated for definitive diagnosis.

Differential Diagnoses

A. Jaundice is a symptom, not a diagnosis.
B. Cancer of pancreas
C. Obstruction of biliary tract
D. Icteric phase of hepatitis
E. Cirrhosis
F. Right-sided heart failure (HF)
G. Chronic hemolysis from prosthetic heart valve

Plan

A. Management depends on primary diagnosis. Most patients can be managed on an ambulatory basis, unless they are unable to maintain hydration or begin to show evidence of severe hepatocellular failure.
B. Cholestyramine 2 to 8 g orally twice a day may be used to help relieve itching. Cholestyramine is ineffective with complete biliary obstruction.

Follow-Up

A. See the patient 2 to 4 weeks after initial diagnosis and referral.
B. Subsequent routine evaluations are related to primary diagnosis.

Consultation/Referral

A. Consult with a gastroenterologist familiar with liver disease and needle biopsy techniques when hepatocellular disease is suspected; when there is evidence of hepatic failure, portal hypertension, or encephalopathy; or when jaundice persists longer than 3 months.
B. Consultation with a gastroenterologist, surgeon, or radiologist experienced in evaluation of jaundice can be very useful when there is clinical suspicion of extrahepatic obstruction.
C. Admission is mandatory when jaundice is complicated by a fever and peritoneal signs indicative of cholangitis. IV antibiotics and prompt surgical consultation are required.

Individual Considerations

A. Pregnancy
   1. Viral hepatitis is the most frequent cause of jaundice in pregnancy.
   2. Intrahepatic cholestasis in pregnancy is associated with modest maternal risks, including increased risk of peripartum bleeding and increased likelihood of subsequent cholelithiasis.
   3. Cholestyramine resin, generally 4 g every 4 to 6 hours, has been reported to afford some relief of pruritus in 50% of affected women, presumably by removing a portion of the bile acids by irreversible binding in the gut.
   4. Pregnant women who take cholestyramine are at increased risk for depletion of vitamin K–dependent coagulation factors and should be followed with serial PT times. Such women should also receive prophylactic vitamin K supplementation. If PT becomes prolonged, medication should be discontinued.
   5. Liver dysfunction and jaundice are common in patients with hyperemesis gravidarum.
B. Pediatrics
   1. Hepatitis predominates as a cause of jaundice.
   2. Neonatal jaundice is more common when the mother is an insulin-dependent diabetic, probably resulting from a higher hematocrit (Hct) developed in utero, especially if oxygen availability is decreased. Newborn jaundice due to liver immaturity is common. It begins on day 2, peaks at 1 week, and disappears in 2 to 3 weeks. About half of all full-term newborns and 90% of premature newborns have some degree of jaundice. Jaundice is usually mild and can be treated with hydration and ultraviolet lamp exposure.
   3. Intense, persistent jaundice suggests liver disease or severe, overwhelming infection.
   4. In Rh isoimmunization infants without appropriate treatment (exchange transfusion), progressive jaundice leads to brain damage (kernicterus), death, or severe handicap (deafness, spasticity, and choreoathetosis).
   5. Acute jaundice in young, healthy individuals suggests acute viral hepatitis.
   6. An overdose of acetaminophen is a common cause of jaundice in the young adult.
C. Geriatrics
   1. The most frequent cause of jaundice in patients older than 65 years is cholelithiasis.
   2. The second most frequent cause of jaundice for patients 65 years and older is cancer, especially of the gallbladder.

3. Painless jaundice in the elderly with weight loss and a mass, but with minimal pruritus, suggests biliary obstruction caused by cancer.

Malabsorption

Cheryl A. Glass

Definition

A. Malabsorption syndrome is a group of signs and symptoms that occur as a result of digestive problems and problems with absorption of nutrients. There may be a resultant decrease in absorption of fat-soluble vitamins A, D, E, and K. Poor absorption of carbohydrates, minerals, and proteins may also occur.
B. The presentation of malabsorption varies from severe overt symptoms with weight loss to discrete oligosymptomatic changes in hematologic/laboratory tests that are found incidentally. Malabsorption can result from congenital defects or from acquired defects, such as bariatric surgery, and may be either global or partial. The degree of nutrient malabsorption from bariatric surgery is dependent on the type of bariatric procedure.

Incidence

A. Incidence is unknown.

Pathogenesis

A. Deficiency of intestinal enzymes: Lactase deficiency
B. Inadequate digestion caused by disease of the pancreas (such as cystic fibrosis [CF]), pancreatic cancer, gallbladder, or liver
C. Change in bacteria that normally live in the intestinal tract
D. Disease of intestinal walls, such as helminths (worms) or parasites, tropical sprue, and celiac disease
E. Surgery that reduces the intestinal tract, decreasing the area for absorption such as bariatric surgery
F. Intolerance to gluten or celiac sprue
G. Atrophic gastritis results in hypochlorhydria and achlorhydria. The body does not produce enough pepsin and hydrochloric acid to release the food-bound vitamin B_{12} from protein.

Predisposing Factors

A. Lactose deficiency
   1. Incidence is increased in African Americans, Indians, and Asians.
   2. Jews typically have onset in adulthood.
B. Family history of malabsorption or CF
C. Use of drugs, such as mineral oil or other laxatives
D. Excess alcohol consumption
E. Travel to foreign countries
F. Intestinal surgery
   1. Partial or total gastrectomy
   2. Small-bowel resections (jejunum, ileum, ileocecal)
   3. Partial or total resection of the pancreas
G. Chronic pancreatitis
H. Advanced age (increased risk for malabsorption and malnutrition)
I. Long-term adherence to a strict vegetarian or vegan diet (exclusion of all forms of animal protein, including eggs and dairy products)
J. HIV infection

Common Complaints

A. Diarrhea stools that are pale, greasy, and copious
B. Foul-smelling stools, frequently with mucus
C. Weight loss despite adequate food intake
D. Gas or vague abdominal discomfort
E. Anorexia

Other Signs and Symptoms

A. Early malabsorption
   1. Minimal weight loss
   2. Softer, more frequent stools
   3. Steatorrhea; stools "float" because of increased trapped gas
   4. Abdominal discomfort
   5. Bloating
B. Later signs: Aforementioned symptoms plus the following:
   1. Marked weight loss
   2. Foul-smelling, bulky, greasy stools
C. Malabsorption of fats and carbohydrates: Previous symptoms plus the following:
   1. Foul-smelling, bulky, greasy, "sticky" stools that may be difficult to flush down the toilet
   2. Ecchymosis
   3. Bone pain
   4. Glossitis
   5. Muscle tenderness
   6. Cramping in lower abdomen after bowel movement (BM)
D. Malabsorption of lactose
   1. Nausea and bloating
   2. Cramps
   3. Diarrhea after ingesting more than customary intake of milk products
   4. Absent or mild weight loss and steatorrhea
   5. Good appetite
E. Edema: With severe protein depletion
F. Ecchymosis and bleeding disorders secondary to vitamin K malabsorption
G. Vitamin malabsorption
   1. Generalized motor weakness (pantothenic acid, vitamin D)
   2. Peripheral neuropathy (thiamine)
   3. Sense of loss for vibration and position (cobalamin)
   4. Night blindness (vitamin A)
   5. Seizures (biotin)

Subjective Data

A. Review the onset, duration, and course of symptoms. Are there any other family members with the same history/symptoms?
B. Ask the patient about dietary intake history.
C. Review any changes in BMs and stool characteristics.
D. Inquire about recent travel to areas known for giardiasis or other parasites.

E. Document weight loss, how much, and over what period of time.
F. Review previous gastrointestinal (GI) surgery, including the bariatric procedures and reversals, small-bowel resections, and partial or total resection of the pancreas.
G. Ask the patient about signs and symptoms of inflammatory bowel disease (IBD), such as easy bruising, paresthesia, and sore tongue.
H. Ask about any irradiation treatment.

Physical Examination

A. Check temperature, pulse, respirations, blood pressure (may have orthostatic hypotension), and weight. Follow serial weight loss and plot on growth charts.
B. Inspect
   1. Observe general appearance, noting wasting and apathetic appearance.
   2. If the patient experiences a BM after the examination, observe the stool for volume, appearance, presence of blood, mucus, and the presence of gross worms/parasites.
   3. Inspect the skin for ecchymosis, jaundice, pallor, surgical scars, stigmata of hyperthyroidism or hepatocellular failure, or signs of Kaposi's sarcoma. Alopecia or seborrheic dermatitis may be present.
   4. Inspect the ears, nose, and throat for glossitis, stomatitis, aphthous ulcers, poor dentition, and goiter.
C. Auscultate
   1. The heart for tachycardia
   2. The abdomen in all four quadrants for bowel sounds noting borborygmi
D. Percuss the abdomen.
E. Palpate
   1. All lymph nodes; look for lymphadenopathy
   2. The abdomen for organomegaly, focal tenderness, masses, distension, and ascites
F. Neurologic examination: Assess for signs of vitamin B_{12} deficiency, including motor weakness, peripheral neuropathy, or ataxia.
G. Rectal examination: Note tenderness, discharge, blood, and stool.

Diagnostic Tests

A. Assessment of stool fat: Qualitative assessment on a single specimen.
B. Quantitative assessment of a 72-hour stool collection while the patient is following a 100 g fat/d diet.
C. Increased fecal fat: Test for celiac disease.
D. Abdominal ultrasound
E. Colonoscopy to evaluate and obtain biopsies
F. Endoscopy to evaluate and obtain biopsies
G. Barium studies
H. Consider CT of the abdomen
I. Endoscopic retrograde cholangiopancreatography (ERCP) helps to document malabsorption due to pancreatic or biliary-related disorders.
J. Breath tests for carbohydrate malabsorption
K. Complete blood count (CBC) and electrolytes
L. Serum iron, vitamin B_{12}, and folate concentrations
M. Prothrombin time (PT): May be prolonged due to vitamin K deficiency
N. Vitamin levels: Vitamins A, D, E, and K may be decreased.
O. Total protein: May be decreased
P. Albumin: May be decreased
Q. Serum amylase
R. Stool for ova and parasites; obtain on alternate days for three or more specimens because parasites are passed intermittently.
S. Serum IgA-used to rule out IgA deficiency
T. Three-stage Schilling test (vitamin B_{12} deficiency)

Differential Diagnoses

A. Malabsorption
B. AIDS
C. Alcoholism
D. Worms or parasites
E. CF
F. Failure to thrive (FTT)
G. Crohn's disease (CD)
H. Tropical sprue
I. Side effect from bariatric surgery
J. Disaccharidase deficiencies (lactase)
K. Fructose intolerance
L. Milk or protein allergy
M. Whipple disease
N. Zollinger–Ellison syndrome
O. Chronic pancreatitis
P. Cirrhosis

Plan

A. General interventions: Treatment depends on underlying cause.
B. Patient teaching: *See Section III: Patient Teaching Guide for this chapter, "Lactose Intolerance and Malabsorption."* ◀
C. Dietary management: In most patients, diet modification, such as gluten-free diet for celiac disease, or dietary supplements restore health.
D. Pharmaceutical therapy
   1. Vitamin supplements: Fat-soluble vitamins A, D, and K are most likely to be depleted. Supplements help prevent malnutrition, even though caloric intake may be replenished.
      a. Vitamin A: 25,000 to 50,000 U/d orally
      b. Vitamin D: 30,000 U/d orally
      c. Vitamin K: 4 to 12 mg/d orally
      d. Vitamin B_{12}: 1,000 g/mo by IM injection
   2. Enzyme replacements: These replace endogenous exocrine pancreatic enzymes and aid in digestion of starches, fat, and proteins. Pancreatic supplements are typically expressed in U.S. Pharmacopeia Convention (USP) units. One international unit (IU) is equivalent to approximately 2 to 3 USP units.
      a. Pancreatin, adults and children: Doses vary with the condition being treated. Oral doses are given before or with meals or each snack. They may also be given in divided doses at 1- to 2-hour intervals throughout the day. **Use with extreme caution for patients with a known hypersensitivity to pork products.**

i. Malabsorption syndrome—8,000 to 24,000 USP units of lipase activity occasionally up to 36,000 units of lipase activity may be required. Considerable dosage variation exists, partly due to the susceptibility of pancreatin to acid–peptic inactivity in the upper GI tract.
ii. Functional indigestion—1,200 to 2,400 USP of lipase activity
b. Pancrelipase (Creon, Pancrease, Zenpep, Viokase): This must be given with each meal or snack.
i. Adults and children older than 4 years: Dosage for pancreatic exocrine dysfunction or for CF is 400 to 2,500 units/kg with meals; titrate dose to desired clinical response. Total daily dose should not exceed 10,000 units/kg body weight/d.
ii. Children aged 1 to 4 years: Dosages for pancreatic exocrine dysfunction or for cystic fibrosis: 1,000 U of lipase/kg/meal orally; dosage should be individualized to the patient's response. Adjust dose according to stool fat and nitrogen content. Dosage range: 1,000 to 25,000 units/kg/meal
3. Antispasmodics
a. Anticholinergic agents are used to reduce the cholinergic stimulation of colonic activity that occurs in response to a meal.
b. Drug of choice: Dicyclomine hydrochloride (Antispas), 10 to 20 mg orally before meals
4. Iron and folic acid supplementation are usually required for celiac disease.
5. Calcium and magnesium supplementation are required after extensive small intestine resection.
6. Antibiotic therapy for bacterial overgrowth
7. Corticosteroids and anti-inflammatory agents to treat regional enteritis

Follow-Up

A. If examination is normal, observe the patient for 1 month and have the patient keep a diary of food intake and weight.
B. For persistent malabsorption, monitor for osteoporosis/bone mass with a dual-energy x-ray absorptiometry (DEXA) scan.

Consultation/Referral

A. Any patient with weight loss of 15 kg is likely to have a life-threatening condition and requires prompt consultation and hospitalization.
B. Consult a gastroenterologist when malabsorption is documented by 72-hour stool fat assessment.
C. Consider a dietary consultation.
D. Refer back to the bariatric surgeon/center, depending on surgical complications from bariatric surgery.
E. Consider a referral for allergy testing for milk and proteins.

Individual Considerations

A. Geriatrics
1. To identify impediments to adequate food intake, question the patient about social isolation, depression, bereavement, physical impairment, poor dentition/edenulous, inability to fix meals, and poverty.
2. Loss of taste is sometimes responsible for poor intake and should be checked.

Nausea and Vomiting

Cheryl A. Glass

Definition

Nausea and vomiting are common symptoms for many conditions and diseases and include several terms to describe the symptoms (see Table 11.19).
A. Hyperemesis gravidarum is a condition of persistent, uncontrollable vomiting that begins in the first weeks of pregnancy and improves by the end of the first trimester; however, it may persist throughout pregnancy.
B. Chronic nausea and vomiting is defined as lasting at least 1 month in duration.
C. Complications of nausea and vomiting include fluid depletion, hypokalemia, and metabolic alkalosis.
D. Vomiting is also considered a protective mechanism to remove harmful ingested substances.

Incidence

A. Nausea and vomiting are very common, and the etiology is dependent on the disease/condition.
B. During pregnancy, 50% to 90% of women experience nausea and/or vomiting; 50% have both nausea and vomiting. Onset after the initial 9 weeks of pregnancy should direct especially careful evaluation for another cause within the differential diagnoses of nausea and vomiting in nonpregnant patients.
C. Hyperemesis gravidarum occurs in 1 in every 0.3% to 2% of pregnancies.
D. Severe hyperemesis requires hospitalization in 0.3% to 2% of pregnancies.
E. Approximately one third of surgical patients have nausea and/or vomiting after general anesthesia.
F. The incidence of nausea and/or vomiting subsequent to cancer treatment is high.

Pathogenesis

A. Protective mechanisms are activated by numerous gastrointestinal (GI) and non-GI causes. Normal function of the upper GI tract involves an interaction between the gut and the central nervous system (CNS).
B. Nausea and vomiting in pregnancy are related to increased hormones, including human chorionic gonadotropin (HCG), estrogen, and progesterone, as well as decreased gastric motility and relative hypoglycemia that results from a night-long fast.

Predisposing Factors

A. Acute nausea and vomiting
1. Medications: Digitalis toxicity, opiate use, chemotherapy agents, drug withdrawal, nicotine/nicotine patches, antibiotics, hormones, and antivirals
2. Ketoacidosis
3. Pregnancy or hormones

TABLE 11.19 Definitions of Terms Used to Describe Nausea and Vomiting

Term	Definition
Vomiting	Forceful oral expulsion of gastric contents associated with contraction of the abdominal and chest wall musculature
Nausea	The unpleasant sensation of the imminent need to vomit, usually referred to the throat or epigastrium; a sensation that may or may not ultimately lead to vomiting
Regurgitation	The act by which food is brought back into the mouth without the abdominal and diaphragmatic muscular activity that characterizes vomiting
Anorexia	Loss of desire to eat; a true loss of appetite
Sitophobia	Fear of eating because of subsequent or associated discomfort
Early satiety	Fear of feeling full after eating an unusually small quantity of food
Retching	Spasmodic respiratory movements against a closed glottis with contraction of the abdominal musculature without expulsion of any gastric contents, referred to as "dry heaves"
Rumination	Chewing and swallowing of regurgitated food that has come back into the mouth through voluntary increase in abdominal pressure within minutes of eating or during eating; rumination may be accompanied by weight loss and bulimia

4. Binge drinking
5. Hepatitis

B. Recurrent or chronic nausea and vomiting
1. Psychogenic vomiting
2. Metabolic disturbances
3. Gastric retention
4. Bile reflux
5. Pregnancy
6. Radiation
7. Gastroparesis

C. Nausea and vomiting with abdominal pain
1. Viral gastroenteritis
2. Acute gastritis
3. Food poisoning
4. Peptic ulcer disease (PUD)
5. Acute pancreatitis
6. Small-bowel obstruction
7. Acute appendicitis
8. Acute cholecystitis
9. Acute cholangitis
10. Acute pyelonephritis
11. Inferior myocardial infarction (MI)

D. Nausea and vomiting with neurologic symptoms
1. Increased intracranial pressure (ICP)
2. Midline cerebellar hemorrhage
3. Vestibular disturbances
4. Migraine headaches
5. Autonomic dysfunction
6. Head trauma
7. Multiple sclerosis

Common Complaints

A. Food aversion
B. Inability to retain food or liquids
C. "Queasy" sensation

Other Signs and Symptoms

A. Increased salivation
B. Bitter taste, "acid brash": Indicates ulcer or small-bowel obstruction
C. Weight loss
D. Dehydration
E. Sweating
F. Fast pulse
G. Pale skin
H. Rapid breathing
I. Light-headedness

Subjective Data

A. Review the onset, duration (acute or chronic problem?), and course of symptoms, including the quality (projectile?) and quantity of emesis. What was the color, taste, and consistency of the emesis? Was blood present?

1. Vomiting bright red blood indicates a hemorrhage—*peptic ulcer.*
2. Dark red blood indicates a hemorrhage—*esophageal or gastric varices.*
3. Coffee-ground material is indicative of digested blood from a slowly bleeding gastric or duodenal ulcer (DU).
4. Vomiting fecal material is a sign of distal *small-bowel obstruction* and blind-loop syndrome.

B. Ask the patient about other symptoms, including pain, fever, diarrhea, and headache.

C. Inquire if other family members are also ill and what are their symptoms.

D. Review the timing of vomiting in relation to meals, time of day, odors, and activity. Does vomiting occur before or after food intake?

E. Ask the patient about medication intake such as antibiotics, chemotherapy, herbals, digitalis, opiates, and birth control pills.

F. Ask about self-image, binge eating, and self-induced emesis.

G. Review any exposure to hepatitis or travel to places with poor sanitation and outbreaks of cholera.

H. Review the patient's medical history for vertigo, head injury, jaundice, diabetes, hypertension, and pregnancy.
I. Inquire about first day of last period and birth control method used.
J. Establish usual weight. Has there been any recent weight change, how many pounds, and over what period of time?
K. Ask about the patient's history of diabetes, gallbladder disease, ulcer disease, or cancer.

Physical Examination

A. Check temperature (if indicated), blood pressure and pulse which should be evaluated both standing and lying down, respirations, and weight.
B. Inspect
  1. Observe general overall appearance of skin for pallor and signs of dehydration. Tenting of skin when it is rolled between your thumb and index finger may indicate dehydration.
  2. Inspect for signs of autonomic insufficiency. Postural hypotension, lack of sweat, or blunted pulse and blood pressure responses to Valsalva's maneuver suggest autonomic dysfunction and a bowel motility problem as the underlying etiology of nausea and vomiting. Postural hypotension indicates marked volume depletion or circulatory collapse.
  3. Oral examination: Inspect mouth, teeth, and gums.
  4. Inspect fontanelles in infants.
C. Palpate
  1. The abdomen for masses, distension, tenderness, signs of peritonitis, and organomegaly
  2. The back; note costovertebral angle tenderness.
D. Percuss the abdomen.
E. Auscultate
  1. The abdomen for bowel sounds in all quadrants
  2. The heart and lungs
F. Perform rectal examination (if indicated).
G. Perform a neurologic examination (if indicated).

Diagnostic Tests

The cause of an acute episode of nausea and vomiting is typically determined through a detailed history and physical examination. Only if the cause is unclear should further testing be performed.

A. Urine: Urinalysis, pregnancy test, culture and sensitivity, if indicated
B. Urinalysis for ketones and specific gravity
C. Serum labs: Multiple chemistry profile, including amylase, electrolytes, blood urea nitrogen (BUN), creatinine, glucose, bilirubin, and transaminase
D. Hepatitis panel
E. Drug screen
F. Upper GI
G. Ultrasonography
  1. Obstetric ultrasound to rule out multiple gestations or molar pregnancy if persistent nausea and vomiting, especially after 16 weeks gestation
  2. Upper abdominal ultrasound, if clinically indicated, to evaluate the pancreas and/or biliary tree
H. Stool for occult blood
I. Endoscopy
J. CT scan
  1. Head CT scan, if indicated
  2. Abdominal CT if appendicitis is suspected
K. Gastric scintigraphy, to rule out gastroparesis if indicated
L. EKG if chest pain/myocardial infarction is suspected

Differential Diagnoses

A. See "Predisposing Factors" section.

Plan

A. General interventions: Assess hydration status. Proceed to intravenous (IV) hydration and antiemetics until ketones clear.
B. Dietary management: See Appendix B, "Nausea and Vomiting Diet Suggestions (Children and Adults)."
C. Pharmaceutical therapy (not an exhaustive list)

> *Antiemetics should not be used in vomiting of unknown etiology in children and adolescents.*

  1. Antiemetics
    a. Dextrose/fructose/phosphoric acid solution (Emetrol); available over the counter (OTC)
      i. Adults: 15 to 30 mL by mouth at 15-minute intervals (not to exceed five doses)
      ii. Children older than 2 years: 5 to 10 mL by mouth at 15-minute intervals (not to exceed five doses)
      iii. Children younger than 2 years or less than 30 lb: Dose is not available.
      iv. Tell the patient not to dilute the drug or take fluids 15 minutes before or after taking the medication.
      v. Diabetics should be instructed not to use without consulting their provider.
      vi. If nausea continues despite medication, contact health care provider.
    b. Promethazine (Phenergan)
      i. Drug of choice for gastroenteritis
      ii. Adults: 25 to 50 mg by mouth or per rectum every 4 to 6 hours
      iii. Children older than 2 years: 12.5 to 25 mg by mouth every 12 hours (usual dose 0.5 mg/lb of body weight, adjusted to age, weight)
      iv. Children younger than 2 years or less than 30 lb: Not recommended
    c. Trimethobenzamide (Tigan)
      i. Used for gastroenteritis and motion sickness
      ii. Adults: 300 mg orally three or four times daily
      iii. Adults: 200 mg intramuscularly (IM) three or four times daily
      iv. Children: Rectal suppositories and oral forms for pediatrics are no longer commercially available in the United States.
      v. Dose adjustment should be considered in elderly patients and with renal impairment (creatinine clearance ≤ 70 mL/min/1.73 m^2).

d. Prochlorperazine (Compazine is no longer available in the United States)

i. Adults: 5 to 10 mg three or four times daily; spansules 15 mg every 12 hours; suppositories 25 mg twice daily

ii. Children 40 to 85 lb: 2.5 mg twice daily, up to a maximum of 15 mg/d

iii. Children 30 to 39 lb: 2.5 mg two or three times a day up to maximum of 10 mg/d

iv. Children younger than 2 years, 20 to 39 lb: 2.5 mg one to two times a day, up to maximum of 7.5 mg/d

v. Children younger than 2 years or less than 20 lb: Not recommended

2. Outpatient IV hydration in pregnancy: 1 L lactated Ringer's solution to correct dehydration and restore electrolyte balance. Check urine ketones after first liter to determine if additional liter is necessary to clear ketones.

3. 5-Hydroxytryptamine$_3$ (5-HT$_3$) antagonists are utilized for nausea related to chemotherapy and postoperative nausea and vomiting. 5-HT$_3$ drugs are available in oral, IV, and transdermal formulations. Consult a prescribing reference for current dosing/formulations:

a. Ondansetron (Zofran)

b. Granisetron (Sancuso and Kytril)

c. Palonosetron (Aloxi)

d. Dolasetron mesylate (Anzemet)

4. Dronabinol (Marinol), cannabinoid 2.5, 5, and 10 mg capsules are indicated for refractory nausea and vomiting associated with chemotherapy. Therapy is individualized before and after chemotherapy.

Follow-Up

A. Tell the patient to call or visit the office in 24 hours to check response and nutritional intake.

B. Tell parents who are giving simple treatment at home to call the office promptly if projectile or prolonged vomiting occurs.

Consultation/Referral

A. ***If overdose is suspected: Contact 1-800-222-1222, the American Association of Poison Control Centers, the local poison control center, or the emergency department immediately.***

B. Hyperemesis gravidarum is the most severe form of nausea and vomiting in pregnancy. Hyperemesis gravidarum may require hospitalization to correct fluid and electrolyte imbalance, and nutritional deficiencies.

C. Consult a physician and hospitalize the patient promptly if there is evidence of bowel obstruction; increased ICP; or another GI, neurologic, or metabolic emergency. **First priority is to rule out acute surgical etiology such as bowel obstruction and peritonitis.**

D. Call for a pediatric consultation immediately for vomiting lasting more than 24 hours, projectile vomiting, vomiting after a fall or head injury, or prolonged vomiting coupled with diarrhea.

E. Call for a psychiatric consultation for suspected psychogenic nausea and vomiting.

F. If postural hypotension occurs, especially in elderly patients, hospital admission for parenteral fluid and electrolyte replacement is indicated.

G. Endocrinologist, gastroenterologist, and surgical consultations for treatment, consideration, and placement of a gastric stimulator for diabetes gastroparesis.

Individual Considerations

A. Pregnancy

1. Determine whether the woman is ingesting nonfood substances, such as starch, clay, or toothpaste, which would indicate pica.

2. Intractable nausea and vomiting require ultrasonography to rule out hydatidiform mole.

3. The only Food and Drug Administration (FDA)-approved drug for treating nausea and vomiting in pregnancy is doxylamine/pyridoxine. Antihistamines, promotility agents (e.g., metoclopramide), Emetrol, promethazine (Phenergan), and prochlorperazine (Compazine) may be used during pregnancy. In cases of refractory to standard therapy, ondansetron and steroids may be considered.

4. Uncorrected hyperemesis gravidarum can result in severe electrolyte imbalance and possible hepatic and renal damage. The major concern for fetal well-being is uncorrected ketosis, which may result in fetal abnormalities or death in early pregnancy.

5. Tell the patient to eat toast or a dry cracker; to eat small, frequent meals and snacks; to drink fluids separately from meals; and to avoid fatty, fried, greasy, or spicy foods and foods with strong odors.

B. Pediatrics

1. The differential diagnosis of vomiting is age dependent.

2. For neonates and young infants, the most frequent diagnostic considerations are the following:

a. Gastroesophageal reflux disease (GERD)

b. Excessive feeding volume

c. Increased ICP/meningitis

d. Food allergy

e. Intestinal obstruction

i. Malrotation without volvulus

ii. Hirschsprung's disease (HD)

iii. Intussusception

iv. Intestinal atresia

v. Pyloric stenosis

3. Older infants and children differential diagnoses include:

a. Gastroenteritis

b. GERD

c. Gastroparesis

d. Mechanical obstruction

e. Munchausen syndrome by proxy

4. Adolescent disorders include the disorders affecting children as well as

a. Appendicitis

b. Inflammatory bowel disease (IBD)

c. Pregnancy

d. Bulimia or psychogenic vomiting

5. Question caregivers regarding the infant's feeding, activity level, irritability, lethargy, and number of wet diapers.
6. Otitis media, pharyngitis, and urinary tract infections (UTIs) may present with nausea and/or vomiting in the pediatric population.
7. Rumination syndrome is a behavioral disorder that is most commonly identified among mentally disadvantaged children and adolescents with cognitive disabilities. The behavior consists of daily, effortless regurgitation of undigested food within minutes of starting or completing ingestion of a meal.

C. Geriatrics

1. Use of the lower dose ranges of an antiemetic is sufficient for most elderly patients due to their susceptibility to hypotension and neuromuscular reactions.
2. Dosages should be increased more gradually in the elderly.

There should be a low threshold for hospitalization of the elderly to treat dehydration and correction of fluid and electrolyte imbalance.

Resources

American Cancer Society: www.cancer.org
Rome Foundation: http://romecriteria.org/criteria

Peptic Ulcer Disease

Cheryl A. Glass

Definition

A. Peptic ulcer disease (PUD) is circumscribed ulceration of the gastrointestinal (GI) mucosa occurring in areas exposed to acid and pepsin. The patient's prior ulcer history tends to predict future behavior and risk of future complications. Complications include bleeding ulcer, perforation, and obstruction.
B. The stomach is divided on the basis of its physiological functions into two main portions. The proximal two thirds, the fundic gland area, acts as a receptable for ingested food and secretes acid and pepsin. The distal third, the pyloric gland area, mixes and propels food into the duodenum and produces the hormone gastrin. "Peptic" lesions may occur in the esophagus (esophagitis), stomach (gastritis), or duodenum (duodenitis).
C. There is often no correlation between the presence of an active ulcer, noted by endoscopy, and symptoms. The disappearance of symptoms does not guarantee ulcer healing.

Incidence

A. The annual incidence of peptic ulcer is estimated to range from 0.1% to 1.8%. The ulcer incidence in *Helicobacter pylori*-infected individuals is about 1% per year. The recurrence rate is 50% to 80% during the 6 to 12 months following the initial ulcer healing, although relapses are not always symptomatic. Some peptic ulcers heal spontaneously, and 2% to 20% of patients have multiple simultaneous ulcers.
B. From 16% to 31% of ulcers are caused by nonsteroidal anti-inflammatory drugs (NSAIDs). Epidemiologic studies show that risks of peptic ulcer and death are three to six times higher among people who take NSAIDs.
C. Cigarette smokers are twice as likely to develop ulcers as nonsmokers.

Pathogenesis

A. Although the precise mechanisms of ulcer formation remain incompletely understood, the process appears to involve the interplay of acid production, pepsin secretion, *H. pylori* bacterial infection, and mucosal defense mechanisms. Excess acid production is the hallmark of duodenal ulcer (DU) disease. Pepsin secretion is also elevated in DU disease.
B. The relation of aspirin and other NSAIDs to ulcer disease is due largely to the drugs' potent inhibition of gastric mucosal prostaglandin synthesis. In addition to prostaglandin inhibition, many NSAID preparations produce acute diffuse mucosal injury by means of a direct erosive effect.

Predisposing Factors

A. *H. pylori* infection is the most common cause of ulceration.
B. Use of NSAIDs, especially aspirin, ibuprofen, and naproxen, is associated with acute erosive gastritis.
C. Smoking
D. Genetic factors: Family history of ulcer disease
E. Age

1. DU occurs between ages 25 and 75 years.
2. Gastric ulcer occurs between ages 55 and 65 years.

F. Gender

1. The ratio of males to females for gastritis is 1:1.
2. The ratio of males to females for peptic ulcers is 2:1.

G. Excessive alcohol consumption, which stimulates acid secretion
H. Medications

1. Corticosteroids potentiate ulcer risk in patients who use NSAIDs concurrently.
2. Anticoagulants
3. Bisphosphonates
4. Spironolactone
5. Selective serotonin reuptake inhibitors (SSRIs)

I. Improper diet, irregular meals, and skipped meals
J. Severe physiological stress

1. Burns
2. Central nervous system (CNS) trauma
3. Surgery
4. Severe medical illness
   a. Cirrhosis
   b. Chronic obstructive pulmonary disease (COPD)
   c. Renal failure
   d. Organ transplantation
   e. Celiac disease
   f. Crohn's disease

K. Other causes

1. Radiation-induced ulcer
2. Chemotherapy-induced ulcer
3. Vascular insufficiency
4. Duodenal obstruction

L. Zollinger–Ellison syndrome
M. Bile reflux
N. Illicit drugs: Crack cocaine

Common Complaints

A. Pain described as aching, boring, gnawing, or burning feeling.
B. Epigastric pain in right upper quadrant (RUQ) and left upper quadrant (LUQ) of the abdomen or occasionally below breast
C. Pain that awakens the patient at night or in early morning
D. Perforated peptic ulcer presents with a sudden severe onset of severe sharp abdominal pain.

Other Signs and Symptoms

A. Asymptomatic
B. GI distress 1 to 3 hours after a meal, on an empty stomach
C. Pain relieved by food, antacids, or vomiting
D. Nausea and vomiting
E. Hematemesis
F. Chest discomfort
G. Blood in stools, "grape jelly" or maroon-colored stools
H. Loss of appetite or weight
I. Weight gain; those with DU may eat more to ease pain.
J. Anemia

Signs and Symptoms of Bleeding

A. Massive bleeding
  1. Acute, bright red hematemesis or large amount of melena with clots in the stool, or "grape jelly" stool
  2. Rapid pulse, drop in blood pressure, hypovolemia, and shock
B. Subacute bleeding
  1. Intermittent melena or coffee-ground emesis
  2. Hypotension
  3. Weakness and dizziness
C. Chronic bleeding
  1. Intermittent appearance of blood
  2. Increased weakness, paleness, or shortness of breath
  3. Occult blood

Subjective Data

A. Ask the patient to describe the onset, duration, type, and location of pain. Does it occur at any special time, for example, before meals, after meals, or during the night?
B. Has the patient had a previous ulcer? What was the treatment; if oral treatment was prescribed, did the patient complete the therapy?
C. Have the patient describe what alleviates pain, such as taking antacids, and what worsens pain, such as use of aspirin, oral steroids, or NSAIDs.
D. Review associated symptoms, such as nausea, vomiting, and heartburn.
E. Ask the patient if any first-degree relatives have ulcers.
F. Inquire whether the patient is a smoker. If so, how much and for how long?
G. Ask the patient about alcohol consumption: How much and for how long?
H. Inquire whether any blood has ever been vomited or passed in stool. If so, have the patient describe it.
I. Take the patient's dietary history, including time of meals, frequency of skipped meals, weight loss, and so forth.
J. Review all medications, including a review of over-the-counter (OTC) and herbal products such as ginkgo biloba.
K. Obtain past medical history of associated diseases, such as cirrhosis, pancreatitis, arthritis, chronic obstructive pulmonary disease (COPD), and hyperparathyroidism.
L. If the patient suspects blood in stool, ask if there has been a change in bowel pattern, presence of abdominal pain or tenderness, and whether the patient recently ingested food such as red beets.

Physical Examination

A. Check temperature (if indicated), pulse, respirations, blood pressure, and weight.
B. Palpate the abdomen for tenderness, guarding, rigidity, masses, and liver or spleen enlargement.
C. Percuss the abdomen for hepatosplenomegaly.
D. Auscultate the abdomen for bowel sounds in all quadrants.
E. Rectal examination
  1. Check for tenderness and masses.
  2. Take stool specimen.

Diagnostic Tests

A. Complete blood count (CBC)
B. Stool for occult blood
C. Coagulation studies
D. Testing for *H. pylori*
  1. Endoscopy with biopsy is the most accurate test.
  2. Rapid urease test is the diagnostic test of choice
  3. Urea breath test (UBT)
  4. Serum test for *H. pylori* antibodies
  5. Stool *H. pylori* antigen testing—more accurate than antibody testing and less expensive
E. Radiography with barium meal
F. Mucosal biopsy, after GI consultation, to rule out cancer.
G. Fasting gastrin level (screen for Zollinger–Ellison syndrome)

Differential Diagnoses

A. PUD
B. Gastroesophageal reflux disease (GERD)
C. Zollinger–Ellison syndrome: Fasting serum gastrin level 500 pg/mL in the presence of acid hypersecretion is diagnostic.
D. Cancer
  1. Gastric lymphoma
  2. Gastric cancer
  3. Pancreatic cancer
E. Pancreatitis (acute or chronic)
F. Myocardial ischemia
G. Abdominal aneurysm
H. Diverticulitis
I. Drug-induced dyspepsia
  1. Theophylline
  2. Digitalis

J. Crohn's disease (CD) involving the stomach or duodenum
K. Gastric infections
L. Cholelithiasis

Plan

A. General interventions: Goals are to alleviate pain, promote healing, limit complications, and prevent recurrences while minimizing costs and side effects of treatment.

1. Encourage the patient to stop taking NSAIDs, unless medically indicated.

a. If NSAID use is unavoidable, the lowest possible dose and duration and cotherapy with a proton pump inhibitor (PPI) based on triple therapy is recommended.

2. Smoking cessation should be highly encouraged at each visit.

▶ **B.** Patient teaching: *See Section III: Patient Teaching Guide for this chapter, "Ulcer Management."*

C. Dietary management: Advise the patient to avoid alcohol, coffee (including decaffeinated), and other caffeine-containing beverages, because they stimulate acid secretion. (See Appendix B, Table B.8.)

D. Medical and surgical management

1. Diagnostic evaluation of the ulcer is by means of endoscopy.

2. Test for *H. pylori.*

a. A single negative *H. pylori* test should be interpreted cautiously, especially in the face of active bleeding. Blood in the stomach can alter the pH indicator in the rapid urease test. False negatives are likely, and additional testing for *H. pylori* is essential.

b. Concurrent use of a PPI, antibiotics, or bismuth will cause a false negative test.

3. Surgery remains an option for treatment of refractory disease and complications. The most serious indications for surgery include brisk bleeding of 6 to 8 units of blood in 24 hours, recurrent bleeding episodes, perforation, gastric outlet obstruction refractory to medical therapy, and failure of a benign gastric ulcer to heal after 15 weeks. Emergency intervention may be required, such as withholding food and oral fluids, starting an IV, placing a nasogastric (NG) tube, oxygen therapy, or blood transfusion. If life-threatening bleeding occurs, treat shock.

E. Pharmaceutical therapy

1. The treatment of peptic ulcer begins with the eradication of *H. pylori* in infected individuals. Empiric therapy for the infection is reasonable for uncomplicated cases in the absence of NSAID use. Documenting infection, even in patients with known ulcers, is an essential step prior to initiating antimicrobial therapy.

a. Triple therapy anti–*H. pylori* regimen: PPI + amoxicillin + clarithromycin

i. PPI-based regimen (choose one):

1) Rabeprazole (Aciphex) 20 mg twice a day—total treatment duration: 7 days

2) Esomeprazole (Nexium) 40 mg once a day—total treatment duration: 10 days

3) Lansoprazole (Prevacid) 30 mg twice a day—total treatment duration: 10 to 104 days

4) Omeprazole (Prilosec) 20 mg twice a day—total treatment duration: 14 days

ii. Amoxicillin 1,000 mg twice a day

iii. Clarithromycin 500 mg twice a day

b. Quadruple therapy—14 days

i. Choose standard-dose PPI, or ranitidine 150 mg, two times daily

ii. Metronidazole (Flagyl) 500 mg four times daily

iii. Tetracycline 500 mg four times daily

iv. Bismuth subsalicylate 525 mg (two chewable tablets) four times daily

2. Antisecretory therapy is the mainstay of therapy in uninfected patients and is used for maintenance therapy in selected cases. Full doses of an H_2 receptor antagonist provide effective initial therapy; however, PPIs are more effective.

3. Patients with uncomplicated, small (less than 1 cm) duodenal ulcer (DU) or gastric ulcer (GU) who have received adequate treatment for *H. pylori* probably are asymptomatic and do not need any further therapy directed at ulcer healing. Maintenance acid suppression with a PPI for 1 year following *H. pyloric* eradication is recommended for patients with a complicated DU. If the ulcer is giant (greater than 2 cm), showing densely fibrosed ulcer beds, or if the patient is a high-risk patient with a protracted prior history, then the patient should be kept on a PPI until a follow-up endoscopy is performed.

a. H_2 receptor antagonists: Split-dose, evening, and nighttime therapy are all effective. In the United States, cimetidine, ranitidine, and famotidine are approved for GU healing. H2 receptor antagonist-based regimens are not Food and Drug Administration (FDA)-approved treatment regimens.

i. Cimetidine (Tagamet) 400 mg orally twice a day or 800 mg at bedtime for 6 to 8 weeks

ii. Ranitidine (Zantac) 150 mg orally twice a day or 300 mg at bedtime

iii. Famotidine (Pepsid) 20 mg orally twice a day or 40 mg at bedtime

iv. Nizatidine (Axid) 150 mg orally twice a day or 300 mg at bedtime

b. PPIs are effective in inducing ulcer healing. The PPIs are the most potent inhibitors of gastric acid secretion. Once-daily dosing is generally sufficient for acid inhibition; however, a second dose may be necessary and should be given before the evening meal. Once-daily PPI dosing inhibits acid output by 66% after 5 days. Optimal dosing is immediately before breakfast.

i. Omeprazole (Prilosec/Zegerid) 20 to 40 mg every morning for 4 weeks

ii. Esomeprazole (Nexium) 20 to 40 mg every morning for 4 to 8 weeks

iii. Lansoprazole (Prevacid) 15 to 30 mg every morning for 4 weeks

iv. Dexlansoprazole (Kapidex) 30 to 60 mg every morning for 4 to 8 weeks
v. Pantoprazole (Protonix) 20 to 40 mg every morning for 4 weeks
vi. Rabeprazole (Aciphex) 20 mg every morning for 4 weeks
vii. Dexlansoprazole (Dexilant) 60 mg every morning for 8 weeks

c. PPIs should not be given concomitantly with prostaglandins, or other antisecretory agents, because of the marked reduction in their effects. An H_2 antagonist can be used with a PPI if given after a sufficient interval between their administrations; the minimal times have not been established. The H_2 antagonist could be given at bedtime for breakthrough symptoms after a morning dose of a PPI.

d. Combination products currently on the market:
i. Omeclamox-Pak—Omeprazole 20 mg (2 caps), amoxicillin 500 mg (4 caps), and clarithromycin 500 mg (2 tabs) per Pak. Take omeprazole 20 mg, amoxicillin 100 mg, and clarithromycin 500 mg twice a day. Treatment is 10 days.
ii. Prevpac—Lansoprazole 30 mg (2 caps), amoxicillin 500 mg (4 caps), and clarithromycin 500 mg (2 caps) per Pak. Take lansoprazope 30 mg, amoxicillin 1,000 mg, and clarithromycin 500 mg twice daily. Treatment is 10 or 14 days.

4. Sucralfate (Carafate) 1 g orally four times daily, 1 hour before meals and at bedtime; maintenance therapy is 1 g twice daily. Sucralfate is not recommended for *H. pylori* or NSAID ulcers.

5. Misoprostol (Cytotec, a prostaglandin analog) is effective for peptic ulcers caused by NSAID use; peptic ulcers respond well to misoprostol 100 to 200 mcg orally four times a day.

Follow-Up

A. Therapeutic trial of lifestyle changes combined with an H_2 receptor antagonist, sucralfate, or omeprazole for 1 to 2 weeks should provide relief. Reevaluate the patient after 2 weeks, and if symptoms are improved, prescribe a full course of 6 to 8 weeks.

B. Reevaluate the patient again at 8 weeks, after the full course of therapy is completed.

C. Consider repeating breath test to confirm eradication of *H. pylori.*

D. Some authorities advocate routine endoscopic or radiologic documentation of healing. However, no studies show this to be cost-effective in uncomplicated cases in which symptoms resolve within 4 to 6 weeks and do not recur.

E. For refractory gastric ulcer—that is, persistent pain after 8 weeks despite a full medical regimen or unresponsive to treatment for *H. pylori*—endoscopic examination and biopsy are needed, especially in patients older than age 40 who are at increased risk of gastric cancer. Barium study is not sufficient, because even malignant ulcers may shrink in size in response to therapy.

F. Evaluate refractory cases for Zollinger–Ellison syndrome, especially when there are multiple ulcers, occurrences in unusual places, marked abdominal pain, or a secretory diarrhea.

G. There is an increased risk of osteoporotic fracture from the long-term use of PPIs.

H. Patients beginning long-term NSAID therapy should first be tested for *H. pylori.*

Consultation/Referral

A. Consult both a surgeon and a gastroenterologist and admit the patient in a hospital when symptoms of hemorrhage, penetration, perforation, or gastric outlet obstruction are present.

B. Refer patients with recurrences or refractory disease to a physician for evaluation for *H. pylori* infection by endoscopy or breath test. If present, eradicate with a 2-week course of triple therapy.

Individual Considerations

A. Pregnancy: The drugs misoprostol and ranitidine are abortifacients. They cross the placental barrier and are excreted in breast milk and are contraindicated in pregnancy or suspected pregnancy. Use in sexually active women of childbearing age should be done with proper warning and detailed patient education.

B. Adults
1. DUs are more common in people between ages 45 and 54 years; gastric ulcers, between 55 and 64 years.
2. Patients older than age 40 years are at greater risk of gastric cancer and should undergo either an upper GI series or endoscopy to document the nature and location of lesions when there is strong clinical suspicion of ulcer disease.
3. Gastritis not associated with reflux is present in 75% of people older than age 50 years.

C. Geriatrics
1. Silent disease is particularly common among the elderly and those using NSAIDs.
2. Lethargy, confusion, slurred speech, agitation, and visual hallucinations have been reported with cimetidine, particularly in the elderly.
3. In the elderly, DU symptoms remain classic with early morning awakening to pain, then quick relief by food or antacids. Gastric ulcer symptoms are less obvious, with burning or gnawing pain experienced in less than 50% of elderly patients.
4. Anemia may be the only symptom of gastric cancer. Cancer must always be considered and confirmed by endoscopy with biopsy.
5. When prescribing an NSAID to the elderly, use the lowest dose, for the shortest period of time, and avoid prescribing a long-acting NSAID, such as indomethacin (Indocin) and piroxicam (Feldene).
6. Due to other medications taken for comorbid health conditions, the elderly are especially

at risk with the combination of NSAIDs and the following:

a. Aspirin
b. Clopidogrel (Plavix)
c. Dabigatran (Pradaxa)
d. Dipyridamole (Persantine)
e. Prasugrel (Effient)
f. Ticlopidine (Ticlid)
g. Warfarin (Coumadin)

Pinworm

Cheryl A. Glass and Audra Malone

Definition

A. Pinworm, *Enterobius vermicularis,* is the most common helminth infection. It is characterized by a white, threadlike worm infestation.

Incidence

A. Pinworm is very common. *Enterobius* occurs worldwide and commonly occurs in family clusters. It has a high incidence of reinfection. Exact data are not available because helminth infestations are not reportable to the Centers for Disease Control and Prevention (CDC).

Pathogenesis

A. The *E. vermicularis* adult nematode, or roundworm, lives in the human rectum or colon and emerges onto the perianal skin to lay eggs. It is transmissible by direct transfer of infective eggs to mouth, or indirectly through clothing, bedding, food, or other articles contaminated with eggs of the parasite. The period of communicability is as long as female nematodes are discharging eggs on perianal skin. Eggs remain infective in an indoor environment, usually 2 to 3 weeks. Humans are the only known hosts; dogs and cats do not harbor *E. vermicularis.*

B. The incubation period is 1 to 2 months or longer, from ingestion of an egg until an adult gravid female migrates to the perianal region.

Predisposing Factors

A. Preschool and school age
B. Member of a family of an infected person
C. Institutional residence
D. Overcrowded living conditions

Common Complaints

A. Intense nighttime anal pruritus
B. Irritability in infants and children

Other Signs and Symptoms

A. Disturbed sleep or insomnia
B. Pruritus vulvae
C. Urethritis
D. Vaginitis
E. Local irritation
F. Secondary infections from scratching
G. Loss of appetite or weight loss
H. Grinding teeth at night

Subjective Data

A. Review the onset, duration, course, and time of symptoms, especially anal itching.
B. Ask the patient about symptoms in other family members.
C. Inquire about genital irritation symptoms in female children.

Physical Examination

A. Check temperature (if indicated), pulse, respirations, blood pressure, and weight.
B. Inspect anus and female genitals for irritation and skin abrasions.

Diagnostic Tests

A. Press sticky side of transparent (not translucent) cellulose tape against perianal folds, and then press tape on glass slide. Eggs will be visible under a microscope.

1. The "tape method" should be conducted on three consecutive mornings.
2. Eggs are most likely to be present on awakening and before the person bathes or uses the toilet.

B. Pinworm eggs may be obtained from a scraping sample from under the fingernails.
C. Order urinalysis to rule out urinary tract infection (UTI).
D. Obtain stool specimen for ova and parasite; adult worms in feces are diagnostic.
E. Serologic tests are not available for diagnosing pinworm infections.

Differential Diagnoses

A. Pinworms
B. UTI
C. Poor hygiene
D. Chemical irritants, soaps, and bubble baths

Plan

A. Patient teaching:

1. *See Section III: Patient Teaching Guide for this chapter, "Roundworms and Pinworms."* ◀
2. Teach the mother how to obtain a specimen from a child.
3. Infected people should bathe or shower in the morning to remove eggs.
   a. Showering is better than taking a bath. Showering avoids potentially contaminating the bath water with pinworm eggs.
   b. Infected people should not co-bathe with others during their time of infection.
4. Use good handwashing habits after using the toilet and before eating or preparing food.
5. Keep fingernails short and avoid nail biting.
6. All household members should be treated as a group when there are multiple instances of infection.
7. Thoroughly launder bedding and clothing to destroy any eggs.

B. Pharmaceutical therapy

1. **Albendazole (Albenza) 400 mg one-time dose and then another single dose 2 weeks later to prevent reinfection. Albendazole is the most common drug for the treatment of pinworms.**
2. Mebendazole (Vermox): 500 mg one-time dose and then another single dose 2 weeks later to prevent reinfection.

a. Mebendazole is available in the United States only through compounding pharmacies.

b. WHO recommends that 1-year-old children be given half of the dose (50 mg) for older children and adults.

3. Pyrantel pamoate (Pyrantel): 11 mg/kg/d for 3 days; do not exceed 1 g/d.

4. It is recommended that all household members be treated at the same time.

Follow-Up

A. If single-dose therapy is not effective, a second course of medication is advised in 2 weeks.

B. Reinfection is common.

Consultation/Referral

A. Consult a physician if the patient is pregnant.

Individual Considerations

A. Pregnancy

1. Anthelmintics are in pregnancy category C; however, the potential risks to the fetus versus benefits should be considered.

2. Breastfeeding should not be withheld during mebendazole therapy.

3. WHO has determined the benefit of pharmaceutical treatment outweighs the risk.

a. WHO allows the use of albendazole in the second and third trimesters of pregnancy.

b. WHO allows the use of pyrantel pamoate in the second and third trimesters of pregnancy.

B. Pediatrics

1. All medications are advised for children.

a. In WHO guidelines for mass prevention campaigns, albendazole can be used in children as young as 1 year.

b. Mebendazole and pyrantel pamoate are on the WHO Model List of Essential Medicines for Children intended for use in children up to 12 years of age.

2. Pinworms may predispose children to developing UTIs.

3. No unusual cleansing other than basic hygiene measures should be undertaken. Excessive zeal in this regard can induce guilt and is counterproductive.

4. The best time to examine a child is 2 to 3 hours after he or she falls asleep.

C. Adults have the lowest incidence of pinworms.

Roundworm

Cheryl A. Glass and Audra Malone

Definition

A. Roundworm, *Ascaris lumbricoides*, is a helminthic parasitic infection of the lumen of the small intestines and sometimes the lungs. Most infections with *A. lumbricoides* are asymptomatic. Roundworms are brownish, are the size and shape of earthworms, and can be seen easily without a microscope. The majority of worms are noted in the jejunum but can be noted from the esophagus to the rectum. Ova can survive for prolonged periods, up to 10 years. The eggs are resistant to normal water purification but can be removed by boiling and water filtration.

Incidence

A. *A. lumbricoides* are very common. Approximately 25% to 33% of the world's population, more than 1.4 billion people, are infected with these human intestinal nematodes. It is the third most frequent helminth infection; only the hookworm and whipworm exceed it. It occurs worldwide, especially in tropical and warm climates. It affects people of all ages but is most common in young children between 3 and 8 years of age.

B. Individuals can be asymptomatic and continue to shed eggs for years. The parasitic eggs are extremely durable in various environments, and each roundworm produces a large number of eggs. Complications secondary to *A. lumbricoides* range from 11% to 67% in infected individuals, with intestinal and biliary tract obstruction the most common serious sequelae. Bowel obstruction or perforation is the highest in children.

C. Many individuals infected with *A. lumbricoides* are also coinfected with other intestinal parasites, including trichuriasis (*Trichuris trichiura*) and hookworm (*Necator americanus* and *Ancylostoma duodenale*).

Pathogenesis

A. *A. lumbricoides* is a large roundworm that infects humans. The nematode measures 15 to 35 cm in length in adulthood. It is contracted by ingesting eggs in contaminated soil through eating the soil (pica), children playing in contaminated soil, eating unwashed fruits and raw vegetables, and drinking water contaminated with feces, or touching food with soil-contaminated hands. Occasionally, transplacental migration of larvae has been reported.

B. The life cycle of *A. lumbricoides* is 4 to 8 weeks, and feces contain eggs about 2 months after ingestion of embryonated eggs. Female roundworms produce 200,000 eggs per day, which are excreted in stool and must incubate in soil for 2 to 3 weeks for the embryo to form and become infectious (second-stage larvae). The interval between ingestion of egg and development of egg-laying adults is approximately 8 weeks. If infection is untreated, adult worms can live 6 to 24 months, resulting in daily excretion of large numbers of ova.

C. The ingested ova hatch in the small intestine (jejunum or ileum) and release larvae. They then may migrate via blood or via the lymphatic system to the heart, lungs, the biliary tree, and occasionally the kidney or brain. It takes approximately 4 days for the larvae to reach the lungs. After maturation, they are passed through the bronchi and the trachea and are subsequently swallowed.

D. Eggs are not shed in the stool until roughly 40 days after the development of pulmonary symptoms.

Predisposing Factors

A. Crowded or unsanitary living conditions

B. Tropical or warm climates, including the southern United States

C. Preschool or early school age (2–10 years)

D. Tend to cluster in families

E. Residence in areas where human feces are used as fertilizer
F. Travelers to endemic areas (Asia, Africa, and South America)
G. Recent immigrants (especially from Latin America and Asia)
H. International adoptees

Common Complaints

A. Asymptomatic
B. Restlessness at night
C. Colicky abdominal pain
D. Frequent fatigue
E. Worms found in bowel movements (BMs) or in bed

Other Signs and Symptoms

A. Transient respiratory symptoms during migration
B. Nausea and vomiting
C. Anorexia and erratic or poor appetite
D. Fever
E. Irritability
F. Diarrhea or constipation
G. Weight loss or gain
H. Dry cough or wheezing, from larvae in lungs
I. Parasites regurgitated or passed through nares of febrile patients
J. Acute transient pneumonitis
K. Acute obstructive jaundice
L. Appendicitis
M. Urticaria
N. Impaired absorption of protein, lactose, and vitamin A
O. Burning chest pain

Subjective Data

A. Review the onset, duration, and course of symptoms.
B. Ask about any problems with pica.
C. Inquire about worms in stool or emesis.
D. Review history of pets treated for worms.
E. Establish normal weight for evaluation.

Physical Examination

A. Check temperature (as indicated), pulse, respirations, blood pressure, and weight. Plot the child's height and weight on a growth curve.
B. Inspect the skin to rule out jaundice and evaluate urticaria.
C. Auscultate
  1. Auscultate the lungs to evaluate the presence of rales, wheezes, diminished breath sounds, and tachypnea.
  2. Auscultate the heart.
  3. Auscultate the abdomen.
D. Palpate the abdomen for distension, tenderness, and masses (worm bolus). Upper right quadrant, lower right quadrant, or hypogastrium tenderness may suggest complications of ascariasis.
E. Percuss the abdomen: Dullness may be noted.

Diagnostic Tests

A. None, if the worm is visualized; they are occasionally passed from the rectum, and nose, and are seen in vomitus.
B. Stool for occult blood, ova, and parasites, and culture.
C. Complete blood count (CBC): Eosinophilia may be noted particularly during the migration of larvae through the lungs.
D. Plain abdominal radiograph
E. Ultrasound/CT to diagnose hepatobiliary or pancreatic ascariasis. Endoscopic retrograde cholangiopancreatography (ERCP) is used for diagnosis and removal.
F. Chest radiography is rarely needed
G. Microscopic wet prep of sputum may be helpful with respiratory symptoms.

Differential Diagnoses

A. Roundworm
B. Asthma
C. Pneumonia
D. Poor nutrition
E. Giardiasis
F. Pancreatitis from other causes
G. Impaired growth/failure to thrive (FTT)
H. Iron-deficiency anemia
I. Appendicitis
J. Bowel obstruction (large or small)
K. Intussusception

Plan

A. Patient teaching:
  1. *See Section III: Patient Teaching Guide for this chapter, "Roundworms and Pinworms."* ◀
  2. Stress the importance of maintaining a clean play area for children.
  3. Stress sanitary disposal of feces.
  4. Explain that household bleach is ineffective in killing eggs *or* worms.
  5. All family members must be treated with medication.
  6. There is no direct person-to-person transmission.
B. Pharmaceutical therapy
  1. Treatment of symptomatic and asymptomatic infections may be achieved by a single dose of the following agents.
    a. Pyrantel pamoate (Antiminth) 11 mg/kg up to a maximum of 1 g given in a single dose. The single dose is 90% effective.
    b. Mebendazole (Vermox) 100 mg twice daily for 3 days or 500 mg as a single dose. Both the single and 3-day treatments are about 95% effective.
      i. The WHO recommends that 1-year-old children be given half of the dose (50 mg) for older children and adults.
    c. Anthelmintic therapy is not usually given at the time of pulmonary symptoms. Dying larvae may increase complications with migrating larvae.
  2. Administer the drug to all family members to decrease risk of spreading infection.
  3. Consider vitamin A supplement if growth is retarded.
  4. Inhaled beta-agonists may be indicated for respiratory symptoms.

Follow-Up

A. Reexamine a stool specimen in 2 weeks to determine if the therapy was successful in eliminating the worms. If the patient is not cured, give a second course of medication.

B. Therapy is effective for adult worms only. Reevaluate in 2 to 3 months for detectable eggs.

C. Endoscopy or laparoscopic extraction of worms may be required with hepatobiliary infestations.

Consultation/Referral

A. Consult with a physician if the patient is pregnant or is considered a surgical risk.

B. Bowel or hepatobiliary obstruction may require surgical or gastroenterologic consultation.

Individual Considerations

A. Pregnancy
- **1.** Anthelmintics are pregnancy category C; however, the potential risks to the fetus versus benefits should be considered.
- **2.** WHO has determined that the benefit of pharmaceutical treatment outweighs the risk.
  - **a.** WHO allows the use of albendazole in the second and third trimesters of pregnancy.
  - **b.** WHO allows the use of pyrantel pamoate in the second and third trimesters of pregnancy.

B. Pediatrics
- **1.** All medications are advised for children.
  - **a.** WHO guidelines for mass prevention campaigns: Albendazole can be used in children as young as 1 year old.
  - **b.** Mebendazole and pyrantel pamoate are on the WHO Model List of Essential Medicines for Children intended for use in children up to 12 years of age.
- **2.** Children are more prone to acute intestinal obstruction because they have smaller diameters of the intestinal lumen and often have large numbers of worms.

C. Adults: Acute intestinal obstruction may develop with heavy infestation.

Ulcerative Colitis

Cheryl A. Glass

Definition

A. Ulcerative colitis (UC) is one of the two inflammatory bowel diseases (IBDs), along with Crohn's disease (CD). UC is limited to the colon; it extends proximally from the anal verge in an uninterrupted pattern to a part of or the entire colon. Extracolonic manifestations also include uveitis, pyoderma gangrenosum, pluritis, erythema nodosum, ankylosing spondylitis, and spondyloarthropathies (Table 11.20).

B. Neither UC nor CD should be confused with IBS, which affects the motility of the colon. Smoking is negatively associated with UC; the relationship is reversed in CD. The general course of UC is intermittent exacerbations and remissions. In severe cases, surgery may result in a cure. The choice of treatment depends on disease activity and extent of pathology, patient acceptability, and mode of drug delivery.

C. Histologically, most of the pathology of UC is limited to the mucosa and submucosa. The extent of UC is defined by the following:
- **1.** Pan-ulcerative (total colitis): Extensive disease with evidence of UC proximal to the splenic flexure. Massive dilation of the colon (toxic megacolon) may lead to bowel perforation.
- **2.** Left-sided disease: Continuous UC that is present from the rectum and the descending colon up to, but not proximal to, the splenic flexure.
- **3.** Proctosigmoiditis: Disease limited to the rectum and sigmoid colon involvement.
- **4.** Ulcerative proctitis: Disease limited to the rectum—usually less than the full rectum.

D. In 2015, The Toronto Consensus Clinical Practice Guidelines for the Management of Nonhospitalized UC published 34 recommendations, including statements on 5-aminosalicylates (5-ASA), corticosteroids, immunosuppresants, anti-tumor necrosis factor (TNF) therapy, and other agents, including probiotics. The guidelines are available at www.gastrojournal.org/article/S0016-5085(15)00303-0/abstract

E. The 2015 Toronto Consensus guideline defined remission and response with UC as:
- **1.** Complete remission: Both symptomatic remission and endoscopic healing defined as follows:
  - **a.** Endoscopic healing: Normal mucosa, vascular blurring, or chronic changes (e.g., inflammatory polyps, scarring) without friability
  - **b. Symptomatic remission: Normal stool frequency (less than or equal to 3/d) and no blood in the stool**
- **2. Symptomatic response: Meaningful improvement in symptoms as judged by both the patient and physician in the absence of remission; response should not be considered a desirable final outcome but is useful to assess early response to treatment.**

Incidence

A. The annual incidence of UC is 10.4 to 12 per 100,000, depending on the country.

B. UC is three times more common than CD.

C. The most common cause of death in patients with UC is toxic megacolon.

D. Adenocarcinoma of the colon develops in 3% to 5% of patients with UC; the risk increases with the duration of the disease.

E. Approximately 6.2% of patients with IBD have a major extraintestinal manifestation.
- **1. Uveitis is the most common—3.8%**
- **2. Primary sclerosing cholangitis—3%**
- **3. Ankylosing spondylitis—2.7%**
- **4. Erythema nodosum—1.9%**
- **5. Pyoderma gangrenosum—1.2%**

Pathogenesis

A. The exact etiology is unknown.

B. UC may be considered an autoimmune disease. Persons with UC often have p-antineutrophil cytoplasmic antibodies (p-ANCAs). Abnormalities of humoral and cell-mediated immunity and/or generalized enhanced reactivity against intestinal bacterial antigen may also be causes of UC.

Predisposing Factors

A. Caucasian
B. Jewish descent
C. 30% more females than males
D. Genetic susceptibility (chromosomes 12 and 16)

Common Complaints

A. Frequent small-volume diarrhea
B. Bloody diarrhea with or without mucus
C. Severe bowel urgency
D. Abdominal cramps and pain with bowel movement (BM)
E. Constipation
F. Anorexia
G. Anemia
H. Nocturnal BMs

Other Signs and Symptoms

A. Tenesmus (rectal urgency/constant feeling of need to pass stool)
B. Abdominal tenderness
C. Arthralgias
D. Fatigue secondary to anemia
E. Failure to thrive (FTT) in children
F. Severe UC
  1. Fever
  2. Tachycardia
  3. Significant abdominal tenderness
  4. Signs of volume depletion

Subjective Data

A. Review the onset, duration, signs, and symptoms (number of stools, presence/absence of blood in the stool, fever, and abdominal pain).
B. Review the patient's recent travel history or camping trips for the presence of intestinal infection.
C. Review the patient's medication history including antibiotics and nonsteroidal anti-inflammatory drugs (NSAIDs one third of patients with exacerbation of UC report recent NSAID use).
D. Review family history for IBD, celiac disease, and colorectal cancer.
E. Review the patient's smoking status.
F. Review the patient's history or contact related to tuberculosis (TB; testing required before biologic therapy).
G. Evaluate if the patient has symptoms of uveitis including light sensitivity, floaters, blurry vision, or pain/tenderness to touch.

Physical Examination

A. Check temperature (if indicated), pulse, blood pressure, and weight. Follow serial weights.
B. Inspection
  1. Observe the general overall appearance for nutritional status, cachexia, and pallor.
  2. Observe the perianal region for the presence of tags, fissures, fistulas, and abscess.
  3. Observe the abdomen for distension and presence of surgical scars.
  4. Examine the eyes for redness, irritation, and ocular complications (episcleritis, scleritis, and uvetis).
  5. Evaluate for the presence of dermatological findings, including erythema nodosum and pyoderma gangrenosum.
C. Auscultation
  1. The heart and lungs
  2. All four quadrants of the abdomen
D. Palpation
  1. Palpate all four quadrants of the abdomen, observing for tenderness, rebound, and guarding.
  2. Evaluate the presence of hepatomegaly.
  3. Perform digital rectal examination to assess for anal strictures and rectal masses.
  4. Palpate the joints for warmth, tenderness, and range of motion.

Diagnostic Tests

A. **Diagnosis is best made with endoscopy and biopsy.**
B. Laboratory tests
  1. Complete blood count (CBC) with electrolytes
  2. Platelet count
  3. Sedimentation rate
  4. C-reactive protein (CRP)
  5. Cytomegalovirus (CMV; chronic immunosuppressive steroids)
  6. HIV
C. Stool testing
  1. Evaluate bacterial, viral, or parasitic causes of diarrhea
  2. Occult blood
  3. Fecal leukocytes
D. Plain abdominal radiograph
E. CT scan
F. MRI
G. Ultrasound
H. Double-contrast barium enema
I. Celiac antibody testing should be considered
J. Intestinal TB testing should be considered

Differential Diagnoses

A. UC
B. Ischemic colitis (especially in the elderly)
C. Toxic megacolon
D. Colon cancer
E. Adenocarcinoma
F. Rectal cancer
G. Radiation colitis
H. Intestinal infections
I. Intestinal lymphoma
J. Chronic diverticulitis
K. Amebiasis

Plan

A. General interventions
  1. See Table 11.20 for the definition of severity of ulcerative colitis.
  2. Severe UC should be managed jointly by a gastroenterologist in conjunction with a colorectal surgeon (Table 11.21).
  3. Stress reduction and stress management may improve symptoms.
  4. Pretreatment screening for TB, using Mantoux (a purified protein derivative [PPD]) skin testing, is

TABLE 11.20 Definition of Severity of Ulcerative Colitis

Mild UC	• ≤4 bloody stools/d with or without blood
	• No systemic toxicity
	• Normal ESR
	• Mild abdominal pain or cramping
Moderate UC	• >4 bloody stools/d
	• No signs of systemic toxicity
	• Pulse <90 beats per minute
	• Temperature <37.5°C (99.5°F)
	• Hemoglobin >10.5 g/dL
	• ESR <30 mm/hr
	• Moderate abdominal pain
Acute severe UC[a]	• ≥6 bloody stools/d or observable massive and significant blood BM *and*
	• 1 or more symptoms of systemic toxicity
	• Tachycardia >90 beats per minute
	• Temperature >37.8°C (100.4°F)
	• Hemoglobin >10.5 g/dL
	• Increased ESR (>30 mm/hr)
Fulminant UC	• >10 stools/d
	• Continuous rectal bleeding
	• Systemic toxicity
	• Tachycardia >90 beats per minute
	• Fever >37.8°C (100.4°F)
	• Anemia requiring blood transfusions
	• Abdominal tenderness and distension
	• Colonic dilation on radiography
	• May lead to toxic megacolon or colonic perforation

[a]Acute severe colitis is defined by Truelove and Witt's Criteria (1955).
ESR, erythrocyte sedimentation rate; UC, ulcerative colitis.

needed before initiation of immunomodulators and thiopurines.

5. Immunization status
   a. Immunizations with inactivated vaccine should be brought up to date and rigorously maintained during treatment, including influenza, meningococcus, and pneumococcus.
   b. Check varicella titers prior to treatment with immunomodulators and reimmunize if titers are low.
   c. The risk of administering live vaccines (polio, rubella and yellow fever) to patients on immuomodulators has not been established; however, most experts avoid live vaccines during treatment.

B. Patient teaching: *See Section III: Patient Teaching Guide for this chapter, "Crohn's Disease."*

C. Dietary management

TABLE 11.21 Management of Mild to Moderate Distal Ulcerative Colitis With Topical Agents

Topical agent	Proximal extent/distribution of agent
Suppository	10 cm
Hydrocortisone foam	15–20 cm
Enema	As far as the splenic flexure

Source: Adapted from the AGA Ulcerative Colitis in Adult Practice Guidelines (2010).

1. Adequate nutrition is critical to promotion of healing. Sufficient protein and calories limit the stress on an inflamed bowel.
2. Many patients with UC have concurrent lactose intolerance. (See Appendix B for lactose-intolerance dietary recommendations.)
3. Decrease dietary fiber during increased disease activity.
4. Low-residue diet may decrease the frequency of BMs.
5. High-residue diet may be helpful in ulcerative proctitis when constipation is the dominant symptom. (See Appendix B, Table B.6.)

D. Pharmacological therapy. Refer to the American College of Gastroenterology Practice Guidelines for full treatment algorithms at http://s3.gi.org/physicians/guidelines/UlcerativeColitis.pdf or the 2015 Toronto Consensus Guidelines for the Management of UC algorithms.

1. The choice of topical agents is guided by the proximal distribution of UC into the bowel, as well as patient preference (see Table 11.21).
2. Stepwise medication approach (see Table 11.5): 5-ASA class of anti-inflammatory drugs is the most common treatment for patients with mild (less than four bloody stools per day) or moderate active disease (more than four bloody stools a day without systemic toxicity).
   a. Sulfasalazine (azulfidine) for mild to moderate UC and remission maintenance
      i. Pediatrics: 50 to 75 mg/kg each 24 hours, divided into three to four doses
      ii. **Reduced absorption of folic acid and digoxin has been reported when administered with sulfasalazine.**
   b. Balsalazide (Colazal) for mild to moderate UC and remission maintenance
      i. Induction: 6.75 g/d, given three times daily dosing
      ii. Maintenance: 2 to 6.75 g/d, given twice a day dosing
      iii. Pediatric dose: 5 years or older: 750 mg, given three times a day for up to 8 weeks
3. Mesalamine for mild to moderate UC and remission maintenance.
   a. Asacol:
      i. Pediatrics: For patients 5 years or older, dosage is weight based (up to a maximum of 2.4 g/d) divided into two daily doses for a duration of 6 weeks.

ii. Two Asacol 400 mg tablets are not interchangeable or substitutable with one mesalamine delayed-release 800 mg tablet.

b. Apriso: 1.5 mg/d orally in the morning

c. Salofalk: 1 to 4 g/d in one or two divided doses

i. Also available as a suppository, rectal suspension, and enema

d. Pentasa: 1 g/d orally in four times a day dosing for up to 8 weeks

i. Also available in a suppository

e. Multi-Matrix System (MMX) marketed as Lialda: Active to moderate UC

i. Induction: 2.4 to 4.8 g/d for up to 8 weeks

ii. Maintenance: 2.4 g/d

iii. *Lialda is not recommended for children younger than 18 years.*

f. Rowasa enema: 4 g/60 mL rectally at bedtime; retain for approximately 8 hours.

g. Mesalamine (Canasa) suppository 1 g/d at bedtime; retain in the rectum for at least 1 to 3 hours. Treat active proctitis for 3 to 6 weeks.

4. Corticosteroids suppress the immune system and are used for moderate to severe UC.

a. Prednisone (Deltasone, Orasone)

i. Induction: 40 to 60 mg/d by mouth for 7 to 14 days followed by gradual taper by 5 mg/wk

ii. Maintenance: 2.5 to 5 mg/wk

b. Budesonide (Entocort EC)

i. Pediatric: For patients 8 to 17 years old who weigh more than 25 kg: 9 mg orally for up to 8 weeks, followed by 6 mg once a day for 2 weeks

5. Immune modifiers are used to decrease corticosteroid dosage.

a. Azathioprine (AZA; Imuran) 2 to 3 mg/kg/d orally

i. Monitoring includes: Complete blood count (CBC), including platelet counts weekly during the first month, twice monthly for the second and third months of therapy, then monthly or more frequently if dosage alteration is necessary.

ii. Thiopurine S-methyltransferase (TPMT) testing: Testing is recommended for consideration to be given to either genotype or phenotype patients for TPMT.

b. 6-Mercaptopurine (6-MP; Purinethol) 1 to 1.5 mg/kg/d orally

i. Patients with little or no inherited TPMT activity are at increased risk for severe Purinethol toxicity and generally require substantial dose reduction.

ii. Pediatrics: 1.0 to 2.0 mg/kg/d orally (maximum of 150 mg/d).

6. Antibiotics

a. Cyclosporine (Neoral, Sandimmune)

i. IV infusion: 2 to 4 mg/kg/d

ii. Can be switched to a doubled oral dose for outpatient therapy

b. Ciprofloxacin (Cipro) 500 mg orally twice a day

c. Metronidazole (Flagyl)

7. Biologic therapy (anti-TNF agents) for moderate to severe UC. **Tuberculin skin test is recommended before therapy. Patients started on infliximab should also be screened for hepatitis B before initiating therapy.**

a. Infliximab (Remicade) infusion therapy has a half-life of approximately 10 days.

b. Adalimumab (Humira) for the treatment of moderate to severe UC.

i. *Pediatrics: Not recommended for those younger than 18 years*

c. Golimumab (Simponi)

i. Initial dosage is 200 mg subcutaneously at week 0

ii. Second dose (week 2): 100 mg

iii. Maintenance dose: 100 mg every 4 weeks

d. Vedolizumab (ENTYVIO)

i. Initial dose: 300 mg IV at weeks 0, 2, and 6

ii. Maintenanc dose: 300 mg IV every 8 weeks of therapy

iii. Discontinue if no evidence of therapeutic benefit by week 14.

G. Indications for the consideration of a total colectomy

1. Failed medical therapy: Refractory UC

2. Severe hemorrhage

3. Fulminate colitis not responsive to treatment

4. Toxic megacolon

5. Obstruction or stricture

6. FTT in children

H. Indications for consideration for elective surgery

1. Long-term steroid dependence

2. Dysplasia or adenocarcinoma found on screening biopsy

3. Disease present 7 to 10 years

Follow-Up

A. Screening colonoscopy is recommended for all patients with UC for 8 to 10 years after the onset of symptoms due to the increase in colonic neoplasia.

B. Patients with extensive UC or left-sided colitis with negative findings on the screening colonoscopy should begin surveillance colonoscopy in 1 to 2 years.

C. Steroids should not be used as maintenance therapy. Patients who require long-term steroids are at increased risk of osteoporosis.

D. Subsequent laboratory monitoring tests are dependent on the prescribed therapy.

E. Anxiety and depression are higher in patients with IBD. Screen for depression at each visit.

Consultation/Referral

A. Gastroenterologist for confirmatory diagnosis with a colonoscopy.

B. Surgeon for severe or fulminant colitis. Toxic megacolon is a life-threatening complication and requires urgent surgical intervention.

C. Patients with ocular complications require an urgent consultation.

D. Patients who have had UC for 8 to 10 years are at risk of colon cancer; therefore, colonoscopy for surveillance is recommended.

Individual Considerations

A. Live vaccinations should not be administered to immunocompromised patients. If required, vaccines should be administered at the time of UC diagnosis.

  1. The flu and pneumonia vaccines should be routinely administered.

  2. Consider administering the human papillomavirus vaccine.

B. Women with IBD have reported to have a high incidence of abnormal Pap smears. Adherence to Pap smear guidelines are recommended by the ACG.

C. Abnormal sperm counts, motility, and morphology are seen with sulfasalazine.

D. Pediatrics

  1. UC is uncommon in persons younger than 10 years.

  2. Fulminant disease occurs more in children than adults.

  3. Children may present with systemic complaints, including fatigue, arthritis, failure to gain weight, and delayed puberty.

Resources

American College of Gastroenterology: http://gi.org

Crohn's and Colitis Foundation of America: www.ccfa.org

Bibliography

Academy of Nutrition and Dietetics. (n.d.). Celiac disease evidence-bases nutrition practice guideline. Retrieved from http://www.adaevidencelibrary.com/topic.cfm?cat=3677

Alexandraki, I., & Smetana, G. W. (2016, October). Acute viral gastroenteritis in adults. *UpToDate.* Retrieved from http://www.uptodate.com/contents/acute-viral-gastroenteritis-in-adults

American Academy of Pediatrics. (2012a). *Ascaris lumbricoides* infections. In L. K. Pickering (Ed.), *Red book: 2012 report of the Committee on Infectious Diseases* (29th ed., pp. 239–240). Elk Grove Village, IL: Author. Retrieved from https://redbook.solutions.aap.org/DocumentLibrary/RB12_interior.pdf

American Academy of Pediatrics. (2012b). Cyclosporiasis. In L. K. Pickering (Ed.), *Red book: 2012 report of the Committee on Infectious Diseases* (29th ed., pp. 299–300). Elk Grove Village, IL: Author. Retrieved from https://redbook.solutions.aap.org/DocumentLibrary/RB12_interior.pdf

American Academy of Pediatrics. (2012c). *Giardia intestinalis* infections. In L. K. Pickering (Ed.), *Red book: 2012 report of the Committee on Infectious Diseases* (29th ed., pp. 333–335). Elk Grove Village, IL: Author. Retrieved from https://redbook.solutions .aap.org/DocumentLibrary/RB12_interior.pdf

American Academy of Pediatrics. (2012d). Hepatitis A. In L. K. Pickering (Ed.), *Red book: 2012 report of the Committee on Infectious Diseases* (29th ed., pp. 361–369). Elk Grove Village, IL: Author. Retrieved from https://redbook.solutions.aap.org/DocumentLibrary/RB12_interior.pdf

American Academy of Pediatrics. (2012e). Hepatitis B. In L. K. Pickering (Ed.), *Red book: 2012 report of the Committee on Infectious Diseases* (29th ed., pp. 369–390). Elk Grove Village, IL: Author. Retrieved from https://redbook.solutions.aap.org/DocumentLibrary/ RB12_interior.pdf

American Academy of Pediatrics. (2012f). Hepatitis C. In L. K. Pickering (Ed.), *Red book: 2012 report of the Committee on Infectious Diseases* (29th ed., pp. 391–395). Elk Grove Village, IL: Author. Retrieved from https://redbook.solutions.aap.org/DocumentLibrary/RB12_interior.pdf

American Academy of Pediatrics. (2012g). Hookworm infections (*Ancylostoma duodenale* and *Necator americanus*). In L. K. Pickering (Ed.), *Red book: 2012 report of the Committee on Infectious Diseases* (29th ed., pp. 411–413). Elk Grove Village, IL: Author. Retrieved from https://redbook.solutions.aap.org/DocumentLibrary/RB12_interior .pdf

American Academy of Pediatrics. (2012h). Pinworm infection (*Enterobius vermicularis*). In L. K. Pickering (Ed.), *Red book: 2012 report of the Committee on Infectious Diseases* (29th ed., pp. 566–567). Elk Grove Village, IL: Author. Retrieved from https://redbook.solutions.aap.org/DocumentLibrary/RB12_interior.pdf

American Academy of Pediatrics. (2012i). Shigella infections. In L. K. Pickering (Ed.), *Red book: 2012 report of the Committee on Infectious Diseases* (29th ed., pp. 645–647). Elk Grove Village, IL: Author. Retrieved from https://redbook.solutions.aap.org/DocumentLibrary/RB12_interior.pdf

American Association for Clinical Chemistry. (2015, February 24). Celiac disease antibody tests. *Lab Tests Online.* Retrieved from labtestsonline.org/ understanding/analytes/celiac-disease/tab/test

American College of Gastroenterology. (2011). Pregnancy and gastrointestinal disorders. *Pregnancy monograph.* Retrieved from http://gi.org/wp-content/uploads/2011/07/institute-PregnancyMonograph.pdf

American College of Obstetricians and Gynecologists. (2009, June). ACOG practice bulletin bariatric surgery and pregnancy. *Obstetrics & Gynecology, 113,* 1405–1413.

American Gastroenterological Association. (2001). American Gastroenterological Association medical position statement: Nausea and vomiting. *Gastroenterology, 120,* 261–262.

American Gastroenterological Association. (2016, July). Peptic ulcer disease. Retrieved from https://www.gastro.org/patient-care/conditions-diseases/peptic-ulcer-disease

Anand, B. S. (2015, January 9). Peptic ulcer disease. *Medscape.* Retrieved from http://emedicine.medscape.com/article/181753-overview

Andersen, S. (2012, August). Beware the irritable bowel deciphering the overlap of symptoms. *ADVANCE for NPs & PAs, 21–24*(3), 32.

Barclay, L. (2010 December 2). American Academy of Pediatrics reviews use of probiotics, prebiotics. *Medscape.* Retrieved from http://www.medscape.com/viewarticle/733463

Basson, M. D. (2013, May 6). Constipation. *Medscape.* Retrieved from http://emedicine.medscape.com/article/184704

Basson, M. D. (2015, November 18). Ulcerative colitis. *Medscape.* Retrieved from http://emedicine.medscape.com/article/183084-overview

Beltrán, B. (2011, June 14). Old-age inflammatory bowel disease onset: A different problem? *World Journal of Gastroenterology, 17,* 2734–2739.

Beth Israel Deaconess Medical Center. (2013). What are the treatments for Crohn's disease? Retrieved from http://www.bidmc.org/CentersandDepartments/Departments/DigestiveDiseaseCenter/InflammatoryBowelDiseaseProgram/CrohnsDisease/WhatarethetreatmentsforCrohnsdisease.aspx

Bleday, R. (2009, May 1). Patient information: Hemorrhoids. *UptoDate.* Retrieved from http://www.uptodate.com/online/content/topic.do?topicKey=digestiv/8271&view=print

Bleday, R., & Breen, E. (2009, May 1). Treatment of hemorrhoids. *UpToDate.* Retrieved from http://www.uptodate.com/online/content/topic.do?topicKey=colosurg/6160&view=print

Bloom, A. A. (2016, April 15). Cholecystitis. *Medscape.* Retrieved from http://emedicine.medscape.com/article/171886-overview

Bonheur, J. L. (2015, October 13). Bacterial gastroenteritis. *Medscape.* Retrieved from http://emedicine.medscape.com/article/176400 -overview

Bousvaros, A., & Leichtner A. (2012, September 17). Overview of the management of Crohn's disease in children and adolescents. *UpToDate.* Retrieved from http://www.uptodate.com/contents/overview-of-the-management-of-crohns-disease-in-children-and-adolescents

Boyce, T. G. (2014, July). Overview of gastroenteritis. Retrieved from http://www.merckmanuals.com/professional/gastrointestinal-disorders/gastroenteritis/overview-of-gastroenteritis

Bressler, B., Marshall, J. K., Berstein, C. N., Bitton, A., Jones, J., Leontiadis, G. I., . . . Fegan, B. (2015). Clinical practice guidelines for the medical management of nonhospitalized ulcerative colitis: The Toronto consensus. *Gastroenterology, 148,* 1035–1058.

Brooks, D. C. (2014, October 4). Overview of abdominal wall hernias in adults. *UpToDate.* Retrieved from http://www.uptodate.com/contents/overview-of-abdominal-wall-hernias-in-adults

Brooks, D. C. (2016, May 3). Overview of treatment for inguinal and femoral hernia in adults. *UpToDate.* Retrieved from http://www.uptodate.com/contents/overview-of-treatment-for-inguinal-and-femoral-hernia -in-adults

Brooks, D. C., Obeid, A., & Hawn, M. (2013, January 25). Classification, clinical features and diagnosis of inguinal and femoral hernias in adults. *UpToDate.* Retrieved from www.uptodate.com/contents/classification-clinical-features-and-diagnosis-of-inguinal-and-femoral-hernias-in-adults?topicKey=SURG%2F3686

Burger, D., & Travis, S. (2011). Conventional medical management of inflammatory bowel disease. *Gastroenterology, 140*, 1827–1837.

Carter, M. J., Lobo, A. J., & Travis, S. P. L. (2004). Guidelines for the management of inflammatory bowel disease in adults. *Gut, 53*(Suppl. 5), V1-V16. Retrieved from http://gut.bmj.com/content/53/suppl_5/vl.extract

Cartwright, S. L., & Knudson, M. P. (2015). Diagnostic imaging of acute abdominal pain in adults. *American Family Physician, 91*, 452–460.

Centers for Disease Control and Prevention. (n.d.). Screening tests at-a-glance. Retrieved from https://www.cdc.gov/cancer/colorectal/pdf/SFL_inserts_screening.pdf

Centers for Disease Control and Prevention. (2011, April 11). Rotavirus. Retrieved from www.cdc.gov/rotavirus/index.html

Centers for Disease Control and Prevention. (2012a, August 17). Recommendations for the identification of chronic hepatitis C virus infection among persons born during 1945–1965. *Morbidity and Mortality Weekly Report, 61(4*), 1–32. Retrieved from https://www.cdc.gov/mmwr/preview/mmwrhtml/rr6104a1.htm?s_cid=rr6104a1_w

Centers for Disease Control and Prevention. (2012b, October 22). Hepatitis C FAQS for the public. Retrieved from https://www.cdc.gov/hepatitis/c/cfaq.htm#cFAQ21

Centers for Disease Control and Prevention. (2013, January 10). Parasites—Hookworms. Retrieved from https://www.cdc.gov/parasites/hookworm/health_professionals/index.html#tx

Centers for Disease Control and Prevention. (2015, February 28). Parasites—Cyclosporiasis (Cyclospora infection). Retrieved from www.cdc.gov/parasites/cyclosporiasis

Centers for Disease Control and Prevention. (2016a, February 3). Parasites—Enterobiasis (also known as pinworm infection). Retrieved from https://www.cdc.gov/parasites/pinworm/health_professionals/index.html

Centers for Disease Control and Prevention. (2016b, July 13). Viral hepatitis—Hepatitis A information. Retrieved from https://www.cdc.gov/hepatitis/HAV/index.htm

Centers for Disease Control and Prevention Vaccines & Immunizations. (2012, November 30). Vaccines and preventable diseases: Rotavirus vaccination. Retrieved from www.cdc.gov/vaccines/vpd-vac/rotavirus/default.htm#ed

Chatoor, D., & Emmnauel, A. (2009). Constipation and evacuation disorders. *Best Practice & Research Clinical Gastroenterology, 23*, 517–530.

Chou, R., & Wasson, N. (2013, June 4). Blood tests to diagnose fibrosis or cirrhosis in patients with chronic hepatitis C infection. *Annals of Internal Medicine, 158*, 807–820 and W-328–W330.

Chowdhury, N. R., & Chowdhury, J. R. (2009, May 1). Diagnostic approach to the patient with jaundice or asymptomatic hyperbilirubinemia. *UpToDate.* Retrieved from http://www.uptodate.com/online/content/topic.do?topicKey=hep_dis/8241&view=print

Ciclitira, P. J. (2009, May 1). Management of celiac disease in adults. *UpToDate.* Retrieved from http://www.uptodate.com/online/content/topic.do?topicKey=mal_synd/5722&view=print

Clinical Practice Committee. (2004). American Gastroenterological Association Institute medical position statement: Diagnosis and treatment of hemorrhoids. *Gastroenterology, 126*, 1461–1462.

Craig, S. (2012, October 26). Appendicitis. *Medscape.* Retrieved from http://emedicine.medscape.com/article/773895

Crocket, J. R., Bastian, L. A., & Chireau, M. V. (2013). Does this woman have an ectopic pregnancy? The rational clinical examination systematic review. *Journal of the American Medical Association, 309*, 1722–1729.

Crohn's and Colitis Foundation of America. (n.d.a). Crohn's disease medication options. Retrieved from http://www.ccfa.org/what-are-crohns-and-colitis/what-is-crohns-disease/crohns-medication.html

Crohn's and Colitis Foundation of America. (n.d.b). Crohn's treatment options. Retrieved from http://www.ccfa.org/what-are-crohns-and-colitis/what-is-crohns-disease/crohns-treatment-options.html

Crohn's and Colitis Foundation of America. (n.d.c). Types of Crohn's disease and associated symptoms. Retrieved from http://www.ccfa.org/what-are-crohns-and-colitis/what-is-crohns-disease/types-of-crohns-disease.html

Crohn's and Colitis Foundation of America. (n.d.d). Types of ulcerative colitis. Retrieved from http://www.ccfa.org/what-are-crohns-and-colitis/what-is-ulcerative-colitis/types-of-ulcerative-colitis.html

Crohn's and Colitis Foundation of America. (2014, February 6). Biologic therapies. Retrieved from http://www.ccfa.org/resources/biologic-therapies.html

Deshpande, P. G. (2015, September 3). Colic. *Medscape.* Retrieved from http://emedicine.medscape.com/article/927760

Dhawan, V. K. (2013, June 17). Hepatitis C. *Medscape.* Retrieved from http://emedicine.medscape.com/article/177792-overview

Dienstag, J. L., & McHutchison, J. G. (2006). American Gastroenterological Association medical position statement on the management of hepatitis C. *Gastroenterology, 130*, 225–230.

Dinning, P. G., & Di Lorenzo, C. (2011). Colonic dysmotility in constipation. *Best Practice & Research Clinical Gastroenterology, 25*, 89–101.

Division of Viral Hepatitis, CDC. (2014). Viral hepatitis surveillance United States, 2014. Retrieved from https://www.cdc.gov/hepatitis/statistics/2014surveillance/pdfs/2014hepsurveillancerpt.pdf

Dora-Laskey, A. (2016, May 18). *Ascaris lumbricoides. Medscape.* Retrieved from http://emedicine.medscape.com/article/788398- overview

Ehlers, A. P., Talan, D. A., Moran, G. J., Flum, D. R., & Davidson, G. H. (2016). Evidence for an antibiotics first strategy for uncomplicated appendicitis in adults: A systematic review and gap analysis. *Journal of the American College of Surgeons, 222*, 309–314.

Emetrol. (2015). Nausea relief for you and your family. Retrieved from http://emetrol.com/otc-nausea-medication/

Fargo, M. V., & Latimer, K. M. (2012). Evaluation and management of common anorectal conditions. *American Family Physician, 85*, 624–630.

Feingold, D., Steele, S. R., Lee, S., Kaiser, A., Boushey, R., Buie, W. D., & Frederick Rafferty, J. (2014). Practice parameters for the treatment of sigmoid diverticulitis. *Diseases of the Colon & Rectum, 57*, 284–294.

Fishman, M. B., & Aronson, M. D. (2012, March 5). History and physical examination in adults with abdominal pain. *UpToDate.* Retrieved from http://www.uptodate.com/contents/history-and-physical-examination-in-adults-with-abdominal-pain

Ford, A. C., Moayyedi, P., Lacy, B. E., Lembo, A. J., Saito, Y. A., Schiller, L. R., . . . Quigley, E. M.; Task Force on the Management of Functional Bowel Disorders. (2014). American College of Gastroenterology monograph on management of irritable bowel syndrome and chronic idiopathic constipation. *American Journal of Gastrenterology, 109*, S2–S26.

Freeman, H. J. (2008). Adult celiac disease in the elderly. *World Journal of Gastroenterology, 14*, 6911–6914.

Gainer, C. L. (2011, September). Helping patients live gluten-free. *Nurse Practitioner, 36*, 14–20.

Gardner, T. B., & Hill, D. R. (2001). Treatment of giardiasis. *Clinical Microbiology Reviews, 14*(1), 114–128.

Ghany, M. G., Nelson, D. R., Strader, D. B., Thomas, D. L., & Seeff, L. B. (2011). An update on treatment of genotype 1 chronic hepatitis C virus infection: 2011 practice guideline by the American Association for the Study of Liver Diseases. *Hepatology, 54*, 1433–1444.

Gisbert, J. P., & Chaparro, M. (2014). Inflammatory bowel disease in the elderly. *Medscape.* Retrieved from http://www.medscape.com/viewarticle/820753

Global RPH. (2016, March 10). TNF inhibitors—Biological response modifiers (BRMs). Retrieved from http://www.globalrph.com/TNF inhibitors.htm

Goebel, S. U. (2013, 2014, July 14). Celiac spruce. *Medscape.* Retrieved from http://emedicine.medscape.com/article/171805-overview

Goebel, S. U. (2014, December 16). Malabsorption. *Medscape.* Retrieved from http://emedicine.medscape.com/article/180785-overview

Green, R. M., & Flamm, S. (2002). AGA technical review on the evaluation of liver chemistry tests. *Gastroenterology, 123*, 1367–1384.

Green, P. H. R., & Cellier, C. (2007). Celiac disease medical progress. *The New England Journal of Medicine, 357*(17), 1731–1744.

Greenberger, N. J. (2013, November). Constipation. *The Merck manual for health care professionals.* Retrieved from http://www.merckmanuals.com/professional/gastrointestinal_disorders/symptoms_of_gi_disorders/constipation.html

Haburchak, D. R. (2016, February 24). Hookworm disease treatment & management. *Medscape Reference.* Retrieved from http://emedicine.medscape.com/article/218805

Hepatitis B Foundation. (2012, February 3). Approved drugs for adults. Retrieved from http://www.hepb.org/patients/hepatitis_b_treatment .htm

HepCnet. (2003, March 7). Drugs & liver damage. Retrieved from http://www.hepcnet.net/drugsandliverdamage.html

Herrine, S. K. (2016, May). Jaundice. *Merck manual professional version.* Retrieved from http://www.merckmanuals.com/professional/hepatic-and-biliary-disorders/approach-to-the-patient-with-liver-disease/jaundice

Heuman, D. M. (2014, April2). Cholelithiasis. *Medscape.* Retrieved from http://emedicine.medscape.com/article/175667-overview

Hill, I. D. (2009, May 1). Management of celiac disease in children. *UpToDate.* Retrieved from http://www.uptodate.com/online/content/topic.do?topicKey=pedigast/9506&view=print

Hofmann, W. P., & Zeuzem, S. (2011, May). A new standard of care for the treatment of chronic HCV infection. *Nature Reviews Gastroenterology & Hepatology, 8,* 257–264.

Hvas, A. M., & Nexo, E. (2006). Diagnosis and treatment of vitamin B_{12} deficiency. An update. *Haematologica/The Hematology Journal, 91,* 1506–1512.

Kagnoff, M. F. (2006). American Gastroenterological Association Institute medical position statement on the diagnosis and management of celiac disease. *Gastroenterology, 131,* 1977–1980.

Kahrilas, P. J., Shaheen, N. J., & Vaezi, M. F. (2008, October). American Gastroenterological Association Medical position statement on the management of gastroesophageal reflux disease. *Gastroenterology, 135,* 1383–1391. Retrieved from http://www.gastrojournal.org/issues?_key-S0016-5085(08)X0010-1

Katz, P. O., Gerson, L. B., & Vela, M. F. (2013, February). Guidelines for the diagnosis and management of gastroesophageal reflux disease. *American Journal of Gastroenterology, 108,* 308–328.

Kelly, C. P. (2013, January 16). Diagnosis of celiac disease. *UpToDate.* Retrieved from http://www.uptodate.com/contents/diagnosis-of-celiac-disease

Kheir, A. E. M. (2012). Infantile colic, facts and fiction. *Journal of Pediatrics, 38,* 34–37.

Kornbluth, A., & Sachar, D. B. (2010). Ulcerative colitis practice guidelines in adults: American College of Gastroenterology, Practice Parameters Committee. *American Journal of Gastroenterology, 105,* 501–523.

Kushner, R. F., & Cummings, S. (2012, July 5). Medical management of patients after bariatric surgery. *UpToDate.* Retrieved from www.uptodate.com/contents/medical-management-of-patients-after-bariatric-surgery

Lanza, F. L., Francis, K. L., Chan, M. D., Eammonn, M. M., Quigley, M. D., & The Practice Parameters Committee of the American College of Gastroenterology. (2009, March). Guidelines for prevention of NSAID-related ulcer complications. *American Journal of Gastroenterology, 104,* 728–738.

Leder, K., & Weller, P. F. (2016, June 16). Ascariasis. *UpToDate.* Retrieved from http://www.uptodate.com/contents/ascariasis

Leder, K., & Weller, P. F. (2009, May 1). Epidemiology, clinical manifestations, and diagnosis of giardiasis. *UpToDate.* Retrieved from http://www.uptodate.com/online/content/topic.do?topicKey=parasite/7013&view=print

Lee, R. M., Lessler, J., Lee, R. A., Rudolph, K. E., Reich, N. G., Perl, T. M., & Cummings, D. A. (2013). Incubation periods of viral gastroenteritis: A systematic review. *BMC Infectious Diseases, 13,* 446. Retrieved from http://doi.org/10.1186/1471-2334-13-446

Lehrer, J. K. (2015, June 16). Irritable bowel syndrome treatment & management. *Medscape.* Retrieved from http://emedicine.medscape.com/article/180389- treatment

Levitt, M. A. (2015, August 28). Management of severe pediatric constipation. *Medscape.* Retrieved from http://emedicine.medscape.com/article/937030-overview

Levitt, M. A. (2011, August 11). Management of severe pediatric constipation. *Medscape.* Retrieved from http://emedicine.medscape.com/937030-overview

Lichtenstein, G. R., Abreu, M. T., Cohen, R., & Tremaine, W.. (2006). American Gastroenterological Association Institute medical position statement on corticosteroids, immunomodulators, and infliximab in inflammatory bowel disease. *Gastroenterology, 130,* 935–939.

Lichtenstein, G. R., Hanauer, S. B., Sandborn, W. J., & The Practice Parameters Committee of the American College of Gastroenterology. (2009). Management of Crohn's disease in adults. *American Journal of Gastroenterology.* Retrieved from http://s3.gi.org/physicians/guidelines/CrohnsDiseaseinAdults2009.pdf

Loc, A. S. F., & McMahon, B. J. (2009). AASLD practice guideline update: Chronic hepatitis B: Update 2009. Retrieved from http://www.aasld.org/sites/default/files/guideline_documents/ChronicHepatitisB2009 .pdf

Longstreth, G. F. (2013, April 5). Approach to the adult with nausea and vomiting. *UpToDate.* Retrieved from http://www.uptodate.com/contents/approach-to-the-adult-with-nausea-and-vomiting

Madoff, R. D., & Fleshman, J. W. (2004). American Gastroenterological Association technical review on the diagnosis and treatment of hemorrhoids. *Gastroenterology, 126*(5), 1463–1473.

Mason, D., Tobias, N., Lutkenhoff, M., Stoops, M., & Ferguson, D. (2004). The APN's guide to pediatric constipation management. *Nurse Practitioner, 29*(7), 13–21.

Mason, J. B., & Milovic, V. (2009, May 1). Overview of the treatment of malabsorption. *UpToDate.* Retrieved from http://www.uptodate.com/online/content/topic.do?topicKey=mal_synd/7320&view=print

Medical Letter®. (March, 2012). Treatment guidelines from the medical letter, drugs for inflammatory bowel disease. *Medical Letter, 10*(15), 19–30.

Medicare.gov. (n.d.). Your Medicare coverage, colorectal cancer screening. Retrieved from www.medicare.gov/coverage/colorectal-cancer-screenings.html

Milovic, V., & Mason, J. B. (2009, May 1). Clinical features and diagnosis of malabsorption. *UpToDate.* Retrieved from http://www.uptodate.com/online/content/topic.do?topicKey=mal_synd/6513&view=print

Moses, S. (2014, May 17). Chronic constipation. Retrieved from http://www.fpnotebook.com/GI/Constipation/ChrncCnstptn.htm

Mounsey, A. L., Halladay, J., & Sadiq, T. S. (2011). Hemorrhoids. *American Family Physician, 84*(2), 204–210.

Natesan, A., & Bury, C. (2015, April). Diverticulitis: Evaluation and management. Retrieved from http://www.ahcmedia.com/articles/135320-diverticulitis-evaluation-and-management

National Digestive Diseases Information Clearinghouse. (2011, January). *Diarrhea.* (NIH Publication No. 11-2749). Retrieved from http://digestive.niddk.nih.gov/ddiseases/pubs/diarrhea/Diarrhea_208.pdf

National Digestive Diseases Information Clearinghouse. (2012, December). *What I need to know about bowel control.* (NIH Publication No.13-6513). Retrieved from http://digestive.niddk .nih.gov/ddiseases/pubs/bowelcontrol_ez/index.aspx

National Digestive Disease Information Clearinghouse. (2014, March 5). Ulcerative colitis. Retrieved from http://digestive.niddk.nih.gov/DDISEASES/PUBS/colitis/index.aspx

National Institute for Health and Clinical Excellence. (2012, October). Crohn's disease, management in adults, children, and young people. *NICE Clinical Guideline, 152.* Retrieved from http://guidance.nice.org.uh/cg152

National Institute of Diabetes and Digestive and Kidney Diseases. (2014, June). Inguinal hernia. Retrieved from www.niddk.nih.gov/health-information/health-topics/digestive-diseases/inguinal-hernia/Pages/facts.aspx

National Institute of Diabetes and Digestive and Kidney Diseases. (2015, September). Hirschsprung disease. Retrieved from https://www.niddk.nih.gov/health-information/health-topics/digestive-diseases/hirschsprung-disease/Pages/ez.aspx

National Institute of Diabetes and Digestive and Kidney Diseases, National Institutes of Health. (2001, July 1). Let's talk about bowel control. Retrieved from http://www.bowelcontrol.nih.gov

National Institute of Diabetes and Digestive and Kidney Diseases, National Institutes of Health. (2013, February 20). Living with bowel control problems. Retrieved from http://www.bowelcontrol.nih.gov/lbc.aspx

Nazer, H. (2016, February 15). Giardiasis. *Medscape.* Retrieved from http://emedicine.medscape.com/article/176718-overview

Nettina, S. (2010). *The Lippincott manual of nursing practice* (9th ed.). Philadelphia, PA: Wolters Kluwer Lippincott Williams & Wilkins.

Neville, H. L. (2012, May 8). Pediatric Hirschsprung disease. *Medscape.* Retrieved from http://emedicine.medscape.com/article/929733-overview

Nguyen, M. C. T. (2011, September 22). Diverticulitis. *Medscape.* Retrieved from http://emedicine.medscape.com/article/173388-overview

NHS Choices. (n.d.). Constipation. Retrieved from http://www.nhs.uk/Conditions/constipation/Pages/Introduction.aspx

Nicks, B. A. (2012, June 6). Hernias. *Medscape.* Retrieved from http ://www.emedicine.medscape.com/article/775630-overview

North American Society for Pediatric Gastroenterology, Hepatology and Nutrition. (2005). Guideline for the diagnosis and treatment of celiac disease in children: Recommendation of the North American Society for Pediatric Gastroenterology, Hepatology and Nutrition. *Journal of Pediatric Gastroenterology and Nutrition, 40*(1), 1–19.

North American Society for Pediatric Gastroenterology Hepatology and Nutrition. (2006). Clinical practice guideline. Evaluation and treatment of constipation in infants and children: Recommendations of the North American Society for Pediatric Gastroenterology, Hepatology and Nutrition. *Journal of Pediatric Gastroenterology and Nutrition, 43,* e1–e13.

Ogunyemi, D. A. (2015, November 14). Hyperemesis gravidarum. *Medscape.* Retrieved from http://emedicine.medscape.com/article/254751-overview#a4

Page, J. (2012). Recent developments in the treatment of chronic hepatitis C. *Journal for Nurse Practitioners, 8,* 225–230.

Paquette, I. M., Varma, M., Ternent, C., Melton-Meaux, G., Rafferty, J. F., Feingold, D., & Steele, S. R. (2016). The American Society of Colon and Rectal Surgeons' clinical practice guidelines for the evaluation and management of constipation. *Diseases of the Colon & Rectum, 59,* 479–492.

Poh, C. H., Navarro-Rodriguez, T., & Fass, R. (2010). Review: Treatment of gastroesophageal reflux disease in the elderly. *American Journal of Medicine, 123,* 496–501.

Qaseem, A., Denberg, T. D., Hopkins, R. H., Humphrey, L. L., Levine, J., Sweet, D. E., & Shekelle, P. (2012). Screening for colorectal cancer: A guidance statement from the American College of Physicians. *Annals of Internal Medicine, 156,* 378–386.

Ramsook, C., & Endom, E. E. (2012, September 12). Overview of inguinal hernia in children. *UpToDate.* Retrieved from www.uptodate.com/contents/overview-of-inguinal-hernia-in-children

Rao, S. S. C., & Meduri, K. (2011). What is necessary to diagnose constipation? *Best Practice & Research Clinical Gastroenterology, 25,* 127–140.

Rather, A. A. (2015, December 1). Abdominal hernias. *Medscape.* Retrieved from http://emedicine.medscape.com/article/189563-overview

Ren, C. J., & Fielding, G. A. (2003). Laparoscopic adjustable gastric banding: Surgical technique. *Journal of Laparoendoscopic & Advanced Surgical Techniques, 13,* 257–263.

Rex, D. K., Johnson, D. A., Adnerson, J. C., Schoenfeld, P. S., Burke, C. A., & Inadomi, J. M. (2009). American College of Gastroenterology guidelines for colorectal cancer screening 2008. *American Journal of Gastroenterology.* Retrieved from www.amjgasro.com

Rivadeneira, D. E., Steele, S. R., Ternent, C., Chalasani, S., Buie, W. D., & Rafferty, J. L. (2011). Practice parameters for the management of hemorrhoids (revised 2010). *Diseases of the Colon & Rectum, 54,* 1059–1064.

RotaTeq (Rotavirus Vaccine, Live, Oral, Pentavalent). (2013). Highlights of prescribing information. Retrieved from http://www.fda.gov/downloads/BiologicsBloodVaccines/Vaccines/ApprovedProducts/UCM142288 .pdf

Rowe, W. A. (2013, June 18). Inflammatory bowel disease. *Medscape* Retrieved from http://emedicine.medscape.com/article/179037-overview

Rubio-Tapia, A., Hill, I. D., Kelly, C. P., Calderwood, A. H., & Murray, J. A. (2013, May). ACG clinical guidelines: Diagnosis and management of celiac disease. *American Journal of Gastroenterology, 108,* 656–676.

Ruiz, A. R. (2014, May). Overview of malabsorption. *The Merck manual for health care professionals.* Retrieved from http://www.merckmanuals.com/professional/gastrointestinal_disorders/malabsorption_syndromes/overview_of_malabsorption.html

Saad, R. J., & Chey, W. D. (2014, February). First-line treatment strategies for *Helicobacter pylori* infection. *Gastroenterology & Endoscopy News,* 1–8. Retrieved from http://www.gastroendonews.com/Review-Articles/Article/06-15/First-Line-Treatment-Strategies-for-Helicobacter-nbsp-pylori-Infection/32678/ses=ogst

Sartor, R. B. (2015, July 6). Antibiotics for treatment of inflammatory bowel diseases. *UpToDate.* Retrieved from http://www .uptodate.com/contents/antibiotics-for-treatment-of-inflammatory-bowel-diseases

Satsangi, J., Silverberg, M. S., Vermeire, S., & Colombel J.-F. (2006). The Montreal classification of inflammatory bowel disease: Controversies, consensus, and implications. *Gut, 55,* 749–753.

Schwarz, S. M. (2011, March 29). Pediatric cholecystitis. *Medscape.* Retrieved from http://emedicine.medscape.com/article927340-overview

Sharma, G. D. (2013, June 17). Cystic fibrosis. *Medscape.* Retrieved from http://emedicine.medscape.com/article/1001602-overview

Shoff, W. H. (2012a, November 16). Cyclospora. *Medscape.* Retrieved from http://emedicine.medscape.com/article/236105-overview

Shoff, W. H. (2012b, November 16). Pediatric ascariasis. *Medscape.* Retrieved from http://emedicine.medscape.com/article/996482-overview

Snyder, J. A., Gurevitz, S. L., Rush, L. S., McKeague, L. C., & Houpt, C.G. (2012, January). Appendicitis review. *Clinician Reviews, 22,* 23–28.

Surawicz, C. M., Brandt, L. J., Binion, D. G., Ananthakrishnan, A. N., Curry, S. R., Gilligan, P. H., . . . Zuckerbraun, B. S. (2013). Guidelines for diagnosis, treatment, and prevention of *Clostridium difficile* infections. *American Journal of Gastroenterology, 108,* 478–498.

Tack, J., Müller-Lissner, S., Stanghellini, V., Boeckxstaens, G., Kamm, M. A., Simren, M., . . . Fried, M. (2011). Diagnosis and treatment of chronic constipation—A European perspective. *Neurogastroenterology and Motility, 23,* 697–710.

Terdiman, J. P., Gruss, C. B., Heidelbaugh, J. J., Sultan, S., & Falck-Ytter, V. T. (2013). American Gastroenterological Association Institiute Guideline on the use of thiopurines, methotrexate, and anti-TNF-α biologic drugs for the induction and maintenance of remission in inflammatory Crohn's disease. *Gastroenterology, 145,* 459–1463.

Thornton, S. C. (2012, September 12). Hemorrhoids. *Medscape.* Retrieved from http://emedicine.medscape.com/article/775407-overview

Truelove, S. C., & Witts, L. J. (1955). Cortisone in ulcerative colitis final report on a therapeutic trial. *British Medical Journal, 2,* 1041–1048.

Turner, T. L., & Palamountain, S. (2009a, May 1). Clinical features and etiology of colic. *UpToDate.* Retrieved from http://www.uptodate.com/online/content/topic.do?topicKey=behavior/2155&view=print

Turner, T. L., & Palamountain, S. (2009b, May 1). Evaluation and management of colic. *UpToDate.* Retrieved from http://www.uptodate.com/online/content/topic.do?topicKey=behavior/4542&view=print

Tyler-Evans, M. E., & Meyer, B. (2009). Post-bariatric surgery: Management considerations for NPs. *American Journal for Nurse Practitioners, 13,* 29–33.

University of Chicago Celiac Disease Center. (n.d.). Gluten free diet. Retrieved from http://www.celiacdisease.net/glutenfree-diet

University of Maryland Medical Center. (2013, June 27). Gallstones and gallbladder disease. Retrieved from http://umm.edu/health/medical/reports/articles/gallstones-and-gallbladder-disease

U.S. Food and Drug Administration. (2011, December). Plavix (clopidogrel bisulfate) tablet detailed view: Safety labeling changes approved by FDA Center for Drug Evaluation and Research (CDER). Retrieved from http://www.fda.gov/Safety/MedWatch/SafetyInformation/ucm225843.htm

U.S. Preventive Services Task Force. (2016, June 21). Screening for colorectal cancer. U.S. Preventive Task Force recommendation statement. *Journal of the American Medical Association, 315,* 2564–2575.

Utah Library of Medicine. (n.d.). Hepatic pathology: Caput medusae. Retrieved from http://library.med.utah.edu/WebPath/LIVEHTML/LIVER061.html

Vargas, H. D. (n.d.). Constipation expanded version. Retrieved from https://www.fascrs.org/patients/disease-condition/constipation-expanded-version

Wagner, J. P. (2015, August 18). Hirschsprung disease. *Medscape.* Retrieved from http://emedicine.medscape.com/article/178493-overview

Wehbi, M. (2011, January 12). Acute gastritis. *Medscape.* Retrieved from http://emedicine.medscape.com/article/175909-overview

Weller, P. F. (2009, May 1). Anthelminthic therapies. *UpToDate.* Retrieved from http://www.uptodate.com/online/content/topic.do?topicKey=antibiot/7691&view=print

Weller, P. F., & Kaplan, S. L. (2015, June 16). Treatment and prevention of giardiasis. *UpToDate.* Retrieved from http://www.uptodate.com/contents/treatment-and-prevention-of-giardiasis

Weller, P. F., & Leder, K. (2016, July 1). Hookworm infection. *UpToDate.* Retrieved from http://www.uptodate.com/contents/hookworm-infection

Wesson, D. E. (2012, December 13). Congenital aganglionic megacolon (Hirschsprung disease). *UpToDate.* Retrieved from http://www.uptodate.com/contents/congenital-aganglionic-megacolon-hirschsprung-disease

World Gastroenterology Organisation Global Guidelines. (2009, June). Inflammatory bowel disease: A global perspective. Retrieved from http://www.worldgastroenterology.org/assets/downloads/en/pdf/guidelines/21_inflammatory_bowel_disease.pdf

World Gastroenterology Organisation Global Guidelines. (2015, September). Irritable bowel syndrome: A global perspective. Retrieved from http://www.worldgastroenterology.org/guidelines/global-guidelines/irritable-bowel-syndrome-ibs/irritable-bowel-syndrome-ibs-english

World Gastroenterology Organisation Practice Guidelines. (2007). Diverticular disease. Retrieved from http://www.worldgastroenterology.org/assets/downloads/en/pdf/guidelines/07_diverticular_disease.pdf

World Health Organization. (2010, September 22). Statement on Rotarix and Rotateq vaccines and intussusception. Retrieved from http://www.who.int/immunization/sage/3_Rotarix_statement.pdf

World Health Organization. (2015, March). *Guidelines for the prevention, care and treatment of persons with chronic hepatitis B.* Geneva, Switzerland: Author.

Young-Fadok, T., & Pemberton, J. H. (2012, November 15). Treatment of acute diverticulitis. *UpToDate.* Retrieved from http://www.uptodate.com/contents/treatment-of-acute-diverticulitis

Zakko, S. F., & Afdhal, N. H. (2015, August 15). Acute cholecystitis: Pathogenesis, clinical features and diagnosis. *UpToDate.* Retrieved from http://www.uptodate.com/contents/acute-cholecystitis-pathogenesis-clinical-features-and-diagnosis

12 Genitourinary Guidelines

Benign Prostatic Hypertrophy

Cheryl A. Glass and Debbie Gunter

Definition

A. Benign prostatic hypertrophy (BPH) is enlargement of the prostate gland that constricts the urethra, causing urinary symptoms. BPH is not believed to be a risk factor for prostate cancer. BPH occurs primarily in the central or transitional zone of the prostate, whereas prostate cancer originates primarily in the peripheral part of the prostate.
B. The voiding dysfunction that results from prostate enlargement and bladder outlet obstruction (BOO) is termed lower urinary tract symptoms (LUTS).

Incidence

A. BPH increases progressively with age. The prevalence of prostatic hyperplasia increases from 8% in men aged 31 to 40 years to 40% to 50% in men aged 51 to 60 years to more than 90% in men older than 80 years.

Pathogenesis

A. The exact cause is unknown; BPH may be a response to the androgen hormone. The process of aging and the presence of circulating androgens lead to the development of BPH. Hyperplasia, in which the normally thin and fibrous outer capsule of the prostate becomes spongy and thick, and the contraction of muscle fibers cause pressure on the urethra. This requires the bladder musculature to work harder to empty urine.

Predisposing Factors

A. Advancing age
B. Race: African American men younger than 65 years may need treatment more often than Caucasian men.
C. Genetic predisposition: Increases with a positive family history of BPH having moderate to severe LUTS
D. Obesity
E. Diabetes
F. High levels of alcohol consumption
G. Physical inactivity

Common Complaints

The clinical manifestations of BPH are LUTS that typically appear slowly and progress gradually over a period of years.
A. Difficulty starting urine flow
B. Dribbling
C. Bladder does not feel like it completely empties
D. Frequency of urination

Other Signs and Symptoms

A. Obstructive symptoms
  1. Hesitancy
  2. Diminution in size and force of urinary stream
  3. Stream interruption (double voiding)
  4. Urinary retention
  5. Straining/Valsalva maneuver to fully empty the bladder
B. Irritative voiding symptoms
  1. Urgency
  2. Frequency
  3. Nocturia
  4. Painless hematuria: An early symptom; may also indicate malignancy
C. Severe late symptoms with untreated BPH
  1. Acute urinary retention
  2. Recurrent urinary tract infections (UTIs)
  3. Hydronephrosis
  4. Loss of renal concentrating ability
  5. Systemic acidosis and renal failure

Subjective Data

A. Have the patient complete the American Urological Association Symptom Score (AUASS) assessment tool at each visit to track symptoms. The AUASS (see Table 12.1) is used to assess the severity of symptoms of BPH.
B. Review the onset, duration, and course of symptoms. The AUASS assessment tool can be used to quantitatively assess BPH symptoms over time.
C. Does the patient have signs of a UTI?
D. Is there any blood in the urine or pain in the bladder region? (Evaluate bladder tumor or calculi.)
E. Does the patient have new symptoms such as bone or back pain, loss of appetite, or weight loss (rule out cancer)?
F. Review the patient's history for medical illness, including diabetes and neurologic problems.
G. Review previous urinary problems, surgeries, infections, treatments, success of treatments, and testing.
H. Review the patient's history of sexual dysfunction and any new sexual partners (sexually transmitted infections [STIs]).

TABLE 12.1 American Urological Association Symptom Score for Benign Prostatic Hypertrophy (BPH)

PATIENT NAME: ______________________ TODAY'S DATE: ______________

(Circle One Number on Each Line)	Not at All	Less Than One Time in Five	Less Than Half the Time	About Half the Time	More Than Half the Time	Almost Always
Over the past month or so, how often have you had a sensation of not emptying your bladder completely after you finished urinating?	0	1	2	3	4	5
During the past month or so, how often have you had to urinate again less than 2 hours after you finished urinating?	0	1	2	3	4	5
During the past month or so, how often have you found you stopped and started again several times when you urinated?	0	1	2	3	4	5
During the past month or so, how often have you found it difficult to postpone urination?	0	1	2	3	4	5
During the past month or so, how often have you had a weak urinary stream?	0	1	2	3	4	5
During the past month or so, how often have you had to push or strain to begin urination?	0	1	2	3	4	5
	None	**Once**	**Two Times**	**Three Times**	**Four Times**	**Five or More Times**
Over the past month, how many times per night did you most typically get up to urinate from the time you went to bed at night until the time you got up in the morning?	0	1	2	3	4	5

Add the score for each number above and write the total in the space to the right. **TOTAL:** __________

SYMPTOM SCORE: 1–7 (Mild); 8–19 (Moderate); 20–35 (Severe)

Quality of Life (QOL)

	Delighted	Pleased	Mostly Satisfied	Mixed	Mostly Dissatisfied	Unhappy	Terrible
How would you feel if you had to live with your urinary condition the way it is now, no better, no worse, for the rest of your life?	0	1	2	3	4	5	6

Source: Used with permission from American Urological Association (AUA) Education and Research Inc.

I. Review the patient's history of urethral trauma, urethritis, or urethral instrumentation that could have led to urethral stricture.

J. Review medications, both prescription and over-the-counter (OTC) drugs, including sinus or cold products, anticholinergic drugs (impair bladder function), and sympathomimetic drugs (increase outflow resistance).

K. Review family history of BPH and prostate cancer.

L. Review fluid intake, especially caffeinated/carbonated drinks.

M. Evaluate how bothersome the symptoms are to the patient's quality of life.

1. How often does he have interrupted sleep to get up to go to the bathroom?
2. How often does he urinate?
3. Does he have to wear an absorptive underwear pad?

Physical Examination

A. Check temperature (if indicated), blood pressure (BP), and weight (if indicated).

B. Inspect

1. Inspect general appearance for discomfort or acute discomfort with urinary retention.

2. Consider having the patient void: Normal urination for a man is the ability to empty the bladder of 300 mL of urine in 12 to 15 seconds.

3. Examine the urethral meatus for discharge.

4. Retract foreskin (if present) and assess for hygiene and smegma.

5. Check the shaft of the penis, glans, and prepuce for lesions.

6. Check inguinal and femoral areas for bulges or hernias; have the patient bear down and cough, and reexamine him.

7. Perform a neurologic examination (evaluate sensory and motor deficits).

C. Palpate

1. Palpate the abdomen for masses or bladder distension.

2. Palpate lymph nodes in the groin for enlargement.

3. Check costovertebral angle (CVA) tenderness.

4. Palpate the testes and epididymides for inflammation, tenderness, and masses.

5. Palpate the scrotum for hydrocele or varicocele.

D. Digital rectal examination (DRE): Use the index finger of the dominant hand for the DRE.

1. Note sphincter tone, nodules or masses, and tenderness. Decreased anal sphincter tone or the lack of muscle reflex may indicate an underlying neurologic disorder.

2. Palpate the two lateral lobes of the prostate gland and its median sulcus for irregularities, nodules, induration, swelling, or tenderness just above the prostate anteriorly; determine whether the rectum lies adjacent to the peritoneal cavity. If possible, palpate this region for peritoneal masses and tenderness.

Diagnostic Tests

A. Urinalysis: Evaluate for infection and hematuria.

B. Urine culture if indicated (patients with BPH are more susceptible to UTIs).

C. Optional studies

1. Prostate-specific antigen (PSA): Reference ranges vary by age and ethnicity and may be elevated with BPH. Recommended in men with at least a 10-year-life expectancy

2. Urodynamic testing, including maximal urinary flow rate

3. Postvoid residual (PVR; as shown by in–out catheterization, radiography, or ultrasound)

4. Cystourethroscopy: Not recommended in the initial routine evaluation visit (may be needed later depending on workup for planning for surgical therapy)

D. The American Urological Association (AUA) recommends that the routine measurement of serum creatinine levels is *not* indicated in the initial evaluation.

Differential Diagnoses

A. BPH: Classifications of BPH from the score of the AUA symptom assessment tool:

1. Mild = total score 0 to 7

2. Moderate = total score 8 to 19

3. Severe = total score 20 to 35

B. Other obstructive causes: Prostate cancer, urethral obstruction, urethral stricture, and vesical neck obstruction

C. Neurogenic bladder

D. Cystitis

E. Prostatitis

F. Bladder calculi

Plan

A. General interventions

1. Have the patient complete a 24-hour voiding chart with assessment of frequency and volume.

2. Any patient with other than mild symptoms needs referral to a urologist to discuss treatment options (surgery or drugs).

3. Monitor the patient with mild symptoms every 3 to 6 months to determine the progression of symptoms. Imaging studies are not routinely necessary in typical cases of BPH unless there is hematuria, an elevated creatinine, or another indication.

4. Treat concurrent UTI and STIs.

B. Patient teaching

1. Patient teaching: *See Section III: Patient Teaching Guide for this chapter, "Prostatic Hypertrophy/Benign."* ◀

2. Patients should be instructed about the hypotensive effect, asthenia, nasal congestion, and effect on ejaculation of the long-acting alpha-1 antagonists. The hypotensive effects can be potentiated by concomitant use of phosphodiesterase-5 (PDE-5) inhibitors sildenafil (Viagra), tadalafil (Cialis), or vardenafil (Levitra).

3. Alpha-1 antagonists have been associated with intraoperative floppy iris syndrome. Patients need to discuss using these medicines with their ophthalmologist before eye surgery (i.e., cataract).

C. Pharmaceutical therapy

1. Five long-acting alpha-1 antagonists are Food and Drug Administration (FDA) approved for the treatment of BPH.

a. Terazosin (Hytrin) 1 to 20 mg/d; side effect increases hypotensive effect with PDE-5 inhibitor. Terazosin requires dose titration to minimize side effects.

b. Doxazosin (Cardura) 1 to 8 mg/d; side effect increases hypotensive effect with PDE-5 inhibitor. Doxazosin requires dose titration to minimize side effects.

c. Tamsulosin (Flomax) 0.4 to 0.8 mg/d; side effect decreases ejaculate volume.

d. Alfuzosin (Uroxatral) 10 mg/d; generally does not cause ejaculation problems.

e. Silodosin (Rapaflo) 8 mg/d; side effect may produce retrograde ejaculation.

2. Prazosin (Minipress), a short-acting alpha-1 antagonist, approved for the treatment of hypertension (HTN). It improves urine flow rates and may be considered for a patient with HTN and urinary symptoms.
3. Two 5-alpha-reductase inhibitors are FDA approved for BPH with an enlarged prostate. The major side effects of these drugs are decreased libido and ejaculatory or erectile dysfunction (ED).
a. The FDA has advised about safety information for the use of the 5-alpha-reductase inhibitors because of an increased risk of being diagnosed with a more serious form of prostate cancer (high-grade prostate cancer).
b. Women who are, or may become, pregnant should not handle the 5-alpha-reductase inhibitors. They are pregnancy category X, known to cause birth defects.
c. Finasteride (Proscar) 5 mg/d
d. Dutasteride (Avodart) 0.5 mg/d
e. Dutasteride–tamsulosin (Jalyn): Each capsule contains 0.5 mg dutasteride and 0.4 mg tamsulosin.
4. Dual-drug combination
5. There are no herbal supplements that have been approved by the FDA for the treatment of BPH; however, patients may report taking saw palmetto. The AUA does not endorse supplements.

Follow-Up

A. See the patient in 2 to 3 weeks to monitor symptoms after specialty referral.
B. PSA testing: Baseline testing should begin at age 40 years. The United States Preventive Services Task Force (USPSTF) recommends that PSA testing be discontinued at age 75 years.
C. PSA is an amino acid glycoprotein specific to prostate disease, but not exclusive to prostate cancer. Once the patient has exhibited an elevated PSA level, repeat the test yearly. Patients who have undergone treatment for prostate cancer are monitored for recurrence by the PSA levels.
D. The concept of "watchful waiting" may be appropriate for patients with mild symptoms. The patient should be seen yearly for evaluation and an examination.

Consultation/Referral

A. Refer to a urologist for any complicated LUTS, including
1. History of prostate cancer
2. Elevated PSA
3. Urethral stricture
4. Spinal cord injury
5. Stroke
6. Recurrent/persistent UTI
B. The presence of microscopic hematuria requires an evaluation of the complete urinary system and needs a referral to a urologist.
C. Refer for procedures after failed medication therapy.
1. Minimally invasive therapy
a. Transurethral microwave therapy (TUMT)
b. Transurethral incision of the prostate (TUIP)
2. Surgical therapies
a. Transurethral resection of the prostate (TURP) is considered the gold standard of surgical treatment of BPH. Sexual dysfunction may occur after a TURP, including decreased libido, impotence, and ejaculatory difficulties. Balloon dilation may be used to reduce symptoms; however, relapse is common.
b. Open prostatectomy
c. Laser procedures
i. Laser vaporization of the prostate
ii. Laser enucleation of the prostate
d. Transurethral needle ablation (TUNA)
e. Photoselective vaporization of the prostate (PVP)

Individual Consideration

A. Geriatrics: Elderly men require special attention because their symptoms may be poorly expressed or confusing.

Resources

Adult Pediatric Urology & Urogynecology: www.adultpediatricuro.com
American Urological Association (AUA): www.auanet.org
National Kidney Urologic Diseases Information Clearinghouse (KNUDIC): kidney.niddk.nih.gov

Chronic Kidney Disease in Adults

Angelito Tacderas and Debbie Gunter

Definition

Chronic kidney disease (CKD) is specifically defined as follows:
A. The persistent and usually progressive reduction in glomerular filtration rate (GFR) less than 60 mL/min/1.73 m^2 and/or
B. Albuminuria: more than 30 mg of urinary albumin per gram of urinary creatinine

CKD is a disorder that leads to progressive kidney damage from a variety of causes, including diabetes, hypertension (HTN), cardiovascular (CV) disease, urinary obstructions, prolonged use of nephrotoxic medications, and inherited diseases such as polycystic kidney disease. Associated comorbidities of CKD include renal osteodystrophy, anemia, metabolic acidosis, and malnutrition. Early recognition of CKD as well as treatment of complications can improve long-term outcomes.

Stages of CKD

A. Stage 1 disease is defined by a normal GFR (greater than 90 mL/min/1.73 m^2) and persistent albuminuria.
B. Stage 2 disease is a GFR between 60 and 89 mL/min/1.73 m^2 and persistent albuminuria.
C. Stage 3 disease is a GFR between 30 and 59 mL/min/1.73 m^2.
D. Stage 4 disease is a GFR between 15 and 29 mL/min/1.73 m^2.
E. Stage 5 disease is a GFR of less than 15 mL/min/1.73 m^2 or end-stage renal disease (ESRD).

Incidence

A. Kidney disease is the ninth leading cause of death in the United States. It is estimated that 80,000 new cases of nondialysis-dependent CKD are diagnosed annually; the incidence of CKD and ESRD has doubled every decade since 1980. The number of patients enrolled in the ESRD Medicare-funded program has increased from approximately 10,000 beneficiaries in 1973 to 661,648 as of December 31, 2013.

B. By age group, CKD is more prevalent among persons older than 60 years (39.4%) than among persons aged 40 to 59 years (12.6%) or persons aged 20 to 39 years (8.5%). CKD prevalence is greater among persons with diabetes than among those without diabetes (40.2% vs. 15.4%) and among persons with CV disease than among those without CV disease (28.2% vs. 15.4%). CKD is higher among persons with HTN than among those without HTN (24.6% vs. 12.5%). In addition, CKD prevalence is greater among non-Hispanic Blacks (19.9%) and Mexican Americans (18.7%) than among non-Hispanic Whites (16.1%).

Pathogenesis

Blood from the renal arteries and their subdivisions is delivered to the glomeruli. The glomeruli form an ultrafiltrate, nearly free of protein and blood elements, which subsequently flows into the renal tubules. The tubules reabsorb and secrete solute and/or water from the ultrafiltrate. The final tubular fluid, the urine, leaves the kidney, draining sequentially into the renal pelvis, ureter, and bladder, from which it is excreted through the urethra. The causes of CKD are traditionally classified by which portion of the renal anatomy is most affected by the disorder.

A. Vascular disease: Vascular disorders of the kidneys may involve partial or complete occlusion of large, medium, or small renal vessels. Examples of macrovascular or large renal vessel disease are renal artery stenosis and atherosclerotic disease. Benign hypertensive arteriolar nephrosclerosis results when chronic HTN damages small blood vessels, glomeruli, renal tubules, and interstitial tissues. Glomerulosclerosis is a severe microvascular or small vessel kidney disease caused by diabetes and uncontrolled HTN in which glomerular function of blood filtration is lost as fibrous scar tissue replaces the glomeruli. Loss of glomerular function leads to proteinuria, hematuria, HTN, and nephrosis, with variable progression to ESRD. Proteinuria occurs because of changes to capillary endothelial cells, the glomerular basement membrane (GBM), or podocytes, which normally filter serum protein selectively by size and charge.

B. Tubular and interstitial disease: As with vascular disease, chronic tubulointerstitial nephritis (CTIN) can be primary or secondary to glomerular damage and renovascular disease. CTIN arises when chronic tubular insults cause gradual interstitial infiltration and fibrosis, tubular atrophy and dysfunction, and a gradual deterioration of renal function, usually over years. Causes of CTIN are immune disorders, infections, reflux or obstructive nephropathy, and drugs. Analgesic abuse nephropathy (AAN) is a type of CTIN caused by cumulative lifetime use of large amounts of certain analgesics such as nonsteroidal anti-inflammatory drugs (NSAIDs).

Predisposing Factors

A. Diabetes
B. HTN
C. CV disease
D. Chronic use of analgesics such as NSAIDs
E. Autoimmune disorder
F. Polycystic kidney disease
G. Urinary tract obstructions such as benign prostatic hypertrophy (BPH) or kidney stones
H. Recurrent urinary tract infections (UTIs)
I. Older than 60 years
J. African American, Native American, or Hispanic ethnicity
K. Smoking
L. Exposure to toxins
M. Family history of kidney disease

Common Complaints

A. For CKD Stages 1 and 2 there are usually no presenting complaints; however, HTN is usually present. CKD is usually identified through routine screening of kidney function and urine tests for microalbumin.

Other Signs and Symptoms

A. In CKD Stage 3, the person will develop CKD complications but will still not usually have identifiable signs/symptoms.

1. HTN
2. Decreased dietary calcium absorption
3. Reduced renal phosphate excretion
4. Elevation of parathyroid hormone
5. Altered lipoprotein metabolism
6. Reduced spontaneous protein intake
7. Anemia
8. Left ventricular hypertrophy
9. Salt and water retention
10. Decreased renal potassium excretion

B. These complications gradually worsen as the person moves to Stage 4 CKD. The person will begin to display signs and symptoms of complications.

1. Changes in bone density
2. Fatigue and pallor related to anemia
3. Edema
4. Decrease in muscle mass

C. As the CKD progresses to Stage 5, in addition to gradual worsening of the signs/symptoms noted in Stages 3 and 4, the person will experience symptoms indicating chronic uremia.

1. Impaired sleep
2. Nocturia
3. Fatigue
4. Anorexia, nausea, vomiting, and weight change
5. Decreased mental acuity
6. Pruritus
7. Edema
8. Respiratory symptoms, including orthopnea and dyspnea

9. Muscle cramps, twitching, and restless legs
10. Peripheral neuropathy

Subjective Data

A. Review the patient's medical history to identify risk factors for CKD (previously noted in "Predisposing Factors" section).
B. Elicit information about how well risk factors such as diabetes mellitus (DM) and HTN are controlled.
C. Review the onset and duration of signs/symptoms of CKD complications and uremia.
D. Review all medications—including all over-the-counter (OTC) medications, especially NSAIDs, and supplements. Obtain specific information about dosing and length of time the drug was used.
E. Elicit smoking history.

Physical Examination

A. Observe general demeanor, attentiveness, and signs of fatigue.
B. Measure
 1. Height, weight, and body mass index (BMI)
 2. Vital signs, including orthostatic blood pressure (BP) and pulse
C. Inspect
 1. Skin for color, moisture, turgor, and signs of scratching because of chronic pruritus
 2. Neck for jugular venous distension
 3. Abdomen for distension
 4. Extremities for edema, muscle mass, and signs of pain disorders such as arthritis
D. Auscultate
 1. Lungs for crackles
 2. Heart for cardiac heave, gallop, or rub
 3. Abdomin or femoral bruit
E. Palpate
 1. Abdomen for masses, distension
 2. Bladder, and assess for flank tenderness
F. Neurologic examination
 1. Assess for sensation and vibratory sense on both feet.

Diagnostic Tests

Laboratory testing is critical in ascertaining the stage, course, chronicity, and complications (and associated comorbid conditions) of CKD.

A. Routine kidney function tests
 1. Serum creatinine
 2. Blood urea nitrogen (BUN)
 3. Urinalysis
 4. Measuring GFR: The severity of CKD should be classified based on the level of the estimated GFR (eGFR). Serum creatinine alone should *not* be used as a measure of kidney function. Kidney function in patients with CKD should be assessed by formula-based estimation of GFR (eGFR), preferably using the four-variable Modification of Diet in Renal Disease (MDRD) equation. Clinicians who do not have access to an automated tool may use a web-based tool, which is available at www.nkdep.nih.gov/professionals/gfr_calculators/index.htm. Calculate eGFRs using the actual MDRD equation:
 eGFR = 186 × (SCr) − 1.154 × (age) − 0.203 × (0.742 if female) × (1.210 if Black)
 (SCr, serum creatinine concentration)
B. Assessing proteinuria
 1. When screening adults at increased risk for CKD, albumin in the urine should be measured in a spot urine sample using
  a. Albumin-specific dipstick
  b. Albumin-to-creatinine ratio
   i. It is usually not necessary to obtain a timed urine collection (overnight or 24 hours).
   ii. First-morning specimens are preferred, but random specimens are acceptable if first-morning specimens are not available.
   iii. In most cases, screening with urine dipsticks is acceptable for detecting proteinuria.
   iv. Standard urine dipsticks are acceptable for detecting increased total urine protein.
   v. Albumin-specific dipsticks are acceptable for detecting albuminuria.
 2. Patients with a positive dipstick test (1 or greater) should undergo confirmation of proteinuria by a quantitative measurement (protein-to-creatinine ratio or albumin-to-creatinine ratio) within 3 months.
 3. Patients with two or more positive quantitative tests spaced apart by 1 to 2 weeks should be diagnosed as having persistent proteinuria and undergo further evaluation and management for CKD.

Other Tests to Determine CKD Complications

A. Complete blood count (CBC)
B. Hemoglobin (Hgb): If Hgb level is less than 12 g/dL in females and less than 13.5 g/dL in adult males, also do blood cell indices, absolute reticulocyte count, serum iron, total iron-binding capacity, percent transferrin saturation, serum ferritin, white blood cell (WBC) count and differential, platelet count, and testing for blood in stool.
C. Lipid profile and triglycerides
D. Comprehensive metabolic profile (serum total protein, serum albumin, glucose, calcium, sodium, potassium, chloride, bicarbonate, BUN, creatinine, alkaline phosphatase, alanine aminotransferase [ALT], aspartate aminotransferase [AST], bilirubin)
E. Prealbumin
F. Phosphorus
G. Parathyroid hormone
H. Urine immunofixation study
I. Antinuclear antibody (ANA), anti-neutrophil cytoplasmic autoantibody (ANCA), complement 3 and complement 4 (C3-C4)
 1. Test is done to rule out autoimmune disorder, lupus, vasculitis, and cancer.
 2. No fasting is needed.
J. Hepatitis B surface antigen (HBsAg) and hepatitis C antibody
K. Anti-GBM antibody
L. Renal ultrasound to rule out postobstructive uropathy
M. Renal Doppler to rule out renal artery stenosis

Differential Diagnoses

Evaluation is meant to determine whether kidney disease is acute or chronic and to determine prerenal, intrarenal, or postrenal causation.

A. CKD
B. Acute kidney disease

Plan

The treatment plan will focus on patients in earlier stages of CKD—Stages 1, 2, and 3. Persons with Stage 4 and 5 CKD need specialized interventions provided by nephrologists and should be referred immediately.

A. General interventions
 1. Provide support to the patient.
 2. Initiate appropriate referrals for a nephrologist, patient education, and social and financial support as soon as possible.
 3. For Stage 4 or 5 CKD, access devices for hemodialysis, such as a primary arteriovenous fistula or graft, require months to mature and should be in place for 6 months before the start of dialysis.

B. Patient teaching: *See Section III: Patient Teaching Guide for this chapter, "Kidney Disease: Chronic."*
 1. Instruct the patient in how kidneys work and how his or her body is affected by the CKD.
 2. Emphasize the importance of following instructions to prevent further kidney damage.
  a. Follow medication management instructions as carefully as possible.
  b. No OTC medications should be taken that are not approved by the provider.
  c. Keeping diabetes and HTN under control is crucial to maintaining kidney function.
  d. Preventing CV complications by lowering cholesterol and BP is more important when you have CKD.
  e. Smoking cessation is an important way to prevent worsening kidney function.
  f. Routine follow-ups with provider are necessary to monitor kidney function. Patients should be educated and encouraged to keep all appointments.
  g. Follow dietary instructions regarding protein, fats, sodium, and minerals.
  h. Dietary intake of protein is usually restricted to 0.8 to 1.0 g/kg/d of high biologic value protein.
  i. Dietary sodium should be restricted to no more than 2 g daily.
  j. Potassium should be restricted to 40 to 70 meq/d.
  k. Calories should be restricted to 35 kcal/kg/d; if the body weight is greater than 120% of normal or the patient is older than 60 years, a lower amount may be prescribed.
  l. Fat intake should be about 30% to 40% of total daily caloric intake.
  m. Phosphorus should be restricted to 600 to 800 mg/d.
  n. Calcium should be restricted to 1,400 to 1,600 mg/d.
  o. Magnesium should be restricted to 200 to 300 mg/d.
 3. Instruct when to notify the provider with urgent signs/symptoms or changes in kidney function.
  a. Changes in urine volume
  b. Anorexia, nausea, and vomiting
  c. Increased edema
  d. Shortness of breath (SOB)
  e. Increased fatigue
  f. Difficulty concentrating
  g. Muscle weakness, cramping, or twitching
  h. Fever
  i. Chest pain

C. Pharmaceutical therapy

General principles of medications used to prevent progression of CKD and to manage symptoms of complications of CKD:

 1. Always prescribe the smallest effective dose of any medication.
 2. Start with a low dose and gradually increase. Dosage intervals may need to be extended.
 3. Monitor the effect of any new medication on kidney function with appropriate follow-up with appropriate laboratory follow-up.
 4. Provide education to the patient of signs/symptoms to report to the provider immediately regarding drug therapy.
 5. Avoid use of nephrotoxic drugs such as radiographic contrast materials, aminoglycoside antibiotics, and NSAIDs to prevent nephrogenic systemic fibrosis. If radiocontrast material use cannot be avoided because the benefit outweighs the risks, protect the kidney with acetylcysteine (Mucomyst) 600 mg orally twice daily on the day of intravenous (IV) contrast.
 6. Immunizations: Some vaccines in usual doses provide protection, while other vaccines require more frequent dosing or larger doses to achieve and maintain protective antibodies. Protective antibody titers may fall and booster doses should be given if appropriate. In general, the recommendations are
  a. Annual influenza vaccination
  b. Pneumococcal vaccine with a single booster dose 5 years after the initial dose
  c. Hepatitis B vaccine series for patients before starting dialysis
 7. HTN control and kidney protection: It is recommended that HTN therapy achieve a goal of BP of 130/80 mmHg or less. Use of an angiotensin-converting enzyme (ACE) inhibitor or angiotensin II receptor blocker (ARB) therapy in early stages of CKD with persons who have proteinuria can preserve kidney function. The clinician should monitor serum potassium on initiation of the therapy. It is common for the serum potassium to initially rise and then return to normal levels in 2 to 3 months. Follow-up serum potassium levels are recommended. In the early stages of CKD, with no proteinuria, the ACE inhibitors and ARBs have not been shown to be effective in

protecting kidney function. HTN control can still be achieved with the ACE/ARB drugs, but other antihypertensive drugs can be used as well.

8. Fluid overload: Occurs when sodium intake exceeds sodium excretion. The combination of sodium restrictions and a loop diuretic, such as furosemide (Lasix), can lower intraglomerular pressure and provide some kidney protection.

9. Hyperkalemia: Hyperkalemia is managed with a low potassium diet in combination with prescribing a loop diuretic such as furosemide. If a patient is on an ACE or ARB, the addition of the loop diuretic will compensate for the elevation of serum potassium related to the ACE/ARB treatment.

10. Metabolic acidosis: Buildup of hydrogen ions causes bicarbonate levels to fall below acceptable levels. Sodium bicarbonate in a daily dose of 0.5 to 1 meq/kg/d is often given. This prevents the symptoms of metabolic acidosis, which can increase muscle mass loss and worsen bone disease.

11. Renal osteodystrophy: The development of renal osteodystrophy is caused by hyperphosphatemia and hypocalcemia that are secondary to decreased kidney function. In order to compensate, the patient will develop secondary hyperparathyroidism. Dietary restriction of phosphate to 800 mg/d is recommended. In Stage 3 CKD, the patient will usually require an oral phosphate binder like calcium carbonate or calcium acetate to prevent hyperphosphatemia. Oral phosphate binders must be taken with meals to be effective. It is imperative to avoid phosphate binders that contain aluminum or magnesium. To suppress parathyroid hormone secretion, the patient is given calcitriol, a vitamin D analog.

12. Anemia: Use of elemental iron 200 mg, such as ferrous sulfate 325 mg three times daily (65 mg elemental iron per dose), is recommended to maintain the percent transferrin saturation greater than 20% and the serum ferritin level greater than 100 ng/mL.

Although primarily used in patients with ESRD, erythropoietic agents (EPO), such as epoetin alfa (Procrit, Epogen) and darbepoetin alfa (Aranesp), are also used to correct anemia in those with CKD who do not yet require dialysis. Dosages of the EPO agents should be prescribed in order to maintain Hgb levels in the range of 11 to 12 g/dL in predialysis patients with CKD.

13. Dyslipidemia: Management of dyslipidemia has been shown to slow progression of CKD. Statins and fibrates are commonly prescribed to lower total cholesterol and low-density lipoprotein (LDL) and triglycerides. The incidence of untoward side effects with statins and fibrates is increased in persons with CKD; therefore, lower dosages and careful monitoring are required.

Follow-Up

A. Regular, consistent follow-up appointments to monitor progression of CKD, management of complications of CKD, and management of comorbidities such as DM and HTN are recommended.

Consultation/Referral

A. Early referral to a nephrologist is recommended for anyone who has CKD. Referral to a nephrologist must be done as quickly as possible for symptomatic patients with Stage 4 or 5 CKD. Consultation with an endocrinologist or HTN specialist may be helpful in cases in which DM and HTN continue to be poorly controlled.

B. After the patient is evaluated as a candidate for kidney transplantation, counseling on renal transplantation should be completed by a nephrologist on what types of transplant are available and how the transplant process works.

C. Referral to a dietitian for nutritional counseling and education to assist the patient to understand and follow complex dietary instructions is recommended.

D. Patients with Stage 4 or 5 CKD need counseling regarding the psychosocial and financial impact of progressive renal disease. Referral to a renal social worker or case manager can help the patient understand his or her health insurance benefits, how the transition to Medicare occurs after the health insurance benefit changes, and to help the patient deal with concerns about work or family life.

E. Patients should be referred to educational and support organizations for further education regarding CKD.

F. Websites

 1. National Kidney Foundation: www.kidney.org

 2. National Kidney Disease Education Program: www.nkdep.nih.gov

Individual Consideration

A. Although renal replacement therapy is widely available, some patients, especially the more debilitated elderly or those who have a terminal illness, may request end-of-life counseling, including advance directives.

Epididymitis

Cheryl A. Glass and Debbie Gunter

Definition

Epididymitis is acute infection of the epididymis, the coiled segment of the spermatic duct that connects the efferent duct from the posterior aspect of the testicle to the vas deferens. Epididymitis is commonly found to develop during strenuous exertion in conjunction with a full bladder. **Testicular torsion should be considered in all cases—this is a surgical emergency.**

A. Acute epididymitis: duration of symptoms lasts less than 6 weeks.

 1. Acute epididymitis often involves the testis (epididymo-orchitis).

B. Chronic epididymitis: duration of symptoms lasts lasts more than 6 weeks.

 1. Inflammation chronic

 2. Obstructive chronic

 3. Chronic epididymalgia

Incidence

A. Epididymitis is the fifth most common urologic diagnosis in men aged 18 to 50 years. There are approximately

600,000 medical visits per year related to epididymitis. An estimated 1 in 1,000 men develop epididymitis annually. Chronic epididymitis may account for up to 80% of scrotal pain noted in the outpatient setting. The mumps, measles, and rubella (MMR) vaccine has markedly reduced the incidence of mumps orchitis.

Pathogenesis

A. The exact pathophysiology is unclear. The cause may be the retrograde passage of infected urine from the prostatic urethra to the epididymis from the ejaculatory ducts and vas deferens. Reflux may be induced by having the patient perform the Valsalva maneuver or may be from strenuous exertion. Pathogens include *Chlamydia trachomatis*, *Neisseria gonorrhoeae*, *Escherichia coli*, *Proteus* species, *Klebsiella* species, *Pseudomonas*, *Mycoplasma* species, and *Treponema pallidum.*

Predisposing Factors

A. Age
- **1.** Age less than 35 years is generally associated with urethritis with the following organisms:
  - **a.** *C. trachomatis* (chlamydia)
  - **b.** *N. gonorrhoeae* (gonorrhea)
- **2.** Benign prostatic hyperplasia (BPH) is more common for men older than 35 years and common organisms include
  - **a.** *E. coli*
  - **b.** *Pseudomonas* species
  - **c.** *Proteus* species
  - **d.** *Klebsiella* species
- **3.** The older populations of men usually have nonsexual epididymitis related to urinary tract instrumentation, surgery, and immunosuppression.

B. Men having sex with men (MSM) who are the insertive partner during anal intercourse have epididymitis with the following organisms:
- **1.** *E. coli*
- **2.** *Pseudomonas*
- **3.** Coliform bacteria

C. Urinary tract infections (UTIs)
D. Tuberculosis (TB; should be considered if there is a history of or recent exposure to TB)
E. Vasectomy
F. Indwelling urethral catheter
G. Urethral stricture
H. Amiodarone—high drug concentrations (dose dependent)
I. Prolonged sitting (sedentary job, travel)
J. Mumps

Common Complaints

A. Swelling and tenderness of the scrotum (usually located on one side)
B. Fever
C. Chronic epididymitis
- **1.** Epididymal pain and inflammation that last more than 6 weeks
- **2.** May be accompanied by scrotal induration

Other Signs and Symptoms

A. Gradual onset of localized, unilateral testicular pain. The patient may get relief with elevation of the scrotum, which *is* a positive **Prehn's sign**.
B. Urethral discharge
C. Dysuria, frequency, urgency
D. Hematuria
E. Fever and chills (in only 25% of adults with acute epididymitis but in up to 71% of children with the condition)

Subjective Data

A. Elicit the onset, duration, and course of the patient's symptoms.
B. Review the patient's history for vasectomy or trauma to the groin.
C. Are there any other symptoms, including fever, dysuria, or discharge?
D. What makes the pain better? Ask about elevating the scrotum.
E. Does the patient's sexual partner(s) have any symptoms or discharge?
F. Has there been any recent instrumentation or catheterization?
G. Is the pain unilateral or bilateral?
H. Review medication history for amiodarone.
I. Does the patient have a recent TB exposure?

Physical Examination

A. Check temperature, blood pressure (BP), and pulse.
B. Inspect
- **1.** Examine the patient generally for discomfort before and during examination.
- **2.** Check the urethral meatus for discharge. Retract foreskin (if present) and assess for hygiene and smegma. Check the shaft of the penis, glans, and prepuce for lesions.
- **3.** Check the inguinal and femoral areas for bulges and hernias; have the patient bear down and cough, and reexamine him.

C. Palpate
- **1.** Palpate testes and epididymides for inflammation, tenderness, and masses. In chronic cases, the epididymis feels firm and lumpy. Vas deferens may be beaded.
- **2.** Check Prehn's sign by elevating the affected hemiscrotum. This action relieves the pain of epididymitis but exacerbates the pain of torsion.
- **3.** Elicit a cremasteric reflex. Stroking the inner thigh should result in rise of the testicle and scrotum on the affected side. A normal cremasteric reflex indicates that testicular torsion is less likely.
- **4.** Palpate the scrotum for hydrocele or varicocele.
- **5.** Check for costovertebral angle (CVA) tenderness.
- **6.** Examine the abdomen for masses, urinary distension, tenderness, and organomegaly.
- **7.** Palpate lymph nodes in the groin.
- **8.** Evaluate for an inguinal hernia.

D. Rectal examination: Check for symmetry, swelling, tenderness, and enlarged prostate.

Diagnostic Tests

A. Gram stain of urethral secretions
B. Urinalysis and urine cultures
C. Urethra swab (before void, after prostate massage) for gonorrhea and chlamydia culture
D. In patients older than 40 years: Express prostatic secretions
E. TB skin test to rule out TB
F. Complete blood count (CBC)

Differential Diagnoses

A. Epididymitis
1. Bacterial
2. Viral epididymo-orchitis (mumps and *Haemophilus influenzae*)
B. Testicular torsion (surgical emergency)
C. Testicular tumor
D. Prostatitis
E. Incarcerated inguinal hernia
F. Orchitis (occurs with parotitis)
G. Trauma
H. Vasectomy side effect
I. Folliculitis
J. Herpes outbreak

Plan

A. General interventions
1. Encourage and stress the importance of adequate fluid intake.
2. Stress importance of taking all antibiotics as directed
B. Patient teaching
► **1.** Offer supportive therapy: Patient teaching: *See Section III: Patient Teaching Guide for this chapter, "Epididymitis."*
C. Pharmaceutical therapy
1. Antibiotic therapy (both partners must be treated for sexually transmitted infection [STI]). Treat empirically until laboratory test results are available.
2. Acute epididymitis should be treated for 10 days (see Table 12.2).
3. Chronic epididymitis should be treated for 4 to 6 weeks for bacterial pathogens, especially chlamydia.
4. Nonsteroidal anti-inflammatory drugs (NSAIDs) for pain management
5. Antitubercular triple therapy consists of rifampin, isoniazid, and pyrazinamide for 6 months.
a. Rifampin (Rifadin) 450 mg orally every day for 2 months; then 900 mg orally every day for an additional 4 months
b. Isoniazid (Laniazid) 300 mg orally every day for 2 months; then 600 mg orally every day for an additional 4 months
c. Pyrazinamide 25 mg/kg/d orally for 2 months only
6. Amiodarone epididymitis usually responds to a dosage reduction or discontinuation.

Follow-Up

A. See the patient in 2 to 7 days depending on severity of infection.
1. Pain typically improves within 1 to 3 days, but may take up to 2 to 4 weeks.
2. Inadequate treatment can result in abscess formation and decreased fertility.
B. Culture urine at end of treatment (test of cure).
C. Failure to recognize and treat both partners for STIs is a potential legal pitfall; test for all STIs and do not just focus on chlamydia and gonorrhea.
D. Consider testing for HIV.
E. Tuberculous epididymitis should be suspected if clinical signs worsen despite appropriate antibiotic therapy.
F. Men older than 50 years should be evaluated for urethral obstruction secondary to prostatic enlargement.

Consultation/Referral

A. Obtain an immediate consultation with a urologist if testicular torsion, scrotal abscess, or failed medical treatment is suspected.
B. Consult physician for the following:
1. Intravenous pyelography (IVP)
2. Doppler ultrasonography
3. Scrotal ultrasonography
4. Radionuclide scrotal imaging
C. Refer for evaluation of pediatric patients for an underlying congenital anomaly.

Individual Considerations

A. Partner: Treat sexual partners for STI. Consider testing for HIV.
B. Pediatric: Epididymitis is rare prepubertally, and testicular torsion is more common in this age group.

TABLE 12.2 The 2015 CDC Recommendation Regimens for Acute Epididymitis

For acute epididymitis all patients should receive: Ceftriaxone 250 mg IM in a single dose *Plus* Doxycycline 100 mg orally twice a day for 10 days
For acute epididymitis most likely caused by enteric organisms, additional therapy can include: Levofloxacin 500 mg orally once a day for 10 days *Plus* Ofloxacin 300 mg orally twice a day for 10 days
For MSM who report insertive anal intercourse and are at risk of both STI and enteric organisms: Ceftriaxone with a fluoroquinolone is recommended.

CDC, Centers for Disease Control and Prevention; IM, intramuscular; MSM, men having sex with men; STI, sexually transmitted infection.

C. Geriatrics
1. Epididymitis in the elderly is often caused by an enlarged prostate gland.
2. Trouble voiding can be an early finding.

Hematuria

Cheryl A. Glass and Debbie Gunter

Definition

A. Hematuria is blood in the urine. Hematuria is a symptom of an underlying disease/condition; however, routine screening is not recommended. Microscopic hematuria is defined as three or more red blood cells (RBCs) per high-power microscope field (HPF) in urinary sediment from two of three properly collected, clean-catch midstream urine specimens.
B. Asymptomatic microscopic hematuria can range from minor findings that do not require treatment to highly significant, life-threatening lesions. Microscopic hematuria is an incidental finding. The American Urological Association (AUA) recommends an appropriate renal or urologic evaluation with asymptomatic microscopic hematuria for patients who are at risk of urologic disease or primary renal disease.
C. If the excretion rate exceeds 1 million RBCs, macroscopic or gross hematuria is noted. Gross hematuria (macroscopic hematuria) is suspected when red or brown urine is present. Glomerulonephritis is associated with brown urine, while bleeding from the lower urinary tract is suggested by pink or red urine. Gross hematuria with passage of clots almost always indicates a lower urinary tract source.

Incidence

A. The prevalence of asymptomatic hematuria is from 1% to 20% of the general population. Less than 3% excrete 10 RBC/HPF. Every disease of the genitourinary (GU) tract can produce hematuria.

Pathogenesis

A. Prerenal pathology
1. Coagulopathy: Hemophilia or idiopathic thrombocytopenia purpura (ITP)
2. Drugs: Anticoagulants, aspirin
3. Sickle cell disease or trait
4. Collagen vascular disease; lupus
5. Wilms' tumor

B. Renal pathology
1. Nonglomerular pathology
a. Pyelonephritis
b. Polycystic kidney disease
c. Granulomatous disease; tuberculosis (TB)
d. Malignant neoplasm
e. Congenital and vascular anomalies
2. Glomerular pathology
a. Glomerulonephritis
b. Berger's disease
c. Lupus nephritis
d. Benign familial hematuria
e. Vascular abnormalities; vasculitis
f. Alport's syndrome; familial nephritis

C. Postrenal pathology
1. Renal calculi
2. Ureteritis
3. Cystitis
4. Prostatitis
5. Benign prostatic hypertrophy (BPH)
6. Epididymitis
7. Urethritis
8. Malignant neoplasm

D. False hematuria
1. Vaginal bleeding
2. Recent circumcision
3. Pigmentation
a. Food: Beets, blackberries
b. Medications: Quinine sulfate, phenazopyridine, and rifampin

E. Other causes
1. Trauma
2. Strenuous exercise (marathons)
3. Fever

Predisposing Factors

A. See "Pathogenesis" section.
B. Risk factors for malignancy
1. Age greater than 35 years
2. Smoking (current use or past history)
3. Chemical exposure (cyclophosphamide, benzenes, aromatic amines)
4. History of pelvic irradiation
5. Prior urologic disease or treatment
6. Chronic urinary tract infections (UTIs)

Common Complaint

A. Pink or red urine (clots may be present) or brown, cola-colored urine on toilet tissue is the common complaint.

Other Signs and Symptoms

A. Pain may or may not be present. Colicky flank pain radiating to the groin suggests a kidney stone. Significant flank pain of renal colic is usually secondary to renal calculi, but may occasionally be associated with passage of clots.
B. Frequency, dysuria, urgency, and suprapubic pain occur with cystitis and inflammatory lesions of the lower urinary tract.
C. Dull flank pain with fever and chills may accompany pyelonephritis.
D. Hesitancy and dribbling of urine suggest BPH.

Subjective Data

A. Elicit the onset, duration, and occurrence (beginning, ending, or during voiding) of hematuria. Describe the color and amount: Is it "pink on tissue" or bright red in the toilet and tissue?
B. Question the patient regarding past medical history of renal disease, systemic disease such as lupus, or sickle cell disease.
C. Review all medications including over-the-counter (OTC) and herbal products. Evaluate specifically for the use of aspirin, ibuprofen, warfarin (Coumadin),

and laxatives containing phenolphthalein. Rifampin and phenazopyridine HCl (Pyridium) can change the color of urine to orange or red.

D. Review other symptoms, such as dysuria, fever, chills, pain, and hesitancy with voiding.

E. Female patients

1. Establish whether the blood was urinary or vaginal (after intercourse or during menstruation).

2. Is the patient postpartum?

3. Is there a history of endometriosis?

F. Does the patient bruise easily? Does the patient have bleeding when flossing or brushing teeth?

G. Has the patient had a recent bout of pharyngitis with a rash, hematuria, edema, or hypertension (HTN [glomerulonephritis])?

H. Has he or she had any recent trauma, car accident, or strenuous exercise (i.e., running a marathon)?

I. Does the patient know if there was any exposure to TB?

J. Is there any family history of kidney disease, stones, and familial nephritis?

K. Does the patient have any current outbreaks of herpes or other sexually transmitted infections (STIs)?

L. Review the patient's smoking history.

M. Review occupational exposure to chemicals or dyes (benzenes or aromatic amines).

N. Review food intake of foods such as beets and blackberries.

O. Does the male patient have any hesitancy and dribbling (signs of prostatic obstruction)?

P. Evaluate if there is rectal bleeding from hemorrhoids from straining with a bowel movement (BM).

Physical Examination

A. Check temperature, blood pressure (BP), and weight in the presence of recent weight gain or edema.

B. Male or female patients

1. Inspect

a. Inspect mouth: Check tonsils for enlargement and gums for petechiae.

b. Examine skin for signs of bleeding or bruises and pallor.

c. Examine for edema.

2. Palpate

a. Check the back and abdomen for costovertebral angle (CVA) tenderness.

b. Check the abdomen for masses, urinary distension, tenderness, and organomegaly.

c. Palpate groin lymph nodes for enlargement.

3. Auscultate

a. The heart and lungs

b. For abdominal bruits

C. Female patients

1. Inspect

a. Direct visualization of the external genitalia for inflammation, ulcerations, nodules, lesions, and hemorrhoids.

b. Ask the patient to bear down to check for cystocele and rectocele.

c. Speculum examination: Observe for atrophic vaginitis, torn tissue, discharge, and friable cervix.

2. Palpate

a. Milk urethra for discharge.

b. Bimanual examination: Check for cervical motion tenderness (CMT) and adnexal masses.

c. Rectal examination: Check for the presence of hemorrhoids.

D. Male patients

1. Inspect

a. Direct visualization of the genitals; check the urethral meatus for discharge.

b. Retract the foreskin (if present) and assess for hygiene and smegma. Check the shaft of the penis, glans, and prepuce for lesions or urethral meatal erosion.

2. Palpate

a. Palpate the testes and epididymides for inflammation, tenderness, and masses; palpate the scrotum for hydrocele or varicocele.

b. Check the inguinal and femoral areas for bulges and hernias; have the patient bear down and cough, and reexamine him.

c. Rectal examination

i. Check for swollen or tender prostate.

ii. Check for the presence of hemorrhoids.

Diagnostic Tests

A. Urinalysis

1. Centrifuge the urine specimen to see if the red or brown color is in the urine sediment or supernatant.

2. If the supernatant is red to brown, test for heme (hemoglobin [Hgb] or myoglobin) with a urine dipstick. Semen is in urine after ejaculation and may cause a positive heme reaction on the dipstick.

3. A positive dipstick must always be confirmed with a microscopic examination.

4. Urine culture and sensitivity

5. Urine cytology

6. Complete blood count (CBC) with differential

7. Blood urea nitrogen (BUN)/creatinine

8. Prothrombin time (PT), partial thromboplastin time (PTT), platelet count, and bleeding time (if indicated)

9. Sickle cell testing (if indicated)

10. CT urography (CTU) is considered the preferred initial imaging in most patients for any unexplained persistent hematuria. CT is considered the best imaging modality for the evaluation of urinary stones, renal and perirenal infections, and associated complications. Intravenous pyelography (IVP) and ultrasound are not as sensitive in the evaluation.

11. Cystoscopy (the combination of a CTU and cystoscopy) provides a complete evaluation.

12. A CT scan of the abdomen or pelvis should be considered with a history of trauma to determine the source of blood.

B. Based on history, consider the following tests:

1. Strep testing to detect poststreptococcal glomerulonephritis

2. Antinuclear antibody to detect lupus nephritis

C. Urologic referral testing includes

1. CTU and cystoscopy

2. MRI if a mass is suspected
3. Renal biopsy

Differential Diagnoses

A. See "Pathogenesis" section for differential diagnoses.

Plan

A. General interventions
1. Investigate and diagnose cause(s). Only a limited workup (electrolytes, CBC) is needed in patients younger than 35 years with normal physical examination.
2. Patients older than 35 years need detailed investigation and referral.
3. Microhematuria with patients on an anticoagulant requires a urologic/nephrology workup regardless of the type or level of anticoagulation.
4. Repeat urinalysis in 2 weeks.

B. Patient teaching
1. There is no one specific treatment for all cases of hematuria.
2. Treatment is aimed at the specific underlying cause, if a cause can be identified.

C. Pharmaceutical therapy: None is recommended for hematuria unless an infection is diagnosed.

Follow-Up

A. For patients at risk of malignancy who have a negative workup:
1. Evaluate in 1 year.
2. After two consecutive negative urinalyses tests, discontinue the follow-up.
3. If gross hematuria occurs after the initial negative urinalysis, repeat a full evaluation.

B. For patients with HTN, proteinuria and/or an increase in creatinine needs to be reevaluated for renal disease.
C. For persistent asymptomatic microhematuria—after a negative workup by the urologist, a yearly urinalysis is needed.
D. For persistent or recurrent asymptomatic microhematuria after the initial negative workup, consider repeating the evaluation within 3 to 5 years.
E. Culture urine for acid-fast bacillus if sterile pyuria and hematuria persist.

Consultation/Referral

A. If all benign causes for hematuria have been ruled out, found conditions treated, and it persists, referral to a urologist or a nephrologist should be made.
B. The presence of significant proteinuria (excretion of more than 1,000 mg per 24 hours), red cell cast or renal insufficiency, or a predominance of dysmorphic RBCs in the urine should prompt an evaluation for renal parenchymal disease by a nephrologist. Red cell casts are considered virtually pathognomonic for glomerular bleeding.
C. New gross hematuria should be promptly reevaluated.

Individual Considerations

A. Women
1. Nonpregnant: Rule out menstruation and sexual activity.
2. Pregnant: Rule out vaginal bleeding such as threatened abortion, abruptio placentae, or placenta previa.
3. Ultrasound can be used to evaluate the pregnant woman. CTU should not be used secondary to the radiation exposure.

B. Pediatrics
1. UTI is the most common cause for hematuria in children. Irritation or ulceration of the perineum or urethral meatus is the next most common cause, followed by trauma.
2. The majority of children who present with gross hematuria have an easily recognizable and apparent cause. The underlying etiology is generally easy to establish by a complete history, physical examination, and urinalysis.
3. Renal ultrasound is the preferred modality for evaluation in children.
4. Cystoscopy is rarely indicated for hematuria in children. It is usually reserved for the child with a bladder mass noted on ultrasound and the child with urethral abnormalities because of trauma.

C. Geriatrics: The risk of malignancy increases among older individuals with a significant history of smoking or analgesic abuse.

Hydrocele

Cheryl A. Glass and Debbie Gunter

Definition

A. Hydrocele is the collection of fluid between layers of the processus vaginalis producing swelling in the scrotum or inguinal area. Cystic masses containing fluid or sperm often develop spontaneously. Inguinal hernia and hydrocele share a similar etiology and pathophysiology and may coexist.

Incidence

A. Incidence is unknown; hydrocele occurs in 6% of the male pediatric population at birth or in the neonatal period. It occurs infrequently in adulthood.
B. Parasitic infection, filariasis, caused by *Wuchereria bancrofti*, is the cause in more than 120 million people worldwide.

Pathogenesis

A. Congenital: Patent processus vaginalis (PPV)
B. Reactive: Inflammatory condition in the scrotum (e.g., trauma, torsion, infection)
C. Idiopathic: Arises over a long period (most common)
D. Hydroceles are believed to arise from an imbalance of secretion and reabsorption of fluid from the tunica vaginalis.

Predisposing Factors

A. Males; most commonly seen in childhood
B. *W. bancrofti* parasite
C. Viral illness
D. Chronic increased intra-abdominal pressure
E. Increased abdominal fluid production

Common Complaint

A. Swollen scrotum is the common indication.

Other Signs and Symptoms

A. Painless swollen scrotum; pain increases with the size of the mass.

B. Rarely does a hydrocele become infected and cause pain.

Subjective Data

A. Elicit the onset, duration, and course of swelling: Is scrotal sac full all day, or does the patient have a flat scrotum in the morning and a gradual increase in fluid during the day?
B. Was the hydrocele noted in the neonatal period?
C. How old is the patient? Has this ever occurred before? If so, what happened, and how was it treated?
D. Review the patient's history for injury to the scrotum.
E. Is there any pain or other symptoms related to hernia with the swelling?
F. Review other symptoms such as discharge, dysuria, fever, or backaches.
G. Review birth control method (vasectomy).

Physical Examination

A. Check temperature (if indicated) and blood pressure (BP).
B. Inspect: Careful examination is necessary to rule out masses and tumor.
- **1.** Examine in the supine and standing positions.
- **2.** Genital examination: Note amount of swelling, symmetry, lesions, discharge, hernias, varices, and color of scrotum.
- **3.** Transilluminate the scrotum to determine if the lesion is cystic, solid, or a varicocele. In a dark room, transillumination light appears as a red glow with serous fluid. If normal, blood and tissue do not transilluminate; however, the bowel may transilluminate.

C. Auscultate
- **1.** Scrotum for bowel sounds to rule out hernia

D. Palpate
- **1.** Check warmth, tenderness, swelling, and any nodularity; if mass is present, check if it has a solid versus cystic feel.
- **2.** Palpate lymph nodes: Supraclavicular, chest, abdomen, and groin
- **3.** Check for inguinal hernia.
- **4.** Palpate the abdomen for masses, rebound, and tenderness.

Diagnostic Tests

A. Laboratory evaluation is not required for the evaluation of hydroceles.
B. Scrotal ultrasonography

Differential Diagnoses

A. Hydrocele: Nontender, smooth, firm; palpation should reveal confinement to the scrotum unless hydrocele has been present for a long time. A hydrocele will transilluminate.
B. Varicocele: Feels like a "bag of worms."
C. Hernia: Herniated bowel makes gurgling sounds upon auscultation of the scrotum.
D. Testicular tumors tend to occur in young men and are the most common tumors in males from ages 15 to 30 years. Consider a tumor if the onset is acute. Tumors feel firm, nontender, and fixed and do not transilluminate. Inguinal lymphadenopathy may also be seen. The patient may complain of heaviness with a tumor.
E. Testicular torsion
F. Orchitis: Rare except with mumps. Orchitis is usually unilateral and is associated with fever, swelling, pain, and tenderness. On occasion, parotitis is absent.
G. Epididymitis: Inflammation is often concurrent with a urinary tract infection (UTI). Epididymis is very tender; scrotal elevation may relieve the pain.
H. Spermatocele: Cystic swelling of the epididymis. It is not as large as a hydrocele, but it also transilluminates.

Plan

A. General interventions
- **1.** Monitor children every 3 months until resolution or until a decision is made to refer to a specialist for evaluation.
- **2.** Factors that indicate surgical repair:
  - **a.** Failure to resolve by age 2 years
  - **b.** Continued discomfort
  - **c.** Enlargement or waxing and waning in volume
  - **d.** Unsightly appearance
  - **e.** Secondary infection

B. Patient teaching
- **1.** Most hydroceles are painless.
- **2.** In adults, if there are no symptoms, it can be left alone and monitored.

C. Pharmaceutical therapy: None is recommended.

Follow-Up

A. Monitor every 3 months.

Consultation/Referral

A. Refer to a urologist for evaluation, as needed.
B. A persistent hydrocele or the association of discomfort may indicate the need for a surgical referral.

Individual Considerations

A. Pediatrics: An infant testicle usually measures 1 cm. The parent may notice a hydrocele that fluctuates slightly in size and usually resolves on its own by 6 months of age.
B. Adults: If an adult experiences a hydrocele, he should be instructed to return for evaluation if the hydrocele becomes larger or uncomfortable, or if it interferes with sexual intercourse.

Interstitial Cystitis

Cheryl A. Glass and Debbie Gunter

Definition

A. Interstitial cystitis (IC) is a chronic condition that results in recurring discomfort or suprapubic pain, pressure in the bladder and surrounding pelvic region, related to bladder filling. IC is also commonly known as painful bladder syndrome (PBS). IC/PBS includes all cases of urinary pain with persistent urge to void or urinary frequency that cannot be attributed to other causes (i.e., infection, stones, or other pathology).
B. The persistent urge to void helps to distinguish the symptoms of IC/PBS from those of overactive bladder

(OAB). IC/PBS affects quality of life related to social activities, lost work productivity, sleep deprivation because of urinary frequency, fatigue, and even depression.

C. The Society for Urodynamics and Female Urology (SUFU) has stated that the symptoms should last more than 6 weeks in order for therapy to begin.

D. IC/PBS patients void to avoid or relieve pain, whereas patients with OAB void to avoid incontinence.

Incidence

A. Actual prevalence is unknown because of the variability of diagnostic criteria. It is not uncommon for patients to experience a lag time of 5 to 7 years before diagnosis. It is estimated that in the United States 3.3 to 7.9 million women older than 18 years are affected by symptoms of IC/PBS. Of these women, however, only 9.7% report being assigned a diagnosis of IC/PBS. The majority of the affected persons are women (10:1 rated over males). The symptom complex is the same for males. IC also occurs in children.

Pathogenesis

A. The pathophysiology of IC/PBS remains unclear. It is not established whether IC/PBS is a localized condition just involving the bladder or whether it is a systemic disease that affects the bladder.

Predisposing Factors

A. In both genders with a higher prevalence in females
B. Mean age of diagnosis is 42 to 45 years
C. Urinary tract infection (UTI)
D. Prostatitis
E. Chronic yeast infections
F. Posthysterectomy or other pelvic surgery
G. Medications
- **1.** Calcium channel blockers
- **2.** Cardiac glycosides

H. Other hypersensitivity conditions that coexist with IC
- **1.** Fibromyalgia
- **2.** Irritable bowel syndrome (IBS)
- **3.** Chronic headaches
- **4.** Vulvodynia
- **5.** Sjögren's syndrome

Common Complaints

A. Mild discomfort to intense pain with bladder filling and/or emptying is the hallmark symptom. The pain is not limited to the bladder/suprapubic area but includes symptoms throughout the pelvic area, lower abdomen, and back.
B. Persistent urge to void/frequency
C. Frequency
D. Urgency
E. Nocturia

Other Signs and Symptoms

A. Combination of urgency and frequency
B. Pressure
C. Increase in symptoms during menstruation
D. Pain during vaginal intercourse
E. Low back pain with bladder filling

Subjective Data

A. Review the onset, frequency, duration, and severity of symptoms.
B. Evaluate if the pain of bladder filling is partially or completely relieved by voiding.
C. Does the patient void frequently in order to maintain a low bladder volume and avoid discomfort versus voiding frequently to avoid urge incontinence (OAB)?
D. Are there any OAB triggers (e.g., citrus, beer, coffee) that exacerbate symptoms?
E. Are symptoms increased after stress, exercise, intercourse, being seated for a long period, or during the menstrual cycle?
F. How much do the symptoms affect the patient's quality of life (e.g., sleep disturbance, loss of work, avoiding activities)?
G. Does the patient have any other chronic pain syndromes such as IBS, chronic fatigue, dyspareunia, or fibromyalgia?
H. Review the patient's surgical history and history of genitourinary (GU) cancers.
I. Any GU trauma or falls onto the coccyx?
J. Review the patient's history of UTIs, urinary retention, and urinary tract stones.
K. Review all medications including over-the-counter (OTC) and herbal products.
L. Administer a pain/symptom evaluation tool at each visit.
- **1.** The Pelvic Pain and Urgency/Frequency Patient Symptom Scale (PUF) is available at defeatic.com/wp-content/themes/bones/library/patient/assets/files/PUF-questionnaire.pdf
- **2.** The Interstitial Cystitis Symptom Index (ICSI) is available at www.essic.eu/pdf/ICSIandICPI.pdf

Physical Examination

A. Temperature (if indicated to rule out infection; fever is not associated with IC) and blood pressure (BP)
B. Inspect
- **1.** Note general appearance for signs of depression and discomfort before and during examination.
- **2.** Inspect the male external genitalia for redness, edema, lesions, and discharge.
- **3.** Inspect female genitalia for discharge, lesions, fissures; inspect cervix for cervicitis.

C. Auscultate
- **1.** The heart and lungs
- **2.** Bowel sounds in all four quadrants

D. Palpate
- **1.** Palpate back; note costovertebral angle (CVA) tenderness.
- **2.** Palpate the abdomen for suprapubic tenderness, rebound masses, or pain.
- **3.** Perform bimanual examination to rule out other infections and pelvic inflammatory disease (PID; tenderness of the cervix, uterus, and adnexa should be absent). During the pelvic examination, evaluate locations of tenderness and trigger points.
- **4.** Males: Complete palpation of external genitalia, prostate, and rectal examination.

E. Percuss
   1. Bladder
   2. Back for CVA tenderness
F. Neurologic
   1. Perform a limited neurologic examination to rule out an occult problem.

Diagnostic Tests

A. Urinalysis with microscopy to exclude hematuria.
B. Urine culture and sensitivity may be ordered even with a negative urinalysis to evaluate low levels of bacteria.
C. Postvoid residual (PVR) volume by straight catheter or ultrasound.
D. Urodynamic testing is not currently considered to have a role in the diagnosis of IC/PBS; however, urodynamic testing should be used for complex presentations.
E. Cystoscopy is usually reserved for gross or microscopic hematuria.
F. Hydrodistension is not required for diagnosis or treatment.
G. Bladder biopsy is not required for diagnosis; however, it is used for exclusion of other disorders.
H. The potassium sensitivity test is not recommended for routine use as results are nonspecific for IC/PBS.

Differential Diagnoses

A. IC
B. UTI
C. IBS
D. Females
   1. Endometriosis
   2. Vulvodynia
E. Males
   1. Chronic prostatitis
   2. Benign prostatic hypertrophy (BPH)

Plan

A. General interventions
   1. Behavior modifications are recommended. Restrict fluids to 64 ounces/d, divided into 16 ounces per meal and 8 ounces between meals.
   2. Progressively timed voiding on a 2- to 3-hour schedule. If the patient is unable to hold urine for this interval, progressively increase urine storage time between void by 15 minutes per week until the goal of a 2- to 3-hour interval is reached.
   3. Kegel exercises should be avoided with IC.
   4. Psychosocial support is an integral part of chronic pain disorders.
B. Patient teaching
   1. Several foods have been identified as bladder irritants, including foods rich in potassium. Patients may try to eliminate foods/drinks and reintroduce them one at a time to identify any items that make their symptoms worse. Examples:
      a. Alcohol
      b. Tomatoes
      c. Spices/spicy foods
      d. Chocolate
      e. Caffeinated beverages
      f. Coffee
      g. Artificial sweeteners
      h. Citrus: Lemons, limes, and oranges (including citrus-flavored beverages)
      i. Cranberries/cranberry juice
C. Pharmacological therapies
   1. Pentosan polysulfate sodium (Elmiron) is the only oral medication approved by the Food and Drug Administration (FDA) for the treatment of IC.
      a. Dosage: 100 mg orally three times daily
   2. Amitriptyline (Elavil) is used in the treatment of other pain syndromes, including IC. May use a self-titrated dose of 25 mg orally every night and increase in increments of 25 mg every week to a maximum dose of 100 mg orally per day.
   3. Bladder instillation
      a. Intravesical dimethyl sulfoxide (DMSO) (Rimso-50) is the only drug approved by the FDA for bladder instillation.
      b. Heparin instillation
      c. Lidocaine instillation
      d. "Bladder cocktail" combination of sodium bicarbonate, heparin, lidocaine, and/or triamcinolone. There are various formulas/combinations.
   4. Medications may be instituted for treating any comorbid depression.
   5. Medications for treating any comorbid infections (e.g., UTIs, sexually transmitted infections [STIs]), inflammatory bowel disease, or endometriosis.
   6. Other medications that have been used for symptomatic relief:
      a. Hydroxyzine hydrochloride (Vistaril, Atarax) 25 to 75 mg orally at bedtime
      b. Gabapentin 300 mg up to 2,400 mg in divided doses. Gabapentin requires careful dose titration because of sedation.
      c. Uro-blue medications for short-term bladder spasms
      d. Nonsteroidal anti-inflammatory drugs (NSAIDs)
   7. Cyclosporine A has been used when other treatments have not provided relief or control of symptoms.
D. Intradetrusor botulinum toxin A (BTX-A)—this therapy may require posttreatment intermittent self-catheterization.
E. Laser or electrocautery if Hunner's ulcers are present
F. Surgical options are available if all other therapies have failed.
G. Therapies that are not recommended/should not be offered include
   1. Long-term antibiotics
   2. High-pressure, long-duration hydrodistention
   3. Systemic steroids
   4. Intravesical resiniferatoxin (ultrapotent capsaicin analog)
   5. Intravesical Bacillus Calmette–Guérin (BCG)
   6. Potassium sensitivity test—not recommended for routine use. It is nonspecific and is a painful test.

Follow-Up

A. Allodynia, the perception of nonnoxious stimuli, such as touch being noxious or painful, may be present; therefore, an adequate pelvic examination may not be possible. Consider empiric treatment and have the patient return for a pelvic examination to finish evaluation.
B. Have the patient keep a 1-day bladder diary before visits to evaluate a pattern of low urine volume frequency characteristic of IC/PBS.
C. As with all medications, start at the lowest dose and titrate/increase doses if there is an improvement in symptoms.

Consultation/Referral

A. Refer to a urologist for more thorough workup and testing.
B. Refer to a pain management specialist if indicated.
C. Electrical stimulation therapy may be considered. The implanted sacral neuromodulation device is FDA approved for the treatment of urinary urgency and frequency but not specifically for the treatment of IC/PBS.

Individual Considerations

A. Pediatrics
  1. The evaluation for interstitial cystitis is essentially the same in children as it is for the adult.
  2. Treatment options are similar to those discussed, including dietary modifications and self-help strategies.

Resources

Adult Pediatric Urology & Urogynecology: www.adultpediatricuro.com
American Urological Association (AUA): www.auanet.org
International Painful Bladder Foundation: www.painful-bladder.org
Interstitial Cystitis Association (ICA): www.ichelp.org
Interstitial Cystitis Network: www.ic-network.com
Pelvic Pain and Urgency/Frequency Patient Symptom Scale: defeatic.com/wp-content/themes/bones/library/patient/assets/files/PUF-questionnaire.pdf
Society of Urodynamics, Female Pelvic Medicine & Urogenital Reconstruction: www.sufuorg.com

Prostatitis

Cheryl A. Glass and Debbie Gunter

Definition

Prostatitis is acute or chronic infection of the prostate gland. Prostatitis is the most important cause of urinary infection in men. Prostatitis constitutes about 2 million outpatient visits a year to urologists and primary care providers. There are four types of prostatitis:
A. Acute bacterial prostatitis (least common)
B. Chronic bacterial prostatitis
C. Chronic prostatitis/chronic pelvic pain syndrome (common in men of any age)
  1. Inflammatory (presence of white blood cells in the semen, expressed prostatic secretions [EPSs], or voided bladder urine postprostatic massage)
  2. Noninflammatory (absence of white cells)
D. Asymptomatic inflammatory prostatitis

Incidence

A. About 50% of adult men in the United States will be treated for prostate conditions during their lifetime.
B. Acute and chronic bacterial prostatitis occurs in about 1 in 10 men.
C. Nonbacterial prostatitis occurs in about 6 in 10 men.
D. Prostatodynia occurs in about 3 in 10 men.

Pathogenesis

A. Nonbacterial prostatitis is an inflammatory condition with an unknown etiology. Infection results in prostatitis in four ways:
  1. Ascending infection of urethra
  2. Reflux of infected urine into the prostate through ejaculatory and prostatic ducts that empty into the prostatic urethra
  3. Hematogenous spread, causing bacterial prostatitis
  4. Invasion by rectal bacteria by direct extension or lymph system spread
B. Causative organisms: *Escherichia coli*, *Klebsiella*, *Pseudomonas*, *Enterococcus*, *Ureaplasma*, *Gardnerella vaginalis*, *Trichomonas vaginalis*, *Chlamydia trachomatis*, *Chlamydia*, *Mycoplasma*, or *Neisseria gonorrhoeae;* cytomegalovirus (CMV), *Mycobacterium tuberculosis*, and fungi have been associated with prostatitis in HIV-infected patients.
C. Incubation period depends on pathogen.

Predisposing Factors

A. More common in younger and middle-aged men
B. Sexual transmission of bacteria
C. Neuromuscular dysfunction
D. Structural voiding dysfunction
E. Benign prostatic hypertrophy (BPH)
F. History of allergies and asthma (increase in nonbacterial prostatitis)

Common Complaints

A. Dysuria
B. Perineal, rectal, or suprapubic pain (chronic pain syndrome)
C. Less urine flow
D. Spiking fever
E. Back pain
F. Sexual dysfunction

Other Signs and Symptoms

A. Acute bacterial prostatitis
  1. Fever and chills, malaise
  2. Acute onset of dysuria
  3. Hesitancy
  4. Urinary frequency and low back pain
  5. Pain with intercourse and with defecation
  6. Initial or terminal hematuria and edema with acute urinary retention
  7. Arthralgia or myalgia
  8. Nocturia
B. Chronic bacterial prostatitis
  1. Usually presents with recurrent urinary tract infection (UTI)
  2. May be asymptomatic between acute episodes; some men have large fluctuation in symptom severity.

3. Perineal, inguinal, or suprapubic pain, or irritative symptoms on voiding such as frequency and urgency
4. Hematuria, hematospermia, or painful ejaculations
5. Prostatic calculi

C. Nonbacterial prostatitis (most common)
1. Vague discomfort or increasing pain: Prostatic, lower back, perineum, groin, scrotum, or suprapubic pain; ejaculatory pain
2. Dysuria, urinary frequency, urgency, hesitancy, and decreased urine flow
3. Penile discharge, especially noted during the first bowel movement (BM) of the day
4. Sexual difficulty
5. Low sperm count
6. Blood or urine in ejaculate

D. Asymptomatic inflammatory prostatitis is found when looking for causes of infertility and testing for prostate cancer.

E. Prostatodynia (cause is unknown)
1. Prostate irritation
2. Pain and discomfort in the prostate, testicles, penis, and urethra
3. Difficulty urinating

Subjective Data

A. Ask the patient to complete the National Institutes of Health Chronic Prostatitis Symptom Index (NIH-CPSI) self-evaluation form (see Table 12.3). The assessment tool evaluates pain, urinary symptoms, and the impact on quality of life.
1. Mild = 0 to 14 total score
2. Moderate = 15 to 29 total score
3. Severe = 30 to 43 total score

An online NIH symptom index that self-scores is available at www.prostatitis.org/symptomindex.html

B. Review the onset, duration, and course of symptoms.

C. Are there any other symptoms such as discharge, pain, hematuria, hesitancy, back pain, or weight loss?

D. Has the patient ever had the same symptoms? If so, how were they treated?

E. Does any sexual partner(s) have any symptoms, lesions, or known sexually transmitted infections (STIs)?

F. Does the patient engage in anal intercourse?

G. Has the patient noted any impaired urinary flow?

H. Has the patient required any recent urethral catheterization or instrumentation?

Physical Examination

A. Check temperature and blood pressure (BP).

B. Inspect
1. Examine the patient generally for discomfort before and during examination.
2. Check the urethral meatus for discharge.
3. Retract foreskin (if present) and assess for hygiene and smegma.
4. Check the shaft of the penis, glans, and prepuce for lesions.

C. Palpate
1. Palpate testes and epididymides for inflammation, tenderness, and masses; palpate scrotum for hydrocele or varicocele.
2. Check back for costovertebral angle (CVA) tenderness.
3. Evaluate for an enlarged tender bladder because of urinary retention.
4. Palpate the abdomen for masses, urinary distension, suprapubic tenderness, and organomegaly.
5. Palpate inguinal lymph nodes; check the inguinal and femoral areas for bulges and hernias; have the patient bear down and cough, and reexamine him.
6. Rectal examination
   a. Before the rectal examination, have the patient obtain a clean-catch urine specimen for culture. Check for symmetry, swelling, tenderness, and enlarged prostate.
   b. In acute prostatitis, rectal examination reveals the prostate gland to be exquisitely tender and boggy.
   c. A fluctuant prostatic mass suggests an abscess that may require surgical intervention.
   d. Perform prostate massage for postmassage urine sample (see Section II: Procedure, "Prostatic Massage Technique: 2-Glass Test").

Diagnostic Tests

A. Acute infection
1. Complete blood count (CBC) with differential
2. Urinalysis and urine culture
3. Culture for STIs
4. Gram stain, culture of EPS
   a. Avoid vigorous massage when obtaining specimen because of the risk of inducing bacteremia.
   b. Gram stain of EPS demonstrates infectious organisms or white blood cells (WBCs) typical of an immune response (greater than 10 WBC/high-power microscope field [HPF] is abnormal). Patients with abnormal WBC but no bacterial growth may have chlamydial or *Ureaplasma* infection and need to be tested or treated empirically.

B. Chronic infection
1. Blood urea nitrogen (BUN)
2. CBC with differential
3. Creatinine

C. Chronic bacterial prostatitis
1. If recurrent infections are confirmed, evaluate for structural or functional abnormality with CT scan.
2. Measure residual urine after voiding.
3. If no urologic abnormalities are found and repeated cultures indicate the same bacterial strain, chronic bacterial prostatitis is likely.

D. Other tests, such as ultrasound, MRI, and biopsies are used as required to rule out other pathology.

Differential Diagnoses

A. Prostatitis
1. Acute: Readily evident by clinical presentation and examination
2. Chronic: More difficult to diagnose. The hallmark symptom is recurrent UTI. It often resembles prostatic hypertrophy, strictures, and prostatic carcinoma.
3. Chronic pelvic pain syndrome

B. Pyelonephritis

C. Epididymitis

TABLE 12.3 National Institutes of Health Chronic Prostatitis Symptoms Index (NIH-CPSI)

Pain or Discomfort

1. In the past week, have you experienced any pain or discomfort in the following areas?

	Yes	No
a. Area between rectum and testicles (perineum)	$\square_1$	$\square_0$
b. Testicles	$\square_1$	$\square_0$
c. Tip of the penis (not related to urination)	$\square_1$	$\square_0$
d. Below your waist, in your pubic or bladder area	$\square_1$	$\square_0$

2. In the past week, have you experienced:

	Yes	No
a. Pain or burning during urination?	$\square_1$	$\square_0$
b. Pain or discomfort during or after sexual climax (ejaculation)?	$\square_1$	$\square_0$

3. How often have you had pain or discomfort in any of these areas over the past week?

$\square_0$ Never
$\square_1$ Rarely
$\square_2$ Sometimes
$\square_3$ Often
$\square_4$ Usually
$\square_5$ Always

4. Which number best describes your *average* pain or discomfort on the days that you had it, over the past week?

☐	☐	☐	☐	☐	☐	☐	☐	☐	☐	☐
0	1	2	3	4	5	6	7	8	9	10

No pain — Pain as bad as you can imagine

Urination

5. How often have you had a sensation of not emptying your bladder completely after you finished urinating, over the past week?

$\square_0$ Not at all
$\square_1$ Less than one time in five
$\square_2$ Less than half the time
$\square_3$ About half the time
$\square_4$ More than half the time
$\square_5$ Almost always

6. How often have you had to urinate again less than 2 hours after you finished urinating, over the past week?

$\square_0$ Not at all
$\square_1$ Less than one time in five
$\square_2$ Less than half the time
$\square_3$ About half the time
$\square_4$ More than half the time
$\square_5$ Almost always

Impact of Symptoms

7. How much have your symptoms kept you from doing the kinds of things you would usually do, over the past week?

$\square_0$ None
$\square_1$ Only a little
$\square_2$ Some
$\square_3$ A lot

8. How much did you think about your symptoms, over the past week?

$\square_0$ None
$\square_1$ Only a little
$\square_2$ Some
$\square_3$ A lot

Quality of Life

9. If you were to spend the rest of your life with your symptoms just the way they have been during the past week, how would you feel about that?

$\square_0$ Delighted
$\square_1$ Pleased
$\square_2$ Mostly satisfied
$\square_3$ Mixed (about equally satisfied and dissatisfied)
$\square_4$ Mostly dissatisfied
$\square_5$ Unhappy
$\square_6$ Terrible

Scoring the NIH-CPSI Domains

Pain: Total of items 1a, 1b, 1c, 1d, 2a, 2b, 3, and 4 = ______

Urinary symptoms: Total of items 5 and 6 = ______

Quality-of-life impact: Total of items 7, 8, and 9 = ______

Calculate and report three separate scores (pain, urinary symptoms, and quality of life).
Calculate and report a pain and urinary score (range 0–31), referred to as the "symptom scale score": mild = 0–9; moderate = 10–18; severe = 19–31.
Calculate and report total score (range 0–43).

D. Anal fistulas and fissures
E. BPH causes urinary retention due to obstruction.
F. Urethral stricture or stone
G. Chronic pain syndromes/back pain

Plan

A. General interventions

1. Patients with acute prostatitis may need hospitalization and intravenous (IV) therapy for severe infection (high fever, increased WBC, dehydration). Less toxic patients may be treated on an outpatient basis.

2. Older men without evidence of infection with lower tract symptoms should have urine cytology to rule out malignancy.

B. Patient teaching

1. Patient teaching: *See Section III: Patient Teaching Guide for this chapter, "Prostatitis."*

2. Having the patient self-massage to reduce symptoms is questionable; the massage of an acutely infected gland is contraindicated because of the risk of bacteremia.
3. Recommend sitz baths two to three times daily.

C. Dietary management
1. Increase fluid intake.
2. Decrease caffeine and alcohol, which can irritate the urethra.

D. Pharmaceutical therapy
1. Analgesics (nonsteroidal anti-inflammatory drugs [NSAIDs]) and stool softeners may be needed.
2. Discontinue or reduce the dosage (if possible) of the patient's anticholinergics, sedatives, and antidepressants because they may impair bladder function.
3. Inpatient: Broad-spectrum penicillin, third-generation cephalosporins with or without aminoglycosides, or fluoroquinolones.
4. Acute outpatient therapy: The usual course of treatment is 14 to 28 days of therapy. Chronic bacterial prostatitis and chronic pain may require 4 to 6 weeks of antibiotic therapy, including fluoroquinolones, trimethoprim, tetracyclines, or macrolides.
5. Low-dose suppressive therapy with an agent that has been shown to be effective may be considered.
6. There are no formal guidelines for the management of chronic bacterial prostatitis or chronic pelvic pain syndrome. Strategies are currently focused on symptomatic relief.
7. Alpha blockers may be used to control symptoms by reducing bladder outlet obstruction (BOO).

Follow-Up

A. See the patient in 2 to 10 days depending on the patient's symptoms and course.
B. Culture urine at completion of drug therapy. Test of cure for antibiotics requires elimination of bacteria from prostatic fluid to prevent chronic flares. Some patients may not achieve cure even after 6 to 12 weeks of therapy.
C. Patients who achieve a partial response may be given a second course of antibiotics. Those failing to demonstrate an organism may benefit from a course of doxycycline or erythromycin for *Chlamydia* and/or *Ureaplasma* coverage.
D. Notify the health department for reportable STIs.

Consultation/Referral

A. Obtain a referral to a urologist for recurrent acute bacterial prostatic infections or infections that persist.
B. Cystoscopy may be required to rule out interstitial cystitis (IC).
C. Urinary retention concomitant with acute prostatitis may require hospitalization.

Individual Considerations

A. Adults
1. Prostatitis is the most common prostate infection in men younger than 50 years.

Resources

American Urological Association (AUA): www.auanet.org
National Institute of Diabetes and Digestive and Kidney Diseases (NIDDK): www.niddk.nih.gov
The Prostatitis Foundation: www.prostatitis.org

Proteinuria

Cheryl A. Glass and Debbie Gunter

Definition

Proteinuria is excess protein (albumin) in urine. Proteinuria may be an incidental finding and have no symptoms. Use of a urine dipstick for screening is acceptable for first detecting proteinuria (see Table 12.4); however, the dipstick should not be used to quantify the amount of urinary protein. Protein concentration is a function of urine volume as well as the quantity of protein present.

The measurement of protein excretion is used to establish the diagnosis and to follow the course of glomerular disease. The normal rate of albumin excretion is less than 20 mg/d; the rate is about 4 to 7 mg/d in healthy young adults and increases with age and an increase in body weight. Persistent albumin excretion between 30 and 300 mg/d is called microalbuminuria. Values of 300 mg/d of protein are considered overt proteinuria or macroalbuminuria.

When proteinuria coexists with hematuria, the likelihood of clinically significant renal disease is high. In patients with diabetes, microalbuminuria usually indicates incipient diabetic nephropathy. In nondiabetics, the presence of microalbuminuria is associated with cardiovascular (CV) disease. Protein is also the cardinal sign of pregnancy-induced hypertension (PIH).

Functional/transient proteinuria is associated with fever, exercise, dehydration, cold exposure, and stress and is not associated with underlying renal disease. Orthostatic proteinuria, a transient proteinuria condition, is related to postural changes that affect the glomerular hemodynamics. Orthostatic proteinuria rarely exceeds 1 g/d. Significant renal disease is not usually found upon further testing and workup.

Persistent proteinuria is defined as greater than 4 mg/m^2/hr of protein in a 24-hour urine collection or greater than 0.02 mg/mg of protein-to-creatinine ratio (PCR) on a spot urine. Persistent proteinuria requires further evaluation to rule out underlying renal pathology.

TABLE 12.4 Dipstick Analysis—Detecting and Quantifying Proteinuria

Dipstick Grade	Quantity of Protein (mg/dL)
Negative	<10
Trace	10–20
1+	30
2+	100
3+	300
4+	1,000

There are three types of mechanisms of persistent proteinuria:

A. Glomerular proteinuria (albuminuria): Because of increased filtration of macromolecules across the glomerular capillary wall. The standard urine dipstick is able to detect glomerular proteinuria. Some causes of glomerular proteinuria include diabetes, hypertension (HTN), nephrotic syndrome, infections including hepatitis, HIV, cytomegalovirus (CMV), malaria, syphilis, and streptococcal infections, chemotherapeutic agents, Alport syndrome, and hemolytic uremic syndrome.

B. Tubular proteinuria: Related to interference with proximal tubular reabsorption. A urinary dipstick is unable to detect tubular proteinuria. Some causes of tubular proteinuria include toxins, pyelonephritis, nonsteroidal anti-inflammatory drugs (NSAIDs), antibiotics, and inherited causes such as Lowe syndrome and Wilson disease.

C. Secretory (overflow) proteinuria: Increased excretion from the tubules secondary to an overproduction of a particular protein, most commonly noted in interstitial nephritis. A urinary dipstick is unable to detect overflow protein.

It is currently recommended that a diagnosis of kidney damage can only be made if at least two measurements are elevated.

Incidence

A. Approximately 6% of males and 7% of females have proteinuria detected by a single routine dipstick test.

B. The incidence of proteinuria found on a urine dipstick in school-age children is approximately 10%. When repeat testing is done, the incidence decreases to 0.1% of school-age children.

C. The prevalence of orthostatic proteinuria is 2% to 5% and is noted more commonly in older children and adolescents.

D. The prevalence of proteinuria is higher in the elderly and in patients with comorbidities.

Pathogenesis

A. Pathogenesis depends on the underlying etiology. An alteration in glomerular filtration that increases excretion (filtration) of plasma proteins occurs. Increased glomerular permeability, increased production of abnormal proteins (Bence Jones protein), decreased tubular reabsorption, surgical traumas, and infections may increase urinary protein. Urinary protein may also be affected by dietary protein intake.

Predisposing Factors

A. Fever

B. Increased exercise

C. Urinary tract infection (UTI)/pyelonephritis

D. Medications
1. Penicillamine
2. NSAIDs
3. Angiotensin-converting enzyme (ACE) inhibitors
4. Aminoglycosides
5. Cisplatin
6. Amphotericin B
7. Quinolones
8. Sulfonamides
9. Cimetidine (Tagamet)
10. Allopurinol (Zyloprim)
11. Antiretroviral drugs can be nephrotoxic.

E. Heavy metal exposure
1. Gold
2. Cadmium
3. Mercury
4. Lead
5. Copper

F. Collagen vascular disease or vasculitis

G. Family history of proteinuria or pyelonephritis

H. HTN

I. Renal disease

J. Congestive heart failure (CHF) or endocarditis

K. Diabetes

L. Lupus

M. Infections
1. HIV
2. Syphilis
3. Hepatitis B and C
4. Group A beta-hemolytic *Streptococcus*
5. Viral infection (e.g., mononucleosis)
6. Malaria

N. Malignancy
1. Lymphoma
2. Hodgkin's disease
3. Breast tumor
4. Lung tumor
5. Colon tumor

O. Heroin use

P. Pregnancy-induced hypertension (PIH)

Q. Radiocontrast media

Common Complaints

A. Asymptomatic

B. Increased weight

C. Decreased urine output

D. Pediatrics
1. Growth failure
2. Deafness or visual impairment suggests hereditary nephritis

Other Signs and Symptoms

A. Edema: Periorbital, presacral, genital, or ankle

B. Nephrotic syndrome: Hypercholesterolemia and hypertriglyceridemia

C. Protein malnutrition: Anorexia and vomiting

D. "Frothy" urine

Subjective Data

A. Review the onset, course, and duration of presenting complaints.

B. Question the patient concerning urinary output, thirst or fluid intake, edema, increase in weight. Establish usual weight history.

C. If a woman, establish the first day of the patient's last period. Is she pregnant? If so, what is the fetus's gestational age? Is there edema, HTN, headache, visual changes (scotoma), hyperreflexia, and/or right upper quadrant pain?

D. Review the patient's past medical history for renal disease, diabetes, congestive heart failure (CHF), systemic disorders such as lupus, and substance abuse.
E. Does the patient have signs or symptoms of a UTI or pyelonephritis?
F. Review the patient's recent history for exertion, emotional stress, surgical trauma, fever, and any acute illness.
G. When was the patient's last evaluation for cholesterol? Is he or she on any special diet?
H. Review medication list, including prescribed and over-the-counter (OTC) medications and herbal products.
I. Review the patient's occupational exposure, smoking history, and risk factors for infectious diseases.

Physical Examination

The patient's physical examination may have few abnormalities unless there are features of multisystem disease.
A. Check temperature (if indicated), blood pressure (BP), pulse, respiration, and weight.
B. Inspect
- **1.** Inspect overall general appearance for edema (pedal, hand, facial, or periorbital edema), butterfly rash (lupus), or ascites.
- **2.** Evaluate for protein wasting.
- **3.** Evaluate for jugular vein distension.
- **4.** *Funduscopic* examination: Evaluate for retinopathy.
- **5.** Inspect for pharyngitis.

C. Auscultate
- **1.** The heart and lungs

D. Palpate
- **1.** Examine the abdomen; evaluate bladder distension, suprapubic tenderness, masses or ascites, abdominal tenderness.
- **2.** Palpate for costovertebral angle (CVA) tenderness.
- **3.** Check deep tendon reflexes, especially in pregnant women.

Diagnostic Tests

A. Urine dipstick is a good screening tool in the outpatient setting.
B. Single-void "spot" urine testing
- **1.** The first urine specimen of the morning is optimal and is guideline recommended. Evaluation of the first morning specimen excludes any postural effect on the protein component.
- **2.** The gold standard for measurement of protein excretion is a 24-hour urine collection, but is now being replaced by the easier-to-obtain and less-complicated spot test. The 24-hour urine is considered impractical for generalized testing, especially in the pediatric population.

C. PCR test or albumin-to-creatinine ratio (ACR) test on a first-morning or a random spot specimen. The PCR or ACR is useful in following trends in the patient's proteinuria.
D. Complete blood count (CBC) and serum electrolytes
E. Serum creatinine (if renal disease is suspected)
F. Lipid profile
G. Blood urea nitrogen (BUN): Serves as an index of renal excretory capacity. Urea is the nitrogenous end product of protein metabolism.
H. Urinalysis, urine culture, and sensitivity (if indicated)
I. Ultrasound of the full urinary tract
J. Screen for diabetes and other testing related to physical findings.
K. Renal biopsy is required to establish the diagnosis in most cases.

Differential Diagnoses

A. See "Predisposing Factors" section.

Plan

A. General interventions
- **1.** Current guidelines for screening for evaluation of albuminuria/proteinuria vary by country, but recommendations include at-risk individuals with diabetes, HTN, obesity, smokers, indigenous populations, family history of chronic kidney disease (CKD), age greater than 50 years, structural renal tract disease, renal calculi, prostatic hypertrophy, vascular disease, and autoimmune disease.
- **2.** Management for nephrotic syndrome includes diet with sodium and protein restriction, loop and distal-acting diuretics, control of cholesterol (low-saturated-fat, low-cholesterol diet), lipid-lowering agents, pneumococcal and influenza vaccines to prevent infections, and use of steroids and immunosuppressive agents as necessary.
- **3.** Patients with hematuria and proteinuria need a 24-hour urine collection for protein and creatinine clearance.

B. Patient teaching
- **1.** Encourage low-fat/low-cholesterol diet if hyperlipidemia is present.
- **2.** Encourage sodium- and protein-restricted diet for nephrotic syndrome.

C. Pharmaceutical therapy: There is no specific drug therapy for excess protein. Use drug therapy appropriate to the underlying medical disease causing proteinuria. In patients with CKD, the administration of ACE inhibitors and/or angiotensin II receptor blocker (ARBs) is aimed at reducing the degree of proteinuria.

Follow-Up

A. If proteinuria is found on a dipstick and the first-morning test results are trace or negative for protein, repeat a first-morning test in 1 year.
B. There is no consensus on how often to screen for proteinuria. Guidelines include annual screening, every 5 years for patients older than 50 years or smokers, and every 3 years for patients who have HTN, obesity, indigenous, or a family history of kidney disease. Monitoring should always include BP, quantitative testing by PCR or ACR, and a serum creatinine.
C. Patient should be assessed at routine examination appointments for vasculitic skin changes, rashes, retinopathy, lymphadenopathy, signs of heart failure, abdominal masses, organomegaly, guaiac stools, prostatic enlargement, and joint inflammation.

Consultation/Referral

A. Consider patient referral if kidney damage is progressing from medical disease (systemic lupus erythematosus, HTN, diabetes).
B. Refer the patient as necessary; HTN is a poor prognostic sign for significant renal impairment.
C. Consultation for diagnostic tests to be considered: Kidney, ureter, and bladder (KUB); intravenous pyelography (IVP); renal ultrasonography; renal biopsy.
D. Referral to a pediatric nephrologist should be considered if a definitive diagnosis is required or a renal biopsy is considered.

Individual Considerations

A. Pregnancy
  1. Protein excretion is considered abnormal in pregnancy when it exceeds 300 mg/24 hr or greater than 0.3 g of protein per gram of creatinine in a random urine specimen. A urine specimen with 1+ protein is considered the cutoff for proteinuria.
  2. The gestational age at which proteinuria is first documented is important in establishing the likelihood of PIH versus other renal diseases. Proteinuria before or early in pregnancy suggests preexisting renal disease.
  3. Monitor urine protein and BP at each prenatal visit and refer the patient if urinary protein remains elevated.
  4. Monitor for intrauterine growth restriction (IUGR).
  5. Proteinuria (or HTN) that persists longer than 3 months after delivery should be followed closely.
B. Pediatrics
  1. The American Academy of Pediatrics recommends that children should be screened on two occasions during childhood:
    a. Before entrance into school
    b. During adolescence
  2. Although there are no set guidelines for children, a child with persistent proteinuria should be initially worked up with a physical examination, BP, urinalysis, serum creatinine, and BUN every 6 to 12 months.
  3. When the child is stable, the follow-up should be done annually.
  4. There are no dietary or physical activity limitations.
C. Geriatrics: Renal function deteriorates in the elderly who may also have coexisting medical conditions (HTN, diabetes) that may cause nephropathy.

Pyelonephritis

Cheryl A. Glass and Debbie Gunter

Definition

A. Pyelonephritis is an acute infection and inflammatory disease of the upper urinary tract (renal pelvis, tubules, and interstitial tissue) of one or both kidneys. Acute pyelonephritis is an ascending urinary tract infection (UTI) that has progressed from the lower urinary tract.
B. Fever has been strongly correlated with the diagnosis of acute pyelonephritis; therefore, patients with clinical symptoms of pyelonephritis in the absence of fever should be evaluated for alternative diagnoses.
C. Acute pyelonephritis characteristically causes some scarring to the kidney and may lead to significant damage, kidney failure, abscess formation, and sepsis. Antibiotic therapy is essential to prevent the progression of pyelonephritis.

Incidence

A. Thirty percent of the female population have at least one UTI in their lifetime.
B. Annual rates of pyelonephritis in women are 15 to 17 cases per 10,000 and three to four cases per 10,000 for men.
C. The incidence of pyelonephritis in pregnancy is 2%. Most cases develop as a consequence of undiagnosed or inadequately treated lower UTI.
D. Upper UTIs are less common and more serious than lower UTIs. After puberty, the prevalence of UTIs increases slightly in females, but remains low in males.
E. After age 65 years, UTIs are more common with an equal incidence in both sexes.

Pathogenesis

A. Pyelonephritis is caused by ascending infection from the bladder, usually caused by *Escherichia coli* (75%–90%) and other gram-negative bacteria including *Proteus mirabilis* (5%), *Klebsiella pneumoniae* (5%), *Enterobacter* (3%), and Group B *Streptococcus* (GBS: 1%). Gram-positive causative agents are less common; 10% to 15% of cases are caused by *Staphylococcus saprophyticus*.
B. Bacteria can also reach the kidneys through the bloodstream from intravenous (IV) drug abuse and endocarditis.
C. In women, the short urethra in close proximity to the perirectal area makes colonization possible. In pregnancy, the increased glycosuria, increase in urinary amino acids, urinary stasis, and the presence of vesicoureteral reflux facilitate bacterial growth.
D. In children, vesicoureteric reflux is the most common pathology.
E. In men, benign prostatic hypertrophy (BPH) causing bladder obstruction is a common pathology.
F. Indwelling catheters increase ascending infections and pyelonephritis.

Predisposing Factors

A. Previous UTI, cystitis, and pyelonephritis
B. Sickle cell disease
C. Diabetes
D. Urinary catheterization
E. Obstruction: Calculi, tumors, and urethral strictures
F. Neurogenic bladder disease: Strokes, multiple sclerosis, and spinal cord injuries
G. Urinary reflux
H. HIV
I. Trauma
J. Chronic constipation (children)
K. Incomplete bladder emptying related to medications (e.g., anticholinergics)
L. Gender
  1. Females
    a. Increased sexual activity, failure to void after intercourse, diaphragms, and spermicides
    b. Pregnancy

c. Atrophic vaginal mucosa predisposes to the colonization of pathogens and UTIs.

2. Males
   a. Homosexuality
   b. Sexual partner with colonization
   c. Obstruction: Prostatic hypertrophy
   d. Age 50 years or older
   e. Acute or chronic bacterial prostatitis

Common Complaints

A. Shaking, chills, and fever
B. Flank pain or tenderness
C. Urinary frequency or urgency
D. Costovertebral angle (CVA) tenderness
E. Guarding
F. Urinary frequency, nocturia, hematuria, and dysuria (not always present in upper tract infections)
G. Blood in urine secondary to hemorrhagic cystitis (unusual in males with pyelonephritis)

Other Signs and Symptoms

A. Adults (particularly the elderly): May be asymptomatic with cystitis
B. Abdominal pain and suprapubic heaviness
C. Pregnancy: Uterine contractions
D. Shortness of breath (SOB)
E. Anorexia
F. Children
   1. Fever may be a child's only presenting symptom
   2. Nausea and vomiting
   3. Irritability
   4. Diarrhea
   5. Abdominal pain/tenderness
   6. Feeding difficulty
   7. Failure to thrive
G. Elderly
   1. Mental status change
   2. Generalized deterioration

Subjective Data

A. Review the onset, course, and duration of symptoms.
B. Are there any problems with voiding such as frequency, urgency, and dysuria?
C. Review the patient's history of fever and any treatment.
D. Are there any other symptoms, odor, and nausea?
E. Have the patient point to the area of the backache. Is it unilateral or bilateral? What makes the backache better?
F. In women, rule out pregnancy; review first day of last menses.
G. Rule out sickle cell disease, diabetes, and multiple sclerosis.
H. Review the patient's previous history of genitourinary (GU) tract problems, stones, UTIs, previous pyelonephritis, any previous testing, and any previous anomalies.
I. Review the strength and character of the urinary stream, especially in older men. Ask if the patient has ever been diagnosed with BPH.
J. Review the patient's history for active herpes lesion. Does urine flow hurt when urine stream begins? Or is the pain noted when urine passes over the lesion?
K. Review drug allergies.
L. Review all medications, including over-the-counter (OTC) and herbal products. Review medications for a recent history of an incomplete course of antibiotics and current use of anticholinergics.

Physical Examination

A. Check temperature, pulse, and blood pressure (BP); note orthostatic hypotension. Tachycardia may or may not be present, depending on associated fever, dehydration, and sepsis.
B. Inspect
   1. Note general appearance for respiratory distress and dehydration.
   2. Inspect the male external genitalia for redness, edema, lesions, and discharge.
   3. Inspect the female genitalia for discharge, lesions, and fissures; inspect cervix for cervicitis.
C. Palpate
   1. Palpate the back; check CVA tenderness (usually unilateral over the involved kidney).
   2. Palpate the abdomen for suprapubic tenderness, rebound masses, or pain.
   3. Perform a pelvic examination to rule out other infections and pelvic inflammatory disease (PID; tenderness of the cervix, uterus, and adnexa should be absent).
D. Auscultate
   1. The lungs and heart
E. Pregnancy
   1. Check fetal heart rate; fetal tachycardia may be present with fever.
   2. Palpate for uterine tenderness and contractions.
   3. Pelvic examination for cervical dilation, if indicated for increased risk of preterm labor
F. Males: Complete palpation of external genitalia, prostate, and rectal examination.

Diagnostic Tests

A. Urine culture and sensitivity should always be performed before initial empiric treatment with antibiotics.
B. Urinalysis for evaluation of pyuria. Pyuria is present in almost all women with acute cystitis and pyelonephritis; its absence strongly suggests an alternative diagnosis.
   1. Leukocyte esterase on dipstick detects pyuria or white blood cells (WBCs).
   2. Significant pyuria is greater than two to five leukocytes per high-power microscope field (HPF).
   3. Urine may need to be obtained from straight in-and-out catheterization if the patient is incontinent or has dementia.
C. Complete blood count (CBC) with differential or WBC, especially with systemic symptoms.
D. Blood culture, if indicated
E. Arterial blood gases (ABGs), if indicated
F. Consider sedimentation rate, especially with severe illness and in the elderly.
G. Culture for gonorrhea and chlamydia, if symptoms are associated with sexually transmitted infections (STIs).

H. Wet prep, if symptoms are associated with STI.

I. Imaging studies are not routinely required for the diagnosis of acute pyelonephritis but can be helpful.

1. CT scan to identify altered parenchymal perfusion, hemorrhage, nonrenal disease, inflammatory masses, and obstruction. CT with contrast medium is considered the imaging modality of choice for nonpregnant women
2. MRI to rule out masses or obstruction
3. Renal ultrasonography
4. Scintigraphy to detect focal renal abnormalities
5. Voiding cystourethrogram
6. Intravenous pyelography (IVP), if indicated

Differential Diagnoses

A. Pyelonephritis
B. Appendicitis/acute abdomen
C. Cholecystitis
D. Pancreatitis
E. Diverticulitis
F. Pneumonia
G. Prostatitis
H. Epididymitis
I. PID
J. Nephrolithiasis

Plan

A. General interventions

1. Optimal therapy for acute uncomplicated pyelonephritis depends on the severity of the illness at presentation.
2. Many severe infections (increased WBC, dehydration or vomiting, high fever) may need hospital admission for intravenous (IV) therapy. Risk factors include older adult, coexisting illness, pregnancy, and uncontrolled vomiting.

B. Patient teaching

1. Give instruction on early recognition of UTIs.
2. Patient teaching: *See Section III: Patient Teaching Guide for "Urinary Tract Infection (Acute Cystitis)."*

C. Dietary management

1. Increase fluids; have the patient drink at least one large glass of water every hour while awake.
2. Encourage the patient to drink cranberry juice to help fight and prevent UTIs. If the taste is objectionable, he or she may mix cranberry juice 1:1 with another juice such as grape juice.
3. There are no dietary restrictions with pyelonephritis.

D. Pharmaceutical therapy

1. Acetaminophen (Tylenol) for fever
2. Urinary analgesic as needed to relieve dysuria. Dysuria is usually diminished fairly quickly after the start of antibiotics.
3. Antiemetics as needed; however, if the patient is not able to tolerate oral fluids, he or she should be hospitalized.
4. Antibiotics: Empiric antibiotic selection should be guided by local antibiotic resistance patterns, allergies, and culture results. Patients with delayed response to therapy should also receive a longer course of antibiotics of 14 to 21 days.

a. Adults

i. First-line therapy: Ciprofloxacin (Cipro) 500 mg twice daily for 7 days, *or* extended-release Cipro XR 1,000 mg once a day for 7 days

ii. First-line therapy: Levofloxacin (Levaquin) 750 mg once daily for 5 to 7 days

iii. Second-line therapy: Trimethoprim and sulfamethoxazole (TMP-SMX; Septra DS, Bactrim DS) 160 mg and 800 mg, respectively, one tablet twice daily for 7 to 10 days. Because of the high rate of resistance of *E. coli*, the empirical use of TMP-SMX should be avoided in patients who require hospitalization.

iv. Alternative therapy: Amoxicillin-clavulanate (Augmentin) 500 mg/125 mg orally twice a day for 14 days *or* Augmentin 250 mg/125 mg orally three times a day for 3 to 7 days.

b. Children younger than 2 years are usually treated for 7 to 14 days. Children older than 2 years who are afebrile and without abnormalities of the urinary tract or have previous episodes of UTIs are usually treated for 5 days.

i. Amoxicillin-clavulanate (Augmentin) 20 to 40 mg/kg orally per day in three doses for 7 to 14 days

ii. Sulfonamide–trimethoprim–sulfamethoxazole (TMP-SMX) 6 to 12 mg/kg trimethoprim and 30 to 60 mg/kg sulfamethoxazole per day orally in two doses for 7 to 14 days

iii. Cephalosporin-cefuroxime (Ceftin) 8 mg/kg/d in one dose for 7 to 14 days

c. Antibiotics that should not be used for pyelonephritis:

i. Nitrofurantoin (Macrodantin) and fosfomycin (Monurol) should not be used to treat pyelonephritis in adults or children; it is excreted in the urine but does not achieve therapeutic serum levels.

ii. Fluoroquinolones are not used in children because of potential concerns about sustained injury to developing joints.

iii. Tetracyclines should not be used in children because of tooth staining.

iv. Fluoroquinolones are not used in pregnancy because of the risk of auditory and vestibular toxicity in the fetus.

v. Aminoglycosides are contraindicated in pregnancy because of the risk of permanent ototoxicity to the fetus.

Follow-Up

A. Follow up with the patient in 24 to 48 hours depending on the evaluation of the initial severity of symptoms.

1. Patients with persistent fever or clinical symptoms after 48 to 72 hours of appropriate antibiotic therapy

should undergo initiation of another class of antibiotics and consider radiologic evaluation.
2. If the patient feels that he or she is not progressing well or is getting worse, evaluate the patient emergently and consider hospital admission and IV antibiotics.
B. Follow-up urine cultures are not needed for patients with acute cystitis or pyelonephritis if symptoms resolved on antibiotics; however, repeat cultures for patients with recurrent symptoms or any complicated course of illness.
C. Women with recurrence of pyelonephritis need further urologic investigation.

Consultation/Referral

A. Consult physician and consider hospitalization for infants with both lower and upper infections, children with pyelonephritis, and children with recurrent infections.
B. Consult or refer the patient to a physician if he or she requires IVP, cystoscopy, or renal biopsy.
C. IV therapy and hospitalization are needed in all cases suggestive of bacteremia in children who are vomiting, children younger than 2 years, and children with documented parenchymal damage.
D. Males with persistent bladder infections need a urologic consultation.
E. Pyelonephritis in men suggests structural problems and needs hospitalization and further evaluation (IVP).
F. Consult an infectious disease specialist for patients with unusual or resistant pathogens.
G. For pregnancy, consultation with an obstetrician is required.

Individual Considerations

A. Pregnancy
  1. Pyelonephritis is the most common urinary tract complication in pregnancy.
  2. Untreated asymptomatic bacteriuria (ASB) is a risk factor for acute cystitis and pyelonephritis in pregnancy.
  3. Based on the higher risk of complications in pregnancy, pyelonephritis has traditionally been treated with hospitalization and IV antibiotics until the woman is afebrile for 48 hours and symptoms improve.
  4. Once the pregnant patient is discharged from the hospital, oral antibiotics should continue for 10 to 14 days of treatment.
  5. A urine culture should be obtained 1 to 2 weeks after completion of therapy and monthly thereafter to monitor for recurrent infection.
  6. Aminoglycosides should be avoided because of the potential risk of ototoxicity following prolonged fetal exposure.
  7. Fluoroquinolones are contraindicated during pregnancy because of the risk of auditory and vestibular toxicity in the fetus.
B. Pediatrics
  1. Always order a urine culture and sensitivity on children suspected of UTI.
  2. Suprapubic aspiration of the bladder should be considered in young infants.
  3. A voiding cystogram should be considered in all children younger than 16 years with a documented UTI.
  4. Indications for hospitalization
    a. Age less than 2 months
    b. Clinical urosepsis or potential bacteremia
    c. Immunocompromised patient
    d. Vomiting or inability to tolerate oral medication
    e. Lack of adequate outpatient follow-up (e.g., no phone, lives far from hospital)
    f. Failure to respond to outpatient therapy
  5. Vesicoureteric reflux is responsible for up to 50% of pyelonephritis in children younger than 6 years.
  6. Assess the child for chronic constipation as a potential cause for urinary obstruction.
C. Males
  1. Consider ordering renal function tests (blood urea nitrogen [BUN] and creatinine).
  2. Men older than 50 years: Consider urologic consultation and IVP.
D. Geriatrics
  1. Patients may need hospitalization for IV antibiotics and hydration.
  2. Bladder or kidney infections may be common in patients with long-term urinary catheters and can lead to septicemia if untreated or unrecognized.
  3. Fluoroquinolone use in the elderly has the potential to cause neuropsychiatric symptoms, including seizures to worsening dementia.

Renal Calculi or Kidney Stones (Nephrolithiasis)

Cheryl A. Glass and Debbie Gunter

Definition

A. Renal calculi, or kidney stones, are caused by the formation of crystals in the urinary system from the kidneys to the bladder. *Nephrolithiasis* refers to renal stone disease; *urolithiasis* refers to the presence of stones in the urinary system. The majority of stones (80%) consist of calcium, usually as calcium oxalate, but they can contain uric acid, struvite (magnesium, ammonium, and phosphate), oxalic acid, phosphate salts, or the amino acid cysteine. Spontaneous passage of a stone is related to the stone size and location. Approximately one half of symptomatic patients require intervention for stone removal. An untreated staghorn (branch shaped) with persistent renal obstruction can destroy renal tissue with potential for life-threatening sepsis.

Incidence

A. Renal calculi are very common in the United States, with a higher incidence noted in males. The overall incidence is rising. At least 12% of men and 7% of women have one symptomatic stone by age 70 years. Initial cases typically occur between ages 30 and 40 years, and the prevalence increases with age. Idiopathic nephrolithiasis

is common in males, whereas primary hyperparathyroidism is more common in females.
B. Most kidney stones pass spontaneously; however, 10% to 30% do not pass and can cause continuing pain, infection, or obstruction.
C. Nephrolithiasis is uncommon in children.
D. Stones because of infection (struvite) are more common in women.
E. The incidence of stones in pregnancy is 1 in every 1,500 to 3,000 pregnancies.
F. The recurrence rate for calculi is 50% within 5 years.

Pathogenesis

A. The formation of uric acid stones requires continued and excessive oversaturation of urine with stone-forming constituents, uric acid, calcium, and oxalate. Dehydration, hyperuricosuria, and significantly acidic urine contribute to uric acid supersaturation and stone formation. Struvite stones form only when the urinary tract is infected with urea-splitting organisms such as *Proteus* species.
B. Hydroureteronephrosis is the most significant renal alteration in pregnancy. Dilatation is greater on the right side than the left because of pressure because of physiological engorgement of the right ovarian vein and dextrorotation of the uterus.

Predisposing Factors

A. Male
B. Dehydration (poor intake and immobility)
C. Chronic obstruction with stasis of urine
D. Hypercalcemia caused by hyperparathyroidism; renal tubular acidosis; multiple myeloma; or excessive intake of vitamin D, milk, and alkali
E. Diet high in purines and abnormal purine metabolism (gout)
F. Pregnancy (1 per 1,500)
G. Chronic infections
H. Foreign bodies
I. Excessive oxalate absorption in inflammatory bowel disease, bowel resection, or ileostomy
J. Previous stone formation
K. Family history of nephrolithiasis
L. Medications
  1. Vitamins A, C, and D
  2. Loop diuretics
  3. Acetazolamide
  4. Ammonium chloride
  5. Calcium-containing medications, including alkali and antacids
  6. Indinavir
  7. Sulfadiazine
  8. Atazanavir
  9. Guaifenesin
  10. Sulfa drugs
  11. Topiramate
  12. Acyclovir
M. Obesity
N. Gastric bypass/bariatric surgical procedures
O. Diabetes

Common Complaints

A. Severe flank and groin pain
B. Blood in urine
C. Asymptomatic (dependent on the size of the stone)

Other Signs and Symptoms

A. Unilateral flank pain that radiates to the groin
B. Sudden onset of colicky pain
C. Hematuria

> *The timing and appearance of hematuria are important. Hematuria seen at the beginning of the urine stream may indicate bleeding in the urethra. Terminal hematuria, or blood in the end of the urine stream, denotes bladder neck or the prostate as the source. Finally, blood throughout the entire urine stream suggests a lesion.*

D. Nausea and vomiting
E. Restlessness
F. Symptoms common with cystitis or inflammatory lesions of the lower tract are usually absent: Frequency, dysuria, urgency, and suprapubic pain.

Subjective Data

A. Review the onset, duration, and course of symptoms.
B. Review other signs and symptoms of urinary tract infection (UTI) or pyelonephritis: Frequency, dysuria, and fever.
C. Have the patient describe pain (colicky); note intensity (use a 1- to 10-point scale, 10 being the worst pain) and the characteristics of pain (constant, intermittent).
D. Has the patient ever had a stone before? How was it treated? What tests were performed? Has the patient ever seen a urologist?
E. Review dietary intake of high animal protein in the diet, milk, and other calcium-containing products for excessive intake.
F. Review the patient's medication history including excessive vitamin C or D supplements, antacids that contain calcium, and other medications noted in the predisposing factors.
G. Ask the patient to describe any hematuria or blood clots passed.
H. Ask about recent trauma to the back or abdomen.
I. Is there a family history of stone formation?
J. Is the patient pregnant?

Physical Examination

A. Check temperature, blood pressure (BP), and pulse (may have tachycardia). Children: Growth measurements to evaluate poor weight gain and/or failure to thrive (congenital and chronic conditions)
B. Inspect
  1. Inspect general appearance for discomfort before and during examination. Patients with renal colic are extremely restless and exhibit active movement on presentation.
  2. During the examination evaluate voluntary guarding of the abdominal musculature.
  3. Inspect external genitalia (male or female) for lesions, discharge, inflammation, and ulcerations.
  4. Assess for peripheral edema.

C. Auscultate
1. The abdomen, noting bruits if present
2. Bowel sounds
D. Palpate
1. "Milk" the urethra for discharge.
2. Palpate the abdomen for masses and tenderness, organomegaly, and suprapubic tenderness.
3. Palpate the groin; check lymph nodes.
4. Palpate the back and abdomen.
5. Check for the presence of costovertebral angle (CVA) tenderness.
E. Perform pelvic or bimanual examination, if indicated, to rule out pelvic inflammatory disease (PID).

Diagnostic Tests

The diagnosis of nephrolithiasis can be made on the basis of clinical symptoms alone, but diagnostic testing is needed to confirm.

A. Laboratory tests
1. Serum blood urea nitrogen (BUN)
2. Creatinine
3. Calcium
4. Uric acid
5. Serum electrolytes; consider fasting serum calcium and phosphorus and parathyroid hormone
6. Pregnancy test (if indicated) to rule out an ectopic pregnancy
B. Stone for analysis
C. Urinalysis
1. Urine dipstick for a gross screen
2. pH determination (pH greater than 7.5 is compatible with infection lithiasis, and a pH less than 5.5 favors uric acid lithiasis)
3. Red cell casts strongly suggest glomerulonephritis.
4. Evaluate urine sediment for crystalluria.
D. Urine culture, if indicated
E. 24-hour urine for creatinine, calcium, uric acid, oxalate, pH, and sodium measurement
1. Patient should be on his or her usual diet before taking 24-hour specimen.
2. Collection should be 1 to 2 months after any interventions, including shock-wave lithotripsy, ureteroscopy, or percutaneous stone removal.
F. Noncontrast helical CT scan is the imaging standard to assess the urinary tract in acute renal colic.
G. Renal ultrasound is the procedure of choice for pregnancy.
H. X-ray of the kidney, ureter, and bladder (KUB) is often ordered with the pelvic CT or ultrasound.
I. Intravenous Pyelography (IVP)
J. Nuclear renal scan

Differential Diagnoses

A. Kidney stone(s): Associated with colicky flank pain radiating to the groin. Significant flank pain of renal colic is usually secondary to renal calculi, but may occasionally be associated with passage of clots.
B. UTI: Passage of large, bulky blood clots implicates the bladder as the source, whereas long, shoestring-shaped specks or thin, stringy clots suggest an upper urinary tract or ureteral origin.
C. Acute abdomen/appendicitis
D. Cholecystitis
E. Pyelonephritis: Associated with dull flank pain with fever and chills. In evaluating urine sediment, the presence of white blood cells (WBCs) and bacteria favors a diagnosis of pyelonephritis or interstitial nephritis.
F. PID
G. Inflammatory bowel disease
H. Urinary tract obstruction
I. Constipation
J. Ectopic pregnancy

Plan

A. General interventions
1. Increase fluids to allow passage of stone. Strain all urine to recover stone for analysis.
2. Reduce possibility of recurrence with dietary modifications.
3. The patient is usually referred for imaging after evaluation of creatinine.
4. Patients can be managed on an outpatient basis with close follow-up if stones are small (less than 6 mm).
B. Patient teaching/dietary management
1. Force fluids to maintain a daily output of 2 to 3 L of urine. Fluid intake that increases urinary production of at least 2 L of urine per day increases the flow rate and lowers the urine solute concentration.
2. Dietary consultation may be needed secondary to stone analysis.
C. Pharmaceutical therapy
1. Pain medication (narcotic and nonnarcotic) is a priority.
a. Nonsteroidal anti-inflammatory drugs (NSAIDs) should be discontinued 3 days before shock-wave lithotripsy to decrease the risk of bleeding.
2. Antibiotics should be given for infection.
3. Antiemetics if needed
4. Other medical/pharmaceutical management depends on the etiology of the stone.
D. Surgical options are dependent on stone size and location.
1. Percutaneous nephrolithotomy is the first treatment option for most patients and is considered the treatment of choice for patients with staghorn calculi.
2. Extracorporeal shock-wave lithotripsy is the least invasive of the surgical methods.
3. Percutaneous nephrostomy should be the last procedure for most patients.
4. Open nephrostomy may also be used.

Follow-Up

A. Reevaluate the patient in 24 hours by phone or in the clinic.
B. Evaluate sooner if pain increases, because of the potential to progress to complete obstruction.
C. Recurrent stone formation is a manifestation of a systemic disease; evaluate for the management of the metabolic abnormality.

Consultation/Referral

A. Patients with severe pain, nausea, and vomiting need hospitalization for intravenous (IV) hydration and pain control. Consult with a physician.
B. Patients with severe symptoms and persistent obstruction beyond 3 to 4 days should be referred for urologic evaluation.
C. Refer to urology for surgical interventions: Lithotripsy, urethroscope interventions, extracorporeal shock-wave lithotripsy, and percutaneous ultrasonic lithotripsy may be indicated. Treatment varies based on the location and size of the stone. Laparoscopy may be indicated for the removal of large or severely impacted ureteral calculi.

Individual Considerations

A. Pregnancy
  1. Urolithiasis is the most common cause of nonobstetrical abdominal pain that requires hospitalization in pregnancy.
  2. Approximately 80% to 90% are diagnosed in the first trimester.
  3. Renal ultrasound is the first-line screening test for pregnant patients. A transvaginal ultrasound may also be performed.
  4. Low-dose CT is reserved for complex cases in the second and third trimesters.
  5. Conservative treatment is used: Bed rest, hydration, and analgesia.
  6. Invasive measures include stent placement, ureteroscopy, and percutaneous nephrostomy.
  7. Upon presentation, rule out
    a. Ectopic pregnancy
    b. Abruptio placentae
    c. Preterm labor
B. Pediatrics
  1. Young children generally do not present with the classic acute onset of flank pain; instead, they may present with abdominal pain. Stone may be detected when abdominal imaging is performed.
  2. Hematuria can present as the sole symptom or in conjunction with abdominal pain.
  3. 10% of children present with symptoms of dysuria and urgency.
  4. Shock-wave lithotripsy and percutaneous-based therapy may be considered in children.

Sexual Dysfunction Male

Nancy Pesta Walsh

Erectile Dysfunction

Definition

Erectile dysfunction (ED), also known as impotence, is the persistent inability to achieve or maintain penile erection sufficient for satisfactory sexual performance. ED occurs with reduced blood flow to the penis or nerve damage as well as psychological triggers. Low self-esteem, performance anxiety, depression, stress, and effects to quality of life occur secondary to ED. ED is noted to be a precursor to symptomatic coronary artery disease (CAD).

Age-associated changes in sexual function in men include delay in erection, diminished intensity and duration of orgasm, and decreased force of seminal emission. ED lasting 3 months or longer should have further evaluation and consideration of treatment.

Multiple male sexual dysfunction questionnaires are available for order through the website www.pfizerpatientreportedoutcomes.com/order-measures sponsored by Pfizer, Inc. The website notes the questionnaires may be ordered free of charge and are available in several translations. Questionnaires include:

A. Erectile Dysfunction Inventory of Treatment Satisfaction (EDITS) used in the evaluation of satisfaction with medical treatment modalities for ED
B. Erectile Hardness Scale (EHS)
C. International Index of Erectile Function (IIEF) is available in two versions. Version 1 is applicable to heterosexual men. Version 2 is edited so that it is applicable to heterosexual and homosexual men. The IIEF assesses five dimensions relevant to sexual function:
  1. Erectile function (six items)
  2. Orgasmic function (two items)
  3. Sexual desire (two items)
  4. Intercourse satisfaction (three items)
  5. Overall satisfaction (two items)
D. Index of Premature Ejaculation (IPE) assesses control over ejaculation, sexual satisfaction, and distress.
E. Premature Ejaculation Diagnostic (PED) tool was developed to screen for premature ejaculation, including control, frequency, minimal sexual stimulation, distress, and interpersonal difficulty.
F. Quality of Erection Questionnaire (QEQ) evaluates satisfaction with the quality of erections, including hardness, onset, and duration.
G. Self-Esteem and Relationship (SEAR) Questionnaire assesses confidence, self-esteem, and relationships.
H. Sexual Health Inventory for Men (SHIM) is a five-item abridged version of the 15-item IIEF.
I. Sexual Quality of Life—Men (SQOL-M) was developed to assess sexual confidence, emotional well-being, and relationship issues. This questionnaire has been validated for men with ED and premature ejaculation.

Incidence

A. ED can occur at any age; however, it is more common in men older than 60 years.
B. It is estimated that 18 to 30 million American men have ED, i.e., approximately 52% of males aged 40 to 70 years.
C. By 2025, it is estimated that 322 million men worldwide will have ED.
D. Men with ED have a 65% to 85% increased risk of subsequent CAD.
E. Reduced libido is estimated as affecting 5% to 15% of men.

Pathogenesis

A. Normal pathology: The dorsal nerve of the penis provides innervation, the dorsal somatic nerve provides sensation, and the autonomic nervous system, via the cavernosal nerves, regulates blood flow to the penis, allowing for erection to occur. The ability to maintain an erection relies on the dorsal nerve, the peripheral nerves, penile vasculature, and biochemical releases within the corpora.

B. Multiple factors may contribute to ED:

1. Vascular (most common)

a. This system is responsible for delivering and trapping the blood in the corporal sinusoids. Usually, the blood flowing in is not the problem; rather, the ED is the result of venous leaking from the corporal sinusoids.

b. Arterial insufficiency contributes to decreased blood flow to the cavernosal sinuses. The cavernosal dysfunction causes difficulty with retaining blood in the penis and makes a patient to sustain an erection.

i. Chronic diseases such as cardiovascular (CV) disease, hypertension (HTN), dyslipidemia, and obesity.

ii. Certain medications can contribute to this physiological effect.

iii. Smoking is also a contributing factor, especially in the presence of existing CV disease, because of the vasoconstrictive effects it causes.

2. Psychological

a. Direct inhibition of the spinal erection center and/or excessive sympathetic nervous system biochemical release occurs, which increases the smooth muscle tone of the penis, preventing erection

i. Age-related decline

ii. Lack of sexual response

iii. Personal intimacy-related issues

iv. Partner-specific intimacy issues

v. Performance anxiety

vi. Depression or life stress related

3. Neurologic

a. Any disease affecting the brain, spinal cord, and cavernous and penile nerves can impair the ability to achieve erection such as spinal cord injury, stroke, or diabetes.

b. Surgery in the pelvic region, including prostatectomy, perineal resection, and sphincterotom.

4. Endocrine

a. Decreased testosterone level

b. Increased prolactin level

c. Hyperthyroidism

d. Hypothyroidism

Predisposing Factors

A. CV disease

B. Diabetes (neurologic and vascular problems)

C. HTN

D. Hyperlipidemia

E. Advanced age (greater than 60 years)

F. Peripheral neuropathy

G. Obesity

H. Neurologic disorders

1. Spinal cord injuries

2. Brain injuries

3. Multiple sclerosis

4. Parkinson's disease

I. Alcohol/tobacco abuse

J. Drug abuse

1. Heroin

2. Cocaine

3. Marijuana

K. Side effect of medication (e.g., serotonin reuptake inhibitors, antihypertensives, antihistamines, diuretics, nonsteroidal anti-inflammatories, muscle relaxants)

L. Surgical/radiation therapy for cancers of the pelvis or pelvic trauma

M. Hypogonadism

N. Psychological and psychiatric disorders

O. Peyronie's disease (deformity of the penis)

P. Obstructive sleep apnea

Q. Physical inactivity

Common Complaints

A. Inability to achieve or sustain an erection

B. Erection is not firm enough for penetration.

C. Absent or delayed ejaculation

D. Inability to control the timing of ejaculation

E. Lack of interest or desire (most common)

F. Pain with intercourse

Other Signs and Symptoms

A. Diminished self-esteem

B. Depression

C. Anxiety

D. Reduced libido

E. Relationship difficulties

F. Premature ejaculation (PE)

Subjective Data

> *History taking for ED includes sexual, medical, surgical, emotional, and medication evaluations.*

A. Sexual history

1. Did the onset of ED coincide with a specific event?

2. How long has the patient had trouble attaining or maintaining an erection?

3. Is he able to obtain an erection in order to penetrate? On a scale of 0 to 10, how hard is the erection?

4. Is the ED getting worse?

5. Is he about to achieve orgasm and ejaculate?

6. How long is the patient able to have intercourse before ejaculation?

7. Is there pain or discomfort with ejaculation?

8. Does the patient have nocturnal or morning erections?

9. How frequently does the patient have sexual activity?

a. Is the activity planned or does it occur spontaneously?

b. How much foreplay occurs?

c. Do the patient and partner agree on the frequency of intercourse?

d. Is the patient's partner satisfied?

10. Has the patient tried any treatment(s) for ED?
  a. What treatments have been tried?
  b. Inquire about his desire to try any particular therapy. Is he opposed to try any particular therapy?

B. Medical history
  1. Does the patient have HTN? When was HTN diagnosed? What is his usual blood pressure (BP)?
  2. Does the patient have diabetes?
    a. Is he insulin dependent?
    b. Does he have any peripheral neuropathy?
  3. Does the patient have heart disease? When was his heart disease diagnosed?
  4. Has the patient ever had cancer, including any surgery, chemotherapy, and radiation?
  5. Does the patient have dyslipidemia? What were the results of his last laboratory tests?
  6. Does the patient smoke? How much, including the number of pack years?
  7. Does the patient drink? How much, how often?
  8. Does the patient have penile curvature (Peyronie's disease)?
  9. Does the patient have any neurologic disorders?

C. Surgical history
  1. Has the patient had any prior surgeries, including pelvic, prostate, or trauma?
  2. Has the patient had any invasive cardiac procedures or surgery?

D. Emotional history
  1. Has the patient ever had a traumatic sexual experience?
  2. Has the patient had a loss of libido?
  3. Does the patient have a history of depression or mood disorders?
  4. Is the patient experiencing any problems related to work and/or family?
  5. Does the patient have any intrapartner problems such as separation or divorce?

E. Medication history: Ask the patient to list all medications currently being taken, particularly substances not prescribed, including herbal products and illicit drugs. Multiple drug classifications have medications that contribute to ED. Review medications from these drug classes:
  1. Nitrates
  2. Antihypertensives (particularly alpha blockers)
  3. Anti-ulcer medications
  4. Lipid-lowering medications
  5. 5-alpha reductase inhibitors (e.g., finasteride or dutasteride)
  6. Antidepressants
  7. Herbal products
  8. Illicit drugs
  9. Caffeine

Physical Examination

A. **Vital signs:** Check BP, height, and weight. Calculate body mass index (BMI).

B. Inspect
  1. Inspect general appearance, noting dyspnea and weakness.
  2. Inspect skin for jaundice, pallor, and diaphoresis.
  3. Inspect legs for edema, cyanosis, and venous stasis.
  4. Perform a *funduscopic* examination.
  5. Evaluate visual field defects (present in hypogonadal men with pituitary tumors).
  6. Inspect for penile plaques (indicates Peyronie's disease).
  7. Inspect the testicles.
    a. Check for presence of atrophy.
    b. Assess asymmetry.
    c. Evaluate the cremasteric reflex by stroking the inner thighs and observe ipsilateral contraction of the scrotum.

C. Palpate
  1. Palpate abdomen for masses, tenderness, bounding pulses, and organomegaly.
  2. Palpate peripheral pulses in legs.
  3. Palpate femoral pulses.
  4. Examine breast to detect gynecomastia.
  5. Palpate the testicles for masses.
  6. Perform a rectal examination to evaluate the prostate.

D. Auscultate
  1. Carotid arteries for bruits
  2. Abdomen for bruits and bowel sounds
  3. Heart for murmurs, rubs, clicks, irregularities, or extra sounds
  4. Femoral bruits (possible pelvic blood occlusion)
  5. All lung fields

E. Observe ipsilateral contraction of the scrotum.

F. Mental status: Assess for depression.

G. Perform a neurologic examination if neurologic etiology is suspected.

Diagnostic Tests

Hormonal testing and treatment of ED should be individualized based on clinical presentation, including libido, premature ejaculation, fatigue, testicular atrophy, and muscle atrophy that suggests a hormonal abnormality.

A. Serum laboratory tests
  1. Lipid profile
  2. Triglycerides
  3. Glucose or hemoglobin A1c (HgbA1C)
  4. Prostate-specific antigen (PSA) testing (if on testosterone replacement)
  5. Hematocrit (if on testosterone replacement)
  6. Testosterone (performed in the morning) and other hormone levels, such as prolactin level, if high index of suspicion for prolactinoma, including visual disturbances or headache.
  7. Urinalysis for protein and glucose

B. Duplex ultrasound of the cavernous arteries and other vascular testing as indicated. Penile perfusion ultrasound may be done to evaluate arterial perfusion of the penis. (Not commonly used.)

C. Nocturnal penile tumescence (NPT) as indicated. This determines the quality and number of nighttime erections. This test is not routinely used and is typically used in younger, more complicated patients.

D. Other tests as indicated for abnormal findings on physical examination

Differential Diagnoses

A. Erectile dysfunction
B. Testosterone deficiency
C. Decreased libido
D. Anorgasmia
E. Peyronie's disease

Plan

A. General interventions
   1. A prolonged erection (priapism) lasting more than 4 hours is a medical emergency often requiring immediate urologic attention.
   2. Lifestyle modifications to include weight loss, increased physical activity, limited alcohol consumption, and smoking cessation.
   3. Control of comorbidities, including cardiovascular (CV) disease, diabetes, and HTN, is desired.
B. Patient teaching
   1. Educate patient about modifying controllable risk factors such as keeping diabetes and HTN under control, diet, exercise, and smoking cessation.
   2. Failure to respond to phosphodiesterase-5 (PDE-5) inhibitor treatment may result from improper instructions or an inadequate dosage of medication. (See Table 12.5 for dosing and side effects.)
   3. The initial administration of an alprostadil intraurethral suppository should be done in the office in order to demonstrate correct administration.
   4. The initial intrapenile administration of alprostadil should be done in the office in order to demonstrate correct administration.
   5. Stepwise therapy for ED includes pharmaceuticals and surgery.
C. Pharmaceutical therapy
   1. **First-line therapy**: Treatment with PDE-5 inhibitors is the first-line therapy for the treatment of ED. PDE-5 inhibitors are not initiators of erection and require sexual stimulation for an erection to occur. The evidence shows that PDE-5 inhibitors improve erections and successful intercourse, with approximately 80% success rate. The use of PDE-5 inhibitors has been extensively studied; however, they are not without side effects. (See Table 12.5 for dosing and side effects.)
      a. Contraindications to PDE-5 inhibitors include high-risk conditions and the concomitant use of nitrites. If the patient develops angina while using a PDE-5 inhibitor, other antianginal agents should be used instead of nitroglycerin.
      b. High-risk patients/conditions are defined as
         i. Unstable or refractory angina
         ii. Refractory angina
         iii. Uncontrolled HTN
         iv. Congestive heart failure (CHF; New York Heart Association classes III and IV)
         v. Myocardial infarction (MI) or a CV accident within the previous 2 weeks
         vi. High-risk arrhythmias
         vii. Hypertrophic obstructive and other cardiomyopathies
      c. Before proceeding to other ED therapies, patients reporting failure of PDE-5 inhibitors should be evaluated to determine whether the medication trial was adequate; evaluate:
         i. Food/drug interactions
         ii. Timing and frequency of dosing
         iii. Lack of adequate sexual stimulation
         iv. Heavy alcohol use
         v. Relationship issues
         vi. Using a licensed PDE-5 inhibitor medication
      d. After evaluation and reeducation and counseling on the medications and partner–partner expectations, titrate to the maximum dosing or prescribe different PDE-5 inhibitor.
      e. Discuss other options for ED if the patient has a contraindication to, or an unsuccessful trial of, PDE-5 inhibitors.
   2. **Second-line therapy:** Pharmaceutical therapy with intracavernous injection is the second-line therapy for the treatment of ED. Penile injection therapy involves injection of alprostadil, a vasoactive drug, into the corpora cavernosa of the penis to expand the blood vessels and increase the blood flow to produce an erection. The most common side effect of alprostadil is burning and a prolonged erection lasting over 4 hours. Hypotension is also a potential side effect. Prolonged erections require medical intervention to reverse the erection.
      a. Alprostadil intercavernal injections are titrated according to patient erection response, within the health care clinic setting. Very specific dosing requirements exist, based upon brand name; create a high potential for priaprism.
      b. Alprostadil (Muse Pellet) urethral pellet: 125 to 250 mcg is to be used before intercourse. Duration of 30 to 60 minutes is followed; use only twice in each 24-hour period.
D. Surgical alternatives
   1. Penile implant is the third-line therapy for the treatment of ED. Penile prostheses (implants) are surgically implanted items, semirigid rods or a hydraulic device to ensure a rigid erection. The prosthesis does not usually affect urination, sex drive, orgasm, or ejaculation. Pain and/or reduced sensation, infection, or mechanical failure may occur from the prosthesis.
   2. Vacuum erection devices are external cylinders used to pump the penis into the cylinder and produce an erection by drawing blood into the penis. An occluding band is then placed at the base of the penis in order to prevent the blood from leaving, with subsequent loss of the erection. **Only vacuum constrictor devices containing a vacuum limiter should be used. The occluding band to maintain the erection should be limited to 30 minutes.**
   3. Penile arterial revascularization is indicated for young men (younger than 45 years) with no known risk factors for atherosclerosis. The goal of the surgery

TABLE 12.5 Dosing and Side Effects of Oral PDE-5 Inhibitors

Dosing Instructions	**Sildenafil Citrate (Viagra)**	**Vardenafil HCl (Levitra)**	**Tadalafil (Cialis)**
Doses	25, 50, and 100 mg doses	5, 10, and 20 mg doses	2.5 and 5 mg—available for continuous daily use 10 and 20 mg doses
Instructions	• Recommended starting dose is 50 mg • Take on an empty stomach • Maximum dosing once a day • Titrate according to patient response/side effects • Effective 30–60 minutes from administration • A heavy fatty meal may reduce or prolong absorption	• Recommended starting dose is 10 mg (5 mg initial dose for the elderly) • Take on an empty stomach • Titrate according to patient response/side effects • Effective from 60 minutes from administration • A fatty meal reduces its effect	• Recommended starting dose is 10 mg • Titrated according to patient response • Maximum dosing once a day • Effective 30–60 minutes from administration • Peak efficacy occurs after 2 hours; efficacy is maintained for up to 36 hours • Not affected by food • Has been approved for continuous, daily use in 2.5 and 5 mg doses • Also prescribed for BPH
Common Side Effects	**Sildenafil Citrate (Viagra)**	**Vardenafil HCl (Levitra)**	**Tadalafil (Cialis)**
Headache	×	×	×
Flushing	×	×	×
Nasal congestion/ rhinitis	×	×	×
Dyspepsia	×	×	×
Priapism	×	Rare	Rare
Myalgia			×
Sinusitis		×	
Backache			×
Limb pain			×
Prolonged erection	×		
Tachycardia		×	
Visual disturbance	Blue-green color tinge to vision, light sensitivity, and blurred vision (lasts 2–3 hours)		
Hypotension with alpha blockers	Should be stable on alpha blocker before initiating a PDE-5 inhibitor; use lowest recommended PDE-5 inhibitor dose	Should be stable on alpha blocker before initiating a PDE-5 inhibitor; use lowest recommended PDE-5 inhibitor dose	Should be stable on alpha blocker before initiating a PDE-5 inhibitor; use lowest recommended PDE-5 inhibitor dose
Sudden vision loss	Discontinue if vision loss occurs	Discontinue if vision loss occurs	Discontinue if vision loss occurs
Sudden hearing loss	Discontinue if hearing loss occurs	Discontinue if hearing loss occurs	Discontinue if hearing loss occurs
Use with nitrates (includes nitroglycerin, isosorbide dinitrate, amyl nitrate, and sodium nitroprusside)	Contraindicated because of hypotension	Contraindicated because of hypotension	Contraindicated because of hypotension

BPH, benign prostatic hyperplasia; PDE-5, phosphodiesterase-5.

is to correct injury by rerouting the blood vessel around a blockage or injured blood vessel. Men with insulin-dependent diabetes or widespread atherosclerosis are not candidates for this surgery.

4. Venous ligation surgery is rarely used. Men with insulin-dependent diabetes or widespread atherosclerosis are also not candidates for venous surgery.

Follow-Up

A. Follow up in 1 to 3 weeks after treatments are initiated to monitor patient satisfaction and the quality of erections.

B. At the time of prescription renewal, patients prescribed PDE-5 inhibitors should have a review of the effectiveness, side effects, and any significant change in health status, including all medications.

Consultation/Referral

A. Patient should be directed to go to the ED if an erection lasts for more than 4 hours.
B. Patients whose CV risk is indeterminant for PDE-5 inhibitors should undergo further evaluation by a cardiologist before receiving therapies for sexual dysfunction.
C. Surgical consultation: Men with penile deformities may require surgical correction.
D. Urologist consultation should be considered for surgical therapies, including implantation of penile prosthesis.
E. Endocrinology consultation for complex endocrine disorders
F. Psychosexual counseling may be considered for the patient and/or couple.
G. Psychotherapy is recommended when ED is related to anxiety and/or depression.

Individual Considerations

A. Adults
  1. A mild prolongation of the QT interval has been observed with vardenafil. The product labeling for vardenafil recommends that caution be used in patients with known history of QT prolongation or in patients who are on current medications that prolong the QT interval.
  2. Testosterone therapy is not indicated in the treatment of ED if the patient has a normal serum testosterone level.
  3. Men who present with sleep disorders should also be questioned about the presence of ED.
  4. In patients with diabetes, PDE-5 inhibitors may fail.
  5. PDE-5 inhibitors are contraindicated in patients with high CV risk and for patients on nitrates.
  6. Men with ED are associated with a higher incidence of CV events.
B. Geriatrics
  1. Dose medications on the lower end for elderly patients:
    a. Sildenafil: Dose at 25 mg for age greater than 65 years. Renal and hepatic dosing required.
    b. Vardenafil: Dose at 5 mg for age greater than 65 years. Renal and hepatic dosing required.
    c. Tadalafil: Renal and hepatic dosing required.

Resources

American Association of Sex Educators, Counselors, and Therapists
1444 I Street, NW, Suite 700
Washington, DC 20005
(202) 449–1099
Info@aasect.org
www.aasect.org

American Society for Reproductive Medicine
1209 Montgomery Highway
Birmingham, AL 35216
205-978-5000
asrm@asrm.org

American Urological Association
1000 Corporate Boulevard
Linthicum, MD 21090
866-746-4282
aua@AUAnet.org

International Society for Sexual Medicine
PO Box 94
1520 AB Wormerveer, The Netherlands
Secretariat@issm.info
www.issm.infor

Society for Sex Therapy and Research
(847)-647–8832
Info@sstarnet.org

Premature Ejaculation

Definition

A. Premature ejaculation (PE) is defined as the inability to control or delay ejaculation, which causes personal distress for the male. Two subtypes exist, based on intravaginal ejaculation latency time (IELT):
  1. Lifelong PE is an IELT of less than 1 minute. Onset is typically from the first sexual encounter. Males have no ability to control the ejaculation.
  2. Acquired PE is an IELT of less than 3 minutes. Onset is at any point in sexual history. The ability to delay ejaculation is decreased or absent.

Two subtypes exist based on personal experience; neither is a true sexual dysfunction.

  3. Variable PE is irregular and not the result of psychogenic cause. Onset is at any point in sexual history. The ability to delay ejaculation is decreased or absent.
  4. Subjective PE is self-reported rapid ejaculation despite normal ejaculation time. Onset is at any point in sexual history. The ability to delay ejaculation is decreased or absent.

Incidence

A. PE is reported in approximately 21% to 31% of males. It is the most common type of sexual dysfunction. Erectile dysfunction (ED) commonly coexists.
B. Approximately 31% of men report problems with sexual function.

Pathogenesis

A. The exact cause is unknown.
B. Organic: Chronic prostatitis, hyperthyroidism, genetic disorders
C. Psychogenic: Relationship problems, psychological preoccupation with performance
  1. Iatrogenic: Nerve damage from surgery or trauma

Predisposing Factors

A. Depression
B. Consumption of alcohol
C. Obesity
D. High blood pressure (BP)
E. High cholesterol
F. Diabetes
G. Obesity

H. Smoking
I. Depression and anxiety medication use

Common Complaints

A. Men
  1. Inability to achieve or sustain erection
  2. Absent or delayed ejaculation
  3. Inability to control the timing of ejaculation
B. Both sexes
  1. Lack of interest or desire (most common)
  2. Inability to become aroused
  3. Pain with intercourse

Other Signs and Symptoms

A. Diminished self-esteem
B. Depression
C. Anxiety
D. ED
E. Reduced libido
F. Relationship difficulties

Subjective Data

A. Include full medical history, sexual history, and psychological, social, and drug history using open-ended questions.
B. Ask
  1. Partner(s)' sexual history
  2. Perceived ejaculatory control
  3. Estimated IELT
  4. Previous interventions used to correct the issue
  5. Impact on personal life and relationships
  6. If the issue has been lifelong or acquired
  7. If a loss of erection occurs before ejaculation, to distinguish ED from PE
C. Screening tools
  1. PE Diagnostic Tool available at www.sexhealthmatters.org/resources/premature-ejaculation-diagnostic-tool
  2. Index of PE available at www.pfizerpatientreportedoutcomes.com/therapeutic-areas/sexual-health/male-sexual-dysfunction

Physical Examination

A. Vital signs: Check BP, pulse, and respiration.
B. Inspect
  1. Thyroid for nodules
  2. Abdomen for surgical scars
  3. Neurologic examination for deficiencies
  4. Lower extremities for hair distribution pattern, lesions, or trauma
  5. Genitalia for abnormalities
  6. Any additional examination should be based on history and previous examination findings.
C. Palpate
  1. Thyroid for nodules
  2. Abdomen for masses or tenderness
  3. Lower extremities for pain and pulses
  4. Neurologic examination of lower extremities
  5. Genitalia for lesions, masses, or pain

Diagnostic Tests

A. Should be based on individual history and physical findings

Differential Diagnoses

A. ED
B. Testosterone deficiency

Plan

A. General interventions
  1. The treatment plan should include the patient and sexual partner.
  2. The patient and partner should be educated about the possible interventions outlined as follows:
    a. Both should be educated in treatment options.
    b. Patient and partner satisfaction is the desired outcome.
B. Patient teaching
  1. Consider the impact of the severity of the issue on the patient, any treatable causes, and patient wishes.
  2. Effectiveness of psychotherapy may diminish over time.
  3. Behavioral therapy: "Stop-and-start" method of ceasing genital stimulation until arousal sensation diminishes, or the "squeeze" method of squeezing the glans prepuce at heightened arousal.
C. Psychotherapy: Recommended for lifelong, acquired, or variable, and is the first-line treatment for subjective PE.
D. Pharmaceutical therapy: Off-label medications include selective serotonin reuptake inhibitors (SSRIs) and eutectic mixture of local anesthetics (EMLA).
  1. Paroxetine 10, 20, or 40 mg/d *or* 20 mg 3 to 4 hours preintercourse
    a. Typically most effective for the indication of PE
  2. Fluoxetine 5 to 20 mg/d
  3. Sertraline 25 to 200 mg/d *or* 50 mg 4 to 8 hours preintercourse
  4. EMLA (lidocaine 2.5%/prilocaine 2.5%) cream: Apply to glans penis 20 to 30 minutes preintercourse.

Follow-Up

A. The patient should be seen in 2 to 4 weeks if medication was started to assess for efficacy. SSRIs typically achieve maximum effect after 1 to 2 weeks.

Consultation/Referral

A. May refer to urologist or sexual health specialist/counselor, particularly if there is provider discomfort with this topic.
B. Psychotherapy: Recommended for lifelong, acquired, or variable, and is the first-line treatment for subjective PE. Referral to a practitioner who specializes in sexual therapy is recommended.

Individual Considerations

A. Adults
  1. Off-label SSRIs should be used with caution for the increased risk of serotonin syndrome.
  2. Off-label EMLA cream used without a condom may result in vaginal wall numbness in the sexual partner.
  3. Prolonged application of EMLA may result in loss of erection if used for 30 to 45 minutes.
B. Geriatrics
  1. Renal and hepatic dosing of paroxetine is required.

2. Hepatic dosing of fluoxetine and sertraline is required.
3. Taper to discontinue any SSRIs is required.

Testicular Torsion

Cheryl A. Glass and Debbie Gunter

Definition

A. Testicular torsion is twisting of the testicle around the vas deferens, with compromise in the blood supply and possible necrosis to the testicles. Testicular torsion is a urologic emergency and is the most frequent cause of testicle loss in the adolescent male population. Approximately 40% of all cases of acute scrotal pain and swelling are diagnosed with testicular torsion. There is often a history of recurrent episodes of testicular pain before torsion.
B. Testicular torsion is most commonly misdiagnosed as epididymitis.
  1. Epididymitis usually presents with gradual onset of pain that is localized posterior to the testes that gradually radiates to the lower abdomen.
  2. These symptoms are rare with torsion.

Incidence

A. Incidence in males younger than 25 years is approximately 1 in 4,000. Although torsion can occur at any age, the largest number of cases occur during adolescence.
B. The bell clapper congenital anomaly is present in approximately 12% of males, and 40% have the abnormality in the contralateral testicle.

Pathogenesis

A. Testicular torsion and torsion of the spermatic cord occur because of abnormal fixation of the testicle to the scrotum, allowing free rotation. The bell clapper deformity allows the testicle to twist spontaneously on the spermatic cord. Venous occlusion and engorgement cause arterial ischemia and infarction of the testicle.

Predisposing Factors

A. Age: More common in adolescence
B. Trauma to testicle
C. Spontaneous occurrence
D. Congenital bell clapper anomaly
E. Exercise
F. Undescended testicle
G. Active cremasteric reflex

Common Complaints

A. Sudden onset of severe unilateral scrotal pain (less than 24 hours)
B. Swelling of scrotal sac
C. High position of the testicle
D. Abnormal cremasteric reflex

Other Signs and Symptoms

A. Sudden onset of testicular pain, may radiate to groin
B. Possible edema
C. Abdominal pain (22%–30%)
D. Nausea and vomiting (50% of cases)
E. Fever (16%)
F. Urinary frequency (4%)

Subjective Data

A. Review the onset, duration, and course of symptoms.
B. Review for a history of prior episodes of intermittent testicular pain that resolved spontaneously.
C. Review abdominal symptoms such as pain, nausea and vomiting, and fever.
D. Review urethral discharge (possible sexually transmitted infection [STI]) and dysuria.
E. Review the patient's history for trauma to the scrotum or testicle.

Physical Examination

A. Check temperature, blood pressure (BP), pulse, and respiration.
B. Inspect
  1. Observe the patient generally for pain before and during examination.
  2. Visualize the scrotal sac for edema, symmetry, lesions, discharge, color (especially for blue dot superior to the affected testicle). Testis is located high in the scrotum as a result of shortening of the cord by twisting.
  3. Check the inguinal and femoral areas for bulges and hernias.
C. Auscultate
  1. Auscultate all four quadrants of the abdomen; note bowel sounds.
  2. Assess the scrotum for bowel noise.
D. Palpate
  1. Palpate the abdomen for masses, rebound, and tenderness or guarding.
  2. Palpate the groin; check the lymph nodes.
  3. Examine for an inguinal hernia.
  4. Genital examination
    a. Check warmth, tenderness, swelling, and any nodularity; if a mass is present, check if it is solid or cystic. The testes should be sensitive to gentle compression, but not tender. They should feel smooth, rubbery, and free of nodules.
    b. Elicit a cremasteric reflex by stroking the inner thigh with a blunt object (reflex hammer or ink pen). The testicle and scrotum should rise on the stroked side. Cremasteric reflex is usually absent in testicular torsion.
    c. Elevate the scrotum; there is usually no relief in pain with torsion. Elevation of the scrotum may improve the pain of epididymitis (Prehn's sign).

Diagnostic Tests

A. Urinalysis: Normal in 90% of cases of testicular torsion
B. Doppler ultrasonography for blood flow and scrotal ultrasonography

Differential Diagnoses

A. Testicular torsion: Firm, tender mass of acute onset in an afebrile young man with a history of prior episodes must be considered to represent torsion until proven otherwise.
B. Epididymitis
C. Orchitis

D. Hydrocele
E. Testicular tumor: Usually a hard, enlarged, painless testicle
F. Acute appendicitis
G. Scrotal/testicular trauma
H. Varicocele

Plan

A. General interventions
  1. Testicular torsion is a urologic emergency requiring surgery.
  2. Immediately refer the patient to a urologist and/or emergency department.
  3. Symptoms for more than 6 hours can indicate testicular necrosis.
  4. The opposite testicle is usually stabilized during the same surgery.
B. Pharmaceutical therapy
  1. None

Follow-Up

A. Patient should follow up with the urologist as directed.

Consultation/Referral

A. All patients with suspected testicular torsion need to be immediately evaluated by a physician and referred to a urologist.

Individual Considerations

A. Pediatrics: Neonatal testicular torsion is rare. The exact mechanism is unknown. The torsion may occur prenatal (at or within 24 hours of delivery) or postnatal (within first 30 days of delivery). On physical examination, a hardened, fixed nontender scrotal mass with a discolored scrotum is noted. Management is controversial because of the lack of data on whether the testis can be salvaged and the risk for concomitant or subsequent torsion of the contralateral side.
B. Geriatrics: In older males, rule out epididymitis, especially with new sexual partners or with symptoms of dysuria and urethral discharge.

Undescended Testes or Cryptorchidism

Cheryl A. Glass and Debbie Gunter

Definition

A. Undescended testicle(s) or cryptorchidism is a testicle that is not within the scrotum and cannot be manipulated from the inguinal canal into the scrotum or is absent. Spontaneous descent of testes usually happens at the end of the first year. Bilaterally absent testicles is anorchia.

Incidence

A. Approximately 10% of males have bilateral cryptorchidism.
B. In unilateral cases, left-side predominance is noted.
C. Between 2% and 5% of full-term and 30% of premature male infants are born with an undescended testicle.
D. 20% to 30% of boys have at least one nonpalpable testis.

Pathogenesis

A. An absent testicle may occur because of agenesis or an intrauterine vascular problem such as torsion. It may also be related to the lack of gonadotropic and androgenic hormones during fetal development. Most undescended testes are a result of a mechanical factor, a hernia sac, or a shortened spermatic artery that impedes the testes' descent into the scrotum.

Predisposing Factors

A. Prematurity; the testes descend into the scrotum at approximately 36 weeks gestation. Most testicles will complete their descent within the first few months of life.
B. Birth weight is the principal determining factor for undescended testes from birth to 1 year of age.
C. Twinning
D. Maternal exposure to estrogen during the first trimester of pregnancy
E. Family history
F. Congenital disorder of testosterone secretion or testosterone action
  1. Kallmann syndrome
  2. Abdominal wall defects
  3. Neural tube defects
  4. Cerebral palsy
  5. Genetic syndromes
    a. Trisomy 18
    b. Trisomy 13
    c. Noonan syndrome
    d. Prader–Willi syndrome
G. Exposure to dibutyl phthalate (endocrine-disrupting chemical)

Common Complaints

A. Empty scrotum
B. Small, flat, undeveloped scrotum
C. Inguinal hernia

Other Signs and Symptoms

A. Absence of testicle noted on newborn examination or by parents during a bath or diaper change

Subjective Data

A. Review the course, duration, and symptoms. Have the testes ever been noticed in the scrotum during a bath or while the baby has been relaxed?
B. Note gestational age and birth weight at delivery (term vs. preterm).
C. Has any health care provider ever noted that the testis was not descended or was absent on examination?
D. Review the maternal history for evidence of an endocrine disturbance during pregnancy.
E. Review family history of congenital abnormalities, genital anomalies, and abnormal pubertal development.
F. Review if the patient has undergone prior inguinal surgery.

Physical Examination

A. Temperature, blood pressure (BP), pulse, and respiration
B. Inspect
  1. Check the scrotum for size, shape, rugae, and any anomaly, particularly hypospadias.
  2. Look for a bulge in the inguinal area.

3. Transilluminate the scrotum to look for testes and note fluid (if present).
   a. To locate the testis, darken the room and shine a bright light from behind the scrotum. In a normal male, the testis stands out as the darker area.

C. Palpate
1. Before you palpate the scrotum, place the thumb and index finger of one hand over the inguinal canals at the upper part of the scrotal sac. This maneuver helps prevent retraction of the testes into the inguinal canal or abdomen.
2. Check each side of the scrotum to detect the presence of the testes and other masses. If either of the testicles is not palpable, place a finger over the upper inguinal ring and gently push toward the scrotum. You may feel a soft mass in the inguinal canal. Try to push it toward the scrotum and palpate it with your thumb and index finger. The testicle of a newborn is approximately 1 cm in diameter.
3. When any mass other than the testicle or spermatic cord is palpated in the scrotum, determine if it is filled with fluid, gas, or solid material. It is most likely to be a hernia or hydrocele. If it is reducible, then transilluminate to differentiate a hydrocele from a hernia.
4. Check the cremasteric reflex: Scrotal sac retracts in response to cold hands and/or abrupt handling (yo-yo reflex).
5. Bimanual digital rectal examination (DRE) may be used to evaluate the nonpalpable testis.

Diagnostic Tests

A. For a unilateral undescended testis without hypospadias, no laboratory studies are needed.
B. Hormone levels (testosterone) may be obtained if both testes are nonpalpable.
C. Karyotype to rule out chromosomal abnormalities
D. Ultrasonography of the abdomen
E. Possible CT of the abdomen

Differential Diagnoses

A. Undescended testis, one or both
B. Anorchia (complete absence)
C. Retractile testis
D. Ectopic testis
E. Ambiguous genitalia: In male-appearing genitals, at least one testis must be palpated; if not, ambiguous genitalia cannot be eliminated. A deep cleft in the scrotum (bifid scrotum) is usually associated with other genitourinary (GU) anomalies or ambiguous genitalia.
F. Tumor: A hard, enlarged, painless testicle may indicate a tumor.

Plan

A. General interventions
1. Refer all children with cryptorchidism by 1 year of age to a surgeon for evaluation.
2. Surgery (orchiopexy) is usually indicated before 18 months, and no later than 3 years of age, secondary to the increased risks of malignancy, infertility, testicular torsion, trauma, and hernia. After orchiopexy, the rate of fertility in these children is about 80% to 90%.

B. Pharmaceutical therapy: Hormonal therapy is carried out by a specialist.

Follow-Up

A. Follow up with surgeon as recommended per surgeon.
B. Monitor the patient's testicles at each well-child visit.

Consultation/Referral

A. A mass that does not transilluminate or reduce with gentle pressure is likely to be an incarcerated hernia. This is a surgical emergency.
B. Refer the patient for urologic recommendations regarding surgery.

Individual Considerations

A. Pediatrics
1. Testicular cancer screening should be done during and after puberty.
2. Examine a child in the tailor's position or with the child sitting on a chair or examination table with legs in "frog position," kneeling, or standing. Note: If the child sits cross-legged, it abolishes the reflex of the cremaster muscle.
3. Examine adolescents while standing and straining.
4. Examination of an adolescent includes evaluation of maturation described by Tanner.

B. Adults
1. Males who have undescended testicles may have an increased risk of developing breast cancer and developing testicular germ cell cancers.
2. Men with a history of undescended testes have an increased incidence of infertility (lower sperm counts, sperm of lower quality, and low fertility rates).
3. Testicular torsion is 10 times higher in undescended testes. Torsion of an intra-abdominal testis can present as an acute abdomen.

Urinary Incontinence

Cheryl A. Glass and Debbie Gunter

Definition

A. Urinary incontinence (UI) is the involuntary loss of urine severe enough to have unpleasant social or hygienic consequences. UI is diagnosed primarily on history; inquire about UI at every interview. UI is a symptom of an underlying disease process in most cases; some cases are reversible with appropriate treatment.
B. Incontinence is not considered a part of normal aging. Morbidity related to incontinence includes urinary tract infections (UTIs), indwelling catheters, falls/fractures, sleep interruption, social withdrawal, and depression.
C. Successful toileting depends on ready access to facilities, motivation to remain dry, mobility and manual dexterity, and the cognitive ability to recognize/react to the urge to void.
D. UI can be divided into the following categories: Functional, urge, overflow, stress, and mixed. Each category

has a unique etiology, pathophysiology, symptoms, and management.

Incidence

A. The exact incidence of UI is unknown. The prevalence of incontinence increases with age.
B. UI is common in children. Daytime urinary continence normally occurs by age 4 years. Successful day-and-night continence is generally achieved by age 5 or 7 years.
  1. Up to 20% of children aged 4 to 6 years have an occasional daytime wetting. Three percent have urinary accidents more than two times per week.
  2. Daytime incontinence, a wetting accident at least once every 2 weeks, decreases with age in the pediatric population.
  3. Overactive bladder (OAB) in children has also been associated with other symptoms, including nocturnal enuresis, constipation, fecal incontinence, a history of UTIs, and poor toilet facilities.
C. The incidence of women identified with the definition of any leakage at least once in the past year ranges from 25% to 51%. The incidence is reported to be 10% when identified with weekly urinary leakage.
D. The prevalence of UI in men is approximately half that of women. The incidence of UI is affected by treatment of prostate disease. Men with incontinence have a higher risk of institutionalization compared with men without UI.
E. The elderly are more frequently affected with UI; 6% to 10% of admissions to long-term care facilities are related to incontinence.

Pathogenesis

UI can be caused by pathologic, anatomic, or physiological factors and differs by type of incontinence.
A. Functional incontinence: Loss of urine because of the inability to get to the bathroom, either caused by problems of mobility or cognition.
B. Urge incontinence/OAB: Inability to delay voiding after the sensation of fullness is perceived. Common causes are detrusor hyperactivity or hyperreflexia associated with disorders of the lower urinary tract, tumors, stones, uterine prolapse, cystitis, urethritis, or impaired bladder contractility. Central nervous system disorders, such as stroke, dementia, parkinsonism, or spinal cord injury, also can be causative factors.
C. Overflow incontinence: Loss of urine associated with an overdistension of the bladder. Common causes are anatomic obstruction by an enlarged prostate, a prolapsed cystocele, acontractile bladder caused by diabetes, spinal cord injury, multiple sclerosis, or suprasacral cord lesions.
D. Stress incontinence: Involuntary loss of urine during coughing, sneezing, laughing, bending over, or other physical activity that increases intra-abdominal pressure. Prostate surgery is the most common cause of stress incontinence in men.
E. Mixed incontinence: Combination of stress and urge incontinence in which the bladder outlet is weak and the detrusor is overactive.

Predisposing Factors

A. Age for both males and females
B. Female: 85% of cases are in women
C. Increased parity
D. Previous genitourinary (GU) surgeries (e.g., prostate surgery, hysterectomy)
E. Restricted mobility
F. Menopause
G. Infections
H. Chronic illnesses (e.g., diabetes)
I. Fecal impactions
J. Excessive urinary output
K. Delirium
L. Dementia
M. Neurologic disorders (e.g., stroke, spinal cord injury)
N. Variety of medications (e.g., antihypertensive medicines, diuretics, sedatives)
O. Pelvic trauma (e.g., episiotomy, forceps delivery)
P. Obesity
Q. Sleep apnea
R. Depression
S. High-impact exercise

Common Complaints

A. Urgency: Sudden and compelling desire to pass urine.
B. Urge incontinence: Involuntary leakage accompanied by urgency with the following precipitating factors.
  1. Hearing running water
  2. Placing hands in water
  3. Trying to unlock the door when returning home
  4. Exposure to a cold environment
C. Stress incontinence: Involuntary leakage with the following precipitating factors:
  1. Exertion
  2. Sneezing/coughing
  3. May experience leakage with little or no activity
D. OAB: Symptoms may occur with or without urge incontinence.
  1. Urgency
  2. Frequency
  3. Nocturia

Other Signs and Symptoms

A. Mixed incontinence: Urge and stress leakage
B. Experiencing leakage with little or no activity
C. Continuous leakage (i.e., dribbling)
D. Daytime frequency
E. Nocturia: Up one or more times a night to void
F. Slow urine stream, intermittent stream, or hesitancy
G. Need to strain to start, maintain, or improve voiding
H. Incomplete emptying sensation
I. Children exhibit holding maneuvers to postpone voiding or suppress urgency.
  1. Standing on tiptoes
  2. Forcefully crossing legs (Vincent's curtsy)
  3. Squatting with hand or heel pressed to the perineum

Subjective Data

A. Question the patient regarding the onset, duration, and severity of the incontinence.

1. Do you ever leak urine/water when you don't want to?

2. Do you ever leak urine when you cough, laugh, or exercise?

3. Do you ever leak urine on the way to the bathroom (urgency)?

4. Do you ever use pads, tissue, or cloth in your underwear to catch urine?

B. Elicit situations when UI is worse, when it is improved, and what stimuli are associated with increasing UI (high fluid intake, high caffeine intake, agitation).

C. Review whether the female patient is pre- or postmenopausal.

D. Review other lower urinary tract symptoms (LUTS) such as nocturia.

E. Review the patient's history of bowel function (e.g., fecal incontinence). If constipation is a problem, abdominal pressure from a large retained stool can cause symptoms, including retention.

F. Review medications, including over-the-counter (OTC) drugs and herbals.

1. Do not prescribe a muscarinic medication with patients when they are currently on other medications with anticholinergic properties.

G. Preview previous continence therapy including surgical treatments.

H. Review the impact of incontinence on quality of life, including work impairment, sexual dysfunction, activities of daily living, sleep, recreational activity, social interaction, and depression.

I. Assess whether the elderly patient has incontinence despite toileting.

J. Review sexual function.

K. Review history and previous treatment for prostate disease.

L. Review other comorbid medical diagnoses such as neurologic disabilities, narrow-angle glaucoma, and diabetes.

1. Do not prescribe a muscarinic medication in a patient with narrow-angle glaucoma unless approved by the treating ophthalmologist.

2. Use caution when prescribing antimuscarinic for OAB with a frail patient.

M. What is the diabetic patient's blood glucose average?

Physical Examination

Both sexes

A. Check temperature (if an infection is suspected), pulse, blood pressure (BP), and respiration.

B. Inspect

1. Look for evidence of cardiac overload: Pedal edema.

C. Auscultate

1. Lungs for evidence of fluid overload: Rales

D. Palpate

1. Abdomen for masses, fullness over bladder, and tenderness

E. Neurologic examination

1. Assess cognitive and functional status, including mobility, transfers, manual dexterity, and ability to toilet in the elderly.

2. Screen for depression.

3. Assess for any change in sensation of the perineal area.

a. Ask the patient if they feel pressure in the bladder or rectal area when they need to urinate or defecate.

b. Ask the patient if they can feel when they are wiping.

c. During the physical exam, assess for perineal sensation.

Females

A. Inspect

1. Assess perineal skin for irritation, thinning, vaginal atrophy, and vaginal discharge.

B. Palpate

1. Perform a bimanual pelvic examination for prolapse, masses, or tenderness.

2. Perform rectal examination for sphincter tone, masses, and fecal impaction.

C. Perform pelvic examination.

1. Remove the top blade of the speculum and evaluate the vaginal wall support.

2. Ask the woman to cough to reevaluate the vaginal wall support.

Males

A. Inspect

1. Inspect the glans penis for abnormalities in urethral meatus. (Hypospadias may cause postvoid dribbling.)

2. Uncircumcised men should be evaluated for phimosis and balanitis.

B. Palpate

1. Perform rectal examination for sphincter tone, masses, fecal impaction, prostate size, and contour.

2. Palpate the scrotum to evaluate masses.

3. Evaluate the presence of an inguinal hernia because straining with a partial urinary obstruction can worsen an inguinal hernia.

Diagnostic Tests

The history, physical examination, and urinalysis are sufficient to guide initial therapy. Other tests include the following.

A. Urine culture and sensitivity if infection is suspected.

B. Urine cytology if hematuria or pelvic pain is present.

C. Cystometry. See Section II: Procedure, "Cystometry: Bedside."

D. Postvoid residual (PVR) by catheterization or ultrasound. A PVR of less than 50 mL is considered adequate emptying and greater than 200 mL is considered inadequate, suggesting either detrusor weakness or obstruction. Indications for PVR:

1. Men with mild to moderate lower urinary symptoms

2. Men with OAB (urgency)

3. Persons with spinal cord injury or Parkinson's disease

4. Persons with prior episodes of urinary retention
5. Persons with severe constipation

E. A serum prostate-specific antigen (PSA) should be considered.

F. Routine urodynamic testing is not recommended.

G. Cystoscopy is not required for incontinence; however, it is indicated for hematuria.

Differential Diagnoses

Eight reversible causes of transient incontinence can be remembered by using the mnemonic: DIAPPERS.

Delirium
Infection (urinary)
Atrophic urethritis and vaginitis
Pharmaceuticals
Psychological disorders, especially depression
Excessive urine output
Restricted mobility
Stool impaction

Plan

A. General interventions

1. Functional UI: Therapy is directed at the cause of the condition, such as overdiuresis, inability to go to the toilet, or poor access to toilet facilities.
2. Behavioral interventions should be reviewed.
   a. A bladder diary (see Table 12.6) may provide information on usual timing and circumstances of UI.
   b. Timed scheduled voiding and/or prompted caregiver scheduled toileting.
   c. Bladder training by systematic ability to delay voiding through the use of urge of inhibition.
   d. Stress incontinence: Kegel perineal exercises may improve UI by 30% to 90%. Exercises using graduated vaginal cones or weights induce pelvic muscle tone and strength, reducing UI.
   e. Overflow UI: Crede's method is used for expressing the bladder, by applying pressure with the hands placed in the suprapubic area after voiding to assist in emptying.
   f. Intermittent catheterization is an option frequently used after other measures have failed or overflow UI.
   g. Weight loss is suggested for obese patients.
   h. Dietary changes including elimination of bladder irritants: Caffeine, citrus/acidic foods, alcohol, and carbonated drinks
   i. Avoid constipation. Discuss measures to prevent constipation.
   j. Reduce excessive fluid intake, with no fluid intake 3 to 4 hours before bedtime if nocturia is a problem.

B. Patient teaching: *See Section III: Patient Teaching Guide for this chapter, "Urinary Incontinence: Women."*

C. Other alternatives

1. Surgical treatment is based on the cause of incontinence.
2. Continence pessaries may benefit women with stress UI.
3. Electrical stimulation may be prescribed to inhibit bladder instability and improve striated and levator contractility and efficiency.
4. Treatment of concomitant constipation is an important step in the treatment of incontinence.
5. Treatment of vaginal atrophy is another important step in the treatment of incontinence.
6. Injection of botulinum toxin (BTX) is an option for treatment of urge incontinence in selected patients.
7. Transurethral bulking agents injected into the submucosal tissues of the urethra or bladder neck are an option for women and men with UI caused by benign prostatic hypertrophy (BPH).
8. Indwelling catheters are not recommended as a management strategy for OAB. Please see *Section III: Patient Teaching Guide for Chapter 12, "Genitourinary Disorders,"* for a copy of the Bladder Control Diary (Table 12.6) to hand out to patients.

D. Pharmaceutical therapy

1. Use of anticholinergic and antispasmodic drugs to decrease reflex bladder contractions and increase bladder capacity (contraindicated in uncontrolled narrow-angle glaucoma, urinary retention, or gastric retention)
   a. Oxybutynin chloride (Ditropan): Tablets and syrup formulation
      i. Adults: 5 mg orally two to three times per day (maximum of 20 mg/d).
      ii. Pediatrics: Indicated for children 5 years of age and older; 5 mg twice a day (maximum of 15 mg/d).
   b. Oxybutynin chloride (Ditropan XL): Extended release tablets
      i. Adults: Initially 5 to 10 mg once a day. May increase the dosage weekly in 5 mg increments (maximum of 30 mg/d).
      ii. Pediatrics: Indicated for children 6 years of age and older. Initially 5 mg once a day. May increase weekly in 5 mg increments (maximum of 20 mg/d).
   c. Oxybutynin chloride (Gelnique): Topical gel
      i. Apply 1 g gel sachet once a day to intact skin.
      ii. Not recommended for children
   d. Tolterodine tartrate (Detrol LA)
      i. 2 to 4 mg orally per day
      ii. Not recommended for children
   e. Fesoterodine (Toviaz): Extended release capsule
      i. 4 mg once a day (maximum of 8 mg/d)
      ii. Not recommended for children
   f. Trospium (Sanctura XR): Extended release capsule
      i. Taken on an empty stomach, 60 mg orally every morning
      ii. Not recommended for children
   g. Darifenacin (Enablex)
      i. 7.5 mg orally once a day
      ii. May increase to 15 mg once a day
      iii. Not recommended for children

TABLE 12.6 Bladder Control Diary

Your Daily Bladder Diary

This diary will help you and your health care team figure out the causes of your bladder control trouble. The "sample" line shows you how to use the diary. Use this sheet as a master for making copies that you can use as a bladder diary for as many days as you need.

Your name: ______________________________

Date: ______________

Time	Drinks		Trips to the Bathroom		Accidental Leaks	Did You Feel a Strong Urge to Go?	What Were You Doing at the Time?
	What kind?	*How much?*	*How many times?*	*How much urine? (circle one)*	*How much? (circle one)*	*Circle one*	*Sneezing, exercising, having sex, lifting, etc.*
Sample	Coffee	2 cups	✓ ✓	(◯) ◯ ◯ sm med lg	◯ (◯) ◯ sm med lg	Yes (No)	Running
6–7 a.m.				◯ ◯ ◯	◯ ◯ ◯	Yes No	
7–8 a.m.				◯ ◯ ◯	◯ ◯ ◯	Yes No	
8–9 a.m.				◯ ◯ ◯	◯ ◯ ◯	Yes No	
9–10 a.m.				◯ ◯ ◯	◯ ◯ ◯	Yes No	
10–11 a.m.				◯ ◯ ◯	◯ ◯ ◯	Yes No	
11–12 noon				◯ ◯ ◯	◯ ◯ ◯	Yes No	
12–1 p.m.				◯ ◯ ◯	◯ ◯ ◯	Yes No	
1–2 p.m.				◯ ◯ ◯	◯ ◯ ◯	Yes No	
2–3 p.m.				◯ ◯ ◯	◯ ◯ ◯	Yes No	
3–4 p.m.				◯ ◯ ◯	◯ ◯ ◯	Yes No	
4–5 p.m				◯ ◯ ◯	◯ ◯ ◯	Yes No	
5–6 p.m.				◯ ◯ ◯	◯ ◯ ◯	Yes No	
6–7 p.m.				◯ ◯ ◯	◯ ◯ ◯	Yes No	
7–8 p.m.				◯ ◯ ◯	◯ ◯ ◯	Yes No	
8–9 p.m.				◯ ◯ ◯	◯ ◯ ◯	Yes No	
9–10 p.m.				◯ ◯ ◯	◯ ◯ ◯	Yes No	
10–11 p.m.				◯ ◯ ◯	◯ ◯ ◯	Yes No	
11–12 midnight				◯ ◯ ◯	◯ ◯ ◯	Yes No	
12–1 a.m.				◯ ◯ ◯	◯ ◯ ◯	Yes No	
1–2 a.m.				◯ ◯ ◯	◯ ◯ ◯	Yes No	
2–3 a.m.				◯ ◯ ◯	◯ ◯ ◯	Yes No	
3–4 a.m.				◯ ◯ ◯	◯ ◯ ◯	Yes No	
4–5 a.m.				◯ ◯ ◯	◯ ◯ ◯	Yes No	
5–6 a.m.				◯ ◯ ◯	◯ ◯ ◯	Yes No	

I used ______________ pads today. I used ______________ diapers today (write number).

Questions to ask my health care team: ______________________________

Let's Talk About Bladder Control for Women is a public health awareness campaign conducted by the National Kidney and Urologic Diseases Information Clearinghouse (NKUDIC), an information dissemination service of the National Institute of Diabetes and Digestive and Kidney Diseases (NIDDK), National Institutes of Health.

Source: National Kidney and Urologic Diseases Information Clearinghouse, National Institutes of Health (NKUDIC, NIH). Retrieved from kidney .niddk.nih.gov/kudiseases/pubs/bcw_ez/insertB.htm

h. Solifenacin (Vesicare)
i. Initially 5 mg orally once a day
ii. May increase to 10 mg daily
iii. Not recommended for children

2. Alpha-adrenergic antagonists stimulate urethral smooth muscle contraction.
a. Imipramine (Tofranil): Used for childhood enuresis
i. Children younger than 6 years: Not recommended
ii. Children older than 6 years: 25 mg initially 1 hour before bedtime
iii. Children 6 to 12 years: 25 mg initially 1 hour before bedtime; increase up to 50 mg after 1 week
iv. Children older than 12 years: 25 mg initially 1 hour before bedtime; may increase up to 75 mg as needed

3. Beta-3 adrenergic agonist: Mirabegron (Myrbetriq)
a. Initially 25 mg once a day
b. May increase to 50 mg once a day
c. Not recommended in children

4. The Food and Drug Administration (FDA) has not approved any medication for stress incontinence.

5. For postmenopausal women, vaginal estrogen may restore urethral mucosa; use the same type, dosage, and patient selection criteria as with estrogen therapy (ET). Systemic estrogen should not be prescribed for UI.

Follow-Up

A. Follow-up is based on the type and cause of UI.

Consultation/Referral

A. When to consult a physician for UI depends on the type and cause of UI. UI is a problem that can be successfully treated.
B. Refer to a specialist for incontinence with abdominal and/or pelvic pain or hematuria in the absence of a UTI, or when surgical treatment is desired.
C. Refer for urodynamic testing, which is considered the gold standard. Testing requires special equipment and training.
D. Refer to a gynecologist or urology clinic practitioner experienced in fitting a continence pessary.
E. Refer to a urologist for hematuria and/or risk factors of bladder cancer.

Individual Considerations

A. Pregnancy: Stress incontinence is frequently associated with pregnancy and is treated with pelvic exercises.
B. Pediatrics
1. UI is most often experienced as enuresis.
2. UI in previously bladder-controlled children requires a thorough workup and referral to a pediatrician.
3. Any child with a suspected neurologic abnormality should be evaluated for an occult neurologic lesion.
4. Dysfunctional voiding is often associated with a psychological comorbidity or behavioral issues.
C. Geriatrics
1. Incontinence in the elderly is a risk factor for falls. Many falls occur en route to the bathroom, especially at night.
2. Incontinence increases social isolation and depression.
3. Functional incontinence is common in older adults with arthritis or Parkinson's or Alzheimer's diseases. Patients are unable to hold their urine until they reach the bathroom and undress. A toileting program usually assists in this situation.
4. Durable medical equipment, such as a bedside commode, should be considered.
5. Antimuscarinic medications may increase confusion.

Urinary Tract Infection (Acute Cystitis)

Cheryl A. Glass and Debbie Gunter

Definition

A. Urinary tract infection (UTI) is an infection of the urinary bladder. UTI is defined as the presence of at least 100,000 organisms per mL of urine in an asymptomatic patient or more than 100 organisms per mL of urine with accompanying pyuria (greater than 7 white blood cells [WBCs]/mL) in a symptomatic patient. Asymptomatic bacteriuria (ASB) when left untreated is a risk factor for acute cystitis (40%) and pyelonephritis in 25% to 30% in pregnancy.
B. UTIs can be divided anatomically into upper and lower tract (cystitis) infections. For a discussion of upper tract infection, see the section in this chapter, "Pyelonephritis."
C. UTIs may be considered uncomplicated or complicated.
1. An uncomplicated UTI is noted in a healthy person with a normal urinary tract system and may be treated with oral antibiotics.
2. A UTI noted in a person with a structural or functional urinary tract system or in a person who is immunocompromised is considered complicated. It may require parental therapy until afebrile.

Incidence

A. Incidence depends on age and gender. The prevalence of UTI in males varies according to age.
1. Young men aged 15 to 50 years rarely develop a UTI.
2. The incidence of a UTI in geriatric males may be as high as in geriatric females (up to 15%).
B. In children, the incidence varies by age and gender. A UTI is the most common cause of fever of unknown origin in pediatrics.
C. More than 50% of women will have one UTI in their lifetime.
1. Prevalence for females increases by 1% per decade and 2% to 4% throughout childbearing years.
2. The incidence of UTIs in pregnancy ranges from 4% to 7%. In pregnancy, the increased incidence is related to both hormonal influence and anatomic

changes that increase the risk of urinary stasis and vesicoureteral reflux.

3. By age 30 years, approximately 50% of women have experienced symptoms of a UTI.

Pathogenesis

A. Bacteria ascend from the perineum through the urethra. The greater susceptibility of younger women and girls is related to a shorter urethra. In older women, it is related to estrogen-mediated dilation of the urethra.

B. The normal male urinary tract has many natural defenses to infection. The greater susceptibility of elderly males is related to problems with the prostate and other urologic disease and can be linked to the instrumentation required for therapy.

C. Gram-negative bacilli are the most common pathogens; 80% to 90% of cases are related to coliform bacteria (*Escherichia coli*). It originates from fecal floras that colonize the periurethral area.

D. Other gram-negative bacteria include *Klebsiella pneumoniae* or *Proteus mirabilis*. *Staphylococcus saprophyticus* (gram-positive coccus) accounts for about 10% to 15% of UTIs.

E. Other pathogens include *Enterobacter*, *Pseudomonas*, *Enterococci*, and *Staphylococci*.

F. The incubation period depends on the pathogen.

Predisposing Factors

A. Female (until elderly, then equal frequency in males and females)
B. Pregnancy
C. Poor hygiene
D. Trauma
E. Instrumentation
F. Sexual intercourse
G. Oral contraceptive or diaphragm use
H. Female patient diagnosed with diabetes (there is no increased risk for diabetic males)
I. Anomalies of the genitourinary (GU) tract
J. Neurologic factors
K. Vesicourethral reflux
L. Obstruction: Stones
M. Foreign bodies
N. Bubble baths and hot tubs
O. Douching
P. Anal intercourse
Q. HIV
R. Uncircumcised penis
S. Catheterization
T. Nosocomial infection
U. Phimosis

Common Complaints

A. Burning on urination
B. Frequency
C. Cloudy or bloody urine
D. Urgency
E. UTI in infants and children
  1. Vague symptoms with or without fever
  2. Gastrointestinal symptoms (vomiting and diarrhea)
  3. Frequent voiding
  4. Incontinence
  5. Dysuria
  6. Suprapubic, abdominal, or lumbar pain
F. Geriatrics
  1. May not present with classic symptoms
  2. Fever
  3. Incontinence
  4. Mental confusion

Other Signs and Symptoms

A. Asymptomatic
B. Frequency, dysuria, bladder spasms, suprapubic discomfort, urgency, and nocturia
C. Suprapubic pain
D. Fever
E. Costovertebral angle (CVA) tenderness
F. Hematuria

Subjective Data

A. Review the onset, course, and duration of symptoms.

B. Does the patient have fever and chills or back or flank pain (unilateral or bilateral)?

C. Are there any other genital problems such as herpes lesions or vaginal discharge?

D. Review the associated factors: Sexual intercourse (specifically review for anal intercourse), douching, or bubble bath.

E. Ask female patients if they use appropriate hygiene practices after urination and bowel movements (BMs).
  1. Wiping from front to back
  2. Frequent changes of hygienic products
  3. Handwashing

F. Is the patient pregnant? If not, what type of birth control does she use?

G. Is there any history of previous UTIs? How often, and how were they treated? Were any tests performed in a workup by a urologist?

H. How much liquid or water does the patient drink every day? Note the amount of caffeine.

I. In older men, review the strength of the urinary flow, dribbling, hesitancy, and so forth.

J. In the postmenopausal woman, review whether she has a known prolapse and/or vaginal atrophy. Does she use any systemic or local estrogen medications?

K. Is there any history of other medical diseases including diabetes or sickle cell disease?

L. Review for the presence of neurologic disorders including spinal cord injury or multiple sclerosis.

M. Does the patient require self-catheterization?

Physical Examination

A. Check temperature, blood pressure (BP), pulse, and respiration. The absence of a fever does not exclude the presence of an infective process.

B. Inspect
  1. General observation of general appearance for discomfort before and during examination

C. Auscultate
  1. Heart and all lung fields

D. Palpate
  1. Palpate the abdomen: Kidneys, masses; assess for suprapubic tenderness.
  2. Palpate the back; note CVA tenderness.
  3. Check for inguinal lymph node enlargement.
  4. Palpate the suprapubic area.
E. Percuss
  1. The bladder and the CVA area for tenderness
F. Females
  1. Pelvic examination
    a. Inspect external genitalia for lesions, Bartholin's gland cysts, irritation, and discharge.
    b. Milk urethra for discharge.
    c. Assess rectal area.
    d. Speculum examination: Evaluate vaginal vault for discharge, cervicitis, and inflammation; evaluate for atrophic vaginal changes and torn tissue.
    e. Bimanual examination: Check for cervical motion, tenderness, and masses.
G. Males
  1. Inspect the penis/urinary meatus for phimosis, lesions, signs of inflammation, and discharge. Retract the foreskin (if present) and assess for hygiene and smegma.
  2. Palpate the testes and epididymides for inflammation, tenderness, and masses.
  3. Rectal examination is mandatory in males: Check for swollen and tender prostate. In patients with suspected acute bacterial prostatitis, palpation should be very gentle because of the potential for bacteremia.

Diagnostic Tests

The diagnosis of a UTI can often be made based on a focused history and the presenting symptoms.

A. Urinalysis: Clean-catch urinalysis may be performed. However, catheterization or suprapubic aspiration may be necessary depending on the patient's age and condition. Examples include pediatrics, elderly, obese, microscopic hematuria or for functionally impaired patients. Catheterization should be reserved for patients with an obstruction or for those who cannot cooperate or collect a clean-catch urine specimen. The percutaneous bladder aspiration is used for young children and infants.

Urinalysis dipstick findings:
  1. Appearance: Should be clear. Cloudy urine may indicate presence of pyuria, pus, blood, cells, phosphate, or lymph fluid.
  2. Odor: Usually faint aromatic odor; ammonia odor indicates *Proteus*, related to food changes; offensive odor indicates bacterial infection.
  3. pH: Normal is around 6 (acid); may normally vary from 4.6 to 7.5. Greater than 7.5 may indicate infection.
  4. Specific gravity: Reflects the kidney's ability to concentrate urine and the body's hydration or dehydration status. Normal is 1.005 to 1.025.
  5. Color: Shows concentration; usually yellow or amber.
    a. Straw color = dilute urine
    b. Dark color = concentrated (dehydrated)
    c. Red or red-brown, to bloody = transfusion reaction, drugs, and bleeding lesions
    d. Yellow brown = bile duct disease, jaundice
    e. Dark brown or black = melanoma or leukemia
  6. Positive leukocyte esterase and nitrates indicate infection.

A negative urine dipstick does not rule out an infection.

B. Microscopic examination of urine findings: White blood cells (WBCs) greater than 2 to 5; WBC/high-power microscope field (HPF); bacteria; positive Gram stain for cocci or rods, yeast, and blood indicates infection.
C. Urine culture and sensitivity
  1. Positive culture standard 10^5 colony-forming units; symptomatic female 10^2; symptomatic males 10^3.
  2. Screening for asymptomatic bacteria is recommended for patients in pregnancy, for elderly males with documented prostatic or urologic abnormalities, for patients with a recent catheterization, and for patients with known stones or documented structural abnormalities.
D. Culture for sexually transmitted infection (STIs) if suspected
E. Wet prep for female, if indicated
F. Imaging
  1. Ultrasound (especially useful in children)
  2. Conventional voiding cystourethrography
  3. Urodynamic evaluation

Differential Diagnoses

A. UTI: Watch for systemic symptoms of pyelonephritis.
B. Vaginal or pelvic infection
C. Prostatitis or epididymitis: Tender, enlarged prostate; tender testicle or scrotum
D. Bladder tumor
E. Interstitial cystitis (IC)
F. Urinary calculi
G. Benign prostatic hypertrophy (BPH): Changes in urinary stream and nocturia
H. Overactive bladder (OAB)/urge incontinence
I. Pelvic organ prolapse
J. Irritant urethritis
K. Consider the possibility that chronic, asymptomatic infections are a potential source of disseminated infection, such as endocarditis. This is particularly likely in the male patient with prostate disease and infection requiring instrumentation.

Plan

A. General interventions
  1. Treatment of acute cystitis is aimed at identifying the underlying cause and initiating treatment as soon as possible.
  2. If antibiotic therapy is initiated, stress the importance of taking all medication as directed, even if symptoms improve before the end of treatment.
B. Patient teaching
  1. Provide patient teaching sheet. Patient teaching: See *Section III: Patient Teaching Guide for this chapter, "Urinary Tract Infection (Acute Cystitis)."* ◀

C. Dietary management

1. Instruct the patient to increase fluids and drink at least one large glass of liquid every hour.

2. Instruct the patient to avoid foods that irritate the bladder: Caffeine, alcohol, tomatoes, citrus, and spicy foods.

3. Encourage the patient to drink cranberry juice to help fight bladder infections. If the patient dislikes the taste of plain cranberry juice, have him or her mix it 1:1 with another juice, such as orange juice.

D. Pharmacological therapy

1. Antibiotics: 3-day course may be efficacious and is less expensive than the traditional 7- to 10-day course of therapy for uncomplicated infections.

2. The antibiotic of choice depends on the specific bacteria found on culture. Empiric antimicrobial therapy should cover all likely pathogens.

3. First-line therapy

a. Nitrofurantoin monohydrate/macrocrystals (Macrobid) 100 mg orally twice a day for 5 days or

b. Trimethoprim/sulfamethoxazole 160 mg/800 mg (Bactrim DS, Septra DS) 1 tablet orally twice a day for 3 days (use when bacterial resistance is less than 20% and patient has no allergy) *or*

c. Fosfomycin (Monurol) 3 g orally in a single dose with 3 to 4 oz of water

4. Second-line therapy

a. Ciprofloxacin (Cipro) 250 mg orally twice a day for 3 days *or*

b. Ciprofloxacin extended-release (Cipro XR) 500 mg orally twice a day for 3 days *or*

c. Levofloxacin (Levaquin) 250 mg orally twice a day for 3 days

5. Alternative therapy

a. Amoxicillin-clavulanate (Augmentin) 875 mg/125 mg orally twice a day for 7 days *or*

b. Amoxicillin-clavulanate (Augmentin) 500 mg/125 mg orally three times per day for 7 days

6. Urinary analgesic if needed

a. Phenazopyridine HCl (Pyridium): 100 to 200 mg tid for 1 to 2 days only when given with an antibiotic. Educate the patient that this drug turns urine orange.

b. Multiple Uro Blue medications are available; take one orally four times a day. Educate the patient that this drug turns the urine blue/green.

7. Drugs of choice for UTI or pyelonephritis in pregnancy

a. Nitrofurantoin (Macrobid) 100 mg: One tablet orally every 12 hours for 5 days

b. Amoxicillin: 500 mg orally every 12 hours for 3 to 7 days

c. Amoxicillin-clavulanate (Augmentin): 500 mg orally every 12 hours for 3 to 7 days

d. Cephalexin (Keflex): 500 mg orally four times a day for 3 to 5 days

e. Cefpodoxime (Vantin) 100 mg twice a day for 5 to 7 days *or*

f. Fosfomycin (Monurol) 3 g orally in a single dose with 3 to 4 oz of water

g. If dysuria is present: phenazopyridine HCl (Pyridium) 200 mg orally three times daily for 2 days when given with an antibiotic.

8. Children younger than 2 years are usually treated for 7 to 14 days; children older than 2 years who are afebrile and without abnormalities of the urinary tract or have previous episodes of UTIs are usually treated for 5 days.

a. Amoxicillin-clavulanate (Augmentin): 20 to 45 mg/kg orally per day every 12 hours

b. Sulfonamide-trimethoprim-sulfamethoxazole (Bactrim, Septra): 6 to 12 mg/kg trimethoprim and 30 to 60 mg/kg sulfamethoxazole per day orally in two doses

c. Cephalosporin-cefixime (Suprax): 8 mg/kg/d in one dose or in divided doses every 12 hours

9. Antibiotics that should not be used in pediatrics or pregnancy include the following:

a. Fluoroquinolones are not used in children because of potential concerns about sustained injury to developing joints.

b. Fluoroquinolones (Category Class C) are contraindicated during pregnancy because of auditory and vestibular toxicity in the fetus.

c. Tetracyclines should not be used in pregnancy (Category Class D) or in children because of tooth staining.

d. Nitrofurantoin is contraindicated in pregnant patients at term, during labor, and during delivery.

10. Consider prophylactic therapy for patients with chronic conditions/recurrent infections.

a. Low-dose antibiotics daily for 3 to 6 months

b. Self-start antibiotics

c. Postcoital antibiotics

11. Quinolones, cephalosporins, and macrolides should be reserved for complicated or resistant infections.

12. Vaginal estrogen should be considered in postmenopausal women with urogenital atrophic changes.

Follow-Up

A. Routine posttreatment urinalysis/culture is not indicated in asymptomatic patients.

B. Have the patient return if symptoms do not resolve at the end of treatment.

C. Have the patient return if the symptoms reoccur within 2 weeks of treatment for a urine culture. Retreatment with a 7-day course of antibiotics using a different agent should be considered.

D. Two UTIs in girls and one UTI in boys should trigger an evaluation to rule out an obstruction, vesicoureteric reflux, and dysfunctional voiding. UTI in children who are severely ill with vomiting and dehydration requires hospitalization and IV antibiotics.

Consultation/Referral

A. Refer all children with more than one UTI to a physician.

B. Young men do not have UTIs very often; a urologic workup may be needed if etiology, such as an STI, cannot be determined.

C. Patients with bacteriuria are also more likely to have identifiable abnormalities on an intravenous pyelography (IVP), including small kidneys, delayed excretion, calyceal dilation and blunting, ureteral reflux, stones, and obstructive lesions.
D. Consultation with a urologist is essential in all forms of prostatitis or in all but the most clear-cut cases of acute scrotum.

Individual Considerations

A. Women
  1. Recurrent infections are common in females.
  2. Repeat urine culture and sensitivity after an antibiotic course is complete (approximately 2–4 weeks after therapy is completed).
  3. If the patient is perimenopausal and has two or fewer UTIs a year, consider patient-initiated therapy to start when symptomatic. Consider topical estradiol cream for atrophic vaginitis. If the patient has three UTIs a year, prescribe a prophylactic single-dose regimen after intercourse. If infections are not related to intercourse, consider urine cultures every 2 months, with extended antibiotic therapy.

B. Pregnancy
  1. The incidence of pyelonephritis in pregnancy is 1% to 2%. Most cases develop as a consequence of undiagnosed or inadequately treated lower UTI.
    a. In the presumptive diagnosis of pyelonephritis in pregnancy, ultrasound of the kidneys and urinary tract should be considered.
  2. Approximately 75% to 80% of pyelonephritis cases occur on the right side, with a 10% to 15% incidence on the left side. A small percentage of cases are bilateral.
  3. Group B *Streptococcus* (GBS) colonization has important implications during pregnancy, contributing to maternal pyelonephritis and preterm birth. Intrapartum transmission may lead to neonatal GBS infection.
    a. Women with documented GBS bacteriuria in the current pregnancy should be treated at the time of labor or rupture of membranes with appropriate intravenous (IV) antibiotics for the prevention of early-onset neonatal GBS disease.
    b. Asymptomatic women with urinary GBS in pregnancy should not be treated with antibiotics for the prevention of adverse maternal and perinatal outcomes.
    c. Women with documented GBS bacteriuria should not be rescreened by genital tract culture or urinary culture in the third trimester, as they are presumed to be GBS colonized.
  4. Current guidelines recommend universal vaginal and rectal screening in all pregnant women at 35 to 37 weeks gestation rather than treatment based on risk factors.
  5. A urine culture screening is recommended for all pregnant women at their first prenatal visit.
  6. Suppressive antibiotic therapy should be instituted in pregnant patients who develop acute cystitis, recurrent or persistent ASB, or pyelonephritis.
  7. Patients with sickle cell hemoglobinopathies are at increased risk of UTI and should be screened more aggressively, possibly benefiting from antibiotic prophylaxis.
  8. Antibiotics that should not be used during pregnancy include
    a. Tetracyclines (adverse effects on fetal teeth/bones and congenital defects)
    b. Quinolones (congenital defects)
    c. Trimethoprim in the first trimester (facial defects and cardiac abnormalities)
    d. Sulfonamides in the last trimester (kernicterus)
    e. Aminoglycosides (permanent ototoxicity in the fetus)

C. Pediatrics
  1. Tetracyclines should not be given to children because of tooth staining.
  2. Fluorinated quinolones may produce cartilage toxicity.
  3. Antibiotic therapy includes amoxicillin, cephalosporins, trimethoprim, and nitrofurantoin.
  4. Children diagnosed with recurrent UTIs should be referred and assessed for sexual abuse.

D. Geriatrics
  1. Patients may not have classic symptoms. Consider UTI if the patient presents with increased urinary incontinence (UI), fever, and mental confusion.

Varicocele

Cheryl A. Glass and Debbie Gunter

Definition

A. Varicocele is engorgement of the internal spermatic veins above the testes. This vascular abnormality is a cause of decreased testicular function. Some varicoceles are easy to identify and may be surgically corrected. The presence of a varicocele does not mean that surgical correction is a necessity.

Incidence

A. Varicocele may occur in 15% to 20% of normal males; 80% to 90% of cases occur on the left side. Up to 35% to 40% of men with a palpable left-sided varicocele may actually have bilateral varicoceles that are identified on physical examination.
B. Right-sided varicocele is uncommon and can indicate retroperitoneal malignancy. Varicocele is the leading known cause of male infertility (40%). Decreased sperm counts, infertility, and testicular atrophy occur in 65% to 75% of varicocele cases. There is no correlation between the size of the varicocele and the degree of infertility.

Pathogenesis

A. The exact pathophysiologic mechanisms for varicoceles are not fully identified. Varicoceles may be because of valvular incompetence or elevated hydrostatic pressure in the spermatic veins. Testicular temperature elevation also appears to play a role in varicocele-induced dysfunction. **New varicoceles in older men may be secondary to renal tumors.**

Predisposing Factor

A. Varicoceles generally manifest at the time of puberty.

Common Complaints

A. Asymptomatic
B. Infertility
C. Pain or discomfort in the scrotum

Other Signs and Symptoms

A. Pain or aching and heaviness in the scrotum
B. Feels like "worms"; scrotum may have bluish discoloration

Subjective Data

A. Note the onset, course, and duration of symptoms. When was the varicocele first noted?
B. Has the scrotum enlarged? If there is enlargement, over what time span? Does it collapse with lying or sitting down?
C. Is there any pain or discomfort?
D. Has there been any history of infertility?

Physical Examination

A. Check vital signs and temperature as indicated.
B. Inspect
  1. The examination should be done when the patient is lying or standing in a warm room. Warm temperature promotes relaxation of the scrotum.
  2. Examine the general appearance of the penis; note scrotal size, shape, and rugae. Varicocele tends to collapse with the patient sitting or supine.
  3. Transilluminate the scrotum to visualize the varicocele.
  4. A large varicocele can easily be identified by inspection.
C. Palpate
  1. Palpate each side of the scrotum for testicular size, presence of varicocele (Valsalva maneuver performed while the patient stands helps to reveal a small varicocele), and absence of vas deferens.
    a. A moderate-size varicocele can be identified by palpation without having the patient perform the Valsalva maneuver.
  2. Palpate the spermatic cord between the thumb and forefingers while the patient performs a Valsalva maneuver.
    a. A small varicocele is identified only when the patient bears down, increasing the intra-abdominal pressure.
    b. Varicocele should significantly diminish in size when the patient assumes the supine position.
  3. Evaluate whether the varicocele can be reduced while the patient is supine.
  4. Palpate the abdomen for hernias, masses, and tenderness.
  5. Rectal examination: Palpate the prostate and seminal vesicles for tenderness and other signs of infection.
D. Auscultate: Listen over the scrotum to assess bowel sounds to rule out hernia.

Diagnostic Tests

A. Scrotal ultrasound with a high-resolution color-flow Doppler is the diagnostic method of choice when clinical examinations are equivocal, but are not indicated for standard evaluation.
B. Semen analysis times two, if indicated
C. CT to evaluate retroperitoneal pathology (e.g., renal cell carcinoma) for
  1. Sudden onset of varicocele
  2. Single right-sided varicocele
  3. Any varicocele that is not reducible in the supine position

Differential Diagnoses

A. Varicocele classifications
  1. Grade I (small): Palpable only on Valsalva maneuver, which increases intra-abdominal pressure and therefore impedes drainage and increases the varicocele size
  2. Grade II (medium): Palpable when standing and bearing down (Valsalva maneuver)
  3. Grade III (large): Visible on inspection alone
  4. Subclinical: Not palpable, vein larger than 3 mm on ultrasound; Doppler reflux on Valsalva maneuver
B. Hernia
C. Epididymitis
D. Hydrocele
E. Testicular tumor: Consider retroperitoneal tumor, especially if presenting symptoms have a sudden onset.

Plan

A. General interventions
  1. Urologic consultation for diagnosis and possible surgery. Surgery should be considered when all of the following conditions are met:
    a. Palpable varicocele on physical examination
    b. Couples with known infertility
    c. Female has normal fertility or potential treatable cause of infertility.
    d. Male partner has abnormal semen parameters or abnormal results from sperm function tests.
B. Patient teaching
  1. If discomfort is present, an athletic supporter should be tried.
  2. If surgery is not indicated, no other interventions are needed.
C. Pharmaceutical therapy: None is recommended.

Follow-Up

A. After surgery, no follow-up is necessary if the patient is taught scrotal self-examination.
B. If no surgery is performed, the patient should be taught self-examination and instructed to return for pain or change in size and shape.
C. Adolescents with varicoceles should be followed with annual objective measurements of testis size and/or semen analyses in order to detect the earliest sign of varicocele-related testicular injury.

Consultation/Referral

A. Refer the patient to a urologist for surgical evaluation. Varicocelectomy is recommended in cases of pain and infertility, and it may be offered in the preadolescent to ensure proper testicular development.

Individual Considerations

A. Adults

1. New onset varicocele in older male may indicate a renal tumor.

B. Pediatrics

1. The young patient with a varicocele should be followed every 6 months or yearly to see how the testis is growing.

Bibliography

Akre, C., Berchtold, A., Gmel, G., & Suris, J. (2014). The evolution of sexual dysfunction in young men aged 18–25 years. *Journal of Adolescent Health, 55*(6), 736–743.

American Academy of Pediatrics. (2011, September, reaffirmed in 2014). Urinary tract infection: Clinical practice guideline for the diagnosis and management of the initial UTI in febrile infants and children 2 to 24 months. *Pediatrics, 128*, 595–610.

American College of Obstetricians and Gynecologists. (2013). Hypertension in pregnancy. Retrieved from http://www.acog.org/Resources-And-Publications/Task-Force-and-Work-Group-Reports/Hypertension-in-Pregnancy

American Urological Association. (n.d.). Guideline on the pharmacologic management of premature ejaculation. Retrieved from https://www.auanet.org/education/guidelines/premature-ejaculation.cfm

American Urological Association. (2010, revised 2014). American Urological Association guideline: Management of benign prostatic hyperplasia (BPH). Retrieved from https://www.auanet.org/education/guidelines/benign-prostatic-hyperplasia.cfm

American Urological Association. (2011, June). The management of erectile dysfunction: An update. Retrieved from https://www.auanet.org/education/guidelines/erectile-dysfunction.cfm

American Urological Association. (2012). Diagnosis, evaluation and follow-up of asymptomatic microhematuria (AMH) in adults: AUA guideline. Retrieved from https://www.auanet.org/education/guidelines/asymptomatic-microhematuria.cfm

American Urological Association. (2013, April). Early detection of prostate cancer: AUA guideline. Retrieved from https://www.auanet.org/education/guidelines/prostate-cancer-detection.cfm

American Urological Association. (2014a, April). Evaluation and treatment of cryptorchidism: AUA guideline. Retrieved from https://www.auanet.org/education/guidelines/cryptorchidism.cfm

American Urological Association. (2014b, September). Diagnosis and treatment of interstitial cystitis/bladder pain syndrome. Retrieved from https://www.auanet.org/education/guidelines/ic-bladder-pain-syndrome.cfm

American Urological Association. (2016, April). Surgical management of stones: American Urological Association/Endourological Society guideline. Retrieved from www.auanet.org/education/guidelines/surgical-management-of-stones.cfm

American Urological Association (AUA). (2016, July). Education and Research Inc. American Urologic Association Symptom Score. Retrieved from https://www.auanet.org

Amin, S. V., Illipilla, S., Hebbar, S., Rai, L., Kumar, P., & Pai, M. V. (2014). Quantifying proteinuria in hypertensive disorders of pregnancy. *International Journal of Hypertension, 2014*, 941408.

Annam, K., Voznesensky, M., & Kreder, K. J. (2016). Understanding and managing erectile dysfunction in patients treated for cancer. *Journal of Oncology Practice, 12*(4), 297–305.

Aora, P. (2015, April 7). Chronic kidney disease. *Medscape*. Retrieved from http://emedicine.medscape.com/article/238798-overview

Associates in Urology. (n.d.-a). Patient questionnaire: AUA Symptom Score (AUASS). Retrieved from www.njurology.com/_forms/auass.pdf

Associates in Urology. (n.d.-b). Sexual health inventory for men (SHIM). Retrieved from http://www.njurology.com/_forms/shim.pdf

Associates in Urology. (n.d.-c). Quality of Life questionnaire. Retrieved from http://www.njurology.com/_forms/qualityoflife.php

Bechis, S. K., Otsetov, A. G., Ge, R., & Olumi, A. F. (2014). Personalized medicine for the management of benign prostatic hyperplasia. *Journal of Urology, 192*(1), 16–23.

Borrelli, S., De Nicola, L., Stanzione, G., Conte, G., & Minutolo, R. (2013). Resistant hypertension in nondialysis chronic kidney disease. *International Journal of Hypertension, 2013*, 929183.

Brusch, J. (2016, March 22). Prevention of urinary tract infections. *Medscape*. Retrieved from http://emedicine.medscape.com/article/2040239-overview#a1

Carrero, J. J., Burrowes, J., & Wanner, C. (2016). A long road to travel: Adherence to dietary recommendations and adequate dietary phosphorus control. *Journal of Renal Nutrition, 26*(3), 133–135.

Centers for Disease Control and Prevention. (2015, June 15). 2015 sexually transmitted diseases treatment guidelines: Epididymitis. Retrieved from https://www.cdc.gov/std/tg2015/epididymitis.htm

Ching, C. B. (2015, December 20). Epididymitis treatment and management. *Medscape*. Retrieved from emedicine.medscape.com/article/436154-treatmemt

Chung, E., Gilbert, B., Perera, M., & Roberts, M. J. (2015). Premature ejaculation: A clinical review for the general physician. *Australian Family Physician, 44*(10), 737–743.

Clemens, J. Q. (2013, February 6). Urinary incontinence in men. *UpToDate*. Retrieved from http://www.uptodate.com/contents/urinary-incontinence-in-men?topicKey=PC%2F14611

Clemens, J. Q. (2015, July 24). Pathogenesis, clinical features, and diagnosis of interstitial cystitis/bladder pain syndrome. *UpToDate*. Retrieved from www.uptodate.com/contents/pathogenesis-clinical-features-and-diagnosis-of-interstitial-cystitis-bladder-pain-syndrome

Clinical Key. (n.d.). Pyelonephritis. Retrieved from https://www.cdc.gov/std/tg2015/epididymitis.htm

Crawford, P., & Crop, J. (2014, May 1). Evaluation of scrotal masses. *American Family Physician, 89*, 723–727.

Cunningham, G. R., & Rosen, R. C. (2013, May 31). Overview of male sexual dysfunction. *UpToDate*. Retrieved from http://www.uptodate.com/contents/overview-of-male-sexual-dysfunction

Curhan, G. C., Aronson, M. D., & Preminger, G. M. (2015, November 11). Diagnosis and acute management of suspected nephrolithiasis in adults. *UpToDate*. Retrieved from www.uptodate.com/contents/diagnosis-and-acute-management-of-suspected-nephrolithiasis-in-adults?topicKey=NEPH%2F7366

Dean, R. C., & Lue, T. F. (2005). Physiology of penile erection and pathophysiology of erectile dysfunction. *Urologic Clinics of North America, 32*(4), 379–395, v.

Deem, S. (2015, December 9). Acute bacterial prostatitis. *Medscape*. Retrieved from emedicine.medscape.com/article/2002872-overview

Deters, L. A. (2015 October 12). Benign prostatic hypertrophy. *Medscape*. Retrieved from emedicine.medscape.com/article/437359-overview

DuBeau, C. E. (2013, January 29). Epidemiology, risk factors, and pathogenesis of urinary incontinence. *UpToDate*. Retrieved from www.uptodate.com/contents/epidemiology-risk-factors-and-pathogenesis-of-urinary-incontinecne?topicKey=PC%2F6875

Feldman, A. (2015, March 18). Etiology and evaluation of hematuria in adults. *UpToDate*. Retrieved from http://www.uptodate.com/contents/etiology-and-evaluation-of-hematuria-in-adults

Fulop, T. (2015, August 11). Acute pyelonephritis. *Medscape*. Retrieved from emedicine.medscape.com/article/245559-overview

Gagnadoux, M. (2016, May 31). Evaluation of proteinuria in children. *UpToDate*. Retrieved from www.uptodate.com/contents/evaluation-of-proteinuria-in-children

Gormley, E. A., Lightner, D. J., Burgio, K. L., Chal, T. C., Clemens, J. Q., Culkin, D. J., . . . Vasavada, S. P. (2014, May). Diagnosis and treatment of overactive bladder (non-neurogenic) in adults: AUA/SUFU guideline. *American Urological Association*. Retrieved from www.auanet.org/content/media/OAB_guideline.pdf

Grabe, M., Bjerklund-Johansen, T. E., Botto, H., Cek, M., Naber, K. G., Pickard, R. S., . . . Wullt, B. (2013). Guidelines on urological infections. *European Association of Urology*. Retrieved from www.uroweb.org/guidelines/online-guidelines

Gulati, S. (2016, February 7). Hematuria. *Medscape*. Retrieved from emedicine.medscape.com/article/981898-overview

Hilz, M. (2015). Assessment and treatment of male and female sexual dysfunction. *Journal of the Neurological Sciences, 357*(1), 498–499.

Hooton, T. M. (2016a, January 5). Acute uncomplicated cystitis and pyelonephritis in men. *UpToDate*. Retrieved from http:// www.uptodate.com/contents/acute-uncomplicated-cystitis-and-pyelonephritis-in-men

Hooton, T. M. (2016b, February 9). Acute complicated cystitis and pyelonephritis. *UpToDate. Retrieved from* http://www.uptodate.com/contents/acute-complicated-cystitis-and-pyelonephritis

Hooton, T. M., & Gupta, K. (2016, May 26). Acute uncomplicated cystitisandpyelonephritisinwomen. *UpToDate*. Retrieved from www.uptodate.com/contents/acute-uncomplicated-cystitis-and-pyelonephritis-in-women?topicKey=ID%2F8063

Inker, L. A., Astor, B. C., Fox, C. H., Isakova, T., Lash, J. P., Peralta, C. A., . . . Feldman, H. I. (2014). KDOQI U.S. commentary on the 2012 KDIGO clinical practice guideline for the evaluation and management of CKD. *American Journal of Kidney Disease, 63*(5), 713–735. doi:10.1053/j.ajkd.2014.01.416

International Society for Sexual Medicine. (2015, January). ISSM patient information sheet on premature ejaculation. Retrieved from http://www.issm.info/images/uploads/ISSM_Patient_Information_Sheet_on_PE_-_website_JAN_2015.pdf

Johnson, E. (2015, May 6). Urinary tract infections in pregnancy. *Medscape*. Retrieved from http://emedicine.medscape.com/article/452604-overview

Kidney Disease Improving Global Outcomes. (2012). KDOQI 2012 clinical practice guideline for the evaluation and management of chronic kidney disease. Retrieved from http://kdigo.org/home/guidelines/ckd-evaluation-management

Kim, E. D. (2013b February 4). History taking in the erectile dysfunction patient. *Medscape*. Retrieved from http://emedicine.medscape.com/article/1980342-overview

Kim, E. D. (2015, October 12). Erectile dysfunction treatment & management. *Medscape*. Retrieved from http://emedicine.medscape.com/article/444220-treatment

Lane, J. (2016, May 16). Pediatric nephrotic syndrome. *Medscape*. Retrieved from emedicine.medscape.com/article/982920-overview

Lee, S. L. (2015, December 8). Hydrocele. *Medscape*. Retrieved from emedicine.medscape.com/article/438724-overview

Lerma, E. V. (2015, December 10). Proteinuria. *Medscape*. Retrieved from emedicine.medscape.com/article/238158-overview

McCabe, M. P., & Connaughton, C. (2014). Psychosocial factors associated with male sexual difficulties. *Journal of Sex Research, 51*(1), 31–42.

National Kidney and Urologic Diseases Information Clearinghouse, National Institutes of Health. Kidney disease. Retrieved from https://www.niddk.nih.gov/health-information/kidney-disease

National Kidney Disease Education Program. (n.d.-a). Glomerular filtration rate (GFR) calculators. Retrieved from https://www.niddk.nih.gov/healthinformation/healthcommunicationprograms/nkdep/lab-evaluation/gfr-calculators/Pages/gfrcalculators.aspx

National Kidney Disease Education Program. (n.d.-b). Manage patients with CKD. Retrieved from https://www.niddk.nih.gov/health-information/health-communication-programs/nkdep/identify-manage/manage-patients/Pages/manage-patients.aspx

National Kidney Foundation. (2012). KDOQI clinical practice guidelines for chronic kidney disease: Evaluation, classification, and stratification. Retrieved from https://www.kidney.org/professionals/guidelines/guidelines_commentaries/chronic-kidney-disease-classification

National Kidney Foundation. (2015). KDOQI clinical practice guideline for hemodialysis adequacy 2015 update. *American Journal of Kidney Disease, 66*(5), 884–930. doi:10.1053/j.ajkd.2015.07.015 Retrieved from www.kidney.org/professionals/guidelines/hemodialysis2015

Nepple, K. G., & Cooper, C. S. (2015, June 19). Etiology and clinical features of bladder dysfunction in children. *UpToDate*. Retrieved from www.uptodate.com/contents/etiology-and-clinical-features-of-bladder-dysfuntion-in-children?topicKey=PEDS%2F6580

Ogunyemi, O. (2015, December 11). Testicular torsion. *Medscape*. Retrieved from http://emedicine.medscape.com/article/2036003-overview

Paco, J. S., & Pereira, B. J. (2016). New therapeutic perspectives in premature ejaculation. *Urology, 88*, 87–92.

Patel, N. D., & Parsons, J. K. (2014). Epidemiology and etiology of benign prostatic hyperplasia and bladder outlet obstruction. *Indian Journal of Urology, 30*(2), 170–176.

Patolia, S. (2015, January 9). Cystitis empiric therapy. *Medscape*. Retrieved from http://emedicine.medscape.com/article/1976451-overview#a1

Preminger, G. M., & Curhan, G. C. (2015, October 21). Nephrolithiasis during pregnancy. *UpToDate*. Retrieved from www.uptodate.com/contents/nephrolithiasis-during-pregnancy?topicKey=NEPH%2F7370

Rajfer, J., Valeriano, J., & Sinow, R. (2013). Early onset erectile dysfunction is usually not associated with abnormal cavernosal arterial inflow. *International Journal of Impotence Research, 25*(6), 217–220.

Rovin, B. (2014, September 14). Assessment of urinary protein excretion and evaluation of isolated non-nephrotic proteinuria in adults. *UpToDate*. Retrieved from www.uptodate.com/contents/assessment-of-urinary-protein-excretion-and-evaluation-of-isolated-non-nephrotic-proteinuria-in-adults

Rovito, M. J., Cavayero, C., Leone, J. E., & Harlin, S. (2015). Interventions promoting testicular self-examination (TSE) performance: A systematic review. *American Journal of Men's Health, 9*(6), 506–518.

Rovner, E. S. (2015, December 9). Interstitial cystitis. *Medscape*. Retrieved from emedicine.medscape.com/article/2055505-overview

Sachdeva, K. (2016, June 3). Testicular cancer. *Medscape*. Retrieved from emedicine.medscape.com/article/279007-overview

Sharp, V. J., Barnes, K. T., & Erickson, B. A. (2013). Assessment of asymptomatic microscopic hematuria in adults. *American Family Physician, 88*(11), 747–754.

Smith, J., & Stapleton, F. B. (2015, June 9). Clinical features and diagnosis of nephrolithiasis in children. *UpToDate*. Retrieved from www.uptodate.com/contents/clinical-features-and-diagnosis-of-nephrolithiasis-in-children?topicKey=PEDS%2F6123

Steiber, A. L. (2014). Chronic kidney disease: Considerations for nutrition interventions. *Journal of Parenteral and Enteral Nutrition, 38*(4), 418–426.

Thadhani, R. (2015, November 30). Proteinuria in pregnancy: Evaluation and management. *UpToDate*. Retrieved from www.uptodate.com/contents/proteinuria-in-pregnancy-evaluation-and-management

The Clinical Advisor. (2013, February 6). Kidney guide features albuminuria testing. Retrieved from www.clinicaladvisor.com/kidney-guide-features-albuminuria-testing/article/279307

The Testicular Cancer Resource Center. (2012, December 5). How to do a testicular self examination. Retrieved from http://tcrc.acor.org/tcexam.html

Turek, P. J. (2016, February 11). Prostatitis. *Medscape*. Retrieved from emedicine.medscape.com/article/785418-overview

Urology Care Foundation. (2016a). ED: Non-surgical management (erectile dysfunction). Retrieved from http://www.urologyhealth.org/urology/index.cfm?article=60

Urology Care Foundation. (2016b). ED: Surgical management (erectile dysfunction). Retrieved from http://www.urologyhealth.org/urology/index.cfm?article=28

Vasavada, S. (2015, October 27). Urinary incontinence. *Medscape*. Retrieved from emedicine.medscape.com/article/452289- overview

Walsh, T. J., Hotaling, J. M., Smith, A., Saigal, C., & Wessells, H. (2014). Men with diabetes may require more aggressive treatment for erectile dysfunction. *International Journal of Impotence Research, 26*(3), 112–115.

Wayment, R. O. (2015, April 17). Pregnancy and urolithiasis. *Medscape*. Retrieved from emedicine.medscape.com/article/455830-overview.

Weinberg, A. E., Eisenberg, M., Patel, C. J., Chertow, G. M., & Leppert, J. T. (2013). Diabetes severity, metabolic syndrome, and the risk of erectile dysfunction. *Journal of Sexual Medicine, 10*(12), 3102–3109.

White, W. M. (2015, December 3). Varicocele. *Medscape*. Retrieved from emedicine.medscape.com/article/438591-overview

Wolfe, J. S. (2013a, February 11). Nephrolithiasis. *Medscape*. Retrieved from emedicine.medscape.com/article/437096-overview

Wolfe, J. S. (2013b, February 11). Nephrolithiasis treatment & management. *Medscape*. Retrieved from emedicine.medscape.com/article/437096-treatment

Zaccardi, J. E. (2013, January 16). Managing UTIs in women. *Clinical Advisor*. Retrieved from http://www.clinicaladvisor.com/features/managing-utis-in-women/article/276373/2

13 Obstetrics Guidelines

ANTEPARTUM

Preconception Counseling: Identifying Patients at Risk

Jill C. Cash and Susan Drummond

A woman's health before conception influences her ability not only to conceive, but also to maintain pregnancy and to achieve a healthy outcome. Some women are unaware that their medical conditions, medications, occupational exposure, or social practices may have negative consequences in the earliest weeks of pregnancy, before the pregnancy test is positive. They do not know that organogenesis begins around 17 days after fertilization. Steps to provide the ideal environment for the developing fetus are most likely to be effective if they precede the traditional initiation of prenatal care.

The goal of preconceptional care is to reduce perinatal mortality and morbidity. Targeting only self-referred women who are planning their next conception or women referred with risk factors can result in a significant number of missed opportunities for primary prevention. Nurses working with women of childbearing age and their families have a responsibility to promote reproductive health during every health encounter. In the United States, the unintended pregnancy rate is nearly 50%; approximately 80% of teen pregnancies are unintended.

The preconception interview is the time to review primary care health issues. Topics of discussion should include status on immunizations; determination of hepatitis status; assessment of rubella immunity; Pap smears; cultures for sexually transmitted diseases (STDs); and reviewing history for chronic diseases, such as diabetes mellitus, hypertension, lupus, and so forth.

When discussing preconception plans, the patient's history, as well as that of her partner, should be evaluated for poor health habits (alcohol, smoking, drug use), exposure to toxic substances (radiation and chemicals), multiple sexual partners (risk of HIV, hepatitis, and sexually transmitted infections [STIs]), and racial or ethnic origin. Preconceptional evaluation should include the following:

A. Maternal age: Preeclampsia occurs at the extreme of ages, insulin-dependent diabetes increases with maternal age, and the risks of Down syndrome and other chromosomal abnormalities increase with age. Advanced maternal age is defined as 35 years of age at delivery. The American College of Obstetricians and Gynecologists (ACOG) recommends counseling on genetic testing options for women of advanced maternal age.

B. Universal carrier screening is available for women who desire to know if they are carriers for an autosomal recessive disorder such as Tay-Sachs disease, sickle cell anemia, or cystic fibrosis. Ideally, this blood test should be done preconceptionally, but it can be performed at any time during the pregnancy. If the screening test is positive, the woman's partner can then be tested.

C. Social issues: Screen every woman for intimate partner violence. Research indicates that most abused women continue to be victimized during pregnancy and that the violence may escalate. Child abuse is also common in homes where there is abuse of adults. This assessment should be done only if the partner is not present. Information should be given to the patient concerning available community, social, and legal resources, and her immediate safety, the safety of her children, and an escape plan should be assessed.

D. Financial issues: Discuss insurance, maternity benefits, work-leave policy, and contingency plans for lost wages because of pregnancy complications with the patient.

E. Environmental and occupational considerations: Routine assessment of hobbies and home and employment environments may identify exposures that have been associated with adverse reproductive consequences that can be minimized in the preconceptual period.

F. Fetal effects are dependent on dose(s) and gestational age at exposure related to the following:

1. Radiation: Fetal effects include microcephaly, mental retardation, eye anomalies, intrauterine growth retardation (IUGR), and visceral malformations. Lead aprons should be used to protect the patient from any radiation exposures.
2. Heavy metals: Mercury exposure is related to brain damage and neuromuscular defects. Lead exposure is related to increased spontaneous abortion, low birth weight, brain damage, and increased premature rupture of membranes (PROM). Cadmium is retained by the fetal liver and kidney and is also associated with fetal craniofacial defects. Nickel is associated with neonatal deaths.

3. Pesticides: Occupations at risk of pesticide exposure include, but are not limited to, the following: Ranch and farm workers (including migrant workers); gardeners (home and professional); groundskeepers; florists; structural pest control workers; hunting and fishing guides; health care workers who deal with contamination; and people employed in pesticide production, mixing, and application. Dioxin is associated with an increased rate of spontaneous abortion, myelomeningocele, and limb defects. The pesticides dichlorodiphenyltrichloroethane (DDT) and dichlorodiphenyldichloroethylene (DDE) are associated with increased abortion, prematurity, low birth weight, and pregnancy-induced hypertension (PIH).

4. Other: Carbon monoxide is associated with increased stillbirths, neurologic deficits, seizures, spasticity, and retarded psychomotor development. Ozone is associated with increased spontaneous abortion and increased structural defects. Anesthetic gases are associated with increased abortion, birth defects, low birth weight, and infertility.

G. Infectious diseases: See Chapter 15, "Sexually Transmitted Infections Guidelines," and Chapter 16, "Infectious Disease Guidelines."

H. Medications: Assess and minimize the risk of exposure to medications by reviewing the patient's use of prescription and nonprescription drugs. Provide the patient with information on the safest choices and the need to avoid drugs associated with fetal risks. Identify all prescription and nonprescription medications taken by the mother and partner to assess for risks to the fetus associated with current medications. Teratogenic defects linked to certain medications may include cleft lip and palate, congenital heart disease, microcephaly, caudal dysplasia, and caudal regression syndrome.

I. Medical problems: Health assessment of potential risk not only to the fetus but also to the woman, should she become pregnant, should be discussed. Care must be taken to identify and counsel all women whose life expectancy could be markedly reduced by pregnancy or whose fetus would have a high likelihood of complications. For example, women with known cardiac problems, epilepsy, transplanted organs, or uncontrolled diabetes and hypertension should be told of the risks associated with pregnancy.

1. Diabetes: Researchers have demonstrated a dose-related response between glycosylated hemoglobin (HgbA1c) during the first trimester of pregnancy and the incidence of congenital defects: The better the glycemic control, the lower the risk of birth defects. The preconceptional plan for diabetes includes the following:

a. Change all patients on oral agents to insulin therapy before pregnancy is attempted.

i. Achieve strict plasma glucose control. The ACOG recommends self-glucose monitoring during pregnancy with the following glucose levels to be met. Goals of blood glucose monitoring during pregnancy:

1) Fasting: Less than or equal to 95 mg/dL

2) Preprandial glucose values less than 100 mg/dL

3) 1-hour postprandial glucose levels less than 140 mg/dL

4) 2-hour postprandial glucose levels less than 120 mg/dL

5) Nighttime glucose levels should not drop below 60 mg/dL. Care should be taken to avoid hypoglycemia during pregnancy.

ii. Reduce the HgbA1c to 6% or less.

iii. Assess the patient for vasculopathy, neuropathy, nephropathy, and retinopathy.

iv. Refer the patient for genetic and nutritional counseling.

v. Enhance the woman's knowledge of diabetes during pregnancy.

J. Nutrition: Dietary evaluation and recommendations of alternatives that may benefit the fetus's development are important components of preconceptional counseling. Evaluation of nutritional status should include assessment of the appropriate weight for the patient's height as well as a discussion of eating habits such as vegetarianism, fasting for religious or personal reasons, eating disorders, and the use of mega vitamins.

K. Obstetric considerations: Preconceptional reproductive history is an important tool for identifying factors that may be amenable to intervention. Review term, preterm, aborted (elective, spontaneous, and therapeutic) pregnancies, as well as a short history on living children. Review the gestational age at delivery of each neonate and any pregnancy and delivery complications. Preterm labor (PTL) has a 30% recurrence risk, and preeclampsia has a 5% to 65% recurrence rate in subsequent pregnancies (Barton & Sibai, 2008). The higher rates are among those with severe features of the disease. In some instances, after preconceptual and genetic counseling, the couple may decide to forego pregnancy or to use assisted reproductive technologies such as donor eggs and/or sperm.

L. Recurrent loss: The workup and counseling for recurrent losses include evaluation for a uterine defect (septal or bicornuate uterus or uterus didelphys), endocrine problem (luteal phase defect or hypothyroidism), chromosomal defect, or presence of antiphospholipid syndrome. Antiphospholipid syndrome is defined as the presence of maternal anticardiolipin antibodies and/or lupus anticoagulant in association with recurrent pregnancy loss, thrombotic events, and/or thrombocytopenia. Approximately 10% of women with unexplained recurrent pregnancy loss test positive for anticardiolipin antibodies and/or lupus anticoagulant. In the nonpregnant patient, thrombosis of a single vessel is the most common complication associated with antiphospholipid syndrome.

M. Lifestyle: Queries regarding a woman's social lifestyle history should seek to identify behaviors and exposures that may compromise reproductive outcome. Although environmental exposures are a frequent concern of couples considering pregnancy, women should be informed that, in general, maternal use of alcohol, tobacco, and other mood-altering drugs is more hazardous for a fetus than most other lifestyle choices.

1. Alcohol: Alcohol is a known teratogen. There is no safe limit of alcohol use during pregnancy. Women should be informed that prenatal alcohol consumption is a preventable cause of birth defects and intellectual disability. Research indicates that as many as 73% of 12- to 34-year-old women expose their fetuses to alcohol at some time during pregnancy.

2. Smoking: Fetal effects of smoking are also related to the dose–response effect. Smoking is associated with an increase in bleeding in pregnancy (abruption and placenta previa), IUGR, preterm birth, low birth weight, stillbirth, respiratory distress in the neonate, and sudden infant death syndrome (SIDS). Counsel the patient on smoking cessation. Suggestions of ways to quit include tapering the use of nicotine (tapering and brand switching to lower tar and nicotine), monitoring smoking behavior, setting a contract to quit smoking, identifying social support or a buddy, and restricting area(s) such as a no-smoking zone. Give the patient positive reinforcement for behavior change and cessation of the use of tobacco.

3. Substance use: If substance exposure is complicated by addiction, structured recovery programs are usually needed to effect behavioral change. Substance use/abuse is teratogenic to the fetus, and cessation of all substances is imperative before, during, and after pregnancy.

N. Exercise: Exercise and recreational activities should be reviewed and discussed relative to safety, including the use of bike helmets, avoiding strenuous exercise, and hyperthermia. The ACOG recommends that maternal heart rate (for pregnant women) not exceed 140 beats per minute (bpm). If the woman is not currently exercising, walking and swimming can be suggested. Heat exposure appears to be teratogenic. Use of saunas or hot tubs and high fevers in the first trimester have been associated with an increased risk of neural tube defects (NTDs).

Preconception counseling helps to identify high-risk patients who need intensive care during pregnancy and delivery, and it identifies women who need referral for medical management, nutritional counseling, genetic counseling, or behavior modification. Prescribe a prenatal vitamin daily for any woman considering pregnancy.

Routine Prenatal Care

Jill C. Cash and Susan Drummond

Initial Prenatal Visit

The initial prenatal visit is a very important visit. A comprehensive health history is obtained; blood is drawn for baseline prenatal laboratory values to be established; and depending on the time, the physical examination may also be performed. Many practitioners have the patient return in 2 weeks to perform the physical examination because of the amount of time needed for the history and collecting blood for laboratory tests. Another variation is to obtain the baseline lab tests (except blood type and Rh factor) after the first trimester (to avoid unnecessary testing in the event the patient should have a miscarriage).

The initial visit is also a time for teaching the pregnant patient (see Exhibit 13.1). Literature and brochures on health promotion (i.e., breast self-examination, dietary recommendations, exercise, and smoking cessation) and information regarding the normal changes, discomforts, and concerns during pregnancy should be provided. The after-hours contact information should also be provided, along with contact information for the labor and delivery. Reassure the patient that as the pregnancy progresses you will answer questions she may have; however, outside resources may also be beneficial for the patient and her family. Encourage the patient to enroll in childbirth education, sibling classes (if applicable), breastfeeding classes, and any other classes of interest to her and her partner.

Important information to cover is the patient's medical and surgical history (including previous obstetric history), family genetic history, psychiatric disorders, contraception history, medications taken since the last menstrual period, menstrual history, social habits (smoking, substance abuse, alcohol), environmental exposures (job, hobbies, etc.), exposure to abuse (mental, physical, sexual), and sources of social support and health promotion (immunizations up to date, etc.).

Laboratory tests that are ordered at the initial examination include the following: Complete blood count (CBC), rubella titer, HIV (with the patient's consent), syphilis (rapid plasma reagin [RPR] or Venereal Disease Research Laboratory [VDRL]), hepatitis B surface antigen, blood type and Rh factor, antibody screen, tuberculosis testing, urine culture and sensitivity, and bacterial vaginosis screen.

Optional tests include HgbA1c, sickle cell screening, thyroid profile, and hepatitis C. Other tests performed with the physical examination include Pap smear and cultures for chlamydia and gonorrhea. Additional tests may be ordered throughout the pregnancy:

A. 15 to 20 weeks gestation: Maternal serum multiple marker screening (quad screen; optional test per patient wishes and father of baby and other family history)

B. 18 to 20 weeks gestation: Obstetric ultrasonography

C. 24 to 28 weeks gestation: Screen all women for gestational diabetes by performing the 1-hour Glucola test, by patient history, or clinical risk factors. Diagnosis of gestational diabetes is determined by the results of the 100-g, 3-hour oral glucose tolerance test (GTT). A positive diagnosis requires two or more of the diagnostic criteria for the 100-g, 3-hour tolerance test for gestational diabetes mellitus (GDM) be met (ACOG, 2013a).

D. 35 to 37 weeks gestation: Vaginal culture for Group B *Streptococcus* infection. American Academy of Pediatrics recommends universal screening for Group B *Streptococcus* infection at 36 weeks gestation.

Neural Tube Defects

In about 90% of cases, NTDs are not expected on the basis of past history. NTDs are associated with multifactorial causes, including environmental factors, undernutrition

EXHIBIT 13.1 **Routine Prenatal Patient Education Topics**

TOPIC	DATES
Prenatal care in your practice: (office visits, blood tests/prenatal handouts)	
Diet/nutrition/weight gain	
Enrolled in WIC program	
Substance use (alcohol, smoking, drugs)	
Domestic violence (history, type of injuries)	
OTC medication use	
Activity: Work and exercise	
Travel	
Clothing	
Personal hygiene	
Cats	
Sexual activity	
Physiological changes during pregnancy	
Fetal development	
Father's role during pregnancy	
Common discomforts/treatments	
Symptoms to report immediately	
Fetal kick counts	
Prenatal classes	
Breastfeeding/bottle feeding	
Circumcision	
Infant supply preparation	
Safety/car safety	
Preparing for delivery	
When to come to the hospital	
Labor and delivery expectations	
Postpartum care	
First days with baby	
Postpartum birth control	
TESTS	
Quad screen; noninvasive prenatal screening	
1-hour DM screen	
Ultrasonography	
Glucose tolerance test if applicable	
Amniocentesis/CVS if applicable	
Group B strep	
Fetal monitoring: Kick counts: ________________	
NST: ________________ BPP: ________________	
(Content discussed can be found in patient handout provided to patient at first prenatal visit.)	

BPP, biophysical profile; CVS, chorionic villus sampling; DM, diabetes mellitus; NST, nonstress test; OTC, over-the-counter; WIC, Women, Infants, and Children.

(lack of folic acid), chromosomal defects, maternal hyperthermia, diabetes, clomiphene citrate (Clomid) induction, and maternal obesity.

In 1996, the Food and Drug Administration (FDA) approved a population-based strategy, effective January 1998, to fortify grain food sources with folic acid. The recurrence risk of NTD is 15% without the use of preconceptional doses of folic acid. Even with the FDA strategy, folic acid supplement of 0.4 mg (400 mcg) per day at least 1 month before conception and during the first trimester of pregnancy is recommended. Women who have had a child with an NTD require higher doses of folic acid, 4 mg daily.

Genetic Screening

Genetic screening is recommended for all women. Genetic counseling for discussion of testing options is recommended if the mother is 35 years or older at the time of delivery, or if she has a family history of any abnormal genetic disorders such as Down's syndrome. The parents choose whether they would like to have genetic testing performed to evaluate the fetus for abnormal chromosomes. The following tests can be performed for genetic screening:

A. Chorionic villus sampling (CVS): Performed at 10 to 12 weeks gestation
B. Amniocentesis: Performed at 15 to 18 weeks gestation
C. Amniocentesis can also be performed to assess for spinal cord defects. The amniocentesis can detect elevated protein levels (alpha-fetoprotein and the presence of acetylcholinesterase) in the amniotic fluid that is present in the event of a spinal cord defect. Therefore, if performing an amniocentesis, information regarding genetic makeup and spinal cord defects can both be determined during the single procedure of the amniocentesis.
D. Noninvasive prenatal screening: Cell-free DNA from the fetus is found in maternal serum and can lead to prenatal identification of pregnancies at high risk of trisomy 13, 18, and 21, as well as detect gender. This screen is a maternal blood test and can be done as early as 10 weeks. A positive screen should be confirmed with a diagnostic test such as CVS or amniocentesis.

Routine Prenatal Visits

The routine schedule of appointments includes a visit every 4 weeks until 28 weeks gestation, every 2 weeks until 36 weeks gestation, and then weekly until delivery.

A. Each visit should document
 1. Weight
 2. Blood pressure (BP)
 3. Fundal height, fetal heart tones, and fetal movement (should be detected by the patient by 20 weeks)
 4. Urine: Protein and glucose
B. Each visit should evaluate and discuss possible problems of pregnancy, such as PTL, vaginal bleeding, and so on. A few questions to ask at each visit include the following:
 1. Have you had any blurred vision, spots before your eyes, or epigastric pain?
 2. Have you had any headaches? If so, evaluate and note source of relief.
 3. Have you had any nausea or vomiting? If so, note source of relief.
 4. Have you had any abdominal pain, contractions, backache, pelvic pressure, or other pain?
 5. Have you had any vaginal bleeding, discharge, or leakage of fluid?
 6. Evaluate fetal movement, noting when movement was first felt (quickening) and daily fetal movement.
 7. Evaluate social support at home and in the work environment.
 8. Assess for substance use/abuse. If the patient smokes, ask about current habits. Teach the patient the effects of smoking on herself and the fetus (bleeding, IUGR, increased risk of miscarriage), and encourage smoking cessation.
 9. Assess nutrition and dietary intake of recommended calories during pregnancy.
 10. Ask the patient about her routine exercise program and tolerance of increased exercise during pregnancy.

Anemia, Iron Deficiency

Jill C. Cash and Susan Drummond

Definition

A. Anemia in pregnancy results from decreased serum iron. The iron-binding capacity is increased. Red blood cells (RBCs) are microcytic and hypochromic. The Centers for Disease Control and Prevention (CDC) and the American College of Obstetricians and Gynecologists (ACOG) define first- and third-trimester anemia as a hemoglobin (Hgb) of less than 11.0 g/dL, hematocrit (Hct) of less than 33%, and second trimester anemia as an Hgb of less than 10.5 g/dL, Hct of less than 32%.

Incidence

A. Anemia is a common medical complication of pregnancy. Iron-deficiency anemia constitutes 75% to 95% of pregnancy-related anemias.

Pathogenesis

A. Increased demand for iron during pregnancy occurs because of increased maternal blood volume. Hgb and Hct decrease during the first and second trimesters because of a greater expansion of plasma volume relative to the increase in RBC mass and usually increase during the third trimester when plasma expansion has ceased.
B. Another 0.5 to 1.0 mg/d of iron is needed for lactation. During most pregnancies, diet alone does not provide the necessary iron.

Predisposing Factors

A. Failure to take oral iron; often because of inability to tolerate oral iron supplements
B. Multiple gestation increases iron requirement and may contribute to increased blood loss at delivery
C. Diet high in phosphorus or foods such as tea, coffee, milk, or soy
D. Low iron and low-protein diet, eating nonfood items (pica)
E. Not eating foods that help with absorption of iron (orange juice, broccoli, strawberries)
F. History of gastrointestinal surgery may cause iron malabsorption (i.e., gastrectomy)
G. Chronic bleeding during pregnancy (i.e., placenta previa, marginal sinus separation of placenta, hemorrhoidal bleeding)
H. Short intervals between pregnancies
I. Race: Non-Hispanic Black females
J. Age: Teenage girls

Common Complaints

A. Tiredness
B. Inability to take prenatal vitamins because of nausea
C. Bleeding problems (see "Predisposing Factors" in this section)
D. Pica

Other Signs and Symptoms

A. Fatigue
B. Pale mucous membranes and skin
C. Tachycardia

Subjective Data

A. Elicit the onset, duration, and course of presenting symptoms.
B. Elicit information about the patient's "typical" dietary intake for meals and snacks, and review pica (eating clay, starch, ice, and other nonnutritive substances).
C. Review the patient's intake of prenatal vitamins and supplemental iron. How often does she take iron? Elicit the reason for skipping the supplemental iron (nausea, constipation), if applicable.
D. Review the patient's history of gastrointestinal surgeries, irritable bowel syndrome (IBS), and Crohn's disease.
E. Review the patient's history for any type of anemia and previous treatment, including blood transfusions.
F. Review pregnancy history for closely spaced pregnancies (two in a calendar year) and multiple gestation.
G. Review the patient's intake of medications for the use of aspirin and other nonsteroidal anti-inflammatory drugs (NSAIDs).

Physical Examination

A. Check pulse and BP: Note postural hypotension and tachycardia.
B. Inspect: General appearance
  1. Inspect the skin, mucous membranes, and conjunctivae for pallor.
  2. Observe the mouth and tongue: Note atrophy of papillae and smooth, beefy red appearance of tongue with anemia.
  3. Note dryness of skin. Inspect texture of nails (brittle, spoon-shaped, concave); inspect the hair for brittleness.
C. Palpate the abdomen for masses; assess fundal height.
D. Auscultate the heart for systolic flow murmurs; auscultate lungs.

Diagnostic Tests

A. Blood work: Hgb/Hct
  1. First trimester: Less than 11 g/dL Hgb or less than 33% Hct
  2. Second trimester: Less than 10.5 g/dL Hgb or less than 32% Hct
  3. Third trimester: Less than 11 g/dL Hgb or less than 33% Hct
B. Peripheral blood smear: Note microcytic and hypochromic RBCs on peripheral smear.
C. Sickle cell screen, if applicable
D. Serum iron: Low with anemia
E. Iron-binding capacity: High iron-binding capacity with anemia
F. Transferrin: Saturation less than 15%
G. Stool for occult blood, if applicable
H. Emesis for presence of blood, if applicable

Differential Diagnoses

A. Iron-deficiency anemia
B. Normal physiological anemia of pregnancy: During normal pregnancy, concentrations of erythrocytes and Hgb usually fall because of the greater increase in plasma volume (increased by 45%) relative to the increase in erythrocyte volume (increased by 25%).
C. Megaloblastic anemia: This condition is commonly associated with iron-deficiency anemia and is rarely seen alone.
D. Hemolytic anemia: Sickle cell anemia, thalassemia, hereditary spherocytosis, and erythrocyte enzyme deficiency
E. Aplastic anemia: Bone marrow failure
F. Hematologic malignancies: Leukemia and lymphoma
G. Clotting factor or other hemostatic deficiencies: von Willebrand's disease, idiopathic thrombocytopenia (ITP), and disseminated intravascular coagulation (DIC)

Plan

A. Do initial evaluation of Hgb and Hct at first prenatal visit; repeat at 24- to 28-week blood draw with diabetes testing.
B. Diet counseling and nutrition consultation: The patient may be eligible for the Women, Infants, and Children (WIC) program, which provides supplemental foods for pregnant women and young children. Ask your local health department for information available in your community.
  1. Advise the patient to take supplemental iron in addition to prenatal vitamins. If she is unable to tolerate prenatal vitamins, suggest a children's chewable vitamin, two tablets daily.
  2. Encourage the patient to continue iron supplementation through the first month postpartum and throughout breastfeeding.
C. Patient teaching: *See Section III: Patient Teaching Guide for this chapter, "Iron-Deficiency Anemia (Pregnancy)."* ◀
D. Pharmaceutical therapy
  1. Prophylaxis: Oral iron supplements are recommended for all gestations with usual dose of 60 mg/d elemental iron, or 325 mg/d ferrous sulfate. Time-release tablets may help, but are more expensive.
  2. Most prenatal vitamins contain supplemental iron. Therefore, if the woman is taking one vitamin daily, she may only need to take two iron tablets. Nausea and vomiting occur in 20% to 25% of patients. These side effects are dose related. Have the patient alter times of administration of the iron supplement to determine when the iron is best tolerated.
  3. Treatment: With iron-deficiency anemia, three times the prophylactic dose of iron should be given, or 325 mg ferrous sulfate three times daily.
  4. Intramuscular (IM) or intravenous (IV) iron may be ordered for the small proportion of patients who do not tolerate oral iron because of gastrointestinal

complaints, malabsorption syndrome, or noncompliance with the oral iron regimen.

Follow-Up

A. Carry out routine prenatal and postpartum follow-up care. When the patient begins taking the recommended dose of supplemental iron, the RBC response can be measured in 2 weeks by an elevation in her reticulocyte count.
B. Repeat Hct after 4 to 6 weeks of therapy.
C. If no improvement is seen in reticulocyte count or Hct after 4 weeks of therapy and the patient has been compliant, another cause of anemia should be investigated.

Consultation/Referral

A. Consider consult with a physician if Hgb is less than 9 g/dL or Hct is less than or equal to 27% and does not improve with the aforementioned treatments.

Gestational Diabetes Mellitus

Jill C. Cash and Susan Drummond

Definition

A. Gestational diabetes mellitus (GDM) is abnormal carbohydrate metabolism diagnosed during pregnancy.

Incidence

A. It is estimated that up to 6% to 7% of pregnancies in the United States are complicated by diabetes mellitus (DM) and approximately 90% of these cases represent women with GDM. It usually resolves after pregnancy.

Pathogenesis

A. Insulin antagonism caused by the placental hormones leads to gestational diabetes. As greater amounts of these hormones are produced with advancing gestation, the diabetogenic effect of pregnancy becomes more pronounced, reaching significant levels in the second trimester. Women with GDM are at risk of later development of type 1 and, more commonly, type 2 diabetes. GDM may actually be the expression of pregnancy-induced stresses on carbohydrate metabolism in the genetically predisposed patient. It is estimated that up to 50% of women with GDM will develop DM within approximately 25 years of the pregnancy. Some women have undiagnosed type 2 diabete before pregnancy.

Predisposing Factors

A. Members of any of the following ethnic groups:
  1. Hispanic American
  2. African American
  3. Native American
  4. South or East Asian
  5. Pacific Islander
B. Maternal age greater than 25 years
C. Obesity (body mass index [BMI]) >30)
D. Family history of diabetes
E. Previous birth of a macrosomic, malformed, or stillborn baby
F. Hypertension
G. Glycosuria at first prenatal visit
H. Gestational diabetes in a previous pregnancy

Common Complaints

A. Common complaints of hyperglycemia include polydipsia, polyuria, fatigue, and blurred vision. However, gestational diabetes is often asymptomatic.

Other Signs and Symptoms

A. Glycosuria
B. Increased thirst
C. Increased urination
D. Size of fetus greater than average for gestational age
E. Frequent candidal infections
F. Rapid weight gain

Potential Complications

A. Ketoacidosis
  1. May develop in GDM
  2. More common in insulin-dependent diabetes
  3. May develop with glucose levels as low as 200 mg/dL
  4. May be present in an undiagnosed diabetic woman receiving beta-mimetic agents (such as terbutaline) for tocolysis or steroids to enhance fetal lung maturity. **Fetal mortality rate is 10% in women who come to the hospital in diabetic ketoacidosis (DKA). Glucose and ketones cross the placenta.**
  5. Therapy hinges on timely, aggressive volume resuscitation and correction of maternal metabolic derangements.
B. Polyhydramnios
C. Increased risk of neonatal morbidity, such as hypoglycemia, hyperbilirubinemia, polycythemia, respiratory distress, because of delayed lung maturity, and/or traumatic birth injury related to shoulder dystocia, which is associated with macrosomia.
D. Increased risk for stillbirth—risk is related primarily to poor glycemic control.

Subjective Data

A. Review previous pregnancy history for two or more spontaneous abortions, previous stillbirths, or unexplained neonatal deaths.
B. Review birth weight (macrosomia) and gestational age of previous children.
C. Review previous pregnancy history for polyhydramnios and/or congenital anomalies.
D. Review the patient's history for a predisposition to infections, especially urinary tract infections (UTIs) and candidal vaginitis and for family history of diabetes.
E. Review previous pregnancy history for gestational diabetes, diet restrictions, and need for insulin therapy.

Physical Examination

A. Check blood pressure (BP), pulse, and weight.
B. Inspect: Perform speculum examination for wet prep, if indicated.
C. Palpate: Check the patient's fundal height each visit after 20 weeks.
D. Auscultate fetal heart tones after 10 to 12 weeks gestation.

Screening/Diagnostic Tests

Women who have risk factors for type 2 diabetes should be screned at the initial prenatal visit.

A. Perform "one-step" 2-hour 75 g (fasting) OGTT or "two-step" 1-hour 50 g (nonfasting) followed by a 3-hour 100 g (fasting) OGTT for positive results.

B. Day curves (fasting blood sugar [FBS] and pre- and postprandial blood glucose testing)

C. Glycosylated hemoglobin (HgbA1c)

D. Urine dipstick for glucose: Early glycosuria needs further evaluation (i.e., HgbA1c, urine culture, random glucose "finger stick")

E. Ultrasonography if fetal size is greater than average for gestational date to rule out twins, congenital anomaly such as atresia, and polyhydramnios.

Differential Diagnoses

A. Gestational diabetes
- **1.** DM (type 1)
- **2.** DM (type 2)

Plan

A. General interventions

1. The American Diabetes Association (ADA) recommends that all pregnant women be screened.

a. Diabetes mellitus screen (DMS): "Two-step" 1-hour 50-g (nonfasting) oral GTT followed by a 3-hour 100-g oral glucose tolerance test (OGTT) for positive results

i. Administer 50-g oral glucose load (fasting not required).

ii. Draw blood for glucose assessment 1 hour after glucose load is given.

iii. Typically performed between 24 and 28 weeks gestation; performed earlier if the patient has glycosuria, risk factors, advanced maternal age, or if fetal size is greater than average for gestational date by fundal height measurement.

iv. Abnormal result is a glucose level of 130 to 140 mg/dL (use your institutional limits).

v. Follow up all abnormal results with a 3-hour GTT; if DMS is greater than 200 mg/dL, the patient may skip GTT and begin dietary modifications and glucose evaluation for insulin needs.

b. Three-hour GTT

i. Draw fasting blood glucose first.

ii. Administer 100-g glucose load.

iii. Draw blood for glucose assessment 1 hour, 2 hours, and 3 hours after glucose load is given.

iv. Plasma or serum glucose results

1) Fasting = 95 mg/dL

2) 1 hour = 180 mg/dL

3) 2 hours = 155 mg/dL

4) 3 hours = 140 mg/dL

v. If two or more values of 3-hour GTT are elevated:

1) Refer the patient for nutritional counseling. Once the patient is on the ADA diet, begin testing her weekly for fasting and 2-hour postprandial blood glucose measurements.

c. "One-step" 2-hour 75-mg OGTT may be performed instead of the "two-step" approach.

2. Antepartum testing

a. For women with well-controlled GDM, there is no national consensus with respect to criteria for initiation and timing of testing. Options include weekly or twice-weekly testing with either the nonstress test (NST) or biophysical profile (BPP) beginning at 32 to 34 weeks.

b. For women with insulin-dependent gestational diabetes or whose condition is *not* well controlled, manage as if the patient had pregestational diabetes. Administer twice weekly testing with either the NST or BPP beginning by 32 weeks. If a patient's diabetes is poorly controlled, consider fetal assessment earlier and more frequently.

3. Serial ultrasonography

a. Evaluate fetal growth, estimate fetal weight, and detect polyhydramnios and malformations.

b. Repeat at 4- to 6-week intervals to assess growth.

c. Macrosomia is a leading risk factor for shoulder dystocia at vaginal delivery and cephalopelvic disproportion. Women with GDM should be counseled regarding the option of a scheduled cesarean delivery when the estimated fetal weight (EFW) is greater than or equal to 4,500 g.

4. Postpartum contraception

a. Low-dose oral contraceptives (OCs) may be used in women with GDM who do not have other risk factors.

b. Rate of subsequent diabetes in OC users is not significantly different from those who do not use OCs.

c. Consider serial measurement of total cholesterol, low-density lipoprotein, high-density lipoprotein, and triglycerides.

5. Notify nursery staff of perinatal diabetes history, especially if the patient has a history of insulin-dependent diabetes, so that the neonate can be carefully monitored for hypoglycemia.

B. Patient teaching: GDM requires intensive patient and family education to help reduce perinatal complications.

1. Exercise

a. If the patient had an active lifestyle before pregnancy, encourage her to continue a program of exercise approved for pregnancy such as walking or swimming for 20 minutes per day.

b. Upper extremity exercise in previously sedentary women with GDM may improve glycemic control.

2. Instruct the patient in self-monitoring blood glucose.

a. Have her take measurement pre- or postprandially, or both. Preprandial values are typically taken if on insulin. Fasting and postprandial values may be taken if the patient is diet-controlled. FBS should be less than 95 mg/dL. Postprandial values should be less than 140 mg/L 1 hour postprandial and less than 120 mg/L at 2 hours postprandial. The HgbA1c goal is less than 6%. Nighttime levels should not decrease lower than 60 mg/dL.

b. If the patient is taking multiple doses of insulin, she may need to take measurements more frequently.

3. *See Section III: Patient Teaching Guides for this chapter, "Gestational Diabetes" and "Insulin Therapy During Pregnancy."*

C. Dietary management: Place the patient on a diet that is prescribed for preexisting diabetes in pregnancy, such as the ADA diet, in the following amounts:

1. Current weight less than 80% ideal body weight (IBW): 35 to 40 kcal/kg/d
2. Current weight 80% to 120% IBW: 30 kcal/kg/d
3. Current weight 120% to 150% IBW: 24 kcal/kg/d
4. Current weight greater than 150% IBW: 12 to 15 kcal/kg/d
5. Dietary consumption 40% to 50% carbohydrate, 20% protein, 30% to 40% fat

D. Pharmaceutical therapy

1. Insulin therapy is recommended if dietary management does not consistently maintain fasting glucose levels of less than 95 mg/dL. Two-hour postprandial values should be less than 120 mg/dL.
2. Oral antidiabetic medications (glyburide and metformin) are being used in women with GDM, although they are not yet approved by the FDA for this indication. Glyburide results in increased insulin secretion and insulin sensitivity at the tissue level. Metformin inhibits hepatic gluconeogenesis and glucose absorption and stimulates glucose uptake in peripheral tissues.
3. In general, insulin therapy in pregnancy is no different from vigorous management of diabetes with insulin in nonpregnant women. Insulin does not cross the placenta.
4. Therapy must respond to the changing insulin requirements during pregnancy; typical starting dosage is 0.7 to 1.0 units/kg/d in divided doses. Women with relatively simple insulin programs when not pregnant may require more complex regimens as the pregnancy progresses.
5. Intensive insulin therapy (as opposed to conventional therapy) is often required in pregnancy
6. Human insulin (Humulin) is preferred to animal or synthetic insulin.
7. Instruct the patient to report glucose values by telephone on at least a weekly basis. Some monitors have a USB port for uploading to a computer where they may be viewed on a website or e-mailed to the provider. Alternatively, patients may opt to fax or telephone in their values.
8. The blood glucose values should be evaluated at least weekly to adjust to the patient's changing needs (see Figure 13.1).

Follow-Up

A. Weekly evaluation of day curves

B. Fetal testing schedule

C. For women who develop diabetes during pregnancy, give the patient a 75-g glucose load to evaluate for the development of type 2 diabetes at the return postpartum visit at 6 weeks after delivery. These women should be screened at least every 3 years from then on. Encourage lifestyle changes to prevent the development of diabetes.

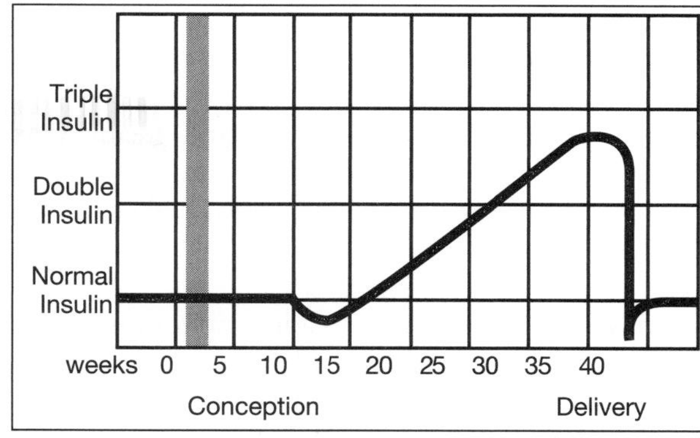

FIGURE 13.1 Insulin requirement during pregnancy.

Consultation/Referral

A. Consult or comanage the patient with a physician as indicated and if GDM is not controlled by diet and exercise.

B. Refer to a dietitian for nutritional consult for carbohydrate counting and to teach the patient dietary and lifestyle changes needed for tight glucose control.

Preeclampsia

Jill C. Cash and Susan Drummond

Definition

Preeclampsia (antiquated term *toxemia*) is hypertension with proteinuria that develops during pregnancy and lasts or develops up to 6 weeks postpartum. In the absence of proteinuria, any of the following can establish the diagnosis: new-onset thrombocytopenia, impaired liver function, renal insufficiency, pulmonary edema, or visual or cerebral disturbances.

Hypertension is defined as the following:

A. Either a systolic BP greater than 140 mmHg or a diastolic BP greater than 90 mmHg or both. The values must be elevated on at least two separate occasions at least 4 hours apart. Severity of hypertension is not necessarily associated with the severity of preeclampsia.

B. Eclampsia, or the occurrence of grand mal seizures, in a patient with preeclampsia.

C. Chronic hypertension in pregnancy is often complicated by superimposed preeclampsia.

Incidence

A. Hypertensive disorders are the most common medical complication of pregnancy, with a reported incidence of up to 10% worldwide. Incidence varies among different regions and countries. The incidence of preeclampsia has increased by 25% in the United States during the past two decades. The risk of recurrent preeclampsia is between 5% and 70%. Women who develop severe features of preeclampsia before 30 weeks gestation have the highest risk of preeclampsia in future pregnancies.

Pathogenesis

A. The etiology of preeclampsia is unknown, although several theories exist. Generalized vascular endothelial damage is a hallmark of the pathophysiologic responses.

Predisposing Factors

A. Nulliparity
B. Chronic hypertension
C. Age extremes (less than 18 years and greater than 35 years)
D. Race (African American women are at higher risk)
E. Diabetes mellitus
F. Renal disease
G. Family history of preeclampsia in a sister or mother
H. Previous pregnancy with preeclampsia
I. Multiple gestation
J. Hydatidiform mole
K. Obesity

Common Complaints

A. Headache unrelieved by analgesics
B. Right upper quadrant (RUQ) pain
C. Severe heartburn unrelieved by antacids
D. Nausea and vomiting
E. Edema: Peripheral and/or facial
F. Visual disturbances
G. Photophobia

Other Signs and Symptoms

A. Hypertension (BP of 140 mmHg systolic or greater or 90 mmHg diastolic or greater that occurs after 20 weeks gestation in a woman without a previous history of hypertension)

> *First-trimester signs of preeclampsia need ultrasonographic evaluation for the presence of a gestational trophoblastic disease (molar pregnancy) as well as the other differential diagnoses.*

B. Proteinuria: Urinary excretion of 0.3 g protein or greater in 24-hour urine specimen
C. Brisk deep tendon reflexes (DTRs) or clonus

Potential Complications

A. Multiple organ involvement
B. HELLP syndrome (hemolysis, elevated liver enzymes, and low platelets)
C. Eclampsia, which may lead to maternal demise
D. Fetal complications: Intrauterine growth retardation (IUGR), oligohydramnios, abruptio placenta

Subjective Data

A. Elicit information about headaches, their onset and duration, the progression of headache, and/or other symptoms.
B. What part of the head hurts? Differentiate headache from sinus headache. Note severity and any relief measure tried (acetaminophen, massage, sleep).
C. Is the headache "new"? Does the patient have a previous history of migraines? Is this like a previous migraine?
D. What are other concurrent symptoms: Nausea, vomiting, RUQ pain, and visual changes?
E. Question the patient about edema. If edema is present, has it significantly worsened over the past few days? Has she been able to wear rings up to this point? Has she had to wear different shoes because of pedal edema?
F. What are the patient's usual weight and today's weight (on the same scales)? Has she gained more than 2 pounds in 1 week?
G. Ask specifics about RUQ pain, sometimes identified as "severe heartburn." Note the duration, severity, and relief measures tried. Have the patient point to the area of discomfort (midsternum or under right breast).
H. Are there any visual disturbances, such as black dots she can't see through?
I. Review other gastrointestinal symptoms such as diarrhea, abdominal pain, and gallbladder attack.
J. Review for signs of fever and thyroid storm.
K. Review the patient's history for seizures.

Physical Examination

A. Check temperature, BP, pulse and respirations, weight, and fetal heart tones.
B. Inspect
  1. Check pedal, hand, and facial edema.
  2. Check fundal height.
C. Palpate
  1. The abdomen, noting any hepatosplenomegaly and RUQ tenderness to the palpation
  2. The lower extremities for pitting edema
D. Percuss
  1. Gently check for liver enlargement.
  2. Perform neurologic examination for hyperreflexia: Check DTR and clonus.
E. Auscultate
  1. The heart and lungs
  2. The fetal heart tone

Diagnostic Tests

A. Complete blood count (CBC) and platelets
B. Liver profile (alanine aminotransferase [ALT] and aspartate aminotransferase [AST])
C. Renal workup
  1. Uric acid, serum creatinine, and urine protein
  2. Urine culture if proteinuria is present to rule out urinary tract infection (UTI)
  3. Collect 24-hour urine for total protein and creatinine clearance.
D. Ultrasonography, if indicated, to rule out IUGR and/or oligohydramnios

Differential Diagnoses

A. Preeclampsia
B. Hyperemesis gravidarum
C. Infection: Appendicitis, gastroenteritis, pyelonephritis, glomerulonephritis, hepatitis, and pancreatitis
D. Acute fatty liver of pregnancy
E. Systemic lupus erythematosus
F. Hemolytic uremic syndrome
G. Hepatic encephalopathy
H. Gastrointestinal disorder: Peptic ulcer and heartburn
I. Thrombotic or idiopathic thrombocytopenia purpura (ITP)
J. Gallbladder disease

K. Chronic hypertension
L. Thyroid storm
M. Gestational hypertension

Plan

A. General interventions
   1. Any patient with an elevated BP should be reassessed in the lateral recumbent position, using proper cuff size, after the patient is allowed to relax for several minutes before BP measurement.
   2. If the patient's BP begins to rise above baseline values:
      a. Advise the patient to maintain a modified bed rest schedule (stop working).
      b. Recommend frequent BP evaluation at home.
      c. See the patient weekly or biweekly for further maternal and neonatal assessment; administer nonstress test (NST) and take biophysical profile (BPP) if appropriate.
   3. If hypertension and proteinuria are present, refer the patient to an obstetrician or perinatologist for further assessment and management. She may need immediate admission to the hospital for inpatient management or delivery.
   4. If the patient has a grand mal seizure, the primary consideration is to protect her. Monitor seizure type and duration. Call for immediate transport to the hospital labor and delivery unit. Place the patient in the lateral recumbent position following the seizure.
   5. Immediately transfer the patient to a hospital for eclampsia after stabilization.

B. Patient teaching
   1. Educate the patient regarding her diagnosis and the importance of controlling her BP to prevent complications.
   2. Stress the importance of bed rest and fetal surveillance with NST or BPP to closely monitor the patient and her fetus to reach the goal of a safe, healthy delivery.
   3. Discuss dietary recommendations for pregnancy. Salt restriction does not stop swelling and high BP problems in pregnancy.

C. Pharmaceutical therapy
   1. Diuretics are *not* prescribed during pregnancy for edema.
   2. Angiotensin-converting enzyme (ACE) inhibitors and angiotensin II receptor blockers (ARBs) are not recommended during pregnancy because of the teratogenic effects on the fetus that may occur such as renal dysgenesis and/or fetal death.
   3. Methyldopa is commonly used during pregnancy to control chronic or superimposed hypertension during pregnancy.
   4. Inpatient therapy is determined by a physician and may include:
      a. Magnesium sulfate for seizure prophylaxis
      b. Hydralazine or labetalol are first-line antihypertensive agents if a patient's diastolic BP is greater than 110 mmHg.
      c. Corticosteroids may be given to enhance fetal lung maturity before delivery in patients between 24 and 34 weeks gestation and may be considered in patients between 23 and 24 weeks gestation.
      d. In preeclampsia with severe features, therapy may include cervical ripening agents, such as prostaglandins or misoprostol, and/or oxytocin induction of labor.
      e. Narcotics may be used for severe headaches.
      f. Diazepam (Valium) and phenytoin (Dilantin) are not recommended for seizures in pregnancy. There is increased risk of recurrent seizures.

Follow-Up

A. The only "cure" for preeclampsia is delivery. See the patient in 1 week after delivery for BP assessment, or sooner if symptoms persist.

Consultation/Referral

A. If the patient is diagnosed with preeclampsia, refer her to a physician for continued care and delivery.

Preterm Labor

Jill C. Cash and Susan Drummond

Definition

A. Preterm labor (PTL) is labor that produces documented cervical changes after 20 weeks and before 37 completed weeks of gestation.

Incidence

A. PTL occurs in approximately 11% of live births in the United States and precedes approximately 70% of the preterm births. It accounts for more than 70% of neonatal mortality.

Pathogenesis

A. Infection and ischemia are common causes of PTL. Infection may originate from several sites, including the bladder, kidney(s), cervix, uterus, gastrointestinal tract, and upper respiratory tract. Ischemia may be caused by decreased oxygen delivery to the uterus because of maternal hypoxia, hypovolemia, or vena caval compression. Overdistension of the uterus in the presence of polyhydramnios or multiple gestation may cause PTL symptoms. However, in most cases, the cause is unknown.

Predisposing Factors

A. Previous PTL or preterm delivery
B. Preterm rupture of membranes (PROM)
C. Uterine anomalies, surgery, and fibroids
D. Multiple gestation
E. History of second-trimester abortion(s)
F. Incompetent cervix
G. History of cone biopsy
H. Recurrent urinary tract and kidney infections
I. Polyhydramnios
J. Macrosomic fetus
K. Maternal age extremes
L. Placenta previa
M. Abruptio placentae
N. Poor nutritional status and low prepregnancy weight
O. Maternal dehydration

P. Maternal race (occurs more frequently in African American population)
Q. Low socioeconomic status
R. Inadequate prenatal care
S. Anemia
T. Substance use/abuse (smoking, drug, alcohol)
U. Vaginal infection
V. Presence of fetal fibronectin, a protein produced by the trophoblast and other fetal tissues, has been noted in cervical–vaginal secretions between 24 and 34 weeks gestation in a subgroup of women who are at increased risk for preterm birth.
W. Short cervical length
X. Short interpregnancy interval

Common Complaints

A. Abdominal pain or cramping
B. Low backache
C. Increase or change in vaginal discharge, "gush" of fluid, loss of mucus plug, and bloody show or vaginal spotting
D. Diarrhea
E. "Something's not right"

Other Signs and Symptoms

A. Pelvic pressure
B. Contractions or period-like cramps

Subjective Data

A. Elicit information about the onset, frequency, duration, and course of cramps; presence or absence of backache; how long these symptoms have existed; and whether symptoms began subsequent to a certain event or activity. What, if anything, makes these symptoms better or worse?
B. Question the patient about color, odor, consistency, and amount of vaginal discharge or bleeding: Was there a spot the size of a quarter or a half-dollar? Has she been wearing a perineal pad? How often does she have to change the pad? Is the pad soaked with blood when she changes it?
C. For fetuses older than 18 weeks gestation, question the patient about frequency of fetal movements.
D. Question the patient about urinary frequency and the presence of urgency or dysuria.
E. Question the patient about recent sexual activity (i.e., has there been recent intercourse?).
F. If the patient complains of diarrhea, ask her if she has a fever and if anyone else in the family is ill.

Physical Examination

A. Check temperature, blood pressure (BP), and fetal heart tones.
B. Inspect: Note general appearance of discomfort.
C. Palpate

- **1.** Abdomen: Note presence, frequency, intensity of uterine contractions, and resting tone. Measure fundal height.
- **2.** Back: Check for costovertebral angle (CVA) tenderness.

D. Auscultate the heart and lungs.
E. Sterile speculum examination: Evaluate rupture of membranes and vaginal discharge or bleeding. **If meconium-stained amniotic fluid is noted, immediately consult a physician and transfer the patient to a hospital. Note whether meconium is thin or thick (thick meconium may be associated with breech presentation).**
F. Bimanual examination: If membranes are not ruptured, perform gentle bimanual examination: Note cervical dilation, effacement, station, cervical position, and softness of cervix.
G. Cervical examination during pregnancy: *See Section II: Procedure, "Cervical Evaluation During Pregnancy: Bimanual Examination."* **Do not perform a digital examination of the cervix if PROM is present without active labor.** ◀

Diagnostic Tests

A. White blood cell (WBC), if indicated
B. Urine dipstick for ketones, leukocyte, esterase, protein, and nitrite
C. Evaluate vaginal discharge for pH with phenaphthazine (nitrazine) tape.
D. Check ferning if discharge is nitrazine positive or if PROM is suspected.
E. Wet prep, if indicated
F. Cervical cultures for sexually transmitted diseases (STDs)
G. Cervical and rectal culture for Group B streptococcus
H. Fetal fibronectin, where available. Candidates for fetal fibronectin testing must meet the following criteria:

- **1.** Intact fetal membranes
- **2.** Cervical dilation less than 3 cm
- **3.** Gestational age 22 0/7th weeks to 34 6/7th weeks
- **4.** Nothing in the vagina in the preceding 24 hours

I. Urine culture
J. Ultrasonography: Fetal biometry and dating, cervical length, amniotic fluid volume, biophysical profile (BPP), placental location, fetal presentation, ruling out fetal anomalies
K. Electronic fetal monitoring for contractions

Differential Diagnoses

A. PTL
B. Preterm, or Braxton Hicks, contractions, with no cervical change
C. Incompetent cervix
D. Preterm rupture of membranes
E. Low back muscle strain
F. Pyelonephritis or urinary tract infection (UTI)
G. Placenta previa
H. Abruptio placentae
I. Gastroenteritis
J. Vaginal infection
K. Maternal dehydration
L. Ketoacidosis

Plan

A. General interventions

- **1.** Regular uterine contractions with cervical dilation or effacement, with pressure on the lower uterine segment, strongly indicates PTL.
- **2.** If the cervix is dilated more than 3 cm with contractions upon presentation, the patient is probably

having PTL. Consult with a physician for hospital admission and tocolysis candidacy.

3. If the patient is symptomatic with a positive fetal fibronectin test, consult with a physician for maternal transfer to a hospital equipped to care for preterm infants.

B. Second trimester: If the patient shows signs and symptoms of PTL, consider diagnosis of incompetent cervix. Refer the patient to a physician for ultrasonography for cervical length and possible cerclage placement.

C. Outpatient management

▶ **1.** Education: *See Section III: Patient Teaching Guide for this chapter, "Preterm Labor."*

2. Outpatient bed rest

3. Outpatient tocolysis therapy

4. Frequent cervical examinations, weekly

5. Prophylactic treatment against infection

6. Administer corticosteroids to enhance fetal lung maturity if less than 34 weeks gestation. Observe the patient for contractions in the office or have her use a uterine monitoring system at home.

7. Fetal fibronectin testing, where available, using American College of Obstetricians and Gynecologists (ACOG) Guidelines

D. Inpatient management of PTL

1. Observation, possibly with IV hydration

2. Cervical cerclage

3. Prophylactic treatment against infection (Group B *Streptococcus* until urine and cervical culture results are available

4. Parenteral tocolysis either to stop PTL or delay delivery long enough to allow transfer to a facility with the ability to care for preterm infants. According to numerous clinical studies, predelivery administration of magnesium sulfate reduces the occurrence of cerebral palsy, and therefore, may be the drug of choice for parenteral tocolysis in the hospital setting.

5. Administer corticosteroids to enhance fetal lung maturity if less than 34 weeks.

6. Transport the patient to a perinatal center for neonatal care.

▶ **E.** Patient teaching: *See Section III: Patient Teaching Guide for this chapter, "Preterm Labor."*

F. Pharmaceutical therapy

1. Tocolytics are generally prescribed from 24 to 34 weeks gestation and may be considered between 23 and 24 weeks gestation. Maintenance therapy with tocolytics is generally ineffective, although short-term use is recommended mainly to allow for the administration of antenatal steroids. Recently, the FDA posted warnings cautioning against the use of maintenance oral terbutaline during pregnancy because of lack of efficacy and potential maternal cardiac risks and death; it should not be prescribed on an outpatient basis. Injectable terbulatine may be used on a short-term basis (48–72 hours) in a hospital setting.

2. Corticosteroids

a. Steroids are given to enhance lung maturity in the fetus.

b. A single rescue course may be considered if the antecedent treatment was given more than 2 weeks prior and the patient is judged to be likely to deliver within the next week.

Follow-Up

A. Depending on the clinical scenario, the patient may need to be seen weekly or biweekly. Fetal fibronectin test may be repeated every 2 weeks, but positive results alone should not be used to exclusively direct management. Repeat cultures as indicated, discontinuing antibiotics if cultures are negative. Encourage close phone contact with the patient regarding questions or concerns.

Pyelonephritis in Pregnancy

Jill C. Cash and Susan Drummond

Definition

A. Pyelonephritis is an infection in one or both kidneys, usually involving the entire urinary tract. **Pyelonephritis may evolve into acute respiratory distress syndrome (ARDS) in pregnancy.**

Incidence

A. The incidence of pyelonephritis in pregnancy is 1% to 2%. Most cases develop as a consequence of undiagnosed or inadequately treated lower urinary tract infection (UTI). Approximately 75% to 80% of pyelonephritis cases occur on the right side, with a 10% to 15% incidence on the left side. A small percentage of cases are bilateral.

Pathogenesis

A. *Escherichia coli* is the main pathogen in pyelonephritis, though *Klebsiella pneumoniae* and *Proteus* species are also important causes of infection. Occasionally, highly virulent gram-negative bacilli, such as *Pseudomonas, Enterobacter,* and *Serratia,* are responsible (more commonly noted in immunocompromised patients). Gram-positive Group B *Streptococcus* may also be responsible. Anaerobes are unlikely pathogens in pyelonephritis except in cases of chronic obstruction or instrumentation.

Predisposing Factors

A. Pregnancy: Because of pregnancy-related anatomic changes in the urinary tract such as dilated ureters caused by smooth muscle relaxation and pressure on the bladder from the enlarging uterus; the immunosuppression of pregnancy may also contribute.

B. History of UTI, cystitis, and pyelonephritis

C. Sickle cell disease

Common Complaints

A. Fever

B. Chills

C. Flank pain or tenderness

D. Urinary frequency or urgency

E. Hematuria and dysuria

Other Signs and Symptoms

A. UTI is associated with urinary frequency, urgency, and dysuria; hematuria; and suprapubic pain.

1. Chemical reactions to deodorant or douches can affect urination.
2. Patients with frequent pyelonephritis do *not* complain of frequency and dysuria.

B. Pyelonephritis is associated with fever, palpitations, dizziness, backache, and urinary frequency.

1. Hematuria may be present, especially if the patient has a history of a previous kidney stone.
2. Dysuria is not always present in upper tract infections.

C. Abdominal pain and uterine contractions, risk of preterm labor (PTL) and birth

D. Shortness of breath (SOB)

Potential Complications

A. Sepsis and septic shock

B. ARDS: Mortality rate—50% to 70%

C. Pulmonary embolus, usually presents as sudden-onset costovertebral angle (CVA) tenderness

Subjective Data

A. Elicit information on the onset, duration, and progression of symptoms.

B. Elicit problems with voiding. Ask the patient about urinary frequency, urgency, and dysuria.

C. Ask the patient if she has experienced preterm contractions.

D. Ask if the patient is complaining of fever or chills.

E. Ask the patient if her urine has a bad odor.

F. Ask the patient if she has felt more tired than usual.

G. Ask the patient if she has felt more nauseated than usual or if she has been vomiting.

H. Does patient have a backache? Note location (unilateral or bilateral) and what, if anything, makes the backache better or worse.

I. Review the patient's history for sickle cell disease, if appropriate; has she been tested?

J. Review prenatal history for recurrent UTIs, previous pyelonephritis, and any abnormalities of the genitourinary (GU) tract.

Physical Examination

A. Check temperature, pulse, respirations, and blood pressure (BP): Fever greater than 100.4°F, tachycardia, tachypnea, hypotension are associated with sepsis, septic shock, and ARDS.

B. Inspect: Note general appearance for respiratory distress.

C. Palpate

1. Back: Check CVA tenderness (right CVA tenderness is more common in pregnancy).
2. Abdomen
   a. Palpate for uterine tenderness and contractions.
   b. Palpate for suprapubic tenderness.

D. Auscultate

1. The lungs and heart
2. The fetal heart rate (FHR)

E. Bimanual examination: Check for cervical dilation

Diagnostic Tests

A. CBC with differential or WBC: Leukocytosis with left shift on differential seen

B. Blood culture, if indicated

C. Respiratory function

1. Arterial blood gases (ABGs), if indicated
2. Pulse oximetry, if indicated

D. Renal function

1. Urinalysis
   a. Check urinalysis for white blood cells (WBCs), red blood cells (RBCs), leukocyte esterase, and/or nitrites.
   b. Glucosuria may be normal in pregnancy because of decreased tubular capacity to reabsorb glucose. If it is consistently noted, further testing is needed.
   c. Proteinuria is *not* normal during pregnancy. All cases warrant further investigation.
2. Urine culture and sensitivity: Greater than 100,000 colonies/mL indicates UTI.
3. Intravenous pyelogram (IVP), if indicated
4. Renal ultrasonography, if indicated

Differential Diagnoses

A. Pyelonephritis

B. Cystitis

C. Urethritis

D. Urethral stricture

E. Urolithiasis

F. Genital infection

G. Chorioamnionitis

H. Septic abortion

I. Postpartum endometritis

J. Muscular strain

K. Pulmonary embolus

L. Severe upper respiratory tract infection

M. Postprocedural dysuria or urinary frequency (i.e., following bladder catheterization or cystoscopy)

N. Chemical irritants

O. Postpartum septic pelvic thrombophlebitis

P. Renal calculi

Plan

A. General interventions

1. Rule out other sources of infection.
2. Assess for PTL.

B. Patient teaching:

1. *See Section III: Patient Teaching Guide for this chapter, "Urinary Tract Infection During Pregnancy: Pyelonephritis."* ◀

C. Dietary management

1. Advise the patient to eat a regular diet as tolerated.
2. Encourage her to drink 8 to 10 glasses of water a day.
3. Warn the patient to avoid beverages with caffeine. Cranberry juice (100%) and cranberry and blueberry capsules are good for urinary tract problems.

D. Pharmaceutical therapy

1. Broad-spectrum antibiotic coverage until cultures and sensitivity results are back
2. Drug of choice
   a. Nitrofurantoin (Macrobid) 100 mg orally every 12 hours for 7 to 10 days
   b. Amoxicillin 500 mg orally every 12 hours for 7 days

c. Augmentin 500 mg orally every 12 hours for 7 days

3. If dysuria is present: Phenazopyridine (Pyridium) 200 mg orally three times daily after meals for 3 days. Warn the patient that phenazopyridine (Pyridium) turns urine orange.

4. Alternative medications

a. Cephalexin (Keflex) 500 mg orally every 12 hours for 7 days

Follow-Up

A. Once antibiotic therapy is initiated, most patients have a decrease in symptoms within 48 hours. By the end of 72 hours, almost 95% of patients are afebrile and asymptomatic. Stress to patients the importance of completing the course of antibiotics regardless of the absence of symptoms.
B. The most likely causes of treatment failure are a resistant microorganism or obstruction; common causes of obstruction in pregnancy are urolithiasis or compression of the ureter by the gravid uterus.
C. Repeat a urine culture at a 2-week follow-up visit.
D. Recurrence rates are very high. After the initial antibiotic therapy course is completed, consider a daily prophylactic dose of an antibiotic, such as nitrofurantoin (Macrodantin) 50 mg to 100 mg by mouth at bedtime, for recurrent infections.
E. Patients receiving prophylactic antibiotics should have their urine screened for bacteria at each subsequent office visit and be questioned about the recurrence of symptoms.
F. If no prophylactic treatment is undertaken, obtain a urine culture if symptoms recur or if urine dipstick is positive for leukocyte esterase or nitrites.

Vaginal Bleeding: First Trimester

Jill C. Cash and Susan Drummond

Definition

Vaginal bleeding during the first trimester of pregnancy may range from spotting to massive hemorrhage (spontaneous abortion). Types of abortion are:
A. Threatened abortion: Vaginal bleeding with absent or minimal pain *and* a closed, long, thick cervix
B. Inevitable abortion: Vaginal bleeding with pain and cervical dilation and/or effacement
C. Spontaneous abortion: The nonviable products of conception are expelled from the uterus spontaneously.
D. Vaginal bleeding may also be related to ectopic pregnancy, implantation of the pregnancy, or cervical inflammation/infection.

Incidence

A. Vaginal bleeding is a common event in pregnancy. Spontaneous abortion, a primary concern in the first trimester, occurs in about 30% of all pregnancies; most occur before the 16th week. Ectopic pregnancy occurs in one of every 200 pregnancies; 75% of pregnancies occurring after failure of tubal sterilization are likely to be ectopic.

Pathogenesis

A. Spontaneous abortion: The pathogenesis varies according to cause. In most cases, it is caused by embryonic death, with resultant decrease in hormone levels and subsequent sloughing of the uterine decidua. Many of the embryonic deaths occur because of chromosomal abnormalities that are incompatible with life.
B. Ectopic pregnancy: Fertilized ovum is prevented or slowed in its progress down the fallopian tube. Pregnancy is implanted outside of the uterus, most commonly in the fallopian tube.

Predisposing Factors

A. Spontaneous abortion: In most cases, the cause is unknown.

1. Advanced maternal age (occurs more often in older women), suggesting that a genetic abnormality in the ovum may contribute
2. Abnormal uterine environment
3. Systemic disease
4. Weight extremes BMI < 18.5 or > 25)
5. Immunologic deficiencies
6. Substance use, including caffeine, alcohol, cigarettes, and cocaine
7. Trauma
8. Previous spontaneous abortion

B. Ectopic pregnancy: Caused by previous damage to the fallopian tube; frequently caused by pelvic inflammatory disease, tubal surgery for infertility, or bilateral tubal ligation.

Common Complaints

A. Spontaneous abortion: Vaginal bleeding occurs that may or may not be associated with cramping or uterine contractions. When a pregnancy is greater than 8 weeks gestation, the presence of uterine bleeding, uterine contractions, and/or pain are indications of a threatened abortion until proven otherwise.
B. Ectopic pregnancy: Vaginal bleeding and pelvic pain occur soon after the first missed period; the patient may be unaware of pregnancy. Sudden, acute, localized abdominal pain is associated with fallopian tube rupture.

Other Signs and Symptoms

A. Threatened abortion: Slight bleeding may be present over several weeks; cramping; no passage of tissue; positive pregnancy symptoms present, including nausea, vomiting, fatigue, breast tenderness, and urinary frequency.
B. Inevitable abortion: Moderate to profuse vaginal bleeding occurs. Tissue may or may not be passed; uterine cramps or abdominal pain occur; symptoms of pregnancy may be decreased or absent.
C. Incomplete abortion: Moderate to profuse vaginal bleeding, sometimes for several weeks, occurs; reports of passage of tissue; painful uterine cramping or "contractions" present; and symptoms of pregnancy often absent.
D. Complete abortion: Patient experiences profuse bleeding, passage of tissue and large clots, abdominal cramping, or uterine contractions.

E. Ectopic pregnancy: Amenorrhea or irregular vaginal bleeding; abdominal pain is usually present, may be unilateral or generalized, and may be associated with vertigo and syncope; shoulder pain, with irritation of phrenic nerve, may be present. Anxiety or palpitations are often noted.

Subjective Data

A. Elicit information about the onset, duration, and progression of symptoms.
B. Ask the patient about vaginal bleeding. When did it start? Is it continuous bleeding, "like a period," or is it spotting? How much bleeding has occurred? How many pads have been saturated? What is the size of the blood spots? Determine the amount of bleeding: How much blood is on Peri-Pad? (a) Scant amount: Less than 1-inch diameter; (b) light amount: Less than a 4-inch diameter; (c) moderate amount: Less than a 6-inch diameter; (d) heavy amount: Saturates the peri-Pad within 1 hour.
C. What is her current method of birth control? Was the birth control method used consistently? Has she had a tubal ligation, or has she recently used an intrauterine contraceptive device (IUD)?
D. Ask the patient the first day of her last menstrual period to date the pregnancy. Did she have a positive pregnancy test? If so, when?
E. Does she have a history of ectopic pregnancy or pelvic inflammatory disease?
F. Question the patient regarding the presence or absence of abdominal and/or back pain. If present, is it a continuous discomfort, or is it intermittent cramping? Was the onset sudden? How severe is the pain?
G. Is she experiencing shoulder pain? This may be referred pain from phrenic nerve irritation because of intraperitoneal bleeding.

Physical Examination

A. Check temperature, pulse, respirations, and BP: Note postural hypotension and tachycardia. Hemodynamic instability may be noted in cases of profuse bleeding; assess vital signs and be alert for hypotension, tachycardia, tachypnea, and/or labored breathing.
B. Inspect
  1. Note general overall appearance of discomfort or pain before, during, and after examination.
  2. Examine Peri-Pad to determine amount of bleeding, if available.
C. Palpate
  1. Perform abdominal examination for rebound tenderness, masses, softness, tenderness, or abdominal wall distension. Sudden, acute, localized abdominal pain with signs of internal hemorrhage suggest rupture of the fallopian tube.
  2. Palpate uterine size. Measure fundal height for consistency with pregnancy dates. If fundal height suggests pregnancy has advanced beyond first trimester, bleeding may be caused by abruption, placenta previa, or rupture of membranes with heavy bloody show.
  3. Check iliopsoas and obturator muscle tests.
D. Auscultate the heart, lungs, and bowel sounds to rule out other abdominal problems.
E. Pelvic examination
  1. Perform sterile speculum examination: Assess color and amount of bleeding. Tissue and the products of conception may be noted at cervical os or in vaginal vault. Assess for Chadwick's sign. The entire fetus may be noted in the vaginal vault; tissues that remain in the uterus may include portions of fetal membranes or placenta. Look for vaginitis/cervicitis and other signs and symptoms of infection that could be causing the bleeding.
  2. Bimanual examination: Check Hegar's sign; elicit this sign cautiously, as a false-positive result may be related to a rough examination. Evaluate cervical dilation; cervical motion tenderness, often present with ectopic pregnancy; and a bulging cul-de-sac, which represents a hemoperitoneum. Adnexal mass is present in 50% of ectopic pregnancies.

Diagnostic Tests

A. Pregnancy test: Quantitative serum beta human chorionic gonadotropin (HCG); serial tests at least 48 hours apart, making sure to perform test at same lab for accurate results
B. Complete blood count (CBC) with differential and platelet count
C. Blood type, Rh, antibody screen, and cross-match if indicated
D. Prothrombin time (PT) and partial thromboplastin time (PTT)
E. Doppler ultrasonography for fetal heart tones, for fetuses greater than 11 weeks
F. Ultrasonography: Transvaginal and/or abdominal

Differential Diagnoses

A. First-trimester vaginal bleeding secondary to
  1. Threatened abortion
  2. Inevitable abortion
  3. Incomplete abortion
  4. Complete abortion
  5. Septic abortion
  6. Ectopic pregnancy: There is strong suspicion of ectopic pregnancy or fallopian tube rupture if symptoms present with a history of fallopian tube damage (i.e., tubal surgery for infertility, previous ectopic pregnancy), pelvic infection, or IUD use.
  7. Hydatidiform mole
  8. Anovulatory bleeding with an antecedent period of amenorrhea
  9. Benign or malignant genital tract lesion
  10. Menstrual bleeding
  11. Genital trauma
  12. Advanced pregnancy with placenta previa or abruptio placentae
  13. Salpingitis
  14. Appendicitis
  15. IUD-related symptoms
  16. Pelvic inflammatory disease

Plan

A. General interventions: Stabilize maternal condition and then determine the cause of bleeding.

1. Threatened abortion: Expectant management. Bed rest is often prescribed. Symptoms either subside, leading to normal gestation, or worsen, leading to inevitable abortion. If bleeding persists without leading to spontaneous abortion, the patient should be evaluated frequently, usually on a weekly basis, by means of ultrasonography to assess fetal viability. The patient should avoid intercourse and should not use tampons to absorb bleeding.

2. Inevitable abortion: Care may include expectant management or preparation for dilation and curettage (D&C).

3. Incomplete abortion: Prepare for suction and possible D&C.

4. Complete abortion: If abortion is complete and the products of conception are delivered with complete membranes present and cessation of bleeding has occurred, no surgical intervention is indicated. In these cases, the tissue specimens must be carefully examined for completeness. Send all specimens to the laboratory for further examination. If there is any question regarding complete passing of the placenta, do serial quantitative HCGs until back to nonpregnant levels.

5. Ectopic pregnancy: Consult with a physician regarding possible medical management with methotrexate or refer the patient to a physician for surgical intervention. The physician may perform culdocentesis to assess for hemoperitoneum. If the patient is in shock, resuscitation with IV fluids should be started immediately by means of two large-bore angiocatheters. IV fluids, such as lactated Ringer's solution or normal saline, should be infused at a rapid rate. The patient is taken to the operating room, where the indicated procedure is one that controls hemorrhage in the shortest period of time. Salpingectomy and/or hysterectomy may be included.

▶ **B.** Patient teaching: *See Section III: Patient Teaching Guide for this chapter, "Vaginal Bleeding: First Trimester."*

C. Pharmaceutical therapy

1. RhQ (D) immune globulin should be administered to any Rh-negative patient.

2. Acetaminophen (Tylenol) or ibuprofen as needed for discomfort.

3. Ectopic pregnancy: Methotrexate is a folic acid antagonist that has been used to inhibit the growth of trophoblastic cells. This chemotherapy is the treatment of choice for ectopic pregnancy when surgery is contraindicated, or in the management of postoperative persistent trophoblast. Refer the patient to a physician to evaluate her for methotrexate or operative intervention. In most cases, operative intervention is required.

Follow-Up

A. Threatened abortion: Follow the patient weekly to assess for interval growth and presence of fetal cardiac motion. Instruct the patient on Peri-Pad count.

B. Spontaneous abortion: Once the uterine contents have been evacuated, follow up with a 6-week postabortion visit, unless the situation warrants an earlier follow-up visit. Contraception needs to be discussed with the patient. Advise her that it is best to wait for two or three menstrual cycles before becoming pregnant again.

C. Ectopic pregnancy: Once the ectopic pregnancy has been removed, the patient should be seen in 2 to 6 weeks for a postoperative examination, unless the situation warrants an earlier follow-up visit. If methotrexate is used, do serial quantitative HCGs until they return to nonpregnant levels.

Consultation/Referral

A. Consult with a physician if the patient has any frank bleeding, signs of fetal compromise, or maternal shock, or if the cause of bleeding cannot be determined.

Vaginal Bleeding: Second and Third Trimesters

Jill C. Cash and Susan Drummond

Definition

Bright or dark red vaginal bleeding during the second or third trimester (more than 12 weeks gestation) may be painless, or it may be associated with uterine contractions or severe abdominal pain. Antepartum bleeding (uterine bleeding after 20 weeks gestation that is unrelated to labor and delivery) occurs in 4% to 5% of pregnancies. Common causes of bleeding include:

A. Low-lying placenta: The edge of the placenta grows into the area of the lower uterine segment near the cervical os.

B. Placenta previa: Implantation of the blastocyst occurs in the lower uterine segment, followed by placental growth. Eventually, the placenta may partially or completely cover the cervix.

C. Abruptio placentae: Partial or premature separation of the placenta takes place.

D. Uterine rupture: Complete uterine rupture extends through the entire uterine wall, and the uterine contents are extruded into the abdominal cavity. Incomplete rupture extends through the endometrium and myometrium, but the peritoneum remains intact. This occurs almost exclusively during labor and/or delivery.

E. Uterine dehiscence: Separation of an old surgical scar

F. Bloody discharge is *not* normal before 37 weeks gestation unless associated with recent sexual intercourse or pelvic examination. Light spotting or bleeding may be caused by recent sexual intercourse, preterm labor (PTL), rupture of membranes, or cervicitis. *Note*: The evaluation of vaginal bleeding before 20 weeks is similar to that in the first trimester.

Incidence

A. Placenta previa: Approximately 1:200 pregnancies, more common in parous women

B. Abruptio placenta: Approximately 1:250 pregnancies

C. Uterine rupture: If uterus is unscarred, incidence is approximately 1:6,000 to 1: 20,000 pregnancies. If uterus has a scar (usually from a previous cesarean section), incidence varies depending on the type and location of the prior uterine incision. If the prior incision was low transverse, the incidence is approximately 0.7% to 2.0% and if the prior incision was classical, the incidence is approximately 1% to 2%.

Pathogenesis

A. Placenta previa: The pathogenesis of placenta previa is unknown. One hypothesis is that the presence of suboptimal endometrium in the upper uterine cavity because of previous surgery or pregnancies promotes implantation of trophoblast in or toward the lower uterine segment. Another hypothesis is that a particularly large placental surface area, as in multiple gestation or in response to reduced uteroplacental perfusion, increases the likelihood that the placenta will cover or encroach upon the cervical os.

B. Abruptio placenta: Abruptio placenta is initiated by bleeding into the decidua basalis. The decidua then splits, and the placenta is sheared off. Blood may move into and through the myometrium, leading to a boardlike uterus.

C. Uterine rupture: Uterine rupture may occur from uterine injury because of previous surgery or trauma.

Predisposing Factors

A. Placenta previa: Late fertilization with delayed implantation, previous uterine scar, advanced maternal age, multiple gestation, large placenta, previous placenta previa, and smoking

B. Abruptio placenta: Hypertension (chronic, gestational, or preeclampsia), cocaine use, trauma, high parity, sudden decompression of overdistended uterus (i.e., when membranes rupture), smoking, chorioamnionitis, abdominal trauma, and cephalic version

C. Uterine rupture: Multiparity, previous uterine incision, tetanic contractions, or prolonged labor, especially with excessive use of oxytocin

Common Complaints

A. Placenta previa: Painless vaginal bleeding, usually in amounts of spotting to frank hemorrhage. Bleeding occasionally is accompanied by cramping or uterine contractions. A "gush" of fluid associated with sudden onset of massive vaginal bleeding may be reported. Painless vaginal bleeding should be treated as a placenta previa until proven otherwise.

B. Abruptio placentae: Firm, tender uterus; high-frequency, low-amplitude uterine contractions

 1. Marginal abruption: Vaginal bleeding may be absent or minimal and bright red; there may be some old, dark blood. Abdominal pain is usually mild.

> *Frank vaginal bleeding with abdominal pain should be treated as an abruption until proven otherwise.*

 2. Moderate abruption: Vaginal bleeding may be moderate or absent. Abdominal pain is usually significant and associated with contractions.

 3. Severe abruption: Vaginal bleeding may be moderate, severe, or absent. Abdominal pain is severe. **The patient may have a concealed placental abruption without vaginal bleeding.**

C. Uterine rupture: Vaginal bleeding is moderate, severe, or absent. The patient may experience a sudden onset of extreme abdominal pain (commonly at the previous uterine scar site).

Other Signs and Symptoms

A. External fetal monitor (EFM) tracings: May exhibit characteristics that are associated with anemia or hypoxemia such as decreased or absent variability, bradycardia, tachycardia, recurrent late or prolonged decelerations, or a sinusoidal pattern.

B. Placenta previa: Uterine resting tone usually relaxed. Fetal status at first examination is usually stable. Recurrence of bleeding is common. First bleeding episode in placenta previa is rarely significant. Second or third bleeding episode is often associated with significant vaginal bleeding.

C. Abruptio placentae: Rupture of membranes reveals blood-stained fluid.

 1. Marginal abruption: Uterine resting tone is usually relaxed. Fetal status on the fetal monitor at first examination is usually stable. Labor progresses rapidly with vaginal bleeding or large amounts of bloody show.

 2. Moderate abruption: Uterine resting tone is hypertonic. At first examination, the fetus is usually alive. Fetal heart rate (FHR) may exhibit characteristics that are associated with hypoxemia or anemia such as decreased/absent variability, tachycardia, bradycardia, recurrent late or prolonged decelerations, or sinusoidal patterns. Labor progresses rapidly with vaginal bleeding or large amounts of bloody show.

 3. Severe abruption: Uterine resting tone is hypertonic or "boardlike." At first examination, the fetus may be dead. If the fetus is alive, EFM is consistent with hypoxemia or anemia as listed earlier.

D. Uterine rupture: Uterine resting tone may be normal or hypertonic. At first examination, fetus is frequently dead or FHR pattern is consistent with hypoxemia or anemia as listed earlier.

Subjective Data

A. Elicit information about the onset, duration, and progression of vaginal bleeding. When did it start? Is it continuous bleeding, "like a period," or is it spotting?

B. Ask: How much bleeding has occurred? How many pads have been saturated? What is the size of the blood spots, the size of a quarter or a half dollar?

C. Elicit information regarding the presence or absence of abdominal pain. If present, review the onset, duration, and progression of pain. Is it a continuous discomfort or intermittent cramping? How severe is the pain? Did it have a sudden onset?

D. Is the patient experiencing shoulder pain? This is likely to be referred pain from phrenic nerve irritation because of intraperitoneal bleeding.

E. Elicit the first day of patient's last menstrual cycle, to date pregnancy.
F. Ask the patient if she feels the baby move, if greater than 18 weeks gestation, and if the movement has been normal this day.

Physical Examination

A. Check temperature, pulse, respirations, and blood pressure (BP); include FHR.
  1. A pregnant patient does not demonstrate signs and symptoms of hypovolemic shock until she has lost 30% of her circulating volume.
  2. Prepare the patient for emergency transport to a hospital even if she is hemodynamically stable.
B. Inspect: Inspect the patient's general appearance related to discomfort and pain. Observe bleeding characteristics and pooling.
C. Palpate
  1. Check for palpable fetal parts on abdominal wall; note fetal movement.
  2. Palpate the uterus for relaxed or hypertonic uterus. Check for contractions. If present, note frequency, duration, and intensity to palpation.
D. Auscultate
  1. The abdomen; check fetal heart tones or EFM for baseline and periodic FHR patterns.
  2. The maternal heart and lungs
E. Perform sterile speculum examination to look for the source of bleeding. **Do not perform vaginal bimanual examination until previa is ruled out.**

Diagnostic Tests

A. Complete blood count (CBC) and platelets
B. Prothrombin time (PT), partial thromboplastin time (PTT), and fibrinogen
C. Blood type, Rh status, and type and cross-match if indicated
D. Fetal cell stain, Kleihauer–Betke test; fetal cell stain can determine the amount of fetal blood in the maternal circulation.
E. Determine if Rh_O(D) immune globulin (RhoGAM) is indicated.
F. Ultrasonography
G. Nonstress test (NST)/electronic fetal monitoring

Differential Diagnoses

A. Placenta previa
B. Abruptio placentae
C. Uterine rupture
D. Ruptured vasa previa
E. Rupture of membranes
F. Normal bloody show
G. Rectal hemorrhoidal bleeding

Plan

A. General interventions
  1. Tocolysis may be considered if the patient has no active hemorrhage and reassuring FHR pattern.
  2. If significant vaginal bleeding is present, the primary goal is to maintain oxygen delivery to the mother and fetus while preparing them for transport. Interventions include maternal positioning to avoid vena caval compression; administering supplemental oxygen; initiating large-bore IV line; delivery of fluid bolus of normal saline or lactated Ringer's solution; keeping a flow sheet of vital signs, assessments, actions, and responses; maintaining continuous recording of FHR and uterine activity on an electronic fetal monitor; and providing emotional support and anticipatory guidance.
  3. If vaginal bleeding is minimal and home management is being considered, discuss risks with the patient and assess her ability to maintain bed rest. Also assess patient's access to transportation in case of a major bleeding episode. Consider the distance from the patient's home to the nearest hospital.
B. Patient teaching: *See Section III: Patient Teaching Guide for this chapter, "Vaginal Bleeding: Second and Third Trimesters."*
C. Pharmaceutical therapy for preterm placenta previa with preterm contractions
  1. Tocolysis options
    a. Terbutaline sulfate (Brethine) 0.25 mg by subcutaneous injection every 15 minutes times three doses if maternal heart rate is less than 120 beats per minute.
    b. Indomethacin 50 mg per rectum followed by 25 mg orally every 6 hours. **Note: Indomethacin should not be given after 32 weeks gestation, and duration of indomethacin therapy should not exceed 72 hours.**
    c. The patient may be admitted to an inpatient antepartum unit for parenteral tocolysis such as magnesium sulfate.
  2. Antenatal steroids may be given if preterm delivery is a possibility within the next week and the estimated gestational age (EGA) is less than 34 weeks.
    a. Betamethasone 12.5 mg may be given by IM injection every 24 hours times two doses.
    b. Dexamethasone 8 mg orally may be given every 12 hours times four doses.
    c. Either regimen may be repeated once a week.
  3. If the patient is Rh-negative, give her Rh_O(D) immune globulin (RhoGAM) IM by injection after each vaginal bleeding episode.
    a. Full-dose Rh_O(D) IM immune globulin, which is adequate

Follow-Up

A. Follow-up depends on patient diagnosis and whether patient hospitalization is needed.

Consultation/Referral

A. Consult a physician for all patients noted to have second- and third-trimester vaginal bleeding.
B. Consult with a physician if the patient has any frank, bright-red bleeding, signs of fetal compromise, or maternal shock, or if the cause of bleeding cannot be determined and/or treated by the practitioner.

POSTPARTUM

Breast Engorgement

Jill C. Cash and Susan Drummond

Definition

A. Breast engorgement is swollen, tender breasts caused by overfilling of milk, increased blood flow, and fluids in the breasts.

Incidence

A. Breast engorgement may affect 40% of postpartum mothers.

Pathogenesis

A. *Primary engorgement* is the result of distension and stasis of the vascular and lymphatic circulations occurring 2 to 4 days following delivery. It is prompted by the decrease in progesterone levels after the placenta is delivered.
B. *Secondary engorgement* occurs because of distension of the lobules and alveoli with milk as lactation is established. It may occur from excessive stimulation of milk production via pumping, taking medications to increase milk supply, or decreased milk extraction from not feeding the baby as often. Without stimulation by suckling and removal of milk, secretion of prolactin decreases and milk production decreases and finally ceases.

Predisposing Factors

A. Engorgement often develops if early feedings are not frequent enough, suckling is inadequate, or breastfeeding is not conducted in a relaxing atmosphere. Engorgement is more likely to develop sooner and more intensely in mothers who have breastfed a prior child.

Common Complaints

A. Swollen, tender breasts
B. Discomfort when breastfeeding
C. A low-grade fever lasting between 4 and 16 hours

Other Signs and Symptoms

A. Pain, tenderness, and redness in one area of the breast are associated with mastitis.
B. Physical examination should not be focused just on breast symptoms but should include a general ruling out of other potential problems such as coexistent urinary tract infection (UTI).

Subjective Data

A. Elicit the onset, duration, and course of symptoms. Review the frequency of breastfeeding and/or use of a breast pump. Is the patient still breastfeeding, or has she stopped because of the discomfort?
B. Exclude other causes of fever, such as UTI, wound infection, and red streaks on one or both breasts, to rule out mastitis.
C. Quantify pain symptoms and relief measures, including heat packs, ice packs, breast binder, and analgesics such as Tylenol.

Physical Examination

A. Check temperature, blood pressure (BP), and pulse.
B. Inspect: Examine the breasts for erythemic streaks. Check the episiotomy or abdominal incision, if indicated.
C. Palpate
  1. Examine the breasts for tenderness, hardness, warmth, and lumps.
  2. Palpate axilla for lymphadenopathy.
  3. Check back for costovertebral angle (CVA) tenderness.

Diagnostic Tests

A. Tests generally are not indicated for breast engorgement.
B. Urine culture or wound culture, if applicable

Differential Diagnoses

A. Breast engorgement
B. Mastitis

Plan

A. General interventions
  1. Encourage the patient to take analgesics before breastfeeding and continue breastfeeding.
  2. Encourage ice packs for discomfort and frequent breastfeeding. There should be *no stimulation* to the breasts other than that provided by the baby when nursing, and the patient should take analgesics for discomfort. Reassure her that engorgement is temporary and usually resolves within 24 to 48 hours.

B. Patient teaching: *See Section III: Patient Teaching Guide for this chapter, "Postpartum: Breast Engorgement and Sore Nipples."* ◀
  1. Educate the patient regarding milk production.
  2. Advise the patient to breastfeed frequently to reduce chances of engorgement.
  3. Provide reassurance and support for the patient to continue breastfeeding through this temporary period of discomfort. Engorgement may last 2 to 3 days before milk supply meets demand; continuation of breastfeeding will resolve discomfort and problems.

C. Pharmaceutical therapy: Acetaminophen (Tylenol) two tablets 500 to 1,000 mg every 4 to 6 hours, or ibuprofen 400 to 600 mg orally 30 to 45 minutes before breastfeeding and as needed.

Follow-Up

A. Follow-up may not be required for engorgement.
B. Lactation consultation if indicated

Individual Considerations

A. Pregnancy loss: It is imperative to discuss breast care and engorgement with women who have a second-trimester termination of pregnancy, have a stillbirth, or experience a neonatal loss.

Endometritis

Jill C. Cash and Susan Drummond

Definition

A. Endometritis is an infection of the endometrium (the interior lining of the uterus) that occurs postpartum.

Endometritis is the most common cause of puerperal fever in obstetrics.

Incidence

A. The incidence of endometritis has been noted to be as high as 38.5% after cesarean section; the incidence is 1.2% after vaginal delivery.

Pathogenesis

During labor and delivery, endogenous cervicovaginal flora enter the uterine cavity. Onset is usually 3 to 5 days after delivery, unless it is caused by beta-hemolytic *Streptococcus*, in which case the onset is earlier and more precipitous. Infection is usually polymicrobial in nature. Undiagnosed or unsuccessfully treated infection of the endomyometrium can progress to involve the entire uterus and may spread to accessory pelvic structures. The main pathway for spread of the infection is the broad ligament. Sources of bacteria may be any one or a combination of the following:

A. Endogenous vaginal bacteria, usually pathogenic only when tissue is damaged
 1. Beta-hemolytic *Streptococcus*
 2. *Streptococcus viridans*
 3. *Neisseria gonorrhoeae*
 4. *Gardnerella*

B. Contamination by normal bowel bacteria
 1. *Clostridium perfringens*
 2. *Escherichia coli*
 3. *Proteus mirabilis*
 4. *Aerobacter aerogenes*
 5. *Enterococcus*
 6. *Pseudomonas aeruginosa*
 7. *Klebsiella pneumoniae*

C. Contamination from environment; *Staphylococcus* is a common organism.

Predisposing Factors

A. Operative delivery: Cesarean section is the major predisposing factor for pelvic infection. The most important determinant of infection for patients undergoing cesarean delivery is the duration of labor.

B. Intrapartum: Prolonged rupture of membranes; numerous vaginal examinations in labor; use of internal monitoring devices during labor; use of instruments in delivery; prolonged labor; and intrauterine manipulation, such as internal rotation or manual removal of placenta, can all lead to endometritis.

C. Postpartum: Retained placental fragments or membranes, improper perineal care, and host resistance also predispose a patient to infection.

D. Anemia: This probably represents a marker for poor nutrition.

E. Obesity

Common Complaints

A. "Feeling ill" with fever or chills
B. Muscle aches
C. Headache
D. Uterine pain and tenderness
E. Foul-smelling lochia

Other Signs and Symptoms

A. Fever (100.4°F–104.0°F)
B. Subinvolution
C. Atonic uterus.
D. Abnormalities of lochia
 1. May be scant and odorless if anaerobic infection
 2. May be moderately heavy, foul, bloody, or seropurulent if aerobic infection
E. Tachycardia

Subjective Data

A. Elicit the onset, duration, and course of symptoms.
B. Review the color, odor, and amount of lochia.
C. Review the patient's pain or discomfort and the relief measures used.
D. Review other body symptoms to rule out other infections such as UTI, breast engorgement, or mastitis.
E. Review labor and delivery events for complications (see Predisposing Factors).

Physical Examination

A. Check temperature, pulse, and blood pressure (BP): The patient may be tachycardic with heart rate of 100 to 140 beats per minute (bpm).

B. Inspect: Observe color, amount, and odor of lochia. Check abdominal incision, if applicable. Check the perineum for lacerations, breakdown of incision, redness, and drainage.

C. Palpate
 1. The abdomen; check uterine tenderness.
 2. The back; check CVA tenderness.

D. Auscultate the heart and lungs.

E. Speculum examination: Inspect the cervix for lacerations, drainage, or redness.

F. Bimanual examination: Check for cervical motion tenderness; palpate adnexa for masses and tenderness; note "heat" of the pelvis.

Diagnostic Tests

A. Complete blood count (CBC) with differential
B. Blood and urine cultures
C. Cervical cultures, to rule out a sexually transmitted infection (STI), if indicated
D. Wet prep, if indicated

Differential Diagnoses

A. Endometritis
B. Sexually transmitted diseases (STDs), such as chlamydia, gonorrhea, or trichomoniasis
C. Septic pelvic thrombophlebitis
D. UTI/pyelonephritis
E. Pneumonitis
F. Extreme breast engorgement: "milk fever"
G. Wound infection

Plan

A. General interventions
 1. Instruct on proper hygiene. Teach the patient proper techniques to prevent infection (perineal area, incision site, breast).
 2. Acetaminophen (Tylenol) for fever as needed

B. Patient teaching: *See Section III: Patient Teaching Guide for this chapter, "Endometritis."*

C. Pharmaceutical therapy
1. Antibiotic therapy
a. Augmentin 500 mg orally four times daily for 10 days
b. If the patient is allergic to penicillin and not breastfeeding, doxycycline 100 mg orally every 12 hours for 7 days
c. If the patient is allergic to penicillin and is breastfeeding, cephalexin (Keflex) 500 mg orally four times daily for 7 days
d. Rocephin/ceftriaxone 250 mg intramuscularly (IM) times one with Flagyl 500 mg orally twice a day for 7 days (if breastfeeding, pump and dispose of breast milk during treatment)
2. If uterus is boggy and/or bleeding is excessive: Methylergonovine maleate (Methergine) 0.2 mg orally every 4 hours for six doses. (Do not give if the patient is hypertensive.)

Follow-Up

A. Call the patient in 24 to 48 hours to evaluate her status.
B. Instruct the patient to call if symptoms do not resolve within 24 hours or if they worsen.

Consultation/Referral

A. Consult with physician if symptoms do not resolve, if they worsen within 24 hours, or if the patient's temperature does not go below 100.0°F after 48 hours on antibiotics. If no significant improvement is seen within 2 to 3 days, the patient may need to be admitted to the hospital.

Secondary Postpartum Hemorrhage

Jill C. Cash and Susan Drummond

Definition

A. Secondary postpartum hemorrhage is blood loss of 500 mL or more after the first 24 hours of delivery and within 6 weeks of delivery.

Incidence

A. Incidence is approximately 0.5% to 2% of women in developed countries.

Pathogenesis

A. Hemorrhage may result from retained placental fragments, subinvolution of the uterus, intrauterine infection, or inherited coagulation defects.

Predisposing Factors

A. Abnormally adherent placenta
B. Prolonged rupture of membranes leading to infection
C. Overdistended uterus from multiple gestation, and polyhydramnios
D. Hematoma

Common Complaints

A. Heavy red bleeding or slow reddish-brown oozing
B. Abdominal pain
C. Loss of appetite
D. Fatigue; cannot get enough rest and is unable to complete self-care and infant-care activities

Other Signs and Symptoms

A. Lochia rubra is bright-red discharge immediately after delivery (1–3 days) and may contain a few small clots. A continuous trickle of bright-red blood suggests a laceration of the cervix or vagina. Saturation of one Peri-Pad in less than 15 minutes (two pads in 30 minutes, or rapid pooling of blood under the buttocks) is considered excessive bleeding and requires immediate attention.
B. Foul odor: Lochia should not be malodorous. Lochia usually has a "fleshy" odor.
C. Boggy uterus: Check the consistency of the uterus, whether it is firm or boggy. If atony is present, support the lower uterine segment, and massage the uterus or do bimanual compression.
D. Faintness
E. Tachycardia
F. Hypotension

Subjective Data

A. Elicit the onset, duration, and course of symptoms.
B. Elicit the amount and color of lochia, including the size of blood clot(s).
C. Review symptoms of infection, including fever and malodorous lochia.
D. Review labor and delivery events, including the date of delivery, use of forceps or vacuum, weight of baby, manual removal of placenta, complications, and postpartum course.
E. Review pregnancy for predisposing factors such as multiple gestation and polyhydramnios (as noted earlier).

Physical Examination

A. Check temperature, blood pressure (BP), pulse, and respirations.
B. Inspect
1. Note color and amount of vaginal bleeding.

Lochia may appear heavier when the woman first stands up because the lochia pools in the vagina while she is recumbent. Once the pooled blood is discharged, lochia flow should return to normal.

2. Inspect episiotomy or abdominal incision.

C. Palpate
1. Check for consistency of uterus, massaging uterus if boggy.
2. Express clots, if applicable.
3. By 2 weeks postpartum, the uterus should have involuted and once again be a "pelvic organ."
4. Check abdominal tension.

D. Speculum examination: Assess cervical lacerations.
E. Bimanual examination: Rule out retroperitoneal hemorrhage.

Diagnostic Tests

A. Complete blood count (CBC) with differential
B. If bleeding is not under control, type and cross-match blood.

C. Coagulation test, if disseminated intravascular coagulation (DIC) is suspected
D. Blood cultures to rule out infection

Differential Diagnoses

A. Late postpartum bleeding
B. Normal postpartum bleeding
C. Postpartum infection

Plan

A. General interventions
- **1.** Perform uterine massage: Support the lower uterine segment during massage to prevent uterine prolapse.
- **2.** Give intravenous (IV) hydration for hypovolemic shock: Hypotension, tachycardia, and faintness.
- **3.** Hospitalization is usually required for postpartum hemorrhage.
- **4.** Encourage breastfeeding (if applicable) to increase uterine contraction.
- **5.** Advise the patient to rest and increase oral fluids.

B. Pharmaceutical therapy
- **1.** Drug of choice: Methylergonovine maleate (Methergine) 0.2 mg orally every 4 hours for six doses. **Do not give if the patient is hypertensive.**
- **2.** For severe hemorrhage
  - **a.** Oxytocin (Pitocin) 10 to 20 units in 250 mL to 1,000 mL IV fluids
  - **b.** Methylergonovine maleate (Methergine) 0.2 mg by IM injection, if the patient has no history of hypertension. Advise the patient to take full course of Methergine even if bleeding stops.
  - **c. Hemabate: 250 mcg; may repeat every 15 to 90 minutes as needed.**
  - **d.** Misoprostol (Cytotec, PGE1); 800 to 1,000 mcg prolonged release (PR)
  - **e.** Continue bimanual compression and notify a physician.
- **3.** If infection is suspected or confirmed antibiotics are prescribed.

Follow-Up

A. Reevaluate the patient 1 week from the date of discharge from the hospital.
B. Repeat hematocrit (Hct)/CBC at postpartum visit.
C. The patient may need iron-replacement therapy, if not already prescribed. If stable at 1-week follow-up visit, have the patient return in 4 to 6 weeks postpartum for routine postpartum examination.

Consultation/Referral

A. Immediately consult or refer the patient to a physician for possible hospitalization for dilation and curettage (D&C).

Mastitis

Jill C. Cash and Susan Drummond

Definition

A. Mastitis is an infection of breast tissue with the potential for abscess formation.

Incidence

A. Mastitis has been estimated to occur in 2% to 10% of breastfeeding mothers. Less than 1% of these require hospitalization. Symptoms seldom appear before the end of the first week postpartum and are most often seen during the first 2 months postpartum.

Pathogenesis

A. During the period of lactation, the breast changes from an essentially nonfunctioning organ to a complex functioning organ of the body. The developing multiductal system becomes a rich environment for the growth of bacteria. The most common offending organism is *Staphylococcus aureus* (95%). The immediate source of the organisms that cause mastitis is almost always the nursing infant's nose and mouth.

Predisposing Factors

Invasion of bacteria in the presence of breast injury, including:
A. Bruising from rough manipulation (pumping) or failing to break the neonate's attachment to the areola and nipple before removing from breast
B. Prolonged breast engorgement
C. Milk stasis in a duct
D. Cracking or fissures of the nipple
E. Poor handwashing

Common Complaints

A. Breast engorgement, usually bilateral
B. Pain in the breast, usually unilateral
C. Fever
D. Red streak(s)
E. Flu-like symptoms: Body aches, headache, malaise, and chills

Other Signs and Symptoms

A. Fever 100.0°F to 104.0°F, rapid rise
B. Exquisitely tender breast tissue
C. Hard mass in the breast
D. Tachycardia and tachypnea
E. Axillary lymphadenopathy

Subjective Data

A. Elicit the onset, duration, and course of symptoms.
B. Note the frequency and length of time of the feeding or pumping.
C. Are there any red streaks on the breasts?
D. Are the nipples cracked and bleeding?
E. Quantify pain symptoms, relief measures tried, and results.
F. Review other symptoms to rule out other infections such as wound infection, episiotomy breakdown, and urinary tract infection (UTI).

Physical Examination

A. Check temperature, blood pressure (BP), pulse, and respirations.
B. Physical examination should not be focused only on breast symptoms, but should include a general ruling out of other potential problems such as coexistent UTI or endometritis.

C. Inspect

1. Visually inspect breasts.
2. Observe breastfeeding for adequacy of latch, suck, swallow, jaw glide, and any clicking.
3. Check episiotomy or abdominal incision to rule out infection.

D. Palpate

1. Perform breast examination.
2. Palpate lymph modes of the neck and axilla.
3. Palpate the abdomen.
4. Check costovertebral angle (CVA) tenderness.

E. Auscultate: Heart and lungs.

Diagnostic Tests

A. Treatment is usually initiated based on symptoms and examination

B. Complete blood count (CBC): Leukocytosis in peripheral smear

C. White blood cell (WBC), culture and sensitivity of breast milk to identify bacteria for persistent signs of infection or if antibiotic treatment is unsuccessful

D. Urine or wound cultures, if applicable

E. Ultrasound considered if breast is not responding to treatment to evaluate for breast abscess

Differential Diagnoses

A. Mastitis: Fever, chills, and malaise in conjunction with unilateral breast pain

B. Breast engorgement: Bilateral presentation of breast discomfort

C. Breast abscess: Discharge of purulent exudate from nipple, masses, or reddened areas that develop a bluish hue of the skin over the area of abscess

D. Clogged milk duct

E. Viral syndrome

F. Inflammatory breast cancer

Plan

A. General interventions: Encourage self-care and support. Advise the family to assist the patient with self-care and infant care during this acute period. The woman may feel extremely ill for the first 24 to 48 hours of therapy and may find it difficult to continue breastfeeding, self-care, and newborn care activities.

B. Patient teaching:

1. ▶ *See Section III: Patient Teaching Guides for this chapter, "Mastitis" and "Postpartum: Breast Engorgement and Sore Nipples."*
2. Advise the patient to continue to breastfeed or pump to maintain milk supply.
3. Stress the importance of continuation of breastfeeding or pumping despite infection.
4. Inform the patient that the breast milk is not infected and it is safe for the newborn to continue to breastfeed. The infection is localized to the breast tissue and will respond quickly with antibiotic therapy.

C. Dietary management

1. There are no dietary restrictions.
2. Have the patient increase fluid intake with increased temperature (at least 10–12 glasses a day).
3. Encourage her to eliminate caffeine, if possible, or use in moderation.

D. Pharmaceutical therapy

1. Antibiotics
   a. Drug of choice: Dicloxacillin 500 mg orally every 6 hours for 10 days
2. Alternative drug therapy
   a. Cephalexin (Keflex) 500 mg orally should be taken four times daily for 10 days.
   b. Concerning methicillin resistant *Staphylococcus aureus* (MRSA), trimethoprim-sulfamethoxazole 1 to 2 tablets twice a day or clindamycin 300 mg orally four times a day for 10 days. Linezolid 600 mg orally twice a day for 10 days may also be used.
   c. For a severe infection, inpatient treatment with vancomycin 30 mg/kg IV twice daily should be used.
3. Advise the patient to complete the full course of antibiotics even if symptoms improve sooner.
4. Candidal vaginitis may develop secondary to antibiotic therapy. The patient should be aware of the signs, symptoms, and treatment plan if it should occur. Use the probiotics *Lactobacillus fermentum* or *Lactobacillus salivarius* with use of antibiotics.
5. Acetaminophen (Tylenol) or ibuprofen for pain management.
6. The patient may require pain medication if acetaminophen (Tylenol) or ibuprofen is not effective. Use acetaminophen with codeine phosphate (Tylenol No. 3) or other narcotic as needed for pain.

Follow-Up

A. Evaluate the patient in 48 hours if a breast abscess is suspected; assess need for surgical consultation.

Consultation/Referral

A. Consult a physician if a breast abscess is suspected, for persistent signs of infection, or if antibiotic treatment is unsuccessful. Treatment of a breast abscess may include surgical incision and drainage of the abscess.

B. Notify the baby's provider if mastitis is diagnosed.

Postpartum Care: 6 Weeks Postpartum Examination

Jill C. Cash and Susan Drummond

History

A. Chart review

1. Antepartum course, including prenatal laboratory data: Pap smear, cervical cultures, maternal blood type and Rh, rubella and syphilis screen, and complete blood count (CBC)
2. Intrapartum course: Length of labor, type of delivery, and any maternal complications
3. Neonatal course: Gestational age, weight, length, cord gases, admission to normal or intensive care

nursery, length of stay in the intensive care nursery, and any neonatal complications

4. Immediate postpartum course: Postpartum recovery, any postpartum complications, laboratory data, and length of hospital stay

B. Interval history
  1. Number of weeks postpartum
  2. General maternal health and well-being, including diet or appetite, bowel and bladder function, level of activity, sleep patterns, and pain or discomfort
  3. Interval problems: Calls to health care provider, visits to emergency room, fever, or illness
  4. Adjustment and role adaptation to the baby: Motherhood, fatherhood, sibling rivalry, psychosocial assessment of depression, family support, housing or financial issues
  5. Resumption of sexual activity: When, problems encountered, comfort measures used, and type of contraception used
  6. Family planning: Previous method of contraception used, success of method, plans to resume contraception, and options for contraception
  7. Status of infant: Breastfeeding or bottle feeding, consolability, sleep patterns, voiding, and stool patterns
  8. Establishment of health care follow-up: Pediatrician appointment and immunizations; referral to Women, Infants, and Children (WIC), public health, and so on, if applicable; or follow-up with nurse practitioner or nurse-midwife

C. Review of relevant systems
  1. Breasts: Cracked or sore nipples, clogged ducts, engorgement, mastitis; breast care practiced
  2. Bladder function: Stress incontinence, dysuria, urinary frequency, and flank pain
  3. Bowel function: Constipation; discomfort, especially if the patient has a history of third-or fourth-degree laceration; relief measures used and results
  4. Perineum: Problems or discomfort at episiotomy site, problems with wound healing, and signs of infection
  5. Lochia: Duration, type, odor, presence of clots; or resumption of menses: Date, duration, and amount
  6. Abdomen: If cesarean delivery, healing of wound, signs of infection; exercises initiated
  7. Legs: Varicosities, heat, swelling, and calf tenderness

Physical Examination

A. Weight, blood pressure (BP), and pulse; temperature, if indicated

B. Inspect:
  1. Examine breast: Examine nipple integrity; assess for drying, cracking, bleeding, blisters.
  2. Examine legs for varicosities and signs of thrombophlebitis.
  3. Examine perineum, healing of episiotomy or lacerations, and abnormalities of Bartholin's gland.
  4. Inspect cesarean section incision for wound integrity and for signs of infection.

C. Auscultate the heart and lungs.

D. Palpate
  1. Abdomen for tenderness, masses, involution of uterus
  2. Breasts for masses, engorgement, inflammation

E. Speculum examination: Note lesions or lacerations of cervix, discharge, signs of infection; obtain Pap smear.

F. Bimanual examination: Check for abnormalities of cervix, uterus, adnexa; status of involution; presence of cystocele or rectocele; and vaginal muscle tone.

G. Rectovaginal examination: Check for integrity of episotomy or laceration if indicated.

H. Psychological examination
  1. See section on "Postpartum Depression" for information on assessment of postpartum blues/postpartum depression.

Diagnostic Tests

A. Pap smear

B. Other tests as indicated; CBC if anemia or hemorrhage is documented or suspected

Differential Diagnoses

A. Well postpartum examination

B. Mastitis

C. Breast engorgement

D. Postpartum blues

E. Postpartum depression

Plan

A. General interventions
  1. This visit may be the last contact the woman has with the health care delivery system for some time. The practitioner should evaluate any problems and provide appropriate consultations, referrals, interventions, counseling, and teaching.

B. Patient teaching
  1. Explain the necessity of a yearly gynecologic examination.
  2. Encourage regular aerobic, abdominal, and Kegel exercises.
  3. Counsel the patient on choice of contraception.
    a. Abstinence
    b. Natural family planning, calendar method
    c. Spermicides
    d. Barrier methods: Condoms, cervical caps, diaphragm
    e. Intrauterine devices
    f. Oral contraceptives
    g. Tubal ligation
    h. Vasectomy
    i. Depo-Provera injection
    j. Contraceptive implants
  4. Explain the benefits of a healthy diet, especially if the patient is breastfeeding.
  5. Discuss breastfeeding, if applicable; answer any questions, and address concerns.
  6. Instruct the patient in breast self-examination, and explain the importance of performing this monthly.
  7. Explain the benefits of an interpregnancy interval of 1 to 2 years.

C. Pharmaceutical therapy—only as indicated from earlier examination.

1. Contraception: See Chapter 14, "Gynecologic Guidelines, Contraception" section.
2. If infection is diagnosed, see section on "Mastitis" or "Endometritis" in this chapter for treatment options.

Follow-Up

A. Administer rubella vaccination if the patient has nonimmune status, administration of vaccine was missed in the hospital stay, and she has not had unprotected intercourse since delivery.

B. If a woman's physical examination and laboratory and Pap tests are normal, she does not require a physical for 1 year.

C. Establish a plan for the woman to obtain Pap smear results (follow-up phone call or letter with results). See the Postpartum Examination sheet (Exhibit 13.2) to use for documentation in the patient's chart.

EXHIBIT 13.2 **Postpartum Examination**

Date: ______

History: Age: ______ G ______ PT ______ P ______ A ______ L ______

Labs: Blood type & Rh: ______ If negative, was RhoGAM workup done and RhoGAM given in the hospital if needed?

Rubella: ______ If nonimmune, was she immunized before hospital discharge? ______

Discharge Hct: ______

Medical and antepartum complications: ______

______

Intrapartum course/complications: ______

______

Delivery: Date: ______ Type: ______ Sex: ______ Birth weight: ______

Apgars: 1 minute: ______ 5 minutes: ______ Neonatal: Gestational age: ______

Complications: ______

Feeding: Breast/bottle: ______ Current infant status: ______

Surgery: BTL: Yes/No ______

If yes, pathology report reviewed: Postpartum complications: ______

Current status: Medical problems: ______

______

Sexual intercourse since delivery/problems: ______

______

Psychosocial/postpartum depression: ______

______

Medications: ______

______

Physical examination: BP: ______ Pulse: ______ Resp. ______ Weight: ______

Breasts: ______

Pelvic: Episiotomy or laceration: ______

Abdomen: ______

Adnexa: ______

Uterus: ______

Vagina: ______

Cervix: ______

Pap smear: Date/results: ______

Plan: Contraception: ______

Referrals: Labs: ______

New prescriptions: ______ Patient Teaching Guides: ______

Other: ______

Signature: ______

BP, blood pressure; BTL, bilateral tubal ligation; Hct, hematocrit.

Postpartum Depression

Jill C. Cash and Susan Drummond

Definition

A. Postpartum depression is a mood disorder characterized by unexplained tearfulness, sadness, irritability, and disturbances in appetite and sleep patterns; inability to care for self or baby; it usually presents within 2 weeks to 3 months postpartum.

Incidence

A. Reported incidence of postpartum depression in the United States is between 8% and 15%.

Pathogenesis

A. It is believed that postpartum depression may be related to psychological, physiological, and cultural factors. The extreme hormonal changes that occur during the postpartum period may contribute. Postpartum thyroiditis is also a suspected factor. However, no confirmed biological cause has been found. Some authorities have suggested that the mother's feeling of "loss of control" over her own life is the underlying precipitating factor.

Predisposing Factors

The following may make a mother more likely to experience postpartum depression:

A. Preterm infant
B. Multiple gestation
C. History of postpartum depression or mental illness
D. Social stressors: Dissatisfaction in the marriage, financial difficulties, and lack of support in the home
E. Age younger than 20 years
F. Single parent
G. Poor relationship with the father of the baby
H. Evidence of significant emotional problems in the past
I. Having experienced separation from one or both parents during childhood or adolescence
J. Having received poor parental support and attention in childhood or having limited social support in adulthood
K. Low self-esteem

Common Complaints

A. Insomnia
B. Poor appetite
C. Tearfulness
D. Fatigue
E. Anxiety
F. Headaches
G. Difficulty concentrating or confusion
H. Feelings of excessive guilt or worthlessness
I. Possible suicidal ideations

Other Signs and Symptoms

A. Mood swings
B. Despondency, social withdrawal, and feeling of inadequacy
C. Guilt
D. Impaired memory
E. Ambivalence about motherhood and baby
F. Inability to care for self and baby
G. Poor grooming of self and/or baby

Subjective Data

A. Elicit the onset, duration, and course of symptoms.
B. Review the patient's medical history for predisposing factors see "Predisposing Factors" in this section.
C. Question the patient regarding her ability to care for her infant, herself, and other family members at home.
D. Review the amount of support in the home. Is she the primary caregiver? Are there any family members or friends who help in the household management, sibling child care, and newborn care?
E. Does the patient get out of bed and dress herself daily?
F. Does the patient have thoughts of harming the infant, herself, or others?

Physical Examination

A. Check temperature, pulse, respirations, and blood pressure (BP).
B. Inspection: Note general overall appearance, including dress, makeup, neatness of hair, tearfulness, and apathy.
C. Observe her interaction with the baby, for example, tone of voice when talking to the baby eye contact, and so on.

Diagnostic Tests

A. Diagnostic tools are available on the Internet, including the Edinburgh Postnatal Depression Scale: www.fresno.ucsf.edu/pediatrics/downloads/edinburghscale.pdf
B. Thyroid panel for diagnosis of depression

Differential Diagnoses

A. Postpartum depression
B. Baby blues: Tearfulness, insomnia, fatigue, headaches, poor appetite, and so on; appearing between the birth and 14 postpartum days
C. Postpartum psychosis: Extreme emotional lability, agitation, delusions, hallucinations, and sleep disturbances
D. Postpartum panic disorder: Extreme anxiety, fear, tightness in the chest, and increased heart rate
E. Postpartum obsessive-compulsive disorder: Obsessive thoughts of harming the child, exaggerated fear of being left alone with the infant, anxiety, depression, and/or unnecessarily vigilant protectiveness of the infant
F. Bipolar disorder

Plan

A. General interventions

1. Assess all patients for postpartum mood disorders at postpartum and all postpartum contacts. See the Blues Questionnaire (Exhibit 13.3) for a sample assessment tool.
2. Early assessment and treatment are very important. Symptoms that are not treated for several weeks may get progressively worse. Patients with severe depression, characterized by suicidal or homicidal ideation, aggressive behavior, delusions, hallucinations, catatonia, poor judgment, or grossly impaired function, are typically hospitalized.
3. Encourage involvement of the patient's partner and immediate family members in the counseling

EXHIBIT 13.3 **Blues Questionnaire**

____________ Days Postpartum: ____________ Date: ____________

Following is a list of words that newly delivered mothers have used to describe how they are feeling. Please indicate HOW YOU HAVE BEEN FEELING TODAY by ticking NO or YES. Then please mark the box that best describes how significant this difference is, if at all from your usual self.

	NO	YES		Much Less Than Usual	Less Than Usual	No Difference	More Than Usual	Much More Than Usual
Tearful			Is this					
Mentally tense			Is this					
Able to concentrate			Is this					
Low spirited			Is this					
Elated			Is this					
Helpless			Is this					
Finding it difficult to show your feelings			Is this					
Alert			Is this					
Forgetful, muddled			Is this					
Anxious			Is this					
Wishing you were alone			Is this					
Mentally relaxed			Is this					
Brooding on things			Is this					
Feeling sorry for yourself			Is this					
Emotionally numb, without feelings			Is this					
Depressed			Is this					
Overemotional			Is this					
Happy			Is this					
Confident			Is this					
Changeable in your spirits			Is this					
Tired			Is this					
Irritable			Is this					
Crying without being able to stop			Is this					
Lively			Is this					
Oversensitive			Is this					
Up and down in your mood			Is this					
Restlessness			Is this					
Calm, tranquil			Is this					

Source: Used with permission from The Royal College of Psychiatrists. Reprinted from Kennerley and Gath (1989).

sessions to assist them in learning ways to assist the patient effectively.

B. Patient teaching

1. Advise the patient that she is not to blame for the condition. Its occurrence is not uncommon and successful treatment is likely.

2. Discuss participation in a support group, interpersonal psychotherapy, or cognitive behavioral therapy.

3. If antidepressants are prescribed, advise the patient that the medication may take 4 to 6 weeks for peak effect. Review the benefits/risks/side effects of the medication prescribed. The risk of suicide may increase after beginning antidepressants; therefore, a follow-up appointment in 1 to 2 weeks is recommended.

C. Pharmaceutical therapy

1. Antidepressants may be ordered for women with moderate to severe symptoms of depression when physical and emotional functioning has been compromised. (Refer to the section "Depression" in Chapter 22, "Psychiatric Guidelines.")
2. Base selection of medication on whether or not the patient is breastfeeding. Selective serotonin reuptake inhibitors (SSRIs) and tricyclic antidepressants are commonly used.
   a. Citalopram (Lexapro) in a single daily dose, usually taken in the morning. Initial dose: 10 mg/d; dosage can be increased at intervals of 1 week to 20 mg.
   b. Sertraline (Zoloft) 50 mg in a single dose at bedtime. Dosage can be increased up to 200 mg/d.
   c. Amitriptyline (Elavil) 75 mg/d in divided doses. Dosage can be increased up to 150 mg/d.

Follow-Up

A. If the patient had risk factors for depression before delivery, a follow-up office visit 3 to 4 days after hospital discharge is suggested.
B. Frequent telephone contact, or several repeat visits, may be necessary during the course of the depression until the symptoms have improved.
C. The risk of suicide may increase after beginning antidepressants; therefore, a follow-up appointment in 1 to 2 weeks is recommended.
D. Assess the patient for suicidal ideation and child neglect at every contact.

Consultation/Referral

A. Assess the need to refer the patient to a psychiatrist, psychologist, or family counselor.
B. Refer to group therapy, interpersonal psychotherapy, and/or cognitive behavioral therapy.
C. Consult a psychiatrist about alternative treatments if no change in signs and symptoms is seen.

Resources

Pacific Postpartum Support Society: www.postpartum.org
Postpartum Support International: www.postpartum.net
Postpartum Support Line: (604) 255–7999

Wound Infection

Jill C. Cash and Susan Drummond

Definition

A. Infection may occur at the site of cesarean section incision, episiotomy, or genital tract laceration. Most wound infections become clinically apparent 5 to 6 days after delivery.

Incidence

A. Rates of infection after cesarean delivery range from five to 30 times greater than vaginal delivery.

Pathogenesis

A. A variety of organisms may be responsible. Examples include *Staphylococcus* or *Streptococcus* species and gram-negative organisms, gram-positive cocci, and *Bacteroides* and *Clostridium* species.

Predisposing Factors

A. Obesity
B. Anemia
C. Malnutrition
D. Smoking
E. Diabetes
F. Substance abuse
G. Susceptible to infection
H. Poor hygiene
I. Lower socioeconomic status
J. Lack of preoperative prophylactic antibiotics

Common Complaints

A. Redness, heat, swelling, and tenderness at site
B. Foul-smelling drainage
C. Elevated temperature

Other Signs and Symptoms

A. Fever and chills
B. Edema
C. Foul-smelling discharge and pus

Subjective Data

A. Elicit the onset, duration, and course of symptoms.
B. Review medical history (see Predisposing Factors); antepartum history for complications such as diabetes; intrapartum complications for prolonged rupture of membranes, fever in labor, use of internal monitoring devices, length of labor, or frequent cervical examinations.
C. Question the patient regarding hygiene at the wound site since delivery, including the frequency of changing Peri-Pads, use of sitz baths, and showering.
D. Question the patient regarding drainage from the wound or episiotomy, noting color, amount, and odor.
E. Review signs and symptoms of breast engorgement and urinary tract infection (UTI).
F. Review vaginal delivery for third- and fourth-degree episiotomy.

Physical Examination

A. Check temperature, pulse, respirations, and blood pressure (BP).
B. **Examination should not be limited to the incision site. A complete physical examination is needed to evaluate breasts, lungs, hematomas, and concurrent UTIs.**
C. Inspect
   1. Examine the incision site (episiotomy or abdomen) for drainage, redness or edema, and intactness.
   2. Inspect bilateral breasts, assessing for erythema, edema, swelling.
   3. Inspect vagina, assessing episiotomy site, lacerations, and hematoma. Evaluate appearance of the lochia.
D. Palpate
   1. Perform breast examination.
   2. Palpate suture line (episiotomy or abdomen). Probe incision with cotton-tipped swab to evaluate for hematoma, cellulitis, and/or pus.
   3. Palpate all abdominal quadrants.
   4. Palpate the vagina to rule out concealed hematoma.
E. Auscultate the heart and lungs.

F. Percuss the back to assess costovertebral angle (CVA) tenderness.

Diagnostic Tests

A. Complete blood count (CBC) with differential
B. Blood culture (optional)
C. Culture of infected area
D. Urinalysis, culture, and sensitivity, if indicated

Differential Diagnoses

A. Wound infection
B. Impending dehiscence. If serosanguinous drainage is noted after the first 24 hours, dehiscence is possible.
C. Episiotomy breakdown

Plan

A. General interventions

1. The wound may need to be opened and cleaned.
2. For an infection at a cesarean section site, wound irrigation and dressing changes several times a day may be necessary.
3. Home health referral may be needed.

▶ **B.** Patient teaching: *See Section III: Patient Teaching Guide for this chapter, "Wound Infection: Episiotomy and Cesarean Section."*

1. Instruct patient on self-care for episiotomy or cesarean section incision site. Instructions on cleaning episiotomy/cesarean incision site should be reinforced.

C. Dietary management

1. No dietary restrictions are recommended; encourage the patient to eat well-balanced meals. Increase protein in the diet for wound healing.
2. Instruct the patient to increase fluid intake; have her drink at least 10 to 12 glasses of liquid a day.

D. Pharmaceutical therapy

1. Augmentin 875 mg twice a day for 7 to 10 days
2. Clindamycin 450 mg every 6 hours for 7 to 10 days; safe for breastfeeding
3. Cefoxitin 1 to 2 g by IM injection or IV infusion every 6 to 8 hours; safe for breastfeeding
4. Acetaminophen (Tylenol) when required for elevated temperature.

Follow-Up

A. Reevaluate the patient in 48 hours to assess wound healing.

Consultation/Referral

A. Consult a physician for evaluation and possible surgical closure.

Bibliography

Abdul-Kadir, R., McLintock, C., Ducloy, A. S., El-Refaey, H., England, A., Federici, A. B., . . . Winikoff, R. (2014). Evaluation and management of postpartum hemorrhage: Consensus from an international expert panel. *Transfusion, 54*(7), 1756–1768.

American Academy of Pediatrics 'Committee on Fetus and Newborn, & American College of Obstetricians and Gynecologists' Committee on Obstetric Practice; Riley, L., Stark, A. R., Kilpatrick, S. J., & Riley, L. E. (2012). *Guidelines for perinatal care* (7th ed.). Elk Grove Village, IL: American College of Obstetricians and Gynecologists.

American College of Obstetricians and Gynecologists. (2005, September). The importance of preconception care in the continuum of women's health care. *ACOG Committee Opinion,* Number 313, reaffirmed 2015.

American College of Obstetricians and Gynecologists. (2006, October). Postpartum hemorrhage. *ACOG Practice Bulletin,* Number 76, reaffirmed 2015.

American College of Obstetricians and Gynecologists. (2008a, July). Anemia in pregnancy. *ACOG Practice Bulletin,* Number 95, reaffirmed 2015.

American College of Obstetricians and Gynecologists. (2008b, June). Medical management of ectopic pregnancy. *ACOG Practice Bulletin,* Number 94, reaffirmed 2014.

American College of Obstetricians and Gynecologists. (2010, August). Moderate caffeine consumption during pregnancy. *ACOG Committee Opinion,* Number 462, reaffirmed 2015.

American College of Obstetricians and Gynecologists. (2012, October). Prediction and prevention of preterm birth. *ACOG Practice Bulletin,* Number 130, reaffirmed 2016.

American College of Obstetricians and Gynecologists. (2013, August). Gestational diabetes mellitus. *ACOG Practice Bulletin,* Number 137, reaffirmed 2015.

American College of Obstetricians and Gynecologists Task Force on Hypertension in Pregnancy. (2013). *Hypertension in pregnancy.* Washington, DC: American College of Obstetricians and Gynecologists.

American College of Obstetricians and Gynecologists. (2014, July). Antepartum fetal surveillance. *ACOG Practice Bulletin,* Number 145.

American College of Obstetricians and Gynecologists. (2015a, September). Nausea and vomiting of pregnancy. *ACOG Practice Bulletin,* Number 153.

American College of Obstetricians and Gynecologists. (2015b, December). Obesity in pregnancy. *ACOG Practice Bulletin,* Number 156.

American College of Obstetricians and Gynecologists. (2016a, October). Management of preterm labor. *ACOG Practice Bulletin,* Number 159.

American College of Obstetricians and Gynecologists (2016b, October). Premature rupture of membranes. *ACOG Practice Bulletin,* Number 160.

American Diabetes Association. (2016). Standards of medical care in diabetes—2016. *Diabetes Care, 39*(Suppl. 1), S4–S5.

Barash, J. H., Buchanan, E. M., & Hillson, C. (2014). Diagnosis and management of ectopic pregnancy. *American Family Physician, 90*(1), 34–40.

Barton, J. R., & Sibai, B. M. (2008). Prediction and prevention of recurrent preeclampsia. *Obstetrics & Gynecology, 112*(2 Pt. 1), 359–372.

Bell, R., Glinianaia, S. V., Tennant, P. W., Rankin, J., & Bilous, R. W. (2012). Peri-conception hyperglycaemia and nephropathy are associated with risk of congenital anomaly in women with pre-existing diabetes: A population-based cohort study. *Diabetologia, 55,* 936–947.

Cash, J. C. (2014). Assessment of the childbearing woman. In J. Weber & J. Kelley (Eds.), *Health assessment in nursing* (5th ed., pp. 665–692). Philadelphia, PA: Lippincott-Raven.

Centers for Disease Control and Prevention. (2010). Prevention of perinatal Group B streptococcal disease. Revised guidelines from CDC. *Morbidity and Mortality Weekly Report, 2010,* 59(RR10); 1–32.

De-Regil, L. M., Peña-Rosas, J. P., Fernández-Gaxiola, A. C., & Rayco-Solon, P. (2015). Effects and safety of periconceptional oral folate supplementation for preventing birth defects. *Cochrane Database of Systemic Reviews, 2015*(2), CD007950.

Hale, T. W. (2014). *Medications and mother's milk* (16th ed.). Amarillo, TX: Hale.

Jovanovic, L., Savas, H., Mehta, M., Trujillo, A., & Pettitt, D. J. (2011). Frequent monitoring of A1C during pregnancy as a treatment tool to guide therapy. *Diabetes Care, 34*(1), 53–54.

Kennerley, H., & Gath, D. (1989). Maternity blues. I. Detection and measurement by questionnaire. *British Journal of Psychiatry, 155,* 356–362. Retrieved from http://bjp.rcpsych.org/content/155/3/356.long

Kuhrt, K., Smout, E., Hezelgrave, N., Seed, P. T., Carter, J., & Shennan, A. H. (2016). Development and validation of a tool incorporating cervical length and quantitative fetal fibronectin to predict spontaneous preterm birth in asymptomatic high-risk women. *Ultrasound in Obstetrics & Gynecology: The Official Journal of the International Society of Ultrasound in Obstetrics and Gynecology, 47*(1), 104–109.

Morbidity and Mortality Weekly Trend. (2013). Preterm births—United States 2006–2010. Retrieved from www.cdc.gov/mmwr/preview/mmwrhtml/su6203a22.htm

Nelson, D. B., Freeman, M. P., Johnson, N. L., McIntire, D. D., & Leveno, K. J. (2013). A prospective study of postpartum depression in 17 648 parturients. *Journal of Maternal–Fetal & Neonatal Medicine: The Official Journal of the European Association of Perinatal Medicine, the Federation of Asia and Oceania Perinatal Societies, the International Society of Perinatal Obstetricians, 26*(12), 1155–1161.

Nettina, S. (Ed.). (2013). *Lippincott manual of nursing practice* (10th ed.). Philadelphia, PA: Wolters Kluwer Health/Lippincott Williams & Wilkins.

Varney, H., Kriebs, J. M., & Gregor, C. L. (2013). *Varney's midwifery* (5th ed.). Sudbury, MA: Jones & Bartlett.

14 Gynecologic Guidelines

Amenorrhea

Rhonda Arthur

Definition

Amenorrhea is absence of menstruation when menstrual periods should occur.

A. Primary amenorrhea

1. No menstrual period by age 14 years in the absence of growth or development of secondary sexual characteristics

2. No menstrual period by age 16 years regardless of the presence of normal growth and development with the appearance of secondary sexual characteristics

B. Secondary amenorrhea: No menstrual period for 6 months in a woman who usually has normal periods, or for a length of time equal to three-cycle intervals in a woman with less-frequent cycles.

Incidence

A. Amenorrhea in a woman who has had menstrual periods is quite common at some time during her reproductive life. Amenorrhea that is a result of agenesis of part of the reproductive system or a chromosomal anomaly is quite rare. See the following for the incidence of each cause.

Pathogenesis

A. Physiological: Pregnancy, breastfeeding, and menopause

B. Disorders of the central nervous system (hypothalamic): Hypothalamic amenorrhea is the most common cause of amenorrhea (28%). There is a deficiency in pulsatile secretion of gonadotropin-releasing hormone (Gn-RH). Examples include a stressful lifestyle (10%); weight loss as in anorexia or bulimia (10%); extreme exercise; medications, such as hormones, as in postpill amenorrhea; hypothyroidism (10%); and major medical disease such as Crohn's disease or systemic lupus erythematosus (SLE).

C. Disorders of the outflow tract or uterine target organ: Abnormalities in the systems of this compartment are uncommon. Examples include Asherman's syndrome from inadvertent endometrial ablation during dilation and curettage (D&C; causes 7% of amenorrhea); and agenesis or structural anomalies of the uterus, tubes, or vagina.

D. Disorders of the ovary: Examples include abnormal chromosomes such as Turner's syndrome (0.5%); normal chromosomes (10%) such as in gonadal dysgenesis or agenesis (there may be no or very delayed Tanner stage); premature ovarian failure (POF); premature menopause, before the age of 40 years; effect of radiation or chemotherapy; and polycystic ovarian (PCO) disease.

E. Disorders of the anterior pituitary: Examples include prolactin tumors (7.5%).

Predisposing Factor

A. The disorder can affect any female between the ages of 14 and 55 years.

Common Complaints

A. "I haven't had a period in months." "I have periods only a few times each year."

B. "I have nipple discharge."

C. "I am 16 years old and have never had a menstrual period."

Other Signs and Symptoms

A. Irregular, infrequent menstrual periods

B. Galactorrhea

C. Pregnancy

D. Excessive hair growth

Subjective Data

A. Review complete menstrual history, including age of onset, duration, frequency, regularity, and dysmenorrhea.

B. Review the patient's pregnancy history.

C. Review the patient's contraception history.

D. Note other medications the patient is taking, such as hormones or antidepressants.

E. Ask the patient if she has had a major medical disease or treatment such as chemotherapy for a childhood cancer.

F. Inquire about any breast discharge.

G. Review the patient's weight pattern.

H. Ask the patient to describe her physical self-image. Does she consider herself obese or fat?

I. Review sources of stress in her life.

J. Discuss exercise pattern and history.

Physical Examination

A. Check height, weight, blood pressure (BP), and pulse.

B. Inspect

1. Note overall appearance. Look at the neck (thyroid). Inspect the breast/genitalia for Tanner staging. See Appendix C: Tanner's Sexual Maturity Stages.

2. Skin assessment: Check for central hair growth, which is androgen-responsive. Areas to inspect for coarse hair include the upper lip, chin, sideburns, neck, chest, lower abdomen, and perineum.

C. Palpate

1. The neck for thyroid enlargement

2. The abdomen for enlarged organs or uterine enlargement compatible with pregnancy

D. Auscultate

1. Auscultate the heart and lungs.

2. If pregnancy is suspected, consider auscultating for fetal heart tones.

E. Pelvic examination

1. Inspect external genitalia. Note pubic hair pattern for Tanner staging. Note any lesions, masses, or discharge.

2. Speculum examination: Inspect vagina and cervix. Note bluish color, which is Chadwick's sign with pregnancy.

3. Bimanual examination: Palpate for softening of the cervical isthmus, which is Hegar's sign for pregnancy. Palpate for size of uterus and for adnexal masses.

Diagnostic Tests

A. Urine: Pregnancy test

B. Serum

1. Serum human chorionic gonadotropin (HCG)

2. Thyroid-stimulating hormone (TSH) to rule out thyroid disease

3. Prolactin: Normal less than 20 ng/mL

4. Follicle-stimulating hormone (FSH): Greater than 40 IU/mL indicates ovarian failure

5. Luteinizing hormone (LH): FSH ratio to rule out polycystic ovaries

C. Vaginal and/or pelvic ultrasonography

D. Genetic testing/karotype analysis in primary amenorrhea

Differential Diagnoses

A. Amenorrhea

B. Pregnancy

C. Constitutional delay

D. Hypothyroidism

E. Polycystic ovary syndrome (PCOS)

F. POF, or early menopause

G. Perimenopause

H. Pituitary adenoma

I. Androgen insensitivity syndrome

Plan

A. General interventions

1. If laboratory values are normal, proceed to progesterone challenge test to rule out hypothalamic amenorrhea.

2. If the patient is pregnant, counsel regarding pregnancy and begin antepartum care.

3. If other laboratory information points to an underlying cause for amenorrhea, treat as appropriate.

▶ **B.** Patient teaching: *See Section III: Patient Teaching Guide for this chapter, "Amenorrhea."*

C. Pharmaceutical therapy

1. Progesterone challenge

a. Micronized progesterone (Prometrium) 300 mg daily or medroxyprogesterone acetate (Provera) 10 mg each day for 5 days.

b. Positive test is any vaginal bleeding. Withdrawal bleeding should occur within 7 to 10 days after finishing the medicine. A late vaginal bleed may be associated with ovulation.

c. In the absence of galactorrhea, with a normal prolactin level, normal TSH, and positive progesterone challenge, further evaluation is unnecessary.

> *All anovulatory patients require therapeutic management. There is a risk of endometrial cancer with unopposed estrogen. There is a short latent period in progression from a normal endometrium to atypia to cancer, even in a young woman.*

A negative withdrawal bleed may be associated with PCOS.

2. Progesterone therapy for hypothalamic amenorrhea

a. Medroxyprogesterone acetate (Provera, Cycrin) 10 mg for 10 days each month

b. Low-dose oral contraceptive pills

c. Clomiphene citrate for women desiring pregnancy

d. Hormone replacement therapy (HRT) for perimenopausal women

Follow-Up

A. Reproductive age: The patient should return after 6 months of treatment with progesterone or oral contraceptive pills. Discontinue the hormones and assess for return of normal periods. If this does not occur, reinstitute progesterone or oral contraceptive therapy.

B. Perimenopausal: Maintain hormonal therapy. The patient should return annually.

Consultation/Referral

A. Refer the patient to a physician if there is no withdrawal bleeding from the progesterone challenge. The problem is either with the outflow track, which is rare, or with the ovarian production of estrogen or hypothalamic production of gonadotropins. This is usually beyond the scope of the nurse practitioner.

B. Refer the patient to a physician if her prolactin level is elevated (greater than 20 mg/mL) for further workup to rule out pituitary adenoma.

Individual Considerations

A. Adolescence

1. Rule out pregnancy. Then determine whether primary or secondary amenorrhea. Refer the patient to a physician for primary amenorrhea.

2. For secondary amenorrhea, complete assessment and evaluation. Assess stress/emotional status, nutritional status, and exercise routine.

3. Refer to a physician if there is no withdrawal bleeding from progesterone challenge test.

4. Refer for evaluation and treatment as indicated for eating, exercise, or psychiatric disorders.

B. Older adults

1. Irregular menses and amenorrhea are common during perimenopause. Provide anticipatory guidance and instructions regarding the need for contraceptive use until menopause is confirmed.

Atrophic Vaginitis

Rhonda Arthur

Definition

A. Atrophic vaginitis is inflammation of the vaginal epithelium due to a lack of estrogen support. Anything that lowers estrogen levels after puberty can result in a loss of vaginal thickness and rugosity and a decrease in the elasticity of the vaginal tissues.

Incidence

A. Atrophic vaginitis is very common. It may occur in three stages of a woman's life: Preadolescence, when breastfeeding a baby, and postmenopause.

Pathogenesis

A. Estrogen maintains the vaginal pH in an acidic range. Lack of sufficient estrogen promotes an increase in vaginal pH that supports the development of bacterial infections. Estrogen loss also results in a decrease in vaginal glycogen and a thin-walled epithelium, promoting friability and inflammation.

Predisposing Factors

A. Preadolescence
B. Breastfeeding
C. Postmenopause
D. Ovarian failure

Common Complaints

A. Vaginal dryness, irritation, and/or bleeding
B. Dyspareunia
C. Dysuria

Other Signs and Symptoms

A. Postcoital bleeding
B. Thin vaginal discharge
C. Vaginal itching

Subjective Data

A. Question the patient regarding onset, duration, and course of symptoms.

B. Is this a new problem? If so, review the use of a new soap, laundry detergent, or hygiene products.

C. Describe the color, amount, and odor of vaginal discharge or bleeding.

D. Determine existence of coexisting vasomotor symptoms, such as hot flashes.

E. Is the patient experiencing dysuria, urinary frequency, vulvar dryness and itching, or dyspareunia? With dyspareunia, question the patient whether the discomfort is due to irritation or pain with deep penetration, or both.

F. Determine whether the patient is breastfeeding and for what length of time.

G. Ask the patient the date of her last menses and if she is having irregular cycles. Determine whether the patient had a hysterectomy with oophorectomy or ovarian failure.

H. Review the number of the patient's sexual partners and any new sexual practices.

I. Review the patient's current medications, including antidepressants.

J. Explore whether she has stopped hormone replacement therapy (HRT).

K. Has the patient tried any self-help measures? Was there any relief?

L. When was the last Papanicolaou (Pap) smear, and what were the results?

Physical Examination

A. Check temperature, pulse, and respirations.

B. Inspect: Observe the patient generally for discomfort before, during, and after examination.

C. Palpate

1. Back: Check for costovertebral angle (CVA) tenderness.
2. Abdomen: Note suprapubic tenderness.

Pelvic Examination

A. Inspect

1. Examine external genitalia for friability, erythema, lesions, condyloma, and amount and color of discharge.
2. Sparse and brittle pubic hair, shrinking of the labia minora, and inflammation of the vulva may be noted in menopausal women.
3. The vulva may appear erythematous, and there may be labial edema.
4. Excoriation may be present if the woman has complained of pruritus.

B. Palpate: "Milk" urethra for discharge to rule out infection.

C. Speculum examination

1. Check rugae, friability of vaginal epithelium, and color and amount of discharge; evaluate cervix for lesions, friability, and erythema.
2. Typical atrophic symptoms on inspection: Thin, friable vaginal epithelium; decreased or absent vaginal rugae; scant vaginal discharge

D. Bimanual examination

1. Check for cervical motion tenderness (CMT), uterine size, and position (if no hysterectomy).
2. Check adnexa for masses.

Diagnostic Tests

A. Routine hormone measurements to evaluate menopause status are not routinely indicated.

B. Urine culture, if applicable
C. Vaginal pH; normal pH range in premenopausal women is 4 to 4.5. Reduced levels of estrogen increase vaginal pH.
D. Pap smear with maturation index. (Vaginal wall maturation index evaluation is controversial.)
E. Wet prep, if applicable
1. Multiple white blood cells (WBCs) indicate inflammation, may show increased bacteria, and may have decreased lactobacillus, suggesting atrophic vaginitis.
2. Test should be negative for *Trichomonas.* Bacterial vaginosis (BV): Whiff test should be negative.
F. Cultures for gonorrhea and chlamydia, if applicable.
G. Ultrasound for uterine lining thickness if applicable (less than 4 or 5 mm suggests loss of estrogenic stimulation).
H. Endometrial biopsy, if indicated.

Postmenopausal vaginal bleeding must be thoroughly investigated to rule out the possibility of endometrial hyperplasia or endometrial cancer.

Differential Diagnoses

A. Atrophic vaginitis
B. Trauma
C. Foreign body in the vagina
D. Urinary tract infection (UTI)
E. Vaginitis from infective cause: Fungus, bacteria, or virus
F. Contact irritation: Latex (condom), spermicide, lubricant
G. Menopause

Plan

A. General interventions
1. Treat any underlying infections (gonorrhea, chlamydia, vaginitis, as diagnosed).
B. Patient teaching
1. *See Section III: Patient Teaching Guides for this chapter, "Atrophic Vaginitis" and "Dyspareunia (Pain With Intercourse)."*
2. Preadolescent girls have amelioration of symptoms with increase of endogenous estrogen as puberty approaches.
3. Women should be reassured that this problem is physical, not emotional.
4. Discuss the benefits of regular sexual activity to decrease problems of atrophic vaginitis. An important reason for decreased sexual activity is unavailability of a partner. Masturbation also facilitates the natural resumption of the production of lubricating secretions by the body. Decline in sexuality is influenced by culture and attitudes as well as physical problems.
5. Symptomatic relief of dryness during sexual activity may be obtained with the use of water-soluble lubricants and adequate foreplay.
6. Vaginal moisturizer may be applied for relief of symptoms.
7. Discuss pregnancy prevention and inform that perimenopausal symptoms do not ensure lack of fertility.
C. Pharmaceutical therapy
1. Calamine lotion may be applied externally for local symptomatic relief.
2. Estrogen therapy (ET)
a. Vaginal hormonal therapy

Absolute contraindications for use of ET also apply to use of topical estrogen (breast cancer, active liver disease, history of recent thromboembolic event). Vaginal estrogen creams are systemically absorbed. As with use of oral and transdermal estrogen, a progestin must be administered to women who have an intact uterus, secondary to the risk of endometrial hyperplasia or cancer.

i. Conjugated estrogen (Premarin) cream 0.625 mg/g: Use 0.5- to 1.0-g applicator inserted intravaginally at bedtime every night for 1 to 2 weeks, then every other night for 1 to 2 weeks, then as needed. Not for daily use if the patient has an intact uterus.
ii. Estradiol (Estrace) 0.1 mg/g: Use one half (2 g) to one (4 g) applicator inserted intravaginally at bedtime every night for 1 to 2 weeks. When vaginal mucosa is restored, maintenance dose is one-quarter applicator (1 g) one to three times weekly in a cyclic regimen. Not for daily use if the patient has an intact uterus.

Vaginal estrogen creams should not be used as a lubricant before intercourse as the hormone can be absorbed through a partner's skin.

Vaginal estrogen creams are systemically absorbed. As with use of oral and transdermal estrogen, a progestin must be administered to women who have an intact uterus, secondary to the risk of endometrial hyperplasia or cancer.

iii. Estradiol (Estring) 7.5 mcg/24 hr; insert one ring in vagina and replace every 90 days.
iv. Estradiol hemihydrate (Vagifem) vaginal tablets 25 mg; insert: One tablet in vagina each day for 14 days, then one tablet twice weekly for 10 weeks.
b. Oral estrogen replacement therapy
i. Conjugated estrogen (Premarin) 0.625 mg orally every day from day 1 through 25, of a month plus conjugated estrogen (Provera) 10 mg orally on days 13 through 25.
ii. See "Menopause" section for other regimens of hormone replacement therapy (HRT).

For long-term ET, consider use of oral or patch methods of delivery if the patient shows additional symptoms of hypoestrogenemia (i.e., hot flashes, night sweats).

Follow-Up

A. Breastfeeding women should be reevaluated following weaning, especially if symptoms persist (i.e., alternate etiology is suspected).
B. Postmenopausal women should be evaluated for additional etiologies (i.e., endometrial hyperplasia) if vaginal bleeding persists beyond 3 to 6 months following a treatment.
C. The patient should return to clinic 1 to 2 months after beginning oral or vaginal drug therapy; the patient then needs to be seen in 3 to 6 months to check side effects, blood pressure (BP), and response to therapy.
D. Perform Pap smears and physical examination per patient health history or risks and guidelines.

Consultation/Referral

A. If bleeding is a symptom in a postmenopausal woman, the practitioner must rule out bleeding of uterine origin. If there is any doubt, consultation for endometrial biopsy or dilation and curettage (D&C) must be obtained.

Individual Considerations

A. Breastfeeding women
  1. Breastfeeding women have amelioration of symptoms as weaning progresses unless an alternate etiology exists.
B. Postmenopausal women
  1. Evaluate the patient for other risks of hypoestrogenemia, such as cardiovascular disease and osteoporosis. Continuous systemic estrogen replacement therapy may be indicated.
  2. Vaginitis in the postmenopausal woman is rarely due to any of the organisms responsible for vaginitis in the premenopausal woman (unless she has new sexual partners). Candidiasis, trichomoniasis, and BV are uncommon after the menstruating years.

Bacterial Vaginosis (or Gardnerella)

Rhonda Arthur

Definition

A. Bacterial vaginosis (BV) is an infection of the vagina caused by an alteration in the normal flora of the vagina, with an increase in anaerobes and gram-negative bacilli as well as a decrease in the *Lactobacillus* flora.

Incidence

A. BV is one of the most common vaginal infections in women of childbearing age and is common in pregnant women. It is not considered exclusively a sexually transmitted infection (STI).

Pathogenesis

A. The main etiologic agent in BV is an increase in anaerobes in the vagina. The reason why this occurs is unknown, but is associated with having multiple sexual partners, douching, lack of condom use, and lack of vaginal lactobacilli. When the normal lactobacilli of the vagina decrease, the vaginal pH is increased. The organisms present in BV cause the level of vaginal amines to be high. These amines are volatilized when the pH is increased, causing the characteristic "fishy" odor.
B. Bacterial vaginitis is primarily polymicrobial, and the pathogens seen include *Bacteroides* species, *Peptostreptococcus* species, *Eubacterium* species, *Mobiluncus* species, *Gardnerella*, and *Mycoplasma hominis*. The incubation period is unknown.

Predisposing Factors

A. History of STIs
B. Multiple sexual partners
C. Intrauterine device (IUD) use
D. Factors that change the normal vaginal flora
  1. Hormonal changes (menses, pregnancy)
  2. Medications: Oral contraceptive use and antibiotic therapy
  3. Foreign bodies in the vagina (tampons, IUDs), semen, and douching

Common Complaints

A. Vaginal discharge (thin, white, gray, or milky)
B. Fishy vaginal odor
C. Postcoital odor

Other Signs and Symptoms

A. Asymptomatic
B. Increase in odor after menses
C. Occasional itching and burning

Subjective Data

A. Elicit onset, duration, and course of presenting symptoms.
B. Review any changes in the characteristics and color of vaginal discharge. Does the patient's partner(s) have any symptoms?
C. Review any symptoms of pruritus, perineal excoriation, burning; signs of urinary tract infection (UTI).
D. Review medication and medical history.
E. Determine whether the patient is pregnant; note the date of last menstrual period (LMP).
F. Question the patient for a history of STIs or other vaginal infections.
G. Review previous infection, treatment, compliance with treatment, and results.
H. Note the last intercourse date.
I. Elicit information about possible foreign body.
J. Review use of vaginal deodorants or sprays, scented toilet paper, tampons, pads, and douching habits.
K. Review change in laundry detergent, soaps, and fabric softeners.
L. Review use of tight restrictive clothing, tight jeans, and nylon panties.
M. Review history for seizures and anticoagulant therapy.

Physical Examination

A. Check temperature, pulse, and respirations.
B. Inspect: Examine external vulva and introitus for discharge, irritation, fissures, lesions, rashes, and condyloma.

C. Palpate

1. Palpate the abdomen for masses or tenderness. Note enlarged or tender inguinal lymph nodes.
2. Palpate the external perineal area for vulvar masses.
3. "Milk" the urethra for discharge.
4. Check for costovertebral angle (CVA) tenderness.

D. Pelvic examination

1. Inspect
   - **a.** Note the color, amount, and odor of discharge.
   - **b.** Inspect the cervix.
     - **i.** BV is a vaginosis rather than a vaginitis. There is usually little or no inflammation of the vaginal epithelium associated with BV.
     - **ii.** BV is associated with a pink, healthy cervix; "strawberry cervix" is seen with cervicitis due to *Trichomonas vaginalis.*
     - **iii.** A red, edematous, friable cervix is seen with *Chlamydia trachomatis.*
2. Speculum examination
   - **a.** Inspect sidewalls for adhering discharge.
   - **b.** The clinical diagnosis of BV requires the presence of three of the following four signs:
     - **i.** Homogeneous, white, adherent vaginal discharge may be present.
     - **ii.** Vaginal fluid pH greater than 4.5. For accurate pH, take smear for testing from the lateral walls of the vagina, not from the cervix.
     - **iii.** A fishy, amine-like odor from vaginal fluid before or after mixing it with 10% potassium hydroxide (positive whiff test). Semen releases the vaginal amines; therefore, there is an increase in odor after intercourse.
     - **iv.** Presence of "clue cells" (squamous vaginal epithelial cells covered with bacteria, causing a stippled or granular appearance and ragged, "moth-eaten" borders) or coccobacilli forms both in the fluid and adheres to the epithelial cells.
3. Bimanual examination: Check for cervical motion tenderness (CMT) and adnexal masses. BV may be a risk factor for pelvic inflammatory disease (PID).

Diagnostic Tests

A. Gram stain (considered the gold standard)

B. BV can be diagnosed by use of clinical criteria; three of the following four are needed to make clinical diagnosis (Amsel's diagnostic criteria [DC]):

1. Vaginal pH: Greater than 4.5 with BV; normal vaginal pH range is 4 to 4.5
2. Clue cells on microscopic examination
3. Homogeneous, thick white discharge that coats the vaginal walls
4. A fishy odor of the vaginal discharge before or after the addition of 10% KOH (wet prep with 10% potassium hydroxide and normal saline prep); microscopic examination of vaginal secretions should always be done

C. Herpes culture, if indicated

D. Urinalysis and culture, if indicated

Differential Diagnoses

A. BV
B. Vulvovaginal candidiasis
C. Trichomoniasis
D. Gonorrhea
E. Chlamydia
F. Presence of foreign body
G. Normal physiological discharge

Plan

A. General interventions

1. Inform the patient regarding other modalities for treating BV. These methods include the following:
   - **a.** Vinegar and water douches: One tablespoon of white vinegar in 1 pint of water. Douche one to two times a week.
   - **b.** *Lactobacillus acidophilus* culture; four to six tablets by mouth daily
   - **c.** Garlic suppositories: One peeled clove of garlic wrapped in a cloth dipped in olive oil inserted vaginally overnight and changed daily

B. Patient teaching

1. *See Section III: Patient Teaching Guides for this chapter, "Bacterial Vaginosis."* ◀
2. BV is not considered an STI.

C. Pharmaceutical therapy

1. Drug of choice
   - **a.** Metronidazole (Flagyl) 500 mg orally twice daily for 7 days *or*
   - **b.** Metronidazole gel 0.75% one applicator (5 g) vaginally at bedtime for 5 days
     - **i.** Metronidazole is less expensive, easier to use, and associated with greater compliance.
     - **ii.** Side effects of metronidazole include sharp, unpleasant metallic taste in the mouth; furry tongue; central nervous system (CNS) reactions, including seizures; and urinary tract disturbances. Advise patients to avoid alcohol while taking metronidazole and 24 hours after completing the medication, or they will experience the severe side effects of abdominal distress, nausea, vomiting, and headache.
     - **iii.** Metronidazole may prolong prothrombin time in patients taking oral anticoagulants.
2. Other medications if the patient is unable to use oral metronidazole
   - **a.** Clindamycin 300 mg by mouth twice daily for 7 days
   - **b.** Metronidazole gel (MetroGel) 0.75% one applicator vaginally twice daily for 5 days
   - **c.** Clindamycin 2% cream one applicator vaginally at bedtime for 7 days

> *Clindamycin cream is oil based and may weaken latex condoms for at least 72 hours after terminating therapy.*

3. Special considerations: Pregnancy
BV has been associated with adverse pregnancy outcomes; therefore, all symptomatic pregnant women and asymptomatic women at high risk for preterm delivery require treatment.
    a. Metronidazole 500 mg orally twice a day for 7 days or 0.75% metronidazole gel 5 g vaginally once daily for 5 days
    b. Clindamycin 300 mg orally twice a day for 7 days

Follow-Up

A. Nonpregnant women: No follow-up is recommended unless indicated. Recurrence is common.
B. Pregnancy: High risk for preterm delivery; pregnant women should be reevaluated 1 month after treatment.
C. Immunocompromised women: Recommendations for treatment of BV in females infected with HIV are the same as for noninfected patients.
D. Partners: Consider treatment of the patient's partner(s) in women with recurrent disease.

Consultation/Referral

A. Refer the patient to a physician for recurrence that is unresponsive to therapies.

Individual Considerations

A. Pregnancy
    1. Clindamycin cream may be associated with increased adverse events in newborns and should not be used during the second half of pregnancy.
B. Partners
    1. Routine treatment of a patient's partner(s) is not recommended at this time because it does not influence relapse or recurrence rates.

Bartholin's Cyst or Abscess

Rhonda Arthur

Definition

A. The Bartholin's glands are small, round, nonpalpable mucus-secreting organs. They are located bilaterally in the posterolateral vaginal orifice. Obstruction of the duct causes the gland to swell with mucus and form a Bartholin's cyst. The cause of obstruction is usually unknown but may be due to mechanical trauma, thickened mucus, neoplasm, stenosis of the duct, or infectious organisms not limited to sexually transmitted infections (STIs). The cyst may become infected, resulting in an abscess. Cysts develop more commonly in younger women, and occurrence decreases with aging; therefore, it is important to rule out neoplasm in women older than 40 years experiencing Bartholin's cyst.
B. The majority of women with Bartholin's cyst are asymptomatic, but large cysts can cause pressure and interfere with walking and sexual intercourse. Abscesses generally develop rapidly over a 2- to 3-day period and are painful. Some abscesses may spontaneously rupture and often reoccur.

Predisposing Factors

A. History of STIs
B. Local trauma

Common Complaints

A. Cysts can be asymptomatic and found incidentally on physical examination.
B. Localized pain/irritation
C. Dyspareunia
D. Difficulty walking or sitting due to edema

Subjective Data

A. Elicit onset, duration, and course of presenting symptoms.
B. Review any changes in the characteristics and color of vaginal discharge. Does the patient's partner(s) have any symptoms?
C. Review any symptoms of pruritus, perineal excoriation, burning; signs of urinary tract infection (UTI).
D. Review the patient's medication and medical history.
E. Determine whether the patient is pregnant; note the date of last menstrual period (LMP).
F. Question the patient for a history of STIs or other vaginal infections.
G. Review previous infection, treatment, compliance with treatment, and results.
H. Note last intercourse date.

Physical Examination

A. Inspect
    1. Examine external vulva and introitus for discharge, irritation, fissures, lesions, and rashes. Bartholin's cyst will appear as a round mass usually near the vaginal orifice causing vulvar asymmetry.
B. Palpate
    1. Bartholin's glands. Cysts are usually unilateral, tense, nontender, and without erythema. An abscess is usually unilateral, tense, erythematous, and painful on palpation.

Diagnostic Tests

A. Culture and sensitivity of purulent abscess fluid
B. Cervical culture for STI (*Neisseria gonorrhoeae* and *Chlamydia trachomatis*)
C. Excisional biopsy in women older than 40 years

Differential Diagnoses

A. Bartholin's cyst
B. Bartholin's abscess
C. Neoplasm
D. STI
E. Sebaceous cyst

Plan

A. General interventions
    1. Reassurance is indicated for women younger than 40 years with asymptomatic cysts. Incision and drainage (I&D) is often required for symptomatic cysts and abscesses. Because cysts and abscesses often reoccur,

surgery to create a permanent opening from the duct to the exterior is often the definitive treatment. Two such surgical methods are placement of a Word catheter or marsupialization. Referral is indicated for I&D and other surgical interventions if the provider is not experienced with the procedures.

Women older than 40 years must be referred for surgical exploration and excision biopsy.

B. Patient teaching

1. Reassure women younger than 40 years that asymptomatic cysts do not need intervention. Rapidly enlarging cysts that are painful or obstruct the vaginal orifice need to be reevaluated.

2. Warm sitz baths three or four times a day may encourage spontaneous rupture of abscess and provide comfort.

C. Pharmaceutical therapy

1. Abscesses are treated with an antibiotic that covers methicillin-resistant *Staphylococcus aureus* (MRSA) such as trimethoprim 160/sulfamethazone 800 mg twice a day or amoxicillin/clavulanate 875 mg bid for 7 days plus clindamycin 300 mg orally four times a day for 7 days.

Follow-Up

A. Follow-up with provider if not improved in 3 to 7 days.

B. Report to care provider if symptoms reoccur.

Consultation/Referral

A. Refer the patient to a physician for recurrence that is unresponsive to therapies.

Individual Considerations

A. Older adults

1. Refer women older than 40 years with cyst for excisional biopsy.

B. Pregnancy: Treatment with antibiotics is recommended due to the risk of complicated infection. Avoid the use of trimethoprin/sulfamethazone during pregnancy. Refer to obstetrics and gynecology (OB/GYN) for recurrence.

Breast Pain

Rhonda Arthur

Definition

A. Benign breast disorders such as mastalgia, mastodynia, and fibrocystic breast changes are characterized by lumps or pain. The lumps may be a physiological nodularity, a ropy thickening, or distended fluid-filled cysts that are mobile. The pain may be cyclic or noncyclic, and it may be unilateral or bilateral.

Incidence

A. This is a very common problem. Fifty percent or more of menstruating women experience breast pain. Two thirds of breast pain is cyclic and occurs in women in their 30s; one third is noncyclic and may occur in women at any age, but it tends to occur in women closer to menopause.

Pathogenesis

A. Dysplastic, benign histologic changes occur in the breast such as hyperplasia of the breast epithelium, adenosis microcysts and macrocysts, duct ectasia, and apocrine metaplasia.

Predisposing Factors

A. Menstruation (related to hormonal changes)

B. Certain medications [combination oral contraceptives (COCs), hormone therapy, antidepressents, and others]

C. Ingesting substances containing methylxanthines (coffee, tea, chocolate, and cola drinks). Methylxanthines have been noted to contribute to breast pain by clinical observation only.

D. Pregnancy

Common Complaints

A. "My breasts are painful, particularly just before my period."

B. "I have lumps in my breasts, and they hurt."

Other Signs and Symptoms

A. Tender breasts with palpation

B. Ropelike masses, usually bilateral, with mobile, well-circumscribed masses that are cystic or rubbery.

Subjective Data

A. Elicit history of pain. Note onset, duration, location, and relation to menstrual period. Ask: Is pain constant or intermittent?

B. What has the patient tried to alleviate the pain? Note what has worked, such as nonsteroidal anti-inflammatory drugs (NSAIDs).

C. Note the patient's family history of breast pain, lumps, or cancer.

D. Has there been trauma such as being hit or having a rough experience during sex?

E. Do her breasts hurt during or after exercise such as running, aerobics, soccer, or basketball?

F. Does she wear a good, supportive, properly fitted bra generally and for sports?

G. Has she had any breast surgery or biopsy?

H. Note medication history such as oral contraceptives.

Physical Examination

A. Inspect

1. Examine the breasts, and note masses; dimples; changes in the skin; changes in the way the nipples are pointed while the patient is in the sitting position with arms in neutral position in lap, above the head, or pressing in on hips.

B. Palpate

1. The breasts; look for hard, fixed, or cystic masses in the breast, under the nipple, in the tail of the breast, and in the axilla. Use a standardized breast examination technique. Compress the nipple for discharge. Measure masses, and describe them in the patient's record. Use a clock face to describe their location.

Diagnostic Tests

A. Mammogram: May be difficult to interpret in women younger than 35 years
B. Ultrasonography to differentiate cystic from solid masses
C. MRI is useful for detecting tissues with increased blood flow but limited by false-positive results.
D. Fine-needle aspiration and biopsy
E. Excisional biopsy for solid lumps
F. Pregnancy test (as indicated)

Differential Diagnoses

A. Fibrocystic breast changes with mastalgia
B. Benign breast masses: Fibroadenoma and duct ectasia
C. Nipple discharge: Duct ectasia, prolactin-secreting pituitary tumors
D. Pain: Costal chondritis, chest wall muscle pain, neuralgia, herpes zoster infection, and fibromyalgia
E. Heart: Angina pectoris
F. Gastrointestinal (GI): Gastroesophageal reflux disease
G. Psychological: Anxiety and depression

Plan

A. General interventions
1. Reassure the patient. Use the term *fibrocystic changes* rather than *fibrocystic disease* to stress the functional nature of the problem. Stress that the pain is real but not caused by a disease state.
B. Patient teaching
▶ **1.** *See Section III: Patient Teaching Guide for this chapter, "Fibrocystic Breast Changes and Breast Pain."*
2. Teach the patient breast self-examination. Encourage monthly breast self-examination. Continue clinical breast examinations annually.
3. "Lumpiness" that varies with the menstrual cycle is not abnormal. Breasts may normally be of different sizes. It is a change that is significant.
4. Consider changing the dose or discontinuing hormone replacement therapy (HRT) for women on HRT with mastalgia.
5. Symptomatic measures to relieve discomfort
a. Good supportive bra, properly fitted. Adolescents whose breasts are maturing and perimenopausal women whose bodies are changing are two groups who often wear improperly fitted bras.
b. Local heat or ice application (whatever works best)
C. Diet
1. Elimination of methylxanthines is a good idea, but the relationship of methylxanthines to breast pain is unproven in research studies.
2. Reduction of dietary fat and sodium intake has also been advocated, but has not been supported by research.
D. Pharmaceutical therapy
1. Diuretic: Spironolactone (Aldactone) 10 mg twice daily premenstrually
2. Oral contraceptive pills: Low-dose estrogen (20 mcg) pills are recommended.
3. Topical nonsteroidal anti-inflammatory gel can be used for local mastalgia.
4. Antiestrogen treatment
a. Danazol (Danocrine) 200 mg daily for 6 months. *Note*: Doses below 400 mg daily may not inhibit ovulation. The patient must use a barrier contraceptive or intrauterine device (IUD) contraceptive measure. Although the side-effect profile is significant, long-term symptomatic relief and histologic changes may be achieved.
b. Tamoxifen citrate 10 mg/d for severe breast pain
5. Vitamins
a. Vitamin E is no longer recommended for treatment of mastalgia.
b. Research has demonstrated mixed results on the benefits of vitamin B_6 and vitamin A.
6. Herbs
a. Flaxseed 25 mg daily may have show benefit in the treatment of cyclic mastalgia.
b. Evening primrose oil (EPO): There is insufficient evidence to recommend EPO for the treatment of mastalgia.

Follow-Up

A. Young women with fibrocystic changes need to be seen after 1 to 2 months of pharmacological therapy to assess for complications and efficacy.
B. Women with atypical hyperplasia on biopsy need close follow-up every 3 to 6 months by a physician.

Consultation/Referral

A. Consult or refer the patient to a physician when breast masses are identified.
B. Consult with a physician and refer the patient to a surgeon if findings include a suspicious mammographic study, an abnormal needle biopsy, or a solid mass per ultrasonogram.

Individual Considerations

A. Pregnancy
1. Consider blocked duct or mastitis with treatment as indicated.
B. Adults
1. Mammography screening for women at average risk according to the American Cancer Society: Mammography is offered annually for women from ages 40 to 64 years, and women should be informed of the risks, benefits, and limitations of regular screening. Women aged 45 to 54 years should have an annual mammogram. Women aged 55 years and older should switch to a mammogram every

2 years but be offered the choice to continue yearly screening.
2. Care should be individualized considering potential risks, benefits, and limitations of screening. High-risk women may benefit from additional screening, including earlier initiation of screening and additional screening modalities such as ultrasound and MRI.
3. When clinical breast examination, mammography, and needle-aspiration biopsy are used, breast cancer detection rates are 93% to 100%.

C. Geriatrics
1. Breast pain should be worked up as possible cancer.

D. Partners
1. Pain may inhibit sexual activity involving the breast.

Cervicitis

Rhonda Arthur

Definition

A. Cervicitis is acute or chronic inflammation of the cervix that is visible to the examiner.

Incidence

A. Incidence is unknown due to multiple etiologies.

Pathogenesis

A. Acute cervicitis is primarily due to infection from the following organisms:
1. Bacteria
a. *Chlamydia trachomatis*
b. *Neisseria gonorrhoeae*
c. Mycoplasma
d. Ureaplasma
2. Viruses
a. Herpes simplex virus type 2 (HSV-2)
b. Human papillomavirus (HPV)
3. *Trichomonas vaginalis*

B. Chronic cervicitis is primarily due to the following:
1. Trauma occurring during childbirth or instrumentation
2. Infection (see earlier)
3. Presence of foreign bodies (i.e., intrauterine devices [IUDs])

Predisposing Factors

A. Vaginal delivery
B. Cervical procedures: Laser, loop, or other excision procedures
C. IUD
D. Sexually transmitted infections (STIs)

Common Complaints

A. Copious mucopurulent vaginal discharge
B. Postcoital bleeding

Other Signs and Symptoms

A. Asymptomatic; may be found on routine gynecologic examination
B. Thick yellow vaginal discharge
C. Dysuria
D. Dyspareunia
E. Vulvovaginal irritation or pruritus

Subjective Data

A. Determine onset, duration, and course of symptoms. Is there any dyspareunia, pelvic pain, fever, or urinary symptoms?
B. Determine characteristics of the vaginal discharge.
C. Review the patient's history of STIs.
D. Review the patient's sexual history to include number of partners and partner symptoms (if any), use of sex toys, and sexual lifestyle.
E. Note the last Papanicolaou (Pap) smear and results. Has the patient ever had an abnormal Pap; if so, how was it treated?
F. Note date of last menstrual period (LMP), use of contraception, and type(s) of contraception.
G. If the patient has recently been pregnant, review her records for cervical cerclage, vaginal delivery with cervical laceration, or other complications.

Physical Examination

A. Check temperature, pulse, and respirations.
B. Inspect
1. Observe generally for discomfort before, during, and after examination.
2. Observe the external vulva for Bartholin's gland enlargement (Bartholin's gland abscess is due primarily to infection by chlamydia), lesions, irritation, fissures, and condyloma.
3. Note color, amount, and odor of vaginal discharge.

C. Palpate
1. Back: Note CVA tenderness.
2. Abdomen: Palpate for enlarged or tender inguinal lymph nodes.

D. Pelvic examination
1. Speculum examination:
a. Inspect cervix for inflammation and ectropion. Cervical ectropion is found in 15% to 20% of healthy young women (especially in teens and with the use of oral contraceptives). It represents columnar epithelium that is found farther out on the ectocervix, causing the cervix to appear granular and red. Presence of cervical erosion, however, suggests advanced cervical pathology. A "strawberry cervix" (petechiae) is highly suggestive of *T. vaginalis*.
b. Check cervix for friability and bleeding when the cervix is touched with a cotton-tipped swab.
c. Assess the vagina and cervix for leukoplakia, lesions, polyps, and discharge.
d. Assess vaginal walls for discharge and rugae.
e. Vesicular or ulcerated cervical lesions warrant testing for syphilis and/or chancroid.
2. Bimanual examination:
a. Check cervical motion tenderness (CMT), adnexal masses, uterine size, consistency, and tenderness.
b. Milk urethra for discharge.
c. Palpate Bartholin's glands.

Diagnostic Tests

A. White blood cell (WBC), if indicated
B. Consider testing for syphilis (rapid plasma reagin [RPR] or Venereal Disease Research Laboratory [VDRL] test)
C. Wet prep
D. Cervical cultures for gonorrhea and chlamydia
E. Pap smear
F. Urine culture and sensitivity, if indicated
G. Herpes culture, if indicated

Differential Diagnoses

A. Cervicitis
B. Chlamydia
C. Gonorrhea
D. Bartholin's gland abscess
E. Cervical neoplasm
F. Cervical polyps
G. HSV-2
H. Urinary tract infection (UTI)
I. Cervical ulceration, or erosion, from trauma: Fingernail, cervical biopsy, postpartum, or sex toys
J. Pelvic inflammatory disease (PID)

Plan

A. General interventions
- **1.** Patients whose culture is negative generally respond to a round of doxycycline therapy, which is the drug of choice for nonchlamydial, nongonorrheal cervicitis.

B. Patient teaching
- **1.** Women should be encouraged to obtain routine care and Pap smear evaluations per guidelines.
- **2.** Patient should have no sexual intercourse for 1 week and avoid reinfection by abstaining from intercourse until sexual partners are adequately treated.
- **3.** Avoid tampons and douches until antibiotics are completed.
- ▶ **4.** Give the patient a teaching sheet. *See Section III: Patient Teaching Guides for this chapter, "Cervicitis."*

C. Pharmaceutical therapy
- **1.** Drug of choice for chlamydia: Azithromycin 1 g orally in a single dose or doxycycline 100 mg twice daily for 7 days. Treat all partners.
- **2.** Drug of choice for gonorrhea: Ceftriaxone (Rocephin) 250 mg by intramuscular (IM) injection plus either a single dose of azithromycin 1 g orally or doxycycline 100 mg orally twice a day for 7 days
- **3.** Drug of choice for herpes simplex virus (HSV): Acyclovir 400 mg three times daily for 7 to 10 days for initial outbreak, acyclovir 400 mg three times a day for 5 days for recurrent outbreak or acyclovir 400 mg twice a day for suppression
- **4.** Drug of choice for *trichomonas*: Metronidazole 500 mg twice daily for 7 days (treat all partners), or 2 g orally in a single dose. Patients should be cautioned to avoid alcohol consumption during and 24 hours after the completion of oral metronidazole due to a disulfiram-like reaction (nausea, vomiting, headache, cramps, and flushing).
- **5.** Drug of choice for UTI: See the section "Urinary Tract Infection (Acute Cystitis)" in Chapter 12.

Follow-Up

A. Recommend "test of cure": Return for repeat testing 3 months after treatment because of high rates of reinfection.
B. Follow up with Pap smear as mandated by guidelines.

Consultation/Referral

A. Refer the patient to a physician for suspected neoplasm and for cervicitis unresponsive to treatment.
B. If the cervix has a suspicious lesion, the patient should be referred for colposcopy and/or biopsy regardless of cytology results. On physical examination, the cervix may be edematous and erythematous and may show exposed columnar epithelium. It may be friable. Reddened areas of the cervix may be seen around the cervical os. The irregularity and friability sometimes differentiate them from eversion; other times colposcopy is required to make the distinction.

Individual Considerations

A. Pregnancy
- **1.** Cervical inflammation is common in early pregnancy.
- **2.** If an STI is diagnosed, nonteratogenic pharmacological therapies must be implemented.

B. Partners
- **1.** A positive STI result warrants treatment of each sexual partner.

Contraception

Rhonda Arthur

Definition

A. Contraception is the intentional prevention of pregnancy by either or both sexual partners. Contraception can be mechanical, chemical, or surgical and is either reversible or nonreversible. Considerations in counseling regarding contraceptive choices include cost, efficacy, safety, and personal considerations such as personal belief systems and ability to use selected method.

The Centers for Disease Control and Prevention's (CDC) U.S. Medical Eligibility Criteria for Contraceptive Use is a formal adaptation of the 1996 World Health Organization's Medical Eligibility Criteria for Contraceptive Use. This valuable document assists health care providers in counseling women and men and assists health care providers to determine safe and effective contraceptive methods individualized to patient preferences and individual health issues. It is available at www.cdc.gov/reproductivehealth/unintendedpregnancy/pdf/legal_summary-chart_english_final_tag508.pdf

Incidence

A. Women frequently visit primary care providers to request contraception and family planning education. There are 61 million women in the United States who are in their childbearing years. Ninety-nine percent of women aged 15 to 44 years have used at least one contraceptive method. Unfortunately, approximately 50% of all pregnancies in the United States are unintended. Consistent use of a reliable and effective contraceptive method can greatly reduce the unintended pregnancy rate. Easy access and education regarding contraceptive use is a keystone in the prevention of unintended pregnancy.

Subjective Data

A. Review complete menstrual history, including age of onset, duration, frequency, regularity, and dysmenorrhea. Review date of last menstrual period (LMP).
B. Review the patient's pregnancy history.
C. Review the patient's contraception and sexual history.
D. Note other medications the patient is taking including over-the-counter (OTC) medications and supplements.
E. Ask the patient whether she has had a major medical disease including hypertension, cardiovascular incident, thromboembolic disease, diabetes, migraine headaches, gallbladder disease, or liver disease.
F. Review substance abuse/use history.
G. Review childhood illness and immunization record.
H. Note allergies.
I. Review pertinent family medical history.

Physical Examination

A. Check height, weight, blood pressure, pulse, and body mass index (BMI).
B. Inspect
  1. Note overall appearance. Look at neck (thyroid). Inspect breast/genitalia for Tanner staging. See Appendix C: Tanner's Sexual Maturity Stages.
  2. Skin assessment: Check for central hair growth, which is responsive to androgens. Areas to inspect for coarse hair include the upper lip, chin, sideburns, neck, chest, lower abdomen, and perineum.
C. Palpate
  1. Palpate the neck for thyroid enlargement.
  2. Palpate the abdomen for enlarged organs or uterine enlargement compatible with pregnancy.
  3. Perform breast examination, palpating for masses. Assess for nipple discharge.
  4. Palpate axilla for masses, and lymphadenopathy.
D. Auscultate
  1. Auscultate the heart and lungs.
  2. If pregnancy is suspected, consider auscultating for fetal heart tones.
E. Pelvic examination
  1. Inspect external genitalia. Note pubic hair pattern for Tanner staging. Note any lesions, masses, or discharge.
  2. Speculum examination: Inspect vagina and cervix. Note any vaginal discharge. Obtain Pap smear and cervical/vaginal cultures as appropriate.
  3. Bimanual examination: Palpate the cervix and check for cervical motion tenderness (CMT). Palpate the size of the uterus and assess for adnexal masses.
  4. Consider rectal examination as indicated.

Diagnostic Tests

A. Urine: Pregnancy test as indicated/urinalysis as indicated
B. Serum: Complete blood count (CBC) if indicated by history
C. Pap smear according to American Society for Clinical Pathology guidelines
D. Vaginal/cervical cultures for sexually transmitted infections (STIs) as indicated

Plan

A. General interventions
  1. Review all methods of contraception available with the patient and partner, if available.
  2. Consider all aspects of the client's history and make recommendations as appropriate.
B. Patient teaching
  1. Review anatomy and physiology of the menstrual cycle and reproduction with all patients.
  2. Review the risks, benefits, costs, use, and efficacy of contraceptive methods. Review perfect use versus typical use of method selected.
  3. Review STI prevention and limitations of STI prevention as related to each method.
  4. Assist the patient in selecting the most appropriate method of contraception with regard to cost, efficacy, health status of the patient, ability to use correctly and consistently, and the patient's personal values.
  5. Warning signs and information as to when to call the care provider should be given to all patients.
  6. All women of childbearing age should be educated on the availability and proper use of emergency contraceptives. *See Section III: Patient Teaching Guide for this chapter, "Contraception: How to Take Birth Control Pills (for a 28-Day Cycle)."* ◀
  7. Provide all patients information on the prevention of STIs.

Methods of Contraception

A. Abstinence: Refraining from sexual intercourse
  1. Advantages: Easy and no cost. Perfect use offers protection against STIs and pregnancy.
  2. Disadvantages: User dependent
B. Barrier methods
  1. Male condom
    a. Advantages: Male condoms are easily accessible (OTC with no prescription needed) and relatively inexpensive. Condoms do not require daily intervention and offer some protections against STIs.
    b. Disadvantages: Male condoms are technique dependent for efficacy. Breakage and spillage can occur. Some condoms are made from latex, and those with latex allergies need to be aware and carefully check the label for latex content. Nonlatex condoms are available. Male condoms are intended for one-time use only.

c. Efficacy with perfect use of male condoms: Approximately 2 in 100 women will become pregnant each year. With typical use of male condoms, approximately 15 in 100 women will become pregnant each year.

2. Female condom

a. Advantages: Female condoms are easily accessible (OTC with no prescription needed) and relatively inexpensive. Condoms do not require daily intervention and offer some protections against STIs.

b. Disadvantages: Female condoms are technique dependent for efficacy. Slippage and spillage can occur. The female condom is intended for one-time use only and may be inserted up to 8 hours before intercourse.

c. Efficacy with perfect use of the female condom: Approximately 5 in 100 women will become pregnant each year. With typical use of the female condom, approximately 21 in 100 women will become pregnant each year.

3. Diaphragm

a. Advantages: Diaphragms are nonhormonal and can be used for years with proper care. May be inserted up to 6 hours before intercourse.

b. Disadvantages: Diaphragms must be properly fitted by an experienced health care provider and are user controlled. Placement is crucial to contraceptive benefit and spermicide must be used. Must be removed within 24 hours due to risk of toxic shock syndrome (TSS). The patient must have fit checked after childbirth and weight gain or loss. Urinary tract infections (UTIs) may be more frequent in diaphragm users, and some women may experience sensitivity or allergy to spermicide. Avoid use during menses.

c. Efficacy with perfect use of the diaphragm: 6 in 100 women will become pregnant each year. With typical use of the diaphragm, 16 in 100 women will become pregnant each year.

4. Cervical cap

a. Advantages: Cervical caps are nonhormonal and can be used for years with proper care. The cervical cap may be inserted and left in place up to 48 hours.

b. Disadvantages: Cervical caps must be properly fitted by an experienced health care provider and are user controlled. Placement is crucial to contraceptive benefit and spermicide must be used. Must be removed within 48 hours due to risk of TSS. The FemCap is made of latex and not appropriate for latex-allergic patients. Some women may experience sensitivity or allergy to spermicide. Avoid use during menses.

c. Efficacy with use of the cervical cap is similar to the diaphragm.

5. Vaginal sponge

a. Advantages: The vaginal sponge is a nonhormonal OTC polyurethane sponge that releases the spermicide nonoxynol-9. It can be used for multiple acts of intercourse over 24 hours.

b. Disadvantages: The vaginal sponge is user-controlled. Some women may experience sensitivity or allergy to the spermicide. Avoid use during menses.

c. Efficacy with use perfects use of the vaginal sponge: Among parous women, 20 in 100 will become pregnant each year, and 9 nulliparous women will become pregnant each year. With typical use, 32 in 100 parous women and 16 nulliparous women will become pregnant each year.

C. Surgery

1. Male sterilization

a. Advantages: Sterilization is a very effective form of contraception. User does not have to remember to do anything before intercourse, and it is not user dependent. Sterilization is permanent.

b. Disadvantages: Sterilization involves a surgical procedure. Insurance may not cover the cost of the procedure.

c. Efficacy with perfect use of male sterilization; 0.1 in 100 women will become pregnant each year. With typical use of male sterilization 0.15 in 100 women will become pregnant each year.

2. Female sterilization is the second most often used contraceptive method in the United States.

a. Advantages: Sterilization is a very effective form of contraception. User does not have to remember to do anything before intercourse, and it is not user-dependent. Sterilization is permanent.

b. Disadvantages: Sterilization involves a surgical procedure. If pregnancy does occur, there is a higher incidence of ectopic pregnancy. Insurance may not cover the cost of the procedure.

c. Efficacy with both perfect and typical use of female sterilization: 0.5 in 100 will become pregnant each year.

D. Intrauterine device (IUD)

1. Hormonal (Mirena)

a. Advantages: Mirena is a very effective form of contraception. Mirena may be left in place for 5 years. User does not have to remember to use before intercourse. Mirena may reduce menstrual flow.

b. Disadvantages: Risks of any IUD include uterine perforation, increased spontaneous abortion, ectopic pregnancy, and pelvic pain and infection. Mirena must be inserted by a qualified health care professional. IUD may be spontaneously expelled.

c. Efficacy with both perfect and typical use of the Mirena: 0.2 in 100 will become pregnant each year.

2. Nonhormonal (ParaGard)

a. Advantages: ParaGard is a very effective form of contraception. ParaGard may be left in place for 10 years. User does not have to remember to use before intercourse.

b. Disadvantages: Risks of any IUD include uterine perforation; increased spontaneous abortion, ectopic pregnancy, and pelvic pain and infection. ParaGard must be inserted by a qualified health care professional. IUD may be spontaneously expelled.

c. Efficacy with perfect use of the ParaGard: 0.6 in 100 women will become pregnant each year. With typical use of the ParaGard, 0.8 in 100 women will become pregnant each year.

Women who are not appropriate candidates for an IUD include those with recent pelvic infections, anatomical uterine abnormalities, and pregnancy. Caution should be exercised when considering an IUD in women who have multiple sexual partners; pelvic inflammatory disease (PID); immunosuppression; undiagnosed, irregular, or heavy menstrual bleeding; abnormal Pap smear; and difficulty obtaining follow-up care. See World Health Organization's IUD Toolkit at www.k4health.org/toolkits/iud

E. Pharmaceutical therapy

1. Progestin-only pills (POPs; also known as mini pills)

a. Advantages: The POP is a safe hormonal alternative for women who cannot take estrogen. It is preferred to combined oral contraceptives (COCs) for lactating women as it is not as likely to decrease milk supply. POPs are rapidly reversible and controlled by women.

b. Disadvantages: The POP cannot be taken if the patient has any contraindications to progestin use. POPs are less effective than COCs and must be taken daily at the same time, requiring strict adherence to regime.

c. Efficacy with perfect use of POPs: 0.3 in 100 women per year will become pregnant. With typical use, 8 in 100 women per year will become pregnant.

2. Injection (Depo-Provera) long-acting depot medroxyprogesterone acetate (DMPA)

a. Advantages: Easy to use. The user only has to remember the injection every 3 months. May decrease vaginal bleeding. DMPA is a safe hormonal alternative for women who cannot take estrogen.

b. Disadvantages: Women cannot use DMPA if they have any contraindications to progesterone use. May cause amenorrhea or irregular vaginal bleeding. May cause increased weight gain. Requires routine (3 months) visits to the provider's office for intramuscular (IM) injections. DMPA does not provide protection against STIs. DMPA is associated with reversible decreased bone mineral density.

c. Efficacy with perfect use of DMPA: 0.3 in 100 women per year will become pregnant. With typical use, 3 in 100 women per year will become pregnant.

d. Depo-Provera should be administered during the first 5 days of the menstrual cycle, or postpartum before resumption of intercourse (preferably after lactation has been established). If this is not possible or if a woman is late for injection, administer pregnancy test and have the patient use condoms for at least 1 week after injection.

3. Contraceptive implant (Nexplanon): Long-acting reversible etonogestrel implant

a. A single-rod subdermal radiopaque implant

b. Advantages: Progestin implant is a safe hormonal alternative for women who cannot take estrogen. A long-acting (3 years) reversible contraceptive.

c. Disadvantages: Women cannot use Nexplanon if they have any contraindications to progestin use. Possible insertion and removal complications

d. The manufacturer strongly recommends that care providers who wish to insert and/or remove Nexplanon participate in training sessions. Only clinicians who have completed the training program are eligible to purchase the product. The link to request this training is www.nexplanon-usa.com/en/hcp/services-and-support/request-training/index.asp

e. Absolute contraindications to progestogen therapy

i. Active thrombophlebitis or thromboembolic disorders

ii. Acute liver disease

iii. Known or suspected cancer of the breast

iv. Pregnancy

v. Undiagnosed, abnormal vaginal bleeding

4. Combined estrogen/progesterone contraceptives: Combined estrogen/progesterone contraceptives come in three delivery methods: Oral pills, a transdermal patch, and a vaginal ring. Advantages and disadvantages and efficacy are similar regarding hormones, but there are some differences in the delivery methods.

a. Advantages: Combined contraceptives are easy to use, convenient, rapidly reversible, and controlled by women. The transdermal patch is only changed weekly, and the vaginal ring is left in place for 3 weeks. In addition to predictable menses, combined contraceptives decrease menstrual flow and length of menses.

b. Disadvantages: Dependent on user, and oral pills must be taken daily. Exposure to hormones may not be suitable for certain women based on health status and risk. See absolute and relative contraindications that are not appropriate for some women in a prescriber's reference guide. Smoking in conjunction with use of combined contraceptive increases cardiovascular risk and should be considered. Does not protect against STIs. Other medications, such as anticonvulsants and antibiotics, may interfere with effectiveness of combined hormonal contraceptives and should be considered in prescribing.

c. Efficacy with perfect use of combined hormonal contraceptive: 0.3 in 100 women per year will become pregnant. With typical use, 8 in 100 women per year will become pregnant.

d. Prescribing considerations: Oral contraceptives come in combination extended cycle, combination monophasic, combination biphasic, combination triphasic, and progestin-only formulations. Side effects can be managed in consideration of pill composition. See prescribing reference guides such as the Monthly Prescribing Reference at www.empr.com. General considerations for pill selection include age, health history/status, and the patient's preference. Because POPs are highly sensitive to consistency in timing, reserve prescriptions of them for women who have contraindications to estrogen. Alternatives for COCs should be considered in women older than 35 years who smoke due to increased risks of thrombolytic events. In asymptomatic adolescents, it is acceptable to prescribe COCs without an initial pelvic examination. For adolescents or anyone who may have difficulty remembering to take a daily pill, consideration should be given to prescription of the vaginal ring, patch, or other methods. See the office's prescriber's reference for complete information on safety side effects and contraindications.

e. Absolute contraindications to estrogen therapy (ET)

- **i.** Acute liver disease
- **ii.** Cerebral vascular or coronary artery disease, myocardial infarction (MI), or stroke
- **iii.** History of or active thrombophlebitis or thromboembolic disorders
- **iv.** History of uterine or ovarian cancer
- **v.** Known or suspected cancer of the breast
- **vi.** Known or suspected estrogen-dependent neoplasm
- **vii.** Pregnancy
- **viii.** Undiagnosed, abnormal vaginal bleeding

f. Relative contraindications to ET

- **i.** Active gallbladder disease
- **ii.** Familial hyperlipidemia

5. Spermicide (foam, film, gel, tablets, and suppositories)

a. Advantages: Spermicide is a nonhormonal OTC preparation and contains nonoxynol-9. It is inexpensive and easily accessible.

b. Disadvantages: Spermicide is user controlled and, if not used consistently, will lead to contraception failure. Some may experience sensitivity or allergy to spermicide. Spermicide has a high failure rate.

c. Efficacy with perfect use of spermicide: 18 in 100 women will become pregnant each year. With typical use of spermicide, 29 of 100 women will become pregnant each year.

F. Natural family planning (NFP)

1. Advantages: NFP is nonhormonal. It has no cost and is easy to use.

2. Disadvantages: NFP is user controlled and depends on regularity of cycle and avoidance of intercourse. Can be complex for user and has a high failure rate. Does not protect against STIs.

3. Efficacy with use: With typical use of the fertility awareness method, 25 in 100 women will become pregnant each year.

Additional information, training, and patient teaching may be found at the following websites: Association of Reproductive Health Professionals (www.arhp.org/Publications-and-Resources/Quick-Reference-Guide-for-Clinicians/choosing/Fertility-awareness), Institute for Reproductive Health (www.irh.org), and Planned Parenthood (www.plannedparenthood.org).

G. Withdrawal

1. Advantages: Withdrawal is nonhormonal, is inexpensive and easily accessible.

2. Disadvantages: Withdrawal is user controlled. Withdrawal has a high failure rate and does not protect against STIs.

3. Efficacy with use: With typical use of withdrawal method, 85 in 100 women will become pregnant each year.

Follow-Up

A. The patient should return in 3 months of initiation of oral contraceptives, ring, and patch to assess blood pressure, use, side effects, and satisfaction. Then yearly visits are recommended for health maintenance.

B. Patients on Depo-Provera injections should return every 3 months for follow-up injection and weight evaluation and then yearly for health maintenance.

C. Patients with a diaphragm should return for refitting with change in weight or postpartum and for routine health maintenance.

Consultation/Referral

A. If the contraceptive method selected is one the practitioner is not experienced in providing (diaphragm, implant, IUD, surgical sterilization), refer to an experienced appropriate provider.

Individual Considerations

A. Adults

1. Discontinue COCs for women aged 35 years and older who smoke.

2. Increased age and obesity increase risk of venous thromobembolism with the use of COCs. COCs should be prescribed with caution and alternative contraceptives should be considered.

3. The health care provider should continue to assess for chronic conditions and medication use and weigh risks and benefits of selected methods.
4. Provide anticipatory guidance regarding the need to use contraceptives until menopause is confirmed to prevent unintended pregnancy.

B. Adolescents
1. A pelvic examination is not required and should not become a barrier to access to contraception. Long-acting reversible contraceptives and methods that require less frequent dosing (patch, ring) promote adherence and continuation and should be encouraged in teens.
2. Education and counseling regarding pregnancy and STI prevention are essential.
3. Many clients have mobile phones with reminder apps that assist in compliance with contraceptive use.

Dysmenorrhea

Rhonda Arthur

Definition

Dysmenorrhea is painful uterine cramping felt primarily in the lower abdomen but also in the lower back and upper thighs.

A. Primary dysmenorrhea: Not associated with pelvic pathology; usually associated with ovulatory cycles. Occurs on the first or second day of the menstrual period; usually worse the first day; affects teens and women in their 20s; is often associated with prostaglandin-induced symptoms of diarrhea, nausea, vomiting, and/or headache.

B. Secondary dysmenorrhea: Painful uterine contractions due to a pathologic etiology such as endometriosis or pelvic inflammatory disease (PID). Primarily occurs in women in their 20s, 30s, and 40s.

Incidence

A. Primary dysmenorrhea is very common, affecting up to 90% of young women to some extent at some time. Dysmenorrhea frequently leads to absenteeism from work or school and impacts limitations on social and sports activities. The incidence of endometriosis is 8% to 30% of women of reproductive age.

Pathogenesis

A. Primary dysmenorrhea is due to myometrial contractions that are caused by prostaglandins in the secretory endometrium. The prostaglandins cause uterine ischemia through platelet aggregation, vasoconstriction, and dysrhythmic contractions.

B. Secondary dysmenorrhea is associated with pathologic conditions such as endometriosis, cervical stenosis, tumors, adhesions, adenomyosis, myomas, polyps, infection (pelvic inflammatory disease [PID]), intrauterine device (IUD)-retained products of conception, or nongynecologic causes. The pain of secondary dysmenorrhea may also be unrelated to menses.

C. In endometriosis, there are islands of endometrium found on peritoneal surfaces of the bladder, broad ligaments, fallopian tubes, ovaries, bowel, and cul-de-sac, as well as distant sites on the abdominal wall, vagina, lung, or other sites.

Predisposing Factors

A. Female
B. Reproductive age
C. Normal menstrual function
D. Cervical stenosis, possibly

Common Complaints

A. "I have painful periods."
B. "My menstrual cramps are terrible, particularly the first day of my cycle."
C. "My cramps are so bad I feel sick to my stomach and have diarrhea."

Other Signs and Symptoms

A. History of menstrual cramps just before the onset of the menstrual period and for the first 24 to 48 hours
B. Pain beginning earlier; associated with intercourse, defecation, and urination; and lasting throughout the menstrual period is associated with endometriosis or adenomyosis.
C. Acute pain may be associated with infection (PID) or ectopic pregnancy.

Subjective Data

A. Obtain a complete menstrual history: Age at menarche; frequency, duration, and regularity of periods; amount of flow in number of perineal pads or tampons used.
B. Ask the patient about the location of the pain; note radiation and associated symptoms such as nausea, vomiting, or diarrhea.
C. Is pain rhythmic or spasmodic (primary) or steady (secondary)?
D. How old was the patient when the pain began? Primary dysmenorrhea usually begins 2 to 3 years after menarche.
E. Inquire about the type of contraception used.
F. Obtain obstetric history.
G. Is the pain related to the menstrual period, or does it occur before or independent of the menstrual period?
H. Does the patient have dyspareunia?
I. Does she have urinary tract infection (UTI) symptoms?
J. What treatments have been tried, and which were effective?

Physical Examination

A. Check height and weight, temperature, blood pressure, and pulse.

B. Inspect
1. Examine the general body habitus for female adipose distribution on the buttocks and thighs.
2. Note breast development (see Tanner's Sexual Maturity Stages in Appendix C).
3. Observe the abdomen for distension.

C. Palpate and percuss
1. Examine the abdomen for masses or tenderness.

D. Auscultate
1. The heart and lungs
2. Abdomen for bowel sounds.
E. Pelvic examination
1. Inspect the external genitalia for pubic hair pattern, lesions, discharge, and odor.
2. Palpate the external genitalia for masses or areas of tenderness.
F. Speculum examination: Inspect the cervix and vagina for discharge, lesions, ectropion, cervical erosion, and IUD string.
G. Bimanual examination
1. Palpate the vagina and cul-de-sac areas for tenderness or masses.
2. Check the cervical position, mobility, and pain with mobility.
3. Check uterine size, mobility, shape, regularity, masses, position, and tenderness.
4. Check the adnexa for masses (cystic or solid) and tenderness.
5. A normal pelvic examination is a significant finding in primary dysmenorrhea and often in endometriosis.

Diagnostic Tests

Primary dysmenorrhea is often diagnosed by history, including symptoms and timing in menstrual cycle and pelvic examination. If secondary dysmenorrhea is suspected and additional information is required, the care provider may consider the following diagnostic tests:
A. Consider pelvic ultrasonography to rule out pelvic pathology.
B. Laboratory studies: Urinalysis, hemoglobin (Hgb), hematocrit (Hct), and white blood cell (WBC)
C. Consider vaginal and cervical cultures for chlamydia and gonorrhea, if infection is suspected
D. Pregnancy test as indicated
E. Papanicolaou (Pap) smear per guidelines

Differential Diagnoses

A. Dysmenorrhea: The patient's history and a normal pelvic examination are used to diagnose primary dysmenorrhea.
B. Complication of pregnancy: Missed or incomplete abortion or ectopic pregnancy
C. Endometriosis or adenomyosis
D. Ruptured ovarian cyst
E. Infection: Endometritis, salpingitis, PID, or pelvic adhesions
F. Fibroid tumors
G. Adhesions
H. UTI
I. Bowel disease: Irritable bowel disease or inflammatory bowel disease

Plan

A. General interventions
1. Support patient concerns and identify reality of discomfort. Identify primary source of pain if other diagnoses exist.
B. Patient teaching:
1. *See Section III: Patient Teaching Guides for this chapter, "Dysmenorrhea (Painful Menstrual Cramps or Periods)" and "Contraception: How to Take Birth Control Pills (for a 28-Day Cycle)."*
2. Educate the patient about the physiology of menstruation.
3. Teach the patient that endometriosis is one of the leading causes of infertility.
4. Encourage activity and exercise, such as walking or swimming.
5. Advise warm baths or heating pads to help relieve some pain.
C. Pharmaceutical therapy
1. Nonsteroidal anti-inflammatory drugs (NSAIDs) are the drugs of choice.
a. They inhibit prostaglandin synthesis in the endometrium, thus decreasing uterine cramping. There is also an analgesic effect.
b. The fenamates have been the most effective, followed by the propionic acid derivatives.
c. The drugs should be started as the menstrual period begins. It is no longer considered the standard of care to begin the drugs a few days before the onset of the menstrual period.
d. Prostaglandin inhibitors relieve dysmenorrhea in 80% of women.
e. Take NSAIDs with food to avoid gastrointestinal (GI) upset and irritation.
2. Medications of choice for dysmenorrhea
a. NSAIDs
i. Arylacetic acid derivatives: Naproxen sodium (Aleve) 200 mg every 8 to 10 hours; naproxen sodium (Anaprox) 275 mg every 6 to 8 hours, or 550 mg every 12 hours; and naproxen sodium (Naprelan) 1 to 1.5 g once daily
ii. Propionic acid derivatives: Ibuprofen (Advil, Motrin, Nuprin) 200 to 800 mg every 4 to 6 hours; ketoprofen (Orudis) 12.5 to 25 mg every 4 to 6 hours. These are over-the-counter (OTC) medications.
iii. Anthranilic acid derivatives: Mefenamic acid (Ponstel) 500 mg initial dose, then 250 mg every 6 hours. The treatment maximum is 2 to 3 days.
iv. Benzeneacetic acid derivatives: Diclofenac potassium (Cataflam) 50 mg three times per day. Initial dose of 100 mg may be given.
b. Hormonal control
i. Oral contraceptive pills: Any combination pill is efficacious. Consider extended cycle dosing to prevent having monthly periods.
ii. Nuvaring
iii. Depo-Provera
iv. Merina
v. Nexplanon
3. Medications of choice for endometriosis
a. NSAIDs
b. Oral contraceptive pills

c. With physician consultation or referral, danazol (Danocrine)
d. With physician consultation or referral, gonadotropin-releasing hormone (Gn-RH) agonists such as nafarelin (Synarel), leuprolide acetate (Lupron, Lupron Depot), and goserelin acetate (Zoladex)

Follow-Up

A. Have the patient return in 3 months. Encourage the patient to undergo the treatment for 3 months to determine the effectiveness.

Consultation/Referral

A. If dysmenorrhea does not respond to NSAIDs or oral contraceptives, consult with a physician for further workup to determine the source of the pain.
B. Consider consultation with obstetrics and gynecology (OB/GYN) for laparoscopy or hysteroscopy to diagnose endometriosis or adhesions. Laser may be used to destroy endometrial implants or to lyse adhesions.

Individual Considerations

A. Pregnancy: Uterine contractions in pregnancy could be preterm labor.
B. Adolescents
  1. Remember that endometriosis can occur in this age group. It is not an extremely rare finding.
C. Adults
  1. Endometriosis can be a disabling condition interfering with work and sexual relationships. It may continue into the perimenopausal period.

Dyspareunia

Rhonda Arthur

Definition

A. Dyspareunia is genital or pelvic discomfort associated with sexual intercourse (entry or deep penetration) and interferes with sexual satisfaction. Dyspareunia may be superficial, relating to vulvar and vaginal pain, or it may be deep, relating to deep, pelvic pain. Vaginismus is the involuntary (often painful) contraction of the pelvic floor muscles in response to pressure or attempted penetration.

Incidence

A. Vaginismus occurs in 1% to 6% of women and dysparunia occurs in 8% to 22% of postmenopausal women.

Pathogenesis

Physical and psychosocial etiologies have been identified.
A. Physical causes
  1. Vulvovaginal anomalies
    a. Thick hymen
    b. Short vagina
    c. Vaginal agenesis
    d. Vaginal septum
  2. Organic dyspareunia
    a. Episiotomy scars
    b. Bartholin's gland cyst
    c. Vulvar dystrophy
    d. Inflammation or infection, sexually transmitted infection (STI)
    e. Vulvovaginal cancer
    f. Pelvic disease
      i. Pelvic inflammatory disease (PID)
      ii. Uterine or ovarian tumors
      iii. Adenomyosis
      iv. Pelvic scarring or adhesions versus endometriosis
  3. Musculoskeletal anomalies
    a. Disk disease
    b. Myofascial pain
    c. Coccygodynia
  4. Extensive prolapse or organ displacement
  5. Urethral syndrome or other urinary tract disorders
  6. Vulvodynia
  7. Gastrointestinal (GI) anomalies
    a. Constipation
    b. Irritable bowel syndrome (IBS)
    c. Inflammatory bowel disease (IBD)
    d. Anorexia
  8. Hormonal factors
    a. Hypoestrogenemia causing atrophic vaginitis
    b. Breastfeeding
    c. Menopause
B. Psychosocial causes
  1. Childhood molestation
  2. Fear of pain, infection, or pregnancy
  3. Pelvic congestion syndrome
  4. Poor partner communication
  5. History of sexual assault, including date rape
  6. Previous trauma during intercourse
  7. Domestic violence

Common Complaints

A. Irritation or burning with intercourse
B. Lack of vaginal lubrication
C. Pain with vulvar or vaginal contact
D. Pain with deep penetration
E. Postcoital bleeding

Other Signs and Symptoms

A. Vulvar pain
B. Vaginal pain or burning
C. Vaginal dryness

Subjective Data

A. Review the onset, duration, and course of presenting symptoms including precise location and timing of pain during intercourse.
B. Review the patient's medical or surgical history for physical causes (see "Pathogenesis" section).
C. Ask: How often does pain occur (with every intercourse, near periods, or in certain sexual positions)? What relief measures have been tried? Is there improvement with using extra lubrication? How much relief was obtained with each measure?
D. Obtain a complete sexual history including the following:
  1. Sexual practices

2. Sexual satisfaction or orgasm
3. Perception of partner satisfaction
4. Age at first coitus
5. History of sexual abuse, molestation, rape
6. Perceptions regarding sexuality
7. Number of sexual partners and preferences
8. Time spent on foreplay
9. History of recent delivery and breastfeeding
10. Age at onset of puberty, date of last menses, and cycle history
11. Current method of birth control and satisfaction with method; previous methods and why they were discontinued
12. Presence of vaginal discharge, odor, dysuria, or other physical symptoms before or after intercourse
13. Medications, including prescription and over-the-counter (OTC) drugs
14. Can the woman insert a tampon without pain?

Physical Examination

A. Check temperature, pulse, respirations, and blood pressure.

B. Inspect: Observe generally for discomfort before, during, and after examination.

> *Look for signs of physical or sexual abuse, cuts, bruises, and lacerations. For pain greatest on deep penile penetration, suspect PID, ovarian cyst, endometriosis, pelvic adhesions, relaxation of pelvic support, or uterine fibroids.*

C. Auscultate
   1. The abdomen for bowel sounds in all quadrants; Auscultation of the abdomen should precede any palpation or percussion due to the changes in intensity and frequency of sounds after manipulation.

D. Palpate
   1. Palpate the abdomen for masses; check for suprapubic tenderness.
   2. Examine the back, assess range of motion. Observe for evidence of disk disease, myofascial pain, and coccygodynia. Palpate for costovertebral angle (CVA) tenderness.

E. Pelvic examination
   1. Inspect: Perform perineal examination for atrophic vaginitis. Atrophic vaginitis presents as red, shiny, smooth vagina (loss of rugae); vaginal thinning; decreased elasticity of vaginal tissues. Vulvar inflammation may be present. Assess discharge and rugae for hormonal support.
   2. Evaluate the patient for vulvovaginitis. Perform vulvar examination for Bartholin's gland enlargement, fissures, condyloma, and herpes. Inspect for anatomic variants: narrowed introitus, congenital malformations (septum), and pelvic relaxation (cystocele and rectocele).

F. Speculum examination: Inspect for cervicitis, friability, and discharge. If the woman can insert a tampon without pain, a mechanical obstruction is unlikely.

G. Bimanual examination: Check cervical motion tenderness (CMT); adnexal masses; and uterine size, consistency, and position.

H. Rectovaginal examination: Palpate uterosacral ligaments for pain and nodularity and other signs of PID and endometriosis. In cases of rectal trauma, cultures may be needed to rule out STIs if anal intercourse is practiced.

Diagnostic Tests

A. **Wet prep to rule out candidiasis, trichomoniasis, and bacterial vaginosis (BV)**

B. Cervical cultures for chlamydia, gonorrhea

C. Viral cultures of lesions, if any

D. Urine culture, if applicable

E. Pelvic ultrasonography, if indicated

F. **Stool culture, if applicable**

G. Sedimentation rate, if indicated by physical

Differential Diagnoses

A. Dyspareunia

B. See "Pathogenesis" section.

Plan

A. General interventions
   1. Detailed physical examination after a thorough history
   2. Patients should be encouraged to involve their partner(s) in assessment, diagnosis, and treatment of dyspareunia.
   3. A secure, trusting relationship must be established with the care provider before many patients feel comfortable discussing sexuality issues. Continuity with one provider is essential.
   4. Patients with dyspareunia should be evaluated for multiple etiologies. Treat underlying pathologies such as musculoskeletal anomalies, pelvic infection, urinary tract infection (UTI), STDs, hormonal deficiencies, and GI etiologies (see specific chapters for treatment plans and drug therapy).

B. Patient teaching
   1. *See Section III: Patient Teaching Guide for this chapter, "Dyspareunia (Pain With Intercourse)."* ◀

C. Pharmaceutical therapy
   1. Refer to specific chapter for therapies related to etiology.
   2. Vulvodynia: Consider the use of topical agents applied to the vulva or vestibule, antihistamine therapy, and/or tricyclic antidepressants.
      a. Lidocaine (Xylocaine) 2% gel applied to vulva, vestibule, and fourchette
      b. Diphenhydramine (Benadryl) 25 to 50 mg orally at bedtime, or 0.1% triamcinolone acetonide cream twice daily for pruritus
      c. Amitriptyline 10 mg orally at bedtime

Follow-Up

A. Perform test of cure for all diagnosed infections, if indicated (see specific infection and therapy).

B. Refer to follow-up plans for specific etiology.

Consultation/Referral

A. Refer the patient to a gynecologist for removal of cysts, endometriomas. Laparoscopy is indicated if endometriosis, adhesions, or an adnexal mass is suspected.
B. Refer the patient to a gynecologist for vulvovaginal anomalies, including thickened hymen, shortened vagina, vaginal agenesis; vaginal dilator therapy may be tried.
C. Refer the patient for sexual therapy consultation for continued complaints without an identifiable physical cause.

Individual Considerations

A. Pregnancy or postpartum
  1. Sexual intercourse may continue throughout pregnancy unless there is pain, bleeding, preterm labor, or premature rupture of the membranes. Alternate positions should be suggested by the provider. Sexual intercourse may resume in the postpartum period when the bleeding has decreased or stopped, incision or episiotomy is healed, and the woman is comfortable upon finger insertion and test of vaginal discomfort.
  2. Breastfeeding causes hormonal changes that may produce a menopause-like state, and extra lubrication is usually required.
B. Partners
  1. Encourage the patient to have partner(s) participate in sexual health counseling.

Emergency Contraception

Rhonda Arthur

Definition

A. Emergency contraception is a prospective method of pregnancy prevention when unprotected intercourse or birth control failure occurs.

Incidence

A. One in nine sexually active women report using emergency contraception, with the highest use rate among women aged 20 to 24 years. The intent is to increase the use of emergency contraception to reduce the number of unintended pregnancies and thus reduce the number of abortions and deliveries of truly unwanted children. More than 43 million women are not using birth control and are at risk of unintended pregnancy.

Pathogenesis

A. Hormones in oral contraceptive pills temporarily disrupt ovarian hormone production and cause an absent or dysfunctional luteal phase hormone pattern. This results in an out-of-phase endometrium that is unsuitable for implantation. Hormone disruption may likewise interfere with fertilization and cause disordered tubal transport. Hormones or minerals (copper) in an intrauterine device (IUD) cause an inflammatory response to occur, which make the endometrium unsuitable for implantation and interfere with fertilization and transport.

Predisposing Factors

A. Rape
B. Failure of other means of birth control, including broken condom, dislodged diaphragm or cervical cap, expelled IUD, lost or forgotten pills
C. Unprotected intercourse

Common Complaints

A. "I'm worried that I might get pregnant because the condom broke."
B. "My diaphragm slipped."
C. "I went on vacation and forgot my pills."

Other Signs and Symptoms

A. Unprotected intercourse

Subjective Data

A. Elicit a menstrual history. When was the patient's last menstrual period (LMP)? Are her periods regular?
B. What form of contraception was used, if any?
C. Has the patient experienced any early signs of pregnancy? If so, discuss.
D. Ask about early symptoms of pregnancy such as frequency of urination, nausea, breast tenderness, and late or missed period.
E. Ask the patient about her feelings or plans if she should get pregnant.

Physical Examination

A. Check blood pressure, pulse, and weight.
B. Inspect abdomen for enlargement compatible with pregnancy.
C. Palpate abdomen for uterine size; if fundus is palpable, measure for fundal height.
D. Auscultate
  1. Heart and lungs
  2. Abdomen. If the uterus is enlarged and is measured to be greater than 11 weeks gestation, attempt to hear fetal heart tones with fetal Doppler.
E. Pelvic examination
  1. Inspect the external genitalia for lesions; note female pubic hair pattern.
  2. Speculum examination: Observe for bluish color of cervix (Chadwick's sign). Observe vaginal discharge; note color and odor.
  3. Bimanual examination: Palpate the cervix for softening associated with early pregnancy. Palpate uterine size.

Diagnostic Tests

A. Pregnancy test: Urine or serum human chorionic gonadotropin (HCG)

Differential Diagnoses

A. Unprotected intercourse, potential for pregnancy
B. Pregnancy
C. Dysfunctional uterine bleeding (DUB)
D. Amenorrhea from anovulation
E. Polycystic ovary syndrome (PCOS)
F. Perimenopause

Plan

A. General interventions

1. Review the patient's past medical history, contraceptive history, date of LMP, estimated date of ovulation, date of unprotected intercourse, and number of hours since the first and most recent unprotected intercourses.

2. Discuss the likely risk of pregnancy.

3. Explore the patient's feeling about continuing pregnancy.

4. Decide whether a physical examination and pregnancy test are needed if there is a possibility of a pregnancy from the previous month.

B. Patient teaching

1. *See Section III: Patient Teaching Guides for this chapter "Emergency Contraception—Levonogesterel" or "Emergency Contraception—Ulipristal Acetate"* based on selected method.

2. Discuss options, risks, failure rates, necessary follow-up, alteration of menstrual period, and warning signs of complications.

3. Discuss interim plan for contraception.

4. Advise the patient to take oral contraceptive pills as prescribed or have an IUD inserted within 96 hours of unprotected intercourse.

5. Treatment is most effective if taken within 72 hours for progestin–estrogen methods and within 120 hours for a progestin antagonist.

6. Treatment is not effective in an already established pregnancy.

7. Educate the patient about the possibility of menstrual cycle disturbance with the next menstrual period.

8. If menstrual bleeding does not begin within 3 weeks, evaluate for possible pregnancy.

9. Emergency contraception is not associated with an increased incidence of abnormal outcome of pregnancy, should pregnancy not be averted. Emergency contraception does not always work.

10. This is not to be used as a primary contraceptive method.

11. Have prescription or pack of pills available for an emergency situation.

12. The IUD should be used only for women at low risk for pelvic inflammatory disease (PID) and when the woman intends to continue use of the IUD for contraception.

C. Pharmaceutical therapy

Choosing the best method for emergency contraception (EC) should be based on day and time of unprotected intercourse; body mass index (BMI); breastfeeding; and recent (within 5 days) use of pill, patch, or ring.

1. IUD—Most effective and can be used up to 120 hours after unprotected intercourse.

a. Copper IUD (ParaGard's CUT 380, Ortho Pharmaceuticals) must be inserted within 5 to 7 days after ovulation in a cycle when unprotected intercourse has occurred. The advantage is that the IUD may be left in place for continuing contraception for 10 years.

b. Mechanism of action: Two ideas have been proposed.

i. IUD leads to endometrial changes that prohibit implantation.

ii. The copper ions have a direct toxic effect on the embryo.

2. Emergency contraception oral formulations

a. Ella (ulipristal acetate) is a progesterone agonist/antagonist that is available only by prescription. Cannot be used in breastfeeding women. May be less effective in women with a BMI greater than 35. May not be as effective as Levonorgestrel emergency contraceptive if the woman has used birth control pills, patch, or ring within the past 5 days.

i. One tablet is taken orally as soon as possible after unprotected intercourse within 120 hours (5 days).

ii. Common side effects are headaches, abdominal pain, and nausea. Less common side effects include dysmenorrhea, fatigue, and dizziness.

iii. Repeated use of ella within the same menstrual cycle is not recommended.

iv. If vomiting occurs within 1 to 3 hours of taking a dose, take another dose.

v. Educate the patient about common side effects such as breast tenderness, abdominal pain, headache, and dizziness.

vi. Because Ella and the progestin component of hormonal contraception bind to receptor sites, women wishing to use hormonal contraception after use of Ella should not do so until 5 days after Ella use, but should be counseled on alternative nonhormonal pregnancy prevention methods.

b. Levonorgestrel emergency contraceptive, commonly called "morning after pill" is available under the brand names "Plan B One-Step," "My Way," and "Next Choice," and is available in one dose (1.5-mg tablet of levonorgestrel). These progestin-only ECs are available unrestricted as over-the-counter medicines. Less effective for women with a BMI greater than 25 and may not be effective for women with a BMI greater than 30.

i. Levonorgestrel 1.5 mg tablet should be taken as soon as possible after unprotected sex (no later than 72 hours).

c. Using a standard packet of oral contraceptives: Two doses of a combination of ethinyl estradiol and norgestrel or levonorgestrel, 12 hours apart. Table 14.1 provides the equivalent dosing that may be used as an emergency contraceptive.

i. Method must be used within 72 hours of unprotected intercourse. Treatment is most effective if taken within 12 to 24 hours.

ii. Side effects of nausea and vomiting with emergency contraception are common. Take each dose with food. Take antiemetic,

TABLE 14.1 Emergency Contraception

Antiprogestin Emergency Contraception Pill			
Directions for antiprogestin pills: Take one pill within 120 hours			
Brand		**Number of Pills per Dose**	
ella		1 white pill	
Progestin-Only Emergency Contraceptive Pill			
Directions for progestin-only pills: Take one dose within 72 hours of intercourse			
Brand	**Number of Pills per Dose**	**Ethinyl Estradiol (mcg)/ Dose**	**Levonorgestrel (mg)/Dose**
Plan B One-Step	1 pill	0	1.5
My Way	1 pill	0	1.5
Next Choice One Dose	1 pill	0	1.5
Combine Oral Contraceptive (COC) Pills for Emergency Contraception			
Directions for COC pills: Take first dose within 72 hours and repeat dose in 12 hours			
Brand	**Number of Pills per Dose**	**Ethinyl Estradiol (mcg)/ Dose**	**Levonorgestrel (mg)/Dose**
Ovral	2 white pills	100	0.50
Lo/Ovral	4 white pills	120	0.60
Nordette	4 orange pills	120	0.60
Levlen	4 orange pills	120	0.60
Triphasil	4 yellow pills	120	0.50
Tri-Levlen	4 yellow pills	120	0.50
Alesse	5 pink pills	100	0.50

dimenhydrinate (Dramamine) 50 mg orally, 30 minutes before dose of medication.

iii. If vomiting occurs within 1 to 3 hours of taking a dose, take another dose.

iv. Educate the patient about common side effects such as breast tenderness, abdominal pain, headache, and dizziness.

Follow-Up

A. Have the patient return in 3 to 4 weeks if she does not have a menstrual period. If she has a menstrual period, recommend that she return in 1 month to assess contraceptive use and offer options.

Consultation/Referral

A. Consult a physician if there is no withdrawal bleed within 4 weeks.

B. Consult or refer the patient to a physician if necessary to insert IUD.

C. Here are several ways patients can find emergency contraception.

1. Not 2 Late is operated by the Office of Population Research at Princeton University and the Association of Reproductive Health Professionals: 888-NOT-2-LATE.

2. Websites

a. Emergency contraception (EC) (you can be included as a provider): ec.princeton.edu

b. Planned Parenthood: www.ppfa.org

Special Considerations

A. Pregnancy: There is no increased incidence of anomalies if pregnancy does occur.

Endometriosis

Rhonda Arthur

Definition

A. Endometriosis is ectopic endometrial tissue that exhibits hormonal responsiveness but is located outside the uterine cavity. Bleeding from this ectopic endometrial tissue causes pelvic inflammation and scarring, resulting in chronic pelvic pain and infertility. Endometrial lesions have been found in the vagina, gastrointestinal (GI) tract (especially the sigmoid colon), thoracic cavity, limbs, and gallbladder.

Incidence

A. The true incidence of endometriosis is unknown. Ranges of 5% to 30% have been cited. Positive family history (mother or sister) increases the risk tenfold. Endometriosis does not have a higher incidence for any particular race or socioeconomic group.

Pathogenesis

A. Retrograde menstruation is the most popular theory for the etiology of endometriosis. Menses are suspected of "flowing backward" through the fallopian tubes, resulting in the "seeding" of endometrial tissue outside the uterus.

Predisposing Factors

A. Positive family history, mother and/or sister

B. History of progressive dysmenorrhea

C. History of prolonged uninterrupted menstrual cycles; first pregnancy at a late age

D. Limited or no prior use of hormonal contraceptives

Common Complaints

A. Pain before period

B. Pain with intercourse

C. Pain with bowel movements; may include constipation from the fear or pain of having a bowel movement (dyschezia)
D. Vaginal spotting and bleeding

Other Signs and Symptoms

A. Dyspareunia and/or pain that radiates to the thigh
B. Chronic, noncyclic pelvic pain
C. Abnormal vaginal bleeding: Premenstrual spotting and dysfunctional uterine bleeding (DUB)
D. Other bowel symptoms: Diarrhea and rectal bleeding
E. Urinary symptoms: Dysuria, urgency, and hematuria

Subjective Data

A. Review the onset, duration, and course of complaints.
B. Question the patient regarding menstrual history: Interval and duration of menstrual cycles and history of dysmenorrhea.
C. Question the patient regarding former use of hormonal contraceptives, including levonorgestrel (Norplant System), birth control pills, medroxyprogesterone (Depo-Provera), and progesterone (Progestasert intrauterine device [IUD]).
D. Question the patient regarding change in bowel patterns or habits or pain with defecation.
E. Question the patient regarding incidence of dyspareunia.
F. Note the patient parity and/or history of infertility.

Physical Examination

A. Check temperature, pulse, respirations, and blood pressure.
B. Inspect
  1. Note general appearance for discomfort before, during, and after examination.
  2. Perform detailed external genitalia examination.
C. Auscultate
  1. Abdomen for bowel sounds in all quadrants. Auscultation of the abdomen should precede any palpation or percussion due to the changes in intensity and frequency of sounds after manipulation.
D. Palpate
  1. Palpate abdomen for masses.
  2. Check for suprapubic tenderness.
  3. Back: Check for costovertebral angle (CVA) tenderness.
E. Pelvic examination
  1. Speculum examination: Inspect the cervix for cervicitis; friability; and discharge color, odor, and amount. Note any cutaneous lesions of the vagina, cervix, and perineum that resemble "powder burn or chocolate spots." Laparoscopic findings frequently reveal "powder burn" lesions of endometrial implants along the uterosacral ligament, pelvic peritoneum, ovaries, sigmoid colon, and other pelvic organs.
  2. Bimanual examination: Check for cervical motion tenderness (CMT), adnexal masses; check uterine size, consistency, position, and mobility.

> *The most common indicator of endometriosis is a fixed retroverted uterus with nodularity felt along the uterosacral ligaments. Palpation of endometrial implants may result in exquisite pain for the patient.*

  3. Rectovaginal examination: Palpate uterosacral ligaments for pain and nodularity. Evaluate for masses and polyps of rectum. A rectal examination is done because the uterus is often fixed in a retroverted position due to endometriosis. The endometrial nodules present on the posterior uterine wall, cul-de-sac, and uterosacral ligament may be distinguished better rectally.

Diagnostic Tests

There are no specific diagnostic tests for endometriosis. Definite diagnosis is done by laparoscopy.
A. Serum beta human chorionic gonadotropin (HCG) to rule out ectopic pregnancy
B. White blood cell (WBC) to rule out infection
C. Cervical culture for chlamydia or gonorrhea, to rule out sexually transmitted infection (STI) and pelvic inflammatory disease (PID)
D. Urine culture, if indicated
E. Transvaginal ultrasonography, to rule out cysts and masses
F. GI series or barium enema, if indicated

Differential Diagnoses

A. Endometriosis
B. Dysmenorrhea
C. Ovarian cysts
D. PID
E. Premenstrual syndrome (PMS)
F. Mittelschmerz
G. Trauma
H. Appendicitis
I. Pregnancy: Normal, missed abortion, or ectopic
J. GI or genitourinary (GU) complaints: Diverticular disease, spastic colon, or urinary tract infection (UTI)

Plan

A. General interventions
  1. After surgical confirmation, the practitioner may comanage endometriosis with a physician.
B. Patient teaching
  1. Treatment goals include prevention of disease progression, alleviation of pain, and establishment or restoration of fertility. Treatment options include the following:
    a. Observation alone
    b. Medical therapy or pharmacological therapy
    c. Referral or consultation for laparoscopic therapy, including laser vaporization and removal of adhesions
  2. Continuation or recurrence of pelvic pain may necessitate assisting the woman to manage her chronic pelvic pain and dysmenorrhea with nonsteroidal anti-inflammatory drugs (NSAIDs) therapy and/or other

non-narcotic chronic pain therapies, such as visualization and biofeedback.

3. Hysterectomy and bilateral salpingo-oophorectomy are the only definitive cures for women who do not wish to conserve their reproductive capacity. This should be considered only as a last resort for failed conservative treatment.

C. Pharmaceutical therapy: Diagnosis must first be confirmed by laparoscopy.

1. Mild endometriosis

a. Combined oral contraceptive (COC) pills are considered the first-line therapy. If the patient experiences pain during the week of withdrawal bleeding, she may take active pills continuously, omitting the placebo pills of the "off week."

Combination oral contraceptives are being used to produce a state of pseudopregnancy that should induce regression of the disease.

b. Medroxyprogesterone acetate 20 to 100 mg daily, norethindrone acetate 5 to 15 mg daily, or megestrol acetate 40 mg daily, or a long-acting progestin (Depo-Provera) 150 mg by intramuscular (IM) injection every 3 months.

2. Moderate to severe complaints

a. Gonadotropin-releasing hormone (Gn-RH) agonist

i. Leuprolide acetate (Lupron) 3.75 mg by IM injection every month

ii. Nafarelin (Synarel) nasal spray twice daily

Use of a Gn-RH agonist, which acts to suppress ovulation, can result in side effects, including hot flashes, mood changes, and other menopausal symptoms. Use is restricted to 6 months to avoid decrease in bone density. Expense of this therapy may preclude its use.

b. Danazol 400 to 800 mg daily for up to 6 months

i. Use of danazol, which acts to produce anovulation and hypogonadotropism, can result in androgenic side effects, including acne, hirsutism, weight gain, and voice changes that may not be reversible.

ii. Other side effects, which are reversible, include decreased breast size, atrophic vaginitis, dyspareunia, hot flashes, and emotional liability.

Follow-Up

A. Patients must return monthly while receiving Gn-RH agonist or danazol therapies to assess for symptom relief and side-effect profile.

Consultation/Referral

A. The workup, evaluation, and medications for endometriosis are expensive. Refer to a gynecologist for initial management. A prudent approach is recommended with a conservative treatment option; evaluate the results before trying another.

B. Refer the patient for a surgical consultation for definitive diagnosis. Endometriosis may be suspected based on symptoms and physical examination. It cannot, however, be confirmed unless actually visualized by laparoscopy.

Individual Considerations

A. Pregnancy

1. Infertility may be a presenting symptom. Treatment may, therefore, be focused on endometriosis abatement and fertility support.

Resource

Endometriosis Association
8585 North 76th Place
Milwaukee, WI 53223
(414) 355 2200
www.endometriosisassn.org

Female Sexual Dysfunction

Nancy Pesta Walsh

Definition

A. Any persistent problem with desire, sexual response, or function, which may affect the patient and her relationship, and occurs for at least 6 months. It is classified into subtypes:

1. Desire disorder: Lack of interest or desire (most common)

2. Arousal disorder: Inability to become aroused during sexual activity; absent or reduced genital sensations

3. Orgasm disorder: Delay, absence, or decreased intensity of orgasm

a. Primary: The patient has never had an orgasm

b. Secondary: The patient has achieved orgasm in the past, but is unable to achieve orgasm at the time of presentation.

4. Pain disorder: Genitopelvic pain/penetration disorder (formerly dyspareunia and vaginismus). This is described as pelvic or vulvovaginal pain during vaginal penetration, anxiety, and/or fear related to the thought of vaginal penetration, or marked tightening of pelvic floor muscles during vaginal penetration.

Incidence

A. Affects an estimated 22% to 43% of women worldwide, and 14% of women aged 45 to 64 years. Only 12% have diagnosable disorders. This includes women who report issues with sexual desire (64%), arousal difficulty (31%), and pain (26%).

Pathogenesis

A. Multiple models exist to describe the phases of normal sexual function.

1. Masters and Johnson—consists of the stages of excitement, plateau, orgasm, and resolution

2. Kaplan and Leif—consists of desire, excitement, and orgasm

3. Basson—consists of emotional intimacy, sexual stimuli, psychological factors, and relationship satisfaction

B. Sexual dysfunction includes various biological, psychological, and social components.

1. Biological factors include aging; medical conditions such as diabetes and hypertension, and declining testosterone or estrogen.
2. Psychological factors include depression or anxiety, history of sexual abuse, childhood trauma, personality disorders, body image disorders, and perceived stress.
3. Social factors include cultural or religious values, relationship issues, career issues, financial hardship, and household responsibilities.

C. Diagnosis is made based on the *Diagnostic and Statistical Manual of Mental Disorders* Fifth Edition (*DSM-5*; 2013) and requires the following: Symptoms must be present for a minimum of 6 months; a woman experiences personal distress; symptoms are not a result of substance or medication use, or medical conditions; and symptoms are not related to a nonsexual medical disorder.

D. Orgasm disorders can be caused by neurologic and/or vascular disease such as spinal cord injury, diabetes, or multiple sclerosis.

Predisposing Factors

A. Emotional

1. Depression
2. Mood disorders
3. Poor body image
4. Low self-esteem
5. Fatigue
6. Stress

B. Poor health status

1. Spinal cord injury
2. Diabetes
3. Premature ovarian failure (POF)
4. Trauma

C. Partner relationship issues

D. Medications that are associated with low sexual desire in women:

1. Serotonin-specific reuptake inhibitors (SSRIs)
2. Anxiolytics
3. Antihistamines
4. Anticholinergics
5. Calcium channel blockers
6. Angiotensin-converting enzyme (ACE) inhibitors
7. Oral contraceptives
8. Anticonvulsants
9. Opiates
10. Illicit drugs

E. History of sexual abuse may contribute to low desire

F. Advancing age

1. Menopausal women affected more frequently. Low sexual desire may result from decreasing hormone levels, specifically testosterone and estrogen levels. Low estrogen levels are also linked to vulvovaginal atrophy and dyspareunia, both of which may decrease sexual desire in women.

Common Complaints

A. Women

1. Absence of orgasm
2. Pain during vaginal penetration
3. Difficulty relaxing pelvic floor muscles to allow vaginal penetration

B. Both sexes

1. Lack of interest or desire (most common)
2. Inability to become aroused
3. Pain with intercourse

C. Men: Common complaints for men are specifically discussed in Chapter 11: Gastrointestinal guidelines.

Other Signs and Symptoms

A. Vaginal discharge

B. Vulvar itching

C. Vulvar pain, described as stinging, burning, irritation, raw sensation

Subjective Data

A. Include full medical, gynecologic, and sexual history, using open-ended questions

1. Assess the patient for signs of depression, anxiety, and sexual concerns.
2. Review the medication list with the patient. Specifically ask about the types of medications that may contribute to low sexual desire:
   a. SSRIs
   b. Anxiolytics
   c. Antihistamines
   d. Anticholinergics
   e. Calcium channel blockers
   f. ACE inhibitors
   g. Oral contraceptives
   h. Anticonvulsants
   i. Opiates
   j. Illicit drugs
3. Assess for medical conditions that contribute to sexual dysfunction, which may include:
   a. Chronic diseases (cardiovascular disease, diabetes, kidney or liver failure)
   b. Neurologic disorders
   c. Hormone imbalances
   d. Alcoholism
   e. Elicit drug use
   f. Evaluate for causes of pelvic pain: Vaginal dryness, vaginal discharge, or vaginal infectious causes (such as STIs, yeast infections, or PID).
4. Evaluate for history of previous pelvic disorders or surgery (fibroids, endometriosis, malignancy, uterine/bladder prolapse, or episiotomy).
5. Evaluate for the degree of distress that this may cause the patient.

B. The use of self-report screening tools is recommended to identify women with low sexual desire. These tools may include:

1. Decreased Sexual Desire Screener

a. Found at www.obgynalliance.com/files/fsd/DSDS_Pocketcard.pdf
2. Brief Sexual Symptom Checklist for Women
a. May be downloaded from www.researchgate.net/figure/277610474_fig1_Figure-2-The-modified-Brief-Sexual-Symptom-Checklist-for-Women-BSSC-W
3. Female Sexual Function Index:
a. Found at www.fsfiquestionnaire.com

Physical Examination

A. Vital signs: Check BP, pulse, and respirations.
B. Inspect
1. Thyroid for presence of nodules
2. Breasts for presence of nipple discharge if history warrants
3. Skin for hirsutism, acne, alopecia, and truncal obesity may indicate hyperandrogenism
C. Palpate
1. Thyroid for presence of nodules
2. May palpate breasts for presence of nipple discharge if history warrants.

Pelvic Examination

A. Inspect
1. Examine external genitalia for erythema, lesions, atrophy, or unusual discharge.
2. Inspect for vulvar dermatoses, such as lichen sclerosus or lichen planus. Lichen sclerosus may look like white skin discolorations or wrinkled patches of skin. Severe cases may have bleeding or ulcerated lesions. Lichen planus may look like purple-colored lesions or bumps with flat tops. Thin white lines or blisters may appear over the lesions.
3. Inspect for pelvic floor prolapse and pelvic floor muscle contraction.
B. Palpate external genitalia for presence of pain.
C. Speculum examination
1. Assess for atrophy (common in postmenopausal women), pelvic floor muscle strength, masses, prolapse, and deep pelvic pain.
D. Bimanual examination
1. Check for cervical motion tenderness (CMT), uterine size, and position.
2. Check adnexa for masses or tenderness.

Diagnostic Tests

A. Laboratory tests should be performed as indicated by the history and physical examination for any medical conditions that may contribute to low desire
B. Pap smear, STI testing, wet prep
C. Serum testing may include thyroid function tests and prolactin levels.
D. Androgen levels and testosterone levels alone are unreliable, unless you suspect a hyperandrogenic condition, as evidenced by hirsutism, acne, alopecia, and truncal obesity.
E. Transvaginal ultrasound may be warranted if pelvic pain upon examination.

Differential Diagnoses

A. Arousal disorder
B. Desire disorder
C. Orgasm disorder
D. Pain disorder
E. Vulvar dermatoses, such as lichen planus or lichen sclerosis
F. Vaginal atrophy
G. Infectious issues, such as STIs, candidiasis, or bacterial vaginosis (BV)
H. Depression or anxiety
I. Cardiovascular disease
J. Diabetes
K. Thyroid disorder
L. Neurologic disorder
M. Hormonal imbalance

Plan

A. General interventions
1. Set realistic goals for treatment.
2. Empower women to take an active role in treatment plan. Encourage discussion about anatomy and sexual function, allowing the women to ask questions as they are comfortable.
3. Office-based therapy may be useful for providers who wish to include this in their practice. The Permission, Limited Information, Specific Suggestion, Intensive Therapy (PLISSIT) model is one office-based counseling model detailed as follows:
a. Permission: Women are given permission for full discussion of the topic.
b. Limited information: The provider gives educational information on sexual function and sexual dysfunction in the form of handouts or videos.
c. Specific suggestion: The provider gives very specific advice tailored to each patient and her presenting issues.
d. Intensive therapy: The provider makes a referral for individual or couples therapy.
B. Patient teaching
1. Educate about normal anatomical and sexual functions.
2. Encourage healthy lifestyle behaviors of diet, exercise, avoiding tobacco, and minimizing stress.
3. Educate patients about the use of vaginal lubricants to assist with vaginal dryness or dyspareunia. KY Jelly or Astroglide: Dose as needed with intercourse.
C. Pharmaceutical therapy is considered when nonpharmacological interventions are not successful.
1. Vaginal estrogen for the treatment of vaginal atrophy:
a. Vagifem: 10 mcg, one tablet in vagina nightly for 2 weeks, then twice a week for maintenance
b. Estring: One ring, placed intravaginally every 3 months
c. Premarin: 0.625 mg/g: Insert 0.5 g/d for 21 days on, 7 days off. May adjust dose based upon patient response
d. Estrace: 100 mcg/g: Insert 2 to 4 g in vagina nightly for 2 weeks, then gradually taper to half the

initial dose for 1 to 2 weeks, then a maintenance dose of 1 g one to three times a week for maintenance. Taper or discontinue at 3- to 6-month intervals

3. Ospemifene
   a. Is a nonestrogen compound for treatment of moderate to severe dyspareunia related to vaginal atrophy in postmenopausal females.
   b. Dosage: 60 mg once per day

Follow-Up

A. As determined by the history and physical examination findings and diagnoses made. Women placed on medications should follow up 1 month after initiating and have routine follow-up at 3- to 6-month intervals to determine if continuation of the medication is necessary.
B. Postmenopausal women with vaginal bleeding should follow up immediately.

Consultation/Referral

A. Refer to any therapist who specializes in sexual problems.
   1. Counseling may include sex therapy or cognitive behavioral therapy (CBT).
B. May refer to pelvic floor therapist for treatment of genitopelvic pain disorders, once other medical conditions have been treated.

Individual Considerations

A. Use of opposing progestin is not necessary when using lowest dose estrogens, though use of estrogen should be the lowest possible effective dose for the shortest duration.
B. Patients with a history of breast cancer: Although risk is low, consult with the patient's oncologist before initiating vaginal estrogen.
C. If using ospemifene (Osphena), use opposing progestin in women with intact uterus. Contraindicated in women with undiagnosed abnormal vaginal bleeding, history of venous thromboembolism, pulmonary embolism, breast cancer, and women of childbearing age.

Resources

American Association of Sexuality Educators, Counselors and Therapists
1444 I Street, NW, Suite 700
Washington, DC 20005
(202) 449–1099
e-mail: info@aasect.org
www.AASECT.org

International Society for the Study of Women's Sexual Health
PO Box 1233
Lakeville, MN 55044
(218)-461–5115
e-mail: info@isswsh.org
www.ISSWSH.org

North American Menopause Society
5900 Landerbrook Drive
Suite 390
Mayfield Heights, OH 44124
(440)- 442–7550
e-mail: info@menopause.org

Society for Sex Therapy and Research
6311 W. Gross Point Rd
Niles, IL 60714
(847)-647–8832
e-mail: info@sstarnet.org
www.SSTARNET.org

Infertility

Rhonda Arthur

Definition

A. Infertility is defined as the inability to conceive within 12 months of unprotected intercourse. Many clinicians use a 6-month time frame if the woman is 35 years of age and older.
B. A woman who has never been pregnant or a man who has never initiated a pregnancy is said to have "primary infertility."
C. If a previous pregnancy has been achieved and the couple is unable to conceive a subsequent pregnancy, the term "secondary infertility" is applied.

Incidence

A. It is estimated that approximately 6.7 million women have impaired ability to become pregnant or carry a baby to term in the United States. Pelvic inflammatory disease (PID) is the leading cause of infertility in the world. About 10% of infertility is unexplained.

Pathogenesis

Infertility may occur in the male (approximately 35%) or female (approximately 55%). Evaluate both partners for
A. Infrequent intercourse
B. Interpersonal problems
C. Medical causes (see Table 14.2)

Predisposing Factors

A. Predisposing factors depend on the etiology.

Common Complaint

A. The common complaint is an inability to achieve pregnancy despite frequent acts of intercourse.

Other Signs and Symptoms

A. Dependent on the pathogenesis and history

Subjective Data

A. Obtain a complete health history, including the following:
   1. Age of both partners
   2. General health of both partners
   3. Complete pregnancy history of the female
      a. Number of pregnancies: Term and preterm
      b. Vaginal deliveries or cesarean sections
      c. Recurrent miscarriages, gestational age(s)
      d. Stillbirths
      e. Dilation and curettage (D&C) for abortions or miscarriages
      f. Cerclage for incompetent cervix
   4. Paternity history of the male
   5. Length of infertility, including prior workup, if any
   6. Coital history
      a. Frequency
      b. Timing and adequacy
      c. Use of lubricants; some may be spermicidal
      d. Postcoital habits: Douching or voiding
   7. Adequacy of intercourse
      a. Penetration of the vagina
      b. Ejaculation by the male

TABLE 14.2 Pathogenesis of Infertility

Male Pathogenesis	Female Pathogenesis
A. Faulty sperm production	**A.** Advanced maternal age
1. Azoospermia from	**B.** Disorder of ovulation/hypothalamic dysfunction
a. Cancer therapy	**1.** Anovulation
b. Adult mumps	**2.** Amenorrhea
c. Sertoli-cell-only syndrome	**3.** Polycystic ovary triad
d. Hypogonadism	**a.** Acne
e. Retrograde ejaculation	**b.** Obesity
2. Oligospermia from	**c.** Hirsutism
a. Varicocele	**4.** Premature ovarian failure
b. Small testicular size	**a.** Autoimmune
B. Reproductive tract anomaly	**b.** Idiopathic
1. Blocked vas deferens	**c.** Cancer therapy
2. Varicocele	**5.** Luteal phase insufficiency
3. Congenital obstruction of epididymis	**6.** Prolactinoma
C. Klinefelter's syndrome	**C.** Ovarian factors
D. Physical and chemical agents' exposure	**1.** Cysts or tumor
1. Coal tar	**2.** Irradiation
2. Radiation	**D.** Tubal disorders/damage/blocked
E. Endocrine disorders	**1.** PID
1. Diabetes	**2.** *Chlamydia trachomatis*
2. Low serum testosterone	**3.** Postpartum infection
3. Pituitary tumors	**4.** Pelvic trauma (motor vehicle accident)
4. Hyperprolactinemia	**5.** Inflammatory bowel disease
F. Testicular infection	**6.** Endometriosis
G. Injury to reproductive organs/tract	**7.** Adhesions
H. Nerve damage/neurologic disease: Spinal cord injury	**E.** Uterine pathology
I. Impotence/erectile difficulty: Performance anxiety	**1.** Congenital anomalies: Duplication
J. Premature ejaculation	**2.** Septate
K. Early withdrawal	**3.** Fibroids
L. Lifestyle factors	**4.** IUD
1. Drugs	**5.** Asherman's syndrome
2. Smoking	**6.** Synechiae
3. Alcohol	**F.** Cervical factors
4. Malnutrition	**1.** Anatomic abnormalities (hood)
M. Antispermatozoa antibodies	**2.** Previous cervical surgery (i.e., conization, which leads to mucus depletion)
N. Medications	**3.** Hostile cervical mucus
1. Antihypertensives	**4.** Presence of sperm antibodies in the cervix
2. Antidepressants	**5.** Infections
3. Antipsychotics	**G.** Lifestyle factors
4. Anti-ulcer agents/antacids	**1.** Drugs
5. Muscle relaxants	**2.** Smoking

(*continued*)

TABLE 14.2 Pathogenesis of Infertility (*continued*)

Male Pathogenesis	Female Pathogenesis
	H. Vaginal factors **1.** Intact hymen **2.** Septum **3.** Absent vagina **4.** Infection **a.** *Trichomonas* **b.** *Candida* **c.** Chlamydia **d.** Mycoplasma **e.** Bacterial vaginosis (BV) **f.** Gonorrhea **g.** *Streptococci* **I.** Medications: Oral contraceptives **J.** Medical problems **1.** Lupus **2.** Hypothyroidism **3.** Diabetes **4.** Antiphospholipid syndrome

IUD, intrauterine device; PID, pelvic inflammatory disease.

B. Obtain a complete menstrual history, including
  1. Age at puberty
  2. Regularity of cycles
  3. Discomfort during menses
  4. Date of last menstrual period (LMP)

C. Obtain a complete gynecologic history including
  1. Contraceptive use
  2. Medical and surgical interventions
    a. D&C
    b. Laparoscopy or endometriosis
  3. Anomalies

D. Take a complete nutritional and exercise history; note eating disorders.
  1. Anorexia nervosa
  2. Bulimia

E. Review female and male reproductive tract infections and treatments for past and present partners.

F. Review each individual's habits.
  1. Smoking: How much, how often, how long
  2. Drugs: How much, how often, how long for each drug
  3. Alcohol: How much, how often, how long
  4. Use of saunas or hot tubs
  5. Exercise, including cycling

G. Take a complete medication history, specifically review for
  1. Antihypertensives
  2. Antidepressants
  3. Antipsychotics
  4. Antiulcer agents or antacids
  5. Muscle relaxants

H. Review for exposure to toxic chemicals, radiation, or known teratogens
  1. Military war exposure
  2. Employment exposure
  3. Residential exposure
    a. Microwaves
    b. Pesticides

I. Inquire about diethylstilbestrol (DES) exposure in utero (for either partner).

J. Review for symptoms of thyroid dysfunction
  1. Weight gain or loss
  2. Change of bowel habits
  3. Intolerance to heat or cold
  4. Appetite changes

K. Review for systemic diseases
  1. Cardiac
  2. Collagen vascular diseases
  3. Diabetes

L. Assess the psychosocial context of the infertility, including personal, emotional, and economic factors; family pressures for children; expectations; timing of pregnancy; consideration of adoption; and stress from failure to conceive.

Signs and Symptoms

A. See the "Pathogenesis" section and information obtained in the "Subjective Data" section regarding past medical history.

B. History of not being able to get pregnant over the past 6 to 12 months is noted.

Physical Examination

Male

A. Check temperature, pulse, respirations, and blood pressure (BP). Obtain height, weight, and body mass index (BMI).

B. Inspect

1. Note general signs and appearance of underandrogenization: Decreased body hair, gynecomastia, and eunuchoid proportions.

2. Test the patient's visual field for possible mass lesion.

3. Examine the penis for hypospadias. Observe urethra for discharge.

C. Percuss: Check deep tendon reflexes (DTRs) for signs of hypothyroidism.

D. Palpate

1. Neck: Examine thyroid.

2. Genitals: Examine the scrotum for testicular size, absence of vas deferens, and presence of varicocele.

E. Rectal examination: Check prostate and seminal vesicles for tenderness and other signs of infection.

Valsalva's maneuver performed while the patient stands helps to reveal small varicocele. Varicocele feels like "a bag of worms" with bluish discoloration visible through the scrotum. Approximately 23% to 30% of infertile males have a varicocele (usually present on the left side). No treatment is necessary if the semen analysis is normal.

Female

A. Check temperature, pulse, respirations, and BP.

B. Inspect

1. Examine breasts for the presence of nipple discharge.

2. Note general signs and appearance of polycystic ovary syndrome (PCOS).

PCOS triad includes acne, obesity, and hirsutism.

C. Auscultate: Abdomen for bowel sounds in all quadrants. Auscultation of the abdomen should precede any palpation or percussion due to the changes in intensity and frequency of sounds after manipulation.

D. Palpate

1. Neck: Examine the thyroid.

2. Abdomen: Note tenderness and masses.

3. Back: Check for costovertebral angle (CVA) tenderness.

E. Percuss: Check DTRs.

F. Pelvic examination

1. Inspect: Perform detailed external peritoneal examination for signs of infection; lesions; or anomalies of clitoris, labia, Skene's gland, Bartholin's gland, vulva, and perineum.

2. Speculum examination

a. Observe length of vagina, position and characteristic of cervix, and any anomalies.

b. Sound the uterus and cervix for stenosis. Observe the characteristics of cervical mucus: Thin and watery or thick and cloudy, odor, or evidence of infection.

3. Bimanual examination: Check uterine size, consistency, contour, mobility, cervical motion tenderness (CMT), and adnexal masses.

A fixed, immobile uterus determined on bimanual examination indicates the presence of pelvic scarring resulting from conditions such as endometriosis and pelvic inflammatory disease (PID).

4. Rectovaginal examination: Palpate uterosacral ligaments for pain and nodularity; evaluate masses and polyps of the rectum.

Diagnostic Tests

A. Male factor: Semen analysis

B. Female (ovarian) factor

1. Basal body temperature (BBT)

2. Serum progesterone measured midway through luteal phase: Serum progesterone greater than 15 ng/mL indicates ovulation.

3. Urinary luteinizing hormone (LH) for surge

4. Follicle-stimulating hormone (FSH): A high FSH, greater than 40 m IU/mL, indicates ovarian failure.

5. Thyroid-stimulating hormone (TSH)

6. Serum prolactin

When nipple discharge is present, check serum prolactin and TSH to rule out hyperprolactinemia and hypothyroidism.

C. Pelvic or uterine factor

1. Hysterosalpingogram (HSG); also done for tubal factor

2. Transvaginal ultrasonography

3. Laparoscopy

D. Other tests

1. Papanicolaou (Pap) smear with maturation index

2. Cultures for gonorrhea and chlamydia

3. Pregnancy test, if amenorrhea is present

4. Complete blood count (CBC), sedimentation rate

5. Mycoplasma culture

6. Wet mount

Differential Diagnoses

A. Infertility

B. Sexual dysfunction

C. Hypothyroidism

D. Hypothalamic dysfunction: Amenorrhea

E. Hyperprolactinemia

F. Menopause

G. Ovarian failure

H. PCOS

I. Asherman's syndrome

J. Tubal occlusion

K. Antisperm antibodies
L. Endometriosis
M. Oligo-ovulation
N. Uterine anomalies: Fibroids, synechiae, and septa
O. Pelvic adhesions

Plan

A. General interventions

1. Semen analysis is the first step in an infertility workup. Semen analysis should be performed in a reputable laboratory. If the first evaluation is abnormal, it should be repeated one time. Normal semen analysis includes the following:

a. Sperm count: Greater than 20 million/mL
b. Volume: 2.6 mL
c. Motility: Greater than 50%
d. Morphology: Greater than 60%
e. Liquefaction: Within 20 to 30 minutes of ejaculation

2. The male physical examination is generally done if semen analysis is abnormal.

3. The male should always be evaluated first before a long and expensive female evaluation is begun.

4. Female evaluation

a. BBT: Followed for several months to evaluate ovulation. Some patients' temperatures dip just before the day of ovulation and then rise. Ovulation and the development of the corpus luteum manifest as an increase in BBT by 0.6°F to 1°F above the patient's baseline temperature (LH surge). The BBT provides presumptive evidence of normal oocyte production and related hormonal change, as well as guidance for the frequency and timing of intercourse.

b. Endometrial biopsy: Sampling of the uterine lining late in the luteal phase. The test is scheduled 10 days after the BBT increase, or 2 to 3 days before the onset of the next menses. A normal secretory endometrium and the absence of inflammation indicate that implantation is feasible.

c. HSG (performed in radiology): Evaluates tubal patency and rules out uterine anomalies. The HSG should be scheduled for the interval between cessation of menstrual flow and ovulation to avoid retrograde flow of menstrual tissue into the tubes and the abdominal cavity.

d. Laparoscopy: Diagnostic if used as the final screening examination for infertility. Performed by a gynecologist, it is usually done in the first 2 weeks of the menstrual cycle to ensure that the patient is not pregnant. Direct visualization of the pelvic organs provides data about degree of adhesion formation, presence of endometriosis or fibroids, and the possibility of surgical repair of damaged tubes.

B. Patient teaching

1. Infertile couples often require extensive counseling, including grief counseling for failure to achieve pregnancy.

2. Teach the patient to take BBT measurements. *See Section III: Patient Teaching Guide for this chapter, "Basal Body Temperature Measurement."*

C. Pharmaceutical therapy

1. Treatment depends on causative factor(s).

2. Prescription medications must be supervised by physician and/or specialist because of possible complications such as ovarian hyperstimulation.

Follow-Up

A. Follow-up depends on causative factor(s).

Consultation/Referral

A. Consultation and referral are required for special testing, surgery, and assisted reproductive therapy.

B. Immediate referral to a physician is necessary for ovarian hyperstimulation.

Individual Considerations

A. Older adults

1. Advancing age increases the risk of age-related infertility. Women aged 35 years and older should be referred to a fertility specialist if unsuccessful in conceiving after 6 months.

2. Women aged 40 years and older should be referred as soon as possible for assisted reproductive therapy.

Menopause

Rhonda Arthur

Definition

A. Physiologic or natural menopause is the cessation of menses for 12 consecutive months due to the loss of ovarian follicular activity. Natural or physiologic menopause is a retrospective diagnosis recognized 12 months after the final menses. Natural menopause is generally experienced in women between 45 and 55 years of age.

B. Natural menopause before the age of 40 years is considered premature.

C. Premature ovarian failure (POF) is the full or intermittent loss of ovarian function before the age of 40 years. POF is thought to be caused by genetics, autoimmune disorders, or surgical or chemical interventions.

D. Induced menopause is the abrupt cessation of menses related to chemical or surgical interventions.

E. Perimenopause is caused by fluctuations in ovarian function in the years preceding menopause. The average onset is usually in a woman's 40s but may occur earlier. Due to fluctuations in ovarian function, pregnancy may still occur and unintended pregnancy should be avoided. Perimenopausal symptoms often last several years, with the average duration being 5 years.

Incidence

A. By the year 2020, it is expected that the number of women in the United States who are older than 51 years will exceed 50 million.

Pathogenesis

A. Physiologic menopause is due to failure of ovarian follicular development and ovarian hormone depletion. The major endocrine changes include the decreasing negative feedback on the hypothalamic–pituitary system with increasing follicle-stimulating hormone (FSH) and luteinizing hormone (LH). When the ovaries cease to produce estrogen, they become unable to respond to FSH, resulting in the cessation of ovulation and menstruation.

Common Complaints

A. Insomnia
B. Absence of menses
C. Urogenital atrophy
  1. Vaginal dryness
  2. Dyspareunia
  3. Dysuria/frequency
D. Vasomotor symptoms such as hot flashes/night sweats
E. Intermenstrual or postcoital spotting/bleeding should be evaluated for pathologic causes.

Subjective Data

A. Determine onset, duration, and course of presenting symptoms.
B. Obtain complete medical history, including medications, and assess for risk of osteoporosis, cardiovascular disease, and breast and endometrial cancer.
C. Obtain complete gynecologic history, including menarche, interval, and duration of menstrual cycles, history of dysmenorrhea, and pregnancy history. Question the patient regarding sexual history and contraceptives used (condoms, pills, diaphragm, intrauterine devices [IUDs]), frequency of method used.
D. What is the patient's current menstrual pattern? Does she think she is pregnant?
E. Review associated symptoms (hot flashes, insomnia, genitourinary symptoms), onset, timing, duration, and impact on daily life.
F. Assess for mood swings and dysphoria.

Physical Examination

A. Check temperature, pulse, respirations, and blood pressure.
B. Inspect: Observe general overall appearance and obtain height, weight, and BMI.
C. Auscultate
  1. Heart
  2. Lungs
  3. Abdomen: Auscultation of the abdomen should precede any palpation or percussion due to the changes in intensity and frequency of sounds after manipulation.
D. Percuss the abdomen for organomegaly.
E. Palpate
  1. Palpate thyroid gland.
  2. Perform clinical breast examination.
  3. Palpate groin for lymphadenopathy.
  4. Palpate the abdomen for masses.
F. Pelvic examination
  1. Inspect: Examine vulva for Bartholin's gland enlargement, fissures, condyloma, herpes, pelvic relaxation, and atrophy.
  2. Palpate: "Milk" the urethra for discharge.
  3. Speculum examination: Inspect for cervicitis and friability. Evaluate vaginal discharge and bleeding for color, amount, and odor. Perform cultures and Papanicolaou (Pap) test as indicated.
  4. Bimanual examination
    a. Check cervical motion tenderness (CMT); evaluate the size, contour, mobility, and tenderness of the uterus. An enlarged or irregular uterus requires additional evaluation.

Over time, it is normal for the postmenopausal uterus to decrease in size.

    b. Palpate the adnexa for tenderness and masses.

Ovaries should not be palpable in postmenopausal women and require further evaluation if masses or ovaries are appreciated.

  5. Rectovaginal examination: Examine stool for occult blood in women older than 50 years

Diagnostic Tests

A. Consider thyroid-stimulating hormone (TSH).
B. Consider qualitative beta human chorionic gonadotropin (HCG).
C. Complete blood count (CBC) if excessive vaginal bleeding
D. Obtain Pap smear as indicated.
E. Endometrial biopsy as indicated for intermenstrual spotting or vaginal bleeding after menopause
F. Transvaginal ultrasonography for enlarged or irregular uterus
G. Additional screening as indicated, such as mammogram, hemoccult, cholesterol, and bone mineral density.
H. FSH greater than 40 international units (IU)/L is consistent with menopause; however, fluctuations in FSH and 17–2 estradiol (E2) may make use of these markers unreliable and are no longer recommended for determining menopausal status.

Differential Diagnoses

A. Menopause
B. Perimenopause
C. Anemia
D. Cardiac abnormalities
E. Leukemia or other cancer
F. Menstrual irregularity for any cause of secondary amenorrhea
G. Pregnancy
H. Psychosomatic illness
I. Thyroid disorders

Plan

A. General interventions
1. Provide reassurance as to the cause of the absence of menses.

B. Patient teaching
1. Discuss common symptoms of menopause.
2. Provide education regarding healthy lifestyle changes: Regular exercise, weight control, smoking cessation, limiting use of drugs and alcohol, and stress reduction.
3. Encourage a healthy diet rich in vitamin D and calcium. Supplement diet with calcium supplements: 1,000 mg/d for women aged 19 to 50 years; 1,200 mg/d for women aged 50 years and older.
a. Vitamin D supplements: 600 IU/d until the age of 70 years and then 800 IU/d for 71 years of age and older. Consider vitamin D serum screening and, if deficient, treat accordingly. See "Vitamin D Deficiency" section in Chapter 21.
4. Encourage water-soluble vaginal lubricants as needed for vaginal dryness. See section on "Atrophic Vaginitis."
5. Avoid warm environments, caffeine, alcohol, spicy food, and emotional upset; these may trigger hot flashes.
6. Encourage sleep hygiene and adequate rest.
7. Discuss the risks and benefits of hormone replacement therapy (HRT).
8. Assess and manage women at increased risk for osteoporosis according to current osteoporosis guidelines.
9. Assess and treat cardiac risk factors including hypertension and lipids as indicated.
10. Give the patient the relevant teaching guide. *See Section III: Patient Teaching Guide for this chapter, "Menopause."*

C. Pharmaceutical therapy
1. HRT
a. All women should be counseled regarding the risk, benefits, limitations, and potential increased risks of HRT. Benefits of HRT include the reduction of hot flashes, insomnia, night sweats, vaginal dryness, mood swings, and depression. Although HRT does reduce the risk of bone loss and fracture, due to potential risks and effective alternative treatments for osteoporosis, it is not recommended for the treatment of osteoporosis (see "Osteoporosis/Kyphosis/Fracture" section in Chapter 21). Risks of HRT include venous thromboembolism and breast cancer. Long-term unopposed estrogen therapy (ET) increases the risk of endometrial cancer. Potential areas of concern with the use of HRT include gallbladder disease and cardiovascular events. The provider should carefully screen and educate the patient before initiating HRT.
b. Estrogen and progesterone are recommended for treatment of moderate to severe vasomotor symptoms and moderate to severe vulvar and vaginal atrophy symptoms. For women with an intact uterus, progesterone is used with ET to reduce the risk of endometrial hyperplasia and cancer. Postmenopausal women without an intact uterus generally are not prescribed progesterone and are treated with estrogen alone.
c. Oral HRT may be given either sequentially or continuously. The sequential regimen is given daily, with progesterone given on days 1 to 12 of the month. It is common to have withdrawal bleed with this regimen. An alternative to this is the continuous regimen in which both estrogen and progesterone are taken daily.
2. Transdermal estrogen
3. Transvaginal estrogen (see Tables 14.3–14.5)
4. Absolute contraindications to use of ET also apply to use of oral and topical estrogen (breast cancer, active liver disease, and/or history of recent thromboembolic event). Vaginal estrogen creams are systemically absorbed. As with use of oral and transdermal estrogen, a progestin must be administered to women who have an intact uterus, secondary to the risk of endometrial hyperplasia or cancer.
5. Absolute contraindications to ET
a. Acute liver disease
b. Cerebral vascular or coronary artery disease, myocardial infarction (MI), or stroke
c. History of or active thrombophlebitis or thromboembolic disorders
d. History of uterine or ovarian cancer
e. Known or suspected cancer of the breast
f. Known or suspected estrogen-dependent neoplasm
g. Pregnancy
h. Undiagnosed, abnormal vaginal bleeding
6. Relative contraindications to ET
a. Active gallbladder disease
b. Familial hyperlipidemia
7. Absolute contraindications to progesterone therapy
a. Active thrombophlebitis or thromboembolic disorders
b. Acute liver disease
c. Known or suspected cancer of the breast
d. Pregnancy
e. Undiagnosed, abnormal vaginal bleeding

Educate the patient to notify the care provider if unusual vaginal bleeding, calf pain, chest pain, shortness of breath, hemoptysis, severe headaches, visual disturbances, breast pain, abdominal pain, or jaundice occur while being prescribed HRT.

D. Nonhormonal pharmacological therapy for vasomotor symptoms
1. Antidepressants
a. Fluoxetine (Prozac) 20 mg/d

TABLE 14.3 Hormone Replacement Therapy

Name	Active Ingredient	Dosage
Estrogen Sequential or Continuous Combined		
Premarin	Conjugated estrogen	0.625 mg/d
Estratab	Esterified estrogen	0.625 mg/d
Menest	Esterified estrogen	0.625 mg/d
Estrace	Micronized estradiol	1.0 mg/d
Ortho-est	Estropipate	0.625 mg/d
Progestin Only for Sequential Regimen		
Amen	Medroxyprogesterone	5–10 mg added to estrogen the first 10–14 days of the month
Cycrin	Medroxyprogesterone	5–10 mg added to estrogen the first 10–14 days of the month
Provera	Medroxyprogesterone	5–10 mg added to estrogen the first 10–14 days of the month
Prometrium	Micronized progesterone	100–200 mg added to estrogen the first 10–14 days of the month
Progestin Only for Continuous Combined Regimen		
Cycrin	Medroxyprogesterone	2.5 mg/d
Provera	Medroxyprogesterone	2.5 mg/d
Combination Packet for Continuous Combined Regimen		
Prempro	0.625 mg conjugated equine estrogen and 2.5 mg medroxyprogesterone	1 tablet orally each day
Activella	1 mg 17-beta estradiol and 0.5 mg norethindrone	1 tablet orally each day
FemHrt	5 mcg ethinyl estradiol and 1 mg norethindrone	1 tablet orally each day

See complete prescribing reference or package insert for dosing, titration, contraindications, and side effects.

TABLE 14.4 Transdermal Replacement Therapy

Delivery	Name	Active Ingredient	Dosage
Transdermal patch	Climara	Estradiol	0.25 mg/d–0.0375 mg/d
			0.05 mg/d
			0.06 mg/d
			0.075 mg/d
			Apply one patch weekly (lower abdomen or upper buttocks)
Transdermal patch	Combipatch	Estradiol 0.05 mg and norethin-drone acetate 0.14 mg/d	Continuous combined regimen of one patch twice weekly for a 28-day cycle (lower abdomen)
		Or estradiol 0.05 mg and noreth-indrone acetate 0.0.25 mg/d	
Transdermal patch	Vivelle		One patch twice weekly to trunk
Gel-Pump	Elestrin	Estradiol	0.06% gel, one pump daily to clean dry skin of upper arm
Gel-Pump	Estrogel	Estradiol	0.75 mg/1.25 g gel, one pump daily to clean dry skin of upper arm
Spray	Evamist	Estradiol	1.53 mg/spray, one spray daily to inside of arm
	Vivelle	Estradiol	0.05/d, 0.1 mg/d

See complete prescribing reference or package insert for dosing, titration, contraindications, and side effects.

TABLE 14.5 **Transvaginal Replacement Therapy**

Delivery	Name	Active Ingredient	Dosage
Cream	Estrace	Micronized 17-beta estradiol	0.1 mg/g, one-half (2 g) to one (4 g) applicator intravaginally at bedtime every night for 1–2 weeks. When vaginal mucosa is restored, maintenance dose is one-quarter applicator (1 g) one to three times weekly in a cyclic regimen.
	Premarin	Conjugated equine estrogen	0.625 mg/g, use 0.5- to 1.0-g applicator inserted intravaginally at bedtime every night for 1–2 weeks, then every other night for 1–2 weeks, then as needed
Ring	Estring	Micronized 17-beta estradiol	7.5 mg/24 hr; insert new ring every 90 days
	Femring	Estradiol acetate	0.05–0.1 mg/d; insert new ring every 90 days
Vaginal tablet	Vagifem	Estradiol acetate	25 mcg once daily for 2 weeks then twice weekly
IUD	Mirena	Levonorgestrel	20 mcg daily

See complete prescribing reference or package insert for dosing, titration, contraindications, and side effects.
IUD, intrauterine device.

b. Venlafaxine (Effexor) 37.5 to 75 mg/d
c. Paroxetine (Paxil) 12.5 to 25 mg/d

2. Anticonvulsant
a. Gabapentin (Neurontin) 300 mg/d and titrate to three or four a day

3. Antihypertensive
a. Clonidine 0.05 to 0.1 mg/twice a day. For nonhormonal pharmacological therapies, review prescribing literature for side effects, titrations, and discontinuation regimens.

E. Nonprescription remedies/herbals

1. Many nonprescription remedies are currently available for the treatment of menopausal symptoms. These remedies include isoflavones (soy and red clover), black cohosh, dong quai, evening primrose oil (EPO), ginseng, licorice, and vitamin E and vitamin C.

2. The provider should review with the patient the lack of standardization and evidence regarding the safety and efficacy of these products. Currently, results of research have been insufficient to support or refute the use of these remedies for the treatment of menopausal symptoms.

Follow-Up

A. Follow up for 3 to 6 months to assess a response to treatment, and then yearly for physical examination, Papanicolaou (Pap) smear, and lipid panel as indicated.

B. Consider discontinuation of HRT in 5 years based on patient response and risks and benefits.

Consultation/Referral

A. Consult a gynecologist if the patient experiences symptoms resistant to treatment or vaginal bleeding from an unknown source.

Pap Smear Screening Guidelines and Interpretation

Rhonda Arthur

The Papanicolau (Pap) smear is a sample of cells taken from the cervix for cytologic evaluation. The Pap smear is a screening test designed to increase detection and treatment of precancerous and early cancerous lesions, and to decrease morbidity and mortality from cases of invasive cervical cancer.

In the United States, approximately 13,000 new cases of cervical cancer will be diagnosed annually. Of these cases, approximately 4,120 deaths will occur. Cervical cancer is the seventh most common cancer in women. There has been a 50% reduction in cervical cancer deaths over the last 30 years due to the use of Pap smear screening.

The following are risk factors for development of cervical cancer:

A. Early age at first intercourse: Younger than 18 years
B. Multiple sexual partners: More than three in a lifetime
C. High parity
D. Lower socioeconomic status
E. Advanced age
F. Compromised immune system: Infection with HIV
G. Smoking
H. Male partner with a history of multiple partners or sexually transmitted infections (STIs)
I. History of STI, especially human papillomavirus (HPV)

Sexually transmitted agents, particularly the HPV strains 16, 18, 31, 33, 39, and 42, are strongly associated with the development of cervical cancer. HPV DNA is present in 93% of cervical cancer and precursor lesions.

J. Diethylstilbestrol (DES) exposure in utero

K. Cervical dysplasia: The risk of carcinoma is 100 times greater in women with dysplasia than in those with a normal cervix.

The Pap smear should include sampling from both the ectocervix and the endocervix to be considered "adequate for interpretation." The ectocervix is the cervical portion extending outward from the external cervical os. The endocervix extends upward from the external os to the internal os, where the cervical epithelium meets the uterine endometrium.

Cervical epithelium is composed of squamous and columnar cells. Squamous epithelium, appearing smooth and pink, lines the vagina and continues upward to cover variable amounts of the ectocervix. Columnar epithelium, darker red and more granular in appearance, lines the endometrium and continues downward to the cervix, lining the endocervical canal. The boundary between squamous and columnar epithelium is called the squamocolumnar junction (or transformation zone) and may occur anywhere on the ectocervix or endocervix.

The squamocolumnar junction may regress at various times as a result of hormonal variation, particularly with sexual activity and during pregnancy, through processes known as epidermidalization and squamous metaplasia. Epidermidalization is an upward growth of squamous cells that replace columnar cells. Squamous metaplasia is the differentiation of columnar cells into squamous cells. The area between the original and new squamocolumnar junction is called the transformation zone. When columnar epithelium is visible on the ectocervix, appearing as a granular, red area, it is referred to as eversion, ectropion, or ectopy. This is often seen in pregnancy or with oral contraceptive use.

Cervical cancer is a progressive disease with a number of histologically definable stages. Invasive cancer of the cervix and its precursors are detectable by cytology before becoming symptomatic and before gross clinical signs appear. When symptoms are present, they usually include (in order of frequency) postcoital spotting; intermenstrual bleeding, especially after exertion; and increased menstrual bleeding. Patients with invasive cancer may experience serosanguineous or yellowish vaginal discharge, which may be foul smelling and intermixed with blood.

Advanced disease may cause urinary or rectal symptoms, including bleeding. On speculum examination, advanced lesions appear as necrotic ulcers; in invasive disease they may extend upward or protrude into the vagina.

▶ *See Section II: Procedures, "Pap Smear and Maturation Index Procedure."*

Bethesda System

The 2001 BethesdaSystem (classification system used to interpret cytologic findings) was updated in 2014. It includes the following information:

A. Specimen type
  1. Conventional versus liquid-based preparation versus other

B. Adequacy of the specimen
  1. Satisfactory for evaluation
  2. Presence or absence of endocervical or transformational zone components
  3. Quality indicators such as obscuring blood or inflammation
  4. Unsatisfactory for evaluation and specific reason

C. General categorization
  1. Negative for intraepithelial lesion or malignancy
  2. Other, such as endometrial cells in women older than 45 years
  3. Epithelial cell abnormality: See "Interpretation/result" that follows.

If an infection is indicated as a Pap smear finding, evaluate the patient and treat her accordingly. Pap smears are not diagnostic of vaginal or cervical infection. Institute therapy for infections confirmed through the use of wet prep and/or cultures as guided by cytologic reading. For example, if Candida *is identified on Pap smear results, evaluate the patient in the office, confirm finding, and treat the patient with appropriate antifungal therapy.*

D. Interpretation/result

Negative for intraepithelial lesion or malignancy (optional to report)
  1. Non-neoplastic cellular variations
  2. Reactive cellular changes associated with
    a. Inflammation
    b. Radiation
    c. Intrauterine device (IUD)
  3. Organisms
    a. *Trichomonas vaginalis*
    b. Fungal organisms
    c. Shift in flora suggestive bacterial vaginosis (BV)
    d. Cellular changes consistent with herpes simplex virus (HSV)
    e. Cellular changes consistent with cytomegalovirus
  4. Other
    a. Endometrial cells (in a woman 45 years or older)

E. Epithelial cell abnormalities
  1. Squamous cell abnormalities
    a. Atypical squamous cells of undetermined significance (ASCUS): Indicates some abnormality but the cause is unclear (infection common).
    b. Atypical squamous cells—high grade (ASC-H): Cannot exclude high-grade squamous intraepithelial lesion.
    c. Low-grade squamous intraepithelial lesion (LSIL): Indicates human papillomavirus (HPV), mild dysplasia, or cervical intraepithelial neoplasia (CIN) I.
    d. High-grade squamous intraepithelial lesions (HSILs): Moderate and severe dysplasia, carcinoma in situ or CIN II, and CIN III
    e. Squamous cell carcinoma

2. Glandular cell

a. Atypical

i. Endocervical cells (not otherwise specify [NOS] or specify in comments)

ii. Endometrial (NOS or specify in comments)

iii. Glandular (NOS or specify in comments)

b. Atypical

i. Endocervical cells favor neoplastic

ii. Glandular cells favor neoplastic

c. Endocervical adenocarcinoma in situ

d. Adenocarcinoma

i. Endocervical

ii. Endometrial

iii. Extrauterine

iv. NOS

F. Other malignant neoplasms: specify

G. Adjunctive testing

H. Computer-assisted interpretation of cervical pathology

I. Educational notes and comments appended to cytology report (optional)

Initial Management of Abnormal Pap Smears

A. ASCUS or LSIL in women aged 21 to 24 years

1. Repeat cytology in 12 months for the next 2 years, with colposcopy after 1 year for HSIL and colposcopy after 2 years if ASCUS or LSIL remains.

2. HPV: Not recommended, but if performed:

a. HPV negative, continue routine screen with Pap test in 3 years

b. HPV positive, annual Pap smear for 2 years with colposcopy after 1 year if HSIL continues and after 2 years if ASCUS or LSIL continues

B. ASC-H is managed with colposcopy.

C. LSIL

1. HPV negative can be managed with repeat cotesting in 1 year or colposcopy.

2. LSIL with positive or no HPV test is managed with colposcopy.

3. Pregnant women with LSIL can be managed with colposcopy or can defer colposcopy until 6 weeks postpartum.

D. HSIL management in women includes either immediate loop excision or colposcopy.

E. Atypical glandular cells (AGC) management for all subcategories except atypical endometrial cells includes colposcopy. For women aged 35 years and older with risk of endometrial neoplasm, endometrial sampling is also indicated.

1. Atypical endometrial cell management includes endometrial and endocervical sampling.

F. Unsatisfactory cytology

1. If HPV unknown or HPV negative, repeat cytology in 2 to 4 months.

2. If HPV positive, either repeat cytology in 2 to 4 months or perform colposcopy.

3. If there are two consecutive unsatisfactory cytology tests, then colposcopy is indicated.

G. Cytology negative but absent or insufficient endocervical/transitional zone component

1. Aged 21 to 29 or 30 years and older with HPV negative, conduct routine screening cytology in 3 years.

2. Aged 30 years and older and HPV unknown, HPV testing is preferred.

3. Aged 30 years and older and HPV positive, conduct cytology + HPV testing in 1 year or immediate genotyping for HPV.

4. See and download ASCCP algorithms* for complete management options at www.asccp.org

The American Society for Colposcopy and Cervical Pathology (ASCCP) has a mobile device application. Look for the mobile application ASCCP Abnormal Cervical Cancer Screening Guidelines on iTunes.

Recommendations

According to the American Cancer Society (ACS), the U.S. Preventative Task Force, ASCCP, and the American College of Obstetricians and Gynecologists guidelines, all women should begin cervical cancer screening at the age of 21 years. Women younger than 21 years should not be screened regardless of the age of sexual initiation. Screening should be performed every 3 years. No woman should be screened annually. Highlights of the recommendations include:

A. Begin screening at the age of 21 years.

B. Women from ages 21 to 29 years should have conventional or liquid-based cytology every 3 years, and no HPV testing should be performed.

C. Women from ages 30 to 65 years should have conventional or liquid-based cytology every 3 years or, to extend testing time, use conventional or liquid-based cytology plus HPV co-test every 5 years. HPV co-testing should not be used in women younger than 30 years.

D. Stop screening at age older than 65 years with adequate screening history. Negative history includes having three consecutive negative cytology results or two consecutive tests with cotesting results in the past 5 years for the patient.

E. Continued regular screening is recommended for women who have had a history of CIN II, CIN III, or adenocarcinoma.

F. Posthysterectomy: Stop screening for total hysterectomy. However, if the patient had a history of high-grade lesions before surgery, then cytology screening every 3 years for the next 20 years is recommended.

G. HPV vaccination screen according to age-specific recommendation.

H. Women who have a high-risk medical history (immunocompromised, HIV positive, DES-exposed in utero,

* *The Journal of Lower Genital Tract Disease,* Volume 17, Number 5, with the permission of ASCCP©, the American Society for Colposcopy and Cervical Pathology, 2013.

or a history of cervical cancer) are not included in the updated routine guidelines.

The Advisory Committee on Immunization practices recommends routine vaccination of females and males aged 11 to 12 years with three doses of quadrivalent HPV vaccine and states the series can be started as young as 9 years of age. Catch-up vaccination is recommended for adolescents and young adults aged 13 to 26 years.

Patient education regarding the prevention of cervical cancer by avoiding exposure to HPV should include reduction or elimination of high-risk activities. These high-risk activities include having sexual intercourse at an early age, having multiple sexual partners, having partners with multiple partners, and having sex with uncircumcised males. Use of condoms can reduce the risk of HPV as well as other STIs. Smoking cessation can also reduce the risk of cervical cancer. Identification and treatment of precancerous lesions can reduce the risk of invasive cervical cancer, so screening according to ACS guidelines should be encouraged.

Treatment Modalities

Treatment is instituted based on the severity of the lesion and the presence of pathology within the columnar epithelium of the endocervix. Treatment options include

A. Observation and repeat cytology
B. Cryotherapy
C. Loop excision of the transformation zone
D. Laser of the transformation zone
E. Cold-knife conization
F. Observation and repeat cytology

Pelvic Inflammatory Disease

Rhonda Arthur

Definition

A. Pelvic inflammatory disease (PID) is an inflammation caused by an infection of the upper genital tract. This inflammation can involve the uterine endometrium (endometritis), fallopian tubes (salpingitis), ovaries (oophoritis), broad ligament or uterine serosa (parametritis), and the pelvic vascular system or pelvic connective tissue.

Incidence

A. Annual incidence is difficult to obtain due to difficulty in definitive diagnosis and reporting.
B. PID is the leading cause of infertility in the world.

Pathogenesis

A. PID is caused by organisms that ascend from the vagina and cervix into the uterus. Menses facilitates gonococcal invasion of the upper genital tract as the luteal phase stimulates gonococcal growth and the cervical mucus barrier is removed. Infection and inflammation spread throughout the endometrium to the fallopian tubes. From there, they extend to the ovaries and peritoneal cavity.
B. The most common organisms cultured from patients with PID are *Chlamydia trachomatis*, *Neisseria gonorrhoeae*, *Mycoplasma hominis*, *Ureaplasma urealyticum*, Bacteroides, *Peptostreptococcus*, *Escherichia coli*, and some endogenous aerobes and anaerobes.
C. The incubation period varies with the infective organism.

Predisposing Factors

A. Age: Rates of PID are higher for women at younger ages. It is highest in the younger than 30-year-old age group (70% incidence under the age of 25 years). Teens are particularly susceptible because they have an immature immune system and larger zones of cervical ectopy with thinner cervical mucus.
B. Sexual activity: Women with multiple sexual partners are three times more likely to develop PID, when compared to women with only one partner.
C. Intrauterine devices (IUDs): IUDs can lead to an iatrogenic development of PID and can promote the spread of vaginal or cervical organisms into the uterus by means of the IUD string.
D. History of PID
E. Menstruation: Supports the development and spread of PID. Women who are not currently menstruating have a decreased risk.
F. History of invasive procedures: These procedures may result in iatrogenic PID. PID is usually seen within 4 weeks of the procedure (dilatation and curettage [D&C], IUD insertion, hysterosalpingogram [HSG], and vacuum curettage abortion).
G. There is an increased incidence of PID in African Americans and non-White women and women in lower socioeconomic groups.
H. Cigarette smoking
I. Frequent vaginal douching

Common Complaints

A. Lower abdominal pain
B. Fever or chills
C. Increased vaginal discharge
D. Nausea and vomiting
E. Low back pain

Other Signs and Symptoms

A. Asymptomatic; vague and nonspecific symptoms
B. Minimal to severe pelvic pain
C. Right upper quadrant pain (25%)
D. Abnormal vaginal bleeding

Subjective Data

A. Determine onset, duration, and course of presenting symptoms.
B. Review the character of vaginal discharge (if any); history of recent dysmenorrhea and/or dyspareunia; any intestinal or bladder symptoms.
C. Question the patient regarding sexual history: Current number of sexual partners; current or most recent sexual activity; and contraceptive used (condoms, pills, diaphragm, IUD) and frequency of method used.

D. Question the patient as to whether her current sexual partner has experienced any symptoms.
E. What is the patient's current menstrual pattern? Does she think she is pregnant? When did the pain begin in relation to her cycle?
F. Review prior pelvic or abdominal surgeries and procedures (HSG, abortion) and when they were done.
G. Review the history and quality of pain: How long, bilateral or unilateral, what makes it better, and what makes it worse (intercourse, Valsalva's maneuver with bowel movement, activity).

Physical Examination

A. Check temperature, pulse, respirations, and blood pressure.
B. Inspect: Observe general overall appearance for discomfort before, during, and after examination.
C. Auscultate abdomen for bowel sounds in all quadrants. Auscultation of the abdomen should precede any palpation or percussion due to the changes in intensity and frequency of sounds after manipulation.
D. Percuss the abdomen for organomegaly.
E. Palpate
  1. Palpate the groin for lymphadenopathy.
  2. Palpate the abdomen for masses.
  3. Palpate the levator ani muscle left and right, the urethra, and the trigone of the bladder.
  4. Perform rebound, involuntary guarding, and jar tests. The jar test is performed by intentionally hitting or jarring the examination table and watching for a pain response. Pelvic discomfort is exacerbated by the Valsalva maneuver, intercourse, or movement. Abdominal or pelvic pain with PID is usually bilateral. About 25% of patients complain of right upper quadrant (RUQ) pain; the pain usually occurs within 7 to 10 days of menses, remains continuously, and is most severe in the lower quadrants.
F. Pelvic examination
  1. Inspect: Examine the vulva for Bartholin's gland enlargement, fissures, condyloma, herpes, and pelvic relaxation.
  2. Palpate: "Milk" the urethra for discharge.
  3. Speculum examination: Inspect for cervicitis and friability. Evaluate vaginal discharge and bleeding for color, amount, and odor. Lower abdominal or pelvic pain is the most common symptom of PID and typically is moderate to severe; however, many women may have subtle or mild symptoms that are not readily recognizable as PID, including abnormal bleeding, dyspareunia, or vaginal discharge.
G. Bimanual examination
  1. Check cervical motion tenderness (CMT); evaluate the size, contour, mobility, and tenderness of the uterus.
  2. Palpate the adnexa for tenderness and masses. Classic PID presentation is lower abdominal and adnexal tenderness and CMT (chandelier sign). The pelvic area may feel hot.
H. Rectovaginal examination: Assess for adnexal thickening and masses.

Diagnostic Tests

A. Complete blood count (CBC) with differential; white blood cell (WBC) greater than 10,500 cell/mm^3
B. Sedimentation rate or C-reactive protein (CRP)
C. Quantitative beta human chorionic gonadotropin (HCG)
D. Rapid plasma reagin (RPR), hepatitis B surface antigen, and HIV if indicated
E. Cultures for gonorrhea and chlamydia
F. Endometrial biopsy
G. Transvaginal ultrasonography
H. Laparoscopy, by referral

Because of the extreme risk of ectopic pregnancy, always test the patient for quantitative beta HCG even if she claims her menses are regular and she is using reliable contraception. Cultures must always be done; lab work (such as HIV) may be done as indicated depending on the patient's history and presentation. Eliciting data in the health history about hysterectomy, previous appendectomy, abortions, and procedures, such as hysterosalpingogram (HSG), may provide exclusionary diagnoses.

I. Diagnostic criteria (DC) for clinical diagnosis of PID.
  1. Minimal criteria: Empiric treatment for PID should be initiated in sexually active women at risk for STDs if they are experiencing one of the following with no other cause identified:
    a. Lower abdominal tenderness
    b. Adnexal tenderness
    c. CMT
  2. Additional routine criteria (one or more of the following support diagnosis of PID)
    a. Oral temperature greater than 101°F
    b. Abnormal cervical or vaginal discharge
    c. Elevated erythrocyte sedimentation rate (greater than 15 mm/hr)
    d. Elevated C-reactive protein
    e. Laboratory documentation of cervical infection with *N. gonorrhoeae* or *C. trachomatis*
  3. Elaborate criteria for diagnosing PID
    a. Histopathologic evidence of endometritis on endometrial biopsy
    b. Tubo-ovarian abscess on ultrasound or radiologic tests
    c. Laparoscopic abnormalities consistent with PID

Differential Diagnoses

A. Gynecologic factors
  1. PID
  2. Ectopic pregnancy
  3. Pelvic endometriosis
  4. Dysmenorrhea
  5. Adenomyosis
  6. Functional ovarian cysts

7. Endometrial polyps or fibroid
8. Pelvic relaxation
9. Anatomic abnormalities

B. Gastrointestinal (GI) factors
1. Acute appendicitis
2. Irritable bowel syndrome
3. Ulcerative colitis, Crohn's disease
4. Diverticulitis
5. Hernia

C. Genitourinary factors
1. Cystitis, urethritis interstitial cystitis
2. Ureteral obstruction
3. Carcinoma of bladder

D. Musculoskeletal factors
1. Myofascial pain
2. Pelvic floor myalgia
3. Spinal injuries or degenerative disease

E. Neurologic factor: Nerve entrapment syndrome

Plan

A. General interventions

1. A low threshold is needed for diagnosis of PID because of the risk of damage to reproductive health. Early treatment with the use of antibiotics of an upper genital tract infection is imperative. Other causes of lower abdominal pain, such as irritable bowel syndrome and endometriosis, are not likely to be impaired by empiric antibiotic therapy. The risk of ectopic pregnancy is 6 to 10 times greater with women with PID compared with uninfected women.

2. Antibiotic therapy should be instituted promptly, based on clinical diagnosis without awaiting culture results, to minimize the risk of progression of the infection and risk of transmission of the organisms to other sexual partners.

3. If a woman with an IUD in place is diagnosed with PID, the IUD does not need to be removed. The woman should receive recommended treatment. If there is no improvement in 48 to 72 hours, the health care provider should consider removing the IUD.

4. Ambulatory patients should be monitored closely and reevaluated within 3 days of initiating antibiotic therapy. A decrease in pelvic tenderness should be observed within 3 to 5 days of initiation of therapy; if not, additional evaluation is warranted.

B. Patient teaching: *See Section III: Patient Teaching Guide for this chapter, "Pelvic Inflammatory Disease."*

1. Male sexual partners (and all partners) of patients with PID must be examined, cultured when possible, and treated empirically for presumptive gonorrheal and chlamydial infection.

2. Women who do not use any contraception are at the greatest risk. Transmission of sexually transmitted infections (STIs) can be minimized with effective use of barrier contraceptives. Spermicides prevent infection with chlamydia and gonorrhea. The use of nonoxynol-9 is protective against *N. gonorrhoeae, Treponema palladium, Trichomonas,* herpes simplex virus (HSV), and *Candida.*

3. Oral contraceptive pills are associated with an increase in chlamydia detection in the cervix, and they protect against symptomatic PID.

C. Pharmaceutical therapy (see Table 14.6)

TABLE 14.6 Centers for Disease Control and Prevention Recommendations for Treating PID

Inpatient Therapy	Ambulatory Therapy
Regimen A[a] Cefotetan 2 g IV every 12 hours *or* cefoxitin 2 g *plus* doxycycline 100 mg IV or orally every 12 hours This regimen is continued for at least 48 hours after clinical improvement and followed by doxycycline 100 mg orally twice daily to complete 14-day total course. **Regimen B**[a] Clindamycin 900 mg IV every 8 hours (15–40 mg/kg/d) **Plus** Gentamicin, loading dose 2.0 mg/kg IV, followed by maintenance dose 1.5 mg/kg IV every 8 hours. Single daily dosing may be substituted. This regimen is continued for at least 48 hours after significant clinical improvement is demonstrated, and it is followed by doxycycline 100 mg orally twice daily to complete a 14-day total course. Alternatively, clindamycin 600 mg orally three times daily may be given to complete a 14-day total course.	**Regimen A** Ceftriaxone 250 mg IM in a single dose *plus* doxycycline 100 mg orally twice a day for 14 days **With or Without** Metronidazole 500 mg orally twice daily for 14 days **Or** Cefoxitin 2 g IM in a single dose and probenecid, 1 g orally administered concurrently in a single dose *plus* doxycycline 100 mg orally twice a day for 14 days *with or without* metronidazole 500 mg orally twice a day for 14 days **Or** Other parenteral third-generation cephalosporin (e.g., ceftizoxime or cefotaxime) *plus* doxycycline 100 mg orally twice a day for 14 days *with or without* metronidazole 500 mg orally twice a day for 14 days

Note: For women or their partners who cannot tolerate doxycycline or tetracycline, erythromycin 500 mg orally four times daily may be used for 10 to 14 days.

[a]When tubo-C is present, many clinicians use clindamycin because it provides more effective anaerobic coverage than doxycycline.

IM, intramuscular; IV, intravenous; PID, pelvic inflammatory disease.

Follow-Up

A. Because of the high risk of reinfection, many clinicians recommend reevaluation in 4 to 6 weeks after completion of therapy. Patients with positive cultures for gonorrhea and chlamydia should be recultured in 7 to 10 days after completing therapy. "Test of cure" is necessary.
B. Hepatitis B immunization should be initiated in previously unvaccinated persons.

Consultation/Referral

Consult a gynecologist if the patient diagnosis is atypical, evidence for a presumptive diagnosis is present, or hospitalization is required. General criteria for hospitalization are the following:
A. Diagnosis is uncertain.
B. Pelvic or tubo-ovarian abscess is suspected.
C. IUD in situ
D. The patient is pregnant.
E. The patient is an adolescent or is believed to be incapable of adhering to outpatient regimen.
F. Outpatient therapy fails; the patient is not better in 48 to 72 hours.
G. The patient cannot be reevaluated in 48 to 72 hours.
H. The patient is HIV positive.
I. There is generalized peritonitis or severe illness.
J. The patient cannot tolerate oral medication therapies.
K. Surgical emergencies cannot be ruled out.

Individual Considerations

A. Pregnancy
   1. Fluoroquinolones are generally contraindicated for pregnant and nursing mothers.
   2. Pregnant women with suspected PID should be hospitalized and treated with parenteral antibiotics.
B. Pediatrics
   1. Fluoroquinolones are generally contraindicated for children and adolescents younger than 18 years.
C. Partners
   1. Sexual partners should be evaluated and treated for STIs.

Premenstrual Syndrome and Premenstrual Dysphoric Disorder

Rhonda Arthur

Definition

A. Premenstrual syndrome (PMS) is a psychoneuroendocrine disorder with a constellation of symptoms that occur in the luteal phase, days 18 to 21, and interfere with a woman's life. This is followed by a symptom-free period. Moderate to severe forms of premenstrual distress are now classified in the American Psychiatric Association's (APA) *Diagnostic and Statistical Manual of Mental Disorders* (*DSM-5;* 2013) as premenstrual dysphoric disorder (PMDD).

Incidence

A. Virtually every menstruating woman experiences some symptoms sometimes. Twenty percent of menstruating women have symptoms serious enough to interfere with their lives, but only 2% to 5% of premenopausal women experience PMDD. Symptoms occur more commonly in women in their 30s and 40s.

Pathogenesis

A. The basis of PMS and PMDD is presumably hormonal. During the luteal phase, progesterone levels increase and estrogen levels decrease, causing a shift in the ratio of these hormones, which contributes to the symptoms experienced during PMS. These hormones are also known to interact with neurotransmitters in the brain, such as serotonin, and these interactions are thought to cause some of the symptoms experienced, such as mood changes and pain thresholds, during PMS and PMDD.

Predisposing Factor

A. Females of reproductive age

Common Complaints

A. Symptoms are temporally related to the menstrual cycle, beginning during the last week of the luteal phase and remitting after the onset of menses.
B. The diagnosis of PMDD requires symptoms to be present in most menstrual cycles over the last year. At least five of the following symptoms including one of the first four listed must be present:
   1. Affective lability, for example, sudden onset of being sad, tearful, irritable, or angry (mood swings)
   2. Persistent and marked anger or irritability
   3. Marked anxiety or tension
   4. Markedly depressed mood and feelings of hopelessness
   5. Decreased interest in usual activities
   6. Easily fatigued or a marked lack of energy
   7. Subjective sense of difficulty in concentrating
   8. Hypersomnia or insomnia
   9. A subjective sense of being overwhelmed or out of control
   10. Marked change in appetite, overeating, or specific food cravings
   11. Physical symptoms such as breast tenderness, headaches, edema, abdominal bloating, joint or muscle pain, and weight gain

Other Signs and Symptoms

A. The symptoms interfere with work, usual activities, or relationships.
B. The symptoms are not an exacerbation of another psychiatric disorder.
C. "I've got PMS; I'm so miserable."
D. Feelings of irritability and emotional lability

Subjective Data

A. Obtain a complete menstrual history.
   1. Age at menarche; frequency, duration, and regularity of periods
   2. Ask about premenstrual symptoms that are physical: Weight gain, edema, acne, nausea, vomiting, constipation, backache, headache, migraine, syncope, breast tenderness, breast enlargement, hot flashes, paresthesia

of hands or feet, aggravation of convulsive disorder, increased appetite, food cravings (sweets, salt, or food in general), and fatigue.

3. Ask about premenstrual symptoms that are emotional: Irritability, emotional lability, anxiety, depression, crying, palpitations, fatigue, aggression, lethargy, and sleep disturbances.

4. Ask particularly about the timing of the symptoms. When do the symptoms begin and end in relationship to the menstrual period? Has the patient kept a calendar of symptoms?

B. Ask about symptoms of dysmenorrhea. Some women confuse menstrual cramps and PMS.

C. Note type of contraception the patient uses.

D. Review her obstetric history, if applicable.

E. Elicit the types of treatment the patient has tried and efficacy of treatment.

F. Ask the patient about the amount and type of exercise she gets. Women with PMS often get little exercise.

Physical Examination

A. Check height, weight, and blood pressure.

B. Inspect

1. Note overall appearance.

2. Inspect thyroid.

C. Palpate

1. The neck, noting thyroid enlargement or nodules

2. The abdomen, noting enlargement, masses, or tenderness

D. Auscultate the heart, lungs, and abdomen.

E. Pelvic examination (if indicated)

1. Inspect the external genitalia for pubic hair pattern, lesions, or discharge.

2. Speculum examination: Check for discharge and lesions.

3. Bimanual examination: Check for size, mobility, shape, and tenderness of the uterus and adnexal area.

4. No physical abnormality or changes are consistent with PMS.

Diagnostic Tests

PMS is diagnosed primarily based on the pattern of symptoms; however, the following diagnostic test should be considered if indicated:

A. Pap smear according to guidelines

B. Screen for sexually transmitted infections (STIs), if indicated

C. Thyroid-stimulating hormone (TSH)

D. Screen for psychiatric disorders as indicated

Differential Diagnoses

A. PMS

B. Major depression

C. Dysmenorrhea

D. Substance abuse

E. Perimenopausal symptoms

F. Sexual dysfunction

G. Fibromyalgia

H. There are rarely major medical problems, but hypothyroidism, hyperthyroidism, anemia, and autoimmune disorders (such as systemic lupus erythematosus [SLE]) must be kept in mind.

Plan

A. General interventions

1. Have the patient keep a menstrual calendar or diary for at least 3 months to document occurrence of symptoms in the luteal phase.

2. Symptomatic treatments: Treatment must be individualized.

B. Patient teaching: *See Section III: Patient Teaching Guide for this chapter, "Premenstrual Syndrome."* ◀

1. Diet: Have the patient eat six small meals a day to even out glucose load. Have her avoid caffeine to decrease irritability and facilitate sleep. Encourage her to avoid simple sugars and eat complex carbohydrates to provide a slow, steady source of energy. She should decrease intake of salt, sugar, and fat. Avoid caffeine and alcohol.

2. Activity: Instruct the patient to increase exercise, preferably aerobic exercise. Suggest exercising every day (walking, swimming, and stretching). Encourage at least 30 minutes of aerobic exercise most days of the week. Encourage stress reduction activities such as imagery or yoga, cognitive behavioral therapy (CBT), support or counseling groups. Encourage smoking cessation as well as adequate sleep and rest.

C. Pharmaceutical therapy

1. Nonsteroidal anti-inflammatory drugs (NSAIDs) for relief of muscular aches, headaches, and menstrual cramps. Follow directions for the particular NSAIDs, whether over-the-counter (OTC) or prescription.

2. Minerals

a. Magnesium 300 to 500 mg/d

b. Calcium 1,200 mg/d

c. Chromium 200 mcg each day

d. Zinc 30 mg each day

3. Vitamins are used to decrease anxiety and irritability, food cravings, painful breasts, depression, fatigue, and lethargy:

a. Vitamin B_6 (pyridoxine) 50 to 150 mg each day (limited benefit)

b. Vitamin E 400 to 600 mg each day (limited benefit)

4. Herbs and biotanics:

a. Vitex Agnus-Castus (Chaste Tree Berry) 30 to 40 mg daily

b. Evening primrose oil (EPO) 500 to 1,000 mg each day (mixed results on effectiveness). This oil contains vitamin E; therefore, do not have the patient take additional vitamin E.

5. See Table 14.7 for other therapies used for PMS.

Follow-Up

A. Follow up every 3 to 4 months to assess or alter treatment and/or therapy.

TABLE 14.7 Medications Used With Premenstrual Syndrome (PMS)

Drug	Dose	Purpose
Diuretics		Decreases edema peripherally and, perhaps, centrally
Spironolactone (Aldactone)	25 mg twice daily as needed	
Antidepressants		Decreases depression and anxiety and improves mood
Fluoxetine (Prozac)	10–40 mg every day or during the luteal phase (individual dose may vary)	
Paroxetine (Paxil)	10–30 mg every day or during the luteal phase (individual dose may vary)	
Sertraline hydrochloride (Zoloft)	25–30 mg every day or during the luteal phase (individual dose may vary)	
Antianxiety Drugs		Decreases anxiety
Alprazolam (Xanax)	0.25 mg three or four times daily during luteal phase as needed	
Buspirone (BuSpar)	7.5–15 mg twice daily	
Miscellaneous Drugs		
Bromocriptine mesylate (Parlodel)	2.5 mg three times daily during breast luteal phase	Used to decrease tenderness; works slowly
Oral contraceptive pills (Yaz[a])	Take on a daily basis	Evens the hormonal milieu, blocks ovulation
Danazol (Danocrine)		Has anti-estrogenic effects. *Consult with a physician.*

[a]Has drospirenone and ethinyl estradiol.

Consultation/Referral

A. Consult a physician if symptoms are severe or not relieved by first-line measures.

Individual Considerations

A. Partners
   1. Encourage the patient to have her partner come to a visit. Partner education and support are helpful.

Vulvovaginal Candidiasis

Rhonda Arthur

Definition

A. Candidiasis (also known as moniliasis) is a common, yeast-like fungal infection of the vulva and vagina. In 90% of the cases, the cause is *Candida albicans* infection.

Incidence

A. Approximately 75% of all women have at least one episode of candidiasis. It is estimated that 50% of these women have recurrences. Yeast has been identified with circumcised males, but symptomatic complaints are more common with uncircumcised males.

Pathogenesis

A. Multiple fungal species cause candidiasis, including *C. albicans* (90%), *C. tropicalis*, *Torulopsis glabrata* (10%), *Candida parapsilosis*, and *Candida krusei*.

B. *C. albicans, C. tropicalis,* or *T. glabrata* are part of the normal flora of the mouth, gastrointestinal (GI) tract, and vagina. They may become pathogenic with changes in the vaginal pH that encourage the overgrowth of the fungus.

C. The incubation period is 96 hours.

Predisposing Factors

A. Diabetes
B. Systemic antibiotic use
C. Pregnancy
D. Oral contraceptive pill use
E. Obesity
F. Warm climate
G. Immunocompromised
H. HIV
I. Wearing tight, restrictive clothing
J. Corticosteroid use
K. Tub bathing
L. Frequent use of hot tubs or whirlpools

Common Complaints

A. Thick white "cheesy" vaginal discharge
B. Itching, mild to intense vulvar pruritus
C. Vaginal or vulvar irritation, red, and swollen
D. Discomfort during and after sexual intercourse

Other Signs and Symptoms

A. Vulvar excoriation
B. Vaginal swelling or inflammation

C. Burning with urination
D. Burning with or during intercourse
E. Increased symptoms near menses

Subjective Data

A. Determine onset, course, and duration of symptoms; note whether the infection is first occurrence, recurrent, persistent, or chronic.
B. Obtain medication history; include antibiotics, steroids, and birth control pills.
C. Review the patient's past medical history, and review systems for evidence of diabetes, HIV, or any immunocompromise.
D. Review hobbies that include the use of hot tubs, whirlpools, or tight exercise clothing.
E. Review the patient's history of wearing polyester underwear, wearing underwear to bed, or wearing tight jeans.
F. Review previous treatment, self-treatment measures, and compliance with previous treatments.
G. Determine whether the patient is pregnant; note first day of last menstrual period (LMP).
H. Review sexual activity and partners. Do the partner(s) have any of the same symptoms, "jock itch," or oral candidiasis?
I. Review the use of vaginal deodorants or spray, scented toilet paper, tampons, pads, and douching.
J. Has there been any change in soaps, laundry detergent, or fabric softeners?
K. Review diet for high sugar content.

Physical Examination

A. Check temperature, pulse, and blood pressure.
B. Inspect
  1. Inspect the vulva for inflammation, fissures, lesions, excoriation, rashes, and condyloma.
  2. Examine the hairline and skin folds for inflammation, irritation, or skin breakdown.
  3. Note skin changes that suggest secondary bacterial infection (erythema, drainage).

> *Inflammation that spares the skin folds is consistent with contact irritation. Inflammation that is within the skin folds suggests candida.*

C. Palpate
  1. Perform external examination for enlarged or tender inguinal lymph nodes, vulvar masses, and lesions.
  2. Back: Assess for costovertebral angle (CVA) tenderness.
D. Pelvic examination
  1. Inspect: Observe side walls of vagina. Note amount, smell, and color of the discharge.

> *Typical discharge with* Candida *is adherent to vaginal side walls and characteristically thick, white, and curd-like (resembles cottage cheese). Side walls may exhibit erythema. The discharge has a musty odor.*

  2. Speculum examination: Inspect the cervix for discharge and friability.
  3. Bimanual examination: Check for cervical motion tenderness (CMT). Palpate for the size of the uterus and for adnexal masses or tenderness.

Diagnostic Tests

A. Wet prep with 10% potassium hydroxide and normal saline prep.

> *Yeast hyphae and/or spores are determined by microscopic examination of vaginal discharge prepared with 10% potassium hydroxide or normal saline. A positive whiff test indicates bacterial vaginosis (BV).*

B. Test discharge with nitrazine paper.

> *The pH with candidiasis remains in the normal range of less than 4.5.*

C. Consider 2-hour glucose testing.
D. Consider testing for gonorrhea and chlamydia.
E. Herpes culture, if lesions present
F. Urinalysis and culture, if indicated

Differential Diagnoses

A. Vulvovaginal candidiasis
B. Vulvar dystrophy
C. Allergic vulvitis
D. BV
E. Urinary tract infection (UTI)
F. Chlamydia
G. Gonorrhea
H. Trichomonas
I. Herpes simplex virus type 2 (HSV-2)
J. Chemical vaginitis
K. Normal physiological discharge

Plan

A. General interventions
  1. Although vaginal candidiasis is treated using over-the-counter (OTC) products, encourage patients with initial presenting symptoms to have an evaluation to rule out other vaginal infections before self-treatment.
  2. Consider treating partners.

> *Although candidiasis is not considered a sexually transmitted infection (STI), it can be sexually transmitted. The partner should be treated in cases of recurrent infections, even if the partner is asymptomatic.*

  3. For recurrent infections, consider fasting and 2-hour postprandial glucose tests for chronic yeast infections.
  4. Consider testing for HIV for chronic yeast infections.

5. Preventive care therapies
   a. Vinegar and water douche may be effective in mild cases: 1 to 2 tablespoons vinegar per quart warm water every 5 to 7 days or twice a day for 2 days.
   b. *Acidophilus* capsules, 4 to 6 tablets daily, especially 2 to 3 days before menses
   c. Vitamin C 500 mg two to four times daily to increase vaginal acidity
   d. Daily yogurt douches or intravaginal applicator full of yogurt twice a day for 1 week. Have the patient use *plain yogurt* with active cultures.

B. Patient teaching: *See Section III: Patient Teaching Guide for this chapter, "Vaginal Yeast Infection."*

1. Patients should be encouraged to present for evaluation whether, after appropriate therapy has been instituted, they continue to have symptoms.
2. Treatment should continue even during menstruation.

C. Pharmaceutical therapy

1. Vaginal antifungal creams: Mild cases may respond to 3 days of therapy; severe cases may require 10 to 14 days. Some of these preparations are available in vaginal suppository form for a 1- or 3-night regimen with proven efficacy.
   a. Clotrimazole (Gyne-Lotrimin, Lotrimin, Mycelex, Mycelex-G) one applicator full at bedtime for 7 days
   b. Miconazole (Monistat) one applicator full at bedtime for 7 days
   c. Butoconazole nitrate (Femstat) one applicator full at bedtime for 7 days
   d. Terconazole (Terazol) one applicator full at bedtime for 7 days
   e. Terconazole vaginal antifungal cream is not available OTC. Imidazole drugs (miconazole, clotrimazole, econazole, butoconazole) are not as effective for non–*C. albicans* infections as are triazole compounds.
2. Oral antifungal agents
   a. Fluconazole (Diflucan) 150 mg orally once. If treatment is not successful, prescription may be refilled one time; if it is still unsuccessful, consider treating the patient's partner and/or glucose testing for diabetes.
   b. Nystatin one tablet (100,000 units) orally or vaginally for 14 days. Nystatin may be taken twice a day or at bedtime.
   c. Ketoconazole (Nizoral) 200 mg orally in single dose:
      i. Dosage may be increased to 400 mg once daily in patients who do not respond to lower dose.
      ii. Treatment is effective for acute infection, but *very expensive.* It causes hepatic toxicity in 5% to 10% of patients; monitor liver function tests. Reserve treatment for long-term suppression of chronic *C. albicans* infection.

Follow-Up

A. The patient who presents with recurrent candidiasis should be evaluated for HIV and/or other immunocompromised etiologies and diabetes.

B. If fasting and 2-hour blood glucose testing is normal, other options for recurrent candidiasis include treatment with clotrimazole one applicator every other week for 2 months. If the patient remains symptom-free, reduce treatment to once each month, in the week before her menstrual period.

C. If recurrent candidiasis persists, request laboratory typing of *Candida* for *T. glabrata* or *C. tropicalis.* If confirmed, treat with prescription of gentian violet-treated tampons. Have the patient use one tampon at bedtime each day for 12 days.

Consultation/Referral

A. Consult or refer the patient to a physician if there is no response to the previous treatments and/or in presence of concurrent systemic disease.

Individual Considerations

A. Pregnancy

1. Pregnancy may lead to an increase in vulvovaginal candidiasis because of the increased glycogen content of the vagina and to the stimulatory effects of estrogen and progesterone on candidal growth. OTC antifungal creams are appropriate for use in this population if there is no rupture of membranes.
2. Candidiasis may be transmitted from infected mother to newborn at delivery.

B. Partners

1. Partners should be evaluated if the patient presents with recurrences. OTC antifungal creams are appropriate for use in this population.

Bibliography

Afaxys, Inc. (2015). Ella full prescribing information. Retrieved from http://www.ellanow.com/pdf/ella-full-prescribing-information.pdf

Akre, C., Berchtold, A., Gmel, G., & Suris, J. C. (2014). The evolution of sexual dysfunction in young men aged 18–25 years. *Journal of Adolescent Health, 55*(6), 736–743.

Alexander, I. M., & Andrist, L. C. (Eds.). (2013). Menopause. In K. D. Schuiling & F. E. Likis (Eds.), *Women's gynecologic health* (2nd ed.). Burlington, MS: Jones & Bartlett.

Aliotta, H. M., & Schaeffer, N. J. (2013). Breast conditions. In K. D. Schuiling & F. E. Likis (Eds.), *Women's gynecologic health* (2nd ed., pp. 377–401). Burlington, MA: Jones & Bartlett.

American Cancer Society. (2015a). American Cancer Society guidelines for the early detection of cancer. Retrieved from http://www.cancer.org/healthy/findcancerearly/cancerscreeningguidelines/american-cancer-society-guidelines-for-the-early-detection-of-cancer

American Cancer Society. (2015b). American Cancer Society recommendations for early breast cancer detection in women without breast symptoms. Retrieved from http://www.cancer.org/cancer/breastcancer/moreinformation/breastcancerearlydetection/breast-cancer-early-detection-acs-recs

American Cancer Society. (2016). What are the key statistics about cervical cancer? Retrieved from http://www.cancer.org/cancer/cervicalcancer/detailedguide/cervical-cancer-key-statistics

American College of Obstetricians and Gynecologists. (2013). New guidelines for cervical cancer screening. Retrieved from http://www.acog.org/-/media/For-Patients/pfs004.pdf?dmc=1&ts=

American College of Obstetricians and Gynecologist. (2015a). *Gynecologic problems: Premenstrual syndrome (PMS)*. Retrieved from http://www.acog.org/-/media/For-Patients/faq057.pdf

American College of Obstetrics and Gynecologists. (2015b). Gynecologic problems: Treating infertility. Retrieved from http://www.acog.org/-/media/For-Patients/faq137.pdf?dmc=1&ts=

American Psychiatric Association. (2013). *Diagnostic and statistical manual of mental disorders* (5th ed.). Arlington, VA: American Psychiatric Publishing.

Annam, K., Voznesensky, M., & Kreder, K. J. (2016). Understanding and managing erectile dysfunction in patients treated for cancer. *Journal of Oncology Practice/American Society of Clinical Oncology, 12*(4), 297–304.

Association of Reproductive Health Professionals. (2008). Managing premenstrual symptoms. Retrieved from http://www.arhp.org/uploadDocs/QRGPMS.pdf#search=%22premenstrual%22

Centers for Disease Control and Prevention. (2015a). 2015 Sexually transmitted diseases treatment guidelines: Bacterial vaginosis. Retrieved from http://www.cdc.gov/std/tg2015/bv.htm

Centers for Disease Control and Prevention. (2015b). 2015 Sexually transmitted diseases treatment guidelines: Pelvic inflammatory disease. Retrieved from http://www.cdc.gov/std/tg2015/pid.htm

Centers for Disease Control and Prevention. (2015c). Human papillomavirus. Retrieved from http://www.cdc.gov/hpv/parents/vaccine.html

Centers for Disease Control and Prevention. (2015d). National Center for Health Statistics: Infertility. Retrieved from http://www.cdc.gov/nchs/fastats/infertility.htm

Centers for Disease Control and Prevention. (2015e). 2015 Sexually transmitted diseases treatment guidelines. Retrieved from http://www.cdc.gov/std/tg2015/default.htm

Chasson, S. (2013). Female sexual dysfunction. In K. D. Schuiling & F. E. Likis (Eds.), *Women's gynecologic health* (2nd ed., pp. 405–421). Burlington, MA: Jones & Bartlett.

Chung, E., Gilbert, B., Perera, M., & Roberts, M. J. (2015). Premature ejaculation: A clinical review for the general physician. *Australian Family Physician, 44*(10), 737–743.

Dean, R. C., & Lue, T. F. (2005). Physiology of penile erection and pathophysiology of erectile dysfunction. *Urologic Clinics of North America, 32*(4), 379–395, v.

Einstein, M. H., & Cox, J. T. (2013). Update on cervical disease. *ObG Management, 25*(5), 42–49.

Faucher, M. A., & Schuiling, K. D. (2013). Normal and abnormal uterine bleeding. In K. D. Schuiling & F. E. Likis (Eds.), *Women's gynecologic health* (2nd ed., pp. 609–646). Burlington, MA: Jones & Bartlett.

Fogel, C. I. (2013). Gynecologic infections. In K. D. Schuiling & F. E. Likis (Eds.), *Women's gynecologic health* (2nd ed., pp. 467–483). Burlington, MA: Jones & Bartlett.

Guttmacher Institute. (2015). Contraceptive use in the United States. Retrieved from http://www.guttmacher.org/fact-sheet/contraceptive-use-united-states

Hilz, M. (2015). Assessment and treatment of male and female sexual dysfunction. *Journal of the Neurological Sciences, 357*(1), 498–499.

International Society for Sexual Medicine. (2014). *ISSM patient information sheet on premature ejaculation*. Retrieved from http://www.issm.info/images/uploads/ISSM_Patient_Information_Sheet_on_PE_-_website.pdf

Ishak, W. W., & Tobia, G. (2013). DSM-5 changes in diagnostic criteria of sexual dysfunctions. Retrieved from http://www.omicsonline.org/dsm-5-changes-in-diagnostic-criteria-of-sexual-dysfunctions-2161-038X.1000122.php?aid=18508

Kingsberg, S. A., & Woodard, T. (2015). Female sexual dysfunction: Focus on low desire. *Obstetrics and Gynecology, 125*(2), 477–486.

Latif, E. Z., & Diamond, M. P. (2013). Arriving at the diagnosis of female sexual dysfunction. *Fertility and Sterility, 100*(4), 898–904.

Massad, L. S., Einstein, M. H., Huh, W. K., Katki, H. A., Kinney, W. K., Schiffman, M., . . . Lawson, H. W. (2013). 2012 updated consensus guidelines for the management of abnormal cervical cancer screening tests and cancer precursors. *Journal of Lower Genital Tract Disease, 17*(5 Suppl. 1), S1–S27.

McCabe, M. P., & Connaughton, C. (2014). Psychosocial factors associated with male sexual difficulties. *Journal of Sex Research, 51*(1), 31–42.

McNeeley, S. G. (2014, July). *Merck manual: Bartholin gland cysts*. Rahway, NJ: Merck Publishing. Retrieved from http://www.merckmanuals.com/professional/gynecology-and-obstetrics/benign-gynecologic-lesions/bartholin-gland-cysts

National Institute of Health. (2014). Vitamin D. Retrieved from http://ods.od.nih.gov/factsheets/VitaminD-HealthProfessional

National Institute of Health. (2016). Calcium. Retrieved from http://ods.od.nih.gov/factsheets/Calcium-HealthProfessional

Nayar, R., & Wilbur, D. C. (2015). The Pap test and Bethesda 2014. "The reports of my demise have been greatly exaggerated" (after a quotation from Mark Twain). *Acta Cytologica, 59*(2), 121–132.

The North American Menopause Society. (2016). Vagina and vulvar comfort: Lubricants, moisturizers, and low-dose vaginal estrogen. Retrieved from http://www.menopause.org/for-women/-em-sexual-health-menopause-em-online/effective-treatments-for-sexual-problems/vaginal-and-vulvar-comfort-lubricants-moisturizers-and-low-dose-vaginal-estrogen

Olshanky, E. (2013). Infertility. In K. D. Schuiling & F. E. Likis (Eds.), *Women's gynecologic health* (2nd ed., pp. 443–465). Burlington, MA: Jones & Bartlett.

Osayande, A. S., & Mehulic, S. (2014). Diagnosis and initial management of dysmenorrhea. *American Family Physician, 89*(5), 341–346.

Paco, J. S., & Pereira, B. J. (2016). New therapeutic perspectives in premature ejaculation. *Urology, 88*, 87–92.

ParaGard. (2014). Prescribing information. Retrieved from http://www.paragard.com/Pdf/ParaGard-PI.pdf

Planned Parenthood. (2014). Morning-*after* pill (emergency contraception). Retrieved from http://www.plannedparenthood.org/learn/morning-after-pill-emergency-contraception

The PLISSIT Model of Sex Therapy. (n.d.). Retrieved from https://coad7404.files.wordpress.com/2014/06/plissitanonsmodel.pdf

Rajfer, J., Valeriano, J., & Sinow, R. (2013). Early onset erectile dysfunction is usually not associated with abnormal cavernosal arterial inflow. *International Journal of Impotence Research, 25*(6), 217–220.

The Society of Obstetricians and Gynaecologist of Canada. (n.d.). Breast pain. Retrieved from https://sogc.org/publications-resources/public-information-pamphlets.html?id=31

Taylor, D., Schuiling, K. D., & Collins Sharp, B. A. (2013). Menstrual cycle pain and disorders. In K. D. Schuiling & F. E. Likis (Eds.), *Women's gynecologic health* (2nd ed., pp. 573–607). Burlington, MA: Jones & Bartlett.

Thomas, H. N., & Thurston, R. C. (2016). A biopsychosocial approach to women's sexual function and dysfunction at midlife: A narrative review. *Maturitas, 87*, 49–60.

Verga, C. A. (2013). Benign gynecologic conditions. In K. D. Schuiling & F. E. Likis (Eds.), *Women's gynecologic health* (2nd ed., pp. 669–700). Burlington, MA: Jones & Bartlett.

Walsh, T. J., Hotaling, J. M., Smith, A., Saigal, C., & Wessells, H. (2014). Men with diabetes may require more aggressive treatment for erectile dysfunction. *International Journal of Impotence Research, 26*(3), 112–115.

Weinberg, A. E., Eisenberg, M., Patel, C. J., Chertow, G. M., & Leppert, J. T. (2013). Diabetes severity, metabolic syndrome, and the risk of erectile dysfunction. *Journal of Sexual Medicine, 10*(12), 3102–3109.

Women's Capital Corporation. (2015, August). PlanB One-Step. Retrieved from http://planbonestep.com/hcp/hcp.aspx

Wright, J. J., & O'Connor, K. M. (2015). Female sexual dysfunction. *Medical Clinics of North America, 99*(3), 607–628.

Zieman, M., Hatcher, R. A., Trussell, J., Nelson, A. L., Cates, W., Hatcher, R. A., & Allen, A. Z. (2015). *Managing contraception for your pocket*. Tiger, GA: Bridging the Gap Foundation.

15 Sexually Transmitted Infections Guidelines

Chlamydia

Jill C. Cash and Robertson Nash

Definition

A. Chlamydia is a sexually transmitted infection (STI).

Incidence

A. The World Health Organization (WHO) estimates 50 million cases worldwide, with more than 4 million cases annually. *Chlamydia* is the most common sexually transmitted organism in the United States. In 2014, the Centers for Disease Control and Prevention (CDC) reported 1,441,789 cases of chlamydia, which is approximately 456 cases per 100,000 population, an increase of 2.8% over 2013. It is not a CDC-reportable infection; however, local health department notification is required.

Pathogenesis

A. *Chlamydia trachomatis* is an intracellular bacterium with parasitic properties. It is transmitted by sexual contact or perinatally when a vaginal delivery occurs through an infected birth canal.

Predisposing Factors

A. History of STIs
B. Multiple sexual partners
C. Early age at first coitus
D. Unprotected intercourse

Common Complaints

A. Up to 80% of those infected are asymptomatic.
B. Mucopurulent cervical, vaginal, or urethral discharge
C. Dysuria
D. Urinary frequency and urgency
E. Pelvic pain (dull or severe)

Other Signs and Symptoms

A. Cervical friability
B. Cervical motion tenderness (CMT)
C. Uterine and/or adnexal tenderness

Subjective Data

A. Elicit history of the onset of symptoms, location, frequency, duration, aggravating and alleviating factors, and associated symptomatology.
B. Question the patient about history of other STIs and sexual habits.

Physical Examination

A. Inspect
  1. Males: Observe for anal and/or urethral discharge.
  2. Female pelvic examination: Observe for anal and/or vaginal discharge.
  3. Female speculum examination: Inspect vaginal wall and cervix for discharge and irritation.
B. Palpate
  1. Males
    a. Palpate inguinal lymph nodes.
    b. Palpate the groin.
  2. Females
    a. Palpate the inguinal lymph nodes.
    b. Bimanual examination
      i. *Milk* urethra.
      ii. Palpate periurethral and Bartholin's glands for exudate.
      iii. Assess for CMT.
      iv. Assess for uterine and adnexal tenderness.

Diagnostic Tests

A. Nucleic acid amplification (NAAT) tests are preferred to culture for diagnosis of *Chlamydia trachomatis*. The Food and Drug Administration (FDA) has approved NAAT tests for both male and female urogenital specimens collected via clean catch. Although not approved by the FDA, NAAT tests are commonly used in practice for the diagnosis of both chlamydia and gonorrhea. It is important to obtain a thorough sexual history from the patient and to screen all orifices used during sexual contact (oropharynx, rectum).
B. Other techniques for obtaining specimens include culture, antigen detections, and genetic probes.

Differential Diagnoses

A. Chlamydia
B. Gonorrhea
C. Urethritis

Plan

A. General interventions for symptomatic patients:
  1. Collect samples immediately for timely treatment. Consider testing for other STIs such as gonorrhea, trichomoniasis, and HIV.
  2. Empirical treatment: People presenting with signs and symptoms of chlamydia and/or gonorrhea should be tested and treated for both infections at the time

of presentation to clinic for care. NAAT swabs should be collected from all orifices exposed to sexual contact, and urine should also be collected and tested. Absent antibiotic allergies, these patients should be treated with both 250 mg ceftriaxone intramuscular (IM) injection and 1 g of azithromycin by mouth, single dose.

B. Patient teaching

1. *See Section III: Patient Teaching Guide for this chapter, "Chlamydia."*

2. Inform the patient of the need for partner notification and treatment. Notification is recommended for any partner with whom the patient has had sexual contact within 30 days of the onset of symptoms or 60 days if asymptomatic.

3. Stress the importance of completing the treatment regimen.

4. Advise the patient to avoid sexual intercourse during treatment and for 7 days following the last day of antibiotic treatment.

C. Pharmaceutical therapy for confirmed infections

1. In cases in which the presence of *C. trachomatis* is demonstrated by NAAT and *N. gonorrhoeae* is not present, the CDC recommends the following regimens:

a. Azithromycin 1 g by mouth in a single dose

b. Doxycycline 100 mg by mouth twice daily for 7 days

2. Alternative regimen

a. Erythromycin base 500 mg by mouth four times daily for 7 days

b. Erythromycin ethylsuccinate 800 mg by mouth four times daily for 7 days

c. Levofloxacin 500 mg orally once daily for 7 days

d. Ofloxacin 300 mg by mouth twice daily for 7 days

Follow-Up

A. The CDC now recommends that all patients followup in 3 months for repeat culture.

Consultation/Referral

A. Consult or refer the patient to a physician when treatment with the recommended dosage fails if patient noncompliance and reexposure have been ruled out.

Individual Considerations

A. Pregnancy

1. Doxycycline, ofloxacin, and levofloxacin are contraindicated during pregnancy.

2. All pregnant women diagnosed with chlamydial infection should be retested in 3 weeks following treatment.

3. For women younger than 25 years of age, those with new partners, and/or those at a high risk for infection, repeat chlamydial testing during the third trimester.

4. All pregnant women diagnosed with chlamydial infection during the first trimester should be retested at 3 weeks following treatment, and again in 3 months after treatment.

5. The CDC recommends the following regimens for pregnant women.

a. Azithromycin 1 g orally in a single dose

b. For those women intolerant to the recommended regimens:

i. Amoxicillin 500 mg by mouth three times daily for 7 days

ii. Erythromycin base 500 mg by mouth four times daily for 7 days

iii. Erythromycin base 250 mg by mouth four times daily for 14 days

iv. Erythromycin ethylsuccinate 800 mg by mouth four times daily for 7 days

v. Erythromycin ethylsuccinate 400 mg by mouth four times daily for 14 days

B. Pediatrics

1. The CDC recommends the following regimens for children.

a. Weighing less than 45 kg: Erythromycin base or ethylsuccinate 50 mg/kg/d by mouth divided into four doses daily for 14 days

b. Weighing 45 kg or more but older than 8 years: Azithromycin 1 g by mouth in a single dose

c. Children 8 years and older: Azithromycin 1 g by mouth in a single dose or doxycycline 100 mg by mouth twice a day for 7 days

C. Adults: Untreated or long-standing chlamydial infection in women may lead to infertility.

Gonorrhea

Jill C. Cash and Robertson Nash

Definition

A. Gonorrhea is a bacterial sexually transmitted infection (STI). Although most commonly seen in both male and female urogenital organs, *Neisseria gonorrhoeae* can thrive in both the oropharnyx and rectum. It is important to complete a thorough sexual history of all patients presenting with concern for exposure to an STI.

Incidence

A. The World Health Organization estimates 2.5 million cases worldwide. Gonorrhea is a Centers for Disease Control and Prevention (CDC)-reportable infection. In 2014, the CDC stated that there were 350,062 cases reported in the United States, which is 111 cases per 100,000 population, an increase of 5.1% since 2013. Male-to-female transmission is estimated at 50% to 90%, while female-to-male transmission is estimated at only 20% to 25%. Women account for two thirds of disseminated gonorrhea with joint infection.

Pathogenesis

A. *N. gonorrhoeae,* a gram-negative diplococcus, is the causative organism. The infection begins with adherence of *N. gonorrhoeae* to the mucosal cells in the genitourinary tract or endocervix. The incubation period is typically 2 to 5 days for urethritis and 5 to 10 days for cervical infection. Rectal and pharyngeal infections are usually asymptomatic. Transmission during vaginal birth is possible and may result in conjunctivitis and blindness in neonates.

Predisposing Factors

A. History of STIs
B. Multiple sexual partners
C. Early age at first coitus

Common Complaints

A. Dysuria
B. Yellow, white, or mucoid urethral discharge in males
C. Greenish, irritating vaginal discharge in females
D. Menstrual irregularities
E. Pelvic pain
F. Fever

Other Signs and Symptoms

A. Asymptomatic
B. Uterine or adnexal tenderness
C. Mucopurulent discharge from endocervix
D. Polyarthralgias
E. Necrotic skin lesions

Subjective Data

A. Elicit history of onset, duration, and location of symptoms. Note aggravating and alleviating factors and associated symptomatology.
B. Question the patient about history of other STIs and sexual habits.

Physical Examination

A. Check temperature.
B. Inspect
  1. Inspect the skin for necrotic skin lesions.
  2. Males: Inspect for anal and/or urethral discharge; elicit latter by milking penis.
  3. Females
    a. Inspect anus and introitus for discharge; milk urethra.
    b. Speculum examination: Inspect vaginal walls and cervix for discharge and irritation.
C. Palpate
  1. Examine joints for effusion and swelling.
  2. Males: Palpate inguinal lymph nodes.
  3. Females
    a. Palpate inguinal lymph nodes.
    b. Palpate periurethral and Bartholin's glands for exudate.
    c. Bimanual examination
      i. Assess for cervical motion, tenderness, and friability.
      ii. Assess for uterine and adnexal tenderness.

Diagnostic Tests

A. Nucleic acid amplification (NAAT) tests are preferred to culture for diagnosis of *N. gonorrhoeae*. The Food and Drug Administration (FDA) has approved NAAT tests for both male and female urogenital specimens collected via clean catch. Although not approved by the FDA, NAAT tests are commonly used in practice for the diagnosis of both gonorrhea and chlamydia. It is important to obtain a thorough sexual history from the patient and to screen all orifices used during sexual contact (oropharynx, rectum).
B. During the septic joint stage, gonococci can be recovered from the joint by aspiration for culture.
C. For persons diagnosed with gonorrhea, testing should also be performed for chlamydia, syphilis, and HIV.

Differential Diagnoses

A. Gonorrhea
B. Chlamydia
C. Arthritis (rheumatoid or osteoarthritis)

Plan

A. General interventions
  1. The U.S. Preventive Services Task Force recommendations include the following:
    a. Screening is not recommended in men and women at low risk for infection.
    b. Screening for infection is recommended for all sexually active, high-risk men and women, including pregnant women.
    c. Prompt diagnosis is needed to begin treatment.
  2. Report positive test results to the health department.
  3. Empirical treatment: People presenting with signs and symptoms of gonorrhea should be tested and treated for both gonorrhea and chlamydia at time of presentation to clinic for care. NAAT swabs should be collected from all orifices exposed to sexual contact, and urine should also be collected and tested.
B. Patient teaching
  1. *See Section III: Patient Teaching Guide for this chapter, "Gonorrhea."* ◀
  2. Stress the importance of completing the medication regimen.
  3. Inform the patient of the need for partner notification and treatment. Notification is recommended for any partner with whom the patient has had sexual contact within 60 days of the onset of symptoms.
C. Pharmaceutical therapy
  1. CDC recommendation: Ceftriaxone 250 mg by intramuscular (IM) injection of a single dose *plus* azithromycin 1 g by mouth, single dose, *or*
  2. If ceftriaxone is not available, CDC recommends: Cefixime 400 mg by mouth in a single dose, *or*
  3. For patients with severe allergy to cephalosporins, the CDC recommends azithromycin 2 g dose orally.
  4. The CDC advised that quinolones no longer be used for treatment of gonorrhea due to the increased bacterial resistance.

Follow-Up

A. The CDC no longer recommends a test of cure; however, patients who continue to exhibit symptoms should have culture performed.

B. All individuals should be closely monitored for treatment failure.
C. Reinforce treatment of all sexual partners within the past 60 days of diagnosis.
D. Providers are advised to report all treatment failures to the local or state public health department within 24 hours.

Consultation/Referral

A. Consult with a physician or refer the patient if treatment with the recommended dosage fails and patient noncompliance and reexposure have been ruled out.

Individual Considerations

A. Pregnancy
- **1.** Pregnant women with *N. gonorrhoeae* infections should be treated with both ceftriaxone 250 mg IM *plus* azithromycin 1 g by mouth, single dose.
- **2.** If unable to tolerate penicillin, consult with infectious disease (ID) provider.
- **3.** Presumed or diagnosed coinfections with chlamydia should be treated with azithromycin.

B. Adults
- **1.** Untreated or long-standing gonorrheal infection in women can lead to infertility.
- **2.** For patients with allergies to cephalosporins, using azithromycin treatment is recommended.

C. Pediatrics
- **1.** Ophthalmia neonatorum prophylaxis—perinatal exposure to the mother's infected cervix during birth can cause a gonococcal conjunctivitis, which can lead to blindness if left untreated. Accordingly, the CDC recommends a single application of erythromycin (0.5%) in each eye of an infant at birth.
- **2.** Sexual abuse should be considered. Suspect chlamydia for conjunctivitis if the infant is 30 days old or younger.
  - **a.** Treatment:
    - **i.** Should the presence of *N. gonorrhoeae* be confirmed, treatment with a single dose of ceftriaxone 25 to 50 mg/kg IM or IV, not to exceed 125 mg, is considered the standard of care.

Herpes Simplex Virus Type 2

Jill C. Cash and Robertson Nash

Definition

A. Herpes simplex is a lifelong, recurring viral disease that is transmitted by direct contact with the secretions or mucosa of an infected individual who is shedding the virus. The virus is usually characterized by painful vesicular lesions that form an ulcer, crust over, and then dry without scarring.

Incidence

A. It is estimated that approximately 776,000 people in the United States are infected with the herpes virus annually. Approximately 15.5% or one out of six, people from 14 to 49 years of age have genital herpes. According to the WHO, more than 500 million people worldwide have herpes simplex, type 2.

Pathogenesis

A. Herpes simplex virus (HSV) is the causative organism. HSV-1 produces oral lesions, and HSV-2 produces genital lesions. Kissing, sexual contact, vaginal delivery, and autoinoculation are all possible routes of transmission. The virus remains dormant, and outbreaks can be stimulated by several factors, including stress, illness, sunlight exposure, and menstruation.

Predisposing Factors

A. Early age at first coitus
B. Multiple sexual partners
C. History of STIs

Common Complaints

A. Dysuria
B. Pruritus
C. Burning
D. Swelling sensation

Other Signs and Symptoms

A. Primary episode
- **1.** Painful, itchy, vesicular, ulcerated, or crusted oral or genital lesion, singly or in clusters
- **2.** Flu-like syndrome: Fever, chills, headache, malaise, and myalgia

B. Recurrent episode: Less painful lesions and little or no systemic symptoms. Recurrent lesions in the same location as the previous outbreak is a significant clinical clue that the lesions are herpetic.

Subjective Data

A. Elicit history of onset of symptoms; their location, frequency, and duration; aggravating and alleviating factors; and associated symptomatology.
B. Question the patient about history of other STIs and sexual habits.

Physical Examination

A. Check temperature.
B. Inspect the head, eyes, ears, nose, throat, and mucous membranes for lesions.
C. Palpate the neck and abdomen for lymphadenopathy.
D. Pelvic examination
- **1.** Assess external genitalia, perineum, and anus for lesions.
- **2.** Assess for inguinal lymphadenopathy.

Diagnostic Test

A. Viral culture

> *Clinical diagnosis is often reliable, but confirmation with viral culture should be attempted. Vesicles should be unroofed or crust removed for most reliable sample.*

- **1.** The preferred methods for HSV testing are either cell culture or polymerase chain reaction (PCR).

Nucleic acid amplification test (NAAT) is considered more sensitive.

2. Viral isolation: Obtain vesicular fluid by swabbing the lesion with a cotton- or Dacron-tipped applicator.

3. Place the applicator in appropriate viral transport medium before drying.

4. Refrigerate until ready for transport.

B. Serology: HSV-specific glycoprotein G2 (HSV-2) and glycoprotein G1 (HSV-1). **Pap smear is not a sensitive test for HSV-2.**

Differential Diagnoses

A. HSV
B. Primary syphilis
C. Chancroid
D. Lymphogranuloma venereum
E. Folliculitis
F. Candidal fissure
G. Vestibular vulvitis
H. Mucocutaneous manifestations of Crohn's disease

Plan

A. General interventions

1. Culture samples immediately to begin treatment.

B. Patient teaching

1. *See Section III: Patient Teaching Guide for this chapter, "Herpes Simplex Virus."*

2. Advise patients to abstain from sexual activity during prodrome or while lesions are present.

3. Condom use should be encouraged when sexually active.

C. Pharmaceutical therapy: The Centers for Disease Control and Prevention (CDC) recommends the following treatment regimens:

1. Primary episode

a. Acyclovir 400 mg by mouth three times a day for 7 to 10 days

b. Acyclovir 200 mg by mouth five times a day for 7 to 10 days

c. Famciclovir 250 mg by mouth three times a day for 7 to 10 days

2. Recurrent episode: Begin during prodrome.

a. Acyclovir 400 mg by mouth three times a day for 5 days

b. Acyclovir 800 mg by mouth twice a day for 5 days

c. Acyclovir 800 mg by mouth three times a day for 2 days

d. Famciclovir 125 mg by mouth two times a day for 5 days

e. Famciclovir 1,000 mg by mouth two times a day for 1 day

f. Famciclovir 500 mg once, followed by 250 mg two times a day for 2 days

g. Valacyclovir 500 mg by mouth two times a day for 3 days

h. Valacyclovir 1 g by mouth once daily for 5 days

3. Daily suppressive therapy

a. Acyclovir 400 mg by mouth twice daily

b. Famciclovir 250 mg by mouth twice a day

c. Valacyclovir 500 mg by mouth twice daily

d. Valacyclovir 1 g by mouth once daily

e. Discontinue after 1 year of continuous use to reassess recurrence rate.

Clients receiving daily suppressive therapy of acyclovir 200 mg should use the lowest dose that provides relief from symptoms. Suppressive therapy has been shown to reduce frequency of recurrences by 75% in clients with more than six recurrences per year. It does not eliminate symptomatic or asymptomatic viral shedding or the potential for transmission.

4. Topical acyclovir, famciclovir (Famvir), and valacyclovir (Valtrex) have had mixed results in clinical trials and are not currently recommended by the CDC.

Follow-Up

A. Follow-up is not recommended unless it is warranted by clinical presentation.

Consultation/Referral

A. Consult or refer the patient to a physician when there is prolonged ulceration unresponsive to therapy.

Individual Considerations

A. Adults

1. Diagnosis is most often made via clinical presentation. Although viral testing is available, empiric treatment is recommended, versus testing and treating (see Other Signs and Symptoms).

2. Patients with HIV may have outbreaks of HSV lesions anywhere on their body. Do not limit diagnosis based on the physical location of lesions.

3. Patients presenting with HSV-1/HSV-2 lesions should be tested for HIV, per CDC recommendations.

4. Failure to isolate HSV does not mean that the patient does not have HSV.

B. Pregnancy

1. Transmission of genital herpes from an infected pregnant patient to the neonate is high, approximately 30% to 50%, when herpes is acquired during the last trimester or near delivery. The risk of transmission is much lower for pregnant patients who have a history of HSV or first acquire the virus during the first half of the pregnancy.

2. All pregnant patients should be questioned and screened for HSV when they are admitted to the hospital for delivery. All women with recurrent genital herpes lesions present at the onset of labor should be delivered by cesarean section to decrease the risk of transmission of the herpes virus to the neonate.

3. Acyclovir and valacyclovir is category B for pregnancy and considered safe to use during pregnancy. These medications can be used for treatment as well as for suppression during pregnancy. The American College of Obstetricians and Gynecologists recommends suppressive therapy beginning at approximately 36 weeks of gestation to prevent an outbreak of lesions and to increase the chance of having a vaginal delivery (see Table 15.1).

TABLE 15.1 Pharmacological Treatment of Herpes in Pregnancy

Antiviral	Acyclovir Dosage	Valacyclovir Dosage
Initial lesion outbreak	400 mg tid for 7–10 days	1 g bid for 7–10 days
Recurrent lesions	400 mg tid for 5 days	500 mg bid for 3 days
Daily suppression from 36 weeks gestation until delivery	400 mg tid	500 mg bid

bid, twice a day; tid, three times a day.

4. Culture lesions if outbreak occurs. Lesion must be crusted for 7 days for vaginal delivery to be an option; otherwise, a cesarean delivery is recommended to avoid transmission of virus to newborn.
5. Pregnant women without genital herpes should be advised to avoid intercourse during the third trimester with partners known or suspected of having genital herpes.
6. Acyclovir allergy: No effective alternatives to acyclovir have been identified.

C. Partners: Symptomatic partners should be evaluated and treated in the same manner as any patient with genital lesions.

D. Pediatrics

1. Transmission of HSV from mother to infant during birth is possible. The CDC recommends treatment of all infants born to mothers whose exposure to HSV was near term. Treatment is acyclovir 20 mg/kg IV every 8 hours for 14 days, unless there is disseminated disease or disease involving the central nervous system. In those cases, treatment should be extended for a total of 21 days.

E. Geriatric

1. Genital herpes is rarely seen in the elderly. Recurrent infection of the buttocks region is not uncommon, especially in females.

Human Papillomavirus

Jill C. Cash and Robertson Nash

Definition

A. The human papillomavirus (HPV) is a sexually transmitted infection (STI). Condyloma acuminata, genital warts, and venereal warts are other names for HPV.

Incidence

A. It is estimated that approximately 79 million Americans are infected with HPV. There are approximately 14 million new infections each year. It is estimated that annually there are 360,000 new cases of genital warts in the United States. Certain strains of HPV are associated with cancer. Annually, in the United States, there are approximately:

12,000 women diagnosed with cervical cancer
3,200 cases of vulvar cancer
735 cases of vaginal cancer
1,048 cases of penile cancer
2,821 cases of anal cancer in women
1,549 cases of anal cancer in men
2,443 oropharyngeal cancers in women
9,974 oropharyngeal cancers in men

Pathogenesis

A. The HPV, a slow-growing DNA virus of the papovavirus family, is the causative organism. More than 70 strains of the virus have been identified, and types 6 and 11 are most associated with genital warts. Types 16, 18, 31, 33, and 35 are of high risk and are associated with cervical neoplasia. Warts may appear as early as 1 to 2 months after exposure, but most infections remain subclinical.

Predisposing Factors

A. Early first coitus
B. Multiple sexual partners
C. History of transmitted infections

Common Complaints

A. Painless genital "bumps" or warts
B. Pruritus
C. Bleeding during or after coitus
D. Malodorous vaginal discharge
E. Dysuria

Other Signs and Symptoms

A. Wart-like growths on genital area that are elevated and rough or flat and smooth
B. Lesions occurring singly or in clusters, from less than 1 mm to cauliflower-like aggregates
C. Papillomas that are pale pink in color

Subjective Data

A. Elicit history of the onset of symptoms, location, frequency, duration, aggravating and alleviating factors, and associated symptomatology.
B. Question the patient about history of other STIs, sexual behaviors, recent change in sexual partner, and partner's history of STIs.

Physical Examination

A. Inspect

1. Inspect external genitalia, perineum, and anus for lesions.
2. Females, speculum examination: Inspect vaginal walls and cervix for lesions.
3. Application of 3% acetic acid whitens lesions (not considered diagnostic by the Centers for Disease Control and Prevention [CDC]).

Diagnostic Tests

A. Visual identification is adequate in most cases.
B. Cytology: Pap smears are useful for screening. Pap results of koilocytosis, dyskeratosis, keratinizing atypia, atypical inflammation, and parakeratosis are all suggestive of HPV.

C. Histology: Colposcopy with directed biopsy is diagnostic for subclinical lesions, dysplasia, and malignancy.

D. DNA typing: Determination of specific strains is useful in diagnosing subclinical infections (the test is costly and false negatives occur).

Differential Diagnoses

A. HPV
B. Condylomata
C. Molluscum contagiosum
D. Carcinoma

Plan

A. General interventions: Make diagnosis promptly to begin treatment.

B. Patient teaching

1. *See Section III: Patient Teaching Guide for this chapter, "Human Papillomavirus."*

2. Explain to the patient that therapy eliminates visible warts but does not eradicate the virus. No therapy has been shown to be effective in eradication of HPV. Ablation of warts may decrease viral load and transmissibility.

3. Advise the patient to abstain from genital contact while lesions are present.

C. Pharmaceutical therapy

1. Therapy is not recommended for subclinical infections (absence of exophytic warts).

2. Trichloroacetic acid (TCA) 80% to 90% solution applied weekly to visible warts by clinician until warts resolve. If unresolved after six applications, consider other therapy. *See Section II: Procedures, "Trichloroacetic Acid/Podophyllin Therapy."*

3. Podophyllum resin (Podophyllin) 10% to 25% in tincture of benzoin compound applied weekly to visible warts by clinician until warts resolve.

a. Application of petroleum jelly on surrounding skin may be used for protection of unaffected areas.

b. Advise the patient to wash off resin after 4 hours. If unresolved after six applications, consider other therapy.

4. Apply TCA 80% to 90% to the warts and allow to dry weekly by clinician until warts resolve.

5. Podofilox, 0.5% solution for home treatment, applied to visible warts by the patient twice daily for three consecutive days, followed by 4 days without treatment. The cycle is repeated up to four times.

6. Imiquimod 5% (Aldara) cream applied to wart at bedtime, left on for 6 to 10 hours, then washed with mild soap. Use daily, three times a week (Monday, Wednesday, and Friday), until wart resolves or up to 16 weeks.

D. Medical/surgical management: Cryotherapy, electrodesiccation, electrocautery, carbon dioxide laser, and surgical excision are options to be considered for patients with large or extensive lesions or refractory disease.

Follow-Up

A. Short-term follow-up is not recommended if the patient is asymptomatic after treatment.

B. The CDC does not recommend more frequent Pap smears for women with external warts.

C. Long-term follow-up should include annual Pap smears and pelvic examinations. Encourage the patient to self-examine genitalia.

Consultation/Referral

A. Consult or refer the patient to a physician when lesions persist after six consecutive treatments or when cervical or rectal warts are diagnosed.

HPV Vaccines

A. There are several HPV vaccines available or in use in the United States, including bivalent (Cervarix), quadrivalent (Gardasil), and nonavalent. The quadrivalent vaccine prevents infection with HPV types 6, 11, 16, and 18, which are most likely to be the cause of genital warts.

B. For both girls and boys, vaccine may start at as young as 9 years of age. The vaccine is recommended for girls and young women aged between 9 and 26 years. For males, the vaccine is recommended for those between 9 and 21 years of age, with an extension of administration until age 26 years for men who have sex with men (MSM) and other immunocompromised males.

C. Administration for children 9 to 11 years of age should be two doses of intramuscular (IM) vaccine, with the second dose given between 6 and 12 months following the first dose. Administration for children of 15 years of age or greater is via a three-dose series of IM injections, with the second dose given 1 to 2 months after the first and the third given 6 months after the first. NOTE: The CDC has no published guidelines for children between 12 and 14 years of age.

D. HPV vaccine is available for those less than 19 years of age via the Vaccines for Children (VFC) program (call CDC-INFO [1-800-232-4636] for more information).

E. Uninsured patients eligible for the vaccine may be able to access patient assistance programs via vaccine manufacturers.

Individual Considerations

A. Pregnancy: Podophyllum and podofilox are contraindicated during pregnancy.

B. Partners:

1. Treatment is recommended if visible lesions are present.

2. Testing sex partners for HPV is not recommended.

3. Sex partners are likely to share HPV. In most cases, the virus is likely to clear without associated health concerns. The risk of HPV warts and cancers increases greatly when the infection does not clear and becomes chronic.

4. Consistent condom usage can lower the chances of acquisition and transmission of HPV virus. However, the virus can infect areas not protected by condoms (that is, female anus during vaginal intercourse and buccal mucosa during oral sex).

C. Adolescents: Education regarding Gardasil vaccine is recommended for girls and boys 9 to 25 years of age for prevention of acquiring the HPV. The vaccination may help to prevent contracting four of the viruses (types 6, 11, 16, and 17) that increase the risk of cervical cancer for women.

D. Geriatric
1. Verrucous carcinoma and vulvar intraepithelial neoplasia (VIN) can be indistinguishable from condyloma. Older women are more likely to have VIN or carcinoma.
2. Diagnosis is made by biopsy; colposcopy is strongly advised.
3. Immunocompetence should be investigated in new or recurrent condyloma.

Syphilis

Jill C. Cash and Robertson Nash

Definition

A. Syphilis is a sexually transmitted infection (STI) characterized by distinct primary, secondary, and tertiary stages that occur over several years or decades. Latent or inactive periods occur between the stages. Early latent is less than 1 year after infection; late latent is more than 1 year after infection. **Health department notification of infection is required by law in all states.**

Incidence

A. In 2014, there were 19,999 reported cases of primary and secondary syphilis in the United States. In 2014, 83% of patients diagnosed were men engaged in sexual activity with other men. There were approximately 458 cases of children born with congenital syphilis in 2014, an increase of 27.5% since 2013.

Pathogenesis

A. *Treponema pallidum,* a spirochete bacterium, is the causative organism that infects the mucous membrane.

Predisposing Factors

A. History of STIs
B. Multiple sexual partners
C. Illicit drug use
D. Prostitution

Common Complaints

A. Genital lesion, generalized rash involving palms and soles, mucous patches, and condyloma latum are common.

Other Signs and Symptoms

A. Primary syphilis
1. Chancre that is painless or minimally painful
2. Round, indurated lesion with little or no purulent exudate
3. Regional bilateral lymphadenopathy

B. Secondary syphilis
1. Generalized maculopapular rash that is nonpruritic and copper colored, on palms or soles; may be erythematous or scaly
2. Mucous patches; painless, white, mucous membrane lesions
3. Generalized lymphadenopathy; flu-like syndrome, including fever, headache, sore throat, and malaise
4. Patchy alopecia

C. Tertiary syphilis
1. Gumma: Locally destructive granulomatous tumors involving various organs or systems; commonly seen on liver but can occur on other organs (heart, brain, skin, bone, testis)
2. Cardiovascular: Aortic involvement, aneurysms, and valve insufficiency
3. Neurologic: Tabes dorsalis and general paresis

D. Latent syphilis: Asymptomatic

Latent phase syphilis manifests itself after treatment failure or no history of treatment. Spirochete can lie dormant for years.

E. Congenital syphilis: Symptoms range from asymptomatic to fatal.

Subjective Data

A. Elicit history of onset, location, frequency, duration of symptoms; aggravating and alleviating factors; and associated symptomatology.
B. Question the patient about history of other STIs, illicit drug use, and sexual habits.

Physical Examination

A. Check temperature, pulse, respirations, and blood pressure.
B. Inspect
1. Inspect the skin; note lesions and rashes.
2. Observe the head; note patchy alopecia.
3. Examine the mouth and throat; note lesions.
4. Inspect the genital and rectal area; note lesions and rashes.

C. Palpate the lymph nodes (neck, supraclavicular, axillary, epitrochlear, and inguinal regions).
D. Auscultate heart and lungs.
E. Neurologic examination
1. Assess sensory functioning.
2. Test cranial nerves, first through twelfth.

Diagnostic Tests

There are two types of tests available for use in the diagnosis and management of syphilis—nontreponemal and treponemal—and knowledge of both is essential. Nontreponemal tests, such as the rapid plasma reagin (RPR), assess for biomarkers typically created by spirochetes. These tests are inexpensive, rapid, and easy to perform. In addition the results are reported as titers, which facilitate monitoring the status of the infection. These are not antibody tests, however. Therefore, it is possible to have a false positive due to several conditions, including autoimmune disease, HIV, pregnancy, older age, and intravenous drug use. Accordingly, the Centers for Disease Control and Prevention (CDC) recommends a confirmatory treponemal test in all cases where the nontreponemal test is positive.

Treponemal tests, such as the treponemal pallidum particle agglutination (TP-PA), are antibody tests. Although more accurate than nontreponemal tests, treponemal tests are more expensive. A further complication of using treponemal tests as screening tools is that a treponemal test is positive for life once a person has had syphilis. Used in isolation, treponemal tests do not reveal whether an infection is active.

Interpretation of treponemal test findings is done in conjunction with findings from nontreponemal tests. Specifically, a fourfold drop in an initial nontreponemal titer indicates successful treatment of syphilis, that is, 1:64 to 1:4. In some cases, titers remain persistent over extended periods (more than 2–3 years); these individuals are referred to as sero-fast.

Evaluate for other STIs for patients presenting with syphilis.

A. Serology: Nontreponemal tests
1. Venereal Disease Research Laboratory (VDRL) test
2. RPR tests
3. HIV: Due to the increased likelihood of false-positive nontreponemal tests in people with HIV, all HIV-infected patients with a positive nontrepomenal test should be followed with a treponemal test, as per "Diagnostic Tests" discussed previously.

Results are reactive (positive) or nonreactive (negative). Titers correlate with active disease and should be quantitative. These tests are equally valid but cannot be compared because of titer differences (RPR is slightly higher than VDRL). All reactive results require confirmation with treponemal tests.

B. Serology: Treponemal tests
1. Fluorescent treponemal antibody absorption (FTA-ABS) test
2. Microhemagglutination assay for antibody to *T. pallidum*

Once FTA-ABS for antibody to T. pallidum, VDRL, and RPR are reactive, these tests usually remain reactive for life.

C. Cerebrospinal fluid (CSF) culture to detect neurosyphilis

D. Microscopy: *T. pallidum* cannot be seen with light microscopy; dark-field microscopic examination of the serous exudate from lesions is the definitive test for syphilis. Properly equipped labs with specially trained personnel must be available for this test.

Differential Diagnoses

A. Syphilis
B. Herpes simplex virus (HSV)

Plan

A. General interventions: Staging of the disease may be difficult but guides management decisions.

B. Patient teaching
1. *See Section III: Patient Teaching Guide for this chapter, "Syphilis."*
2. Advise the patient to abstain from sexual activity until treatment is completed.
3. Inform the patient of Jarisch–Herxheimer reaction (fever, headache, myalgia) that may occur within the first 24 hours of treatment. Antipyretics may be prescribed.
4. Discuss the importance of partner notification.
5. Stress the importance of complying with the follow-up regimen.

C. Pharmaceutical therapy: The CDC recommends the following treatment regimens.
1. Primary syphilis, secondary syphilis, early latent syphilis.
   a. Adults: Benzathine penicillin G 2.4 million units injected intramuscularly (IM) in a single dose
   b. Pediatrics: Benzathine penicillin G 50,000 units/kg, up to the adult dose of 2.4 million units, injected IM in a single dose
2. Late latent syphilis, latent syphilis of unknown duration, late syphilis (manage with expert consultation)
   a. Adults: Benzathine penicillin G 7.2 million units total, administered as three doses (2.4 million units each) injected IM at 1-week intervals
   b. Pediatrics: Benzathine penicillin G 50,000 units/kg, up to the adult dose of 2.4 million units, injected IM for three total doses at 1-week intervals
3. Neurosyphilis (manage with expert consultation)
   a. Adults: Aqueous crystalline penicillin G, 18 to 24 million units daily, 3 to 4 million units administered intravenously (IV) every 4 hours for 10 to 14 days
   b. Adults: Procaine penicillin 2 to 4 million units injected IM daily, plus probenecid 500 mg by mouth four times a day, both for 10 to 14 days
   c. Pediatrics: Penicillin desensitization, then treatment with recommended regimen
4. Primary syphilis, secondary syphilis, latent syphilis, late latent syphilis in (nonpregnant) patient with penicillin allergy: Doxycycline 100 mg by mouth twice daily for 2 weeks, or tetracycline 500 mg by mouth four times daily for 2 weeks
5. Latent syphilis of unknown duration, late syphilis: Treat with aforementioned regimen for infections of less than 1-year duration. If greater than 1 year, treat with aforementioned regimen for 4 weeks.
6. For pregnant patients with penicillin allergy, penicillin treatment after desensitization is recommended for the following reasons:
   a. Penicillin is effective for preventing transmission and treating the infected fetus.
   b. Doxycycline and tetracycline are contraindicated in pregnancy.
   c. Erythromycin may not cure the infected fetus.

Follow-Up

A. Primary and secondary syphilis: Clinical and serologic examinations should be conducted at 6, 12, and 24 months. Absence of fourfold decrease in RPR titer at 3 months is indicative of treatment failure.

B. Latent syphilis: Clinical and serologic examinations should be conducted at 6, 12, and 24 months. Absence of fourfold decrease within 12 to 24 months is indicative of treatment failure.

C. Tertiary syphilis: Minimal evidence regarding follow-up exists. Follow-up largely depends on nature of lesions.
D. Neurosyphilis: CSF examination should take place every 6 months until cell count is normal.

Consultation/Referral

A. Consult or refer the patient to a physician when the recommended treatment fails and patient noncompliance and reexposure have been ruled out, or when neurosyphilis is diagnosed.

Individual Considerations

A. Pregnancy
  1. Draw blood samples for RPR/VDRL from all prenatal patients.
  2. Women in communities with high prevalence of syphilis and/or with high-risk behavior should be tested twice during the third trimester: Once at 28 to 32 weeks, and again at delivery.
  3. Any woman having a fetal death at greater than 20 weeks should be tested for syphilis.
  4. Administer appropriate regimen of penicillin for the patient's stage of syphilis. Consider a second dose of penicillin 1 week after the initial treatment.
  5. Patients who are allergic to penicillin should be desensitized and treated with penicillin during pregnancy.
  6. Follow-up: Perform serologic tests monthly until adequacy of treatment has been ensured.
  7. The Jarisch–Herxheimer reaction may predispose women to premature labor or fetal distress if treatment occurs in the second half of the pregnancy. Advise these patients to immediately seek medical attention if they experience uterine contractions or changes in fetal movement.
  8. All pregnant women diagnosed with syphilis should be offered HIV screening.
B. Pediatrics
  1. Congenital syphilis is caused by untreated infection or treatment failure in the mother.
  2. Refer the patient to a physician for infectious disease consultation.
  3. Medication therapy: See "Pharmaceutical therapy" noted previously.
C. Partners: Identify at-risk partners who have had sexual contact with the patient within these time frames:
  1. Primary syphilis: 3 months plus duration of symptoms
  2. Secondary syphilis: 6 months plus duration of symptoms
  3. Early latent syphilis: 1 year
D. Geriatric
  1. Dementia, tremors, and pupillary changes are the result of long-term untreated syphilis.
  2. The CSF should be tested using the FTA-ABS test. The VDRL is usually not adequate.
  3. Syphilis is uncommon in the elderly in developed countries; however, it is very common worldwide.

Trichomoniasis

Jill C. Cash and Robertson Nash

Definition

A. Trichomoniasis is a sexually transmitted infection (STI). Nonsexual transmission by means of fomites is possible but rare.

Incidence

A. Trichomoniasis is not a Centers for Disease Control and Prevention (CDC)-reportable infection. Therefore, its exact incidence is unavailable. The CDC estimates that 3.7 million people have the infection.

Pathogenesis

A. *Trichomonas vaginalis,* a flagellated protozoan, is the causative organism.

Predisposing Factors

A. History of STIs
B. Multiple sexual partners

Common Complaints

A. Copious, yellow-green, or watery gray vaginal discharge
B. Vaginal odor
C. Dysuria
D. Dyspareunia
E. Postcoital spotting or bleeding
F. Abdominal discomfort
G. Pruritus

Other Signs and Symptoms

A. Asymptomatic
B. Perineal irritation

Subjective Data

A. Elicit history of the onset, location, frequency, duration of symptoms, and aggravating and alleviating factors; note associated symptomatology.
B. Question the patient about history of other STIs or vaginal infections, changes and characteristics of vaginal discharge, and recent change in sexual partner.

Physical Examination

A. Check temperature.
B. Inspect: Inspect introitus for discharge and irritation.
C. Speculum examination
  1. Inspect the vaginal walls for discharge and irritation.
  2. Inspect the cervix for discharge, erythema, punctate hemorrhages (strawberry-patch cervix), and friability.

D. Bimanual examination
1. Assess for cervical motion tenderness (CMT).
2. Palpate for uterine and adnexal tenderness.

Diagnostic Tests

A. Wet prep: Perhaps the most common diagnostic tool, intended to visualize presence of motile, flagellated trichomonads. Increased number of white blood cells (WBC) (greater than 0.10 per high-power field) may be present. As per the CDC, the sensitivity of wet-mount analysis is low (51%–65%) in vaginal specimens and even lower in male urine samples.
B. NAAT methods are the current standard, and are reportedly three to five times more accurate than wet-mount microscopy. New tests using vaginal, endocervical, and urine samples are becoming commercially available.
C. Pap smear: Report may include trichomonads, but sensitivity is low.
1. If trichomonads are noted on Pap smear, the patient should be reexamined and diagnosis confirmed with a wet prep.
D. Vaginal pH is usually greater than 4.5.
E. The potassium hydroxide/wet prep "whiff test" may be positive.

Differential Diagnoses

A. Trichomoniasis
B. Bacterial vaginosis
C. Vulvovaginal candidiasis
D. Chlamydia
E. Gonorrhea
F. Pelvic inflammatory disease
G. Foreign-body vaginitis

Plan

A. General interventions: Prompt diagnosis helps to initiate treatment.
B. Patient teaching
1. *See Section III: Patient Teaching Guide for this chapter, "Trichomoniasis."*
2. Advise the patient to abstain from sexual activity until treatment is complete.
3. Advise the patient to avoid alcohol consumption during and 24 hours after metronidazole treatment due to the possible Antabuse effect from the medication.
4. Inform the patient that urine may darken in color during treatment.
5. Inform the patient of a possible metallic taste in the mouth during treatment.
C. Pharmaceutical therapy
1. **Drug of choice: Metronidazole 2 g orally in a single dose or tinidazole 2 g orally in a single dose. Advise patients that alcohol and alcohol-containing products should be avoided at least 24 to 48 hours after the last dose of metronidazole is taken.**
2. Alternative regimen: Metronidazole 500 mg by mouth twice daily for 7 days. Expected cure rate from either regimen is 95%.
3. Treatment failure: The CDC recommends retreatment with metronidazole 500 mg by mouth twice daily for 7 days.
4. If repeated failure occurs, treat with metronidazole 2 g by mouth four times daily for 3 to 5 days.
5. Metronidazole gel is unlikely to achieve therapeutic levels in the urethra or perivaginal glands. It is a considerably less efficacious treatment than oral preparations and is *not* recommended for use.

Follow-Up

A. Immediate follow-up is not recommended if the patient is initially asymptomatic or symptoms are relieved by treatment. Due to concern of resistance, a 3-month follow-up for sexually active women is recommended.

Consultation/Referral

A. Failure to clear infection with single-dose therapy should be followed with a 7-day course of metronidazole 500 mg twice daily for 7 days for the patient and sexual partner(s).
B. Should treatment with the previous regimen fail in a patient felt to be adherent with medication and not subject to reinfection, consult with or refer the patient to a physician for assessment of metronidazole susceptibility.

Individual Considerations

A. Pregnancy
1. First trimester: Metronidazole is contraindicated.
2. Palliative treatment: Clotrimazole 1% vaginal cream one applicator full daily at bedtime for 7 days is suggested.
3. Second and third trimesters: Metronidazole 2 g by mouth, one time
4. Lactation: Metronidazole 2 g by mouth one time; discontinue breastfeeding during and 24 hours after treatment. Pumping and discarding milk is recommended.
B. Partners: Recommended treatment is metronidazole 2 g orally, one time.
C. Geriatric
1. Uncommon pathogen in postmenopausal women
2. Symptoms are vulvar irritation with discharge
3. Diagnose with wet prep
4. Treat with metronidazole 1 g in the morning and 1 g in the evening
D. Patients with HIV
1. Screen all women at first visit and annually for trichomoniasis. Treatment for trichomoniasis—multiple dose therapy: Metronidazole 500 mg twice a day for 7 days

Bibliography

American College of Obstetricians and Gynecologists Committee on Practice Bulletins. (2007). ACOG Practice Bulletin. Clinical management guidelines for obstetrician-gynecologists. No. 82 June 2007 reaffirmed in 2016. Management of herpes in pregnancy. *Obstetrics and Gynecology, 109*(6), 1489–1498.

Borhart, J., & Birnbaumer, D. M. (2011). Emergency department management of sexually transmitted infections. *Emergency Medicine Clinics of North America, 29*(3), 587–603.

Centers for Disease Control and Prevention. (2015a). Chlamydia. Retrieved from www.cdc.gov/std/chlamydia/default.htm

Centers for Disease Control and Prevention. (2015b). Genital herpes—CDC fact sheet. Retrieved from https://www.cdc.gov/std/herpes/stdfact-herpes.htm

Centers for Disease Control and Prevention. (2015c). Genital HPV infection—Fact sheet. Retrieved from https://www.cdc.gov/std/hpv/stdfact-hpv.htm

Centers for Disease Control and Prevention. (2015d). Gonorrhea. Retrieved from www.cdc.gov/std/gonorrhea/default.htm

Centers for Disease Control and Prevention. (2015e). Incidence, prevalence, and cost of sexually transmitted infections in the United States. Retrieved from https://www.cdc.gov/std/stats/sti-estimates-fact-sheet-feb-2013.pdf

Centers for Disease Control and Prevention. (2015f). Reported STDs in the United States: 2014 National data for chlamydia, gonorrhea, and syphilis. Retrieved from www.cdc.gov /std/stats14/std-trends-508.pdf

Centers for Disease Control and Prevention. (2015g). Sexually transmitted diseases treatment guidelines, 2015. Retrieved from https://www.cdc.gov/std/tg2015

Kao, T., & Manczak, M. (2013). Family influences on adolescents' birth control and condom use, likelihood of sexually transmitted infections. *Journal of School Nursing, 29*(1), 61–70.

Mark, H., Jordan, E.T., Cruz, J., & Warren, N. (2012). What's new in sexually transmitted infection management: Changes in the 2010 guidelines from the Centers for Disease Control and Prevention. *Journal of Midwifery & Womens Health, 57*(3), 276–284.

O'Connor, C., & Shubkin, C. (2012). Adolescent STIs for primary care providers. *Current Opinion in Pediatrics, 24*(5), 647–655.

Richardson, K. K., & Shannon, M. T. (2012). STI screening & treatment in pregnancy. *Nurse Practitioner, 37*(12), 30–37.

16 Infectious Disease Guidelines

Cat Scratch Disease

Cheryl A. Glass and Jill C. Cash

Definition

A. Cat scratch disease (CSD) is a lymphatic infection occurring 3 to 14 days after a dermal abrasion from a cat scratch. Infection causes unilateral regional adenitis; however, CSD manifestations may also include visceral organ, neurologic, and ocular involvement. There are two phases of symptoms.

- **1.** Oroya fever: Symptoms include fever, headache, muscle aches, abdominal pain, and severe anemia.
- **2.** Verruga peruana: Symptoms include skin lesions/nodular growths that then emerge as red to purple vascular lesions. The lesions are prone to bleeding and ulceration.

Incidence

A. Incidence is less than 25,000 new cases every year; it is believed to be relatively common. More than 90% of cases have had a history of recent contact with cats, often kittens, which are usually healthy. Multiple cases have been observed in families, presumably resulting from contact with the same animal. There is no documentation of human-to-human transmission. Persons who are immunocompromised are more susceptible to the systemic manifestations. Dissemination to the liver, spleen, eye, or central nervous system (CNS) occurs in 5% to 14% of individuals.

B. CSD occurs worldwide.

C. Most cases, 70% to 90%, of CSD occur in the fall and winter months in the United States.

D. CSD is more common in patients younger than 21 years.

E. Approximately 1% of diagnosed cases have no history of an animal scratch.

Pathogenesis

A. *Bartonella henselae* is considered to be responsible for most cases of CSD. *B. henselae* is a fastidious, slow-growing, gram-negative bacterium. Most transmission occurs from feline bites or scratches as well as cat licking to nonintact skin. About 40% of cats carry *B. henselae* at some time in their lives. Other vectors that may be involved in the transmission of *B. henselae* to humans include dogs, monkeys, *Ixodes* ticks, and fleas from cats or kittens.

B. The incubation period for lesions to appear is 7 to 12 days after abrasion; lymphadenopathy appears 5 to 50 days (median = 12 days) after appearance of the primary lesion.

Predisposing Factors

A. Exposure to domestic and outside cats

B. Immunocompromised

Common Complaints

A. Swollen lymph glands (regional lymph node, groin, axillary, and cervical areas). The predominant sign is regional lymphadenopathy in an otherwise healthy person.

B. Low-grade fever

C. Body aches

D. Fatigue

E. Anorexia

Other Signs and Symptoms

A. A skin papule appears 3 to 10 days after inoculation, often found at the presumed site of inoculation. The papule progresses through the erythematous, vesicular, and popular crusted stages. The papules are generally nonpruritic.

B. Headache

C. Extreme fatigue (anemia)

D. Abdominal pain in the presence of hepatosplenomegaly

E. Arthropathies of the knee, wrist, ankle, and elbows

F. Visual

- **1.** Unilateral eye redness/conjunctivitis is the most common ocular manifestation.
- **2.** Loss of vision
- **3.** Visual disturbances
- **4.** Ocular pain (i.e., foreign-body sensation)
- **5.** Serous discharge

G. Central nervous

- **1.** Changes in level of consciousness (LOC)
- **2.** Persistent high fever
- **3.** Seizures within 6 weeks of lymphadenopathy

H. Cardiac

- **1.** Murmur
- **2.** Dyspnea

Subjective Data

A. Review onset and duration of symptoms.

B. Elicit the history of abrasion caused by a kitten/cat or other vectors.

C. Ask the patient about other symptoms such as low-grade fever and body aches.
D. Rule out other illness with review of symptoms (such as pharyngitis and mononucleosis).
E. Ask about visual loss (painless, unilateral visual loss is present with neuroretinitis).
F. Has the patient had a febrile seizure?

Physical Examination

A. Check temperature, pulse, respirations, and blood pressure.
B. Inspect
- **1.** Examine the skin for scratches, bite marks, erythema, or rash.
- **2.** Conduct an ear, nose, and throat examination.
- **3.** Conduct an eye examination if indicated.
  - **a.** Visual examination: Snellen chart
  - **b.** Funduscopic examination
    - **i.** The optic disc appears edematous.
    - **ii.** Exudates frequently surround the macula.
    - **iii.** The funduscopic examination may need to be deferred if photophobia is present.

C. Auscultate
- **1.** Heart
- **2.** Lungs

D. Palpate
- **1.** Palpate lymph nodes: Preauricular, cervical, axillary, epitrochlear, and inguinal nodes. Unilateral tender lymph nodes (usually singular) are palpable near the scratch site. The area around the affected lymph nodes is typically tender, warm, erythematous, and indurated.
- **2.** Abdomen to rule out organomegaly.
- **3.** Breast: Examine if indicated: Mastitis is rare.

Diagnostic Tests

A. Usually none; CSD is often diagnosed by history and physical examination alone. Presenting symptoms may indicate further testing, including
- **1.** Complete blood count (CBC) with differential
- **2.** Sedimentation rate
- **3.** Bartonella antibody testing
- **4.** Disseminated polymerase chain reaction (PCR) assay

B. Warthin–Starry silver impregnation stain of lymph node, skin, or conjunctival tissue.
C. Biopsy of lymph node (when malignancy is suspected).
D. Culture and sensitivity of any aspirated fluid or blood cultures. Cultures should be held for 21 days since *B. henselae* is a slow-growing bacterium. Trench fever, Carrion's disease, and endocarditis can also be diagnosed with serology.
E. Abdominal ultrasound or CT in the presence of hepatomegaly, splenomegaly, or hepatosplenomegaly on physical examination.
F. The cat-scratch skin test is no longer recommended.

Differential Diagnoses

A. CSD
B. Infectious mononucleosis
C. Kawasaki disease (KD)
D. Lyme disease
E. Malignancies that involve lymph nodes such as lymphoma/Hodgkin's disease
F. Fever of unknown origin (FUO)
G. Trench fever
H. Carrion's disease
I. Endocarditis

Plan

A. General interventions
- **1.** Management is usually treatment of symptoms. CSD is self-limiting with slow resolution in 2 to 4 months.
- **2.** Prescribe analgesics for pain.
- **3.** Rest is advised.
- **4.** Ice may be applied to the affected nodes.
- **5.** About 10% of nodes will suppurate and require aspiration. However, lymph node aspiration is not recommended unless to relieve severe pain. During aspiration, the needle should be moved around in several locations because microabscesses often exist in multiple septated pockets. Incision and drainage are not recommended because of the potential of chronic sinus tract formation.

B. Patient teaching
- **1.** The lymphadenopathy usually regresses within 2 to 4 months but may persist for up to 1 year.
- **2.** Patient education on cats includes the following:
  - **a.** People should avoid playing roughly with cats.
  - **b.** Stray cats should not be handled by children or immunocompromised people.
  - **c.** Testing cats is not recommended. Cats do not need to be removed or destroyed.
  - **d.** Always cleanse animal bites or scratches immediately with soap and water to prevent or reduce the transmission of CSD.
  - **e.** Control fleas (fleas have been found to have *B. henselae*).
- **3.** If there are any signs of an infection after a cat bite/scratch, the patient should be seen by his or her health care provider.
- **4.** Disease is not contagious: There is no person-to-person transmission.
- **5.** No vaccination is currently available.

C. Pharmaceutical therapy
- **1.** Antibiotic therapy is not essential for patients with normal immune systems. Symptoms are usually self-limiting.
- **2.** Acetaminophen (Tylenol) as needed
- **3.** Nonsteroidal anti-inflammatory drugs (NSAIDs) as needed
- **4.** Oral corticosteroids for individuals with atypical symptoms

5. Antibiotics may be prescribed if the patient is acutely ill with systemic symptoms, particularly immunocompromised individuals; with hepatosplenomegaly, visual, cardiac, or neurologic symptoms; or with large, painful adenopathy.

a. Azithromycin (Zithromax) dosing for lymphadenitis:

i. For patients weighing more than 45.5 kg, prescribe 500 mg on day 1, followed by 250 mg for 4 days.

ii. For patients weighing less than 45.5 kg, prescribe 10 mg/kg on day 1, followed by 5 mg/kg for 4 days.

b. Clarithromycin (Cipro) may be used as an alternative to azithromycin for lymphadenitis.

i. For patients weighing more than 45.5 kg, prescribe 500 mg twice a day for a 7- to 10-day course.

ii. For patients weighing less than 45.5 kg, prescribe 15 to 20 mg/kg divided into two doses for a 7- to 10-day course.

c. Rifampin may be used as an alternative for lymphadenitis.

i. In children, prescribe 10 mg/kg every 12 hours to a maximum dose of 600 mg/d for a 7- to 10-day course.

ii. In adults, prescribe 300 mg twice a day for a 7- to 10-day course.

d. Trimethoprim-sulfamethoxazole may be used as an alternative for lymphadenitis.

i. In children, prescribe trimethoprim 8 mg/kg/d, sulfamethoxazole 40 mg/kg/d in two divided doses for 7 to 10 days.

ii. In adults, prescribe one double-strength tablet twice a day.

e. For hepatosplenic disease and prolonged fever, use rifampin (as previously noted) for 10 to 14 days and add a second agent such as azithromycin or gentamicin.

i. Azithromycin (as previously noted) for an entire 10- to 14-day course

ii. Gentamicin loading dose 2 mg/kg, then 1.5 mg/kg over 8 hours; dose based on normal renal function and adjusted with monitoring

f. Neurologic disease/neuroretinitis: Patients diagnosed with neuroretinitis or neurologic disease should be prescribed with doxycycline 100 mg twice a day plus rifampin 300 mg orally twice a day (bid). Treatment should be prescribed for 4 to 6 weeks for neuroretinitis and 10 to 14 days for other neurologic disease. Consult with a physician. Consult with the ophthalmologist since the patient will require close monitoring.

g. Endocarditis: The optimal antibiotic therapy and optimal duration of therapy for *Bartonella* endocarditis are unknown. Consult with a physician.

Follow-Up

A. Reevaluate the patient in approximately 6 to 8 weeks if mild symptoms.

B. Reevaluate in 10 days if placed on antibiotics.

C. CSD is not reportable to the health department or the Centers for Disease Control and Prevention (CDC).

Consultation/Referral

A. Complications are rare; refer the patient to a physician, including specialists (neurologist, cardiologist, and ophthalmologist) if infection is systemic or unresponsive to antibiotics.

1. Hearing loss

2. Neurologic disability

3. Digit or limb amputations

4. Skin scarring

B. Patients diagnosed with neuroretinitis should be referred to an ophthalmologist for comanagement.

C. Infectious disease consult should be ordered for patients diagnosed with serious infections such as trench fever, Carrion's disease, and endocarditis.

Individual Considerations

A. Pediatrics

1. If neuroretinitis is diagnosed in children less than 8 years of age, treatment should include azithromycin or trimethoprim-sulfamethoxazole in place of doxycycline.

Cytomegalovirus

Cheryl A. Glass and Jill C. Cash

Definition

A. Cytomegalovirus (CMV) is in the herpesvirus family, which includes varicella-zoster virus (chickenpox) and infectious mononucleosis (Epstein–Barr virus [EBV]). Differences in CMV genotypes may be associated with differences in virulence. CMV is responsible for a viral infection with a high rate of asymptomatic excretion. Shedding of the virus takes place intermittently. CMV can be isolated in cell culture from urine, pharynx, respiratory secretions, human milk, tears, saliva, semen, cervical secretions, and body fluids such as blood and amniotic fluid. Cytomegalic cells can be found in tissue, including the lung, liver, kidney, intestine, adrenal gland, and the central nervous system (CNS).

B. CMV persists in latent form after a primary infection, and reactivation can occur years later, particularly under conditions of immunosuppression, transplantation, and pregnancy. CMV is one of the **TORCH** infections (toxoplasmosis, other [i.e., hepatitis and syphilis], rubella, CMV, and herpes infections).

C. The most common illness caused by CMV is retinitis.

Incidence

A. CMV is found worldwide in all ages, races, and ethnic groups. Seropositivity increases with age, ranging from 40% to 100% depending on geography, cultures, child-rearing practices, and socioeconomic status. Approximately 50% of blood donors have been exposed to CMV, and 10% carry CMV in white blood cells

(WBCs). The incidence of horizontal transmission of CMV occurring in settings such as day care ranges from 10% to more than 80% from the exposure to saliva and urine. Another increase in CMV is noted in adolescence secondary to sexual activity.

B. CMV is the most common congenital infection in the United States. The incidence of congenital vertical transmission of CMV ranges from 0.2% to 2.5%. Most newborns appear normal and are asymptomatic; however, 5% to 15% of congenitally infected newborns will have symptoms at delivery. Prenatal CMV infections occur from contact with maternal cervicovaginal secretions during delivery or from breast milk ingestion. Preterm infants are at greatest risk of acquiring CMV from breast milk.

C. Combination antiretroviral therapy (ART) has reduced the risk of CMV in people with HIV by 75%.

D. The risk of CMV is the highest in HIV patients when their CD4 cell counts are below 50 cells/μL. CMV is rare if the CD4 count is more than 100 cells/μL.

E. The most common illness caused by CMV is retinitis.

Pathogenesis

A. Human CMV, a DNA virus, is a member of the herpesvirus group. This virus is transmitted both horizontally (by direct person-to-person contact with virus-containing secretions) and vertically (from mother to infant before, during, or after birth). Infections have no seasonal correlation.

B. The incubation period for horizontally transmitted CMV infections in households is unknown. Primary CMV infection usually manifests itself within 4 to 7 weeks and may persist as long as 16 to 20 weeks after initial infection. CMV disease is most likely 30 to 60 days after transplant.

C. CMV remains in a person for life; there is no treatment that will permanently eliminate CMV infection.

Predisposing Factors

A. Exposure to young children (especially those in day care centers)

B. Sexual contact (cervicovaginal secretions and semen)

C. Blood transfusions: Patients with impaired immune function (e.g., bone marrow and organ transplant recipients, premature babies) are at risk for CMV infection from contaminated transfused blood.

D. Hospital or occupational exposure: Universal precautions are considered adequate to prevent transmission of CMV within hospitals. Nosocomial transmission from person to person has not been documented. Isolation is not recommended.

E. Pregnancy: Pregnant health care workers are not restricted from caring for CMV-infected patients and should follow universal precautions.

F. Transplacental transmission

G. Ascending infection from the cervix

H. Tissue or organ transplantation

I. Household spread among family members; a young child is most frequently the index case.

J. Breast milk

Common Complaints

A. Mononucleosis-like syndrome

B. Fever

C. Overwhelming fatigue

D. Pharyngitis

E. Ulcerative lesions in the mouth

F. Loss of vision (retinal detachment may occur in up to 50% to 60% in the first year after diagnosis)

Other Signs and Symptoms

A. Mothers: Asymptomatic or mononucleosis-like syndrome

B. Fetuses
- **1.** Intrauterine growth retardation (IUGR)/small for gestational age
- **2.** Nonimmune hydrops fetalis
- **3.** Microcephaly noted on ultrasound
- **4.** Intracerebral calcification

C. Infants after congenital exposure
- **1.** Asymptomatic
- **2.** Skin
  - **a.** Jaundice at birth
  - **b.** Petechiae and purpura of the skin
- **3.** Hepatosplenomegaly
- **4.** Anemia
- **5.** Thrombocytopenia
- **6.** Eyes: Chorioretinitis, retinal hemorrhage, optic atrophy
- **7.** Seizure disorders
- **8.** Feeding difficulties

D. Children with congenital exposure
- **1.** Asymptomatic
- **2.** Development: Developmental delays, learning disability, and mental retardation
- **3.** Ears: Progressive hearing loss (usually unilateral). Universal hearing screening programs may identify some of the otherwise asymptomatic infants.
- **4.** Loss of vision

E. Adults
- **1.** Visual changes: Floaters or loss of visual fields on one side
- **2.** Retinitis
- **3.** Arthralgias
- **4.** Nausea, abdominal cramping, and vomiting (includes hematemesis)
- **5.** Prolonged fever
- **6.** Mild hepatitis
- **7.** Headache
- **8.** Gastritis presents with abdominal pain and colitis presents as a diarrheal illness. CMV may infect the gastrointestinal (GI) tract from the oral cavity through the colon. The typical manifestation of disease is ulcerative lesions. In the mouth, these may be indistinguishable from ulcers caused by herpes simplex virus (HSV) or aphthous ulceration.

F. Immunocompromised persons
- **1.** Bacterial: Pneumonia, retinitis, myocarditis, and aseptic meningitis
- **2.** Anemia
- **3.** Thrombocytopenia

Subjective Data

A. Review onset of presenting signs, symptoms, and their duration.

B. Review the patient's history for recent upper respiratory infection (URI) and mononucleosis-like symptoms.

C. Elicit information concerning contact with any person known to be CMV infected.

D. Review history for other family members with similar symptoms.

E. Ask the patient about any occupational exposure.

F. Review the patient's exposure to children in day-care centers.

G. Review recent blood transfusions and/or organ transplantation.

H. Determine the patient's history for risk factors or presence of HIV.

- **1.** If known HIV, does the patient know his or her last viral load CD4 count?
- **2.** Is the patient taking ART? When were the antivirals started?

I. Ask family members if the patient has been confused, lethargic, or withdrawn or has exhibited personality changes (CMV encephalitis, dementia).

Physical Examination

A. Check temperature, pulse, respirations, blood pressure, and weight (document serial weight loss).

B. Inspect

- **1.** Inspect skin for jaundice and petechiae.
- **2.** Evaluate age-appropriate developmental tasks.
- **3.** Conduct a detailed eye examination.
  - **a.** CMV infection may appear as yellow-white areas with perivascular exudates and hemorrhage, having a "cottage cheese and ketchup" appearance at either the periphery or the center of the fundus.
    - **i.** Differentiating suspected CMV retinitis and cotton wool spots is essential. Cotton wool spots appear as small, fluffy white lesions with indistinct margins and are not associated with exudates or hemorrhages.
  - **b.** Evaluate field of vision.
- **4.** Perform ear, nose, and throat examination.

C. Auscultate

- **1.** Heart
- **2.** Lungs

D. Palpate

- **1.** The abdomen, noting organomegaly
- **2.** Pregnancy: Palpate fundal height and evaluate for suspected IUGR.

E. Neurologic examination

- **1.** Assess all cranial nerves.
- **2.** Sensation (deficits may occur without loss of vibratory sense and proprioception)
- **3.** Deep tendon reflexes
- **4.** Motor skills and coordination
- **5.** Gait
- **6.** Conduct hearing test

Diagnostic Tests

A. Viral culture of specimen from urine, cervix, vagina, nasopharynx, and saliva

- **1.** Viral culture is the best means of diagnosing acute CMV infections, although it does not distinguish between primary and recurrent disease. Urine contains high titers of the virus because CMV is relatively stable in urine.

B. Complete blood count (CBC) with differential: Differential WBC count reveals increased lymphocytes, many of which are atypical.

C. Total direct and indirect serum bilirubin

D. Liver function: Alanine aminotransferase (ALT) and aspartate aminotransferase (AST)

E. Serology for CMV immunoglobulin G (IgG) and immunoglobulin M (IgM): Only the recovery of the virus from a target organ provides unequivocal evidence that the disease is caused by CMV infection. However, a fourfold or greater rise in IgG-specific antibody titer is usually considered evidence of acute infection.

F. Immunocompromised patients, especially transplant recipients, may be monitored for viral surveillance weekly using surrogate markers for viremia (polymerase chain reaction [PCR]).

G. Chest x-ray if indicated

H. CT scan if indicated to evaluate abnormalities of the brain in the presence of an abnormal neurologic examination, seizures, and microcephaly

I. Sensorineural hearing evaluation

Differential Diagnoses

A. CMV

B. Other TORCH infections

C. HIV

D. Viral: Autoimmune hepatitis or hepatitis A to E

E. Enteroviruses

F. Fever of unknown origin (FUO)

Plan

A. General interventions

- **1.** Provide support for the patient and family.
- **2.** Contact social services if long-term support will be required for these infants/families.
- **3.** Rest is vital.

B. Patient teaching

- **1.** Patients with splenomegaly should avoid activity that may increase the risk of injury to the spleen, such as contact sports and heavy lifting.
- **2.** Mothers infected with CMV should be discouraged from breastfeeding because CMV is secreted in breast milk. CMV-specific IgM antibodies are present in only 80% of patients with primary CMV infections and in 20% of patients with recurrent infections; therefore, a negative result does not exclude the diagnosis of CMV.
- **3.** Isolation is not required.
- **4.** Use universal precautions, especially good handwashing.
- **5.** Do not share eating or drinking utensils, drinks, or food with toddlers or young children.

6. Educate about the importance of ART in treating CMV.

a. Patients with CMV retinitis may require lifelong suppressive therapy to prevent blindness. Vision loss will not return to pre-CMV status.

b. Report visual deterioration immediately.

C. Pharmaceutical therapy

1. Drug of choice: Ganciclovir (Cytovene) for CMV retinitis is the treatment both for adults and for children older than 3 months; treatment is divided into an induction and a maintenance phase.

a. The safety of ganciclovir in pregnancy has not been established.

b. Patients receiving ganciclovir should have blood counts monitored closely due to dose-dependent bone marrow suppression. Monitor for leukopenia, neutropenia, anemia, or thrombocytopenia. Stop ganciclovir when neutrophil counts are less than 500/mm^3. Growth factors may be necessary.

c. The dose should be decreased in patients with impaired renal function. Monitor creatinine.

d. Ganciclovir induction: 5 mg/kg per dose intravenously (IV) administered over 1 hour every 12 hours for 14 to 21 days, depending on the clinical and virologic response. Oral ganciclovir should not be used for induction.

e. Ganciclovir maintenance.

i. A single daily dose of 5 mg/kg may be administered IV every other day or 5 days a week, skipping the weekend.

ii. Oral ganciclovir 1 g orally three times a day may be used for maintenance/prophylaxis in some patients, but poor oral availability makes it less effective than IV administration.

iii. Ganciclovir has been associated with bone marrow suppression, such as leukopenia. This may be addressed with prescribing hematopoietic growth factors.

f. Although ganciclovir has appeared to be beneficial in the treatment of some congenitally infected infants, its use is controversial and is considered mainly for high-risk patients with severe congenital CMV.

g. Newborns: 6 mg/kg per dose administered IV over the course of 1 hour. Ganciclovir has been administered in clinical trials for infants at 6 mg/kg IV for 6 weeks.

2. Alternative drug therapy: Foscarnet (Foscavir)

a. Used in ganciclovir-resistant CMV retinitis and herpes simplex disease.

b. Use in children is limited, and the safe dose has not been established.

c. The safety of foscarnet in pregnancy has not been established.

d. Foscarnet is nephrotoxic. Meticulous attention must be paid to renal function. Small changes in creatinine require new calculation for renal clearance. Obtain a 24-hour serum creatinine at baseline and discontinue if serum creatinine is less than 0.4 gL/min/kg.

e. Patients must be well hydrated.

f. Foscarnet

i. Foscarnet induction: 60 mg/kg IV every 8 hours or 90 to 120 mg/kg IV every 12 hours for 14 to 21 days for the induction of CMV retinitis.

ii. Foscarnet maintenance: 90 to 120 mg/kg IV per day as a single infusion. Infusion rate should not exceed 1 mg/kg/min.

3. Cidofovir (Vistide)

a. Cidofovir induction: 5 mg/kg IV once a week for 2 weeks

b. Cidofovir maintenance: 5 mg/kg IV every 2 weeks

c. Probenecid is given on the day of the IV infusion in order to reduce the renal uptake of cidofovir.

4. CMV immunoglobulin intravenous: Initial dose is 150 mg/kg followed by gradually reduced doses once every 2 weeks for 16 weeks. Currently available antiviral agents do not cure CMV disease in HIV-infected patients.

5. Immune globulin (Ig) or CMV hyperimmune globulin CytoGam may be utilized for passive immunoprophylaxis, especially in bone marrow and organ transplant recipients, to help develop antibodies and protect against CMV infection.

6. CMV vaccines are currently in clinical trials.

Follow-Up

A. Retinitis is the most common manifestation of CMV disease; patients with CNS, GI, or pulmonary disease should be assessed with a dilated retinal examination to detect subclinical retinal disease.

B. The patient should be seen for reports of excessive bruising or bleeding, jaundice, or abnormal CNS functioning.

C. Monitor CBC, serum creatinine, and electrolytes (especially calcium and magnesium) every week.

Consultation/Referral

A. Consultation with an infectious disease specialist is indicated for acute infection, especially for immunocompromised patients.

B. Antivirals have many adverse effects and are best managed by a physician who has experience using these drugs.

C. Consultation with a hematologist is needed in severe cases, especially with hemolytic anemia and thrombocytopenia.

D. Consultation with a neurologist is indicated for meningitis, encephalitis, polyneuritis, and Guillain–Barré syndrome.

E. Consultation with an ophthalmologist is needed on an emergent basis for a dilated retinal examination due to the risks of blindness. Serial dilated retinal examinations should be done after ART induction therapy and monthly thereafter.

F. Consultation with a perinatologist is indicated for pregnant patients. Evaluation may include ultrasonography, amniocentesis, and percutaneous umbilical blood sampling (PUBS).

G. Refer to a gastroenterologist for an endoscopic evaluation with tissue biopsies.

Individual Considerations

A. Pregnancy

1. Routine maternal screening for CMV infection is not recommended during pregnancy. Laboratory tests that are currently available generally cannot conclusively determine whether a primary CMV infection has occurred during the pregnancy.

2. Between 55% and 85% of pregnant women are immune to CMV, with a higher prevalence of immunity in lower socioeconomic populations.

3. Susceptible pregnant women have a 2% to 2.5% risk of acquiring primary CMV during pregnancy. Those with prior immunity have a 1% chance of reactivation of latent infection.

4. Amniocentesis for PCR to detect CMV DNA is the preferred diagnostic approach for detecting the infected fetus.

5. Recovery of CMV from the cervix or urine of women at or before the time of delivery does not warrant a cesarean section.

B. Perinatal transmission of CMV occurs by four routes:

1. In utero transplacental infections

2. Ascending infections from the cervix

3. Exposure to infected secretions from the lower genital tract during delivery

4. Ingestion of infected breast milk

Because CMV is spread by intimate contact with infectious secretions, handwashing after exposure to secretions is particularly important for pregnant health care workers.

C. Pediatrics

1. Routine screening for CMV is not recommended for internationally adopted children.

2. Up to half of all neonates exposed to CMV in the lower genital tract during delivery become infected. Intrapartum or postpartum CMV acquisition does not result in adverse outcomes or sequelae except in very-low-birth-weight infants. Viral excretion from intrapartum or postpartum exposure begins at 3 to 9 weeks of life; thus, the initial viral cultures are negative.

3. The child with congenital CMV infection should not be treated differently from other children and should not be excluded from school or child-care institutions as the virus is frequently found in many healthy children.

4. Sensorineural hearing loss is the most common sequelae following congenital CMV infection. Evaluate for hearing loss at each pediatric visit.

D. Adults

1. Occupational exposure: Risk often appears to be greatest for child-care personnel who care for children younger than 2 years.

2. Routine serologic screening for child-care staff is not currently recommended.

3. Pregnant personnel who may be in contact with CMV-infected patients should be counseled regarding the risk of acquiring CMV infection and about the need to practice good hygiene, particularly handwashing. There is no need for routinely transferring personnel to other work situations.

E. Geriatrics

1. CMV colitis can be life-threatening for the immunocompromised older patient with chronic renal disease.

2. Monitor for symptoms such as bloody diarrhea. Consider colonoscopy with biopsy for diagnosis.

Encephalitis

Cheryl A. Glass and Jill C. Cash

Definition

A. Encephalitis is the inflammation of cerebral tissue caused by viral agents or other toxins. The syndrome of acute encephalitis shares many clinical features with acute meningitis. Patients with either syndrome present with fever, headache, and altered states of consciousness. In most cases of encephalitis, there is some concomitant meningeal inflammation, in addition to the cephalitic component, a condition commonly referred to as meningoencephalitis.

Incidence

A. Incidence is unknown. Japanese encephalitis (JE) occurs in annual epidemics in Asia during the rainy season. The prevalence of JE (arbovirus) is related to ecologic and climatic conditions that affect the natural transmission cycles during summer months (June–September).

B. Arboviruses (Eastern or Western equine, St. Louis, and West Nile virus [WNV]) cause disease when mosquitoes are active, whereas walking in the woods or marshy areas with high tick populations might suggest other viral encephalitides such as Colorado tick fever or nonviral etiologies such as Lyme disease or Rocky Mountain spotted fever (RMSF).

C. Herpes encephalitis has the highest morbidity and mortality of the common viral encephalitides and may occur at any time. The mortality rate for untreated patients is 70%; less than 5% of survivors have normal neurologic function. Herpes simplex virus (HSV) type 1 is the most common cause of sporadic encephalitis. The most important viral etiology to rule out is HSV, because this clinical entity is usually fatal if left untreated. Survival and recovery from neurologic sequelae are related to the mental status at the time of acyclovir initiation.

D. Encephalopathy is the most common central nervous system (CNS) manifestation of HIV infection, occurring in 65% of patients with HIV/AIDS.
E. Mortality depends on the etiological agent. Morbidity related to the severity of sequelae also varies according to the causative agent.

Pathogenesis

A. JE is the most common form of epidemic viral encephalitis. For the past several years, WNV has been the most common cause of proved viral encephalitis in the United States. Encephalitis may occur as a secondary infection from mumps, varicella (chickenpox), rubella, rubeola, rabies, herpes simplex types 1 and 2, Epstein–Barr virus (EBV), HIV, and influenza. Postinfectious encephalitis, in contrast to viral encephalitis, typically occurs either as the initial infection is resolving or may appear following subclinical illness that was not appreciated by the patient.
B. The incubation period depends on the pathogen.
C. Tick-borne diseases include Russian spring–summer encephalitis and Powassan encephalitis.

Predisposing Factors

A. Military personnel and travelers
B. Age extremes are highest risk
C. Exposure to vectors
  1. Mosquitoes
  2. Ticks
  3. Bat
  4. Raccoon
  5. Feral dogs/cats
  6. Sandflies
D. HIV positive
E. Herpes
F. Rodent-borne arenavirus: Exposure to the secretions of mice, rats, and hamsters
G. Occupational exposure
  1. Laboratory workers
  2. Health care workers
  3. Veterinarians
H. Recreational activities (camping/hunting)
I. Recent vaccination

Common Complaints

A. Severe headache. A person with encephalitis has a severe headache throughout the entire head. Over the course of about 48 hours, the person may show a lack of energy and then lapse into a coma.
B. Stiff neck
C. Mental changes: Altered mental status, altered behavior, and personality changes
D. Decreased level of consciousness (LOC)
E. Fever

Other Signs and Symptoms

A. CNS symptoms
  1. Nuchal rigidity
  2. Irritability
  3. Hemiparesis: Weakness or paralysis on one side of body
  4. Flaccid paralysis: Consider WNV infection.
  5. Seizures
  6. Exaggerated deep tendon reflexes
  7. Ataxia
  8. Nystagmus
B. Photosensitivity
C. Swollen or protruding eyes
D. Malaise
E. Nausea and/or vomiting
F. Dysphagia with rabies
G. Parotitis: Consider mumps encephalitis.
H. Maculopapular rash
I. Tremors

Subjective Data

A. Review the onset, duration, and course of all symptoms.
B. Rule out recent history of chickenpox, rubeola, herpes, or other infections.
C. Ask the patient about recent travel.
D. Question the patient regarding recent mosquito or animal bites (rule out rabies).
E. Elicit a detailed sexual history.
F. Does the patient have HIV?
G. Ask about recent recreational activities, including camping, spelunking, or hunting.

Physical Examination

A. Check temperature, pulse, respirations, and blood pressure.
B. Inspect
  1. Observe general overall appearance.
  2. Conduct an eye examination.
  3. Examine the skin for rash, vesicles, or bites.
    a. Maculopapular rash is seen in approximately half of patients with WNV.
    b. Grouped vesicles in a dermatomal pattern suggest varicella zoster.
    c. Classic herpetic skin lesions suggest herpes encephalitis.
  4. Assess dehydration status.
  5. Observe for seizure activity.
  6. Observe for tremors of the eyelids, tongue, lips, and extremities, which may suggest the possibility of St. Louis encephalitis or West Nile encephalitis.
C. Auscultate
  1. Lungs and monitor breathing pattern
  2. Heart
D. Palpate
  1. The lymph nodes: Preauricular, posterior auricular, submental and sublingual, anterior cervical chains, and supraclavicular nodes
  2. The mastoid bone
E. Neurologic examination
  1. Assess LOC.
  2. Assess the patient for personality changes.
  3. Assess for meningeal signs.
    a. Signs of meningeal irritation include nuchal rigidity.

b. Positive Brudzinski's and Kernig's signs
   i. Brudzinski's sign: Place the patient supine and flex the head upward. Resulting flexion of hips, knees, and ankles with neck flexion indicates meningeal irritation (see Figure 16.1).
   ii. Kernig's sign: Place the patient supine. Keeping one leg straight, flex the other hip and knee to a bent knee to form a 90° angle. Slowly extend the lower leg. This places a stretch on the meninges, resulting in pain and spasm for the hamstring muscle. Resistance to further extension can be felt (see Figure 16.2).

4. Check deep tendon reflexes (exaggerated and/or pathologic reflexes).

Diagnostic Tests

A. CBC with differential, electrolytes, glucose, blood urea nitrogen (BUN), and creatinine
B. Polymerase chain reaction (PCR) tests for viruses
C. Serology for arboviruses
D. Lumbar puncture for the following:
   1. Protein (elevated)
   2. Glucose (usually normal)
   3. White cell count (increased)
   4. Red cell count (usually negative in a nontraumatic tap)
   5. Culture (viral and bacterial): Detection of virus-specific IgM antibody in cerebrospinal fluid (CSF) is diagnostic.
E. EEG

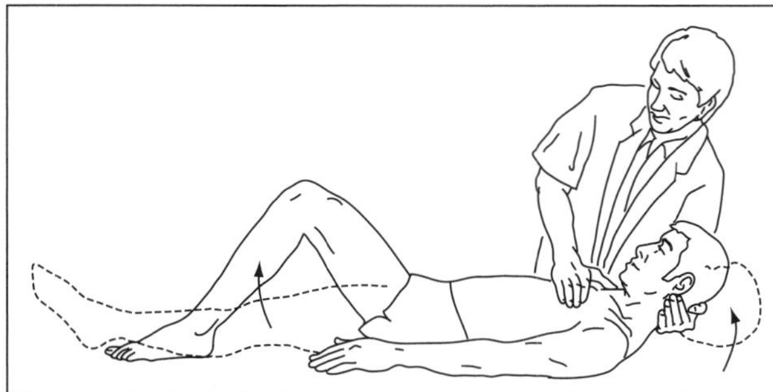

FIGURE 16.1 Brudzinski's sign.

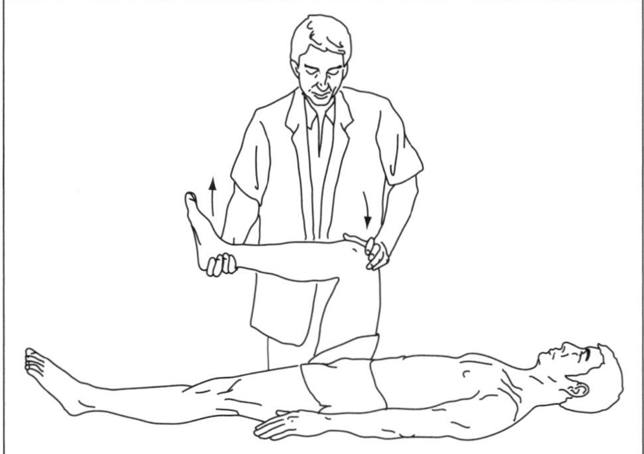

FIGURE 16.2 Kernig's sign.

F. CT scan: Useful to rule out space-occupying lesions or brain abscess
G. MRI: Sensitive for detecting demyelination
H. Brain scan: Imaging studies (CT scan, MRI, brain scan) may be normal early; later, nonspecific abnormalities are seen.
I. Stool or throat cultures may be helpful if enteroviruses are suspected.
J. Skin lesions and urine may be cultured for herpes simplex and cytomegalovirus (CMV).
K. Brain biopsy is the diagnostic standard.

Differential Diagnoses

A. Encephalitis
B. WNV
C. St. Louis virus
D. Chickenpox
E. Measles: Rubeola or rubella
F. Herpes
G. Rabies
H. Influenza
I. Mumps
J. Meningitis
K. Brain abscess
L. Tuberculosis
M. Syphilis
N. Intracranial hemorrhage
O. Trauma
P. Toxic ingestion
Q. Fungal meningitis
R. RMSF/tick-borne diseases
S. Cerebral bacterial infections
T. Toxoplasmosis
U. Lyme disease
V. Cat scratch disease
W. CMV
X. Nonparalytic poliomyelitis

Plan

A. General interventions: If encephalitis is suspected, hospitalization is recommended for further diagnostic studies and evaluation.
B. Patient teaching
   1. Prevention of vector-borne encephalitis involves mosquito and tick avoidance, use of insect repellents, and vaccination.
   2. The JE vaccine is an inactivated vaccine derived from infected mouse brain and is recommended for expatriates living in Asia and for certain travelers. It is also recommended for the following:
      a. Persons who will be residing in areas where JE virus is endemic or epidemic.
      b. Travelers planning prolonged stays (more than 30 days) in endemic areas during the transmission season, especially with activities such as bicycling, camping, or other unprotected outdoor activities in rural areas.
   3. If rabies is suspected, the domestic animal should be observed for 10 days to detect rabid behavior. If there is no indication of rabies, the animal should be immunized.

Animals that show rabid behavior or wild animals should be sacrificed and their brains submitted to the local/state health department for pathology testing.

C. Pharmaceutical therapy

1. Empiric treatment for HSV-1 should always be initiated as soon as possible if the patient has encephalitis without explanation due to the high mortality and morbidity. Acyclovir 10 mg/kg is administered IV (given over 1 hour) every 8 hours for 14 to 21 days.

2. Antibiotics for bacterial etiology (refer to diagnosis-specific chapters).

3. Anticonvulsants for seizures.

4. Other pharmaceutical therapies depend on specific causal agent.

5. Initiate short courses of corticosteroids to control brain edema.

6. If rabies is suspected: Human rabies immune globulin (Ig) should be given 20 U/kg dose.

Follow-Up

A. Follow-up varies and is specific to causal agent.

B. Long-term management of patients with neurologic sequelae includes rehabilitation services, home care, or nursing home placement for convalescent care.

Consultation/Referral

A. Refer the patient to a physician and/or hospital. Consultations include a neurologist, infectious disease specialist, and neurosurgeon for managing elevated intracranial pressure.

Individual Considerations

A. Adult travelers

1. Advise patient to take mosquito bed nets and aerosol insecticide sprays to reduce the risk of mosquito bites at night.

B. Inactivated JE vaccine series

1. Adults: Three doses of 1.0 mL each, administered subcutaneously on days 0, 7, and 30. An abbreviated schedule of 0, 7, and 14 days can be used when the longer schedule is precluded by time constraints.

2. Children 1 to 3 years: Three doses of 0.5 mL each, administered subcutaneously on days 0, 7, and 30. The abbreviated schedule days (0, 7, 14) are the same.

No data are available on vaccine safety and efficacy in infants younger than 12 months.

C. Geriatrics

1. Elderly patients may be at risk for severe disease.

2. WNV encephalitis occurs primarily in patients older than 65 years.

3. Encephalitis should be considered in all elderly patients who have progressive mental confusion.

4. Herpes simplex encephalitis in the elderly may present in an atypical fashion:

a. Progressive amnestic cognitive disorder

b. Behavioral changes

c. Progressive mental confusion

d. Focal neurologic deficits, which mimic stroke

H1N1 Influenza A (Swine Flu)

Cheryl A. Glass and Jill C. Cash

Definition

A. H1N1 influenza A, swine flu, is an influenza A virus that causes a highly contagious respiratory disease. H1N1 has been reported worldwide and was designated a phase 6 global pandemic status by the WHO in 2009.

B. Persons with flu-like symptoms should promptly contact their health care providers. If an antiviral is warranted, it should ideally be started within 48 hours from the onset of symptoms. Viral pneumonia is the primary sign of clinical deterioration.

Incidence

A. The WHO declared the 2009 H1N1 pandemic over as of August 2010. However, this strain of flu still continues to circulate with other seasonal flu strains.

B. Influenza activity remained low and began increasing in late December 2015.

Pathogenesis

A. H1N1 is a new subtype of influenza A (A/H1N1) virus that is spread by human-to-human transmission. The swine flu is also transmitted by pig-to-person; however, persons cannot be infected with the H1N1 virus from consuming pork.

B. The primary mode of transmission is through exposure to viral strain respiratory secretions from respiratory droplets (coughing or sneezing) and direct contact of contaminated surfaces. H1N1 is also noted to be spread through contaminated diarrheal stools.

C. The infectious period is considered to be 1 day before the onset of fever until 24 hours after fever ends.

Predisposing Factors

A. Age

1. Children younger than 5 years, especially those younger than 2 years

2. Adults 25 to 64 years who have medical conditions that place them at high risk for influenza-related complications

3. Adults aged 65 years or older

B. Pregnant women

C. Women up to 2 weeks postpartum

D. Crowded conditions

E. Institutions such as nursing homes

F. Occupational exposure: Teachers and health care workers

Common Complaints

A. Clinical manifestations of H1N1 influenza depend on the age and previous experience with the influenza virus. Rapid-onset respiratory illness is the most common complaint.

1. Cough

2. Sore throat

3. Dyspnea/wheezing

4. Rhinorrhea

B. Abrupt onset of fever and/or chills (temperature of 100°F [37.8°C] or greater)
C. Headache
D. Body aches
E. Altered mental status
F. Children
  1. Apnea
  2. Tachypnea
  3. Cyanosis
  4. Dehydration
  5. Extreme irritability
  6. Febrile seizure

Other Signs and Symptoms

A. Joint pain
B. Diarrhea (common with H1N1)
C. Vomiting (common with H1N1)

Subjective Data

A. Review the onset, course, and duration of symptoms, especially fever and respiratory symptoms.
B. Review symptoms of other family members or coworkers who are also ill. Is the onset of acute febrile respiratory illness within 7 days of close contact with a person with a confirmed case of H1N1?
C. If pregnant, establish gestational age.
D. Review for recent travel location and use of cruise ships/planes.
E. Evaluate living conditions for exposure risks.
F. Is the patient a smoker?
G. Review all medications, including over-the-counter (OTC) and herbal products. Has the patient taken any medications for the symptoms?
H. Does the patient have a history of asthma or chronic obstructive pulmonary disease (COPD)?
I. Is the patient immunocompromised (i.e., HIV, transplant recipient, chemotherapy)?
J. What other medical comorbidities, such as diabetes, does the patient have?

Physical Examination

A. Check temperature, pulse, respirations, and blood pressure.
B. Inspect
  1. Observe general overall appearance for pallor and for any respiratory distress.
  2. Assess hydration status inspecting skin turgor and mucous membranes.
  3. Conduct an eye, ear, nose, and throat examination.
  4. Children
    a. Observe for seizure activity.
    b. Note level of activity (playful vs. lethargic).
C. Auscultate
  1. Lung fields, observing for wheezing and crackles
  2. Heart
D. Palpate
  1. Neck
  2. Lymph nodes: Preauricular, posterior auricular, submental and sublingual, anterior cervical chain, and supraclavicular nodes
E. Neurologic examination
  1. Assess level of consciousness (LOC).
  2. Assess for nuchal rigidity.
  3. Assess for meningeal signs.
    a. Signs of meningeal irritation include nuchal rigidity.
    b. Positive Brudzinski's and Kernig's signs (refer to Figures 16.1 and 16.2).
      i. Brudzinski's sign: Place the patient supine and flex the head upward. Resulting flexion of both hips, knees, and ankles with neck flexion indicates meningeal irritation.
      ii. Kernig's sign: Place the patient supine. Keeping one leg straight, flex the other hip and knee to a bent knee to form a 90° angle. Slowly extend the lower leg. This places a stretch on the meninges, resulting in pain and spasm for the hamstring muscle. Resistance to further extension can be felt.

Diagnostic Tests

Testing is not necessary for all patients who present with influenza-type symptoms.
A. Rapid influenza antigen testing
B. Respiratory swab for H1N1 testing for detection by real-time reverse transcriptase polymerase chain reaction (PCR)
C. Viral culture
D. Complete blood count (CBC) with differential (not a required test)
E. Imaging (rule out complications)
  1. Chest x-ray
  2. CT chest imaging for complications

Differential Diagnoses

A. Influenza
  1. H1N1 A (swine flu)
  2. Influenza A
  3. Influenza B
  4. Avian flu (H5N1)
B. Pneumonia
C. Bronchitis
D. Mononucleosis
E. Respiratory syncytial virus (RSV)
F. Early HIV
G. Severe acute respiratory syndrome (SARS)
H. Meningitis

Plan

A. General interventions
  1. Management usually focuses on treatment of symptoms and is supportive.
    a. Bed rest
    b. Increased fluids
    c. Antipyretics and analgesics for fever and myalgias
    d. Encourage patients to stay home (self-isolate) if they become ill and avoid touching the eyes, nose, and mouth.
  2. Community precautions
    a. Avoid close contact with those who are sick.

b. Wash hands often or use alcohol-based hand gels.
c. Use of face masks may be advisable or required.
d. Droplet precautions should be used and maintained for 7 days after onset of illness or until symptoms have resolved.

B. Pharmaceutical therapy
1. Coverage for the H1N1 swine flu is now included in the seasonal influenza vaccination available in both an inactivated influenza vaccine (IIV), previously called trivalent inactivated vaccine (TIV), and a live attenuated influenza vaccine (LAIV). The influenza vaccine should be administered as prophylaxis before flu season (generally October–March). All patients older than 6 months should be encouraged to receive an annual flu vaccine.
a. The live, attenuated influenza available as a nasal mist is available for target age populations for use in children older than 5 years through adults up to 49 years of age. **The American Academy of Pediatrics (AAP) policy recommendations note that healthy children older than 2 years can receive either the IIV or the LAIV.**
b. A high-dose influenza vaccine is available for adults older than 65 years.
c. The most current information available on the flu vaccines is noted on the Centers for Disease Control and Prevention (CDC) website (www.cdc.gov).
2. Antiviral therapy

Antivirals started within the first 48 hours confer the greatest benefit.

a. Neuraminidase inhibitors oseltamivir (Tamiflu) and zanamivir (Relenza) are used for both treatment and chemoprophylaxis of the H1N1 influenza A virus.
b. In December 2012, the Food and Drug Administration (FDA) expanded the use of Tamiflu for use in children as young as 2 weeks of age.
c. Zanamivir (Relenza) is only approved for children older than 7 years.
d. Amantadine and rimantadine antivirals are not recommended for H1N1 because of resistance to other influenza strains.
e. The WHO recommends that patients with underlying medical conditions and pregnant women should receive treatment with oseltamivir (oral) or zanamivir (inhaled) as soon as possible after symptom onset without waiting for laboratory test results.
f. Antiviral therapy recommendations vary by type of influenza, age group, renal function, and risk factor. In order to prescribe the most current antiviral therapy, refer to the CDC website for the most up-to-date recommendations (www.cdc.gov) and to the current AAP *Red Book: Report of the Committee on Infectious Diseases.*
g. Oseltamivir should not be administered with an LAIV within 2 weeks before or 48 hours after treatment.
3. Acetaminophen or ibuprofen as needed for fever and myalgia.
4. Health care providers should refrain from recommending cough suppressants and OTC cough medicines for young children because of associated morbidity and mortality. The CDC noted in 2009 that, in response to safety concerns, manufacturers of cough and cold medications for children voluntarily changed labels stating that the medications should not be used for children younger than 4 years.

Follow-Up

A. Schedule a follow-up visit within 7 to 10 days if symptoms do not improve.
B. Monitor patient for pulmonary and neurologic complications.
C. The local and state health departments are the point of contact for information about current influenza activity.

Consultation/Referral

A. Refer the patient to a physician or neurologist for any complications.

Individual Considerations

A. Pregnancy
1. Pregnancy predisposes the patient to an increased risk for influenzal pneumonia.
2. Flu vaccine may be given to patients in high-risk populations. Because of the risk of influenzal pneumonia, many physicians recommend that pregnant women be vaccinated when an epidemic threatens.
3. Immunization of pregnant women is considered safe at any stage of pregnancy.
4. Zanamivir is the antiviral of choice for pregnancy because of limited systemic absorption.
5. Oseltamivir is used in pregnancy for women with asthma secondary to a higher risk for complications.
6. Both oseltamivir and zanamivir are pregnancy category C drugs.
7. Breastfeeding is not contraindicated during influenza.

B. Pediatrics
1. Influenza A/H1N1 vaccine should be offered/administered before flu season (as early as September) to children with asthma and chronic lung problems or those who are immunosuppressed.
2. Infants who are ill with H1N1 influenza A should continue to breastfeed.
3. Aspirin or aspirin-containing products (e.g., bismuth subsalicylate—Pepto-Bismol) should not be given to children and young adults with viral illnesses before 21 years of age due to the increased risk of Reye's syndrome.

4. Reye's syndrome has been associated primarily with influenza B, but it is also associated with influenza A infections.

5. Amantadine HCl and rimantadine HCl are not effective against H1N1 infections and are not FDA approved for use in children younger than 1 year.

C. Adults: Persons with high-exposure occupations, such as teachers, health care workers, police, and firefighters, should consider yearly immunization. Vaccine should be offered/administered to persons with chronic metabolic diseases, renal dysfunction, HIV infection, and immunosuppression.

Resource

Centers for Disease Control and Prevention: www.cdc.gov/flu/professionals

Influenza (Flu)

Cheryl A. Glass and Jill C. Cash

Definition

A. Influenza is a common, acute, viral infection that is a self-limiting, febrile illness of the respiratory tract. Illness is spread person to person primarily by respiratory secretions that can be spread from infected persons through sneezing, coughing, talking, and self-inoculation of secretions through direct contact routes. Influenza is one of the top 10 causes of death in the United States when it occurs with pneumonia.

Incidence

A. Epidemics occur yearly, primarily in the winter months, in both the northern and southern hemispheres. Travelers should be reminded that the flu season is different by hemisphere and can occur on cruise ships. Attack rates may be as high as 10% to 20% of the population. Mortality is highest in the geriatric population older than 65 years, except during pandemics when 50% of influenza deaths occur in individuals younger than 65 years. Extraordinarily high attacks have occurred in the institutionalized and semiclosed populations.

Pathogenesis

A. Influenza A and B are viruses that have the ability to undergo periodic antigenic changes of their envelope glycoproteins, the hemagglutinin and neuraminidase. Among influenza A viruses that infect humans, there are three major subtypes of hemagglutinins (H1, H2, and H3) and two subtypes of neuraminidases (N1 and N2). Influenza A outbreaks typically start abruptly, peak over 2 to 3 weeks, and last approximately 2 to 3 months. H1N1 (swine flu) is an influenza A virus.

B. The avian flu was the N5N1 and H7N7 viral infection associated with recent exposure to dead or ill poultry. Following exposure, the incubation period for human H5N1 infection is 7 days or less. Clusters of human-to-human transmission of avian flu had a typical incubation period of 3 to 5 days.

C. Influenza B outbreaks are generally less extensive and less severe. Outbreaks associated with the B virus have been reported in schools, military camps, nursing homes, and cruise ships.

D. *Haemophilus influenzae* is a gram-negative coccobacillus. *H. influenzae* is an invasive bacterial disease that can cause meningitis, otitis media, sinusitis, epiglottitis, septic arthritis, occult febrile bacteremia, cellulitis, pneumonia, and empyema; occasionally, this virulent organism causes neonatal meningitis.

E. The incubation period for *H. influenzae* is between 18 and 72 hours to 5 days after exposure. The exact period of communicability for *H. influenzae* is unknown, but it may be for as long as the organism is present in the upper respiratory tract.

Predisposing Factors

The primary mode of spread is via exposure to viral strain respiratory secretions from respiratory droplets (coughing or sneezing) and direct contact of contaminated surfaces.

A. Adults

1. Aged older than 65 years (dependent on the viral strain)

2. Pregnancy

3. High-exposure jobs: Teachers, health care workers, police, and firefighters

4. Recent illnesses or state that has lowered resistance (stress, excessive fatigue, poor nutrition)

5. Immunosuppression from drugs, illness, or chronic illness (transplant recipients, lung disease, heart disease, rheumatoid arthritis)

6. Crowded living conditions, including military camps and institutions such as nursing homes

7. Travel in endemic areas

8. Avian flu: Exposure to dead or ill poultry

B. Pediatrics

1. Chronic pulmonary disease, including bronchopulmonary dysplasia/chronic lung disease, asthma, cystic fibrosis, or any condition that compromises the respiratory function

2. Congenital heart disease or abnormalities

3. Children younger than 5 years

Common Complaints

A. Clinical manifestations of influenza depend on age and previous experience with the influenza virus. Children cannot verbalize symptoms such as myalgias and headache. Respiratory symptoms may be less prominent at the onset of illness in children and adults.

B. Rapid-onset respiratory illness is the most common complaint.

C. Abrupt onset of fever and/or chills (children tend to run higher fevers)

D. Joint pain

E. Headache

F. Conjunctivitis (avian flu)

Other Signs and Symptoms

A. Upper respiratory congestion (watery eyes, clear nasal drainage, headache, sore throat, and hoarseness)

B. Malaise or fatigue

C. Anorexia
D. Swollen lymph nodes
E. Nonproductive cough (persisting for weeks)
F. Muscle aches
G. Gastrointestinal (GI) symptoms (children tend to have more nausea, vomiting, and poor appetite)
H. Febrile seizures
I. Otitis media

Subjective Data

A. Review the onset, course, and duration of symptoms, especially myalgia and malaise.
B. Query the patient when his or her last flu vaccination was received.
C. Review symptoms of other family members or coworkers who are also ill.
D. Check immunization status. For children, note whether *H. influenzae* b (Hib) vaccination is up to date.
E. Review for recent travel location and use of cruise ships/planes.
F. Evaluate living conditions for exposure risks.
G. Is the patient a smoker?
H. Review all medications, including over-the-counter (OTC) and herbal products. Has the patient taken any medications for the symptoms?
I. Does the patient have a history of asthma or chronic obstructive pulmonary disease (COPD)?
J. Is the patient immunocompromised (i.e., HIV, transplant recipient, chemotherapy)?
K. What other medical comorbidities, such as diabetes, does the patient have?

Physical Examination

A. Check temperature, pulse, respirations, and blood pressure.
B. Inspect
- **1.** Observe overall appearance for pallor and for any respiratory distress.
- **2.** Assess hydration status.
- **3.** Conduct an eye, ear, nose, and throat examination.
- **4.** Children
  - **a.** Observe for seizure activity.
  - **b.** Note level of activity (playful vs. lethargic).

C. Auscultate
- **1.** Lung fields, observing for wheezing and crackles
- **2.** Heart

D. Palpate
- **1.** Neck
- **2.** Lymph nodes: Preauricular, posterior auricular, submental and sublingual, anterior cervical chain, and supraclavicular nodes

E. Neurologic examination
- **1.** Assess level of consciousness (LOC).
- **2.** Assess for nuchal rigidity.
- **3.** Assess for meningeal signs:
  - **a.** Signs of meningeal irritation include nuchal rigidity.
  - **b.** Positive Brudzinski's and Kernig's signs (refer to Figures 16.1 and 16.2).
    - **i.** Brudzinski's sign: Place the patient supine and flex the head upward. Resulting flexion of both hips, knees, and ankles with neck flexion indicates meningeal irritation.
    - **ii.** Kernig's sign: Place the patient supine. Keeping one leg straight, flex the other hip and knee to a bent knee to form a 90° angle. Slowly extend the lower leg. This places a stretch on the meninges, resulting in pain and spasm for the hamstring muscle. Resistance to further extension can be felt.

Diagnostic Tests

Usually none is required. However, if the patient appears ill, consider the following:
A. Complete blood count (CBC; white blood cells [WBC])
B. Viral RNA cultures: Obtain during the first 72 hours of illness because the quality of virus shed subsequently decreases rapidly. There is some evidence that a throat sampling yields an improved specimen. Nasopharyngeal secretions obtained by swab or aspirate should be placed in an appropriate transport medium for culture.
C. Rapid antigen test (usually less sensitive in the detection of influenza A than the polymerase chain reaction [PCR]; a negative rapid diagnostic test should be confirmed with a viral culture or other means)
D. Monospot test (monospot test is negative with the flu and positive with mononucleosis.)
E. Chest radiograph (only if pneumonia is suspected)
F. Sputum culture (complications only)
G. Lumbar puncture (complications only)
H. Rapid plasma reagin (RPR) test (for high-risk HIV factors): Negative RPR to rule out syphilis
I. PCR assay (can differentiate between influenza subtypes; it offers high sensitivity and specificity but is not readily available for clinical use)

Differential Diagnoses

A. Influenza
- **1.** Influenza A
- **2.** Influenza B
- **3.** Avian flu (H5N1)
- **4.** H1N1 (swine flu)

B. Pneumonia
C. Bronchitis
D. Mononucleosis
E. Respiratory syncytial virus (RSV)
F. Early HIV
G. Severe acute respiratory syndrome (SARS)
H. Meningitis

Plan

A. General interventions
- **1.** Management is usually treatment of symptoms.
- **2.** Encourage flu vaccine for patients in susceptible populations before flu season.
- **3.** *H. influenzae*, including both type b and nontype b infection and cases in fully or partially immunized children, should be reported to the Centers for Disease

Control and Prevention (CDC) through the local and state public health departments. See Chapter 1, "Health Maintenance Guidelines," for Hib immunization information.

4. Influenza-associated pediatric deaths should be reported to the CDC through the state health department.

5. Patients should expect to have a persistent cough and malaise after initial acute phase. Health care providers should refrain from recommending cough suppressants and OTC cough medicines for young children because of associated morbidity and mortality. The CDC noted in 2009 that, in response to safety concerns, manufacturers of cough and cold medications for children voluntarily changed labels stating the medications should not be used for children younger than 4 years.

▶ **B.** Patient teaching: *See Section III: Patient Teaching Guide for this chapter, "Influenza (Flu)."*

C. Pharmaceutical therapy

> *Influenza can alter the metabolism of certain medications, especially theophylline, possibly resulting in the development of toxicity from high serum concentrations.*

1. Acetaminophen (Tylenol) as needed for fever.

2. Nonsteroidal anti-inflammatory drugs (NSAIDs) are given as needed for body aches.

3. Antivirals started within the first 48 hours confer the greatest benefit. Antiviral therapy recommendations vary by type of influenza, age group, renal function, and risk factor. In order to prescribe the most current antiviral therapy, refer to the CDC website for the most up-to-date recommendations (www.cdc.gov/flu/professionals/antivirals/antiviral-summary-clinicians.htm) and to the current American Academy of Pediatrics (AAP) *Red Book: Report of the Committee on Infectious Diseases.*

4. Zanamivir (Relenza) is not recommended for persons with underlying airway disease, including asthma or COPD. Zanamivir is for uncomplicated acute illness due to influenza A or B in adults and children 7 years and older who have been symptomatic for no more than 2 days. Zanamivir is only approved for children older than 7 years.

5. Oseltamivir (Tamiflu) is for adults and adolescents 13 years of age or older who have been symptomatic for no more than 2 days. Special dosing is required for children who are younger than 13 years and/or weigh less than 80 oz. In December 2012, the Food and Drug Administration (FDA) expanded the use of oseltamivir for children as young as 2 weeks of age.

6. Vaccination.

a. The CDC's Advisory Committee on Immunization Practice (ACIP) and the AAP recommend annual influenza vaccination for all children aged 6 months to 18 years.

b. Flu vaccine should not be administered to persons allergic to eggs.

c. The vaccine should be administered in the autumn before the flu season, at least 6 weeks before the onset of the season.

d. Immunization is the major means of influenza prevention. Each year the vaccine is produced with influenza strains. The vaccine may be trivalent or quadrivalent formulations.

e. Two types of administration of the vaccine are available.

i. Inactivated influenza vaccine (IIV), previously called trivalent inactivated vaccine (TIV), is administered intramuscularly.

ii. Live attenuated influenza vaccine (LAIV) is administered intranasally. The CDC Advisory Committee has voted that the "nasal spray" flu vaccine should *not* be used during the 2016 to 2017 flu season. This decision was made due to studies showing the LAIV was less effective than IIV.

iii. Check on the CDC website for the current *Morbidity and Mortality Weekly Report* (*MMWR*) for the current recommendations on vaccines for prevention and control of influenza. The FDA has approved Flublok, which is made by Protein Sciences Corporation for the 2016 to 2017 season.

iv. A high-dose influenza vaccine is also available for adults older than 65 years.

f. The recommended site of vaccination in adults and older children is the deltoid muscle. The anterolateral aspect of the thigh is the preferred site for flu vaccine for small children.

g. Oseltamivir (Tamiflu) should not be administered with an LAIV within 2 weeks before or 48 hours after treatment.

Follow-Up

A. Schedule a follow-up visit within 7 to 10 days if symptoms do not improve.

B. Monitor the patient for pulmonary and neurologic complications.

C. Local and state health departments are the points of contact for information about current influenza.

Consultation/Referral

A. Refer the patient to a physician or neurologist for any complications.

Individual Considerations

A. Pregnancy

1. Pregnancy predisposes the patient to an increased risk for influenzal pneumonia.

2. The flu vaccine may be given to patients in a high-risk population. Because of the risk of influenzal pneumonia, many physicians recommend that pregnant women be vaccinated when an epidemic threatens.

3. Immunization of pregnant women is considered safe at any stage of pregnancy. Inactivated vaccine is safe for breastfeeding mothers and their children.
4. Zanamivir is the antiviral of choice for pregnancy because of limited systemic absorption.
5. Oseltamivir is used in pregnancy for women with asthma secondary to a higher risk for complications.

B. Pediatrics
1. Influenza vaccine should be offered/administered before flu season (as early as September) to children with asthma or chronic lung problems, or those who are immunosuppressed.
2. The most common pediatric complication of influenza is otitis media. However, in young infants, influenza can produce a sepsis-like picture and occasionally can cause croup or pneumonia.
3. Aspirin or aspirin-containing products (e.g., bismuth subsalicylate—Pepto-Bismol) should not be given to children and young adults with viral illnesses before 21 years of age due to the increased risk of Reye's syndrome.
4. Reye's syndrome has been associated primarily with influenza B, but it is also associated with influenza A infections.
5. Amantadine HCl and rimantadine HCl are not effective against influenza B infections and are not FDA approved for use in children younger than 1 year.
6. An increased incidence of convulsions has been reported in children with epilepsy who receive amantadine.

C. Adults: Persons with high-exposure occupations, such as teachers, health care workers, police, and firefighters, should consider yearly immunization. Vaccine should be offered/administered to persons with chronic metabolic diseases, renal dysfunction, HIV infection, and immunosuppression.

D. Geriatrics
1. Influenza vaccine is recommended yearly for patients over the age of 60 years. The vaccine should be offered to nursing home residents, especially those with a history of cardiopulmonary disease. Factors that contribute to more severe infections include decreased lung compliance and decreased respiratory muscle strength.
2. Pneumococcal pneumonia and influenza are significant causes of mortality and morbidity in the elderly.

Resource

Centers for Disease Control and Prevention: www.cdc.gov/flu/professionals

Kawasaki Disease

Cheryl A. Glass and Jill C. Cash

Definition

A. Kawasaki disease (KD) is an acute febrile illness associated with generalized vasculitis. It was formerly known as mucocutaneous lymph node syndrome. KD is the leading cause of acquired heart disease in U.S. children. Death results from myocardial infarction with coronary occlusion due to thrombosis or progressive stenosis. Approximately 75% of fatalities occur within 6 weeks of the onset of symptoms, but myocardial infarction and sudden death can occur months to years after the acute episode.

B. Although a febrile seizure may occur, there is no evidence that links KD with autism or a long-term seizure disorder.

C. Long-term prognosis is unknown. Second episodes rarely occur in previously affected children. Cardiac problems are the primary cause of morbidity and mortality from pericardial effusion, myocarditis, aneurysms, ectasia (coronary artery larger than normal for the child's age), and myocardial infarction. Current American Heart Association (AHA) guidelines stratify KD by its risk of myocardial infarction:
1. Risk Level I—Normal coronary arteries on all imaging studies
2. Risk Level II—Transient coronary artery ectasia or dilation that resolves by 8 weeks after disease onset
3. Risk Level III—Small to medium coronary artery aneurysms
4. Risk Level IV—Large (greater than 6 mm) aneurysms and coronary arteries with multiple complex aneurysms without obstruction
5. Risk Level V—Coronary artery aneurysms with obstruction documented on angiography

D. For children presenting with a rash and a persistent fever (greater than 5 days) the diagnosis of KD should be held at the forefront for workup for confirmation of KD secondary to the long-term cardiovascular sequelae. Diagnostic criteria: Diagnosis of typical syndrome requires fever of at least 5 days duration, plus four of the following:
1. Mucous membrane changes
2. Extremity changes
3. Cervical lymphadenopathy of at least 1 cm in size is the least consistent feature of KD. When present, it tends to involve the anterior cervical nodes overlying the sternocleidomastoid muscle.
4. Rash
5. Bilateral nonexudative conjunctivitis: Present in more than 90% of patients

Incidence

A. Peak age of occurrence in the United States is between 18 and 24 months. Approximately 80% of patients are younger than 5 years. Children older than 8 years rarely have the disease. KD has been noted worldwide and affects all races. Approximately 2% of patients experience KD a second time months to years later.

B. Approximately 1 in 5 children will develop coronary artery aneurysms.

C. The risk of myocardial infarction is greatest the first 2 years after onset of KD.

Pathogenesis

A. Etiology is unknown; it may be caused by viruses or bacteria such as Group A *Streptococci*. A microbial agent is favored because of the disease's acute, self-limited course and community-wide outbreaks.
B. The incubation period is unknown.

Predisposing Factors

A. Age: Children younger than age 5
B. Gender: Incidence higher in boys than in girls (2:1)
C. Asian and Pacific Island ancestry
D. Siblings of children with KD (possibly genetic)
E. Epidemics generally occur during the winter and spring seasons

Common Complaints

A. Long-term fever (1–2 weeks) that does not respond to antibiotics. The fever ranges from 101°F to above 104°F. Fever may rise and fall for up to 3 weeks.
B. Bilateral bulbar conjunctival injection without exudate.
C. Red, tender hands and soles of feet on Days 3 to 5 following fever.

Classic finding is swollen, indurated, erythematous, and tender palms. Desquamation of the fingers and toes occurs approximately 1 to 2 weeks after onset of the fever, and a deep groove may cross the nails (Beau's lines).

D. Cracked, red, dry lips; tongue may appear coated, slightly swollen, and look like a strawberry; mouth ulcers
E. Irritability
F. Decreased food/fluid intake
G. One or more gastrointestinal (GI) symptoms (vomiting, diarrhea, or abdominal pain)
H. One or more respiratory symptoms (rhinorrhea or cough)

Other Signs and Symptoms

A. Tachycardia (disproportionate to fever), gallop rhythms, and EKG changes, including sinus tachycardia, QRS/QT prolongation, diffuse T-wave inversions, ventricular arrhythmias, and atrioventricular (AV) conduction defects, are suggestive of myocarditis.
B. Pericarditis (often subclinical): Coronary aneurysms have been detected as early as 3 days after onset of symptoms, but in most cases they appear 1 to 2 weeks later. Carditis can occur at any time during the first 3 weeks of illness and generally resolves by 6 to 8 weeks.
C. Polymorphous rash that may be maculopapular, scarlatiniform, morbilliform, erythema marginatum, or rarely vesiculopustular; frequently confluent in the perineum, where it undergoes desquamation. **Rash involves the entire body, especially in the perineal region.**
D. Swollen cervical lymph node(s). Patient may have a singular enlarged lymph node, usually a cervical node, up to 1.5 cm.
E. Joint pain
F. Weakness
G. Urethritis with sterile pyuria (70% of cases)
H. Mild anterior uveitis (25%–50% of cases)
I. Arthritis or arthralgia
J. Photophobia

Subjective Data

A. Review onset, course, and duration of symptoms, especially fever.
B. Elicit the initial site of the rash and the progression to other body areas.
C. Determine if the patient has had any new medication and contact exposures.
D. Rule out other family members with similar symptoms.
E. Review the patient's history for recent strep infection.
F. Take a thorough history of symptoms and medication or treatment type and duration.

Physical Examination

A. Check temperature, pulse, respirations, and blood pressure.
B. Inspect
  1. Inspect skin, especially hands, feet, and nails.
    a. Rash—polymorphous that may be maculopapular, scarlatiniform, morbilliform, erythema marginatum, or rarely vesiculopustular; frequently confluent in the perineum. (Bullae and pustules are not diagnostic of KD.)
    b. The rash involves the entire body; only the face is spared.
    c. Fine desquamation in the groin area can occur in the acute phase.
    d. Check the nail beds for detachment (periungal lifting) and transverse grooves across the finger and toenail beds (Beau's lines).
    e. Observe for facial swelling.
  2. Conduct a thorough eye examination.
    a. Bilateral bulbar conjunctival injection without exudate
  3. Conduct a thorough ear and nose examination.
  4. Perform an oral examination.
    a. Red fissured lips with edema.
    b. Tongue may appear coated and slightly swollen (generally in the first 4–5 days)—strawberry tongue after the membrane is shed.
    c. Posterior pharynx and palate—erythematous
  5. Check hydration status.
C. Auscultate
  1. Heart: A persistent resting tachycardia and the presence of an S3 gallop are often noted.
  2. Lungs
D. Palpate
  1. Palpate the lymph nodes, especially the cervical area.
    a. Primarily noted in the anterior cervical nodes overlying the sternocleidomastoid muscles
    b. Size: At least 1.5 cm

c. Lymphadenopathy is the least common clinical symptom but may be present and most prominent in an older child.
2. Check the joints for swelling and tenderness.
3. Males: Check for testicular swelling.
4. Evaluate for splenomegaly.

Diagnostic Tests

No laboratory study proves diagnosis; diagnosis rests on clinical features and exclusion of the other illnesses in the differential diagnosis.

A. Complete blood count (CBC) with differential: Neutropenia
B. Erythrocyte sedimentation rate (ESR): Elevated
C. C-reactive protein (CRP): Elevated
D. Uric acid
E. Platelet count: Elevated platelet count (1 week after onset)
F. Serum transaminase: Elevated
G. Serum albumin
H. Specialty tests: Quantitative serum immunoglobulins, antinuclear antibody (ANA), rheumatoid factor (RF), Venereal Disease Research Laboratory (VDRL) test, immune complexes, and complement levels
I. Urinalysis: Proteinuria and sterile pyuria
J. Echocardiogram
K. EKG
L. Angiography may be needed
M. Chest radiograph

Differential Diagnoses

A. KD
B. Streptococcal scarlet fever
C. Rubeola
D. Cat scratch fever
E. Drug reaction
F. Rocky Mountain spotted fever (RMSF)
G. Infectious mononucleosis
H. Toxic shock syndrome
I. Other febrile viral exanthemas
J. Syphilis
K. Lyme disease
L. Juvenile rheumatoid arthritis
M. Stevens–Johnson syndrome
N. Staphylococcal scalded skin syndrome
O. Adenovirus

Plan

A. General interventions

1. The most severe sequela is the development of a coronary artery aneurysm; therefore, prevention and early detection are important.

2. Initial therapy should be started within 10 days of illness, which reduces the risk of coronary artery aneurysm fivefold. Management is initially aimed at reducing inflammation.

3. Use of intravenous immunoglobulin (IVIG) therapy has drastically reduced the incidence and morbidity and mortality of cardiovascular aneurysm.

B. Patient teaching

1. Teach parents which signs and symptoms indicate when to contact the office: Arthralgias, chest pain, and palpitations.

2. Disease is not communicable by means of person-to-person contact; therefore, patients do not need to be isolated from other family members.

C. Pharmaceutical therapy

1. The American Heart Association (AHA) and the American Academy of Pediatrics (AAP) recommend the following: IVIG (2 mg/kg) administered as a single infusion over 8 to 12 hours within the first 7 to 10 days of the illness shortens the duration of fever and decreases the frequency of coronary artery aneurysms and other abnormalities. **IVIG is considered the gold standard for treatment of KD.**

2. Up to 20% of patients who receive the IVIG single infusion and aspirin may have a recurrent fever and require retreatment with IVIG 2 g/kg within 24 to 48 hours of persistent fever.

3. The AHA and the AAP recommend initial use of aspirin (acetylsalicylic acid [ASA]) 80 to 100 mg/kg/d given orally four times a day until afebrile. The maximum ASA dose should not exceed 4 g/d. Then ASA 3 to 5 mg/kg should be given orally per day for 6 to 8 weeks for its antiplatelet action.

4. Aspirin is continued until laboratory markers for acute inflammation (e.g., platelet count and ESR) return to normal, unless cardiac abnormalities are detected by echo.

5. Aspirin should be rapidly discontinued upon exposure to or sign of varicella or influenza due to the increased risk of Reye's syndrome.

6. Analgesic and antipyretic medications, such as acetaminophen (Tylenol) or ibuprofen, as needed for pain and inflammation.

7. The role of glucocorticoids remains unclear for treatment of KD. A single pulsed dose of IV methylprednisolone to the single dose of IVIG (2 mg/kg) does not significantly reduce the incidence of cardiac abnormalities.

8. Scheduled routine immunizations of inactivated childhood vaccines may be given at recommended intervals except for live virus vaccines such as varicella-containing vaccines and measles for children who have received IVIG. Varicella and measles vaccination may be given for an outbreak if the child's exposure is high and as long as the vaccination is repeated in at least 11 months after administration of IVIG.

9. Ibuprofen should be avoided in children taking aspirin because it may antagonize the antiplatelet effect of the aspirin.

Follow-Up

A. The prognosis of patients following KD depends on the severity of cardiac involvement. Refer the patient to a pediatric cardiologist or physician for follow-up.

Consultation/Referral

A. Consult with a physician if fever persists longer than 5 days and KD is suspected.
B. Refer all affected children to a pediatric cardiologist for coronary artery evaluation.
C. Long-term management of KD is based on the extent of coronary artery abnormalities—risk level.

Individual Considerations

A. Pediatrics
  1. Most children are hospitalized for diagnostic evaluation and supportive care. Older children with mild disease may be managed on an outpatient basis.
  2. Yearly influenza vaccination is indicated in patients 6 months to 18 years of age who require long-term aspirin therapy, because there is an increased risk for children taking aspirin of development of Reye's syndrome.
  3. Children should have limited physical activity during convalescence. Restrictions should be prescribed by the cardiologist.

Resources

AAP: www.healthychildren.org/English/health-issues/conditions/infections/Pages/Kawasaki-Disease.aspx
AHA Scientific Statement: Diagnosis, treatment, and long-term management of KD. Available at: circ.ahajournals.org/content/110/17/2747.full.pdf+html
KD Foundation: www.kdfoundation.org

Lyme Disease

Cheryl A. Glass and Jill C. Cash

Definition

A. Lyme disease is a multisystem infection that may be acute or chronic. Lyme disease is the leading vector-borne disease in the United States.
B. Morbidity from Lyme disease usually involves neurologic/cognitive dysfunction and rheumatic conditions, causing arthralgias. Approximately 15% to 55% of untreated or inadequately treated patients develop some symptoms of post-Lyme disease symptoms. Posttreatment Lyme disease syndrome (PTLDS) includes cognitive disturbances, fatigue, joint/muscle pain, headaches, hearing loss, vertigo, mood disturbances, paresthesias, and difficulty sleeping.
C. Proposed criteria for PTLDS include the presence of fatigue, musculoskeletal pain, and/or cognitive difficulties within 6 months of the diagnosis and persistence of symptoms for at least 6 months after completion of accepted antibiotic therapy.

Incidence

A. There is an increased incidence of Lyme disease in southern New England and in the eastern mid-Atlantic states as well as a lower incidence in the upper Midwest. Lyme disease is less common on the West Coast, especially northern California. There is a seasonal increase between the months of April and October; more than 50% of cases occur in June and July. In the United States, the incidence is highest among children aged 5 to 9 years and in adults aged 45 to 54 years.

Pathogenesis

A. *Borrelia burgdorferi*, a spirochete bacterium, is the infectious agent and is carried by the *Ixodes dammini* deer tick on the East Coast and midwestern areas of the United States. Vector transmission is usually from the deer tick to humans. Rodents and pets can also harbor deer ticks.
B. The spirochete enters the bloodstream at the time of tick feeding. The incubation period is 3 to 32 days, or about 1 to 3 weeks after bite. Late manifestations occur several months to more than 1 year later.

Predisposing Factors

A. People of all ages are affected.
B. Recreational exposure
  1. Hiking
  2. Golfing
  3. Hunting
  4. Soccer
C. Gardening
D. Exposure to rodents such as field mice and domestic pets, which may also carry the ticks

Common Complaints

A. Flu-like symptoms
B. Fatigue
C. Headache
D. Joint pain

Other Signs and Symptoms

A. Stage 1: Acute (early localized)
  1. Rash: Erythema migrans

About 80% of infected persons develop a characteristic expanding erythematous rash, erythema migrans. It usually begins as a red macule at the site of the tick bite and spreads out to form a large annular lesion with red secondary outer rings, an intense red outer border (measuring at least 5 cm), and some clearing at the site of the bite. Appearance is a "bull's-eye" shape. The lesion is generally painless and not pruritic.

  2. Body aches
  3. Fever or chills
  4. Swollen lymph nodes
B. Stage 2: Disseminated infection (early disseminated)
  1. Malaise, debilitating fatigue
  2. Headache
  3. Photophobia
  4. Mild neck stiffness
  5. Joint or muscle pain
  6. Migratory arthralgia
  7. Rash: Diffuse erythema
  8. Itching
  9. Transient heart block
    a. In 5% to 10% of cases, patients have cardiac involvement: A transient heart block ranging from asymptomatic, first-degree atrioventricular

(AV) block to complete heart block with fainting. Cardiac phase lasts 3 to 6 weeks.

10. Bell's palsy
    a. A unilateral or bilateral Bell's palsy is the most common cranial nerve deficit.
11. Mild encephalopathy

C. Stage 3: Chronic (late disease)
1. Prolonged arthritis
    a. Approximately 60% of complaints evolve into frank arthritis. Onset of arthritis is variable but averages 6 months from the time of initial infection. The knee is the most common site and the pattern continues to be oligoarticular.
2. Chronic neurologic deficits
3. Distal paresthesia
4. Radicular pain
5. Memory loss

Subjective Data

A. Review the onset, course, and duration of symptoms.
B. Ask the patient about any recent outdoor activities, such as camping, hiking, gardening, or other activities. Less than half of the people infected remember a tick bite. A history of a tick bite is not necessary for diagnosis.
C. Have other family members had similar symptoms?
D. Review thorough history of medications.
E. Review any history of rash and course of spread.
F. Rule out late symptoms associated with Lyme disease such as arthritis, memory loss, and distal paresthesia.
G. Has the patient been previously treated for Lyme disease or Rocky Mountain spotted fever (RMSF)?

Physical Examination

A. Check temperature, pulse, respirations, and blood pressure.
B. Inspect
1. Observe general overall appearance.
2. Observe rash pattern and type.
3. Inspect the skin; observe for target-like pattern.

C. Palpate
1. Palpate the lymph nodes and mastoid bones.
2. Examine the joints for tenderness, swelling, and range of motion.

D. Auscultate
1. Heart
2. Lungs

E. Neurologic examination: Evaluate for signs of meningeal irritation by means of Brudzinski's sign and Kernig's signs (refer to Figures 16.1 and 16.2).
1. Brudzinski's sign: Place the patient supine and flex the head upward. Resulting flexion of both hips, knees, and ankles with neck flexion indicates meningeal irritation.
2. Kernig's sign: Place the patient supine. Keeping one leg straight, flex the other hip and knee to a bent knee to form a 90° angle. Slowly extend the lower leg. This places a stretch on the meninges, resulting in pain and spasm for the hamstring muscle. Resistance to further extension can be felt.

Diagnostic Tests

A. Complete blood count (CBC) with differential
B. Sedimentation rate
C. Serum antibody (enzyme-linked immunosorbent assay [ELISA]) testing for *B. burgdorferi* (not present for several weeks)
D. Western blot if ELISA is positive
E. Lyme titer or culture for spirochete (after 20 days of signs and symptoms)
F. Arthrocentesis for joint effusion
G. Polymerase chain reaction (PCR) testing
H. Alanine aminotransferase (ALT) and aspartate aminotransferase (AST) (may be mildly elevated)
I. Creatine phosphokinase
J. Lumbar puncture indicated for the presence of manifestations of meningitis

Differential Diagnoses

A. Lyme disease
B. Insect or spider bite
C. RMSF
D. Cellulitis
E. Arthritis
F. Bacterial meningitis
G. Chronic fatigue syndrome (CFS)
H. Viral syndrome
I. Nummular eczema
J. Tinea corporis (ringworm)

Plan

A. General interventions
1. **Prophylactic therapy after a tick bite is generally not advised.** It takes 24 hours from the time of tick contact with the skin to transmit the spirochete.
2. Start prophylactic treatment with doxycycline for tick bites that are "swollen."
3. Wait for the development of symptoms (e.g., erythema migrans) and treat promptly if the patient becomes symptomatic.
4. There is no evidence of the existence of "chronic Lyme disease." Some symptoms (fatigue, arthralgia, headaches) may last for several months; however, long-term antibiotic treatment has not proven to be effective and can contribute to a host of other adverse problems.

B. Patient teaching
1. Patient teaching: *See Section III: Patient Teaching Guide for this chapter, "Lyme Disease and Removal of a Tick."* ◀
2. Not all neurologic signs and symptoms may completely resolve (such as headache, photophobia, Bell's palsy, and third-stage symptoms).
3. Patients with active Lyme disease should not donate blood because spirochetemia occurs in early Lyme disease. Patients who have been treated for Lyme disease in the past can be considered for blood donation.
4. Currently there is no vaccine for Lyme disease. The vaccine was withdrawn in early 2002. Previously vaccinated patients are not protected against Lyme disease.

5. Nonspecific symptoms may persist for months after treatment of Lyme disease. There is no evidence that the complaints represent ongoing active infection or need repeated antibiotics.
   a. Headache
   b. Fatigue
   c. Arthralgias

C. Pharmaceutical therapy
1. Early localized Lyme disease
   a. Doxycycline: 14- to 21-day antibiotic course (warn patient regarding photosensitivity)
      i. Adults: 100 mg, orally, twice daily
      ii. Children older than 8 years: 2 mg/kg orally twice daily (maximum 100 mg dose)
   b. Amoxicillin: 14- to 21-day antibiotic course
      i. Adults: 500 mg orally three times a day
      ii. Children: 50 mg/kg (maximum of 1.5 g/d) orally divided into three doses
   c. Cefuroxime (Ceftin): 14- to 21-day antibiotic course
      i. Adults: 500 mg twice a day
      ii. Children: 30 mg/kg (maximum 1,000 mg/d), divided into two doses
2. Lyme carditis
   a. Ceftriaxone (Rocephin): 75 to 100 mg/kg (maximum of 2 g/d), intramuscular (IM) or intravenous (IV) infusion for 14 to 28 days
   b. Penicillin: 300,000 U/kg (maximum of 20 million U/d) given by IV infusion in divided doses every 4 hours for 14 to 28 days
3. Neurologic manifestations
   a. Facial nerve paralysis: Use oral regimen for early disease for 21 to 28 days.
   b. Lyme meningitis
      i. Ceftriaxone (Rocephin): 14- to 28-day antibiotic course
         1) Adults: 2 g IM or IV infusion once a day
         2) Children: 50 to 75 mg/kg (maximum of 2 g/d), IM or IV infusion
      ii. Penicillin: 14- to 28-day antibiotic course
         1) Adults: 18 to 24 million U/d IV divided into 6 daily doses
         2) Children: 200,000 to 400,000 U/kg (maximum 18–24 million U/d) IV divided into six daily doses
   c. Possible alternatives for Lyme meningitis: Doxycycline 100 mg by mouth or IV infusion for 14 to 21 days
4. Lyme arthritis
   a. Same oral regimen as early localized Lyme disease for a total of 28 days
   b. Ceftriaxone (Rocephin): 75 to 100 mg/kg (maximum of 2 g/d), IM or IV infusion for 14 to 28 days
   c. Penicillin: 300,000 U/kg (maximum of 20 million U/d) given by IV infusion in divided doses every 4 hours for 14 to 28 days.
5. Pregnant women
   a. For localized early Lyme disease, amoxicillin 500 mg three times daily for 21 days
   b. For disseminated early Lyme disease or any manifestation of late disease, penicillin G 20 million U/d for 14 to 21 days
   c. For asymptomatic seropositivity, no treatment is necessary.
6. The Jarisch–Herxheimer reaction, with increased fever, chills, and malaise, can occur transiently when antibiotic therapy is initiated. Nonsteroidal anti-inflammatory drugs (NSAIDs) may be beneficial, and the antimicrobial agent should be continued.

Follow-Up

A. Follow-up depends on the stage of disease.
B. Repeat Lyme titer in 1 to 2 months to determine the need for continuation of antibiotic therapy.

Consultation/Referral

A. Referral to a physician is indicated when the patient with strong clinical evidence of Lyme disease fails to respond to prescribed antibiotics.
B. Consultation with a physician is particularly important for those patients with refractory neurologic deficits or debilitating arthritis.
C. Consultation with a rheumatologist is needed for patients with persistent arthritis or fibromyalgia occurring after Lyme disease.

Individual Considerations

A. Pregnancy
1. Maternal–fetal transmission of infection with subsequent injury to the fetus has been reported. Antibiotic treatment should be instituted promptly in symptomatic patients.
2. Tetracyclines are contraindicated in pregnancy. Otherwise, therapy is the same as for nonpregnant persons.
3. There is no causal relationship between maternal Lyme disease and congenital malformations.
4. There is no evidence that Lyme disease can be transmitted in breast milk.

B. Pediatrics
1. Erythema migrans is the most common manifestation of Lyme disease in children.
2. Carditis occurs rarely in children.
3. The Academy of Pediatrics (AAP) recommends that children not be exposed to products containing more than 30% N, N-diethyl-m-toluamide (DEET) due to potential neurotoxicity.
4. The AAP also recommends that insect repellents not be used around children younger than 2 months.
5. DEET repellent should not be applied to children's hands.

Resources

American Lyme Disease Foundation: www.aldf.comlymedisease.org

American Lyme Disease Foundation. Lyme Disease Tick Map [Mobile application software]. Retrieved from www.aldf.com/lyme-disease

Meningitis

Cheryl A. Glass and Jill C. Cash

Definition

A. Meningitis is an acute inflammation of the meninges, or membranes lining the brain and spinal cord. A virus or noninfectious insult, such as blood in the subarachnoid space, causes aseptic meningitis. Three baseline clinical features have been independently associated with an adverse outcome—hypotension, altered mental status, and seizures.

B. Vaccines are available for three types of bacteria that cause meningitis:

  1. *Neisseria meningitidis*: Polysaccharide or conjugate vaccines are available.

  2. *Streptococcus pneumonia*: Pneumococcus vaccine

  3. *Haemophilus influenzae* type b (Hib) vaccine

C. Bacterial meningitis is a severe infection with associated complications including brain damage, hearing loss, neurologic/learning disabilities, and digit or limb amputations. Mortality rate varies in part with the organism and if it is a nosocomial or a community-acquired infection.

Incidence

The attack rate of bacterial meningitis in the United States is 0.6 to 4 cases per 1,000,000 persons. It occurs in approximately 1.2 million cases annually worldwide. It is also considered to be one of the top 10 infectious causes of death. It is estimated that meningococcal meningitis, which is the bacterial form, can cause severe brain damage and is fatal in 50% of cases that are not treated. The most common organisms causing bacterial meningitis are presented here.

A. Neonates

  1. Group B *Streptococcus*

  2. *Escherichia coli*

  3. *Listeria monocytogenes*

B. Ages 2 to 18 years

  1. *N. meningitidis* with portal entry in the nasopharynx

  2. *S. pneumoniae*

  3. Hib

  4. Remaining cases are caused by Group B *Streptococcus* and *L. monocytogenes.*

C. Adults up to age 60 years

  1. *S. pneumoniae*

  2. *N. meningitidis*

  3. *H. influenzae*

  4. *L. monocytogenes*

  5. Group B *Streptococcus*

D. Adults 60 years and older

  1. *S. pneumoniae*

  2. *L. monocytogenes*

  3. *N. meningitidis*

Acute meningitis due to infectious causes usually does not recur. However, a small number of patients with acute meningitis may develop recurrent attacks between intervals of good health. Chronic meningitis is arbitrarily defined as meningitis lasting 4 weeks or more.

Pathogenesis

A. An acute inflammation of the meninges can be caused by *S. pneumoniae*, Group B *Streptococci*, *H. influenzae*, *L. monocytogenes*, *N. meningitidis*, gonococci (rare), *Mycobacterium tuberculosis*, *E. coli*, pol herpes, gram-positive anaerobes, and *Bacteroides,* and as a sequelae of Lyme disease and varicella (chickenpox).

B. The incubation period is variable, depending on the pathogen, usually 1 to 10 days. Transmission occurs from person to person through droplets from the respiratory tract and requires close contact.

Predisposing Factors

A. Peak demographics

  1. Children 4 years of age or younger (peak attack rate: Younger than 1 year)

  2. Adolescents

  3. Freshman college students living in dormitories

B. Attendance at day care, school, camps, and the military

C. Sequela of Lyme disease

D. Odontogenic infection

E. Sequela of otitis media, bacterial sinusitis, *H. influenzae* type B infection, and varicella

F. Sickle cell disease, asplenia, Hodgkin's disease, and antibody deficiencies

G. Review history for sexually transmitted and HIV infection

H. Penetrating wound, head trauma, spinal tap, surgery, or anatomic abnormality

I. Occupational exposure such as laboratory personnel

J. Travel exposure

K. Maternal infection and fever at the time of delivery

L. Lumbar epidural steroid injections

M. Immunosuppression

Common Complaints

A. Classic triad

  1. Nuchal rigidity

  2. Fever

  3. Altered mental status

Other Signs and Symptoms

A. Neonates or infants

  1. Decreased level of consciousness (LOC)

  2. High-pitched cry

  3. Irritability, inconsolability

  4. Fever and/or temperature instability

  5. Poor feeding and/or vomiting

  6. Bulging fontanelles

  7. Seizures

  8. Respiratory distress syndrome

  9. Hypotonia

B. Children or adults

  1. Sudden onset of a severe, constant headache affecting the entire head that worsens with movement; central nervous system (CNS) symptoms (nuchal rigidity, nausea and/or vomiting, confusion, lethargy, decreased LOC)

  2. Fever or chills

3. Backache
4. Photophobia
5. Difficulty swallowing
6. Facial and eye weakness and sagging eyelids
7. Seizures
8. Rash: The type of rash—macular, maculopapular, petechial, or purpuric—is dependent on the virus/organism.
9. Anorexia

C. Chronic meningitis: Usually have subacute onset of symptoms including fever, headache, and vomiting

Subjective Data

A. Review the onset, course, and duration of symptoms, including a progressive petechial or ecchymotic rash.
B. Determine current or recent history of ear infections, upper respiratory infection (URI), sinus infection, and chickenpox exposure.
C. Ask the patient about any recent dental procedures, extractions, and gum procedures.
D. Review the patient's recent history of tick bite and any treatments.
E. Review the patient's recent history of Hib immunization.
F. Evaluate a history of serious drug allergies.
G. Evaluate a history of recent head trauma/fracture.
H. Evaluate full history for ventriculoperitoneal shunt and other cranial surgery/procedures.
I. Review history for use of lumbar epidural steroid injections for pain.
J. Review all medications, including over-the-counter (OTC) and herbal products. Determine recent use of antibiotics.
K. Review for a history of illicit drug use, especially the intravenous (IV) route.
L. Review any recent travel locations.
M. Neonates: Review pregnancy, labor, and deliver history for treatment for Group B *Streptococcus* (GBS).

Physical Examination

A. Check temperature, pulse, respirations, and blood pressure.
B. Inspect
1. Observe general overall appearance.
2. Examine the skin for the presence of a petechial or ecchymotic rash.
3. Complete an ear, nose, and throat examination.
4. Examine mouth and teeth for dental diseases and disorders.
5. Assess the patient for dehydration.
6. Observe the patient for seizure activity.
7. Assess level of pain.
8. Inspect for cranial nerve palsies.

C. Auscultate
1. Lungs, monitor breathing pattern
2. Heart

D. Palpate
1. Neck: Palpate the lymph nodes.
2. Head: Palpate the fontanelle in children.
3. Palpate the mastoid bones.
4. Abdominal examination: Hepatosplenomegaly

E. Neurologic examination
1. Perform a complete neurologic examination.
2. Evaluate for signs of meningeal irritation by means of positive Brudzinski's and Kernig's signs:
a. Brudzinski's sign: Place the patient supine and flex the head upward. Resulting flexion of both hips, knees, and ankles with neck flexion indicates meningeal irritation (refer to Figures 16.1 and 16.2).
b. Kernig's sign: Place the patient supine. Keeping one leg straight, flex the other hip and knee to a bent knee to form a 90° angle. Slowly extend the lower leg. This places a stretch on the meninges, resulting in pain and spasm for the hamstring muscle. Resistance to further extension can be felt.

Diagnostic Tests

The definitive diagnosis is from bacteria isolated from cerebrospinal fluid (CSF) and the presence of elevated protein and low glucose in the CSF.

A. Lumbar puncture to obtain CSF for analysis
1. Gram stain
2. Absolute neutrophil count
3. CSF protein
4. CSF glucose
5. Culture and sensitivity
6. White blood cells (WBCs [pleocytosis])

B. Laboratory tests
1. Complete blood count (CBC) with differential
2. Metabolic panel, including electrolytes, glucose, blood urea nitrogen (BUN), and liver profile
3. Coagulation profile
4. Platelet count
5. Blood cultures × 2

C. Cultures of petechial or purpuric lesion scraping and synovial fluid
D. MRI or CT scan, with and without contrast (a screening CT is not necessary in the majority of the patients)

Differential Diagnoses

A. Meningitis
1. Bacterial etiology
2. Viral etiology
3. Fungal etiology
4. Aseptic meningitis
5. Chronic meningitis

B. Neonatal sepsis or pneumonia
C. Lyme disease
D. Herpes
E. Dementia
F. Gonorrhea
G. Otitis media
H. Dental abscess
I. Chickenpox
J. Sinusitis
K. Mastoiditis
L. Intracranial abscess

M. Encephalitis
N. Subarachnoid hemorrhage

Plan

A. General interventions

1. Treat aggressively because the progression of disease is often rapid. Antibiotic therapy should be initiated immediately after blood cultures are drawn and the results of the lumbar puncture if the clinical suspicion is high.

2. Dexamethasone should be given shortly before or at the same time as the antibiotics if clinical/laboratory evidence suggests bacterial meningitis.

3. Maintain hydration.

4. In addition to standard precautions, droplet precautions are recommended until 24 hours after initiation of effective antimicrobial therapy.

5. Chemoprophylaxis is warranted for people who have been exposed directly to a patient's oral secretions through close social contact, such as sharing of toothbrushes or eating utensils as well as child care and preschool contact within 7 days before the onset of the disease in the index case. Throat and nasopharyngeal cultures are of no value in deciding who should receive chemoprophylaxis and are not recommended.

6. Airline travelers with 8 hours of contact, who are seated directly next to an infected person, should receive prophylaxis.

B. Patient teaching

1. If a child suddenly develops a severely stiff neck along with fever and irritability, he or she needs medical help immediately.

2. Advise close contacts of the patient with meningococcal and *H. influenzae* meningitis that prophylactic treatment with rifampin (Rifadin) may be indicated; they should check with their health care providers or the local public health department.

C. Pharmaceutical therapy

1. Dexamethasone therapy should be considered when bacterial meningitis in infants and children (older than 1 month) is diagnosed or strongly suspected on the basis of the CSF tests, *H. influenzae* type B meningitis, and pneumococcal or meningococcal meningitis.

a. Dexamethasone should be administered 15 to 20 minutes before the first dose of antibiotics.

b. The recommended dexamethasone regimen is 0.4 mg/kg every 12 hours for a total of two doses by IV infusion for the first 2 days of antibiotic treatment. A regimen of 0.15 mg/kg every 6 hours for 4 days is also appropriate.

2. Antibiotic therapy: Broad-spectrum coverage should be initiated until culture results are available. The doses vary by the organism. All antibiotics should be administered IV for at least 7 days. Empiric therapy may require adjustment after the culture results.

a. Cefotaxime and ceftriaxone are commonly used as empiric therapy with *S. pneumoniae*, *N. meningitidis*, and *H. influenzae*. Vancomycin may be added to cefotaxime or ceftriaxone if renal function is normal until culture and susceptibility results are available.

b. Listeria has traditionally been treated with ampicillin or penicillin G, and gentamicin may be added for its synergistic effect.

c. *Pseudomonas aeruginosa* is often resistant to most commonly used antibiotics. Ceftazidime has been the most consistently effective cephalosporin therapy.

3. Chemoprophylaxis in adults includes rifampin, ceftriaxone, ciprofloxacin, and azithromycin.

4. Vaccinations: Polysaccharide (alone or conjugate) meningococcal vaccines are licensed in the United States. Two types of vaccines protect against meningococcal serogroups A, C, W, and Y: Meningococcal polysaccharide vaccine (MPSV4) and meningococcal conjugate vaccine (MenACWY). Recommendations include the following:

a. MPSV4 is administered in a single 0.5 mL dose intramuscularly. For children younger than 18 months, two doses administered 3 months apart are recommended. MPSV4 can be given concurrently with other vaccines but administered at a different site. In school-aged children and adults, MPSV4-induced protection persists for at least 3 to 5 years. MPSV4 is the only meningococcal vaccine licensed for people older than 55 years.

b. MenACWY recommendations:

i. Preferred vaccine for people 2 months to 55 years who have received this vaccine previously, or require multiple doses

ii. All children/teens aged 11 through 18 years: The first dose is recommended between 11 and 12 years, with a booster at 16 years of age.

iii. Children 2 months to 23 months with complex disorders.

iv. First-year college students younger than 22 years of age, living in a residential hall

v. People 2 months old or older at risk during an outbreak caused by a vaccine serogroup A, C, W, or Y meningococcal disease

vi. People 2 months of age or older traveling to a country at risk for meningitis (Mecca, Saudi Arabia)

vii. Microbiologists who work in a laboratory are at risk of meningitis.

viii. U.S. military recruits

ix. Anyone taking the drug eculizumab (Soliris)

x. Anyone whose spleen has been damaged or removed

xi. Persons diagnosed with the rare immune disorder "persistent complement component deficiency"

c. MPSV4 and MenACWY do not provide protection for the prevention of serogroup B meningococcal disease. New vaccines are available to protect from meningococcal serogroup B: Trumenba and Bexsero.

d. Immunizations with the pneumococcus, Hib, and influenzae vaccines also protect against bacterial meningitis.

Follow-Up

A. Have the patient return to the clinic in 2 to 3 days if conditions (e.g., otitis media) are not significantly improved with antibiotic therapy.

B. Follow-up is dependent on symptoms. Schedule a return visit after completion of antibiotics or 2 to 3 weeks after initial examination.

C. Sequelae associated with meningococcal disease occur in 11% to 19% of patients.

1. Hearing loss

2. Neurologic disability

3. Digit or limb amputations

4. Skin scarring

D. Bacterial meningitis is a disease notifiable to the local health department. All presumptive, probable, and confirmed cases should be reported.

Consultation/Referral

A. Neonate: Consult with a physician if the patient is younger than 3 months. Neonates need hospitalization.

B. Child: Consult with a physician.

1. Exceptions: Localized, nonserious infections. Child should be active, playful, drinking, and voiding.

2. The child needs immediate consultation with a physician if lethargic and inconsolable.

Individual Considerations

A. Pregnancy

1. The Academy of Pediatrics (AAP) lists the following indications for selective intrapartum chemoprophylaxis in GBS-positive women:

a. Preterm labor and delivery

b. Preterm rupture of membranes

c. Rupture of membranes greater than 18 hours before delivery

d. Intrapartum fever

e. Multiple gestation

f. Previous offspring with invasive GBS disease

2. Maternal: Culture introital or vaginal and anorectal samples for GBS, using a selective medium such as Todd–Hewitt broth. Vaginal colonization of Group B *Streptococcus* occurs in 5% to 40% of pregnant women, of whom 40% to 70% transmit GBS to their offspring.

3. The most significant problem associated with pregnancy is exposure of the fetus to GBS in the maternal genital tract. In 2002, the Centers for Disease Control and Prevention (CDC), the AAP, and the American College of Obstetricians and Gynecologists recommended universal perinatal screening for vaginal and rectal GBS colonization at 35 to 37 weeks gestation.

4. Treat patients with positive urine culture only because recolonization occurs frequently. Antibiotics should be administered to women in labor for preterm labor, premature rupture of membranes, positive GBS cultures (past or present), and preterm premature rupture of membranes in labor.

B. Pediatrics

1. Neonatal sepsis occurs in approximately 1% to 2% of cases. In the United States, the risk of developing *H. influenzae* type B invasive disease during the first 5 years of life is about 1:200.

2. Neonatal GBS infections *usually* present as early onset in the first 2 days of life and as late onset in newborns up to 3 months of age.

3. The premature neonate is at the highest risk for development of symptomatic neonatal disease.

4. Neonates often appear normal at delivery, only to develop a fulminant infection with rapid deterioration. Because of the severity and fulminant course of neonatal GBS infections, the primary focus is on preventing the vertical transmission of the organism.

5. Infants up to 2 years old may have meningitis without a stiff neck.

6. All infants with meningitis should undergo careful follow-up examinations, including tests for hearing loss and neurologic abnormalities.

C. Adults

1. Immunization with the pneumococcal vaccination has been shown to decrease the incidence of bacterial meningitis.

D. Geriatrics

1. Increased mortality rate for these patients secondary to the comorbid conditions.

Mononucleosis (Epstein–Barr)

Cheryl A. Glass and Jill C. Cash

Definition

A. Infectious mononucleosis is an acute, infectious viral disease caused by Epstein–Barr virus (EBV). EBV is also known as human herpesvirus 4. There are three classic symptoms: Fever, pharyngitis, and lymphadenopathy. The spread is via intimate contact between susceptible persons and asymptomatic EBV shedders through the passage of saliva.

B. Oral shedding may occur for 6 months after the onset of symptoms before its latency phase.

C. The fatigue related to EBV may last several months.

Incidence

A. Antibodies to EBV have been demonstrated in all population groups with a worldwide distribution. Approximately 90% to 95% of adults are EBV seropositive. Incidence is unknown; it occurs primarily in adolescents and young adults. The peak incidence of infection is noted in the 15- to 24-year age range. The majority of patients with primary EBV recover uneventfully.

Pathogenesis

A. EBV, human herpesvirus 4, is the primary agent of infectious mononucleosis. EBV persists asymptomatically for life in nearly all adults and is associated with the development of B-cell lymphomas, T-cell lymphomas, and Hodgkin's lymphoma in certain patients.

B. The incubation period is 30 to 50 days, with an average of 11 days; it is communicable during the acute phase, which may be prolonged. Acute symptoms resolve in 1 to 2 weeks. Pharyngeal excretion may persist for up to 18 months following clinical recovery. It is estimated that once infected with EBV, the virus may be intermittently shed in the oropharynx for decades.

C. EBV has also been isolated both in the cervix and in male seminal fluid, suggesting the possibility of sexual transmission.

D. EBV has also been noted in breast milk.

Predisposing Factors

A. Age 12 to 40 years, with peak incidence between 15 and 24 years of age

B. Exposure through oropharyngeal secretions (kiss, cough, shared food)

C. Roommates

D. Intrafamilial transmission to siblings

Common Complaints

A. Infectious mononucleosis is characterized by the following triad of symptoms:

- **1.** Fever
- **2.** Tonsillar pharyngitis (with exudate possibly having a white, gray-green, or necrotic appearance)
- **3.** Lymphadenopathy (usually posterior cervical chains—typically symmetric)

Other Signs and Symptoms

A. Fatigue: May be persistent and severe

B. Generalized aches

C. Appetite loss

D. Headache

E. Hepatosplenomegaly: Mild hepatitis is encountered in approximately 90% of individuals; splenomegaly is noted in approximately 50%. Jaundice is uncommon.)

F. Otitis media (infants and children)

G. Abdominal complaints and diarrhea (infants and children)

H. Upper respiratory symptoms (more prominent in young infants)

Subjective Data

A. Review signs, symptoms, and course and duration of symptoms, specifically the triad of pharyngitis, fever, and lymphadenopathy.

B. Assess the patient for recent upper respiratory infection (URI) and sore throat.

C. Inquire about any contact with persons known to have mononucleosis and other infections such as strep infections.

D. Review the patient's history for other family members with similar symptoms.

E. Carefully review medications. A mononucleosis syndrome with atypical lymphocytosis can be induced by drugs including

- **1.** Phenytoin
- **2.** Carbamazepine
- **3.** Antibiotics such as isoniazid and minocycline

Physical Examination

A. Check temperature, pulse, respirations, and blood pressure.

B. Inspect

- **1.** Conduct ear, nose, and throat examination, especially tonsils and palate.
  - **a.** Pharynx shows lymphoid hyperplasia, erythema, and edema.
  - **b.** Tonsillar exudates are present in about 50% of the cases.
  - **c.** Tonsillar pillars may touch "kissing tonsils" and may lead to airway compromise.
  - **d.** Evaluate for petechiae at the junction of the hard and soft palate.
  - **e.** Evaluate for oral hairy leukoplakia (OHL) on the lateral portions of the tongue. OHL appears as white corrugated painless plaques that cannot be scraped from the surface. (EBV-related malignancies as well as HIV may present with OHL.)

C. Auscultate

- **1.** Heart
- **2.** Lungs

D. Palpate

- **1.** Lymph nodes, especially anterior and posterior cervical chains, axilla, and groin. Firm, tender, and mobile lymph nodes are indicative of mononucleosis; lymphadenopathy is usually symmetric and presents in the posterior cervical chain more than the anterior chain.
- **2.** Abdomen, especially the spleen. Splenomegaly is noted in 50% of cases. Hepatomegaly and tenderness are noted in 10% of cases.

E. Percuss

- **1.** Abdomen, especially the spleen area.

F. Neurologic examination

- **1.** Evaluate for facial nerve palsy or symptoms of meningitis. See "Meningitis" in this chapter.

Diagnostic Tests

A. White blood cell (WBC) count with differential and a heterophile test.

> *A positive heterophile antibody test is diagnostic of EBV.*

B. Throat swab for rapid strep; if negative, send for culture.

C. Monospot test—not recommended for general use. Results may reflect a false positive/negative result. Results do not confirm the absence of EBV infection since the heterophile antibodies detected by this test are often not present in children.

D. Viral capsid antigen (VCA):

- **1.** Anti-VCA immunoglobulin M (IgM): Appears early and disappears in 4 to 6 weeks.

2. Anti-VCA immunoglobulin G (IgG): Appears in the acute phase of infection, peaks at 2 to 4 weeks, declines, and remains positive for a person's lifetime.
3. EBV nuclear antigen: Performed by immunofluorescent test, not sensitive early in acute phase but appears 2–4 months after onset and remains positive for life.
4. Elevated antibody levels are not diagnostic of recent infection and can be present for years.

E. Cold agglutinin titer: Cold agglutinin titer is markedly elevated in the setting of hemolysis (greater than 1:1,000).
F. Liver function tests: Abnormal liver function tests in a patient with pharyngitis strongly suggest the diagnosis of infectious mononucleosis (80%–90% of cases have elevated liver enzymes).
G. Abdominal ultrasound is performed if indicated for splenomegaly.

Differential Diagnoses

A. Mononucleosis
B. Streptococcal pharyngitis (Group A beta-hemolytic *Streptococcus*)
C. Viral syndrome
D. Hodgkin's disease
E. Hepatitis
F. Cytomegalovirus (CMV)
G. Secondary syphilis
H. Chronic fatigue syndrome (CFS)
I. Acute HIV
J. Toxoplasmosis
K. Adenovirus
L. Rubella
M. Acute HIV
N. Human herpesvirus type 6 (HHV-6; roseola)
O. HHV-7

Plan

A. General interventions
1. Make certain that the patient does not have an upper airway obstruction from enlarged tonsils and lymphoid tissue.
2. Treat concurrent infections.
3. Isolation is not required with good handwashing and prevention of the spread of pharyngeal secretions.
4. Bed rest is unnecessary.
5. There is no commercially available vaccine to prevent EBV infection.
6. Splenic rupture is rare but potentially life-threatening, occurring in one to two cases per thousand. It occurs between the 4th and 21st day of symptomatic illness, but can be the presentation symptom. The typical manifestations are abdominal pain and/or a falling hematocrit.

B. Patient teaching
▶ 1. Patient teaching: *See Section III: Patient Teaching Guide for this chapter, "Mononucleosis."*
2. Prolonged communicability may persist for up to 1 year.

C. Pharmaceutical therapy
1. Acyclovir is not recommended for infectious mononucleosis.
2. Antibiotic therapy is reserved for concurrent infections such as streptococcal pharyngitis.
3. Administer analgesics, such as acetaminophen or nonsteroidal anti-inflammatory drugs (NSAIDs), for fever, body aches, and malaise.
4. Corticosteroids may be considered in the presence of overwhelming infections including mononucleosis-related airway obstruction or other complications, such as severe hemolytic or aplastic anemia.

Follow-Up

A. Examine the patient every 1 to 2 weeks.
B. Initial monospot test may be negative.
C. If splenomegaly is present, schedule an appointment to reevaluate the patient before the release for contact sports. **Splenomegaly puts patients at risk for rupture secondary to blunt trauma (i.e., sports and motor vehicle accidents).**
D. Patients with the classic triad symptoms of mononucleosis should also have a diagnostic test for strep since the presenting symptoms are so similar.

Consultation/Referral

A. Consult a physician for marked tonsil enlargement and difficulty swallowing or symptoms lasting longer than 2 weeks. An emergent consultation with an otolaryngologist may be required.

Individual Considerations

A. Pregnancy: Intrauterine infection with EBV is rare.
B. Pediatrics: Primary EBV in young infants and children is common and frequently asymptomatic. Ampicillin and penicillin may cause morbilliform rashes.
C. Geriatrics: Older adults may not present with the classic triad of symptoms.
1. Lymphadenopathy is not as common with older patients.
2. Pharyngitis and myalgia are the most frequent complaints.
3. Fever may be prolonged, lasting several weeks.

Mumps

Cheryl A. Glass and Jill C. Cash

Definition

A. Mumps is an acute systemic viral illness. The viral illness is self-limited. Humans are the only natural host to the mumps virus. Mumps is highly contagious for patients who are not immune by vaccination or through maternal antibodies.
B. The hallmark sign of mumps is the unilateral swelling of one or more salivary glands. The parotid glands are typically involved unilaterally, then bilaterally. The swelling is visible under the ears and chin.
C. Mumps is spread by respiratory droplets, saliva, direct contact, or fomites. Current literature indicates that patients should be isolated for approximately 5 days from the onset of symptoms.
D. Central nervous system (CNS) involvement is the most common extrasalivary complication of mumps.

Meningitis and encephalitis from mumps have a good prognosis and usually resolve with complete recovery.

E. There is no specific treatment for mumps except supportive therapy; mumps is most often treated on an outpatient basis.

F. Immunization: The vaccine is a live-attenuated measles–mumps–rubella (MMR) vaccine or the measles–mumps–rubella–varicella (MMRV). The Centers for Disease Control and Prevention (CDC) recommends two doses of MMR vaccine.

1. First dose given between 12 and 15 months of age.
2. Second dose given between 4 and 6 years of age.
3. Persons born after 1957 who have no laboratory evidence of immunity or documentation of vaccination of the MMR after 12 months of age should receive at least one MMR vaccination.
4. The CDC recommends two doses of MMR for health care workers, students entering college, and international travelers.
5. The MMR vaccine should be given 1 month before or 1 month after any other live attenuated vaccines such as varicella.
6. Common side effects of the MMR vaccination include low-grade fever, skin rash, itching, hives, redness and swelling at the immunization site, and weakness.
7. Severe adverse side effects of the MMR vaccination include seizures; encephalopathy; thrombocytopenia; joint, muscle, and nerve pain; gastrointestinal (GI) disorders; and conjunctivitis.
8. MMR vaccine may be given with other vaccines at different injection sites and given in separate syringes.

Incidence

A. Mumps occurs worldwide.

B. The highest incidence is among Blacks.

C. Males and females are affected equally with parotitis.

D. Symptomatic meningitis is more common in males (3:1 ratio over females).

Pathogenesis

A. Mumps is caused by the *Rubulavirus*, a specific RNA virus. *Rubulavirus* is in the genus *Paramyxovirus* and is a member of the Paramyxoviridae family. The *Rubulavirus* shares morphologic features with the human parainfluenza; however, there is no cross-immunity between the two.

B. Mumps shares characteristics with other pediatric illnesses, including measles and rubella.

C. Mumps has an incubation of 16 to 18 days. Incubation can be as early as 7 days and as late as 23 days. Infectious period is approximately 3 days before to 9 days after the onset of symptoms. The illness lasts an average of 7 to 10 days.

Predisposing Factors

A. Lack of immunization

B. International travel

C. Immune deficiencies

D. Age groups

1. Primary school ages
2. High school ages
3. College ages
4. Occupational exposure

E. Crowded settings such as day care and military bases

Common Complaints

A. Asymptomatic (20%–30%)

B. Prodromal symptoms may last 3 to 5 days and include

1. Low-grade fever
2. Headache
3. Anorexia
4. Malaise
5. Myalgias

C. About 48 hours after the prodromal period, the most common symptom is parotitis (30%–40%) caused by the direct viral infection of the ductal epithelium.

1. Unilateral initially, then bilateral parotitis
   - a. Tenderness/pain with pressure
   - b. Edema (may last for 10 days)
2. Males
   - a. Unilateral orchitis (uncommon in males under 10 years of age but occurs in 33% of postpubertal males)
   - b. Bilateral orchitis only occurs in about 10% of cases.
   - c. Orchitis develops within 1 to 2 weeks of parotitis.
   - d. High fever
   - e. Severe testicular pain accompanied by swelling and scrotal erythema
   - f. Nausea, vomiting, and abdominal pain with orchitis
3. Females: Oophoritis (7%)
4. Aseptic meningitis (usually presents within the first week after parotid swelling)
   - a. Headache
   - b. Fever
   - c. Nuchal rigidity
   - d. Nausea and vomiting

Other Signs and Symptoms

A. Earache on the same side as the parotitis

B. Acute pancreatitis (5% incidence)

1. Abdominal distention
2. Pain
3. Fever (usually low grade)
4. Nausea and vomiting

C. Thyroiditis

D. Mastitis

E. Encephalitis (5 cases per 1,000 mumps cases)

Potential Complications

A. Meningitis

B. Encephalitis

C. Gonadal atrophy (20%–50% in postpubertal males)

D. Sterility (rare)

E. Guillain–Barré syndrome

F. Sensorineural deafness (0.5–5 cases per 100,000 cases)

1. Up to 20% is bilateral deafness
2. Often deafness is permanent

G. Impaired renal function/glomerulonephritis
H. Miscarriage if pregnant

Subjective Data

A. Review the onset and duration of symptoms.
B. Rule out similar symptoms in other family members.
C. Review the patient's immunization history.
D. Determine any new contact exposures.
E. Determine if the patient is pregnant.
F. Ask patient to list all medications, including over-the-counter (OTC) and herbal products.

Physical Examination

A. Check temperature, pulse, respirations, and blood pressure.
B. Inspect
  1. Visually inspect the face, under/behind the ears, and chin for edema.
  2. Conduct an ear, nose, throat, and mouth examination.
  3. Make a visual inspection of the scrotum.
C. Palpate
  1. Palpate the parotid glands.
  2. Palpate the neck and lymph glands, especially the cervical chains.
  3. Palpate the abdomen.
  4. Gently palpate the scrotum.
D. Auscultate
  1. Lungs (at risk for pneumonia)
  2. Heart (at risk for myocarditis)
E. Neurologic examination
  1. Assess hearing (may be unilateral loss).
  2. Evaluate for signs of meningeal irritation by means of Brudzinski's and Kernig's signs. How to perform and note positive Brudzinski's and Kernig's signs (refer to Figures 16.1 and 16.2):
    a. Brudzinski's sign: Place the patient supine and flex the head upward. Resulting flexion of both hips, knees, and ankles with neck flexion indicates meningeal irritation.
    b. Kernig's sign: Place the patient supine. Keeping one leg straight, flex the other hip and knee to a bent knee to form a 90° angle. Slowly extend the lower leg. This places a stretch on the meninges, resulting in pain and spasm for the hamstring muscle. Resistance to further extension can be felt.

Diagnostic Tests

A. Serum amylase level increase supports the diagnosis
B. Serum lipase
C. Mumps immunoglobulin M (IgM) and immunoglobulin G (IgG) (not required if the patient has a classic presentation of parotitis)
D. Other tests as indicated for presenting symptoms of complications

Differential Diagnosis

A. Mumps
B. Cytomegalovirus (CMV)
C. Parainfluenza virus 1 and 3
D. Influenza A
E. HIV
F. Bacterial infection
G. Drug reaction
H. Coxsackievirus
I. EBV
J. Adenovirus
K. Bacterial infections, particularly *Staphylococcus aureus*

Plan

A. General interventions
  1. There is no medication prescribed for the mumps.
  2. Symptomatic treatment recommended for comfort.
  3. Patients with complications, such as severe nausea/vomiting, may be hospitalized for intravenous hydration.
  4. Monitor for severe complications such as meningitis or pancreatitis. Hospitalization may be required.
  5. Notify the local public health department of active cases of the mumps.
B. Patient teaching
  1. The Academy of Pediatrics (AAP) and the Centers for Disease Control and Prevention (CDC) recommend that infected children not attend school/child care until 5 days after parotid swelling begins to subside.
  2. Stress universal precautions. The mumps virus can be found in the saliva, throat, and urine of the person infected.
    a. Practice good handwashing techniques.
    b. Use droplet precautions: Cover the mouth and nose with a tissue when coughing and sneezing and dispose of the tissue immediately.
    c. Do not share food or drink with the person with mumps.
  3. Encourage rest.
  4. Apply warm or cold packs to parotid gland for comfort.
  5. Add scrotal elevation/support and ice pack compresses.
C. Dietary management
  1. There is no special diet for the mumps. However, one should avoid acidic fluids and liquids, such as orange juice. Acid-containing foods may cause pain and difficulty swallowing with parotitis.
  2. Encourage drinking of fluids.
D. Pharmaceutical therapy
  1. Antiviral agents are not indicated for the mumps.
  2. Immunoglobulin has not been shown to be effective as a postexposure therapy.
  3. Analgesics, such as acetaminophen or ibuprofen, are prescribed for headache and parotitis.

Follow-Up

A. Follow-up is determined by patient's needs, severity of symptoms, and the presence of complications.
B. Notify the local health department if mumps occurs in a child-care setting. Persons exempted from vaccination

for medical, religious, or other reasons should be excluded for school/day care until at least 26 days after the onset of parotitis in the last person with mumps in the affected family.

Consultation/Referral

A. Consult with a physician for evaluation and need for hospital admission for complications.

Individual Considerations

A. Pregnancy
  1. There is no evidence that the mumps causes congenital abnormalities.
  2. Vaccinated women should avoid pregnancy for 3 months after immunization.
  3. Termination of pregnancy is not indicated if the MMR vaccination is given during pregnancy.
B. Pediatric
  1. Infants born to mothers who have mumps a week before delivery may have clinically apparent mumps at birth or mumps may develop in the neonatal period.

Parvovirus B19 (Fifth Disease, Erythema Infectiosum)

Cheryl A. Glass and Jill C. Cash

Definition

A. Parvovirus B19, also known as "fifth disease," is considered one of the TORCH (toxoplasmosis, other [i.e., hepatitis and syphilis], rubella, cytomegalovirus, and herpes) infections.
B. In children, parvovirus B19 can cause erythema infectiosum (EI), a mild febrile illness with rash. EI is also referred to as "fifth disease" since it represents one of six common childhood exanthems, each named in the order of dates they were first described. In contrast, patients with underlying hemolytic disorders can develop a transient aplastic crisis (TAC). Parvovirus B19 is an acute, communicable, viral infection that is spread by means of respiratory droplet and transplacental transmission. It can be associated with chronic hemolytic anemia and, in pregnancy, has been associated with nonimmune fetal hydrops and fetal death in 2% to 6% of cases.
C. Parvovirus B19 is the only infectious cause of TAC in over 80% of patients with sickle cell disease.
D. The polyarthropathy associated with parvovirus B19 typically lasts 1 to 3 weeks; however, the arthritis may be prolonged, and parvovirus should be considered in the differential diagnosis of newly diagnosed rheumatoid arthritis.
E. Parvovirus B19's rash may be confused with rubella.
F. There is no vaccine that can prevent parvovirus B19 infection.

Incidence

A. Parvovirus B19 is extremely common, but the true incidence is unknown. Parvovirus occurs worldwide. It is more common in children, and outbreaks are more usual in late winter and early spring. Up to 60% of the infections occur during school. Because less than 1% of teachers who are pregnant during EI outbreaks are expected to experience an adverse fetal outcome, exclusion of pregnant women from employment in child care or teaching is not recommended.

Pathogenesis

A. Human parvovirus B19 belongs to the *Erythrovirus* genus within the Parvoviridae family. Human parvovirus B19 is a DNA virus with preference to erythroid precursor cells. The virus replicates in the erythroid progenitor cell of the bone marrow and blood, leading to inhibition of erythropoiesis, which can result in symptoms of anemia. The parvovirus-associated rash is presumed to be at least partially immune mediated.
B. The incubation period for initial symptoms to develop is 4 to 14 days after exposure; the rash usually lasts 5 days, but it can last as long as 21 days. Parvovirus B19-specific immunoglobulin M (IgM) antibodies are detected at days 10 to 12 and can persist for up to 5 months. Rash and joint symptoms occur 2 to 3 weeks after acquisition of infection.
C. The annual seroconversion rate among pregnant women without parvovirus B19 is 1.5%.

Predisposing Factors

A. The only known host for parvovirus B19 is humans.
B. Exposure to school-aged (through junior high) and day care populations
C. Occupational exposure for teachers (20%), day care workers and homemakers (9% each), and health care workers
D. Exposure to close contact or crowded conditions.

Common Complaints

A. Clinical presentation is influenced by the infected individual's age and hematologic and immunologic status.
B. Approximately 25% of infected individuals are asymptomatic, and 50% have nonspecific flu-like symptoms of malaise, muscle pain, and fever.
C. Classic symptoms
  1. Red rash on the face that spreads to the rest of the body. **Erythematous, macular rash on cheeks produces "slap-cheek" pattern.**
  2. Arthritis: Joint pain most frequently affects the hands, followed by the knees and wrists. Joint symptoms are more common in adults and may be the sole manifestation of infection. Joint pain is more common in women. The arthritis associated with acute parvovirus B19 infection does not cause joint destruction.
  3. Edema

Other Signs and Symptoms

A. Adults: Chronic arthropathy
B. Child
  1. Bright red rash on cheeks; may be confused with rubella
  2. Maculopapular rash on trunk and extremities; may be pruritic
  3. Circumoral pallor

4. Malaise
5. Headache
6. Sore throat and pharyngitis
7. Conjunctivitis
8. Diarrhea

C. Fetus
1. Nonimmune hydrops fetalis
2. Stillbirth
3. Anemia

Subjective Data

A. Review the onset, duration, and course of symptoms.

B. Elicit the initial site of rash and progression to other body areas.
1. Determine if the rash is pruritic, especially on the soles of the feet.

C. Elicit job exposure for schoolteachers and day-care workers.

D. Determine if the patient is pregnant.

E. Determine whether the patient has had any new medication or contact exposures.

F. Rule out other family members with similar symptoms.

G. Ask about pain in the joints (usually in the hands, feet, or knees).

H. Review all medications, including over-the-counter (OTC) and herbal products.

Physical Examination

A. Check temperature, pulse, respirations, and blood pressure.

B. Inspect
1. Observe rash pattern.
a. Erythematous malar “slapped-cheek sign” rash on the face is the typical facial erythema. **The facial rash is the most recognized feature.**
b. “Lacy”-patterned rash over the chest, back, buttocks, arms, and legs.
2. Conduct an ear, nose, and throat examination.

C. Palpate
1. Blanch rash area: Rash over extremities blanches with pressure, heat or cold, and sunlight.
2. Palpate spleen: Splenomegaly is a hallmark sign.
3. Palpate lymph nodes: Enlarged lymph nodes, especially the posterior cervical nodes, are indicative of infection.
4. Assess joints for tenderness, swelling, and range of motion.

Diagnostic Tests

A. Complete blood count (CBC) with differential: Hallmark laboratory finding is the dramatic decrease or absence of measurable reticulocytes.

B. Parvovirus IgG and IgM antibodies—approximately 30% to 60% of adults have positive antibodies.

C. Polymerase chain reaction (PCR) test

D. Pregnancy test if necessary

E. Fetal assessment
1. Ultrasonography to evaluate for fetal hydrops. Fetal ascites and pleural and pericardial effusions are evident on ultrasonogram (nonimmune hydrops fetalis).
2. Percutaneous umbilical blood sampling (PUBS) to evaluate for fetal infection and anemia may be performed.

Differential Diagnoses

A. Parvovirus B19 (fifth disease)
B. Rubella
C. Aplastic crisis
D. Other viral infection
E. Contact dermatitis
F. Medication allergies
G. Chronic anemia

Plan

A. General interventions
1. Management is usually supportive treatment of symptoms
2. Analgesics for joint pain
3. Antipyretics for temperature
4. Starch bath for pruritus
5. Self-limiting without treatment
6. Immunosuppressed patients respond well to intravenous immunoglobulin (IVIG)
7. Aplastic crises may require transfusion

B. Patient teaching
1. Educate pregnant and immunocompromised patients to avoid exposure.
2. Routine infection control practices minimize the risk of transmission, including handwashing and droplet precautions. Avoiding sharing food or drinks may partially prevent the spread of parvovirus B19.
3. Disease is most communicable before rash; it is not communicable after rash outbreak.

C. Pharmaceutical therapy
1. Acetaminophen (Tylenol) for fever
2. Nonsteroidal anti-inflammatory drugs (NSAIDs) for symptomatic relief
3. Ig prophylaxis is not recommended by the Centers for Disease Control and Prevention (CDC) at this time.
4. There is no vaccine to prevent parvovirus B19.

Follow-Up

A. None is recommended as the disease is self-limiting for low-risk population.

Consultation/Referral

A. The incidence of acute parvovirus B19 in pregnancy is 3.3% to 3.8%. Refer pregnant patients to a perinatologist for fetal evaluation for acute exposure in pregnancy.

B. Consult or refer the patient to a physician immediately for exposure of immunocompromised patients, who might require a blood transfusion.

Individual Considerations

A. Pregnancy
1. A positive IgG antibody and a negative IgM indicate maternal immunity, and the fetus is therefore protected from infection. A positive IgM antibody is consistent with acute parvovirus infection.
a. If testing is negative for IgG and IgM after recent parvovirus exposure, PCR testing for maternal parvovirus B19 DNA should be performed.
2. Parvovirus B19 is not teratogenic. Fetal risks are related to the trimester of exposure. Nonimmune hydrops fetalis occurs secondary to hemolysis and inadequate production of erythrocytes. Other risks include spontaneous abortion, intrauterine growth restriction, stillbirth, and neonatal death.
3. Women who are diagnosed with acute infection beyond 20 weeks gestation should receive periodic ultrasounds (although serial ultrasounds are commonly performed).
4. Intrauterine blood transfusion may be performed if severe anemia is confirmed.
5. Delivery and postnatal management of the hydropic infant should occur in a tertiary care center. The majority of hydropic infants require respiratory assistance and mechanical ventilation.

B. Pediatrics
1. Neonates who had hydrops attributed to parvovirus B19 in utero do not require isolation if the hydrops is resolved by delivery.
2. Most children born to mothers who develop parvovirus B19 infection in pregnancy do not appear to suffer long-term sequelae; the infection does not appear to cause long-term neurologic morbidity.
3. Children with abnormal red blood cells (sickle cell disease, hereditary spherocytosis, thalassemia) can develop transient aplastic anemia and may require multiple transfusions.
4. Children may attend child care or school once the rash appears since they are no longer contagious.

C. Adults
1. Patients may have arthritis and arthralgias lasting months to years after exposure.
2. Adults may initially be asymptomatic.
3. Immunocompromised patients may develop severe, chronic anemia.
4. Working women with young children may benefit from prenatal testing and limiting exposure in pregnancy.

Rheumatic Fever

Cheryl A. Glass and Jill C. Cash

Definition

A. Acute rheumatic fever (ARF) is an autoimmune inflammatory process that occurs as sequelae of a Group A beta-hemolytic streptococcal (GAS) tonsillopharyngitis. Rheumatic fever is a preventable disease through the detection and adequate treatment of streptococcal pharyngitis.

B. The individual who has had an attack of rheumatic fever is at very high risk of developing recurrences after subsequent GAS pharyngitis and needs continuous antimicrobial prophylaxis to prevent such recurrences (secondary prevention). The most significant complication of ARF is rheumatic heart disease, which occurs after repeated bouts of acute illness.

Incidence

A. The incidence of rheumatic fever is 19 per 100,000 worldwide, but lower in the United States (2–14 cases per 100,000) following ineffectively treated cases of Group A streptococcal (GAS) upper respiratory infections (URIs). ARF is most common among children 5 to 15 years. It is relatively rare in infants and uncommon in preschool-aged children. The incidence of first episodes falls steadily after adolescence and is rare after 30 years of age. The disease does not seem to have a major racial predisposition. About 20% of children diagnosed with rheumatic fever have a positive history of pharyngitis and only 35% to 60% recall having any upper respiratory symptoms within the preceding 3 months.

B. Cardiac involvement is the most serious complication. Morbidity due to congestive heart failure (CHF), stroke, and endocarditis is common among individuals with rheumatic heart disease, and about 1.5% of persons with rheumatic carditis die of the disease annually. Mitral stenosis and Sydenham chorea are more common in females who have gone through puberty.

Pathogenesis

A. Rheumatic fever is caused by a preceding infection with GAS and *Streptococcus pyogenes.* Nonsuppurative inflammatory lesions of the joints, heart, subcutaneous tissue, and central nervous system (CNS) characterize ARF. The incubation period is between 1 and 5 weeks and 6 months after GAS pharyngitis.

Predisposing Factors

A. Group A pharyngitis, untreated or inadequately treated
B. Age 5 to 15 years
C. Crowded living conditions
D. Occupational exposure: Teachers, health care providers, and military personnel
E. Most common in tropical countries
F. Gender: More common in females

Common Complaints

A. Sore throat (generally of sudden onset), pain on swallowing

B. Joint pain/arthralgias to frank polyarthritis is usually symmetrical and involves large joints such as the knees, ankles, elbows, and wrists. Joints feel warm, swollen, and inflamed. **Polyarthritis is the most common manifestation. Both synovitis and periarticular inflammation occur, especially in the knees and ankles. There may be erythema of the overlying skin.**

C. Fever varies from 101°F to 104°F.

Other Signs and Symptoms

A. Fatigue
B. Appetite loss
C. Sydenham chorea (more common in girls): Chorea, a CNS disorder lasting 1 to 3 months, is purposeless, involuntary, rapid movements often associated with muscle weakness, involuntary facial grimaces, speech disturbance, and emotional liability. Sydenham chorea usually resolves with permanent damage but occasionally lasts 2 to 3 years.
D. Subcutaneous nodules are firm, painless nodules that are seen or felt over the extensor surface of certain joints, particularly elbows, knees, and wrists; in the occipital region; or over the spinous processes of the thoracic and lumbar vertebrae. The skin overlying them moves freely and is not inflamed.
E. Erythema marginatum is an evanescent, nonpruritic, pink rash with pale centers and round or wavy margins; lesions vary greatly in size and occur mainly on the trunk and extremities and are usually not seen on the face. Erythema is transient, migrates from place to place, and may be brought out by the application of heat.
F. Enlarged lymph nodes
G. Headache
H. Carditis: Development of new heart murmurs, cardiomegaly, and CHF
I. Pericarditis, pericardial friction rub, and/or pericardia effusion
J. Aortic regurgitation, manifested by
  1. Palpitations
  2. Dyspnea on exertion
  3. Angina at rest

Subjective Data

A. Review a recent history (1–3 months) of sore throat and the onset, duration, severity, and treatment of symptoms.
B. Complete a drug history. Did the patient finish the prescribed antibiotics? Does the patient take aspirin? **Use of aspirin can mask signs of inflammation and tends to prolong the course of the disease.**
C. Assess the patient for signs and symptoms of rheumatic and scarlet fever.
D. Discuss the patient's history of heart problems, chest pain, or shortness of breath.
E. Evaluate the onset and complaints of chorea: Fidgeting, clumsiness, uncoordinated erratic facial movements, including grimaces, grins, and frowns.
F. Tongue movements. Ask if the movements and other symptoms disappear with sleep.
G. Review symptoms of joint pain.

Physical Examination

A. Check temperature, pulse, respirations, and blood pressure.
B. Inspect
  1. Inspect joints for swelling and warmth.
  2. Observe for signs of chorea (symptoms noted previously).
  3. Conduct a dermal examination, especially the trunk and proximal aspects of the extremities. Individual lesions of erythema marginatum are evanescent, moving over the skin in wavy patterns or with indented margins. The lesions may be macular and can develop and disappear in minutes, appearing to change shape while being examined.
  4. Complete an ear, nose, mouth, and throat examination. Evaluate tonsillopharyngeal erythema with or without exudates. Observe for beefy, red, swollen uvula.
C. Auscultate
  1. Auscultate the heart. Note any heart murmur, pericardial friction rub, or effusion. Characteristic murmurs of acute carditis include the high-pitched, blowing, holosystolic, apical murmur of mitral regurgitation and a high-pitched, decrescendo, diastolic murmur of aortic regurgitation heard in the aortic area. The features of CHF include tachycardia, a third heart sound, rales, and edema.
  2. All lung fields. Note shortness of breath.
D. Palpate
  1. Neck lymph nodes
  2. Extremities: Apical and radial pulses
  3. Abdomen
E. Neuromuscular examination for chorea
  1. Have the patient stick out his or her tongue for observation of a "bag of worms" when protruded.
  2. Have the patient grip your hand—with chorea he or she will be unable to maintain a grip; rhythmic squeezing results.
  3. Observe for the spooning sign—a flexion at the wrist with finger extension when the hand is extended.
  4. Observe for the pronator sign—the palms turn outward when held above the head.

Diagnostic Tests

A. No single specific laboratory test can confirm the diagnosis of ARF. The throat culture remains the criterion for confirmation of GAS infection.
  1. If a rapid antigen detection test is negative, obtain a throat culture.
  2. Because of the high specificity, a positive rapid antigen test confirms a streptococcal infection.
B. Erythrocyte sedimentation rate (ESR) is usually elevated at the onset of ARF.
C. C-reactive protein (CRP) is usually elevated at the onset of ARF.
D. EKG or echocardiography. ***Note*: Prolonged PR interval.**
E. Chest radiograph can reveal cardiomegaly and CHF.
F. Echocardiography may demonstrate valvular regurgitant lesions.
G. Tests that may rule out differential diagnoses include rheumatoid factor (RF), antinuclear antibody (ANA), Lyme serology, blood cultures, and evaluation for gonorrhea.

Differential Diagnoses

A. Rheumatic fever: Jones criteria (updated in 2015)
  1. Requires two major criteria or one major plus two minor criteria to support the diagnosis of ARF in a patient with evidence of a preceding GAS infection.

2. Patients with a history of ARF are at risk of repeat episodes of ARF with GAS and more likely to have cardiac involvement. These patients require two major, one major plus two minor, or three minor criteria for the diagnosis of recurrent ARF. Criteria are as follows:

a. Major criteria

i. Carditis (based on clinical criteria) (50%–70% seen)

ii. Polyarthritis (35%–66% seen)

iii. CNS involvement (Sydenham chorea—neurologic disorder exhibiting abrupt, nonrhythmic, involuntary movements, muscle weakness, emotional disturbance) (rare in adults, seen in 10%–30%)

iv. Erythema marginatum (uncommon, rare in adults, less than 6% seen)

v. Subcutaneous nodules (uncommon, rare in adults, 0%–10% seen)

b. Minor criteria

i. Arthralgia

ii. Fever

iii. Elevated ESR or CRP level

iv. Prolonged PR interval

3. There are three exceptions to the aforementioned criteria in which criteria do not need to be met for the diagnosis of ARF. Those three exceptions include:

a. Chorea as only symptom

b. Indolent carditis for patients who present months after acute GAS infection

c. Recurrent ARF for patients with a history of ARF-associated carditis or rheumatic heart disease

4. Criteria may also be modified for moderate- to high-risk populations.

B. Juvenile rheumatoid arthritis

C. Rheumatoid arthritis

D. Gonococcal arthritis

E. Septic arthritis

F. Sickle cell anemia

G. Infective endocarditis

H. Leukemia

I. Gout

J. Huntington's chorea

K. Kawasaki disease (KD)

L. Systemic lupus erythematosus

M. Lyme disease

N. Reiter's syndrome

O. Scarlet fever

Plan

A. General interventions

1. Bed rest is a traditional part of ARF therapy and is especially important with carditis. Bed rest is needed throughout the acute illness and should continue until the ESR has returned to normal for 2 weeks.

B. Patient teaching

1. Reinforce the need to take the complete prescribed course of antibiotics for strep infections.

2. Adequate treatment for a streptococcal pharyngitis or skin infection is the best prevention against rheumatic fever. Strep infections are contagious, but rheumatic fever is not.

3. Chorea is usually managed conservatively in a quiet nonstimulatory environment. Valproic acid is the preferred agent if sedation is needed. Although there is no conclusive evidence of their efficacy, intravenous immunoglobulin (IVIG), steroids, and plasmapheresis have all been used successfully in refractory chorea.

4. Diuretics are the mainstay of carditis/heart failure.

C. Pharmaceutical therapy

1. Antibiotic treatment in patients who present with ARF is necessary regardless of the throat culture results to minimize the possible transmission of the rheumatogenic streptococcal strain. The drug of choice is penicillin, but erythromycin or sulfadiazine may be used in patients who are allergic to penicillin. Use of long-acting intramuscular penicillin G avoids compliance problems of oral regimens.

a. Benzathine penicillin G

i. Adults

1) Primary prophylaxis for treatment of GAS pharyngitis: 1.2 million units intramuscularly (IM) in a single dose

ii. Pediatrics

1) Primary prophylaxis: Children less than or equal to 27 kg: 600,000 units IM in a single dose

2) Children less than 27 kg: 600,000 units

3) Children more than 27 kg: 1.2 million units IM in a single dose

b. Penicillin V—drug of choice for GAS pharyngitis

i. Adults

1) Primary prophylaxis: 500 mg by mouth two to three times a day for 10 days

ii. Pediatrics

1) Primary prophylaxis: Children less than 27 kg: 250 mg by mouth two to three times a day for 10 days

2) Children more than 27 kg: 500 mg orally two to three times a day for 10 days

c. Amoxicillin

i. Adults: Primary prophylaxis: 500 mg orally in two divided doses for 10 days

ii. Pediatrics: 50 mg/kg/d orally in two divided doses for 10 days

d. Cephalexin

i. Adults: 500 mg orally twice daily for 10 days

ii. Pediatrics: 25 to 50 mg/kg/d orally in two divided doses (maximum 1,000 mg/d) for 10 days

e. Patients with severe hypersensitivity to beta-lactam antibiotics:

i. Azithromycin

1) Adults: 500 mg orally on day 1 and 250 mg once a day on days 2 to 5
2) Children: 12 mg/kg orally on day 1, then 6 mg/kg once a day on days 2 to 5

ii. Clarithromycin

1) Adults: 250 mg orally twice a day for 10 days
2) Pediatrics: 7.5 mg/kg/d given orally every 12 hours for 10 days; do not exceed maximum dose of 250 mg/d

iii. Clindamycin

1) Adults: 300 mg orally three times a day for 10 days
2) Pediatrics: If less than 70 kg: 7 mg/kg/dose (maximum 300 mg /dose) orally three times a day for 10 days. If greater than 70 kg: 300 mg orally three times a day for 10 days

2. Codeine is the analgesic of choice for arthritis symptoms.

3. Aspirin (Anacin, Ascriptin, Bayer acetylsalicylic acid [ASA], Bayer Buffered ASA) is the first-line anti-inflammatory therapy. It is used in patients with moderate to severe arthritis and carditis without heart failure. Treatment is administered for 1 to 2 weeks but may be administered for 6 to 8 weeks.

a. Adults: 4,000–8,000 mg/kg/d divided every 4 to 6 hours for 1 to 2 weeks. Treatment may be extended if needed.

b. Pediatrics: 80 to 100 mg/kg/d by mouth divided every 4 hours for 1 to 2 weeks. Treatment may be extended if needed.

4. Cardiac involvement with confirmed rheumatic fever

a. Heart failure—antibiotics + diuretic + angiotensin-converting enzyme inhibitors + steroid therapy

b. Atrial fibrillation—antibiotics + digoxin

c. Valve leaflet or chordae tendineae rupture—antibiotics and full assessment for an emergent valve replacement.

5. Severe chorea—antibiotics + anticonvulsants

6. Secondary antibiotic prophylaxis for procedures for chronic established changes of the heart valves

Follow-Up

A. The test of cure is a negative throat culture.

B. Pharyngitis patients with a history of rheumatic fever and those who are symptomatic and have a household member with documented GAS infection should receive immediate treatment without need for prior testing.

C. Since 2007, **the American Heart Association (AHA) no longer recommends prophylaxis for infective endocarditis in most patients.** The AHA prophylaxis for systemic bacterial endocarditis is available at www.inesss.qc.ca/fileadmin/doc/INESSS/Outils/Guides_antibio_II/endocardite_2012_web_EN.pdf

D. The major complication is cardiac valve disease. Rheumatic fever accounts for the largest number of aortic regurgitation cases. Continuous streptococcus prophylaxis in patients with prior rheumatic fever is the major means of preventing cardiac sequelae.

E. The patient with carditis should be followed every 6 months and by a cardiologist with an echocardiography every 1 to 2 years.

Consultation/Referral

A. Consult and comanage the patient with a physician.

B. Consult an ear, nose, and throat (ENT) specialist if indicated for patients with intact tonsils and recurrent symptomatic strep infections for consideration of tonsillectomy.

C. Consultation with a cardiologist may be required to manage heart blocks and CHF.

D. Consultation with a neurologist or psychiatrist may be required to confirm the diagnosis of chorea and to assist in its management.

Individual Considerations

A. Pediatrics

1. Highest risk group; rare in children younger than 5 years.

B. Adults

1. Cases are rare for patients older than age 40 years.

2. Cases of arthritis following a streptococcal infection that are not supported by the Jones criteria are called poststreptococcal reactive arthritis. Many of these patients will have one major and two minor symptoms and are considered to have ARF.

C. Pregnancy

1. Penicillin G is pregnancy category B. Fetal risk is not confirmed in humans but has been shown in some studies in animals.

2. Erythromycin is pregnancy category B.

3. Aspirin products are pregnancy category D. As fetal risk has been shown in humans, use only if the benefits outweigh the risk to the fetus.

Rocky Mountain Spotted Fever

Cheryl A. Glass and Jill C. Cash

Definition

A. Rocky Mountain spotted fever (RMSF) is a systemic febrile illness with characteristic rash from the bite of an infected tick. It can involve the skin; central nervous, cardiac, and pulmonary systems; gastrointestinal (GI) tract; and muscles. Ticks need 6 to 10 hours of feeding to transmit RMSF; therefore, early discovery and removal of ticks is a preventative measure.

B. In the United States, RMSF is a reportable disease and the most severe rickettsial illness.

C. Long-term sequelae are common with severe RMSF including

1. Paraparesis
2. Hearing loss
3. Peripheral neuropathy
4. Seizures
5. Bowel incontinence
6. Cerebellar and vestibular dysfunction
7. Blindness

Incidence

A. RMSF is the most common rickettsial infection in the United States. The prevalence of RMSF is in the southeastern and southern central states. Although RMSF is more common in rural and suburban locations, it does occur in urban areas. The incidence varies by geographic area. RMSF is more common in the spring and early summer, but has been seen in the cold weather months in the southern United States.
B. People of all ages can be infected.
C. African Americans have a higher case-fatality rate, possibly due to the difficulty of distinguishing the rash in highly pigmented skin.

Pathogenesis

A. *Rickettsia rickettsii* is the infectious agent and is transmitted by a tick vector. *Rickettsia* also infects rodents, squirrels, and chipmunks. Up to one third of patients with proven RMSF do not recall a recent tick bite or tick contact. RMSF is not transmitted by person-to-person contact.
B. The incubation period is usually about 1 week, but it ranges from 2 to 14 days after the tick bite. It appears to be related to the size of the rickettsial inoculum.
C. Principal recognized vectors:
  1. *Dermacentor variabilis* (American dog tick)
  2. *Dermacentor andersoni* (Rocky Mountain wood tick)
  3. *Amblyomma americanum* (Lone Star tick)
  4. *Rhipicephalus sanguineus* (brown dog tick)

Predisposing Factors

A. Outdoor activities (hunting, hiking, camping)
B. Tick bite: The tick must attach and feed for 4 to 6 hours before transmitting the infection.
C. Age is not a predisposing factor, but the disease is more common in children and young adults.
D. Exposure to heavy brush areas
E. Contact with dogs and other animals with ticks
F. Transmission has occurred on rare occasion by blood transfusion.
G. Blood transmission is rare

Common Complaints

In early phase, most patients have nonspecific signs and symptoms that may include
A. Fever
B. Sudden onset of severe headache
C. Children may present with prominent abdominal pain that may be mistaken for acute appendicitis, cholecystitis, or bowel obstruction.
D. Rash (90%) usually occurs between days 3 and 5 of illness. The typical RMSF rash begins as a pink maculopapular eruption on the ankles and wrists. The rash then spreads both centrally and to the palms of hands and soles of the feet. By the fourth day, the rash spreads centripetally and becomes petechial and papular. Hemorrhagic, ulcerated lesions may follow. In a small percentage, onset of the rash is delayed (past 5 days) and/or is atypical (e.g., confined to one body region). **Urticaria and pruritus are not characteristic of RMSF, and their presence makes the diagnosis unlikely.**
E. Malaise
F. Myalgias
G. Nausea with or without vomiting

Other Signs and Symptoms

A. Deep cough
B. Edema, especially in children
C. Bleeding
D. Conjunctivitis
E. Retinal abnormalities
F. EKG abnormalities
G. Seizures
H. Dehydration

Subjective Data

A. Review the onset, course, and duration of symptoms.
B. Elicit information about a recent tick bite or removal.
C. Ask the patient about any recent outdoor activities such as camping, hiking, and so on.
D. Rule out similar symptoms in other family members.
E. Review any history of rash and course of spread.
F. Elicit a history of mental or neurologic changes including seizures.
G. Rule out other symptoms associated with Lyme disease such as arthritis, memory loss, and distal paresthesia.
H. Review the patient's recent history of blood transfusion.

Physical Examination

A. Check temperature, pulse, respirations, and blood pressure.
B. Inspect
  1. Conduct an ear, nose, and throat examination.
  2. Inspect the skin, especially on the wrist, palms, ankles, and soles of the feet.
  3. Note the presence of petechiae.
  4. Conduct an eye examination and evaluate periorbital edema and petechial conjunctivitis.

C. Auscultate
  1. Perform a complete heart evaluation.
  2. Auscultate all lung fields.

D. Palpate
  1. All lymph nodes
  2. The mastoid bones

E. Neurologic examination
  1. Assess level of consciousness (LOC).
  2. Evaluate the patient for signs of meningeal irritation, such as nuchal rigidity and positive Brudzinski's and Kernig's signs (see Figures 16.1 and 16.2).

Diagnostic Tests

A. Antibody titers: A fourfold rise in antibody titer is the diagnostic gold standard for RMSF. Antibodies typically appear 7 to 10 days after the onset of the illness.
B. Complete blood count (CBC) with differential
C. Platelet count: As the illness progresses, thrombocytopenia becomes more prevalent and may be severe.
D. Electrolytes

E. Liver function studies
F. Bilirubin
G. Skin biopsy: 3 mm punch biopsy
H. Lumbar puncture may be indicated.
I. Rickettsial blood cultures are highly sensitive and specific; however, they require specialized laboratories.

Differential Diagnoses

A. RMSF is commonly mistaken for an undifferentiated viral illness during the first few days of illness
B. Viral meningitis
C. Lyme disease
D. Mononucleosis
E. Atypical measles
F. Viral hepatitis
G. Parvovirus B19 (fifth disease)

Plan

A. General interventions

1. Early treatment is necessary; never delay initiation of antimicrobial treatment to confirm clinical suspicion of the disease. This is a life-threatening disease.

2. Antibiotic therapy (see "Pharmaceutical therapy"). If penicillin or a cephalosporin is administered empirically in the first few days of the illness, the subsequent rash may be incorrectly diagnosed as a drug reaction.

3. Hospitalization should be considered for most patients, especially children.

B. Patient teaching

▶ **1.** Patient teaching: *See Section III: Patient Teaching Guide for this chapter, "Rocky Mountain Spotted Fever and Removal of a Tick," and Section II: Procedure, "Tick Removal."*

2. RMSF is not transmissible by person-to-person contact; therefore, isolation is not necessary.

3. Relapse of the illness may occur; the patient should report recurrence of symptoms immediately.

4. Patients who report tick bites should be advised to inform their health care provider if any systemic symptoms, especially fever and headache, occur in the following 14 days.

5. All pets should be treated for ticks.

C. Pharmaceutical therapy

> *The diagnosis of RMSF can rarely be confirmed or disproved in its early phase; the cornerstone of management is empiric therapy based on clinical judgment and the epidemiologic setting.*

1. Drug of choice: Doxycycline 100 mg orally or intravenous (IV) every 12 hours for 5 to 7 days for adults or children weighing more than 45 kg. Doxycycline 2.2 mg/kg IV (maximum dose 100 mg/dose) or orally every 12 hours is the dosage for smaller children.

a. Doxycycline 200 mg initial loading dose IV may be given for critically ill patients.

b. Doxycycline is the drug of choice in adults except for pregnant women.

c. Tetracyclines can cause dental staining when administered to children younger than 8 years. Most experts consider the risk of morbidity from rickettsial diseases greater than the minimal risk of dental staining from one short course of doxycycline.

2. Alternative drug therapy: Chloramphenicol (Chloromycetin)

a. Chloramphenicol requires frequent serum platelet counts and complete blood counts (CBCs).

b. Not available in oral form in the United States.

c. Use of chloramphenicol should be considered only in rare cases, such as severe allergy to doxycycline or in pregnancy if the mother's life is in danger.

d. Use of chloramphenicol is associated with a higher risk of fatal outcome.

3. Prophylactic therapy with doxycycline or another tetracycline is not recommended following tick exposure.

4. Severe doxycycline or tetracycline allergy in patients should be discussed with the patient. Consider consulting with allergy/immunology specialist. If not life-threatening, administer doxycycline in a controlled setting or consult for rapid doxycycline desensitization with an allergy/immunology specialist. Anaphylactic reactions have been reported, but rare.

5. Asymptomatic patients with seropositive results for tickborne rickettsial disease should not be treated with antibiotics because antibodies may remain positive for several years after infection.

Follow-Up

A. See the patient 24 to 48 hours after initial visit and again at the end of antibiotic therapy (unless following lab for chloramphenicol therapy). RMSF progresses rapidly. Approximately 10% of outpatients are subsequently admitted to the hospital.
B. The patient must be seen for any alteration in mental status, stiff neck, severe headaches, nausea and vomiting, severe weakness, dizziness, or high fever.
C. Hospitalization is indicated in patients who are severely ill or have complications, such as seizures, hypotension, or marked GI symptoms.
D. Several rickettsial diseases, including RMSF, are nationally notifiable diseases and should be reported to state and local health departments.

Consultation/Referral

A. Consult a physician for any suspected signs of RMSF because the patient is in danger of vascular collapse and disseminated intravascular collapse.
B. Consultation with an infectious disease specialist is advised.

Individual Considerations

A. Pregnancy: Tetracyclines should not be used in pregnancy. Limited data exist for the use of doxycycline during pregnancy. Data on the risks of treatment during pregnancy are unlikely to have a substantial teratogenic risk. Prophylactic use of tetracycline is not recommended. Chloramphenicol is an alternative for RMSF; however, precautions should be used for possible gray baby syndrome. Short-term use of doxycycline is considered safe during lactation and, per the American Academy of Pediatric Committee on Drugs, is "compatible with breastfeeding."

Roseola (Exanthem Subitum)

Cheryl A. Glass and Jill C. Cash

Definition

A. Roseola is a benign viral illness. It is the most common exanthem in infants and young children aged 1 to 3 years. Roseola can often be diagnosed by its classic presentation of a sudden onset of a high fever, up to 104°F, lasting 3 to 4 days. The pink-red macules and papules on the trunk and extremities occur after the patient's fever defervesces. The high fever associated with roseola often triggers a febrile seizure. Up to 15% of children will experience their first febrile seizure with roseola.

Incidence

A. Incidence is unknown; 90% of cases involve children younger than 2 years. Human herpesvirus type 6 (HHV-6) has been isolated in Kaposi sarcoma (caused by HHV-8), in which roseola may contribute to tumor progression. HHV-6 may facilitate oncogenic potential in lymphoma and has been associated with chronic fatigue syndrome (CFS).

Pathogenesis

A. HHV-6 is the causative organism. The two variants of HHV-6 are A and B. The genomes of HHV-6A/B have been sequenced. Nearly all primary infections in children appear to be caused by HHV-6B. In the primary infection, replication of the virus occurs in the leukocytes and the salivary glands. It is present in the saliva. HHV-6 and HHV-7 are spread by respiratory droplets. The communicable period is most likely during the febrile phase.

B. The incubation period is 5 to 15 days.

C. Like other herpesviruses, HHV-6 remains latent in most patients who are immunocompetent. Following the acute primary infection, HHV-6 remains latent in lymphocytes and monocytes and has been found in low levels in many tissues. The HHV-6 virus is a major cause of morbidity and mortality in patients who are immunosuppressed, particularly in patients with AIDS and in those who are transplant recipients.

Predisposing Factors

A. Classic age: 9 to 12 months (age range: 2 weeks to 3 years)

B. Attendance at day care centers

C. Transplacental infection in about 1% of cases

D. Immunosuppression

Common Complaints

A. Primary infection with HHV-6 may be asymptomatic or it may cause the exanthem subitum/roseola syndrome.

B. Child with high fever (up to 105°F) for several (1–3) days: Abrupt onset of fever followed by rose-pink maculopapular rash with rapid resolution of both is characteristic of roseola. Rash appears after fever is resolved.

C. Rosie pink rash on chest and body: Rash typically begins on the trunk or chest and spreads to the arms and neck, with mild involvement of face and legs; rash can last several hours to 2 days and fades quickly.

D. Characteristic enanthem (Nagayama spots) consists of erythematous papules on the mucosa of the soft palate and the base of the uvula (usually present on the fourth day).

Other Signs and Symptoms

A. Drowsiness

B. Seizures (secondary to high fever)

C. Bulging anterior fontanelle (rare)

D. Encephalopathy (rare)

E. Irritability

F. Mild diarrhea

G. Otitis media

H. Respiratory distress

I. Patients who are immunocompromised may have malaise and central nervous system (CNS) and other organ system involvement.

Subjective Data

A. Ask the parent or caregiver to describe the progression and color of the rash, onset, and duration of all symptoms.

B. Ask about the patient's temperature history and the treatments administered.

C. Review other symptoms such as coryza, cough, sore throat, and watery eyes (rules out roseola).

D. Review family history of others with similar symptoms.

E. Review the patient's history of febrile seizures.

F. Complete a drug history for possible allergic reaction.

G. Inquire regarding recent measles–mumps–rubella (MMR) immunization.

Physical Examination

A. Check temperature, pulse, respirations, and blood pressure.

B. Inspect

1. Inspect the skin. Observe for the presence of erythematous pink-red 3 to 5 mm maculopapular rash on chest and body: Rash typically begins on the trunk or chest and spreads to the arms and neck, with mild involvement of face and legs.
2. Observe the patient for seizure activity.
3. Conduct an ear examination for inflamed tympanic membranes to rule out otitis media.
4. Observe for the presence of periorbital edema, which is common in the febrile phase of infection.

5. Conduct a nasal examination; coryza is generally not a presenting symptom of roseola.
6. Conduct an oral/throat examination to evaluate for the presence of characteristic enanthem Nagayama spots appear as erythematous papules on the mucosa of the soft palate and the base of the uvula.

C. Auscultate
1. Heart
2. Lungs; cough may be present

D. Palpate
1. Palpate the head and the anterior fontanelle (if applicable).
2. Palpate the neck and the cervical, suboccipital, and postauricular lymph nodes.

E. Neurologic examination
1. Check for nuchal rigidity.

Diagnostic Tests

A. None is required unless the diagnosis is unclear.
B. Rule out testing.
1. Complete blood count (CBC) with differential
2. Urinalysis and culture for urinary tract infection (UTI)
3. Chest radiograph for pneumonia
4. Blood cultures
5. Cerebrospinal fluid (CSF) examination if indicated

C. Skin biopsy (rarely performed unless the diagnosis is unclear and there are other complicating medical factors).

Differential Diagnoses

A. Roseola
B. Allergic reaction
C. Cytomegalovirus (CMV)
D. RMSF
E. Fifth disease (parvovirus B19)
F. Scarlet fever
G. Meningococcemia
H. Fever of unknown origin (FUO)
I. Pneumococcemia
J. Herpes simplex
K. Otitis media
L. Rubella
M. Enterovirus
N. Epstein–Barr virus (EBV)
O. Measles

Plan

A. General interventions
1. Encourage fluids to prevent dehydration (popsicles, Jell-O, clear fluids).
2. Monitor for lethargy, decreased fluid intake, cough, and irritability.

B. Patient teaching
1. Treatment is supportive.
2. Advise parents/care provider that controlling temperature and providing supportive care is essential. Avoiding high fever, greater than 104°F, is imperative.
3. Discomfort and body aches are often related to fever.

C. Pharmaceutical therapy
1. At present, there is no antiviral therapy available for HHV-6 infection.
2. Acetaminophen (Tylenol) as needed for fever.
3. Acute or chronic antiseizure medications are not recommended for infants who have had a febrile seizure secondary to roseola.

Follow-Up

A. None is required unless other problems occur; resolution is usually rapid.
B. See the patient immediately for the following:
1. Twitching or other signs of seizure
2. Refusal to drink liquids or signs of dehydration
3. Loud and persistent crying; does not stop when consoled
4. Listlessness and stiff neck

Consultation/Referral

A. Consult and/or refer the patient to a physician if febrile seizures/neurologic signs are present.

Individual Considerations

A. Pediatrics: Children with roseola are often playful without change in appetite, even with high fever.

Rubella (German Measles)

Cheryl A. Glass and Jill C. Cash

Definition

A. Rubella, also known as German measles and 3-day measles, is primarily known as a childhood disease. Rubella is considered one of the TORCH (toxoplasmosis, other [i.e., hepatitis and syphilis], rubella, cytomegalovirus, and herpes infections) infections and is highly contagious. The disease is preventable by immunization. Passive immunity is acquired from birth to 6 months of age from maternal antibodies.

B. The goal of immunization is to prevent congenitally acquired rubella. Routine immunization is achieved by using the measles-mumps-rubella (MMR) or the MMR combined with varicella (MMRV) vaccine. The rubella vaccine is a live-attenuated virus.

C. Immunization schedule recommended by the American Academy of Pediatrics (AAP):
1. First immunization is given between 12 and 15 months of age.
2. Second immunization is given at 4 to 6 years of age when the child is entering school.
3. People who have not received the second immunization at school entry should receive their second immunization as soon as possible but optimally no later than 11 to 12 years of age.

Incidence

A. Rubella is no longer endemic in the United States as a result of an intensive vaccination campaign. The Centers for Disease Control and Prevention (CDC) declared rubella to be eliminated from the United States in 2004. Incidence is unknown. Peak season for rubella is late winter and spring.

B. The rubella vaccination is given only in about half of the world's population. Congenital rubella syndrome causes 15% of all birth defects in Russia.
C. Congenital defects occur in up to 85% of infants if maternal rubella infection occurs during the first 12 weeks of gestation.

Pathogenesis

A. Rubella virus is an enveloped, positive-stranded RNA virus classified as Rubivirus in the Togaviridae family. Humans are the only source of infection. The virus is spread by nasopharyngeal, airborne respiratory droplets and transplacental routes.
B. The incubation period for postnatally acquired rubella ranges from 14 to 23 days (usually 16–18 days). It is communicable 1 week before and 4 days after rash and illness. The neonate born with congenital rubella is often highly infectious and should be isolated. Neonates may continue to shed the virus for 1 year or longer.

Predisposing Factors

A. Age 5 to 9 years
B. Transplacental transmission
C. Never received rubella vaccine
D. Attendance at schools and day-care centers
E. Compromised immune system

Common Complaints

A. Low-grade fever
B. Swollen glands: Posterior auricular, suboccipital, and posterior cervical lymphadenopathy is frequently present 24 hours before rash develops.
C. Rash: Light pink to red macular rash that starts on the face and moves down the body to the trunk. The facial rash clears as the extremity rash erupts. The macular lesions rapidly become papular lesions and fade in 3 to 4 days. Exanthematous lesions remain discrete and pink, in contrast with the rash of rubeola, which is deep red and becomes confluent (Koplik's spots). Exanthem of rubella is usually preceded by 1 to 5 days of prodrome symptoms and generally last 3 days, but may persist for as long as 5 days.

Other Signs and Symptoms

A. Headache
B. Sore throat
C. Mild coryza
D. Cough
E. Malaise
F. Conjunctivitis
G. Forchheimer spots in the soft palate
H. Transient polyarthralgia and polyarthritis (older children, adolescents, and women)
I. Itching
J. Asymptomatic

Subjective Data

A. Review the onset, duration, and course of symptoms.
B. Rule out similar symptoms in other family members.
C. Review the patient's immunization history (especially recent immunization of MMR or MMRV vaccines).
D. Determine any new medications or contact exposures.
E. Review any history of rash and the course of spread.
F. Determine if the patient is pregnant.
G. If a fever is present, has the patient experienced a febrile seizure?

Physical Examination

A. Check temperature, pulse, respirations, and blood pressure.
B. Inspect
  1. Conduct an ear, nose, and throat examination.
  2. Inspect the mouth for Koplik's spots. Forchheimer spots are reddish spots on the soft palate seen during the prodrome or first day of the rash.
  3. Inspect the skin.
C. Auscultate
  1. Heart
  2. Lungs
D. Palpate
  1. Check the lymph nodes, especially the anterior/posterior cervical chains in neck.

Diagnostic Tests

A. Blood or urine
  1. Latex agglutination
  2. Enzyme immunoassay (enzyme-linked immunosorbent assay [ELISA])
  3. Passive hemagglutination
  4. Fluorescent immunoassay tests
B. Rubella titer (test initially and repeat 2 to 4 weeks after exposure)

> *Serologic rubella titer less than 8 indicates nonimmunity. Rubella titer greater than 1:32 indicates immunity from a past infection. A fourfold rise in the titer (about 2 weeks after exposure) indicates infection.*

C. Pregnancy test if indicated
D. Tissue culture of throat

Differential Diagnoses

A. Rubella (German measles)
B. Rubeola
C. Parvovirus
D. Scarlet fever
E. Allergic reaction, contact dermatitis
F. Roseola
G. Infectious mononucleosis
H. Toxoplasmosis

Plan

A. General interventions
  1. Primary prevention is through immunization.
  2. Vaccinating adolescents and adults in college reduces the chance of outbreaks and helps to prevent congenital rubella syndrome.

3. Generally, the course is mild; however, rest is encouraged.
4. Treatment is supportive. Have the patient increase oral fluid intake.
5. Reinforce respiratory and nasal discharge precautions (droplet precautions); encourage good handwashing.
6. Immunize patients preconceptually; advise them to use a method of birth control for at least 4 weeks or longer after immunization.
7. Rubella cases should be reported to the local health department.
8. Health care professionals should be immunized.

B. Patient teaching
1. Patient/children should not return to work or school for 7 days after the onset of the rash.
2. Pregnant patients with documented rubella infection should be counseled about the risk of fetal infection and/or compromise.
3. Children with congenital rubella should be considered contagious until they are at least 1 year of age, unless nasopharyngeal and urine culture are negative consecutively for rubella virus; infection control precautions should be considered in children up to 3 years who are hospitalized for congenital cataract extraction.
4. Febrile seizures may occur in children 12 to 24 months of age.

C. Pharmaceutical therapy
1. Acetaminophen (Tylenol) for fever and headache
2. Antihistamines: Diphenhydramine (Benadryl) for pruritus
3. Limited data indicate that intramuscular immunoglobulin (Ig) in a dose of 0.55 mL/kg may decrease clinically apparent shedding and the rate of viremia significantly in exposed susceptible people. The absence of clinical signs in a woman who has received intramuscular Ig does not guarantee that infant infection is prevented. The CDC recommends limiting the use of Ig to women with known rubella exposure who decline pregnancy termination.
4. Live-virus rubella vaccine administered within 3 days of exposure has not been demonstrated to prevent illness.
5. Glucocorticoids, platelet transfusion, and other supportive measures are reserved for patients with complications such as thrombocytopenia or encephalopathy.

Follow-Up

A. The disease is self-limiting and has no sequelae (except congenital exposure).
B. Repeat titer 3 to 4 weeks after exposure.
C. Rubella is a disease reportable to the local or state health department.

Consultation/Referral

A. Refer the patient to an obstetrician if the patient is pregnant.

Individual Considerations

A. Pregnancy
1. Rubella infection has few consequences for an adult, but it presents significant problems for a fetus. Rubella's viral teratogenic effects include cardiovascular malformation, deafness, mental retardation, cataracts, glaucoma, microcephaly, and microphthalmos.
2. If maternal infection occurs during the first trimester, 50% of the fetuses infected may abort or have complications. Approximately 30% to 50% of fetuses that acquire rubella in the first month of gestation suffer cardiac anomalies. Neural deafness is a common sequela when infection occurs in the second gestational month.
3. The rubella vaccine is a live, attenuated virus; therefore, it is *not* safe to give in pregnancy. Immunization may be given postpartum; instruct the patient to avoid pregnancy for the next 4 weeks or longer. The rubella vaccine may be given to a woman if she is breastfeeding.
4. Routine prenatal screening for rubella immunity should be undertaken. If a woman is found to be susceptible, the rubella vaccine should be administered during the immediate postpartum period before discharge.
5. Breastfeeding is not a contraindication to postpartum immunization of the mother.

B. Pediatrics
1. The infected neonate must be kept in isolation in the nursery. The neonate may continue to spread the virus for 1 year or longer.
2. Cardiac and eye defects are most frequent when maternal infection occurs before 8 weeks gestation; hearing loss and growth retardation are observed in maternal infections up to 16 weeks gestation.
3. Other reported abnormalities include jaundice, hepatosplenomegaly, thrombocytopenia, and dermal erythropoiesis (blueberry muffin lesions).
4. The Advisory Committee on Immunization Practices (ACIP) currently recommends that all children receive two doses of MMR vaccine, separated by at least 28 days, administered on or after the first birthday.

Rubeola (Red Measles)

Cheryl A. Glass and Jill C. Cash

Definition

A. Rubeola (red measles), also known as hard measles, is a highly communicable viral disease. The disease is preventable by immunization. Passive immunity is acquired from birth to between 4 and 6 months of age if the mother is immune before pregnancy. Immunity after measles infection is thought to be lifelong.
B. Modified measles occurs in patients who received the serum immunoglobulin (Ig) postexposure to the measles virus. The incubation period may be up to 21 days. Their symptoms are generally milder.

C. Atypical measles occurs in patients who had the original killed-virus measles immunization that has incomplete immunity. Their symptoms are similar to the clinical presentation for patients who have not been vaccinated and have initial exposure.

1. The killed-virus vaccine was administered between 1963 and 1967.

2. In 1967 the live-attenuated vaccine replaced the killed-virus measles vaccine.

D. In the United States, the measles vaccine is currently available in two formulations: The trivalent measles–mumps–rubella (MMR) vaccine and the measles–mumps–rubella–varicella (MMRV).

Incidence

A. Incidence is unknown; widespread measles vaccination has led to its virtual disappearance in the United States. In 2014, the WHO noted that globally there were 114,900 measles deaths. Most of those deaths occurred in children younger than 5 years. In 2014, approximately 85% of the world's children received one dose of the measles vaccine by their first birthday.

B. In temperate areas, the peak incidence of infection occurs during late winter and spring.

C. About 5% of all measles cases are due to vaccine failure.

D. There is an increased incidence in two populations: Children younger than 5 years and college students who have not been immunized.

E. Rubeola is rarely encountered in pregnancy; however, the reported mortality of congenital measles is 32%.

F. One in every 1,000 patients with measles will develop acute encephalitis. Most fatalities from measles are from respiratory tract complications or encephalitis.

G. Patients with defects in cell-mediated immunity (AIDS, lymphoma, or other malignancies) are at risk for severe, progressive measles infection.

H. A generalized immunosuppression that follows measles frequently predisposes patients to complications such as otitis media and bronchopneumonia. Laryngotracheobronchitis (croup) and diarrhea occur more commonly in young children. Two rare neurologic syndromes are associated with measles:

1. Acute disseminated encephalomyelitis may occur soon after the initial clinical manifestations of measles have resolved.

2. Subacute sclerosing panencephalitis presents 7 to 10 years after the initial infection.

Pathogenesis

A. Paramyxovirus (an RNA virus) is the causative agent and is spread by respiratory droplet, direct skin contact, or transplacental passage. The incubation period lasts 7 to 14 days from exposure to onset. It is communicable a few days before fever to 4 days after rash appears. The measles virus replicates locally, spreads to regional lymphatic tissues, and is then thought to disseminate to other reticuloendothelial sites via the bloodstream.

B. The virus remains active and contagious in the air or on infected surfaces for up to 2 hours.

Predisposing Factors

A. Age less than 5 years and not immunized

B. Schools: College age and not immunized with two doses. In 1989, the United States adopted a two-dose strategy; revaccination with MMR vaccine is recommended for all students and their siblings.

C. Late winter and early spring

D. Transplacental passage; presents clinically in the first 10 days of life

E. Crowded living conditions

F. Measles has been attributed to poor nutritional status and vitamin A deficiency.

Common Complaints

A. Suspected case: Febrile illness accompanied by a rash

B. Clinical case: The patient is usually very ill with a fever and the three Cs: cough, coryza, and conjunctivitis. The patient generally recovers rapidly after the first 3 to 4 days.

1. Fever greater than 101°F and often exceeding 104°F

2. Respiratory symptoms: Coryza and cough. The cough may persist for 1 to 2 weeks after the measles infection.

3. Conjunctivitis

C. Rash: Macular rash develops on the face and neck; then lesions become maculopapular and spread to the trunk and extremities in 24 to 48 hours. The rash may appear red brown or purple red at the hairline. The rash lasts 4 to 7 days.

D. Koplik's spots on buccal mucosa: Koplik's spots are pathognomonic for measles—bluish-gray specks or "grains of sand" on a red base.

E. Probable case meets clinical case definition but is not linked epidemiologically to a confirmed case and lacks serologic or virologic proof of disease.

F. Confirmed case meets the laboratory criteria for measles or meets the clinical case definition and is epidemiologically linked to a confirmed case.

Other Signs and Symptoms

A. Loss of appetite

B. Bronchitis

C. Photophobia

D. General lymphoid involvement

E. Myalgia

F. Pruritus

G. Diarrhea

Subjective Data

A. Review the onset and duration of symptoms such as cough, conjunctivitis, coryza, and Koplik's spots.

B. Rule out similar symptoms in other family members.

C. Review the patient's immunization history.

D. Determine any new medications or contact exposures.

E. Review any history of rash and the course of spread.

F. Elicit the presence of chest pain, ear pain, and confusion (signs of complications).

G. Determine if the patient is pregnant.
H. Review the patient's history of tick bite (recent camping, hiking, and so forth).

Physical Examination

A. Check temperature, pulse, respirations, and blood pressure.
B. Inspect
  1. Conduct an eye examination: Nonpurulent conjunctivitis with lacrimation is not uncommon. Photophobia may be present.
  2. Conduct an ear examination: Otitis is a complication noted with the measles.
  3. Conduct a nasal examination: Coryza is one of the classic triad of symptoms.
  4. Conduct a throat examination: Pharyngitis encompasses all complications of the measles.
  5. Examine the mouth for Koplik's spots; they appear on buccal mucosa within 12 hours. Koplik's spots are tiny (1–3 mm) bluish-white spots on an erythematous base that cluster adjacent to the molars on the buccal mucosa. Koplik's spots often begin to slough when the exanthem appears.
  6. Conduct a dermal examination. The characteristic rash is maculopapular and blanches; it begins on the face and spreads centrifugally to involve the neck, upper trunk, lower trunk, and extremities. The lesions may become confluent, especially in the face, where the rash develops first. The palms and soles of the feet are rarely involved. Some petechiae may be present with the rash.
C. Auscultate
  1. Lungs
  2. Heart
D. Palpate
  1. Palpate the neck and lymph nodes.
  2. Generalized lymphadenopathy and splenomegaly are uncommon.
E. Neurologic examination
  1. Check for nuchal rigidity.
  2. Complete a mental status examination.

Diagnostic Tests

A. Serologic procedures are not routinely done; however, leukopenia and T-cell cytopenia often occur and thrombocytopenia may also be seen.
B. Antibody titer at the onset of the rash; repeat antibody titer every 3 to 4 weeks.
  1. Rubeola immunoglobulin G (IgG) and immunoglobulin M (IgM) antibody levels. The WHO has recommended that the diagnosis of measles be confirmed with laboratory testing.
  2. Serum IgM alone is the standard test to confirm the diagnosis of measles. At least a fourfold increase in antimeasles antibody titer is indicative of infection.
C. Chest x-ray if indicated: May show interstitial pneumonitis.

Differential Diagnoses

A. Rubeola (red, or 7-day measles)
B. During the prodromal period, measles may resemble a common cold, except a fever is present.
C. Rubella (German measles)
D. Roseola (exanthem subitum)
E. Rocky Mountain spotted fever (RMSF)
F. Scarlet fever
G. Mononucleosis
H. Drug reaction
I. Kawasaki disease (KD)
J. Parvovirus B19
K. Toxic shock syndrome
L. Mycoplasma pneumoniae
M. Respiratory viruses:
  1. Rhinoviruses
  2. Parainfluenza
  3. Influenza
  4. Adenovirus
  5. Respiratory syncytial virus (RSV)
N. Dengue fever should be ruled out for international travelers.

Plan

A. General interventions
  1. Primary prevention is through immunization.
    a. In order for vaccination to be considered adequate for school outbreaks, two doses of measles vaccine must have been administered after the age of 12 months and separated by at least 28 days.
    b. Those who are properly vaccinated may reenter school immediately after vaccination.
    c. International travelers should receive one or two doses of the measles vaccine before travel.
  2. Encourage the patient to rest.
  3. The patient must be isolated 4 days from the onset of the rash, up to 21 days.
  4. Encourage respiratory and nasal discharge precautions. The cough may persist for up to 2 weeks after the measles.
  5. There is no specific treatment for rubeola.
    a. Otitis media and pneumonia, both due to bacterial superinfection, should be treated with appropriate antibiotics.
    b. Intravenous (IV) hydration may be required secondary to dehydration from diarrhea or vomiting.
  6. Monitor the patient for signs of complications.
B. Patient teaching
  1. Tell the patient to avoid bright lights with photophobia; may need sunglasses.
  2. Reinforce the need to comply with immunization schedule.
C. Pharmaceutical therapy
  1. Vitamin A is recommended by the WHO and the United Nations Children's Fund (UNICEF) to all children with measles in areas where vitamin A deficiency is prevalent or where the mortality from measles exceeds 1%. Vitamin A treatment can help prevent eye damage and blindness. It has been shown to reduce the number of deaths by 50%.

a. Children younger than 6 months: 50,000 IU/d for 2 consecutive days
b. Children 6 months to 11 months: 100,000 IU/d for 2 consecutive days
c. Children 12 months of age and older: 200,000 IU/d for 2 consecutive days
d. For children with ophthalmologic evidence of vitamin A deficiency, a third dose of vitamin A dosage should be repeated in 2 to 4 weeks utilizing the age-specific dosing.

2. Treatment for exposed persons
a. Give live measles vaccine if exposure was within 72 hours. Dose is 0.5 mL by subcutaneous injection in the outer aspect of the upper arm.
b. Give immunoglobulin (Ig) 0.25 mL/kg/dose (0.5 mL/kg for patients with HIV) by intramuscular (IM) injection (maximum dose is 15 mL) to induce passive immunity and to prevent or modify symptoms within 6 days of exposure for the following high-risk groups:
i. Immunocompromised
ii. Infants 6 months to 1 year of age
iii. Infants younger than 6 months who are born to mothers without measles immunity
iv. Pregnant women
c. If Ig dose exceeds 10 mL, divide dose into several muscle sites to reduce local pain.
d. **Do not give Ig with the live measles vaccine.**
e. Measles is susceptible to ribavirin. Further studies are needed to determine whether this treatment should be recommended. **Ribavirin is not Food and Drug Administration (FDA) approved for the treatment of measles.**

3. Live measles virus vaccine should be given (except in pregnant women) approximately 3 months after Ig administration as long as patient is at least 15 months of age at that time and there is no contraindication to vaccination.
4. Children and adolescents with symptomatic HIV infection who are exposed to measles should receive Ig 0.5 mL/kg regardless of vaccination status.
5. Exposure to measles is not a contraindication to vaccination. Available data suggest that live measles virus vaccine, if given within 72 hours of measles exposure, provides protection in some cases. If the exposure does not result in infection, the vaccine should induce protection against subsequent measles infection.

Follow-Up

A. See the patient daily for mental status examination and examination of chest to rule out complications such as encephalitis and pneumonia.
B. Follow-up is needed 3 to 4 days after the onset of exanthem.
C. Investigate immune status of the family and other immediate contacts; prescribe vaccine if necessary.
D. Rubeola cases should be reported to the local health department since one case is considered an outbreak.

Consultation/Referral

A. Refer the patient to a physician if fever lasts over 4 days; this is indicative of complications. Hospitalization may be indicated for treatment of measles complications (e.g., bacterial superinfection, pneumonia, dehydration, or croup).

Individual Considerations

A. General
1. A history of anaphylaxis after ingestion of gelatin is associated with an increased risk of anaphylaxis from the MMR or measles vaccine. This history should warrant a skin test for gelatin allergy.
2. Individuals with anaphylaxis, excluding contact dermatitis, from neomycin should not receive these vaccines because they contain a small amount of this antibiotic.
3. A history of anaphylaxis after egg ingestion is *not* a contraindication to measles immunization.

B. Pregnancy
1. Susceptible pregnant women who are exposed to rubeola should receive the Ig (see "Pharmaceutical Therapy" section) in an attempt to modify or prevent the infection.
2. Although no increase in risk of birth defects has been observed in mothers who were given live measles or MMR vaccine during pregnancy, there is a theoretical risk of such events. Measles vaccine is a live attenuated vaccine and is contraindicated in pregnancy.
3. Measles in the mother during delivery does not necessarily lead to measles in the neonate. Congenital measles (defined by the appearance of the measles rash within 10 days of birth) and postnatally acquired measles (rash appears within 14–30 days of birth) have been associated with a spectrum of illnesses ranging from mild to severe disease.
4. Measles vaccine may be administered postpartum to nonimmune mothers.

C. Pediatrics
1. Ig 0.25 mL/kg should be given to infants delivered from mothers with measles in the last week of pregnancy or the first postpartum week.
2. Children without evidence of measles immunity are recommended not to be admitted to school until the first dose of MMR has been administered.
3. A childhood maintenance visit between 11 and 12 years is recommended to update vaccinations.
4. Concern has been raised periodically about the possible link between receipt of MMR/MMRV and autism. A number of studies have now been performed that fail to demonstrate any such association.
5. Pediatric immunization:
a. Children older than 6 months: 1.5 mL in the outer aspect of the upper arm. Trivalent MMR vaccine should be used unless contraindicated in adults and children older than 12 months.

Scarlet Fever (Scarlatina)

Cheryl A. Glass and Jill C. Cash

Definition

A. Scarlet fever is an acute infectious disease with vascular response to bacterial exotoxin usually associated with Group A streptococcal (GAS) pharyngitis. Scarlatina may be present with pharyngitis. Scarlet fever is known as scarlatina in older literature references.
B. Scarlet fever is a nonsuppurative (inflammation without pus) complication of GAS. Development of the scarlet fever rash requires prior exposure to *Streptococcus pyogenes*.
C. There is no vaccine available for the prevention of scarlet fever.

Incidence

A. Scarlet fever is uncommon in children younger than 2 years. Highest incidence is in children 4 to 8 years of age. By the time children are 10 years old, 80% have developed lifelong protective antibodies against streptococcal pyrogenic exotoxins.

Pathogenesis

A. GAS and some strains of *Staphylococcus* are spread by respiratory droplet means and occasionally by direct physical contact from infected wounds, skin, or burns.
B. The incubation period is 12 hours to 4 days. It is communicable during the incubation period and clinical illness (around 10 days) and is no longer infectious after 24 hours of antibiotic therapy.
C. Exotoxin-mediated streptococcal infections range from localized skin disorders (e.g., bullous impetigo) to the systemic rash of scarlet fever to the uncommon but highly lethal streptococcal toxic shock syndrome.

Predisposing Factors

A. Strep throat pharyngitis; family history of recurrent strep infections
B. Direct physical contact with sputum or infected skin
C. Crowded situations (e.g., schools, institutional settings) or unsanitary living conditions
D. Occurs year-round but peaks in the winter and spring
E. Age: Children 5 to 15 years of age

Common Complaints

A. Abrupt onset of fever
B. Headache
C. Sore throat
D. Bright-red rash
E. Nausea and vomiting
F. Pruritus follows with the desquamating rash

Other Signs and Symptoms

A. Day 1: High fever (as high as 103°F–104°F), red sore throat, swollen tonsils (may have exudate), enlarged lymph nodes in neck, cough, and vomiting. Fever peaks by the second day and gradually returns to normal in 5 to 7 days. Fever abates within 12 to 24 hours after initiation of antibiotic therapy.
B. Day 2: The characteristic rash appears 12 to 48 hours after onset of fever. Bright red rash on the face, except around the mouth. **Bright red rash blanches on pressure, has a rough sandpaper texture, and appears first on flexor surfaces, then rapidly becomes more generalized. The rash lasts 4 to 10 days followed by desquamation of the hands and feet that disappears by the end of 3 weeks. Rash is typically present on the face, which usually has a flushed appearance with circumoral pallor. The rash is most marked in the skin folds. The rash often exhibits a linear petechial character in the antecubital fossae and axillary folds, known as Pastia's lines.**
C. Day 3
   1. Strawberry tongue; rash on the body increases and then spreads to neck, chest, back, then the entire body.
   2. Strawberry tongue appears as a thick, white coat with hypertrophied red papillae 24 to 48 hours after infection.
D. Days 4 to 5: The white coating disappears from the tongue.
E. Day 6: Rash fades and skin begins to peel; continues for 10 to 14 days; the palms of the hands and the soles of the feet are usually spared.

Subjective Data

A. Ask the patient/parent about the onset and progression of the rash, its color and duration, and all other symptoms.
B. Review other symptoms related to complications, such as ear pain, chest pain, and edema.
C. Review family history and possible contact with infected wounds or others with similar symptoms of pharyngitis.
D. Determine any new medications or contact exposures.
E. Determine if the patient is allergic to penicillin.
F. Review patient's recent history of impetigo.

Physical Examination

A. Check temperature, pulse, respirations, and blood pressure.
B. Inspect
   1. Conduct an ear and nose examination.
   2. Inspect the mouth and throat.
      a. Exudative tonsillitis preceding scarlet fever is often accompanied by erythematous oral mucous membranes, along with petechiae, and punctuate red macules on the hard and soft palate and uvula (i.e., Forchheimer spots).
      b. Day 1 or 2, a white coating covers the dorsum of the tongue with reddened papillae projecting through white before becoming a strawberry red tongue.
      c. Distinctive facial finding: Circumoral pallor
   3. Inspect the skin.
      a. Note the texture of the rash: "sandpaper" quality secondary to small 1- to 2-mm papular elevations.

b. The red rash starts on the head, with the soles of the feet and the palms spared.
c. The rash is most marked in the skin folds of the inguinal, axillary, antecubital, and abdominal areas and about pressure points.
d. The rash associated with scarlet fever may have a linear petechial characteristic known as Pastia's lines in the antecubital and axillary folds.
e. The erythematous rash blanches with pressure.
f. The rash desquamates with the fingers and toes most pronounced.

C. Auscultate
1. Heart
2. Lungs

D. Palpate
1. Abdomen for organomegaly
2. Lymph nodes in the neck: Tender and bilateral cervical nodes noted.

Diagnostic Tests

A. Throat culture remains the criterion standard for confirmation of GAS upper respiratory infection (URI). Vigorously swab the posterior pharynx, tonsils, and any exudates with a cotton or Dacron swab under strong illumination; avoid the lips, tongue, and buccal mucosa.
B. Rapid antigen detection testing via strep throat swab
C. White blood cells (WBCs) in scarlet fever may increase to 12,000 to 16,000 per mm^3, with a differential up to 955 polymorphonuclear lymphocytes.

Differential Diagnoses

A. Scarlet fever: Staphylococcal scarlet fever can be differentiated from streptococcal scarlet fever in the following ways:
1. There is no circumoral pallor or strawberry tongue with staphylococcal scarlet fever.
2. The erythematous skin is often painful or tender with staphylococcal infection.
3. Desquamation of the superficial epidermis occurs as with the streptococcal illness; if the superficial skin separates and sloughs after only a few days, the patient should be classified as having scalded skin syndrome. Desquamation, one of the most distinctive features of scarlet fever, begins 7 to 10 days after the resolution of the rash and may continue up to 6 weeks.

B. Kawasaki disease (KD): KD needs to be carefully differentiated from scarlet fever; KD has additional signs of conjunctivitis, cracking lips, and diarrhea.
C. Rubeola
D. Rubella
E. Toxic shock syndrome
F. Drug reaction

Plan

A. General interventions
1. Have the patient rest with no work or school. Patients should not return to work or school until they have completed a full 24 hours of antibiotics.
2. Prepare the patient for skin desquamation. The desquamating rash is self-limited but may take over 2 weeks for resolution. Skin emollients may be used.
3. Throat cultures on other household members may be necessary.
4. Acetaminophen (Tylenol) for temperature and pain relief

B. Patient teaching: Reinforce the need to comply with full antibiotic treatment even if the symptoms resolve.
C. Pharmaceutical therapy

The goal of antibiotic therapy is the prevention of acute rheumatic fever, acute glomerulonephritis, and other complications.

1. Tetracyclines and sulfonamides should not be used.
2. Drug of choice for streptococcal infections is penicillin by mouth or intramuscular injection. Azithromycin and erythromycin may be substituted for patients with penicillin allergies.
a. Adults
i. Penicillin V (Pen-Vee K): 250 mg orally three or four times daily for 10 days.
ii. Penicillin G benzathine (Bicillin L-A): 1.2 million units by intramuscular (IM) injection in one dose.
iii. Erythromycin (erythromycin ethylsuccinate [EES], E-mycin, or Ery-Tab): 250 mg every 6 hours orally before meals, or 500 mg orally every 12 hours before meals for 10 days.
b. Children
i. Children younger than 12 years: Penicillin V (Pen-Vee K) 25 to 50 mg/kg/d orally divided into three or four doses for 10 days; do not exceed 3 g/d.
ii. Children older than 12 years: Administer penicillin V as adults.
iii. Children less than 27 kg: Penicillin G benzathine 600,000 units IM as one dose.
iv. Children greater than 27 kg: Administer penicillin G benzathine as in adults.
v. Amoxicillin is often used in place of oral penicillin in children, since the taste of the oral suspension is more palatable. Administration of 50 mg/kg (maximum 1,000 mg) in a single dose orally for 10 days is as effective as oral penicillin V or amoxicillin given in multiple times per day for 10 days. **However, strict adherence on once-daily dosing must be ensured.**
vi. Erythromycin (E-mycin or Ery-Tab): 30 to 50 mg/kg four times a day for 10 days.
vii. Azithromycin 12 mg/kg once a day to a maximum of 500 mg/dose for 5 days (Food and Drug Administration [FDA] approval for 5-day therapy).

3. Antihistamines may be used to control pruritus that follows the desquamating rash.

Follow-Up

A. No follow-up is needed for patients with uncomplicated illnesses. Patients should return if they continue to have fever and increased throat or sinus pain.
B. Consider KD if fever persists more than 4 days.

Consultation/Referral

A. Refer the patient to a physician (i.e., ear, nose, and throat [ENT] or infectious disease specialist) for complications, such as unresolved otitis media, sinusitis, bacteremia, rheumatic fever, and glomerulonephritis.
B. Consult a dermatologist if the diagnosis is unclear.

Toxoplasmosis

Cheryl A. Glass and Jill C. Cash

Definition

A. Toxoplasmosis is caused by an intracellular protozoan parasite, *Toxoplasma gondii.* Cats are the primary host in which *T. gondii* can complete its reproductive cycle. Humans are the intermediate host. Toxoplasmosis is acquired through contact with infected cat feces, by eating raw or undercooked meat, and by eating soil-contaminated fruit or vegetables. In less developed countries, contaminated unfiltered water is an important source of infection, as is a transfusion or organ transplantation from an infected donor (rare).
B. Emphasis should not be placed on prior exposure to cats, since patients can acquire toxoplasma without direct contact with felines. Toxoplasmosis is one of the TORCH (toxoplasmosis, other [i.e., hepatitis and syphilis], rubella, cytomegalovirus, and herpes infections) infections. Toxoplasmosis causes central nervous system (CNS) disease in patients with AIDS and has perinatal consequences. Latent infection can persist for the life of the host.
C. There are three genotypes of *T. gondii*, types I, II, and III. Genotype II is generally responsible for congenital toxoplasmosis in the United States.
D. There is no vaccination available for the prevention of toxoplasmosis.

Incidence

A. Toxoplasmosis has a worldwide distribution. There is no association with cat ownership. The incidence of seropositivity in adults ranges from 9% (United States) to 85% (Europe). Adults most commonly acquire toxoplasmosis by environmental exposure, that is, ingestion of infectious oocysts usually from soil contamination with feline feces.
B. Once a person is infected, the parasite lies dormant in neural and muscle tissue and will never be eliminated. Approximately 50% of all pregnant women in the United States have been previously infected and are immune, whereas those who keep cats as pets have a higher seropositivity rate. The rate of primary infection during pregnancy ranges from 1 to 8 per 1,000.
C. The global annual incidence of congenital toxoplasmosis is approximately 190,100 cases, which poses a global health burden. The severity of congenital infection is dependent on the gestational age at the vertical transmission. The greatest risk to the fetus is vertical transmission in the first trimester. Thirty percent of exposed fetuses acquire the infection; however, 85% of live infants appear normal at birth.
D. Approximately 225,000 cases of toxoplasmosis are reported each year in the United States.
E. *T. gondii* is the third most common lethal foodborne disease in the United States.

Pathogenesis

A. *T. gondii* is the causative agent and an intracellular protozoan parasite. *T. gondii* is worldwide in distribution; cats, birds, and domesticated animals serve as reservoirs. *T. gondii* is recognized as a major cause of opportunistic infection in AIDS.
B. The incubation period is estimated to be on average 7 days (4- to 21-day range).
C. Routine screening for toxoplasmosis in pregnancy is not currently recommended.
- **1.** Maternal toxoplasmosis infection is acquired orally.
- **2.** Fetal infection results from transmission of parasites via the placenta (vertical transmission).
- **3.** Neonatal infection may also occur during vaginal delivery.

Predisposing Factors

A. Food sources
- **1.** Eating raw or undercooked meats, especially mutton, lamb, and pork
- **2.** Drinking unpasteurized goat milk
- **3.** Eating raw shellfish

B. Exposure to contaminated soil or garden, kitty litter, and cats
C. Immunocompromised state
- **1.** HIV infection/AIDS
- **2.** Cancer therapy
- **3.** Transplant recipients
- **4.** Prescribed immunosuppressive drugs

D. *T. gondii* has been documented as being acquired from blood or blood product transfusion and organ (i.e., heart) or bone marrow transplant from a seropositive donor with latent infection
E. Poor sanitary conditions
F. Consumption of contaminated unfiltered water
G. Occupational exposure
- **1.** Working with meat
- **2.** Landscaper

H. Travel to underdeveloped country

Common Complaints

A. 80% to 90% of acute *T. gondii* infectious hosts are asymptomatic.
B. Bilateral, symmetrical, nontender cervical adenopathy.
C. 30% of symptomatic patients have generalized lymphadenopathy.

Other Signs and Symptoms

A. Usually subclinical infection
- **1.** Fever

2. Arthralgia, malaise, and myalgia
3. Headache
4. Sore throat/pharyngitis
5. Skin rash: Diffuse nonpruritic maculopapular rash
6. Hepatosplenomegaly
7. Chorioretinitis: Ocular pain and loss of visual acuity (most frequent, permanent manifestation of toxoplasmic infection)

B. Pregnancy
1. Intrauterine growth retardation (IUGR) or low birth weight
2. Hydrocephaly
3. Microcephaly
4. Anemia

C. CNS toxoplasmosis
1. **Headache, dull and constant, is an almost universal symptom of cerebral lesions in AIDS patients.**
2. Fever
3. Lethargy
4. Altered mental state
5. Seizures
6. Weakness
7. Hemiparesis
8. Cranial nerve disturbances
9. Sensory abnormalities
10. Movement disorders
11. Neuropsychiatric manifestations: Toxoplasmosis is a significant factor in the causation of mental retardation and blindness.

Subjective Data

A. Review onset, course, and duration of symptoms.
B. Determine if the patient is pregnant.
C. Review presence of an indoor cat and contact with kitty litter.
D. Rule out other illnesses with review of symptoms such as pharyngitis (mononucleosis).
E. Elicit initial site of rash and progression to other body areas.
F. Determine any new medications and contact exposures.
G. Rule out other family members with similar symptoms.
H. Review HIV status.
I. Review ingestion of raw/rare or undercooked meats, raw shellfish, and unpasteurized goat milk.
J. Review recent travel to an underdeveloped country (untreated water).
K. Review occupational exposure.

Physical Examination

A. Check temperature, pulse, respirations, and blood pressure.
B. Inspect
1. Conduct ear, nose, and throat examination and careful funduscopic examination.

A funduscopic examination may reveal yellow-white areas of retinitis with fluffy borders. Diagnosis of ocular toxoplasmosis is based on observation of characteristic retinal lesions in conjunction with toxoplasma-specific serum immunoglobulin G (IgG) or immunoglobulin M (IgM) antibodies.

2. Complete a dermal examination.

C. Auscultate
1. Heart
2. Lungs

D. Palpate
1. Palpate all lymph nodes, especially cervical nodes. Lymph nodes are usually smaller than 3 cm in size and nonfluctuant.
2. Abdomen
3. Joints, noting swelling, erythema, or pain with examination.

E. Neurologic examination: Conduct a mental status evaluation.

Diagnostic Tests

A. Enzyme-linked immunosorbent assay (ELISA) is the most commonly employed test due to overall performance and cost for toxoplasmosis IgG and IgM antibody titer. Maternal infections usually are confirmed by a fourfold rise in the serum IgG.
B. Serial titers: No single level of IgG antibody can be used to determine the duration of the infection. IgG-specific antibodies achieve peak concentration 1 to 2 months after exposure and remain positive indefinitely.
C. Complete blood count (CBC) with differential
D. HIV (rule out)
E. Pregnancy test if indicated
F. Culture: Tissue smears, tissue section, and body fluids for presence of *T. gondii* may be considered in neonates. It takes 3 to 6 weeks to confirm the diagnosis.
G. CT scan or MRI (usually superior to CT scan)

Differential Diagnoses

A. Toxoplasmosis
B. Epstein–Barr virus (EBV)
C. Cytomegalovirus (CMV [CMV retinitis])
D. Cat scratch disease
E. Tuberculosis
F. Syphilis
G. Sarcoidosis
H. Hodgkin's disease
I. Lymphoma
J. Viral syndrome
K. HIV
L. Mononucleosis
M. Pneumocystis carinii pneumonia
N. Varicella zoster
O. Fungal infection of eye

Plan

A. Patient teaching: **Handwashing is the single most important measure to reduce transmission of *T. gondii*.** Patient teaching: *See Section III: Patient Teaching Guide for this chapter, "Toxoplasmosis."* ◀
B. Pharmaceutical therapy

1. Treatment is rarely necessary because most clinical illnesses resolve spontaneously; the exception is during pregnancy.
2. Treatment is usually given for 2 to 4 weeks.
   a. Nonpregnant adults: One of two regimens is typically prescribed:
      i. Pyrimethamine: 100 mg loading dose then 25 to 50 mg by mouth daily; *plus* sulfadiazine 2 to 4 g/d by mouth in divided doses; *plus* leucovorin calcium (folinic acid) 10 to 25 mg by mouth daily.
      ii. Pyrimethamine: 100 mg loading dose, then 25 to 50 mg by mouth daily; *plus* clindamycin 300 mg by mouth four times a day; *plus* leucovorin calcium (folinic acid) 10 to 25 mg by mouth daily.
   b. Pregnancy: Despite the lack of evidence of treatment efficacy, prenatal treatment is usually offered to pregnant women who are diagnosed with toxoplasmosis.
      i. Spiramycin alone: 1 g orally every 8 hours without food. The drug is available in the United States for use in pregnancy from Rhone-Poulenc (Montreal, Quebec) if an Investigation New Drug number is obtained from the FDA under the "compassionate use" pathway.
      ii. Three-week course of pyrimethamine 50 mg once a day orally or 25 mg twice a day; *and* sulfadiazine 3 g/d orally divided into two or three doses *alternating* with a 3-week course of spiramycin 1 g orally three times a day until delivery.
      iii. Pyrimethamine 25 mg once per day by mouth *and* sulfadiazine 4 g/d orally divided into two to four doses until term.
      iv. Leucovorin calcium (folinic acid) 10 to 25 mg/d orally is added during pyrimethamine and sulfadiazine administration to prevent bone marrow suppression.
   c. Children
      i. Trimethoprim-sulfamethoxazole 150 to 750 mg/m^2/d in two divided doses daily
      ii. For children 1 month of age or older: Dapsone 2 mg/kg (maximum of 25 mg, orally every day; *plus* pyrimethamine 1 mg/kg orally every day; *plus* leucovorin 5 mg orally every 3 days)
   d. Persons with compromised immune system:
      i. Trimethoprim 10 mg/kg/daily *plus* sulfamethoxazole 50 mg/kg/daily by mouth. May be considered as a nonpyrimethamine alternative for AIDS patients if unable to tolerate usual adult therapy noted previously.
      ii. Administering dapsone with pyrimethamine appears to provide effective chemoprophylaxis in HIV patients seropositive for *T. gondii* who have CD4 cell counts lower than 200. However, rash, fever, and hemolytic anemia are common adverse effects, often necessitating cessation of therapy.
      iii. For AIDS patients, after primary therapy, lifelong prophylaxis for recurrence of toxoplasmosis is required for as long as they are immunosuppressed.

Follow-Up

A. Follow up in 1 week to evaluate for secondary complications.

B. Pyrimethamine is a folic acid antagonist that can cause dose-related bone marrow suppression with resultant anemia, leukopenia, and thrombocytopenia. Sulfadiazine is another folic acid antagonist, works synergistically with pyrimethamine, and can cause bone marrow suppression and reversible acute renal failure. Patients should return for laboratory monitoring (complete blood count [CBC] and platelet counts) weekly.

Consultation/Referral

A. Consultation is needed for all patients; comanage with a physician/specialist.

B. Refer the patient to an obstetrician if she is pregnant.

C. Ophthalmologist medication recommendation depends on the size of the eye lesion, the location, and the characteristics of the lesion (active acute vs. chronic not progressing).

Individual Considerations

A. Pregnancy
   1. Routine prenatal screening is not the standard of care secondary to costs. Many women have antibodies before pregnancy that protect the fetus.
   2. Transplacental infection increases the incidence of first-trimester spontaneous abortion, IUGR, preterm birth, neonatal anomalies, and stillbirth.
   3. Pyrimethamine is a folic acid antagonist and should not be given in the first trimester.
   4. Sulfadiazine should not be given in the third trimester secondary to the increased incidence of jaundice in the neonate.
   5. Transmission of toxoplasmosis in breast milk has not been demonstrated. Pyrimethamine is excreted in breast milk; however, the WHO and the Academy of Pediatrics (AAP) classify it as compatible with breastfeeding.

B. Pediatrics
   1. 70% to 90% of affected infants with congenital infection may be asymptomatic at birth or may present with low birth weight, enlarged liver and spleen, jaundice, and anemia.
      a. Signs of congenital toxoplasmosis at birth can include maculopapular rash, generalized lymphadenopathy, hepatomegaly, splenomegaly, jaundice, and thrombocytopenia.
      b. Cerebral calcifications may be demonstrated by radiography, ultrasound, or CT of the head.
      c. Characteristic retinal lesions (chorioretinitis) develop in up to 85% of young adults after

untreated congenital infection. Acute ocular involvement manifests as blurred vision.

d. Ocular disease can become reactivated years after the initial infection in health and immunocompromised people.

2. Complications including visual impairment from chorioretinitis or learning disabilities or mental retardation damage may develop several years later.

3. Treatment consists of drug therapy for the first year of life (see "Pharmaceutical therapy" section), which appears to limit further CNS injury but does not reverse the prenatal damage already sustained by the neonate.

4. Corticosteroids also may be administered to infants with chorioretinitis.

C. AIDS patients

1. Patients with AIDS who have antibodies to *T. gondii* and a CD4 count of 100 cells/mm^3 should be considered at high risk for the development of clinical disease. Reactivation of latent infection in the CNS is a common HIV- and AIDS-related complication.

2. Patients with a CD4 count less than 100 cells/mm^3 should receive prophylaxis against toxoplasmosis.

3. Serology in HIV-infected patients is used mainly to identify those at risk for developing toxoplasmosis. Therefore, all HIV-positive patients should be tested for the presence of IgG antibodies.

Varicella (Chickenpox)

Cheryl A. Glass and Jill C. Cash

Definition

A. Varicella, commonly called chickenpox, is a viral disease with a vesicular rash that occurs in crops. It manifests as a generalized, pruritic, vesicular rash. Varicella-zoster virus (VZV) infection causes two clinically distinct forms of disease: Varicella (chickenpox) and herpes zoster (shingles).

1. Primary VZV results in the diffuse vesicular rash of chickenpox.

2. VZV remains dormant in the sensory nerve roots for life. Reactivation of the virus is known as shingles.

a. With shingles, the virus migrates along sensory nerve via dermatomes. The symptoms include pain, sensory loss, and neurologic complications.

b. A diagnostic clue of shingles is sensory symptoms that do not cross the midline.

c. Postherpetic neuralgia is a prolonged complication from shingles.

B. Varicella is considered one of the TORCH (toxoplasmosis, other [i.e., hepatitis and syphilis], rubella, cytomegalovirus, and herpes infections) infections. Varicella infection can be fatal for an infant if the mother develops varicella from 5 days before to 2 days after delivery. A newborn is protected for several months from chickenpox if the mother had the disease before or during pregnancy. Infant immunity diminishes in 4 to 12 months.

C. There are two available vaccines for the prevention of varicella. The measles–mumps–rubella–varicella (MMRV) and a monovalent varicella vaccine are currently available. The Academy of Pediatrics (AAP) notes that the quadrivalent MMRV is preferred to giving two separate injections secondary to the additional pain and the risk of the child falling behind in his or her immunization schedule.

1. Both the monovalent and the quadrivalent immunizations carry a risk of febrile seizures. A personal or family history of seizures is considered a precaution for the administration of the MMRV.

2. The AAP also advises that with personal or family history of seizures, the measles–mumps–rubella (MMR) and the varicella vaccine should be administered as separate immunizations. Varicella vaccine may be given simultaneously with MMR vaccine, but separate syringes and injection sites must be used. If not given simultaneously, the interval between administration of varicella vaccine and MMR should be at least 28 days apart.

Incidence

A. Infants are generally protected in the first few months through passive immunity. The peak incidence shifting from children younger than 10 years to children between 10 and 14 years of age demonstrates the highest incidence following the implementation of universal immunization in 1995. Varicella tends to be more severe in adolescents and adults. Hemorrhagic varicella is much more common among immunocompromised patients. Immunity is generally considered lifelong.

B. The rate of herpes zoster after varicella vaccination was 2.6/100,000 according to the 1998 Centers for Disease Control and Prevention (CDC) unpublished data. The incidence of herpes zoster after natural varicella infection among healthy children less than 20 years old is 68/100,000; for all ages, the incidence is 215/100,000.

C. Varicella incidence has greatly declined since the chickenpox vaccine has become available in the United States. It is predicted that varicella deaths, outbreaks, and hospitalizations have been greatly reduced.

D. Seasonal incidence of VZV peaks in the months of March through May.

E. The rate of chickenpox is 5 persons per 1,000.

F. After the primary infection, the risk of shingles increases with age. The lifetime risk of herpes zoster infection is 15% to 20%.

G. The incidence of congenital varicella is 1% to 2% if the maternal infection occurs before 20 weeks gestation.

Pathogenesis

A. VZV, herpesvirus 3, is a member of the herpesvirus family. Humans are the only source of infection for this highly contagious virus infecting over 90% of susceptible household contacts. Person-to-person transmission occurs primarily by direct contact with a patient with varicella or zoster, and it occasionally occurs by airborne droplet spread, from respiratory secretions spread onto the conjunctival or nasal/oral mucosal, and from direct contact with vesicular zoster lesions. In utero infections also occur from transplacental passage of the virus during maternal varicella infection.

B. The incubation period is 14 to 16 days. It is communicable 1 to 2 days to 1 week before macular eruption and until lesions crust over (about 1 week).

Predisposing Factors

A. Exposure to someone with the varicella virus
  1. Direct contact with skin lesions or by respiratory tract secretions
  2. Direct contact with patients with shingles can induce chickenpox in susceptible health care workers.
B. Compromised immune system
C. Nosocomial transmission is well documented in pediatric units, but transmission is extremely rare in newborn nurseries.
D. Late winter and early spring

Common Complaints

A. Low-grade fever
B. Mild malaise
C. Skin lesions or rash: Characteristic rash is pruritic, vesicular exanthem occurring in crops that begin on the head and neck and progress to involve the trunk and extremities. Blisters collapse within 24 hours to 1 week and crust over to form scabs. Skin eruptions appear almost anywhere on the body, including the scalp; penis; and inside the mouth, nose, throat, and vagina.
D. Itching
E. Myalgia 1 to 4 days before onset of rash

Other Signs and Symptoms

A. Children may have a mild prodrome to bacterial infections.
B. Adults may develop varicella pneumonitis. (The risk of pneumonitis is higher in smokers than in nonsmokers.)
C. Cough
D. Headache
E. Respiratory symptoms: Cough and chest discomfort. Respiratory symptoms usually develop shortly after cutaneous eruption. Respiratory failure in pregnancy can be rapid.
F. Abdominal pain lasting 1 to 2 days

Subjective Data

A. Review the onset, duration, and course of symptoms.
B. Elicit exposure information when noting characteristic rash, the time it started, spread of the rash or lesions, and characteristic changes.
C. Review any pulmonary or nervous system problems, such as seizures, that occur as complications.
D. Determine if the person has HIV, is immunocompromised, or is pregnant.
E. Determine the caregiver's immunity status to varicella.
F. Review the patient's immunization history.
G. Review all medication, including over-the-counter (OTC) and herbal products.

Physical Examination

A. Check temperature, pulse, respirations, and blood pressure.
B. Inspect
  1. Conduct a dermal examination, especially the hairline.
  2. Inspect the buccal mucosa.
  3. Conduct an ear, nose, and throat examination and a detailed eye examination.
  4. Shingles: Note location of lesions; they usually involve only one to three dermatomes.
C. Auscultate
  1. Heart
  2. Lungs
D. Palpate
  1. Neck and lymph nodes.

Diagnostic Tests

A. Diagnosis is usually determined by the appearance of the skin eruptions, and laboratory tests are not necessary.
B. Enzyme-linked immunosorbent assay (ELISA)
C. Tissue culture of vesicular fluid or tissue biopsy (requires up to a week for result).
D. Varicella immunoglobulin G (IgG) and IgM: VZV-specific IgM is present within 5 days of onset of the rash and lasts 4 to 5 weeks. A significant increase in varicella IgG antibody by standard serologic assay can confirm a diagnosis retrospectively. These antibody tests are not as reliable in immunocompromised people.
E. Pregnancy test if indicated; if positive, order the following:
  1. Anti-VZV IgG to establish immunity
  2. Tzanck smear of suspicious lesions
  3. Culture lesion for herpes simplex
F. Polymerase chain reaction (PCR) of vesicular swabs or scrapings, scabs for crusted lesions, or tissue biopsy.
G. Chest x-ray, if indicated, to rule out pneumonia.
H. Genotyping of the virus is available free of charge through a specialized CDC reference lab. The CDC reference lab contact number is 404-639-0066. Merck & Company (contact number 1-800-672-6372) also performs genotyping through a safety research program.

Differential Diagnoses

A. Varicella (chickenpox)
B. Herpes simplex
C. Scabies
D. Impetigo
E. Coxsackievirus
F. Insect or spider bite
G. Drug reaction
H. Secondary syphilis
I. Measles
J. Rubella
K. Rocky Mountain spotted fever (RMSF)
L. Scabies

Plan

A. General interventions

1. Avoid contact with persons infected with chickenpox. Patients with varicella should avoid contact with others. Health care workers should be immune to varicella. Determine immunity status with varicella IgG antibody titer if status unknown.

2. Strict isolation should be enforced. Varicella is contagious 1 week before outbreak and until the lesions crust over (about 1 week). Isolation is a precaution until the vesicles dry.

3. Order oatmeal baths (Aveeno) for comfort. Spray starch may also be sprayed on lesions to assist with severe itching.

B. Patient teaching

▶ **1.** Patient teaching: *See Section III: Patient Teaching Guide for this chapter, "Chickenpox (Varicella)."*

2. Lesions that can be covered pose little risk to a susceptible person because transmission usually occurs from direct contact with the fluid from the lesion. Clothing or a dressing should cover lesions until they have crusted.

3. Scarring can occur from secondary infection of lesions; encourage good handwashing and no scratching.

C. Pharmaceutical therapy

1. Children with varicella should not receive salicylates, such as aspirin, or salicylate-containing products due to the increased risk of Reye's syndrome. Acetaminophen (Tylenol) may be used as needed for fever.

2. Acyclovir therapy is *not* recommended routinely for treatment of uncomplicated varicella in otherwise healthy children.

3. Acyclovir is recommended if it can be initiated within the first 24 hours after the onset of rash in the following groups:

a. Otherwise healthy, nonpregnant individuals 13 years of age or older

b. Children older than 12 months with a chronic cutaneous or pulmonary disorder, and those receiving long-term salicylate therapy

c. Children receiving a short, intermittent, or aerosolized course of corticosteroids (if possible, discontinue corticosteroids)

4. If therapy can be initiated within the first 24 hours of rash onset, prescribe oral acyclovir 20 mg/kg/dose in four divided doses for 5 days (maximum dose is 800 mg/dose four times daily); the usual dose for adults is 800 mg four times a day. Patients on oral acyclovir should be well hydrated during therapy.

5. Acyclovir by intravenous (IV) infusion is recommended for treatment of immunocompromised patients and patients with serious complications such as varicella pneumonia or encephalitis. Acyclovir IV dosage is 10 mg/kg every 8 hours for 7 days.

6. Varicella-zoster immune globulin (VZIG) is no longer available. The only manufacturer of this product has ceased production.

7. Systemic antipruritic: Diphenhydramine HCl (Benadryl)

a. Adults: 25 to 50 mg every 4 to 6 hours (maximum adult dosage 300 mg/d)

b. Children

i. Not recommended for neonates.

ii. Children younger than 6 years: Dosage must be individualized.

iii. Children 6 to 12 years of age: 12.5 to 25 mg every 4 to 6 hours (maximum children dosage 150 mg/d)

8. Varicella vaccine may be given simultaneously with MMR vaccine, but separate syringes and injection sites must be used. If not given simultaneously, the interval between administration of varicella vaccine and MMR should be at least 1 month.

9. Antihistamines are helpful in the symptomatic treatment of pruritus.

10. The use of corticosteroids for patients with shingles to prevent postherpetic neuralgia is controversial.

11. Treatment for postherpetic neuralgia includes gabapentin, pregabalin, tricyclic antidepressants, phenytoin, carbamazepine, cimetidine, and topical capsaicin.

Follow-Up

A. No follow-up is necessary in uncomplicated cases.

B. Have the patient return to the office for any secondary skin infections, conjunctival involvement, central nervous system (CNS) problems such as encephalitis and meningitis, or pneumonia.

Consultation/Referral

A. Refer the patient to a physician if pregnant; varicella pneumonia in pregnancy is a medical emergency.

Individual Considerations

A. Pregnancy

1. Varicella vaccine should not be administered to pregnant women.

a. Women are advised not to get pregnant for at least 1 month following the varicella immunization.

b. A pregnant mother or household member is not a contraindication for immunization for a child in the household.

2. When postpubertal females are immunized, pregnancy should be avoided for at least 1 month after immunization.

3. VZIG: Maternal therapy's aim is to reduce maternal morbidity; whether it protects the fetus is unknown.

4. Reporting by telephone of inadvertent immunization when the varicella-zoster-containing vaccine is given during pregnancy is encouraged: 1-800-986-8999 or via the Internet at www.merckpregnancyregistries.com/varivax.html

5. Maternal complications of active varicella infection may include preterm labor, encephalitis, and varicella pneumonia. Mortality rate in gravid females is 10%. The profound maternal hypoxia that occurs in varicella pneumonia is associated with increased risk of spontaneous abortion and stillbirth.

6. Fetal complications of active varicella infection may include intrauterine growth retardation (IUGR), limb reduction defects, and eye defects.

7. Acyclovir is a category B drug based on the Food and Drug Administration (FDA) drug classification in pregnancy. IV acyclovir is recommended for the pregnant patient with serious complications of varicella. VariZIG or intravenous immunoglobulin (IVIG) can be used during pregnancy for susceptible women who are exposed to VZV.

B. Pediatrics

1. Varicella can develop between 1 and 16 days of life in infants born to mothers with active live varicella at delivery.

2. Neonates usually have no prodrome or mild signs and symptoms with slight malaise and low-grade fever. Neonatal varicella is a serious illness associated with up to a 25% mortality rate. Complications include conjunctival involvement, secondary bacterial infection, viral pneumonia, encephalitis, aseptic meningitis, myelitis, Guillain–Barré syndrome, and Reye's syndrome.

3. Children entering day-care facilities and schools should have received varicella vaccine or have evidence of immunity.

4. Children with varicella should not receive salicylates or salicylate-containing products due to the risk for Reye's syndrome.

5. Children with varicella who have been excluded from child care may return when all lesions have dried and crusted.

C. Adults

1. Adult patients usually have a prodrome and more severe illness than children. Adults have a 25% increased risk of mortality.

2. Shingles (reactivated chickenpox) appears as grouped vesicular lesions distributed in one to three sensory dermatomes, sometimes accompanied by pain localized to the area. Systemic symptoms are few.

3. A recommendation for varicella vaccination includes persons at high risk for exposure, which include adolescents and adults who live in households with children.

D. Immunocompromised: IV antiviral therapy is recommended for immunocompromised patients, including patients being treated with chronic corticosteroids. Therapy initiated early in the course of illness, especially within 24 hours of rash onset, maximizes efficacy. Oral acyclovir should not be used to treat immunocompromised children with varicella because of poor bioavailability.

West Nile Virus

Cheryl A. Glass and Jill C. Cash

Definition

West Nile Virus (WNV) disease is a mosquito-borne viral illness caused by one of the most widely distributed arthropod-borne (arbovirus) viruses. WNV is a member of the genus *Flavivirus* group, meaning it is a single-strand RNA virus. WNV is transmitted from infected animal hosts, typically wild birds, to humans via the most common types of mosquitoes. Once a patient recovers from WNV disease, he or she is thought to have a lifelong immunity to the disease. There is no immunization for WNV.

The two categories of WNV disease are nonneuroinvasive and neuroinvasive.

A. Nonneuroinvasive disease is less severe and often presents as a febrile illness.

B. Neuroinvasive disease leads to encephalitis, meningitis, and flaccid paralysis and requires much more intensive treatment.

Incidence

A. WNV is a reportable disease that allows the Centers for Disease Control and Prevention (CDC) to maintain significant surveillance data and statistics. In 2016, WNV cases were reported in 48 states, with the highest number of cases reported in Texas, California, Colorado, and Mississippi.

B. Approximately 20,000 new cases occur in North America each year, with 1 in 150 patients developing severe neurologic disease; 3% to 15% of those developing severe neurologic disease will die.

C. WNV was first noted in North America in 1999. WNV is endemic in the Middle East, Africa, and Asia.

D. Human WNV infections usually begin in midsummer and decline in September, correlating with peak mosquito activity. Mosquito bites are most likely to occur during peak feeding times during dawn and dusk. Prolonged contact or multiple mosquito bites increase the risk of developing WNV.

Pathogenesis

A. Mosquitoes are infected with WNV when feeding on an infected animal host. Wild birds are the most common source of infection, although other animals, such as horses and chickens, can be animal hosts. The virus is delivered to the human via mosquito bite when the mosquito's saliva is deposited in the human skin cells. The virus replicates in the skin cells and migrates to the lymph nodes and various organs. Infected immune cells are able to transverse the blood–brain barrier and infect the brain parenchyma leading to encephalitis and meningitis. The typical incubation period for WNV is 3 to 14 days.

Predisposing Factors

A. Time of year: Late summer and early fall

B. Region: Living in or traveling to a region with a higher number of reported cases

C. Work or recreational outdoor exposure

D. Homelessness

E. Age: Most likely to occur in children and young adults with most serious disease occurring in the elderly and infants

Common Complaints

A. Nonneuroinvasive WNV

1. Up to 80% of persons are asymptomatic

2. Fever
3. Headache
4. Myalgia
5. Arthralgias
6. Fatigue
7. Gastrointestinal (GI) symptoms: Nausea, vomiting, and diarrhea
8. Maculopapular rash: Usually noted on chest, back, and arms and occurs in 20% to 50% of patients. The presence of the rash represents a decreased risk of neuroinvasive disease.

Other Signs and Symptoms

A. Abdominal pain
B. Eye pain
C. Irregular heart rhythm

Potential Complications

A. Meningitis: Stiff neck, photophobia, focal neurologic deficits, and higher fever (up to 104°F)
B. Encephalitis: Mental status changes, stupor, confusion, coma, movement disorders, focal neurologic deficits, personality changes, higher fever (up to 104°F), and seizures
C. Flaccid paralysis: Cranial nerve palsy, vertigo, dysarthria, dysphagia, respiratory failure
D. Other rare complications:
1. Cardiac dysrhythmia
2. Myocarditis
3. Rhabdomyolysis
4. Optic neuritis
5. Uveitis
6. Chorioretinitis
7. Orchitis
8. Pancreatitis
9. Hepatitis

Subjective Data

A. Review the onset, course, and duration of symptoms, especially fever, rash, headache, and myalgia.
B. Ask patient to describe any neurologic symptoms, changes in mental status, stiff neck, photophobia, and seizures.
C. Review symptoms of other family members or coworkers who are also ill.
D. Ask the patient to recall what activity brought about or preceded his or her symptoms.
E. Ask patient what steps he or she has taken to treat symptoms at home.
F. Review the patient's medical history for any chronic illnesses.
G. Review all medications, including over-the-counter (OTC) and herbal products.
H. Review history of mosquito bites and any preventive steps taken such as use of insect repellent.
1. Outdoor work activities
2. Outdoor recreational activities
3. Review recent travel
I. Evaluate living conditions for exposure risks

Physical Examination

Patients presenting with neurological symptoms should be quickly assessed and referred to a neurologist for immediate evaluation of symptoms.

A. Check temperature, pulse, blood pressure, and respirations.
B. Inspect
1. Observe general overall appearance noting weakness, difficulty breathing, or changes in affect, speech, or level of consciousness (LOC).
2. Assess hydration status.
3. Ophthalmic examination: Assess the presence of papilledema.
4. Inspect the face for muscle weakness or drooping.
5. Dermal inspection for the presence of a maculopapular rash, especially on the abdomen, back, and arms.
6. Children
a. Observe for seizure activity
b. Note LOC (playful vs. lethargic)
C. Auscultate
1. Heart for dysrhythmias
2. All lung fields for adventitious breath sounds
D. Palpate
1. Skin for signs of dehydration—poor skin turgor
2. The neck and lymph nodes: Preauricular, posterior auricular, submental and sublingual, anterior cervical chain, and supraclavicular nodes
3. Abdomen for tenderness and/or organomegaly
E. Mental status and neurologic examination
1. Administer mental status examination to look for confusion, stupor, and changes in LOC.
2. Complete cranial nerve testing: Focus on visual fields, extraocular movement (EOM) of a transient downbeat nystagmus, facial muscle movement and strength, and gag reflex.
3. Muscle strength testing and testing for sensation in all extremities
4. Test reflexes
a. Deep tendon reflexes
b. Babinski reflex is performed by running the reflex hammer up the midline of the sole of the foot from heel to the base of the toes (both feet are tested).
i. A normal reaction is for the toes to either remain still or else to curl downward.
ii. A positive Babinski is noted when the big toe points upward and the other toes fan out *except for infants.*
5. Assess for meningeal signs.
a. Signs of meningeal irritation include nuchal rigidity.
b. Assess for positive Brudzinski's and Kernig's signs (refer to Figures 16.1 and 16.2).
6. Brudzinski's sign: Place the patient supine and flex the head upward. Resulting flexion of both hips, knees, and ankles with neck flexion indicates meningeal irritation.

7. Kernig's sign: Place the patient supine; keeping one leg straight, flex the other hip and knee to a bent knee to form a 90° angle. Slowly extend the lower leg. This places a stretch on the meninges, resulting in pain and spasm for the hamstring muscle. Resistance to further extension can be felt.

Diagnostic Tests

A. **WNV immunoglobulin M (IgM) antibody capture enzyme-linked immunosorbent assay (MAC-ELISA) is the gold standard diagnostic test.** A positive result would indicate WNV.
B. If there is concern that the illness could have been caused by another type of flavivirus, an additional test, the plaque reduction neutralization test, is used to identify false-positive MAC-ELISA test results.
C. Complete blood count (CBC) with differential: Will show increased leukocytes.
D. For patients with neuroinvasive disease
  1. Lumbar puncture—positive for WNV—will show pleocytosis, increased lymphocytes, increased protein, and normal glucose. The MAC-ELISA test should be performed on cerebrospinal fluid (CSF) when lumbar puncture is completed.
  2. Imaging: MRI of the brain and spinal cord is the preferred imaging test. MRI may show meningeal inflammation and bilateral lesions.
  3. EEG: May show generalized slowness.

Differential Diagnoses

A. Nonneuroinvasive WNV
  1. WNV
  2. Other viral causes of febrile illness
B. Neuroinvasive WNV
  1. Other viral causes of encephalitis: St. Louis equine encephalitis, California encephalitis, Western and Eastern encephalitis
  2. Acute poliomyelitis
  3. Postpolio syndrome
  4. Guillain–Barré syndrome
  5. Multiple sclerosis
  6. Vertebrobasilar stroke

Plan

A. General interventions
  1. WNV should be reported to the health department for surveillance purposes. Special populations may be subject to follow-up.
  2. Care is primarily supportive, treating symptoms such as fever, nausea/vomiting, and diarrhea.
  3. Neuroinvasive disease: Patients presenting with neurological symptoms should be quickly assessed and referred to a neurologist for immediate evaluation and treatment of acute symptoms.
B. Patient teaching
  1. Educate about expected signs and symptoms of WNV acute febrile illness.
  2. Explain signs and symptoms that would require immediate medical evaluation such as mental status changes, stiff neck, and neurological symptoms.
  3. Instruct the patient to rest as needed. The patient may expect fatigue to continue for up to 3 weeks.
C. Dietary management
  1. There are no specific dietary recommendations for WNV.
  2. Encourage the patient to drink plenty of fluids to prevent dehydration.
  3. If the patient is experiencing nausea and vomiting, meals should be light and nonspicy and should be taken in smaller amounts more frequently.
D. Pharmaceutical therapy
  1. Utilize supportive therapy such as acetaminophen for fever, antiemetics for nausea and vomiting, and antidiarrheal medications for diarrhea.

Follow-Up

A. Follow-up would be determined by the patient's needs, severity of acute symptoms, and risk of complications.

Consultation/Referral

A. Neuroinvasive disease: Refer to neurologist immediately.
  1. For longer term relief from neuroinvasive disease, the patient may benefit from a referral to a neuropsychologist, rehabilitation specialist, physical therapist, occupational therapist, and/or speech therapist.
B. Consider an infectious disease specialist if there is difficulty with identifying the infectious agent.

Individual Considerations

A. Pregnancy
  1. There has been no causal relationship found between WNV during pregnancy and fetal abnormalities. A small number of infants, born to women who developed WNV within 3 weeks before delivery, were found to have symptomatic WNV disease shortly after birth.
  2. If WNV is diagnosed during the last few weeks of pregnancy, a detailed examination of the newborn should be completed and steps taken to monitor for signs and symptoms of the disease in the days and weeks after the birth.
  3. All cases of WNV in pregnant women should be reported to the health department so that the cases can be followed to determine the outcome of the pregnancies.
  4. The virus has been found in breast milk and, in rare cases, breastfeeding has been linked to development of WNV in infants. The benefits of breastfeeding outweigh the risks of WNV disease; therefore, mothers should be encouraged to breastfeed.
  5. Pregnant women can use insect repellent products containing N-diethylmetatoluamide (DEET) without adverse effects.

B. Pediatrics

1. Infants are more likely to suffer a more serious illness with WNV. A thorough assessment and educating the parent to recognize important signs and symptoms are crucial.

2. The Academy of Pediatrics (AAP) recommends that insect repellents should not be applied to children younger than 2 months.

C. Geriatrics

1. Older adults are more likely to suffer more serious illness and are more likely to develop neuroinvasive disease. Close attention should be given to the mental status examination and neurologic examination of the elderly.

Zika Virus Infection

Jill C. Cash

Definition

A. Zika virus is an arthropod-borne virus that is transmitted by the *Aedes* species mosquito. The virus is in the same family as the dengue virus, yellow fever virus, and West Nile virus. It was initially found in the rhesus monkey in 1947 and then detected in humans in 1952 in Uganda and Tanzania. The Zika virus infection has been documented in Africa, Southeast Asia, the Pacific Islands, and has now spread to the Americas. Mosquito-borne transmission has not been reported in the United States; however, cases of infection have been reported in male and pregnant and nonpregnant female travelers who were exposed in other countries from the mosquito-borne illness.

B. Congenital microcephaly is a known pregnancy complication of Zika viral infection. Vertical transmission to the fetus occurs from the primary infected mother or can occur from the infected male to noninfected female.

Incidence

A. The first case of congenital microcephaly in the United States was reported in January 2016 in Hawaii in which the pregnant woman had lived in Brazil during her pregnancy.

B. In Texas, there has been documentation of sexually transmitted Zika virus infection in February 2016.

C. During the months of January through June 2016, reports from New York City show that approximately 3,605 travelers were exposed to the Zika virus in other countries and 182 of those patients tested positive for the Zika virus in the United States.

Pathogenesis

A. Incubation period is unknown; however, it is thought to be within a few days to 7–12 days.

B. The Zika virus is transmitted to humans by an infected mosquito that bites the person.

C. The virus is detected in urine, blood, semen, saliva, female genital secretions, breast milk, amniotic fluid, and cerebral spinal fluid.

D. The virus can be transmitted by maternal–fetal transmission, sex (vaginal, anal, and oral), blood transfusion, organ transplantation, and exposure in the laboratory from body fluids.

Predisposing Factors

A. Recent travel to Brazil or other countries at high risk for Zika virus. See the Centers for Disease Control and Prevention (CDC) website for a listing of countries: www.CDC.gov

B. Exposure to body fluids from documented infected person

C. Sexual contact with person confirmed with Zika virus

D. Vertical transmission from infected mother

Common Complaints

Two or more of the following symptoms appear; symptoms may be mild and/or may not be recognized by the patient.

A. Acute-onset low-grade fever

B. Maculopapular pruritic rash

C. Arthralgia of small joints (hand and feet)

D. Conjunctivitis (nonpurulent)

Other Signs and Symptoms

A. Headache

B. Malaise

C. Retro-orbital (eye) pain

D. Asthenia

E. Less common symptoms may include gastrointestinal symptoms (nausea, vomiting, diarrhea, abdominal pain, and mucous membrane ulcers).

Subjective Data

A. Inquire whether the patient has traveled outside of the United States in areas that are high risk for Zika virus, such as Brazil, Sint Eustatius, and Argentina. Refer to the CDC website for current updated list of areas infected with Zika virus: www.CDC.gov

B. Has the patient had sexual contact with another person who could possibly be infected with the Zika virus? If so, were condoms used?

C. What are the patient's current symptoms? When did symptoms begin and how have they progressed?

D. Has the patient had low-grade fever, joint pain, headache, eye pain, muscle weakness?

E. Does the patient have any gastrointestinal symptoms (nausea, vomiting, abdominal pain)?

F. Has the patient noted any skin rash or irritation?

G. What has the patient used for symptoms that have presented? Did the treatment(s) improve symptoms? Has the patient taken any medications before the appointment to help with fever or pain?

Physical Examination

A. Check vital signs: Temperature, blood pressure (B/P), pulse, respirations

B. Inspect

1. Skin for rash. Note if maculopapular, pruritic rash is present.

2. Eyes for erythema, drainage. Perform ophthalmic examination. Note eye pain.

C. Auscultate
1. Heart
2. Lungs
D. Palpate
1. Abdomen for tenderness, rebound tenderness, masses
2. Back for costovertebral angle (CVA) tenderness
3. Joint examination should be performed in hands, feet, and other joints in which the patient is complaining of joint pain.
E. Neurological examination
1. Perform neurological examination if Guillain–Barré syndrome is suspected. See Chapter 19, Neurological Guidelines, "Guillain-Barré Syndrome" for assessment.

Diagnostic Tests

A. Complete blood count (CBC)—usually normal
B. The Food and Drug Administration (FDA) has issued two diagnostic tests for Zika virus: Zika immunoglobulin M (IgM) antibody capture enzyme-linked immunosorbent assay (MAC-ELISA) and Trioplex real-time reverse transcriptase polymerase chain reaction (PCR) assay. Only certain laboratory centers are qualified to run these complex tests.
C. Clinicians are encouraged to contact the state or local public health department for testing instructions. The FDA website may be used for further instructions.
D. The Zika virus is a nationally notifiable condition. All state, local, and territorial health departments must notify the CDC of positive results.

Differential Diagnoses

A. Zika virus
B. Other viruses (dengue fever, parvovirus, rubella, enterovirus, adenovirus)
C. Group A *Streptococcus*
D. Measles
E. Malaria
F. Leptospirosis
G. Guillain–Barré syndrome

Plan

A. General interventions
1. There is no vaccine or treatment available for Zika virus.
2. Treatment is recommended for presenting symptoms such as low-grade fever, joint pain, and so on.
3. Mosquito bite prevention is highly recommended to avoid this virus.
4. Confirmation of the diagnosis is essential for proper care and management.
5. Pregnant women should avoid traveling to areas at high risk for Zika virus.
6. Sexual contact should be avoided with patients diagnosed with Zika virus.
B. Patient teaching
1. Patient teaching: *See Section III: Patient Teaching Guide for this chapter, "Zika Virus Infection."*
2. Advise travelers to avoid going to areas that are high risk for Zika virus, such as Brazil. Refer to the CDC website for a list of countries at risk for the Zika virus: www.CDC.gov
3. The *Aedes* mosquito is most active during daytime hours, but precautions must also be used at dusk and nighttime.
4. Educate the patient regarding preventive measures for the Zika virus.
a. Advise patients to wear loose, long-sleeved, light-colored clothing (shirts and pants) to avoid mosquito bites. Treat clothing with insecticide, such as permethrin.
b. Apply insect repellent that contains N-diethylmetatoluamide (DEET) when outside.
c. Apply insect repellent after sunscreen.
d. If traveling in exposed areas, use mosquito bed nets while sleeping if areas are not screened in or screens are not used in windows. Treat bed nets with insecticide.
e. Avoid mosquito insect breeding areas, such as standing water (pools, water-filled buckets, etc.). Empty out containers with standing water.
f. Advise women to avoid becoming pregnant while traveling to high-risk areas as well as avoiding pregnancy up to 8 weeks after travel.
5. Practice safe sex, using condoms, or abstain from sexual activity with patients diagnosed with Zika virus.
6. Pregnant women confirmed with the Zika virus should use condoms or abstain from sex for the duration of the pregnancy.
7. Men with confirmed Zika virus should use condoms or abstain from sex for at least 6 months after the onset of the virus.
8. Couples in which the man has traveled to a high-risk area but did not develop symptoms should use condoms or abstain from sex for at least 8 weeks to prevent spreading potential virus.
C. Pharmaceutical therapy
1. There is no medication currently available for the prevention or the treatment of Zika virus.
2. The CDC recommends using analgesics such as acetaminophen (Tylenol) for the treatment of arthralgia and fever.
3. Nonsteroidal anti-inflammatory drugs (NSAIDs) and aspirin should be avoided due to the risk of dengue infection and risk of hemorrhage.

Follow-Up

A. Depending on symptoms, the patient should be reevaluated in 24 to 48 hours either by office visit or phone.
B. If the patient has myalgia, joint pain, and fever or if symptoms worsen or new symptoms present, advise the patient to return for a follow-up evaluation.
C. If the patient begins having muscle weakness and/or symptoms of Guillain–Barré syndrome, the patient should make a follow-up appointment immediately with the provider or go to the emergency department

for evaluation. See Chapter 19, Neurologic Guidelines, "Guillain–Barré Syndrome" for assessment and patient education.

D. Blood work that is sent to the laboratory for screening for the Zika virus may take up to 3 weeks for final interpretation of results. Advise the patient that precautions should be taken while waiting on results.

E. All positive results are reportable to the CDC.

Consultation/Referral

A. Consult with collaborating physician if a patient presents with complaints relating to Zika virus.

B. Consider referral to infectious disease specialist for evaluation and management.

Individual Considerations

A. Pediatric

1. Presenting symptoms in children may be the same as in adults. Other symptoms may include poor feeding, irritability, difficulty walking or bearing weight, and joint pain with active/passive movement of joint.
2. Neurologic complications (brain ischemia, myelitis, meningoencephalitis) have been documented in children who were exposed to the virus in utero.

B. Pregnancy

1. Congenital microcephaly and fetal loss have been reported in newborns exposed to the Zika virus in utero.

C. Adults

1. Guillain–Barré syndrome has been documented as a complication of Zika virus. Further evaluation is necessary if Guillain–Barré is suspected.

Bibliography

Akhter, K. (2015). Cytomegalovirus. *Medscape.* Retrieved from www.emedicine.medscape.com/article/215702-overview

Albrecht, M. A. (2016a). Epidemiology, clinical manifestations, diagnosis and management of mumps. *UpToDate.* Retrieved from www.uptodate.com/contents/epidemiology-clinical-manifestations-diagnosis-and-management-of-mumps?topicKey=ID%2F8310

Albrecht, M. A. (2016b). Vaccination for the prevention of shingles (herpes zoster). *UpToDate.* Retrieved from www.uptodate.com

Anderson, W. E. (2014). Varicella-zoster virus. *Medscape.* Retrieved from emedicine.medscape.com/article/231927-overview

Armstrong, C. (2010). Practice guidelines: AHA guidelines on prevention of rheumatic fever and diagnosis and treatment of acute streptococcal pharyngitis. *American Family Physician, 81*(3), 346–359. Retrieved from www.aafp.org/afp/2010/0201/p346.html

Aronson, M. D., & Auwaeter, P. G. (2016). Infectious mononucleosis in adults and adolescents. *UpToDate.* Retrieved from www.uptodate.com/contents/infectious-mononucleosis-in-adults-and-adolescents?topicKey=ID%2F8318

Basarab, M., Bowman, C., Aarons, E. J., & Cropley, I. (2016). Zika virus. *British Medical Journal, 352,* i1049.

Biggs, H. M., Barton Behravesh, C., Bradley, K. K., Dahlgren, F. S., Drexler, N. A., Dumler, J. S., & . . . . Traeger, M. S. (2016). Diagnosis and management of tickborne Rickettsial diseases: Rocky Mountain spotted fever and other spotted fever group Rickettsioses, Ehrlichioses, and Anaplasmosis—United States. *MMWR Recommendations & Reports, 65*(2), 1–44.

Centers for Disease Control and Prevention. (2012). Summary of rationale for Varicella vaccination. Retrieved from www.cdc.gov/vaccines/vpd-vac/varicella/rationale-vacc.htm

Centers for Disease Control and Prevention. (2013). Parasites—Toxoplasmosis (Toxoplasma infection). Retrieved from www.cdc.gov/parasites/toxoplasmosis

Centers for Disease Control and Prevention. (2014a). About Epstein–Barr virus (EBV). Retrieved from www.cdc.gov/epstein-barr/about-ebv.html

Centers for Disease Control and Prevention. (2014b). Cat-scratch disease. Retrieved from www.cdc.gov/healthypets/diseases/cat-scratch.html

Centers for Disease Control and Prevention. (2015a). Bartonella infection (cat scratch disease, trench fever, and Carrion's disease). For Health-Care Providers. Retrieved from www.cdc.gov/bartonella/clinicians/index.html

Centers for Disease Control and Prevention. (2015b). Fifth disease. Retrieved from www.cdc.gov/parvovirusb19/fifth-disease.html

Centers for Disease Control and Prevention. (2015c). Lyme disease. Retrieved from www.cdc.gove/lyme/treatment/index.html

Centers for Disease Control and Prevention. (2015d). Measles (rubeola). Retrieved from www.cdc.gov/measles/hcp/

Centers for Disease Control and Prevention. (2015e). Meningococcal disease. Retrieved from www.cdc.gov/meningococcal/about/prevention.html

Centers for Disease Control and Prevention. (2015f). Tick removal. Retrieved from www.cdc.gov/ticks/removing_a_tick.html

Centers for Disease Control and Prevention. (2015g). West Nile virus. Retrieved from www.cdc.gov/westnile/index.html

Centers for Disease Control and Prevention. (2016a). ACIP votes down use of LAIV for 2016–2017 flu season. Retrieved from www.cdc.gov/media/releases/2016/s0622-laiv-flu.html

Centers for Disease Control and Prevention. (2016b). Immunizations and pregnancy vaccines chart. Retrieved from www.cdc.gov/vaccines/pregnancy/pregnant-women/index.html

Centers for Disease Control and Prevention. (2016c). Influenza (flu). Retrieved from www.cdc.gov/flu

Centers for Disease Control and Prevention. (2016d). Frequently asked flu questions 2016–2017 influenza season. Retrieved from www.cdc.gov/flu/about/season/flu-season-2016-2017.htm

Centers for Disease Control and Prevention. (2016e). Meningitis. Retrieved from www.cdc.gov/meningitis/index.html

Centers for Disease Control and Prevention. (2016f). Vaccine information statement: Meningococcal ACWY vaccines (MenACWY and MPSV4) VIS. Retrieved from www.cdc.gov/vaccines/hcp/vis/vis-statements/mening.html

Centers for Disease Control and Prevention. (2016g). West Nile virus neuroinvasive disease incidence by state—United States, 2015 (as of January 12, 2016). Retrieved from www.cdc.gov/westnile/statsmaps/preliminarymapsdata/incidencestatedate.html

Centers for Disease Control and Prevention. (2016h). Zika virus. Retrieved from www.cdc.gov/zika

Chen, S. S. P. (2013a). Measles clinical presentation. *Medscape.* Retrieved from emedicine.medscape.com/article/966220-clinical

Chen, S. S. P. (2013b). Measles treatment & management. *Medscape.* Retrieved from emedicine.medscape.com/article/966220-treatment

Cunha, B. A. (2015). Infectious mononucleosis. *Medscape.* Retrieved from emedicine.medscape.com/article/222040-overview

Cunha, B. A. (2016). Rocky Mountain spotted fever. *Medscape.* Retrieved from emedicine.medscape.com/article/228042-overviewencephalitis and emedicine.medscape.com/article/234009-overview

Cunha, B. A. (2015). West Nile encephalitis. *Medscape.* Retrieved from www.emedicine.medscapecom

Defendi, G. L. (2014). Mumps. *Medscape.* Retrieved from reference.medscape.com/article/966678-overview

Domingo, P., Pomar, V., de Benito, N., & Coll, P. (2013). The spectrum of acute bacterial meningitis in elderly patients. *BMC Infectious Diseases, 13,* 108.doi: 10.1186/1471-2334-13-108

Edwards, M. S. (2016). Rubella. *UpToDate.* Retrieved from www.uptodate .com

Fact sheet on Zika virus disease (updated on June 2, 2016). (2016). *Weekly Epidemiological Record, 91*(24), 314–316.

Farrar, F. (2013). West Nile virus: An infectious viral agent to the central nervous system. *Critical Care Nursing Clinics of North America, 25,* 191–203.

Fiebelkorn, A. P., & Goodson, J. L. (2015). Measles (Rubeola). In G. W. Brunette, The yellow book: CDC health information for international travel 2016 (pp. 258–261). New York, NY: Oxford University Press. Retrieved from wwwnc.cdc.gov/travel/yellowbook/2016/infectious-diseases-related-to-travel/measles-rubeola

Friel, T. J. (2016). Epidemiology, clinical manifestations, and treatment of cytomegalovirus infection in immunocompetent adults. Retrieved from www.uptodate.com

Galloway, J., & Cope, A. P. (2015). The ying and yang of fever in rheumatic disease. *Clinical Medicine, 15*(3), 288–291.

Gewitz, M. H., Baltimore, R. S., Tani, L. Y., Sable, C. A., Shulman, S. T., Carapetis, J., . . . Kaplan, E. L.; American Heart Association Committee on Rheumatic Fever, Endocarditis, and Kawasaki Disease of the Council on Cardiovascular Disease in the Young. (2015). Revision of the Jones criteria for the diagnosis of acute rheumatic fever in the era of Doppler echocardiography: A scientific statement from the American Heart Association. *Circulation, 131*, 1806–1818.

Gibofsk, A. (2016). Acute rheumatic fever: Clinical manifestations and diagnosis. *UpToDate*. Retrieved from www.uptodate.com

Gilbert, R., & Petersen, E. (2016). Toxoplasmosis and pregnancy. *UpToDate*. Retrieved from www.uptodate.com

Gluckman, S. (2016). Viral encephalitis in adults. *UpToDate*. Retrieved from www.uptodate.com

Hasbun, R. (2014). Meningitis. *Medscape*. Retrieved from emedicine .medscape.com/article/232915-overview.

Hemmert, A. C., & Gilbreath J. J. (2016). The current state of diagnostics for meningitis and encephalitis. *Medical Laboratory Observer, 48*(7), 12–14.

Hilton, L. (2016). Zika virus: Top mosquito repellent recommendations. *Contemporary Pediatrics, 33*(6), 14–16.

Hu, L. (2016). Clinical manifestations of Lyme disease in adults. *UpToDate*. Retrieved from www.uptodate.com

Immunization Action Coalition. (n.d.). Healthcare personnel vaccination recommendations. Retrieved from www.vaccineinformation.org

Jordan, J. A. (2013). Clinical manifestations and pathogenesis of human parvovirus B19 infection. *UpToDate*. Retrieved from www.uptodate .com/contents/clinical-manifestations-and-pathogenesis-of-human -parvovirus-b19-infection?topicKey=ID%2F8272

Journal Watch Specialities. (n.d.). FluMist: Intranasal flu vaccine. Retrieved from infectious-diseases.jwatch.org/cgi/content/full/2003/808/3

Kawasaki Disease Foundation. Retrieved from www.kdfoundation.org

LoBue, P. (2015). Tuberculosis. In G. W. Brunette, *The yellow book: CDC health information for international travel 2016* (pp. 258–261). New York, NY: Oxford University Press. Retrieved from wwwnc.cdc.gov/travel/ yellowbook/2016/infectious-diseases-related-to-travel/tuberculosis

Lockwood, C. J. (2016). Zika virus and microcephaly. *Contemporary OB/ GYN, 61*(2), 6–9.

Lupton, K. (2016). Zika virus disease: A public health emergency of international concern. *British Journal of Nursing, 25*(4), 198–202.

Meyerhoff, J. O. (2014). Lyme disease. *Medscape*. Retrieved from emedicine.medscape.com/article/330178-overview

National Vaccine Information Center. (n.d.). Quick facts mumps. Retrieved from www.nvic.org/vaccines-and-diseases/Mumps.aspx

Newburger, J. W., Masato, T., Burns, J. C., & Takahashi, M. (2016). Kawasaki disease. *Journal of the American College of Cardiology, 67*(14), 1738–1749.

Nicoteri, J. A. L. (2013). Adolescent pharyngitis: A common complaint with potentially lethal complications. *Journal for Nurse Practitioners, 9*, 295–300.

Nishimura, R. A., Otto, C. M., Bonow, R. O., Carabello, B. A., Erwin, J. P., Guyton, R. A., . . . Thomas, J. D. (2014). Practice guideline, 2014 AHA/ACC guideline for the management of patients with valvular heart disease: A Report of the American College of Cardiology/ American Heart Association Task Force on Practice Guidelines. *Journal of the American College of Cardiology, 63*(22), e57–e185. Retrieved from www.onlinejacc.org/content/63/22/e57

O'Connell, J., & Sloand, E. (2013). Kawasaki syndrome and streptococcal scarlet fever: A clinical review. *Journal of Nurse Practitioners, 9*, 259–264.

O'Malley, P. A. (2016). Zika virus. *Clinical Nurse Specialist: The Journal for Advanced Nursing Practice, 30*(4), 194–197.

Oster, A. M., Russell, K., Stryker, J. E., Friedman, A., Kachur, R. E., Petersen, E. E., . . . Brooks, J. T. (2016). Update: Interim guidance for prevention of sexual transmission of Zika virus—United States, 2016. *Morbidity & Mortality Weekly Report, 65*(12), 323–325.

Palomo, A. M. (2016). Zika virus: An international emergency? *Journal of Public Health Policy, 37*(2), 133–135.

Petersen, E. E., Polen, K. D., Meaney-Delman, D., Ellington, S. R., Oduvebo, T., Cohn, A., . . . Rivera, M. (2016). Update: Interim guidance for health care providers caring for women of reproductive age with possible Zika virus exposure—United States. 2016. *Morbidity & Mortality Weekly Report, 65*(12), 315–322.

Petersen, L. R. (2016). Epidemiology and pathogenesis of West Nile virus infection. *UpToDate*. Retrieved from www.uptodate.com

Pichichero, M. E. (2016). Complications of streptococcal tonsillopharyngitis. *UpToDate*. Retrieved from www.uptodate.com

Plourde, A. R., & Bloch, E. M. (2016). A literature review of Zika virus. *Emerging Infectious Diseases, 22*(7), 1185–1192.

Practice Bulletin no. 151. (2015). Cytomegalovirus, parvovirus B19, varicella zoster, and toxoplasmosis in pregnancy. *Obstetrics & Gynecology (Serial Online), 125*(6), 1510–1525.

Riley, L. E., & Fernandes, C. J. (2016). Parvovirus B19 infection during pregnancy. *UpToDate*. Retrieved from www.uptodate.com

Rowley, A. H., & Ryan. S. F. (2013). Kawasaki disease. *Clinician Reviews, 23*, 34–38.

Russell, K., Blanton, L., Kniss, K., Mustaquim, D., Smith, S., Cohen, J., . . . Burns, E. (2016). Update: Influenza activity—United States, October 4, 2015—February 6, 2016. *Morbidity & Mortality Weekly Report, 65*(6), 146–153.

Saccomano, S. J., & Ferrara, L. R. (2013). Infectious mononucleosis. *Clinician Reviews, 23*, 42–49.

Salinas, J. D. (2016). West Nile virus. *Medscape*. Retrieved from emedicine. medscape.com

Salvaggio, M. R. (2013). Human herpesvirus 6 infection differential diagnoses. *Medscape*. Retrieved from emedicine.medscape.com/article /219019-differential

Sanchez, E., Vannier, E., Wormser, G. P., & Hu, L. T. (2016). Diagnosis, treatment and prevention of Lyme disease, human granulocytic anaplasmosis, and babesiosis: A review. *Journal of the American Medical Association, 315*(16), 1767–1777.

Savva, G. M., Pachnio, A., Kaul, B., Morgan, K., Huppert, F. A., Brayne, C., & Moss, P. A. (2013). Cytomegalovirus infection is associated with increased mortality in the older population. *Aging Cell, 12*, 381–387.

Shapiro, E. D. (2016). Lyme disease: Clinical manifestations in children. *UpToDate*. Retrieved from www.uptodate.com

Sotoodian, B. (2016). Scarlet fever. *Medscape*. Retrieved from www .medscape.com

Spach, D., & Kaplan, S. (2016). Treatment of cat scratch disease. *UpToDate*. Retrieved from www.uptodate.com.

Sundel, R. (2016). Kawasaki disease: Clinical features and diagnosis. *UpToDate*. Retrieved from www.uptodate.com

Thorner, A. (2016). Treatment and prevention of pandemic H1N1 influenza ("swine influenza"). *UpToDate*. Retrieved from www.uptodate.com

Torgerson, P. R., & Mastroiacovo, P. (2013). The global burden of congenital toxoplasmosis: A systematic review. *Bulletin of the World Health Organization, 91*(7), 501–508.

Tremblay, C., & Brady, M. T. (2016). Roseolainfantum (exanthema subitum). *UpToDate*. Retrieved from www.uptodate.com

Tunkel, A. R. (2016). Clinical features and diagnosis of acute bacterial meningitis in adults. *UpToDate*. Retrieved from www.uptodate.com

Wallace, M. R. (2014). Rheumatic fever. *Medscape*. Retrieved from emedicine.Medscape.com

White, S. W. (2013). Roseolainfantum. *Medscape*. Retrieved from emedicine.medscape.com/article/1133023-overview

World Health Organization. (2015). Meningococcal meningitis fact sheet. Retrieved from www.who.int/mediacentre/factsheets/fs141/en/

World Health Organization. (2016). Measles fact sheet. Retrieved from www.who.int/medicentre/factsheets/fs286/en

World Heart Federation. (2014). Rheumatic heart disease. Retrieved from www.world-heart-federation.org

Wormser, R. J., Dattwyler, E. D., Shapiro, J. J., Halperin, A. C., Steere, A. C., Klempner, M. S., . . . Nadelman, R. B. (2006). The clinical assessment, treatment, and prevention of Lyme disease, human granulocytic anaplasmosis, and babesiosis: Clinical Practice Guidelines by the Infectious Diseases Society of America. *Clinical Infectious Disease, 43*(9), 1089–1134.

17 Systemic Disorders Guidelines

Chronic Fatigue Syndrome (Systemic Exertion Intolerance Syndrome)

Julie Adkins

Definition

A. Fatigue is one of the most common symptoms confronting the practitioner in an office practice. A patient with chronic fatigue is characterized as having fatigue with multiple associated symptoms for longer than 6 months in which these symptoms have a profound impact on daily activities and are moderate to severe symptoms that occur over half the time. The fatigue is not relieved by rest.

Incidence

A. Fatigue accounts for 1% to 3% of visits to generalists as an isolated symptom or diagnosis. Psychiatric disorders are involved in less than 50% of cases. Chronic fatigue has a reported frequency in excess of 20%. Fatigue is seen predominantly four times more in women than in men and the highest prevalence is in people aged 40 to 59 years, but it can affect people of all ages, including teens and children.

Pathogenesis

A. Fatigue is a sensitive but nonspecific indicator of underlying medical and/or psychological pathology. It is reportedly more often due to unknown cause or to psychiatric illness than to physical illness, injury, medications, drugs, or alcohol.

Predisposing Factors

A. Hyperthyroidism
B. Hypothyroidism
C. Cardiac disease: Congestive heart failure (CHF)
D. Neurally mediated hypotension
E. Infections: Endocarditis, hepatitis
F. Respiratory disorders: Chronic obstructive pulmonary disease (COPD) and sleep apnea
G. Anemia
H. Arthritides and related disorders
I. Cancer
J. Alcoholism
K. Side effects from drugs such as sedatives and beta-blockers
L. Psychological conditions such as insomnia, depression, anxiety, and somatization disorder
M. Female gender
N. Virus, such as Epstein–Barr virus and herpes virus

Common Complaints

A. Sudden onset of fatigue, with other symptoms
B. Unrefreshing sleep
C. Extreme exhaustion lasting more than 24 hours after physical or mental exercises
D. Loss of memory and concentration
E. Joint pain that moves around without swelling or redness
F. Muscle fatigue
G. Swollen lymph nodes in neck/armpits

Other Signs and Symptoms

A. Headache with new pattern and intensity
B. Overexertion
C. Poor physical conditioning
D. Stress
E. Undernutrition and poor appetite
F. Emotional problems: Depression, anxiety, and somatization disorder

Subjective Data

A. Review history for onset, duration, and course description of the fatigue.
B. Ask the patient about significant losses, low self-esteem, and occurrence of crying spells and suicidal thoughts. High prevalence of depression and suicide is present in this patient population.
C. Ask the patient about a history of any abuse of hypnotic drugs, alcohol, or tranquilizers.
D. Review medications, both over-the-counter (OTC) and prescription drugs.
E. Review the patient's medical history for cardiac, thyroid, and other medical conditions.
F. Review sleep and insomnia history.
G. Review history for family illness, new baby, or postpartum.
H. Establish last menses to rule out pregnancy.
I. Review exercise patterns.
J. Review diet with 24-hour recall.

K. Elicit history of fever, night sweats, weight loss, and enlarged lymph node(s).
L. Inquire about recent major life changes, such as moving or a change in job.
M. Establish usual weight, and review recent weight gain or loss, over what period.
N. Review any recent infections, flu, or mononucleosis.
O. Review high-risk sexual practices and intravenous drug use to rule out HIV exposure.
P. Review recent history for transfusion of blood products to rule out hepatitis or HIV exposure.
Q. Obtain history of the patient's daily living and working habits.

Physical Examination

A. Check temperature, pulse, respirations, blood pressure, and weight; check for postural hypotension.
B. Inspect
  1. Observe general overall appearance. Skin: Conduct dermal examination for changes in pigmentation, purpura, dryness, rashes, jaundice, pallor, splinter hemorrhages, or petechiae.
  2. Eyes: Conduct a funduscopic examination to rule out Roth's spots and tuberculoma.
  3. Check sclerae for icterus.
  4. Throat: Inspect pharynx for petechiae at the junction of the hard and soft palates to rule out mononucleosis.
  5. Extremities: Inspect the joints for inflammation.
C. Ausculate
  1. Heart
  2. Lungs
D. Percuss the abdomen for organomegaly, masses, ascites, and hepatic tenderness.
E. Palpate
  1. Palpate the neck, to rule out goiter.
  2. Palpate all lymph nodes (neck, axilla, and groin) for size, degree of tenderness, and distribution.
  3. Complete clinical breast examination for masses.
  4. Palpate the abdomen for organomegaly, masses, and ascites.
  5. Palpate the joints for tenderness.
  6. Assess the genitalia for masses and tenderness, to rule out infection.
F. Neurologic examination: Complete mental status assessment
G. Rectal examination: Assess for masses, prostatic pathology, and occult blood.

Diagnostic Tests

A. Complete blood count (CBC) with differential and peripheral smear
B. Erythrocyte sedimentation rate (ESR)
C. Calcium, albumin, blood urea nitrogen (BUN), and creatinine
D. Glucose
E. Transaminase (aminotransferase): Viral hepatitis is associated with elevation in transaminase.
F. HIV serum test
G. Thyrotropin-stimulating hormone (TSH) to rule out hyperthyroidism or hypothyroidism
H. Heterophile test to rule out acute mononucleosis
I. Monospot
J. Epstein–Barr virus
K. Sleep study

Differential Diagnoses

A. Chronic fatigue syndrome (CFS). According to the 2015 Institute of Medicine Criteria, CFS must have the following three symptoms[a]:
  1. Decreased ability to engage in pre-illness activities such as work, social, educational, or personal activities. Must last 6 months, along with symptoms of severe fatigue that is not improved with rest.
  2. Post exertional malaise
  3. Unrefreshed sleep
  Must have one of the two of the following symptoms:
    a. Cognitive impairment or
    b. Orthostatic intolerance
B. Hypercalcemia
C. Mild renal failure
D. Early diabetes mellitus
E. Hypothyroid or hyperthyroidism
F. Cardiac disease
G. Anemia
H. Anicteric hepatitis
I. Connective tissue disease
J. Immune hyperactivity
K. Disturbed sleep
L. Occult neoplasm
M. Infection: History of fever, sweats, weight loss, and diffuse adenopathy. These symptoms also suggest HIV, especially with high-risk behaviors (see "Human Immunodeficiency Virus" section).

Plan

A. General interventions
  1. Find out the patient's view of his or her illness before proceeding with patient education.
  2. Manage underlying disease (refer to specific chapters).
  3. Managing CFS can be as complex as the illness itself. There is no cure and symptoms vary over time. Treating the most disruptive symptoms first is paramount and then monitoring medications and supplements, managing activities and exercise, and improving health and quality-of-life issues are the primary goals.
  4. Cognitive behavioral therapy and exercise therapy have been shown to be beneficial to the patient.
  5. Evaluate the patient for the possibility that he or she is confusing focal neuromuscular disease with generalized lassitude.

---

[a] Retrieved from Institute of Medicine of the National Academies. *Beyond Myalgic Encephalomyelitis/CFS: Redefining an Illness*. Report brief, January 2015. Reprinted with permission from the National Academies Press, Copyright 2015 National Academy of Sciences.

B. Patient teaching
  1. Discuss and review the evidence for the diagnosis, and offer a careful explanation of symptoms. Many patients think they have a medical problem producing fatigue symptoms.
  2. Review the diagnostic criteria for depression (see Chapter 22, "Psychiatric Guidelines"), and describe the neurochemical mechanisms by which depression leads to fatigue. Refer the patient for individual counseling or group therapy.
  3. Review the idiopathic nature of CFS and its nonprogressive nature. Inform the patient that it has a gradually improving clinical course and has the chance of full recovery. Symptoms are self-limited, usually clearing within 12 to 18 months. Research shows that people with chronic fatigue 2 years or less are more likely to improve than the person for whom it has taken more time to diagnose.
  4. Encourage the patient to begin a gentle exercise program and to engage in life's activities.
  5. Provide nutritional education.

C. Pharmaceutical therapy
  1. For postural hypotension
    a. Increase dietary sodium
    b. Antihypotensive agent: Fludrocortisone 0.1 mg daily
  2. Low-dose antidepressant therapy for disordered sleep
    a. Amitriptyline HCl 25 mg every bedtime
    b. Imipramine HCl 25 to 50 mg at bedtime; may increase dosage up to 300 mg daily
    c. Doxepin HCl 10 to 20 mg every bedtime
    d. Short-term hypnotic: Zolpidem (Ambien) 5 to 10 mg at bedtime
  3. Nonsteroidal anti-inflammatory drugs (NSAIDs) for symptomatic relief of myalgia, arthralgia, or headache
  4. Correct anemia with iron supplements, if applicable.

Follow-Up

A. Follow up in 2 weeks to reevaluate status and then monthly depending on signs and symptoms.

B. Follow up closely whether the patient is depressed

Consultation/Referral

A. Consult a physician if no improvement is seen with therapies. Emphasize the legitimacy of the patient's symptoms and summarize the workup, its rationale, and its findings.

B. Refer the patient to a mental health professional as indicated by depression and/or suicidality.

Individual Considerations

A. Adults
  1. Fatigue is most often explained by common factors such as overexertion, poor physical conditioning, inadequate quantity or quality of sleep, obesity, undernutrition, stress, and emotional problems.

B. Pediatrics
  1. Between 0.2% and 2.3% of children and adolescents suffer from CFS. It is more prevalent in adolescents than in younger children and is more likely to develop after an acute flu-like illness or mononucleosis. Gradual onset may also occur.

Resource

Fact sheets may be obtained with information about child, adolescent, and adult CFS at the Centers for Disease Control and Prevention at www.cdc.gov.

Chronic Fatigue Immune Dysfunction Syndrome (CFIDS) Association
PO Box 220398
Charlotte, NC 28222-0398
800-442-3437
Available 24 hours a day, 7 days a week

Fevers of Unknown Origin

Julie Adkins

Definition

A. The criteria for fevers of unknown origin (FUO) are an illness of at least 3-week duration, fever greater than 101.0°F (38.3°C) on several occasions, and remaining undiagnosed after 1 week of study in the hospital. Because of cost factors, the criterion requiring 1 week of hospitalization is often bypassed.

Incidence

A. In adults, infections account for 30% to 40% of the cases. Cancer accounts for 20% to 30% of the cases of FUO. In children, infections are the most common cause of FUO, accounting for 30% to 50% of the cases; cancer is a rare cause of FUO in children. Autoimmune disorders occur with equal frequency in adults and children. Infection, cancer, and autoimmune disorders combined account for 20% to 25% of FUO in patients who have been febrile for 6 months or longer. Various miscellaneous diseases account for another 25%. Approximately 50% of FUO remain undiagnosed but have a benign course, with symptoms eventually resolving. Between 5% to 15% of FUO cases defy diagnosis even after exhaustive studies.

Pathogenesis

There are five categories of causes of FUO.

A. Infection: Most common systemic infections are tuberculosis (TB) and endocarditis.

B. Neoplasms: Most common are lymphoma and leukemia.

C. Autoimmune disorders: Most common are Still's disease, systemic lupus erythematosus (SLE), and polyarteritis nodosa.

D. Miscellaneous causes: These include hyperthyroidism, thyroiditis, sarcoidosis, Whipple's disease, familial Mediterranean fever, recurrent pulmonary emboli, alcoholic hepatitis, drug fever, factitious fever, and others.

E. Undiagnosed FUO

Predisposing Factors

A. Upper respiratory infection

B. Urinary tract infection

C. Viral illnesses

D. Drug allergy, especially to antibiotics
E. Connective tissue disease
F. Tuberculosis
G. HIV
H. Parasite infection

Common Complaints

A. The patient feels "sick all over," with malaise and fatigue.
B. The patient has chills all over the body with high fever.

Other Signs and Symptoms

A. Tachycardia
B. Sensation of warmth or flushing
C. Piloerection
D. Myalgias
E. Mild inability to concentrate, confusion, delirium, or even stupor
F. Labial herpes simplex outbreak, or fever blisters
G. Children: Seizures

Subjective Data

A. Review the onset, course, and duration of symptoms.
B. Review family, occupational, and social history.
C. Review sexual practices, including monogamy and oral, rectal, and vaginal sexual habits; recreational habits; and any new changes.
D. Elicit information regarding use of intravenous drugs.
E. Review if the patient has had this illness before. How was it treated?
F. Review travel during the last month.
G. Review any new hobbies, changes at home or work, or other new events.
H. Review the patient's history for contact with any friends or family members who have been sick and do not seem to be getting any better.
I. Review the patient's history for eating any uncooked meat and dietary changes during the past month.
J. Review the child's history specifically for febrile seizures.
K. Review for risk factors for thrombophlebitis (see Chapter 10, "Cardiovascular Guidelines").

Physical Examination

A. Check temperature, pulse, respirations, blood pressure, weight, and height.
B. Inspect
  1. Conduct funduscopic examination to rule out retinopathy, Roth's spots, and choroidal tubercles.
  2. Examine the ears, nose, and throat. Inspect the mouth.
  3. Observe the skin and mucous membranes.
  4. Perform transillumination of sinus cavities for evidence of sinusitis.
  5. Inspect body for skin rashes or wounds.
C. Auscultate
  1. Heart for murmurs and rubs
  2. Lungs for rales, consolidation, and effusion
D. Percuss
  1. Sinuses for tenderness
  2. Chest for consolidation
  3. Abdomen
E. Palpate
  1. Neck, axilla, and groin for lymphadenopathy
  2. Thyroid gland
  3. Abdomen for organomegaly, masses, tenderness, guarding, rebound, suprapubic tenderness, and costovertebral angle (CVA) tenderness
  4. Musculoskeletal system for bone or joint swelling, tenderness, increased warmth; check lower extremities for evidence of phlebitis, asymmetrical swelling, calf tenderness, and palpable cord
  5. Elderly: Palpate scalp for tender arteries.
  6. Infants: Palpate fontanelles.
F. Neurologic examination
  1. Assess for signs of meningeal irritation (Brudzinski's and Kernig's signs) and presence of focal deficits.
  2. Conduct mental status examination.
G. Genitorectal examination, if applicable
  1. Female: Conduct pelvic examination for cervical discharge, adnexal masses, lesions, and pelvic inflammatory disease (PID) symptoms.
  2. Male: Conduct prostate and testicular examination for tenderness and masses; check penis for discharge, rash, and lesions.
  3. Both: Conduct rectal examination for discharge, tenderness, and masses; check stool for occult blood specimen.

Diagnostic Tests

A. Complete blood count (CBC) with differential
B. Sedimentation rate
C. Urinalysis and urine culture
D. Blood glucose
E. Liver function test
F. Blood cultures
G. Consider serology for suspected infections or pathology (refer to Chapter 16, "Infectious Disease Guidelines"). Suspected infections include Epstein–Barr virus, Q fever, Lyme disease or other tick-borne diseases, hepatitis, syphilis, and cytomegalovirus (CMV).
H. Suspected collagen disease: Antinuclear antibodies (ANAs) and rheumatoid factor
I. Suspected TB: Tuberculin skin test, sputum, and urine cultures
J. Immunologic studies: Enzyme-linked immunosorbent assay (ELISA), Western blot test, and antistreptolysin O (ASLO) titer
K. Suspected mononucleosis: Heterophile antibody test
L. Suspected Salmonella: Widal's test
M. Suspected thyroiditis: Thyroid profile
N. Suspected malaria or relapsing fever: Direct examination of blood smears
O. Imaging: Depends on suspected infection
  1. Chest, sinus radiographic films
  2. Gastrointestinal (GI) studies: Proctosigmoidoscopy, evaluate gallbladder function

3. CT scan of abdomen and pelvis, abdominal ultrasonography
4. MRI is better than CT scan for detecting lesions of the nervous system.

P. Suspected embolism: Ventilation–perfusion (V/Q) scan

Q. Suspected endocarditis or atrial myxoma: Echocardiography

R. Radionuclide studies: Gallium scan and radium-labeled immunoglobulin are useful in detecting infection and neoplasm.

S. Laparotomy in the deteriorating patient if the diagnosis is elusive despite an extensive evaluation. Any abnormal finding should be aggressively evaluated: Headache necessitates a lumbar puncture to rule out meningitis; biopsy any skin from an area of rash to look for cutaneous manifestations of collagen vascular disease or infection; enlarged lymph nodes should be aspirated or biopsied and examined for cytologic features to rule out neoplasm and send for culture.

Differential Diagnoses

A. FUO
B. Systemic and localized infections
C. Neoplasms
D. Autoimmune disorders
E. Thrombophlebitis
F. Miscellaneous causes (see "Definition" section)

Plan

A. General interventions: Observe the patient taking his or her own temperature to document the presence of a fever to make sure the temperature is not self-induced.
   1. Treatment should be directed toward the underlying cause once a diagnosis is made.

B. Patient teaching
   1. Instruct the patient to keep a record of temperatures, preferably rectal, taken each evening, when elevations are most likely to occur.
   2. Reassure the patient that there is nothing abnormal about temperatures in the range of 97.0°F to 99.3°F.
   3. Instruct the patient on use of physical cooling aids, such as exposure of skin to cool ambient temperature, bedside fan, and sponging with cool water or alcohol.
   4. Explain to the patient that immersion in an ice water bath may be indicated for hyperthermic emergencies.

C. Pharmaceutical therapy
   1. Start therapeutic trials if a diagnosis is strongly suspected.
      a. Antituberculous drugs for TB
      b. Tetracycline for brucellosis
      c. If the patient shows no clinical response in 2 weeks, stop therapy and reevaluate.
   2. Symptomatic antipyretic therapy: Salicylates or acetaminophen every 4 hours.

Follow-Up

A. Follow up in 24 to 48 hours.

B. Indications for admission to the hospital: Fever remains elevated beyond 101°F for weeks, and ambulatory diagnostic efforts have been unsuccessful.

Consultation/Referral

A. Consult with a physician for diagnosis and comanagement if indicated.

B. Refer the patient to a specialist (infectious disease) if unable to differentiate definitive diagnosis.

Individual Considerations

A. Pregnancy
   1. Refer the patient for perinatal consultation.
   2. High fevers early in the first trimester have been associated with an increase in neural tube defects.
   3. Maternal fevers may cause fetal tachycardia.

B. Pediatrics
   1. Toxic-appearing infants and children should be hospitalized and given parenteral antibiotic therapy following prompt diagnostic testing that includes white blood cell (WBC); urinalysis; and cultures of blood, urine, and cerebrospinal fluid. Consult a physician.
   2. Infants under 28 days regardless of appearance are generally hospitalized and given parenteral antibiotic therapy following prompt diagnostic testing with WBC, urinalysis, and cultures.
   3. Aspirin products should not be given to children due to the risk of Reye's syndrome.
   4. Consider inflammatory bowel disease in older children and adolescents.

C. Geriatrics
   1. Common causes of FUO include TB, Hodgkin's lymphoma, and temporal arteritis.
   2. Elderly patients commonly present with nonspecific symptoms.

Human Immunodeficiency Virus (HIV)

Beverly R. Byram

Definition

A. AIDS is a chronic, life-threatening condition caused by the HIV. HIV is a retrovirus that targets helper T (CD4) cells and contains a viral enzyme called reverse transcriptase that allows the virus to convert its ribonucleic acid (RNA) to DNA then integrate and take over the cell's own genetic material. Once taken over, the new cell begins to produce new HIV retrovirus. This process kills the CD4 cells that are the body's main defense against illness. This interferes with the body's ability to fight off infection—bacteria, viruses, and fungi—that causes the disease. AIDS is the term used to define a severely compromised immune system.

Incidence

A. According to the Centers for Disease Control and Prevention (CDC), by the end of 2012, there were approximately 1.2 million persons living with HIV in the United States. Approximately 12.8% of those were unaware of their HIV status. In 2014 an estimated 45% of those living with HIV were African American, 29% White, and 23% Hispanic. Asians/Pacific Islanders and American Indians/Alaskan Natives each represent 3%.

B. The largest population living with HIV comprises men having sex with men (MSM), followed by persons infected by high-risk heterosexual contact, those infected by intravenous drug users (IVDUs), and those exposed through both MSM and IVDU.

C. The widespread use of antiretroviral therapy has altered the course of HIV disease. In 2012, HIV was reclassified as a chronic illness. More than 50% of deaths in HIV-positive persons on highly active antiretroviral therapy (HAART) are related to conditions other than AIDS. The U.S. Preventive Services Task Force (USPSTF) recommends HIV screening for all people between the ages of 15 and 75 years as well as younger and older people at high risk of HIV infection.

D. Due to the rapidity of changing technology and knowledge, refer to the websites for the newest statistics.

Pathogenesis

A. HIV belongs to a subgroup of retroviruses called lentiviruses or "slow" viruses. The course of infection of the virus is characterized by a long interval between infection and the onset of serious symptoms. CD4 cells are the primary target of the HIV.

B. Primary HIV infection is followed by a burst of viremia during which the virus is easily detected in peripheral blood per HIV polymerase chain reaction (PCR) viral load (VL). During the "window period," the first 2 to 6 weeks following the infection, persons may test negative for the HIV antibody with the enzyme-linked immunosorbentassay (ELISA) and Western blot tests. During this time, the person can be highly infectious to sexual partners. In this time of early infection with high VL, the CD4 cells can decrease by 20% to 40%. Within 2 to 4 weeks after the exposure to the virus, up to 70% of infected patients experience a flu-like illness related to acute infection. The immune system fights back to reduce the HIV levels with killer T cells (CD8) that attack and kill the infected cells. The patient's CD4 cell count may rebound by 80% to 90%. A patient can remain symptom-free for a long time, often years. During this time, there is low-level replication of HIV but an ongoing deterioration of the immune system. Enough of the immune system remains intact to prevent most infections. The patient is infectious during this time.

C. The final phase of HIV occurs when a sufficient number of CD4 cells are destroyed and when production of new CD4 cells cannot match destruction. Patients exhibit fatigue, fever, and weight loss. This failure of the immune system leads to AIDS.

D. An HIV-infected person can live an average of 8 to 10 years before developing clinical symptoms. HIV disease is not uniformly expressed in all people. A small portion of patients develop AIDS and die within months of infection. Approximately 5% of infected patients, known as "long-term nonprogressors," have no signs of disease after 12 or more years.

E. Most AIDS-defining conditions are marked by a CD4 count of less than 200 cells or the appearance of one or more of the opportunistic infections (OIs). Bacteria, viruses, or fungi that would not cause illness in a healthy immune system cause OIs. These infections are often severe and sometimes fatal.

Predisposing Factors

A. Gay or bisexual men or prostitutes
B. Needle sharing by IVDU
C. Perinatal infection: Mother-to-child transmission
D. Open wound and mucous membrane exposure to body fluids of infected person
E. Recipients of transfusion of contaminated blood or blood products (rare since 1985)

Common Complaints

A. Fatigue: Often severe
B. Fever: Longer than 1 month
C. Night sweats: Drenching
D. Loss of appetite
E. Weight loss
F. Rash

Other Signs and Symptoms

A. Lymphadenopathy: Enlarged lymph nodes often involving at least two noncontiguous sites
B. Anemia
C. Neutropenia
D. Thrombocytopenia
E. Cough
F. Dyspnea
G. Asymptomatic whitish patches on sides of tongue: Hairy leukoplakia
H. Thrush: Oral candidiasis
I. Odynophagia: Esophageal candidiasis, cytomegalovirus (CMV) esophagitis
J. Chronic vaginal candidiasis
K. Skin changes: Rashes, dry skin, and seborrheic dermatitis
L. Purplish, nonblanching nodules found on the skin, mucous membranes, and viscera: Kaposi's sarcoma
M. Muscle wasting
N. Chronic diarrhea: Longer than 1 month
O. Hepatosplenomegaly
P. Cardiomyopathy
Q. Chronic bacterial infections, including community-acquired pneumonias
R. Tuberculosis
S. Sexually transmitted infections (STIs)
T. Peripheral neuropathy
U. Dementia
V. Children: Failure to thrive

Subjective Data

A. Review symptoms: Onset, course, and duration.
B. Ask about previous HIV testing including dates and reasons for testing.

C. Past medical history: Hospitalizations, comorbidities, immunizations, normal weight, pain, chronic lymph node disorders, and any changes of skin overlying lymph nodes

D. Past surgical history

E. Sexual history: Number of partners in the past year, number of lifetime partners, any previous partner known to be HIV positive or have STIs, and any previous partner known to have been incarcerated.

- **1.** Women: History of abnormal Paps, contraception, and condom use with partner
- **2.** Men: MSM, heterosexual, bisexual, receptive anal intercourse, and condom use

F. Past mental health history: Past and current mental health diagnosis and treatment.

G. Substance use: Tobacco, alcohol, and drugs

H. History of IVDU: Needle sharing and when last used drugs

I. Transfusion or blood product history before 1985

J. Lived or traveled outside of the United States: When and for how long

K. Assess the presence of persistent fever with no localizing symptoms.

L. Assess the patient's support system: Who knows the diagnosis?

Physical Examination

A. Height, weight, blood pressure, pulse, respiratory rate, and temperature

B. General observation: General appearance, including fat distribution signs of wasting

C. Inspect

- **1.** Skin: Evaluate for rashes, seborrhea, folliculitis, moles, Kaposi's sarcoma, warts, herpes, dry skin, skin cancer, fungal infections, molluscum contagiosum, jaundice, and needle marks.
- **2.** Head and neck; head, eyes, ears, nose, and throat (HEENT).
  - **a.** Assess visual acuity
  - **b.** Retina examination for abnormal findings—cotton wool spots, and the like
  - **c.** Evaluate sclera for icterus
  - **d.** Oral examination for thrush, hairy leukoplakia, mucosal Kaposi's sarcoma, gingivitis, aphthous ulcers, and dental health

D. Auscultate

- **1.** Pulmonary auscultation for air movement and abnormal breath sounds
- **2.** Cardiac evaluation for normal and abnormal heart sounds

E. Palpate

- **1.** Palpate the thyroid.
- **2.** Lymphatic evaluation of regional versus generalized swelling: Specific location, size, and texture of nodes
- **3.** Palpate the abdomen to evaluate the presence of hepatosplenomegaly, masses, tenderness, pain, or rebound tenderness.
- **4.** Breast examination (female)

F. Rectal/vaginal examination

- **1.** Both genders: Inspect for the presence of ulcers and warts in the vagina, perineum, and rectum.
- **2.** Females: Perform bimanual examination, Pap smear, obtain specimens for STI testing, and perform a digital rectal examination. Consider anal cytology if abnormal Pap smear.
- **3.** Males: Testicular examination, digital rectal examination, anal cytology if MSM

G. Neurologic examination

- **1.** Assess mental status.
- **2.** Assess cranial nerves, including gait, strength, deep tendon reflexes, evaluation of proprioception, vibration, pinprick, temperature, and sensation in distal extremities.

H. Psychiatric examination: Screen for depression.

Diagnostic Tests

A. Repeat HIV testing if the patient does not have a confirmed lab copy of diagnosis

B. Complete blood count (CBC), with differential, including platelets

C. Complete chemistry profile

D. Fasting lipid profile

E. Venereal disease research laboratory (VDRL) test and rapid plasma reagin (RPR) test

F. Serologies for toxoplasmosis

G. CD4/CD8 cells and CD4/CD8 ratio

H. HIV RNA viral load (VL)

I. HIV-resistance genotype and integrase strand transfer inhibitors (INSTI) genotype if under previous exposure

J. HLA-B 5701 (risk of abacavir hypersensitivity reaction syndrome)

K. Hepatitis serologies: Hepatitis A virus (HAV) serology (antibody), hepatitis B virus (HBV) complete serology profile, and hepatitis C virus (HCV) serology (antibody)

L. Cultures for gonorrhea/chlamydia (GC)/chlamydia—anal, vaginal, and oral

M. Urinalysis

N. Pap smear

O. Anal cytology with MSM; recommended for women with abnormal Pap smear

P. Tuberculosis (TB) screening: T-spot, QuantiFERON, or purified protein derivative (PPD). Chest x-ray yearly in case of a history of TB treatment. Refer to a TB clinic if screening is positive.

Differential Diagnoses

A. HIV

B. Other diseases that lead to immune suppression or are related to symptoms

C. Cancer

D. Chronic infections

E. Toxoplasmosis, other (syphilis, varicella-zoster, parovirus B19), rubella, cytomegalovirus and Herpes (TORCH) infections

F. Syphilis

G. Tuberculosis

H. Endocarditis

I. Infectious enterocolitis

J. Bowel disorders: Antibiotic-associated colitis, inflammatory bowel disease, or malabsorptive symptoms
K. Endocrine diseases
L. Neuropathy
M. Alcoholism
N. Liver disease
O. Renal disease
P. Thyroid disease
Q. Vitamin deficiency
R. Chronic meningitis

Plan—Clinical Guidelines per National Institutes of Health: AIDSinfo.NIH.gov

A. General interventions
1. Refer and comanage the patient with HIV/AIDS clinician.
2. Identify and treat substance abuse.
3. Explain to the patient that at each visit you will review history, conduct a physical examination, and run laboratory studies to assess health status.
4. Discuss health habits: Smoking, nutrition, and exercise.
5. Discuss treatment plan.
a. Highly active antiretroviral therapy (HAART)
b. Therapy for opportunistic infections (OIs) and malignancies
c. Prophylaxis for OIs: *Pneumocystis carinii* pneumonia (PCP) and mycobacterium avium complex (MAC) according to CD4 count
d. Managing side effects of medications and comorbidities
e. Immunizations

B. Patient teaching
1. Discuss living with HIV disease.
2. Discuss transmission prevention strategies: Safer sex practices and condom use.
3. Provide contact information for AIDS service organizations (ASOs).
4. Discuss the patient's concerns, including notification of sexual partner(s) and needle-sharing partner(s).
5. *See Section III: Patient Teaching Guide for this chapter, "Reference Resources for Patients With HIV/AIDS."*

C. Discuss birth control and family-planning issues. Offer preconception counseling.

D. Pharmaceutical therapy
1. Treatment with HAART: Always consult with an infectious disease HIV/AIDS specialist for treatment options.
a. HAART: At this time there are 25 individual medications from seven classes of drugs as well as 14 pills that are combinations of two to four of these medications. Recommendations are a minimum of three drugs from a minimum of two classes (Public Health Service Task Force Guidelines for the Use of Antiretroviral Agents in HIV-1 Infected Adults and Adolescents). Classes:
i. Nucleoside/nucleotide reverse transcriptase inhibitors (NRTIs)
ii. Non-nucleoside reverse transcriptase inhibitors (NNRTIs)
iii. Protease inhibitors (PIs)
iv. Integrase inhibitors (INIs)
v. Fusion inhibitors (FIs)
vi. Entry inhibitors (EIs)
vii. Pharmacokinetic enhancer
viii. Combination antiretrovirals
2. Prophylaxis and treatment for OIs. May discontinue prophylaxis if sustained an immune reconstitution on HAART.
a. PCP. Prophylaxis if CD4 count less than 200 or patient has oral candidiasis
i. First line: Bactrim DS (TMP-SMZ) 1 tablet three times weekly or 1 tablet daily (if toxoplasmosis positive)
ii. Alternatives: Dapsone, atovaquone, and aerosolized pentamidine
b. MAC prophylaxis if CD4 count is less than 75.
i. First line: Zithromax 1,200 mg weekly
ii. Alternative: Clarithromycin
3. Managing side effects of HAART and complications of HIV therapy: Multiple complications of long-term HIV infection and treatment with HAART
a. Lipodystrophy syndrome, bone marrow suppression, cardiovascular disease, CNS side effects, gastrointestinal (GI) intolerance, hepatic failure, hepatoxicity, hyperlipidemia, insulin resistance, diabetes, lactic acidosis/hepatic steotosis, nephrotoxicity, osteonecrosis, osteopenia, peripheral neuropathy, nephrolithiasis, urolithiasis, crystalluria, hypogonadism, and psychiatric complications
4. Immunizations
a. Hepatitis A and B series—if not immune, recommended dosing as per renal failure
b. Tetanus—Tdap
c. Pneumococcal vaccine—13 followed by 23 per recommendations
d. Yearly influenza vaccines
e. HPV vaccine series for women and men up to age 27 years

Follow-Up

A. Schedule return visit within 4 weeks after initial visit to discuss staging HIV/AIDS, living with HIV/AIDS, and to start HAART regimen.
B. Purified protein derivative (PPD) yearly unless there is a history of positive PPD, then yearly chest x-ray
C. Pap smear
1. Initially, if normal, repeat in 6 months, then yearly if remains normal
2. If abnormal, follow the guidelines by the American Society of Colposcopy and Cervical Pathology (ASCCP).
D. Some clinicians advocate for anal Pap smears for men but there are no set guidelines at present.

Consultation/Referral

A. Refer the patient to a specialist in HIV for management of continued care and pharmacological therapy.

B. Refer the patient to a nutritionist for baseline evaluation and diet counseling.
C. Refer pregnant women to a perinatologist.
D. Ophthalmology examination yearly for cytomegalovirus (CMV) screening and vision changes
E. Dental referral
F. Hepatology referral if chronic, active hepatitis B and/or C

Individual Considerations

A. Adults
1. Preconception counseling: Clinical Guidelines per National Institutes of Health—AIDSinfo.NIH.gov
2. Preconception counseling: The goal is to avoid transmission of HIV to partner and fetus. Use ovulation kits (basal body charts) to determine the most fertile time for pregnancy.
a. Discordant couples
i. HIV-positive female and HIV-negative male
1) Self-insemination (methods: syringe, turkey baster, cervical cap)
2) Use of preexposure prophylaxis (PrEP) for HIV-negative partner
ii. HIV-positive male and HIV-negative female
1) Sperm washing/IVF: Very expensive; often cost-prohibitive
2) HIV-positive male partner on HAART and HIV viral load (VL) as close to undetectable as possible
3) Unprotected sex during ovulation times only and no other
4) Use of PrEP for uninfected partner
iii. HIV-positive male and HIV-positive female: Avoid superinfection
1) Both partners on HAART and VL as close to undetectable as possible
2) Unprotected sex during ovulation times only and no other

B. Pregnancy: Clinical Guidelines per National Institutes of Health—AIDSinfo.NIH.gov
1. Antepartum
a. HAART starting at 10 to 12 weeks of gestation or maintaining treatment if already on pregnancy-approved HAART.
b. Goal of therapy is undetectable HIV-VL.
c. Sustiva should not be used in pregnancy during first trimester.
d. Vaginal delivery can be offered if HIV-VL is less than 1,000.
2. Intrapartum
a. Continue oral HAART.
b. Zidovudine intravenously (IV) 2 mg/kg in the first hour and then 1 mg/kg throughout delivery if VL is not detectable.
c. C-section if HIV-VL greater than 1,000
3. Postpartum
a. HAART for mother is continued depending on immunologic status.
b. Infant receives zidovudine 2 mg/kg every 12 hours for the first 4 weeks of life if mother has undetectable HIV-VL. If mother's VL is unknown or the aforementioned is undetectable, the baby should receive combination therapy.
c. Breastfeeding is contraindicated.

C. Pediatrics: Clinical Guidelines per National Institutes of Health—AIDSinfo.NIH.gov
1. Perinatal transmission in the United States has been reduced to less than 2% due to HAART.
2. Infants born to HIV-infected mothers test positive for HIV antibody ELISA test. Transplacentally acquired antibody may persist in the child for up to 18 months.
3. Clinical and laboratory evaluation of the child must be done postpartum. Initial HIV-RNA-VL testing should be done at birth, 14 to 21 days, 1 to 2 months, and 4 to 6 months postpartum.
4. Children who are HIV positive from vertical transmission should be followed by pediatric infectious disease clinicians.
5. All routine immunizations are recommended for HIV-infected children except for severely immunocompromised HIV-infected children who should not receive live-virus vaccines.

D. Prophylaxis
1. PrEP is a prevention method for HIV-negative partners.
a. Truvada is FDA approved for use as PrEP for heterosexual and MSM-HIV negative partners.
i. One tablet is taken daily to reduce the risk of infection.
ii. Those taking PrEP should be monitored for potential side effects.
2. Postexposure prophylaxis (PEP): Clinical Guidelines per National Institutes of Health—AIDSinfo.NIH.gov
a. Depending upon exposure type and severity, postexposure antiretroviral therapy (ART) should be started as quickly as possible and be taken for 4 weeks postexposure.
b. Expert consultation should be obtained as quickly as possible. (National HIV/AIDS Clinician's Consultation Center PEPline: 1-888-448-8765)
c. Follow with occupational health for regular clinical assessment and labs.
d. Perform HIV testing: Baseline, 6 weeks, 3 months, 6 months, and 1 year.
e. HIV testing with HIV-RNA-VL if an illness compatible with seroconversion illness occurs (fever, lymphadenopathy, pharyngitis, rash).
f. Advise transmission precautions during first 3 to 6 months postexposure (use condoms, refrain from donating blood, discontinue breastfeeding).

Resource

National HIV/ AIDS Clinician's Consultation Center: Warmline 800-933-3413
PEPline 888-448-4911
Perinatal HIV Hotline 888-448-8765

Idiopathic (Autoimmune) Thrombocytopenic Purpura

Julie Adkins

Definition

A. Idiopathic thrombocytopenic purpura (ITP) is an autoimmune disorder in which an immunoglobulin G (IgG) autoantibody is formed that binds to platelets. Platelets help your blood clot by clumping together to plug small holes in damaged blood vessels. The platelet count is less than 150,000 mm^3.

Incidence

A. Acute ITP occurs commonly in childhood, frequently precipitated by a viral infection. It is seen in children of 1 to 6 years of age and middle-aged adults of 30 to 40 years of age. There is a 2:1 female-to-male predominance. The adult form is usually a chronic disease (greater than 6 months) and seldom follows a viral infection.

Pathogenesis

A. ITP results from production of antiplatelet antibodies that leads to peripheral destruction and sequestration of platelets. It is not clear which antigen on the platelet surface is involved. Platelets are not destroyed by direct lysis. Destruction takes place in the spleen, where splenic macrophages with Fc receptors bind to antibody-coated platelets. The primary cause of long-term morbidity and mortality is hemorrhage, whether spontaneous or accident-induced trauma.

Predisposing Factors

A. Infections
B. Chronic alcoholism
C. Sepsis
D. AIDS
E. Immune disorders, such as systemic lupus erythematous (SLE)
F. Drug use
G. Chronic lymphocytic leukemia (CLL)
H. Pregnancy

Common Complaints

A. Purple spots and bruises on skin
B. Nosebleeds
C. Mouth and gum bleeding

Other Signs and Symptoms

A. Purpura, petechiae, and hemorrhagic bullae in the mouth
B. Tendency to bleed easily—easy bruising
C. Menorrhagia—abnormal heavy menstruation
D. No systemic illness: The patient feels well and is not febrile

Subjective Data

A. Determine when the patient or caregiver first noticed symptoms; note whether the symptoms have changed or progressed.
B. Rule out pregnancy as a cause of nosebleeds.
C. Ask whether the patient is feeling well except for the bleeding or bruising.
D. Determine whether the patient has a fever.
E. Obtain medication history for over-the-counter (OTC) and prescribed medications.
F. Determine the patient's history of immune disorders, recent infections, alcoholism, and pregnancy.
G. Establish usual weight and any recent weight loss.

Physical Examination

A. Check temperature, pulse, respirations, blood pressure, and weight.
B. Inspect
  1. Observe general appearance.
  2. Conduct dermal examination for purpura and petechiae.
  3. Conduct eye examination; check sclera for hemorrhages.
  4. Examine the mouth for dental caries and poor hygiene, mouth petechiae, and hemorrhagic bullae.

C. Palpate
  1. The abdomen, liver, and spleen.

Normally, the spleen should not be palpable.

  2. Palpate the cervical, axillary, and groin lymph nodes for adenopathy.

D. Percuss
  1. Abdomen
  2. Liver
  3. Spleen

E. Auscultate
  1. Heart
  2. Lungs
  3. Abdomen for bowel sounds and bruits

Diagnostic Tests

A. Platelet count

The major concern during the initial phase is risk of cerebral hemorrhage when platelet count is less than 5,000 platelets/μL.

B. IgG

Increased levels of IgG appear on the platelet count in the presence of thrombocytopenia.

C. Complete blood count (CBC) with differential and peripheral smear

Peripheral smear shows normal white blood cells (WBCs) and red blood cells (RBCs), platelets low in count with large size.

D. Bleeding time is prolonged.
E. Coagulation tests: Prothrombin time (PT), partial thromboplastin time (PTT), and fibrinogen—usually normal. Platelet-associated antibodies may be detected.

Coagulation studies are normal.

F. Bone marrow aspiration, per specialist

Bone marrow may appear normal or have increased megakaryocytes (early form of platelets) with thrombocytopenia.

Differential Diagnoses

Thrombocytopenia may be produced in two ways: By abnormal bone marrow function or by peripheral destruction of platelets.

A. Abnormal bone marrow function
  1. Aplastic anemia
  2. Hematologic malignancies
  3. Myelodysplasia: This can be ruled out only by examining the bone marrow.
  4. Megaloblastic anemia
  5. Chronic alcoholism

B. Non bone marrow disorders
  1. Immune disorders
    a. ITP
    b. Drug induced from medications being taken
    c. Secondary to CLL and SLE
    d. Posttransfusion purpura
  2. Hypersplenism resulting from liver disease
  3. Disseminated intravascular coagulation (DIC)
  4. Thrombotic thrombocytopenic purpura
  5. Sepsis
  6. Hemangiomas
  7. Viral infection
  8. AIDS
  9. Pregnancy
  10. Hypothyroidism

Plan

A. General interventions: Comanage the patient with a physician for medication therapy.

B. Patient teaching
  1. Instruct the patient to avoid trauma; advise that the patient cannot participate in *contact sports.*
  2. Instruct the patient to avoid salicylates; they impair platelet function.
  3. Prednisone therapy benefits
    a. Prednisone increases platelet count by increasing platelet production.
    b. Long-term therapy may decrease antibody production.
    c. Bleeding often diminishes 1 day after beginning prednisone.
    d. Platelet count usually begins to rise within a week; responses are almost always seen within 3 weeks.
    e. About 80% of patients respond to treatment and the platelet count usually returns to normal.

C. Medical or surgical management
  1. Splenectomy is the most definitive treatment. Most adults ultimately undergo splenectomy.
  2. Splenectomy is indicated if patients do not respond to prednisone initially or require unacceptably high doses to maintain an adequate platelet count.

D. Pharmaceutical therapy
  1. Initial treatment
    a. Prednisone 1 to 2 mg/kg/d
      i. High-dose therapy should be continued until the platelet count is normal, and the dose should then be gradually tapered.
      ii. In most patients, thrombocytopenia recurs if prednisone is completely withdrawn.
      iii. High-dose therapy should not be continued indefinitely in an attempt to avoid surgery.
  2. Alternative drug therapy
    a. High-dose intravenous immunoglobulin 400 mg/kg/d for 3 to 5 days is highly effective in rapidly raising the platelet count.
      i. This treatment is expensive, costing approximately $5,000 or more.
      ii. The beneficial effect lasts only 1 to 2 weeks.
      iii. This therapy should be reserved for emergency situations such as preparing a severely thrombocytopenic patient for surgery.
    b. Thrombopoietin receptor agonists: Drugs that boost platelet production such as romiplostim (Nplate) and eltrombopag (Promacta). The medications stimulate the bone marrow to produce more platelets. Side effects include headache, dizziness, nausea, vomiting. There is also an increased risk of blood clots.
  3. Platelet transfusions are an option rarely used. Transfusions may be necessary in emergency situations along with intravenous methylprednisolone and intravenous immune globulin.
  4. Avoid aspirin, nonsteroidal anti-inflammatory drugs (NSAIDs), or warfarin, which interfere with platelet function and blood clotting.

Exogenous platelets survive no better than the patient's own platelets. In many cases, platelets survive less than a few hours. This therapy is reserved for cases of life-threatening bleeding in which enhanced hemostasis for even an hour may be of benefit.

Follow-Up

A. The patient must be monitored very closely by a physician. Perform daily to weekly platelet counts; frequency depends on the severity and course.

B. Prognosis for acute ITP: 80% respond and fully recover within 2 months; 15% to 20% progress to chronic ITP.

C. Prognosis for chronic ITP: 10% to 20% recover fully; remainder continue to have low platelet counts and may see a remission or relapse over time.

D. The principal cause of death from ITP is intracranial hemorrhage.

Consultation/Referral

A. After diagnosis, refer the patient to a hematologist.

Individual Considerations

A. Pregnancy
1. Rule out hemolysis, elevated liver enzymes, low platelets (HELLP) syndrome, infection, and DIC as causes of thrombocytopenia.
2. There is an increased incidence of spontaneous abortions and hemorrhage at the time of delivery from genital tract injury.
3. Antepartum management: Conduct fetal blood sampling and testing when the mother has a known history of ITP.
4. Intrapartum management
a. Avoid fetal hypoxia, which can decrease the fetal platelet count.
b. Avoid prolonged labor.
c. Conduct continuous fetal monitoring.
d. Epidural anesthesia may be used if the platelet count is at least 100,000 cells/mm^3.
5. Postpartum management: Breastfeeding is not recommended because of the possible transmission of antiplatelet antibodies through breast milk.
B. Pediatrics
1. ITP is frequently precipitated by a viral infection.
2. It usually has an acute course that is self-limited.
C. Geriatrics
1. ITP is uncommon in this population; there is usually another cause for low platelets in geriatrics.
2. Persons older than 60 years must be evaluated for other causes such as myelodysplastic syndromes, acute leukemia, or bone marrow infiltration.
3. Persons with ITP aged 70 years or older are at risk of spontaneous bleeding and adverse events of treatment.

Iron-Deficiency Anemia (Microcytic, Hypochromic)

Julie Adkins

Definition

A. Microcytic anemia is characterized by small, pale red blood cells (RBCs) and depletion of iron (Fe) stores. The hematocrit (Hct) is less than 41% in males, with a hemoglobin (Hgb) less than 13.5 g/dL. In females, the Hct is less than 37% with an Hgb less than 12 g/dL.

Incidence

A. Iron deficiency is the most common cause of anemia worldwide; it is particularly prevalent in women of childbearing age. It is estimated to occur in 20% of adult women, 50% of pregnant women, and 3% of adult males in the United States.

Pathogenesis

A. Anemia is acquired; it develops slowly and in stages. Iron loss exceeds intake so that stored iron is progressively depleted. As stored iron is depleted, a compensatory increase in absorption of dietary iron and in the concentration of transferrin occurs. Iron storage can no longer meet the needs of the erythroid marrow; the plasma-transferring level increases and the serum iron concentration declines, resulting in a decrease in iron available for RBC formation.

Predisposing Factors

A. Female with heavy menses
B. Chronic blood loss, gastrointestinal (GI) blood loss
C. Family history or personal history of anemia
D. Poor diet, including strict vegetarian diets. Vegetarian diets do not include iron-rich foods.
E. Excessive cow's milk intake (children who drink greater than 16 to 24 oz a day). Excessive cow's milk intake interferes with iron absorption and irritates the intestinal lining
F. Closely spaced pregnancies
G. Lactation
H. Pica
I. Chronic hemoglobinuria due to an abnormally functioning cardiac valve
J. Chronic aspirin use or nonsteroidal anti-inflammatory drug (NSAID) use
K. Repeated blood donation
L. Decreased iron absorption due to gastric surgery
M. Taking too many antacids that contain calcium
N. Post-gastric bypass surgery
O. GI diseases such as celiac disease, irritable bowel syndrome (IBS), ulcerative colitis, Crohn's disease, and peptic ulcer disease
P. Chronic kidney disease
Q. Frequent blood donations

Common Complaints

A. Fatigued all of the time
B. Heart feels like it is racing, beating hard
C. Out of breath on exertion
D. Loss of appetite
E. Nausea and vomiting
F. Headaches throughout day
G. Weak and dizzy

Other Signs and Symptoms

Clinical presentation depends on severity, patient's age, and the ability of the cardiovascular and pulmonary systems to compensate for the decreasing oxygen-carrying capacity of the blood.

A. Initial: Exercise-induced dyspnea and mild fatigue symptoms may be minimal until the patient has significant anemia.
B. As Hct falls, dyspnea and fatigue increase.
1. Malaise
2. Drowsiness
3. Sore tongue and mouth
4. Skin pallor
5. Pale mucous membranes and conjunctiva
6. Pale nail beds
7. Tachycardia
8. Palpitations
9. Tinnitus
10. Pica symptoms (craving ice or clay)

11. Brittle nails
12. Hair loss

C. Severe anemia
1. Atrophic glossitis, cheilitis (lesions at the corner of the mouth)
2. Koilonychia (thin concave fingernails with raised edges)

Subjective Data

A. Inquire about onset, course, and duration of symptoms.
B. Ask the patient about past history of GI bleeding.
C. Take careful history of GI complaints that might suggest gastritis, peptic ulcer disease, or other conditions that might produce GI bleeding.
D. Ask if there has been a change in stool color or bleeding from hemorrhoids.
E. In menstruating women, ask about blood loss during menses.
F. Ask about dietary intake of iron-rich foods.
G. Inquire about pica habits, intake of non-food items such as clay, dirt, detergent, and the like.
H. Obtain medication history, especially use of aspirin and other nonsteroidal anti-inflammatory drugs (NSAIDs).
I. Rule out history of anemia, blood-clotting problems, sickle cell disease, glucose-6-phosphate dehydrogenase (G6PD) deficiency, or other hereditary hemolytic disease.
J. Review occupation and activities with exposure to lead or lead paint.
K. Has the patient experienced palpitations, chest pain, dizziness, or shortness of breath?

Physical Examination

A. Check temperature, pulse, respirations, blood pressure, and weight. Check for postural hypotension. Children: Plot weight, height, and head growth parameters on growth chart (see Table 17.1).
B. Inspect
1. Inspect general appearance; the patient may be pale, lethargic, or without overt signs if anemia is mild.
2. Conduct eye examination; check conjunctivae for paleness.
3. Examine oral mucosa, corners of the mouth (for cheilitis); note appearance of the tongue (atrophy of the papillae; smooth, shiny, beefy red appearance), angular stomatitis, or pale gums.
4. Examine the skin for dryness and perfusion.
5. Examine nails for brittleness, flattening, ridges, and concave or spoon shape.

C. Auscultate
1. Heart for systolic flow murmurs.

D. Palpate
1. Abdomen for tenderness and enlargement of the liver and spleen.

E. Percuss
1. Abdomen

F. Rectal examination: Assess for masses and obtain stool for occult blood.

TABLE 17.1 Normal Hemoglobin and Hematocrit Values for Children

Age (Years)	Hgb (%)	Hct (%)
1–2	>11.0	>33.0
2–5	>11.2	>34.0
5–8	>11.4	>34.5
8–12	>11.6	>35.5
12–18	>12.0	>36.0

Hct, hematocrit; Hgb, hemoglobin.

Diagnostic Tests

A. Initial
1. Complete blood count (CBC) with differential and peripheral smear
2. Serum ferritin level, serum iron, total iron-binding capacity (TIBC), reticulocyte count, RBC indices
3. Serum iron concentration: Absent iron storage equals ferritin value less than 30 ng/mL.
4. Urinalysis
5. Stool for occult blood

B. Follow-up
1. TIBC: Serum TIBC and serum ferritin rise.
2. Hct 3 to 4 weeks after treatment. Treatment should continue for at least 4 to 6 months after the Hct returns to normal.
3. GI series, if indicated.
4. Endoscope, if indicated.
5. Ultrasonography, if indicated.

Differential Diagnoses

A. Iron-deficiency anemia
B. Inadequate intake of iron
C. Any condition that causes acute or chronic blood loss
D. Hemolytic diseases such as sickle cell and G6PD deficiency
E. Anemia of chronic disease (thalassemia, sideroblastic anemias)
F. Lead poisoning
G. Neoplasm

Plan

A. General interventions
1. Identify source of anemia.
2. Discuss dietary sources of iron-rich foods.
3. Infants should be ingesting formula enriched with iron and iron-enriched cereals.

B. Patient teaching
1. Stress the importance of dietary intake of foods high in iron, which is absorbed better than most vitamins. Vitamin C increases absorption of iron. Suggest taking with a glass of orange juice or vitamin C supplement.
2. Tea and milk reduce iron absorption. Avoid large consumptions.
3. Provide iron supplements as indicated.
4. Encourage the patient to stop smoking if applicable.

C. Pharmaceutical therapy
1. Oral iron replacement
a. Adult
i. Begin 6-month trial of ferrous sulfate tablets 300 to 325 mg three times daily before meals or with orange juice or vitamin C 250 mg 1 hour before meals. Food decreases iron delivery by 50%.
ii. Iron supplement (Slow Fe) one time-release capsule daily or Niferex 150 Forte daily.
iii. If the patient has been prescribed an antacid, oral iron supplements should be taken 2 hours before or 4 hours after taking the antacid to avoid absorption interaction.
b. Children
i. Liquid iron 3 mg/kg/d in a single dose
ii. Chewable vitamin with an iron supplement one tablet every day for mild cases
2. Alternative drug therapy: Parenteral iron is indicated if the patient cannot tolerate or absorb oral iron or if iron loss exceeds oral replacement.
a. Iron dextran injection (Imferon)
b. Iron sorbitex injection (Jectofer)
i. Parenteral iron therapy is expensive.
ii. It is associated with significant side effects: Anaphylaxis, phlebitis, regional adenopathy, serum sickness-type reaction, and staining of intramuscular injection sites.
iii. Dose is based on the patient's weight.
iv. Do not administer parenteral iron along with oral iron.

Follow-Up

A. Follow-up of adults is variable, depending on the source of blood loss. Manage signs of anemia.
B. It is advisable to see the patient after 3 to 4 weeks, both to monitor the hematologic response and to answer questions about the medication, which may result in improved compliance.
C. If the patient's Hgb level has increased by 1.0 g/dL in 3 to 4 weeks, continue iron supplementation for an additional 3 to 6 months. The Hct should return to normal after 2 months of iron therapy. However, keep taking iron supplements for another 6 to 12 months to replace the body's iron storage in the bone marrow.
D. Determine the effectiveness of iron replacement therapy during the first 2 weeks of therapy by checking the reticulocyte count.

Consultation/Referral

A. Refer the patient to a physician for the following.
1. Hgb is not increased by 1.0 g/dL after 1 month of treatment.
2. The therapeutic trial should not be continued beyond 1 month because the Hgb concentration has not increased and patient compliance with recommended regimen is not a factor.
3. There is a steady downward trend in Hct despite treatment.
4. There is a significant drop in Hct over previous readings (rule out lab error first).
5. Laboratory findings show Hgb less than 9.0 g/dL or Hct less than 27%. Suspect underlying inflammatory, infectious, or malignant disease.
B. Refer the patient for nutrition consultation, if indicated.

Individual Considerations

A. Pregnancy
1. Check Hct at initial prenatal visit, 28 weeks, and 4 weeks after initiating therapy.
2. Laboratory findings of Hgb greater than 13 g/dL and Hct greater than 40% may indicate hypovolemia. Be alert for signs of dehydration and preeclampsia.
3. Counsel the patient on proper diet and refer him or her to a dietitian.
4. Recommend one to two iron tablets a day in addition to prenatal vitamins containing iron.
5. If unable to tolerate vitamins, recommend children's Chewable Flintstones vitamins with iron, two orally, daily.
B. Pediatrics
1. Place medication in back of mouth to reduce staining of teeth.
2. All infants must be on iron-fortified formula or breast milk.
3. Inform caregiver not to give cow's milk to infants younger than 12 months old.
4. Educate parents about iron-rich foods that are age-appropriate: Cereals, bran, dried fruit, red meat, and beans.
5. Obtain height and weight of infants and children, plot on growth chart, and compare with previous parameters.
C. Adults
1. Bleeding is the usual cause of anemia in adults. In adult men and postmenopausal women, bleeding is usually from the GI tract.
2. In premenopausal women, menstrual loss may be the underlying cause of anemia.
3. Smokers may have higher Hgb levels; therefore, anemia may be masked if standard Hgb levels are used.

Lymphadenopathy

Julie Adkins

Definition

Lymphadenopathy is enlargement of a lymph node, manifested in benign, self-limiting diseases and in those that are incurable and fatal. Only small lymph nodes in the neck, axilla, and groin are palpable in normal individuals. Palpable nodes in other regions, or any node exceeding 0.5 cm in size, are potentially abnormal. The body has approximately 600 lymph nodes.

There are different categories of lymphadenopathy:
A. Localized adenopathy
B. Hilar adenopathy

C. Generalized lymphadenopathy
D. Other lymphatic abnormalities that present in other ways, such as lymphangitis, lymphadenitis, and lymphedema

Incidence

A. Lymphadenopathy is a very common presenting symptom. Age is an important diagnostic factor: In patients younger than 30 years, the cause proves to be benign in 80% of cases; in patients older than age 50, the rate of benign disease falls to 40%. In primary care patients with unexplained lymphadenopathy, approximately three fourths of patients will present with localized lymphadenopathy and one fourth with generalized lymphadenopathy. Lymphadenopathy in children is commonly caused by benign self-limiting diseases, such as viral disease.

Pathogenesis

A. Inflammation and infiltration are responsible for pathologic enlargement. Localized lymphadenopathy may represent the spread of disease from an area of drainage. The left supraclavicular node is referred to as the "sentinel" node, which is in contact with the thoracic duct and drains much of the abdominal cavity. The right supraclavicular node drains the mediastinum, lungs, and esophagus. Generalized lymphadenopathy often results from infection, malignancy, hypersensitivity, and metabolic disease.

Predisposing Factors

A. Factors posing high risk for HIV infection
  1. Homosexuality and bisexuality
  2. Intravenous drug abuse
  3. Hemophilia, conditions requiring multiple transfusions
  4. Prostitution
  5. Haitian ancestry
B. Occupational exposure
C. History of pharyngitis, upper body infections (head and neck), or intraoral infection
D. Exposure to animals: Cats, sheep, cattle, rodents, deer ticks
E. Travel to the southwest United States
F. Exposure to bird droppings
G. Lacerations sustained from gardening
H. Exposure to tuberculosis (TB)
I. History of sexual exposure resulting in sexually transmitted infections (STIs)
J. History of tobacco abuse
K. Cancer
L. Medications
  1. Anticonvulsant drugs that cause skin rash, fever, hepatosplenomegaly, and eosinophilia (e.g., phenytoin [Dilantin])
  2. Hydralazine
  3. Para-aminosalicylic acid
  4. Allopurinol

Common Complaints

A. Sore throat
B. Fever
C. Fatigue and malaise
D. Loss of appetite
E. Loss of weight
F. Swollen, painless lumps in neck, axilla, supraclavicular, iliac, and inguinal areas

Other Signs and Symptoms

A. May feel "good" except for finding enlarged lymph node
B. Node location(s): For inguinal enlargement, rule out conditions that may resemble inguinal or femoral lymphadenopathy—Hernias; ectopic testicular, endometrial, or splenic tissue; lipomas; varices; and aneurysms. If inguinal area is painful and tender, it is most frequently caused by STIs.
C. Skin rash
D. Bruising or petechiae
E. Pruritus
F. Erythema of skin or scalp
G. Skin eruption
H. Night sweats
I. Abdominal pain, enlarged and tender abdomen
J. Joint pain

Subjective Data

A. A comprehensive and detailed history is necessary for diagnosis (see "Predisposing Factors" section).
B. Review the onset, course, and duration of symptoms.
C. What does the patient note with respect to location, tenderness or painfulness, softness or hardness, and mobility of lymph nodes? Has the patient noticed more than one enlarged lymph node?
D. Review the patient's history of intravenous drug use. Review risk factors for HIV.
E. Review history for hobbies, specifically gardening and camping, and occupation (see "Lyme Disease" and "Toxoplasmosis" in Chapter 16, "Infectious Disease Guidelines").
F. Review medications: Prescription, over-the-counter (OTC), and herbal remedies.
G. Determine whether the patient has a fever or a known valvular heart disease.
H. Review any other associated symptoms or signs.
I. Review any recent exposure to family and friends with infections. Has the patient had recent immunizations?
J. Review recent dental problems or abscessed teeth.
K. Note whether the patient is a smoker. If so, how much, for how long, and when did the patient quit smoking?
L. Review the patient's history for recent cat scratches (see "Cat Scratch Disease" in Chapter 16, "Infectious Disease Guidelines").
M. Review the patient's history for recent travel.
N. Review the patient's history for new sexual partners, to rule out STIs.
O. Review usual weight and any recent weight loss, noting how much and over what period of time.
P. Elicit information about similar symptoms in the past, when they occurred, how they were treated (antibiotics, biopsy), and the success of the treatment.
Q. Elicit information about alcohol intake, noting how much, how long, and whether the patient has quit and how long ago.

Physical Examination

A. Check temperature, pulse, respirations, blood pressure, and weight.

B. Inspect

1. Conduct a funduscopic examination.

2. Examine the eyes, ears, nose, and throat.

3. Conduct a dermal examination, and check mucous membranes for a primary inoculation site; this may be a clue to a diagnosis of cat scratch disease (CSD).

C. Auscultate

1. Heart and lungs

D. Palpate

1. Palpate the abdomen.

2. Conduct a clinical breast examination. Palpate mass to determine if it is a lymph node, if applicable.

3. Palpate all nodal areas for localized and generalized lymphadenopathy.

a. Hard, fixed nodes suggest metastasis, and a biopsy should be taken promptly. Size alone is not itself diagnostic; any node larger than 3 cm suggests neoplastic disease.

4. Palpate the scalp in the elderly for the tender arteries of cranial arteritis.

5. Palpate the neck for thyroid gland tenderness or masses.

6. Musculoskeletal system examination

a. Assess and palpate for bone or joint swelling, tenderness, and increased warmth.

b. Examine lower extremities for evidence of phlebitis: Asymmetric swelling, calf tenderness, and palpable cord.

E. Percuss

1. Sinuses for tenderness, and transilluminate for evidence of sinusitis.

F. Genital–rectal examination

1. Conduct careful external evaluation for herpetic lesions, masses, discharge, erythema, chancroid, scabies, and pediculosis.

2. "Milk" urethra for discharge.

3. Note any folliculitis if the patient regularly shaves the genital area.

4. Female pelvic examination: Look for cervical discharge, cervical motion tenderness, adnexal tenderness, and mass or "heat" in the pelvis.

5. Males: Examine the prostate and testicles for tenderness and masses, and the penis for discharge and rash.

6. Examine the rectum for discharge, tenderness, masses, and fistulas.

Diagnostic Tests

A. Complete blood count (CBC) with differential

B. Peripheral blood smear: The most useful laboratory test: (It may be helpful in the diagnosis of chronic leukemia, infectious mononucleosis, and other viral illnesses.)

C. Blood chemistries

D. Liver function tests, especially alkaline phosphatase

E. Angiotensin-converting enzyme (ACE)

F. Antinuclear antibody (ANA) and rheumatoid factor

G. RPR and microhemagglutination assay for antibody to *Treponema` pallidum* (MHA-TP), to rule out syphilis

H. Heterophile test, to rule out mononucleosis

I. ELISA and Western blot, to rule out HIV

J. Uric acid: Elevations may reflect lymphoma or other hematologic malignancies

K. Blood cultures

L. Urethral or cervical cultures and smears

M. Throat culture

N. Chest x-ray

O. Mammogram with ultrasonography of suspicious breast area, if indicated

P. After consultation

1. Abdominal ultrasonography or CT scan, if indicated

2. Biopsy or fine-needle aspiration: Fine-needle aspiration is used to obtain a cytologic diagnosis of a suspected cancer. False negative results may occasionally occur.

3. Lymph node biopsy: Lymph node biopsy is the definitive test to confirm or rule out a suspected neoplastic process.

4. Mediastinoscopy

Q. Tuberculin skin testing of purified protein derivative (PPD) and the ACE determination can facilitate assessment.

1. If the patient tests *negative for ACE and PPD* and is Caucasian, then bronchoscopy and mediastinoscopy may be necessary to rule out lymphoma. If the patient tests *positive for ACE but negative for PPD*, then the probability is very high that sarcoidosis is the cause.

2. If the patient tests *negative for ACE but positive for PPD*, then primary TB is likely.

Differential Diagnoses

A. There are four general categories for lymphadenopathy.

1. Infections

a. Mononucleosis

b. AIDS or AIDS-related complex (ARC): Generalized adenopathy in an asymptomatic HIV-infected patient indicates a high risk of progression to AIDS. The lymphadenopathy represents follicular hyperplasia in response to HIV infection.

c. Toxoplasmosis

d. Secondary syphilis

2. Hypersensitivity reactions

a. Serum sickness

b. Phenytoin and other drugs

3. Metabolic diseases

a. Hyperthyroidism

b. Lipidoses

4. Neoplasia

a. Leukemia

b. Hodgkin's disease, advanced stages

c. Non-Hodgkin's lymphoma

B. Causes can be isolated by site of the enlarged nodes (see Table 17.2).

TABLE 17.2 Causes of Lymphadenopathy by Site of Enlarged Nodes

Anterior Auricular Viral conjunctivitis Trachoma Posterior auricular Rubella Scalp infection **Submandibular or Cervical (Unilateral)** Buccal cavity infection Pharyngitis (can be bilateral) Nasopharyngeal tumor Thyroid malignancy **Cervical (Bilateral)** Mononucleosis sarcoidosis Toxoplasmosis pharyngitis **Supraclavicular (Right)** Pulmonary malignancy Mediastinal malignancy Esophageal malignancy **Supraclavicular (Left)** Intra-abdominal malignancy Renal malignancy Testicular or ovarian malignancy	**Axillary** Breast malignancy Breast infection Upper extremity infection **Epitrochlear** Syphilis (bilateral) Hand infection (unilateral) **Inguinal** Syphilis Genital herpes Lymphogranuloma venereum chancroid Lower extremity or local infection **Any Region** Cat scratch fever Hodgkin's disease Leukemia Metastatic cancer Sarcoidosis Granulomatous infections **Hilar Adenopathy** Sarcoidosis (unilateral or bilateral) Fungal infection (histoplasmosis, coccidioidomycosis) Lymphoma (unilateral or bilateral) Bronchogenic carcinoma (unilateral or bilateral) Tuberculosis (unilateral or bilateral)

Plan

A. General interventions
   1. Pay careful attention to nodal history and characteristics on physical examination.
   2. Make a careful assessment to establish the palpable mass is a lymph node. Chronicity alone is not always serious.

B. Patient teaching: As indicated by the particular disease process causing the lymphadenopathy. See the relevant guidelines.

C. Pharmaceutical therapy: Dependent on the diagnosis

Follow-Up

A. Follow the patient closely to evaluate resolution of lymphadenopathy and disease process.

B. Follow-up depends on the diagnosis.

Consultation/Referral

A. Consultation with a physician may be useful if a period of observation is needed.

B. Refer the patient to a specialist after initial workup, if indicated.

C. Refer the patient to an oncologist or oncologic surgeon if the patient is suspected of having a malignancy, to consider the need for biopsy or best approach to obtaining a tissue diagnosis.

Individual Considerations

A. Pediatrics
   1. Palpable nodes in the anterior cervical triangle of the neck are common in children and usually suggest infection as a cause.
   2. Kawasaki disease is seen among children and young adults; it is also known as mucocutaneous lymph node syndrome (see Chapter 16, "Infectious Disease Guidelines").

B. Adults
   1. Hodgkin's lymphoma is one of the most common cancers of young adults.

C. Geriatrics
   1. Regional lymphadenopathy occurs often when carcinomas metastasize to lymph nodes in the elderly.

Pernicious Anemia (Megaloblastic Anemia)

Julie Adkins

Definition

A. Pernicious anemia is a megaloblastic, macrocytic, normochromic anemia caused by a deficiency of intrinsic factor in the gastric juices produced by the stomach, which results in malabsorption of vitamin B_{12} necessary for DNA synthesis and maturation of red blood cells (RBCs). There is production of abnormally large and oval red cells with a mean corpuscular volume in excess of 100 fL (femto-liters). The anemia can be severe, with hematocrit (Hct) as low as 10% to 15%.

Incidence

A. Pernicious anemia is common in people of northern European descent. Both sexes are equally affected. It is most prevalent in Scandinavian and English-speaking populations. It usually occurs in the fifth and sixth decades of life; it is rarely seen in persons younger than 35 years, but it can occur in individuals in their 20s. There is an increased incidence in those with other immunologic disease.

Pathogenesis

A. Pernicious anemia is possibly due to an autoimmune reaction involving the gastric parietal cell that results in nonproduction of intrinsic factor and atrophy of gastric mucosa. Vitamin B_{12} deficiency can result from inadequate intake, impaired absorption, increased requirements as in pregnancy, or faulty utilization. Poor intake is rare, occurring most often in strict vegetarians. You get this vitamin from eating foods such as meat, poultry, shellfish, eggs, and dairy products (U.S. National Library of Medicine, 2013).

Predisposing Factors

A. People of northern European descent
B. Ages 50 to 60 years
C. Immunologic disease
D. Loss of parietal cells following gastrectomy
E. Overgrowth of intestinal organisms
F. Crohn's disease
G. Ileal resection or abnormalities
H. Fish tapeworm
I. Congenital enzyme deficiencies
J. Diet: Strict vegetarian diets
K. Medications such as aminosalicylate sodium
L. Alcoholism
M. Hashimoto's thyroiditis
N. Addison's disease, Graves' disease, myasthenia gravis, or type 1 diabetes

Common Complaints

> *Classic presentation involves sore tongue and numbness and tingling in the extremities, hands, or feet.*

A. Weakness and dizziness
B. Tongue is sore, red, and shiny
C. Numbness, burning, tingling sensation of arms or legs
D. Feel heart "jumping out of skin"
E. Edema of lower extremities
F. Anorexia
G. Diarrhea

Other Signs and Symptoms

A. Dyspnea on exertion
B. Pallor
C. Fatigue
D. Tachycardia
E. Exercise intolerance
F. Angina
G. Glossitis
H. Mucositis
I. Peripheral paresthesia
J. Palpitations
K. Abdominal tenderness, organomegaly
L. Advanced stages: Dementia and spinal cord degeneration

Subjective Data

A. Inquire about onset, duration, and course of presenting symptoms.
B. Ask the patient to describe usual bowel habits. Has there been any blood in stools?
C. If gastrointestinal (GI) complaints are present, inquire about presence of red, burning tongue; abdominal complaints; and/or presence of diarrhea or constipation.
D. If neurologic complaints are present, inquire about the presence of pins-and-needles paresthesia and weakness, unsteadiness due to proprioceptive difficulties, lethargy, and fatigue.
E. Inquire about dietary intake, using a 24-hour recall.
F. Ask about alcohol consumption: How much? How long?
G. Obtain medication history: OTC and prescription drugs.
H. Obtain past medical history, specifically if the patient has a history of gastrectomy, resection of ileum, or other GI disorders.
I. Review usual weight and recent loss.

Physical Examination

A. Check temperature, pulse, respirations, blood pressure, weight, and height for children; plot on graph.
B. Inspect
  1. Observe general, overall appearance; observe walking.
  2. Conduct oral examination for characteristic red, shiny tongue.
  3. Conduct dermal and eye examinations for color: Affected patients are slightly icteric.
  4. Evaluate the look of the person related to age: Affected patients show premature aging or graying.
C. Auscultate
  1. Heart sounds and lungs
  2. The abdomen for bowel sounds
D. Palpate
  1. Palpate the abdomen for masses.
  2. Evaluate pedal edema.
E. Percuss
  1. The abdomen for tenderness and organomegaly
F. Neurologic examination
  1. Assess DTRs and mental status.
  2. Assess for paresthesia involving hands and feet.
  3. Observe for gait disturbances.
  4. Ask the patient to perform finger-to-nose test. Poor finger–nose coordination may be seen.
  5. Observe Romberg's test. Elicit Babinski's sign. Positive Romberg's and Babinski's signs may be present.
  6. Assess for memory loss. Differentiate among mild forgetfulness, dementia, or altered thought processes.

Diagnostic Tests

A. Complete blood count (CBC) with differential and peripheral smear: Macroovalocytes and hypersegmented neutrophils may be present on peripheral blood smear. (They are absent in the setting of concurrent iron deficiency.)
B. Serum vitamin B_{12} level: Less than 100 pg/mL
C. Serum folic acid levels, serum iron, serum ferritin, and TIBC

D. Serum intrinsic factor antibody
E. Lactate dehydrogenase (LDH)
F. Urinalysis
G. Stool for occult blood
H. Oral Schilling test with and without intrinsic factor
I. GI radiographic studies
J. Gastric analysis: Achlorhydria is found on stimulation testing
K. Bone marrow aspiration
L. A woman with low B_{12} levels may have a false positive Pap smear due to vitamin B_{12} effects on the epithelial cells.

Differential Diagnoses

Differential diagnosis of anemia by red cell morphology can be undertaken (mean corpuscular volume [MCV], mean corpuscular hemoglobin concentration [MCHC]). Common causes of each type of anemia are as follows:

A. Normochromic, normocytic: Normal MCV = 80 to 100, MCHC = 32% to 36%
- **1.** Aplastic anemia
- **2.** Chronic disease
- **3.** Early iron deficiency
- **4.** Hemolysis
- **5.** Hemorrhage

B. Microcytic: MCV = 50 to 82, MCHC = 24 to 32
- **1.** Chronic disease
- **2.** Iron deficiency
- **3.** Thalassemia

C. Macrocytic: MCV greater than 100, MCHC greater than 36
- **1.** Antimetabolites
- **2.** Folic acid deficiencies
- **3.** Vitamin B_{12} deficiencies
- **4.** Chronic alcoholism

Plan

A. General interventions
- **1.** Most common method of determining vitamin B_{12} deficiency is by serum vitamin B_{12} assay.
- **2.** Most common method of demonstrating folate deficiency is by measurement of serum folic acid levels.
- **3.** Red cell indices and peripheral smear should be done to determine classification of anemia to facilitate workup.
- **4.** Red cell distribution width (RDW) determination can assist in detecting red cell heterogeneity previously available only by examination of the peripheral smear. The RDW determination overcomes the problems of detecting coexisting microcytic and macrocytic anemias.

B. Patient teaching
- ▶ **1.** *See Section III: Patient Teaching Guide for this chapter, "Pernicious Anemia."*
- **2.** Neurologic symptoms usually improve with treatment; however, some neurologic deficits may not be reversible.

C. Pharmaceutical therapy
- **1.** Vitamin B_{12} (cyanocobalamin or hydroxocobalamin) 100 mg intramuscularly or subcutaneous administration daily for 1 week.
  - **a.** Decrease the frequency and administer a total of 2,000 mg during the first 6 weeks of therapy (weekly for 1 month).
  - **b.** Maintenance treatment requires lifelong administration of 100 mg intramuscular injection monthly depending on B_{12} levels. Some people may require lifelong administration at different intervals such as every 2 weeks.
  - **c.** Nascobal (intranasal cyanocobalamin) one spray in one nostril one time per week.
- **2.** Recommended daily allowance for vitamin B_{12}
  - **a.** Neonates and infants up to 6 months: 0.3 mcg/d
  - **b.** Children older than 6 months to 1 year: 0.5 mcg/d
  - **c.** Children 1 to 3 years: 0.7 mcg/d
  - **d.** Children 4 to 6 years: 1.0 mcg/d
  - **e.** Children 7 to 10 years: 1.4 mcg/d
  - **f.** Adults and children older than 11 years: 2.0 mcg/d
  - **g.** Pregnant women: 2.2 mcg/d
  - **h.** Breastfeeding women: 2.6 mcg/d
- **3.** Concomitant iron supplementation during first month of therapy. Rapid blood cell regeneration increases iron requirements and can lead to iron deficiency.

Follow-Up

A. The patient must be seen in 2 weeks to determine response to treatment: Increased reticulocyte count and increased Hct; diminution in neurologic signs and symptoms.
B. Evaluate the patient monthly when giving vitamin B_{12} injections.
C. Endoscopy every 5 years is used to rule out gastric carcinoma. People with pernicious anemia may have gastric polyps and are more likely to develop gastric cancer and gastric carcinoid tumors.
D. Check the patient every 6 months for Hct, and check his or her stool for occult blood.
E. Hct value rises 4% to 5% per week in uncomplicated cases.

Consultation/Referral

A. Refer the patient to a dietitian.
B. Rapid reticulocytosis should be seen following treatment; it peaks in 7 to 10 days.
C. Consult a physician if no change is seen.

Individual Considerations

A. Pregnancy
- **1.** Lactovegetarians and ovolactovegetarians do well in pregnancy.
- **2.** Vegetarian women who eat neither eggs nor milk products should take vitamin B_{12} supplements during pregnancy and lactation.

B. Pediatrics
- **1.** Congenital disorder usually is seen before 3 years of age.

C. Adults

1. Disorder rarely is seen in patients younger than age 35 years.

D. Geriatrics

1. Disorder most commonly is seen in the geriatric population.

2. Follow up elderly patients with assessment of cardiovascular symptoms 48 hours after initiating therapy.

3. Rapid blood cell regeneration increases iron requirements and can lead to iron deficiency.

Bibliography

The AIDS Infonet. (2013). Reliable, up-to-date treatment information. Retrieved from www.aidsinfonet.org

AIDSmeds. (2012a, August 28). Treatment for HIV & AIDS. Retrieved from http://www.aidsmeds.com/list.shtml

AIDSmeds. (2012b, November 13). Currently approved drugs for HIV: A comparative chart. Retrieved from http://www.aidsmeds.com/articles/DrugChart_10632.shtml

American Academy of HIV Medicine. (2010). *Fundamentals of HIV medicine for the HIV specialist.* Washington, DC: Author. Retrieved from http://www.AAHIVM.org

American Society for Colposcopy and Cervical Pathology. (2012). Consensus guidelines 2012: Updated consensus guidelines for the management of abnormal cervical cancer screening tests and cancer precursors. Retrieved from http://www.asccp.org/guidelines

Americans Society of Hematology. (2016). Iron deficiency anemia. Retrieved from www.hematology.org

Angeline, M. E., Gee, A. O., Shindle, M., Warren, R. F., & Rodeo, S. A. (2013). The effects of vitamin D deficiency in athletes. *American Journal of Sports Medicine, 41*(2), 461–464.

The Body. (n.d.-a). Approved HIV medications by class. Retrieved from http://www.thebody.com/index/treat/classes.html

The Body. (n.d.-b). First steps to HIV/AIDS treatment. Retrieved from http://www.thebody.com/index/treat/first.html

The Body. (n.d.-c). HIV/AIDS medication basics. Retrieved from http://www.thebody.com/content/art40488.html

The Body. (n.d.-d). HIV drug-drug interactions. Retrieved from http://www.thebody.com/index/treat/interactions.html

The Body. (n.d-e). Side effects of HIV/AIDS and HIV medications. Retrieved from http://www.thebody.com/index/treat/side_effects.html#general

The Body. (2016). The complete HIV/AIDS resource. Retrieved from http://www.thebody.com

Brown, H. (2013). Managing pernicious anemia. *Independent Nurse, 18*(02), 22–24.

Centers for Disease Control and Prevention. (2012a, June). Monitoring selected National HIV prevention and care objectives by using HIV surveillance data-United States and 6 U.S. dependent areas-2010. HIV Surveillance Supplemental Report. Retrieved from https://www.cdc.gov/hiv/topics/surveillance/reports

Centers for Disease Control and Prevention. (2013a, January). HIV testing trends in the United States, 2000– 2011. Retrieved from https://www.cdc.gov/hiv/pdf/ testing_trends.pdf

Centers for Disease Control and Prevention. (2013b, April 15). HIV surveillance report: Diagnoses of HIV infection in the United States and dependent areas, 2011. Retrieved from https://www.cdc.gov/hiv/pdf/statistics_2011_HIV_Surveillance_Report_vol_23.pdf

Centers for Disease Control and Prevention. (2013c, November). HIV in the United States: At a glance. Retrieved from https://www.cdc.gov/hiv/basics/statistics.html

Centers for Disease Control and Prevention. (2013d, May 13). HIV among African American gay and bisexual men. Retrieved from https://www.cdc.gov/hiv/risk/racialethnic/bmsm/facts/index.html

Centers for Disease Control and Prevention. (2014a). Chronic fatigue syndrome (CFS). Retrieved from www.cdc.gov/cfs

Centers for Disease Control and Prevention. (2014b, December 11) Recommendations for HIV Prevention with Adults and Adolescents with HIV. Retrieved from https://www.cdc.gov/hiv/guidelines/personswithhiv.html

Centers for Disease Control and Prevention. (2016a). HIV/AIDS statistics overview. Retrieved from www.cdc.gov/hiv/statistics/overview

Centers for Disease Control and Prevention. (2016b). Opportunistic infections. Retrieved from www.cdc.gov/hiv/basics/livingwithhiv/opportunisticinfections.html

Centers for Disease Control and Prevention. (2016c). Updated guidelines for antiretroviral postexposure prophylaxis after sexual, injection drug use, or other nonoccupational exposure to HIV—United States, 2016. Retrieved from stacks.cdc.gov/view/cdc/38856

Chan-Trak, K. (2015). Fever of unknown origin. Retrieved from http://emedicine.medscape.com/article/217675

Christley, Y. J., & Martin, C. R. (2012). Perinatal perspective on chronic fatigue syndrome. *British Journal of Midwifery, 20*(6), 389–393.

Correia, L., Sodre, F., Garcia, G., Sabino, M., Brito, M., Kalil, F., & Noya-Rabelo, M. (2013). Relation of severe deficiency of vitamin D to cardiovascular mortality during acute coronary syndromes. *American Journal of Cardiology, 111*(3), 324–327.

Friedman, J. J., Chen, Z., Ford, P., Johnson, C., Lopez, A., Shander, A., & van Wyck, D. (2012). Iron deficiency anemia in women across the life span. *Journal of Women's Health, 21*(12), 1282–1289.

Günthard, H. F., Saag, M. S., Benson, C. A., del Rio, C., Eron, J. J., Gallant, J. E., . . . Volberding, P. A. (2016). Antiretroviral drugs for treatment and prevention of HIV infection in adults: 2016 recommendations of the International Antiviral Society-USA Panel. Journal of the American Medical Association, 316(2), 191–210. Retrieved from https://www.iasusa.org/content/antiretroviral-drugs-treatment-and-prevention-hiv-infection-adults-2016-recommendations

Horowitz, H. (2013). Fever of unknown origin or fever of too many origins? *New England Journal of Medicine, 368*(3), 197–199.

Institute of Medicine. (2015). *Beyond myalgic encephalomyelitis/chronic fatigue syndrome: Redefining an illness.* Washington, DC: National Academies Press.

International AIDS Society–USA. (n.d.). Antiretroviral treatment of adult HIV infection. Retrieved from https://www.iasusa.org/content/antiretroviral-drugs-treatment-and-prevention-hiv-infection-adults-2016-recommendations

Kahanov, L., Eberman, L. E., & Grammer, S. (2012). Diagnosis and treatment of idiopathic thrombocytopenic purpura. *International Journal of Athletic Therapy & Training, 17*(2), 25–28.

Kanwar, V. (2016). Lymphadenopthy. Retrieved from www.emedicine.medscape.com

Kessler, C. (2015). Immune thrombocytopenic purpura (ITP). Retrieved from emedicine.medscape.com

Mayo Clinic. (2014). Chronic fatigue syndrome. Retrieved from www.mayoclinic.org

Mayo Clinic. (2016). Idiopathic thrombocytopenia purpura (itp). Retrieved from www.mayoclinic.org

Motyckova, G., & Steensma, D. (2012). Why does my patient have lymphadenopathy or spleenomegaly? *Hematology/Oncology Clinics of North America, 26*(2), 395–408.

National HIV/AIDS Clinician's Consultation Center. Retrieved from http://nccc.ucsf.edu/

Panel on Antiretroviral Guidelines for Adults and Adolescents. (2016, July 14). *Guidelines for the use of antiretroviral agents in HIV-1-infected adults and adolescents.* Washington, DC: Department of Health and Human Services. Retrieved from https://aidsinfo.nih.gov/contentfiles/lvguidelines/AdultandAdolescentGL.pdf

Panel on Antiretroviral Therapy and Medical Management of HIV-Infected Children. (2016, March 1). *Guidelines for the use of antiretroviral agents in pediatric HIV infection.* Washington, DC: Department of Health and Human Services. Retrieved from https://aidsinfo.nih.gov/contentfiles/lvguidelines/pediatricguidelines.pdf

Panel on Opportunistic Infections in HIV-Infected Adults and Adolescents. (2013b, May 7). *Guidelines for the prevention and treatment of opportunistic infections in HIV-infected adults and adolescents: Recommendations from the Centers for Disease Control and Prevention, the National Institutes of Health, and the HIV Medicine Association of the Infectious Diseases.* Society of America. Washington, DC: Department of Health and Human Services. Retrieved from https://aidsinfo.nih.gov/contentfiles/lvguidelines/adult_oi.pdf

Panel on Treatment of HIV-Infected Pregnant Women and Prevention of Perinatal Transmission. (2016, October 26). *Recommendations for use of antiretroviral drugs in pregnant HIV-1-infected women for maternal health* and *interventions to reduce perinatal HIV transmission in the United States.* Washington, DC: Department of Health and Human Services. Retrieved from http://aidsinfo.nih.gov/contentfiles/lvguidelines/perinatalgl.pdf

Park, S., Kang, J., Roh, J., Huh, H., Yeo, J., & Kim, D. (2013). Secondary syphilis presenting as a generalized lymphadenopathy: Clinical mimicry of malignant lymphoma. *Sexually Transmitted Diseases, 40*(6), 490–492.

POZ.com HIV Drug Chart. Retrieved from https://www.poz.com/drug_charts/hiv-drug-chart

Short, M., & Domagalski, J. (2013). Iron deficiency anemia: Evaluation and management. *American Family Physician, 87*(2), 98–104.

Stabler, S. (2013). Clinical practice: Vitamin B_{12} deficiency. *New England Journal of Medicine, 368*(2), 149–160.

U.S. Food and Drug Administration. (n.d.). Antiretroviral drugs used in the treatment of HIV infection. Retrieved from http://www.fda.gov/ForPatients/Illness/HIVAIDS/Treatment/ucm118915.htm

U.S. National Library of Medicine. (2013a, March 12). Iron deficiency anemia. Retrieved from https://www.ncbi.nlm.nih.gov/pubmedhealth/PMHT0022011

U.S. National Library of Medicine. (2013b, March 12). Pernicious anemia. Retrieved from https://www.ncbi.nlm.nih.gov/pubmedhealth/PMHT0022012

U.S. Preventive Services Task Force Recommendation Statement. (2013, April) Screening for HIV. Retrieved from http://www.uspreventiveservicestaskforce.org/uspstf13/hiv/hivfinalrs.htm

Weiss, S. (2012). Oral involvement of systemic diseases. *Clinical Advisor for Nurse Practitioners, 15*(6), 25–30.

World Health Organization. (2012, July). *Guidance on oral pre-exposure prophylaxis (PrEP) for serodiscordant couples, men and transgender women who have sex with men at high risk for HIV: Recommendations for use in the context of demonstration projects.* Geneva, Switzerland: Author. Retrieved from http://www.who.int/hiv/pub/gidanceprep/en

Yancey, J., & Thomas, S. (2012). Chronic fatigue syndrome: Diagnosis and treatment. *American Family Physician, 86*(8), 741–746.

18 Musculoskeletal Guidelines

Neck and Upper Back Disorders

Julie Adkins

Definition

A. Nonspecific disorders: Self-limited, usually benign disorders with unclear etiology, such as regional upper back and neck pain and shoulder pain adjacent to the neck. Pain can occur as a result of injury or through strain or poor posture over time.
B. Degenerative disorders: Consequences of aging or repetitive use, or a combination thereof, such as degenerative disk disease and osteoarthritis (OA).
C. Potentially serious neck or upper back disorders: Fractures, dislocation, infection, tumor, progressive neurologic deficit, or cord compression. Examples include muscle strains, overuse injuries, sports injuries, auto accidents; all can result in muscular irritation of the shoulder girdle, causing upper back pain.
D. There are three general types of neck pain:
1. Acute—lasts less than 4 weeks
2. Subacute—lasts 4 to 12 weeks
3. Chronic—lasts 3 months or longer

E. There are seven vertebrae of the cervical spine that surround the spinal cord and canal. The neck includes skin, neck muscles, arteries, lymph nodes, thyroid gland, parathyroid gland, esophagus, larynx, and trachea. Any condition affecting these tissues of the neck can cause neck pain.

Incidence

A. Exact numbers are unknown. Neck pain is common among adults but can occur at any age. In the course of a year, 15% of U.S. adults have neck pain that lasts at least one full day at a minimum, ranging from a mild nuisance to excruciating pain. The pain can go away in a few days or weeks or more constantly radiate to other body parts. Neck pain and upper back disorders can cause headaches or occipital neuralgia.

Pathogenesis

Cervical strain is irritation and spasm of the upper back and cervical muscles. The upper portion of the trapezius and the levator scapulae muscles, rhomboid major and minor muscles, and the long cervical muscles are most often affected. Neck pain can be identified by location:
A. C1 and C2: At the top of the cervical spine, these control the head; irritation may cause headaches.
B. C3 and C4: Regulate the diaphragm that is instrumental in breathing. C4 can radiate pain to the lower neck and shoulder.
C. C5: If impinged or irritated, shoulder pain and weakness can affect the top of the upper arms.
D. C6: If impinged or irritated, weakness can affect the biceps and the wrists. Pain, tingling, and numbness can radiate through the arm to the thumb.
E. C7: Compression causes weakness of the back of the upper arm or pain can radiate down the back of the arm and into the middle finger.
F. C8: Compression causes weakness with the handgrip as well as numbness and tingling down the arm to the little finger.

Predisposing Factors

A. Whiplash-like injuries
B. Cervical strain
C. Cervical arthritis
D. Holding your head in a forward posture or odd position
E. Sleeping on a pillow too high or too flat
F. Stress/tension

Common Complaints

A. Aching neck
B. Tightness and tenderness in neck area
C. Stiffness and tightness in shoulders
D. Stiff neck and a headache on awakening

Other Signs and Symptoms

A. Limited range of motion (ROM)
B. Back pain: Guarding with cervical motion
C. Numbness in upper extremities
D. Muscle weakness

Subjective Data

A. What are presenting symptoms? Note pain, numbness, weakness, or stiffness.
B. Was there any type of injury, either recently or in the past?
C. Is the pain located primarily in the neck, upper back, or shoulder? Is there any radiation noted?
D. How do these symptoms limit the patient's activity?

E. How long can the patient sit, stand, walk, or do overhead work?
F. Is the patient able to lift? If so, how much weight is bearable? Compare with normal weight.
G. How long has the patient had these symptoms?
H. How have the symptoms evolved, from the beginning of discomfort until now?
I. If the patient has a previous history of a similar or the same pain, what therapy was used in the past and what were the results?
J. Does the patient have any medical problems?

Physical Examination

Infection may include severe cervical spasms (nuchal rigidity), elevated temperature, chills, hypotension, and tachycardia.

A. Check temperature, blood pressure, and pulse.
B. Inspect: Observe stance and gait. Note the patient's coordination and use of extremities.
C. Ausculate
- **1.** Heart
- **2.** Lungs

D. Palpate
- **1.** Palpate trigger points in upper back, paracervical, and rhomboid muscles.
- **2.** Palpate for any bony tenderness in neck, shoulders, and upper back.
- **3.** Perform ROM tests.
- **4.** Assess the patient for reduced ipsilateral and contralateral bending of the neck.
- **5.** Check for fracture, or inability to move the neck due to pain, and severe cervical midline vertebral pain. Note tenderness, the patient holding head for stability; look for possible neurologic deficits.

E. Assess deep tendon reflexes (DTRs) bilaterally.
- **1.** Biceps reflex tests fifth and sixth cervical nerve root.
- **2.** Brachioradialis reflex tests fifth and sixth cervical nerve root.
- **3.** Triceps reflex tests seventh and eighth cervical nerve root.

F. Shoulders: Test muscle strength in shoulders. Ask patient to shrug shoulders against resistance. Test abduction of upper extremities.
G. Elbows: Abduction, elbow flexion, or supination tests fourth and fifth cervical disks.
H. Wrists: Check for weakness of radial wrist extension, indicating fifth and sixth cervical disk problems. Check for weakness of elbow extension and ulnar wrist flexion, indicating seventh cervical nerve impairment. Check weak finger abduction and adduction, indicating seventh and eighth cervical nerve impairment.
I. Measure circumference at forearm and upper arm for muscle atrophy. Dominant arm is 1/4 inch greater than nondominant arm.
J. Sensory: Test light touch, pinprick, pressure sensations in forearm and hand. Possible cervical spinal cord compromise is indicated by paresthesia of upper extremities, weakness of upper or lower extremities, and difficulty walking.
K. Percuss back, spine, and neck areas. Tumor is indicated by tenderness to vertebral percussion and cachexia.

Diagnostic Tests

A. Nontraumatic neck pain should have radiographic studies performed on patients with the following criteria:
- **1.** Age more than 50 years with new symptoms
- **2.** Concern of infection
- **3.** Unexplained symptoms, such as weight loss, fever, or chills
- **4.** Neurologic symptoms that continue to progress
- **5.** Concern or history of malignancy

B. Radiography of cervical spine. Testing may include:
- **1.** X-ray: Recommended for nontraumatic pain in all patients older than 50 years with new symptoms.
- **2.** MRI: Recommended if symptoms are worsening or signs of neurologic disease, symptoms longer than 6 weeks, or concern over malignancy or infection.
- **3.** CT of spine
- **4.** Myelogram
- **5.** Electromyography (EMG): Useful for more pain experienced in extremities than in the neck.
- **6.** Nerve conduction studies: Evaluates nerve damage.
- **7.** Bone scan

Differential Diagnoses

A. Regional neck pain
B. Cervical strain
C. Cervical arthritis
D. Cervical nerve root compression with radiculopathy
E. Rotator cuff tendinitis
F. Rotator cuff tendon tear
G. Postlaminectomy syndrome
H. Spinal stenosis
I. Torticollis, which may be present at birth or caused by injury or disease

Plan

A. General interventions
- **1.** Correct posture and lifestyle modifications (exercise, strengthening, etc.) are imperative for the patient to remain free of pain. Patient education and therapy depend on individual diagnosis.

B. Patient teaching
- **1.** Teach the patient to use local applications of cold packs during the first 3 days of acute complaints and hot pack applications thereafter.
- **2.** Encourage the following changes in lifestyle:
  - **a.** Sitting straight with shoulders held high
  - **b.** Sleeping with the head and neck aligned with the body and a small pillow under the neck
  - **c.** Driving with shoulders slightly shrugged, using arm rests
  - **d.** Avoiding carrying objects with a strap over shoulders
- **3.** Encourage daily stretching exercises, including shoulder roll, scapular pinch, and neck stretches.
- **4.** Have the patient perform ROM exercises daily.
- **5.** Advise the patient to avoid extremes of ROM, prolonged periods in one position, and any other aggravating activity.

6. Explain relaxation techniques and stress reduction.
7. Massage may be useful to help relax muscles in back and neck.
8. Provide the patient teaching sheet; Patient teaching: *See Section III: Patient Teaching Guide for this chapter, "RICE Therapy and Exercise Therapy," if applicable.*

C. Pharmaceutical therapy
1. Nonprescription medications: Acetaminophen or nonsteroidal anti-inflammatory drugs (NSAIDs), topical pain relief patches, muscle rubs
2. Prescription medications: NSAIDs and/or muscle relaxants for nighttime use
a. Motrin (ibuprofen) 400 to 800 mg orally three times a day as needed. Use prescribing precautions found in prescribing literature.
b. Aleve (naproxen) 200 to 500 mg twice a day as needed. See Monthly Prescribing Reference (2016) for guidance on prescribing.
c. Flexeril (cyclobenzaprine) 5 to 10 mg orally three times a day as needed. Use of flexeril for periods longer than 2 to 3 weeks is not recommended. Dosing should be considered for patients with liver impairment and/or elderly patients. Advise patients that driving and the use of machinery is not recommended while taking this medication. Monthly Prescribing Reference (2016) for guidance on prescribing.
d. Soma (carisoprodol) 250 to 350 mg orally three times a day as needed. Precautions should be given for no driving or use of machinery while taking this medication. Use caution in patients with compromised liver and/or kidney function. Soma should not be used for long-term use greater than 2 to 3 weeks. See Monthly Prescribing Reference (2016) for guidance on prescribing.
3. Trigger injections of cortisone and anesthetics may be used as necessary.

Follow-Up

A. Evaluate the patient after 2 weeks of conservative treatment. If pain continues after 2 to 3 weeks despite adequate therapy, order radiography and physical therapy. Treatment options include ultrasonography, massage, and gentle cervical traction beginning at 5 pounds for 5 to 10 minutes once a day. Soft cervical collar may be worn while doing physical work.

Consultation/Referral

A. Consult or refer the patient to a physician if there is still no improvement after adequate time for healing and no relief is noted with physical therapy and medications.

Individual Considerations

A. Adults
1. Neck and upper back problems are more commonly seen in adults.

B. Pediatrics
1. Sports are the primary cause for head and neck/spinal injuries in children. Football, cheerleading, hockey, and gymnastics are the sports most commonly seen in athlete head/ spinal injuries.

C. Geriatrics
1. Precautions should be used when treating older adults with NSAIDs. Use prescribing literature for guidance. Consider using lower dose medications for older patients. Long-term medications should also be taken into consideration for interactions between medications.

Plantar Fasciitis

Julie Adkins

Definition

A. Plantar fasciitis is an inflammatory condition in the plantar fascia (foot) that causes pain in the arch of the foot and radiates to the heel. The plantar fascia connective tissue runs across the bottom of the foot and connects the bottom of the tuberosity of the calcaneous to the heads of the metatarsal bones.

Incidence

A. Plantar fasciitis is the most common cause of heel pain in the United States. Plantar fasciitis is seen in both men and women, most often affecting active men aged 40 to 60 years.

Pathogenesis

A. Repetitive small tears in the plantar fascia causing collagen breakdown at the medial tubercle of the calcaneus.

Predisposing Factors

A. Athletes: Overuse injury from running
B. Tight or weak muscles/tendons (Achilles tendon, heel cord, gastrocnemius, soleus muscle)
C. Poor arch support/improper footwear (poor support in shoes)
D. Anatomic abnormalities (low arch support, flat foot, high arch, tibial torsion, overpronated foot, leg length discrepancy, forefoot varus, thinning of fat pad)
E. Overweight/obesity

Common Complaints

A. Severe, stabbing foot pain in the bottom of the foot, especially first thing in the morning
B. Burning pain when walking
C. Stiffness in foot/heel
D. May be worse in the morning, improve during the day, and then get painful at the end of the day
E. Increased foot pain with walking after long periods of standing or sitting.

Other Signs and Symptoms

A. Both heels may be affected.
B. Pain is located at the medial tubercle of the calcaneus, medial of the longitudinal arch.
C. Heel spurs may or may not be present.
D. Pain worsens with standing for long periods of time.

Subjective Data

A. Ask the patient when pain began, when it occurs, and how long it lasts.

B. Does pain occur with walking, running, and standing?
C. Is pain constant, stabbing pain? Rate pain on a pain scale of 1 to 10.
D. Locate pain site; Does pain radiate into toes or leg?

Physical Examination

A. Check pulse and blood pressure.
B. Inspect
  1. Examine feet bilaterally.
  2. Note swelling, discoloration, or rash.
C. Auscultate
  1. Heart
  2. Lungs
D. Palpate
  1. Palpate both feet, noting tenderness at point tenderness. Point tenderness will be noted over insertion on medial heel (calcaneus medial tubercle).
  2. Perform passive dorsiflexion of toes and ankle. Have the patient stand on tips of toes to see if this elicits pain.

Diagnostic Tests

A. X-ray may be performed but is often normal and not needed. Perform if tumor, spur, or fracture is suspected.
B. MRI should be ordered if thickening of proximal plantar fascia is noted or rupture of proximal fascia suspected.

Differential Diagnoses

A. Plantar fasciitis
B. Heel pain
C. Heel spur

Plan

A. General interventions
  1. Conservatory treatment includes no long periods of standing for the next 6 to 8 weeks.
  2. Proper foot care and support recommended.
B. Patient teaching
  1. Shoe arch supports are imperative for relief. New shoes may provide this support or additional arch supports may be needed to insert into the shoe to provide adequate support.
  2. Suggest getting proper shoe fitting for running if the patient is an athlete.
  3. The patient should avoid walking on hard surfaces and never go barefoot, even indoors. Avoid wearing sandals and flip-flops.
  4. Ice therapy may help with pain control and swelling.
  5. For severe cases, a corticosteroid lidocaine injection 1 to 1.5 mL injected directly into the most tender area on the sole of the foot may be helpful.
  6. Exercises
    a. Roll foot arch with a tennis ball or a frozen bottle of water for 20 to 30 minutes each evening to help stretch the plantar fascia.
    b. Perform calf stretches against a wall; leaning forward against the wall, extending one leg behind you and one leg in front of you, stretch the leg, and reverse.
C. Pharmaceutical therapy
  1. Nonsteroidal anti-inflammatory drugs (NSAIDs) such as ibuprofen (Motrin) 800 mg three times daily or naproxen (Naprosyn) 500 mg by mouth twice a day for comfort.

Follow-Up

A. Recommend follow-up in 4 weeks following treatment. Pain should slowly improve with aggressive treatment management. The patient must be compliant with instructions given for improvement. May take 6 to 12 months for complete resolution.
B. Complications of foot, knee, hip, or back problems may occur if change of gait occurs to minimize pain with walking.
C. If pain worsens, consider diagnostic workup (x-ray or MRI).

Consultation/Referral

A. Refer to a podiatrist if conservatory treatment therapy fails after 6 weeks.

Individual Considerations

A. None

Sciatica

Julie Adkins

Definition

A. Sciatica is a sharp or burning pain, usually associated with numbness that radiates down the posterior or lateral leg that can result in neurosensory and/or motor deficits. Sciatica indicates abnormal function of the lumbosacral nerve roots or one of the nerves in the lumbosacral plexus.

Incidence

A. The prevalence of sciatica in the general population is 40%, though only 1% have any neurosensory or motor deficits. The most common cause of sciatica is herniated disks, 95% of which occur at the L4 to L5 or L5 to S1 level.

Pathogenesis

A. Pressure on the nerve from a herniated disk, from bony osteophytes, a compression fracture, or any other extrinsic pressure (e.g., pelvic mass or epidural process, "wallet sciatica") causes progressive sensory, sensorimotor, or sensorimotor visceral loss. Typically, sciatica affects only one side of the body. The nerve may be "pinched" on the inside or outside of the spinal canal as it passes into the leg.

Predisposing Factors

A. Inflexibility
B. Obesity
C. Trauma
D. Bony osteophytes
E. Herniated or slipped disc
F. Piriformis syndrome
G. Spinal stenosis
H. Spondylolisthesis

Common Complaints

A. Pain around the buttocks area may occur suddenly or develop gradually.
B. Pain often associated with numbness traveling down the lateral or posterior leg
C. Numbness
D. Paresthesia

Other Signs and Symptoms

A. Difficulty walking with affected leg
B. Positive straight leg raises
C. Decreased sensation

Subjective Data

A. Elicit information on onset of symptoms, duration, and what makes pain better or worse.
B. Inquire about previous episodes of pain or trauma.
C. Have the patient point to the area of pain, numbness, or tingling.
D. Are symptoms unilateral or bilateral?
E. Question the patient about loss of bowel or bladder control or other deficits and/or changes.
F. Does the patient notice leg weakness or difficulty walking?

Physical Examination

A. Check pulse and blood pressure.
B. Inspect gait and movement of back and extremities.
C. Palpate spinous processes.
D. Examine flexion and extension of spine. Assess sensation, deep tendon reflexes (DTRs), muscle strength, and motor weakness of lower extremities.
E. Examine neurologic function of back and lower extremity.
  1. Straight leg raising sign is positive.
  2. Dorsiflexion of ankle is positive.
  3. Check for loss of sensation in radicular pattern. Light-touch pinprick and two-point discrimination are not present.
  4. Look for decrease or loss of DTRs.
  5. Check muscle strength of lower extremities.
  6. Check motor weakness.
  7. Check for cauda equina syndrome, indicated by urinary retention, radicular symptoms, and saddle anesthesia.

> *Cauda equina syndrome is a surgical emergency, characterized by bowel and bladder dysfunction; saddle anesthesia at the anus, perineum, or genitals; and widespread or progressive loss of strength in the legs or gait disturbances.*

F. Percuss for tenderness over the spinous processes.

Diagnostic Tests

A. Radiography, when red flags for fracture, cancer, or infection are present
B. CT scan or MRI, when cauda equina, tumor, infection, or fracture is suspected; MRI is test of choice for patients with prior back surgery.

Differential Diagnoses

A. Sciatica of unknown etiology
B. Lumbosacral strain
C. Herniated disk
D. Bony osteophytes, spinal stenosis
E. Compression fracture
F. Neoplasm of spine
G. Pelvic mass
H. Epidural process causing progressive sensory, sensorimotor, or sensorimotor visceral loss
I. Meralgia paresthetica

Plan

A. General interventions
  1. Care for these patients should evolve over a three-step process. See the following.
B. Patient teaching
  1. Step 1 (2–4 days)
    a. Bed rest for severe radiculopathy only.
    b. Limit walking and standing to 30 to 40 minutes each day.
    c. Recommend application of heat or cold packs to site as needed.
  2. Step 2 (7–14 days)
    a. Reevaluate neurologic and back examination; tell the patient "Let pain be your guide" when resuming normal daily activities.
    b. Have the patient perform gentle stretching exercises.
    c. Encourage walking on flat surfaces.
    d. Educate the patient regarding proper care of the back, with regard to exercises, posture, and so forth.
    e. Provide handouts on back exercises/stretches for the patient.
    f. Physical therapy may be implemented at this time if no significant improvement is noted.
  3. Step 3 (2–3 weeks)
    a. Reevaluate the patient, noting degree of improvement with examination.
    b. Continue muscle toning and reconditioning exercises.
    c. If improvement is noted, gradually increase physical activities.
    d. Reinforce healthy care of the back.
    e. Continue physical therapy until the patient can perform exercises without assistance or until released by the physical therapist.
C. Pharmaceutical therapy
  1. Nonsteroidal anti-inflammatory drugs (NSAIDs) as needed: Naproxen (Naprosyn) 500 mg initially, followed by 250 mg every 6 to 8 hours.
  2. Acetaminophen may also be used as needed, especially if the patient is not able to tolerate ibuprofen.
  3. For more severe pain not relieved by NSAIDs, consider acetaminophen (Tylenol) with codeine for short duration. Narcotics should not be used for more than 2 weeks.

4. Muscle relaxants: Muscle relaxants should not be used for more than 2 weeks.

a. Cyclobenzaprine (Flexeril) 10 mg one to three times daily

b. Muscle relaxants place patients at risk for drowsiness. Warn the patient not to mix medications with alcohol because it may potentiate the medication.

Follow-Up

A. Initial follow-up is needed in 1 to 2 weeks. See the Plan section for recommendation of stepwise approach.

Consultation/Referral

A. If cauda equina syndrome is suspected, prompt referral to a physician is necessary.
B. If pain is severe enough that narcotics are needed, consult with a physician.
C. If bilateral sciatica is associated with vertebral collapse, osteoporosis, neoplasia, and/or vascular disease, consult with a physician.

Individual Considerations

A. Pregnancy

1. Sciatica pain is common due to physiological changes of the pelvis as pregnancy progresses to term.
2. Avoid use of NSAIDs.
3. Physical therapy may be used as indicated.

B. Adults

1. For adults older than 50 years presenting with no prior history of backache, consider a differential diagnosis of neoplasm. Most common metastasis is secondary to primary site of breast or prostate, or to multiple myeloma. Pain is most prominent in the recumbent position and rarely radiates into buttock or leg.

C. Geriatrics

1. Bilateral sciatica is associated with vertebral collapse, osteoporosis, neoplasia, and/or vascular disease. Refer the patient to a physician immediately.
2. Use caution when prescribing medications for pain to the elderly due to the risk for drowsiness and potential falls.

Sprains: Ankle and Knee

Julie Adkins

Definition

Sprains are ligament stretching or partial tears from forceful stress on the joint. Sprains are categorized as the following:
A. Grade 1: Microscopic tears without ligament tearing or joint instability
B. Grade 2: Partial tearing of involved ligaments and laxity of joint with moderate function loss
C. Grade 3: Ligament tearing with severe function loss and joint instability

Incidence

A. *Ankle* sprains are among the most common injuries seen in primary care. It is estimated that more than 628,000 ankle sprains occur in the United States each year.
B. *Knee* injuries are among the 10 most common causes of occupational injury and worker compensation claims.

Pathogenesis

A. Sudden stress to a supporting ligament causes ligament stretching or tearing. Sprains are usually the result of jumping, falling, or rotating a joint.
B. Ankle sprains are most often inversion sprains with symptoms on the lateral side of the joint.
C. Eversion injuries affect the medial side.
D. Knee sprains most often involve the patellofemoral joint.

Predisposing Factors

A. Previous injury to ankle or knee
B. Athletic activities
C. Patellofemoral instability

Common Complaints

A. "I twisted my ankle or knee."
B. "I stepped off of a step and came down on the side of my foot."
C. Swelling, pain, weakness of ankle or knee from a previous injury.

Other Signs and Symptoms

A. First degree: Minimal pain; mild to moderate pain with stress, little swelling; minimal tenderness with palpation; little functional loss; unimpaired weight bearing or walking; internal microdamage with full continuity
B. Second degree: Moderate pain with range of motion (ROM); swelling; marked tenderness on palpation; moderate loss of function; difficulty with weight bearing or walking; mechanical dissociation with partial loss of continuity
C. Third degree: Severe pain, especially with passive inversion; severe swelling, marked tenderness; marked decrease in ROM; intolerant of weight bearing or walking; joint instability; discoloration of skin; complete rupture of a ligament

Subjective Data

A. Inquire about history of trauma.
B. Have the patient describe the injury: Time, place, activity, predisposing factors, and time the symptoms developed.
C. Determine if the symptoms are acute or chronic.
D. Inquire about the type and location of the pain.
E. Have the patient describe the pain and what conditions aggravate or relieve the pain.
F. Ask if there are symptoms of popping, clicking, locking, recurrent swelling, or giving way of the joint.
G. Ask if there is pain or other symptoms elsewhere, such as low back, hip, or leg.
H. Explore history of any previous ankle or knee injury.
I. Determine if the current injury was evaluated and treated previously.

J. Have the patient describe ability to bear weight on the extremity and to tolerate ROM.
K. Review the patient's medical history for arthritis, gout, cancer, autoimmune disorders, or metabolic disease.

Physical Examination

A. Check temperature, pulse, respirations, and blood pressure.
B. Inspect
 1. Observe ambulation. Note overall appearance and facial grimaces during examination.
 2. Inspect injured area for swelling, discoloration, and deformity. Compare injured side to uninjured side.
C. Palpate
 1. Palpate the injured site for tenderness.
 2. Palpate the joints above and below the injured site.
 3. Perform ROM (active and passive) and resisted ROM to evaluate strength.
 4. Check for catching or locking of the knee on extension.
 5. Assess neurovascular status of the knee or ankle and distal extremity.
 6. *Ankle*: Palpate for tender sulcus in anterolateral aspect on inversion of the ankle. Assess for pain aggravated by forced ankle inversion. Perform isometric test of plantar flexion and eversion. Perform anterior drawer test, talar tilt test.
 7. *Knee:* Palpate for tenderness on the medial and lateral joint line. Perform McMurray's test to detect a torn meniscus (*see the Section II: Procedure, "Evaluation of Sprains"*). Symptoms of sprained knees include:
  a. Meniscus tear: Locking of knee with flexion and giving way of knee
  b. Collateral ligament tear or strain: Pain at lateral or medial sides
  c. Anterior cruciate tear: Popping sound at injury site and immediate swelling
  d. Posterior cruciate tear or strain: Pain in interior knee
  e. Patellofemoral syndrome: Popping or snapping, pain under patella with motion, and pain on stairs or hills
  f. Tendinitis: Pain over patellar tendon
  g. Prepatellar bursitis: Swelling over patella with inability to kneel due to swelling
  h. Nonspecific effusion: Effusion worse with exercise
 8. *See Section II: Procedure, "Evaluation of Sprains."*

Diagnostic Tests

A. Radiography of extremity, if fracture is suspected.
B. MRI, if mechanical symptoms and effusion persist.
C. Bone scans or MRI are usually reserved for those who have failed to respond after 6 to 12 weeks of therapy.

Differential Diagnoses

A. Ankle sprain
 1. Fracture
 2. Acute dislocation
 3. Infection
 4. Ligament strain
 5. Tendinitis or tenosynovitis
 6. Nonspecific foot or ankle pain
B. Knee sprain
 1. Fracture
 2. Dislocation
 3. Septic arthritis
 4. Infected prepatellar bursitis
 5. Inflammation
 6. Tumor
 7. Meniscus tear
 8. Collateral ligament tear
 9. Anterior cruciate tear
 10. Posterior cruciate tear
 11. Collateral ligament strain
 12. Cruciate ligament strain
 13. Patellofemoral syndrome, or chondromalacia
 14. Effusion, nonspecific
 15. Patellar tendinitis
 16. Prepatellar bursitis
 17. Nonspecific knee pain

Plan

A. General interventions
 1. Reinforce the degree of injury and the need to take care of the extremity to prevent further damage.
 2. Prescribe an exercise program to prevent stiffness, restore function, improve ROM and restore normal flexibility and strength.
 3. A mild ankle sprain may require 3 to 6 weeks of rehabilitation, a moderate sprain may require 2 to 3 months of rehabilitation, and a severe sprain may require 8 to 12 months of therapy to return to full activity.
B. Patient teaching
 1. *See Section III: Patient Teaching Guide for this chapter, "RICE Therapy and Exercise Therapy"; "Ankle Exercises" or "Knee Exercises."*
C. Pharmaceutical therapy
 1. Drug of choice
  a. NSAIDs to reduce pain and inflammation
  b. Consider one of the following: Aspirin, ibuprofen, indomethacin, or piroxicam. Do not use these medications in the long term.
  c. If there is increased risk for bleeding, acetaminophen with codeine may be used for pain.
 2. Injectable medication
  a. Methylprednisolone acetate (Depo-Medrol) may be used if symptoms continue to be present 6 to 8 weeks after injury.
  b. Repeat injection in 4 to 6 weeks if symptoms have not been reduced by 50%.

Follow-Up

A. Schedule initial follow-up in 2 weeks to evaluate current therapy or sooner if problems arise.
B. Follow-up appointments should be scheduled according to treatment/therapy.

Consultation/Referral

A. Refer the patient to a physician if fracture is suspected.
B. Refer to physical therapy as needed.
C. Refer the patient to a physician or orthopedic surgeon if therapy is unproductive and symptoms have not begun to regress within 6 weeks.

Individual Considerations

A. Pediatrics: In prepubertal or peripubertal patients, knee ligaments usually do not tear. Instead, the growth plate may open up on one side. This age group needs stress radiography to check for fracture of the growth plate.

Bibliography

American Orthopedic Foot and Ankle Society. (2016). Plantar fascitis. Retrieved from www.aofas.org/footcaremd/conditions/ailments-of-the-heel/pages/plantar-fascitis.aspx

Bettin, C., Richardon, D., & Donley, B. (2015). Ligamatous injuries of the ankle: Sprained ankle. *Sports Injuries*, 1753–1761. doi:10.1007/978-3-642-365569-0_136

Carter, D., & Amblum-Almer, J. (2015). Analgesia for people with acute ankle sprain. *Emergency Nurse: The Journal of the RCN Accident and Emergency Nursing Association, 23*(1), 24–31.

Cleveland Clinic. (2015). Sciatica. Retrieved from www.clevelandclinic.com/medicalpubs/diseasemanagement/low-back-pain

Gross, A. R., Paquin, J. P., Dupont, G., Blanchette, S., Lalonde, P., Cristie, T., . . . Bronfort, G.; Cervical Overview Group. (2016). Exercises for mechanical neck disorders: A Cochrane review update. *Manual Therapy, 24*, 25–45.

Hirsch, B. P., Webb, M. L., Bohl, D. D., Fu, M.,Buerba, R. A., Gruskay, J. A., & Gracer, J. N. (2014). Improving visual estimates of cervical spine range of motion. *American Journal of Orthopedics, 43*(11), 261–265.

Janssen, K. W., van der Zwaard, B. C., Finch, C. F., van Mechelen, W., & Verhagen, E. A. (2016). Interventions preventing ankle sprains; previous injury and high-risk sport participation as predictors of compliance. *Journal of Science and Medicine in Sport/Sports Medicine Australia, 19*(6), 465–469.

Javanshir, K., Amiri, M., Mohseni Bandpei, M. A., De las Penas, C. F., & Rezasoltani, A. (2015). The effect of different exercise programs on cervical flexor muscles dimensions in patients with chronic neck pain. *Journal of Back and Musculoskeletal Rehabilitation, 28*(4), 833–840.

Jun Ho, K., Han Suk, L., & Sun Wook, P. (2015). Effects of the active release technique on pain and range of motion of patients with chronic neck pain. *Journal of Physical Therapy, 27*(8), 2461–2464.

Kalaci, A., Cakici, H., Hapa, O., Yanat, A. N., Dogramaci, Y., & Sevinç, T. T. (2009). Treatment of plantar fasciitis using four different local injection modalities: A randomized prospective clinical trial. *Journal of the American Podiatric Medical Association, 99*(2), 108–113.

Karls, S. L., Snyder, K. R., & Neibert, P. J. (2016). Effectiveness of corticosteroid injections in the treatment of plantar fasciitis. *Journal of Sport Rehabilitation, 25*(2), 202–207.

Keating, J.F. (2014). Acute knee ligament injuries and knee dislocations. *In G. Bentley, European surgical orthopedics and traumatology: The EFORT textbook* (2014th ed.,. pp. 2949–2971. Berlin, Germany: Springer.

Kovacs, F. M., Seco, J., Royuela, A., Melis, S., Sánchez, C., Díaz-Arribas, M. J., . . . Abraira, V. (2015). Patients with neck pain are less likely to improve if they experience poor sleep quality: A prospective study in routine practice. *Clinical Journal of Pain, 31*(8), 713–721.

Lewis, R. A., Williams, N. H., Sutton, A. J., Burton, K., Din, N. U., Matar, H. E., . . . Wilkinson, C. (2015). Comparative clinical effectiveness of management strategies for sciatica: Systematic review and network meta-analyses. *The Spine Journal: Official Journal of the North American Spine Society, 15*(6), 1461–1477.

Mau, H., & Baker, R. T. (2014). A modified mobilization-with-movement to treat a lateral ankle sprain. *International Journal of Sports Physical Therapy, 9*(4), 540–548.

Mayo Clinic. (2014). Plantar fascitis. Retrieved from www.mayoclinic.org

McNerney, J. (2015). Treatment of lateral ankle instability. *Podiatry Management, 34*(7), 135–146.

Mitchell, H., Rothenberg, M. D., & Graf, B. (2016). Evaluation of acute knee injuries. *Postgraduate Medicine, 93*(3), 75–86.

Monthly Prescribing Guide (2016, Spring). Retrieved from www.empr.com

Podolsky, R., & Kalichman, L. (2015). Taping for plantar fasciitis. *Journal of Back and Musculoskeletal Rehabilitation, 28*(1), 1–6.

Poquet, N., & Lin, C. W. (2016). Management strategies for sciatica (PEDro synthesis). *British Journal of Sports Medicine, 50*(4), 253–254.

Savage, N. J., Fritz, J. M., & Thackeray, A. (2014). The relationship between history and physical examination findings and the outcome of electrodiagnostic testing in patients with sciatica referred to physical therapy. *Journal of Orthopaedic and Sports Physical Therapy, 44*(7), 508–517.

Shashua, A., Flechter, S., Avidan, L., Ofir, D., Melayev, A., & Kalichman, L. (2015). The effect of additional ankle and midfoot mobilizations on plantar fasciitis: A randomized controlled trial. *Journal of Orthopaedic and Sports Physical Therapy, 45*(4), 265–272.

Shim, J. (2016). Causes of upper back pain. Retrieved from www.spine-health.com

Steffens, D., Hancock, M. J., Pereira, L. S., Kent, P. M., Latimer, J., & Maher, C. G. (2016). Do MRI findings identify patients with low back pain or sciatica who respond better to particular interventions? A systematic review. *European Spine Journal: Official Publication of the European Spine Society, the European Spinal Deformity Society, and the European Section of the Cervical Spine Research Society, 25*(4), 1170–1187.

U.S. National Library of Medicine. (2013). Plantar fasciitis. Retrieved from http://www.ncbi.nlm.nih.gov/pubmedhealth/PMH0004438

van Ochten, J. M., van Middelkoop, M., Meuffels, D., & Bierma-Zeinstra, S. M. (2014). Chronic complaints after ankle sprains: A systematic review on effectiveness of treatments. *Journal of Orthopaedic and Sports Physical Therapy, 44*(11), 862–871, C1.

Xie, P., Qin, B., Yang, F., Yu, T., Yu, J., Wang, J., & Zheng, H. (2015). Lidocaine injection in the intramuscular innervation zone can effectively treat chronic neck pain caused by MTrPs in the trapezius muscle. *Pain Physician, 18*(5), E815–E826.

Zhou, B., Zhou, Y., Tao, X., Yuan, C., & Tang, K. (2015). Classification of calcaneal spurs and their relationship with plantar fasciitis. *Journal of Foot and Ankle Surgery: Official Publication of the American College of Foot and Ankle Surgeons, 54* (4), 594–600.

19 Neurologic Guidelines

Alzheimer's Disease

Jill C. Cash and Julie Adkins

Definition

A. Alzheimer's disease is a permanent, progressive decline in several dimensions of cognitive functioning, including memory disturbance, that severely interferes with the person's everyday living but produces no decrease in level of consciousness (LOC). Insidious onset, gradually progressive decline in intellectual functioning, and absence of other specific causes of dementia are also present.

Incidence

A. The prevalence of Alzheimer's disease was 44 million people throughout the world in 2015 and is expected to double by the year 2050. Among the elderly, approximately 40% of those older than 85 years of age are affected. Of all types of dementias, Alzheimer's dementia includes 70% of those affected, with the other 30% affected by atypical dementia. Alzheimer's disease is the sixth leading cause of death in the United States.

Pathogenesis

A. The disease is a degenerative process involving cell loss from the basal forebrain, cerebral cortex, and other areas in which plaques and tangles build up and block the cell processes that are needed to survive, thereby destroying the nerve cells. Death of the nerve cells causes memory loss, changes in personality, and other signs and symptoms of Alzheimer's disease.

B. Obesity has been identified as a major risk factor for developing Alzheimer's disease because it increases adipokine dysregulation, which causes release of the proinflammatory adipokines and decreases anti-inflammatory adipokines.

Predisposing Factors

A. Advanced age older than 50 years
B. Severe head trauma
C. Abnormal genetic makeup, such as Down syndrome
D. Positive family history of Alzheimer's disease
E. Obesity

Common Complaint

A. Significant memory loss

Other Signs and Symptoms

The 10 warning signs of Alzheimer's disease:

A. Memory loss interrupting daily living
B. Loss of all intellectual capacities such as following plans, solving problems, and so on
C. Difficulty completing daily tasks at home or work
D. Confusion with time or place
E. Having problems understanding visual images or spatial relationships
F. Difficulty with speaking or writing words
G. Losing things and not being able to retrace steps to find them
H. Poor judgment in daily routine
I. Withdrawal from work or social activities
J. Change in mood or personality (www.alz.org/national/documents/checklist_10signs.pdf)

Subjective Data

> *Family members are a good resource for obtaining an accurate history.*

A. Determine onset, course, and duration of symptoms.
B. Note loss of immediate, recent, or remote memory, such as trouble remembering appointments, difficulty recalling recent events, and inability to find personal belongings.
C. Determine the patient's ability to make reasonable judgments such as answering the phone when it rings and so forth.
D. Is the patient able to carry on daily functions of living, including cooking meals and cleaning house?
E. Discuss the patient's sleep–wake cycle.
F. Assess the patient for decreased appetite, lack of pleasure in usual activities, melancholy mood, or other symptoms associated with depression.
G. Note language difficulties and problems expressing self.
H. Note any recent physical illness.
I. Review the patient's medication history.
J. Discuss alcohol intake and abuse factors.
K. Review past medical history of head trauma, hypertension, cerebrovascular accident (CVA), cancer, metabolic problems, neurologic disease, infections, gastric surgery (vitamin B_{12} deficiency), and emotional or psychiatric problems.

Physical Examination

A. Check blood pressure, pulse, respirations, and weight.

B. Inspect

1. Inspect overall appearance for hygiene and nutritional status.

C. Auscultate

1. Heart

2. Lungs

D. Neurologic examination

1. Perform a complete neurologic examination.

2. Perform the standardized Mini-Mental State Examination (MMSE) screening tool, available at www.uml.edu/docs/mini%20Mental%20State%20Exam_tcm18-169319.pdf.

3. The clock-draw test (CDT) may also be administered and used as a screening tool. The CDT is available at www.rehabmeasures.org (see Section II: Procedure, "Clock-Draw Test").

Rule out other specific causes of dementia, including cerebrovascular disease.

Diagnostic Tests

A. Complete blood count (CBC)

B. Chemistry profile

C. Thyroid function studies

D. Folate and vitamin B_{12} levels

E. Homocysteine

F. Methylmalonic acid

G. Vitamin D level

H. Venereal Disease Research Laboratory (VDRL) for syphilis

I. CT scan of brain

Differential Diagnoses

A. Alzheimer's disease

B. Drug interactions

C. Delirium

D. Depression

E. Cerebrovascular disease

Plan

A. General interventions

1. Identify the stage of impairment:

Stage 1: No impairment—No evidence of symptoms

Stage 2: Very mild decline—No symptoms of dementia, has memory lapses

Stage 3: Mild decline—Difficulty in memory and concentration

Stage 4: Moderate decline—Impairment with complex tasks, trouble solving math problems, forgetting personal history

Stage 5: Moderately severe decline—Unable to remember phone number, address, confusion on the day of the week, difficulty with decisions on dressing self properly, and so forth

Stage 6: Severe decline—Difficulty with personal history, difficulty with naming family members, spouse, difficulty with dressing self, behavior changes, may wander and get lost

Stage 7: Very severe decline—Unable to communicate appropriately with others, requires assistance with activities of daily living (ADL), abnormal reflexes, difficulty swallowing

2. Provide supportive measures for patient and family. Explain to family and the patient findings of examination and possible treatment options.

3. Treatment may include treating coexisting diseases, thyroid disease, and vitamin B_{12} deficiency.

4. Discuss therapy options such as musical therapy, occupational therapy, and mind-stimulating activities. Cognitive stimulation has been shown to slow down the degenerative process.

5. Environment: Ensure that the patient has a safe environment; measures may need to be taken for environmental safety such as locks on doors, alarms on doors, relinquishing driving privileges, and so on.

6. Exercise: Daily exercise should be encouraged.

B. Patient teaching

1. Educate patients, family, and the community about preventive measures for developing Alzheimer's disease. Obesity is a major risk factor; lifestyle changes, such as dietary/caloric restriction, eating a healthy diet, exercise, mental stimulation, and socialization, can all help to decrease the risks of developing Alzheimer's disease.

2. Support groups are encouraged for the patient, spouse, and/or family. Therapy sessions for each may be beneficial.

3. Patient support group: Alzheimer's Association: www.alz.org; 24/7 Helpline: 1-800-272-3900

4. Families needing legal and financial advice should seek this out early and not wait for a crisis. Alzheimer's Disease Family Relief Program: 800-437-2423

C. Pharmaceutical therapy

1. Cholinesterase inhibitors

a. Rivastigmine (Exelon) 1.5 to 6 mg twice a day or patch starting at 4.6 mg/24 hr and then titrate up to 9.5 mg/24 hr. May be increased to the maximum effective dose of 13.3 mg/24 hr as indicated.

b. Donepezil (Aricept) 5 mg at bedtime, then 10 mg/d may be given after 1 month.

c. Galantamine (Razadyne) 4 mg twice a day with meals for 4 weeks, then may titrate to max of 12 mg twice a day. For missed doses, the patient will need to retitrate doses. Razadyne ER: 8 mg once daily. After 4 weeks, may increase to 16 mg once daily, up to maximum of 24 mg daily titration.

2. *N*-methyl-D-aspartate (NMDA) receptor antagonist

a. Memantine (Namenda) 5 mg daily, titrate up each week by 5 mg; 5 mg twice daily to maximum of 20 mg twice daily. Use titration pack for the first 4 weeks. Severe renal impairment should not exceed 5 mg twice daily.

3. Assess the patient for secondary behaviors of dementia. Psychosis, delusions, hallucinations, anxiety, depression, and insomnia may occur and should be treated accordingly. Cognitive and behavioral interventions should be initiated in assisting the patient in controlling these behaviors. The benefits and risks must be weighed, and pharmacological treatment may be necessary for those patients exhibiting extreme, aggressive behaviors with irritability and/or insomnia. Treatment with antipsychotics is very controversial because of the side effects and extreme complications that may occur with these medications.
4. Treatment of depression: Nortriptyline (Pamelor) 30 to 50 mg daily, sertraline (Zoloft), paroxetine (Paxil), or escitalopram (Lexapro). Monitor selective serotonin reuptake inhibitor (SSRI) for weight loss, decrease in seizure threshold, tremors. Do not use with monoamine oxidase inhibitors (MAOI). Monitor coumadin and lithium levels closely.

Follow-Up

A. Follow-up is variable, depending on patient status and needs of the patient and family. Follow-up is recommended every 3 months to follow progression of disease. If medications are being introduced, monitor the patient monthly.

Consultation/Referral

A. Consider visiting nurse, social worker, occupational and/or physical therapy.
B. Consult a physician for medication treatment for secondary behavioral symptoms.

Individual Considerations

A. Adults
1. Alzheimer's disease should be considered at early ages in adults to avoid risk factors.
2. Lifestyle and dietary changes should be encouraged in adults to prevent risks of developing Alzheimer's disease. Exercising, eating a healthy diet, and maintaining a healthy weight (body mass index [BMI]) can decrease risks factors for developing Alzheimer's disease.

B. Geriatrics
1. Alzheimer's disease is primarily seen in this population.
2. Long-term prognosis: Average patient lives 7 to 10 years after early symptoms, but life span while demented can be 20 years or more.
3. The use of probiotics in the elderly has been shown to improve the anti-inflammatory properties of the gut. However, behavioral changes should be monitored closely.

Bell's Palsy

Jill C. Cash and Julie Adkins

Definition

A. Bell's palsy, also known as idiopathic peripheral facial palsy, is characterized by an acute onset of unilateral facial paralysis. The facial nerve affected is the seventh *cranial nerve, which travels in the skull beneath the ear to the muscles on each side of the face. Each facial nerve controls the muscles, which controls eye blinking and closing and facial expressions such as smiling and taste sensations from the tongue.* Bell's palsy affects only one of the paired facial nerves, but in rare cases, it can affect both sides.

Incidence

A. Bell's palsy has an incidence of 40,000 Americans a year. It accounts for approximately 75% of all cases of facial paralysis. Approximately 5% of those affected experience recurrence. Both sexes are affected, as well as all ages, but less common before the age of 15 years and after the age of 60 years.

Pathogenesis

A. The pathogenesis of Bell's palsy is unknown, but some possible etiologies include genetic, metabolic, autoimmune, and vascular causes. An increasing body of evidence reveals that Bell's palsy may be a virally induced neuritis. A triggering event or stressor induces activation of a latent virus, most likely herpes simplex virus or herpes zoster virus, present within the geniculate ganglion of the facial nerve. Viral activation results in re-expression of dormant viral particles and neural inflammation, leading to entrapment, ischemia, and degeneration of the facial nerve.

Predisposing Factors

A. Diabetes
B. Pregnancy
C. Recent infection
D. Positive family history
E. Hypertension
F. Hypothyroidism

Common Complaints

A. Acute onset of unilateral facial weakness with inability to close one eye
B. Sagging of one eyelid
C. Loss of nasolabial fold
D. Mouth drawn to affected side

Other Signs and Symptoms

A. Ipsilateral retroauricular pain with or preceding paralysis
B. Hyperacusis or hypersensitivity to sound
C. Dysgeusia, or perversion of taste, in the anterior two thirds of the tongue
D. Facial paresthesia
E. Drooling
F. Decreased tearing

Subjective Data

A. Elicit onset, duration, and course of symptoms.
B. Have the patient describe all neurologic symptoms present.
C. Note associated symptoms such as disruption of taste and disturbances in visual function or hearing.
D. Note predisposing factors such as trauma, infection, or pregnancy.

E. Review the patient's family history for presence of Bell's palsy.
F. Review the patient's medical history; especially note cerebrovascular or cardiac risk factors. A focused history should include contraindications to use of steroids.

Physical Examination

A. Check temperature, pulse, respiration, and blood pressure.
B. Inspect
  1. Note facial appearance.
  2. Observe symmetry of eyes. Check corneal reflex (decreased).
  3. Assess the skin for lesions. Assess in and behind ears for zosteriform lesions.
  4. Ears: Complete ear examination to rule out infection
  5. Mouth and nose
C. Auscultate
  1. Heart
  2. Lungs
D. Neurologic examination
  1. Perform a complete neurologic examination; test all cranial nerves.
  2. Assess paralysis of all the muscles supplied by one facial nerve. Paralysis may be of varying degrees and need not be complete.

> *Subjective decreased sensation may be present in the trigeminal distribution.*

Diagnostic Tests

A. Lyme titer: Positive in patients with secondary facial weakness from Lyme disease
B. Skull radiography, CT scan, or MRI: Negative in Bell's palsy, but may show evidence of fracture line, bony erosion by either infection or neoplasm, stroke, or tumor
C. Electromyographic (EMG) studies: Occasionally performed to predict prognosis and progression. EMG is reserved for severe cases of paralysis lasting longer than 1 week.
D. Lumbar puncture: Indicated only when other conditions are suspected. Cerebrospinal fluid (CSF) should be sent for cytology.

Differential Diagnoses

A. Bell's palsy
B. Sjögren's syndrome
C. Stroke
D. Lyme disease
E. Sarcoidosis
F. Ramsay Hunt syndrome, herpes zoster oticus
G. Acoustic neuroma
H. Middle ear disease such as purulent otitis media or neoplasms
I. Guillain–Barré syndrome
J. Parotid gland tumor
K. Carcinomatous meningitis

Plan

A. General interventions
  1. The condition is usually short term (3–4 weeks) and may be managed with steroids and acetaminophen as needed for discomfort.
  2. Physical therapy may be beneficial for muscle weakness and strengthening muscles.
  3. Ensure the patient gets reassurance and emotional support.

> *Recovery may take 3 to 6 months or longer and is complete in approximately 80% of the cases.*

B. Patient teaching
  1. *See Section III: Patient Teaching Guide for this chapter, "Bell's Palsy."* ◀
  2. Provide eye protection by means of the following.
    a. Apply methylcellulose drops as needed and ocular lubricant (Lacri-Lube) at bedtime.
    b. Tape eye closed, especially at night.
    c. Wear dark glasses when outdoors to minimize exposure.
  3. Application of heat/cold packs may be useful for pain as needed.
C. Pharmaceutical therapy
  1. Prednisone: Adults take 80 mg every day with breakfast for first 3 days, then decrease dosage to 40 mg for 3 days, then to 20 mg daily for 3 days, then stop.

> *Recent studies suggest that a brief course of prednisone conveys modest benefits with minimal risks.*

  2. Acyclovir 400 mg five times a day for 10 days. Consider acyclovir for patients without renal insufficiency and with no other contraindications to therapy.
  3. Analgesics, such as acetaminophen, when necessary (prn) for ear pain.

Follow-Up

A. For patients with severe symptoms, follow-up in 3 to 4 days, then again in 2 weeks.
B. If symptoms worsen or do not resolve within 4 weeks, have the patient return to the clinic.

Consultation/Referral

A. Consult a neurologist for the following:
  1. Failure to resolve significantly after 4 to 6 weeks. Only 5% to 8% report distressing residual signs and symptoms, including contracture of facial muscles at rest and synergistic mass innervation because of defective nerve regeneration, manifested as either crocodile tears secondary to abnormal secretory fibers intended for the salivary glands or ipsilateral eyelid shutting.
  2. Other cranial nerve involvement or other abnormalities on neurologic examination
  3. Recurrence of facial palsy: About 5% to 7% of patients experience recurrence of symptoms. Known causes of recurrent palsy include sarcoidosis, diabetes, leukemia, and infectious mononucleosis.
  4. Bilateral facial palsies

B. Consult an ophthalmologist for persistent ocular pain or development of a corneal abrasion or ulceration.
C. Consult an otolaryngologist if decompression is considered.

Individual Considerations

A. Pregnancy: The incidence of Bell's palsy is increased in pregnancy, with the highest incidence in the third trimester or immediately postpartum. May treat with prednisone during pregnancy.

Carpal Tunnel Syndrome

Jill C. Cash and Julie Adkins

Definition

A. Carpal tunnel syndrome (CTS) is a nerve entrapment condition of the median nerve of the wrist.

Incidence

A. CTS occurs in approximately 1% of the general population. It is primarily seen in 30- to 60-year-old adults. Women and older people are more likely to develop the condition.

Pathogenesis

A. CTS occurs from compression of the median nerve in the carpal canal. Compression occurs because of swelling of the flexor tenosynovium; the pressure blocks the nerve fibers, which produces numbness and discomfort in the digits/hands. Repetitive flexion and extension of the wrists create increased pressure in the carpal canal.
B. Potential causes of CTS include blunt trauma or structural changes; tumors; systemic diseases, such as rheumatoid disorders, diabetes mellitus, thyroid disorders, endocrine diseases, and so forth; mechanical overuse syndrome; and infectious diseases, such as tuberculosis (TB) and leprosy. Consider multifactorial causes of CTS. Heredity is likely an important factor as the carpal tunnel may be smaller in some people or anatomic differences change the amount of space of the nerve; therefore, this trait can run in families.

Predisposing Factors

A. Women
B. Hobbies or jobs that require repetitive wrist or hand movement and the use of vibratory tools
C. Pregnancy
D. Heredity

Common Complaints

A. Pain
B. Tingling/numbness/burning, primarily in the thumb and index, middle, and ring fingers; sensations in the wrists, hands, and fingers that radiates up into the forearm
C. Dropping things because of weakness and numbness or loss of proprioception
D. Nighttime symptoms that are worse than daytime symptoms

Other Signs and Symptoms

A. Paresthesia in wrists, hands, and fingers
B. Localized pain of radial three digits of the hand
C. Weakness with grasp
D. Decreased dexterity
E. Night pain in wrists
F. Referred pain to elbow and/or shoulder
G. Long-term pressure in the carpus can produce ischemic changes and may lead to axonal death, muscular atrophy, and pain. Long-term nerve compression may produce irreversible changes.

Subjective Data

A. Determine onset, duration, and course of presenting symptoms.
B. Note the progression of symptoms since the initial occurrence.
C. Assess whether the symptoms increase with hand or wrist activity and decrease with the joint at rest.
D. Identify what factors precipitate symptoms, what makes symptoms worse, and what alleviates symptoms.
E. Inquire whether the patient awakens at night with numbness and tingling sensations.
F. Have the patient describe the pain, and note if radiation is present. Are symptoms bilateral?
G. Note the patient's occupation, hobby, and/or daily routines that require hand or wrist use.
H. Identify what treatment and/or relief measures have been used, and note results.

Physical Examination

A. Inspect
  1. The hands for deformities. Note wasting or atrophy.

B. Palpate
  1. Perform sensory motor evaluation of the hand and arm.
  2. Perform Tinel's test: Tap over transverse carpal ligament; result is positive if tingling in fingers is noted.
  3. Perform Phalen's test: Have patient place elbows on flat surface and hold forearms in vertical position, then flex wrists; result is positive if pain, numbness, or tingling is noted within the next 60 seconds.

Diagnostic Tests

A. Electromyogram (EMG)
B. Nerve conduction velocity studies
C. If an underlying systemic illness or condition exists, consider the following:
  1. Erythrocyte sedimentation rate (ESR)
  2. Blood glucose
  3. Thyroid profile
  4. Inflammatory disease studies

Differential Diagnoses

A. CTS
B. Peripheral neuropathy
C. Cervical spondylosis and cervical disc herniation
D. Brachial plexus lesion
E. Trauma
F. Thenar atrophy and neuropathy

G. Osteoarthritis
H. Neurologic disorders: Polyneuritis, multiple sclerosis (MS), tumors, and so on

Plan

A. General interventions
1. Help the patient identify causative agents, eliminate activity if possible, decrease repetitive use, or use alternative methods to accomplish the same task.
2. Advise resting arms and wrists as much as possible.
3. Encourage daily stretching exercises.
4. Give instructions on applying wrist splints, especially at bedtime, while sleeping.
B. Patient teaching
1. Instruct the patient on splinting wrists.
2. Demonstrate stretching exercises.
3. Stress the importance of rest and elimination of the causative activity.
C. Pharmaceutical therapy
1. Nonsteroidal anti-inflammatory drugs (NSAIDs) as needed. Ibuprofen (Motrin) 600 to 800 mg by mouth three times daily or naproxen (Naprosyn) 500 mg by mouth twice a day.
2. Vitamin B_6 100 mg/d
3. Consider corticosteroid injections in carpal canal (40 mg/mL with 1% lidocaine 1 mL).

Follow-Up

A. Depending on treatment, consider follow-up in 1 month to evaluate status.

Consultation/Referral

A. Refer the patient to a surgeon for severe symptoms that could require carpal tunnel release.
B. Consider occupational therapy consult.

Individual Considerations

A. Pregnancy: CTS is the most frequent complaint during pregnancy. About 15% of the cases will progress and continue several months postpartum.

Dementia

Jill C. Cash and Julie Adkins

Definition

A. Neurocognitive disorders are characterized by deficits in cognitive function, with a significant decline from a previous level of function. Decline may be evident in one or more areas of function, including attention, language, memory, visuospatial skills, or executive function (complex tasks such as organizing, sequencing, judgment, and reasoning).
B. Neurocognitive disorders include Alzheimer's disease, vascular dementia, Lewy body dementia, and other dementias (frontotemporal dementia, Parkinson's dementia, HIV dementia, neurosyphilis, and Korsakoff's dementia).
C. Clinical features that differentiate these disorders:
1. Alzheimer's disease
a. Gradual onset and a course of progressive decline
b. Memory, language, and visuospatial deficits
c. Depressive symptoms, which may precede diagnosis
d. Delusions, hallucinations, agitation, and apathy
2. Vascular dementia
a. Abrupt onset and a stepwise course of progression
b. Aphasia
3. Lewy body dementia
a. Visual hallucinations and delusions
b. Extrapyramidal symptoms (muscle rigidity, parkinsonism)
c. Fluctuating mental status
d. Increased sensitivity to antipsychotic medications
4. Frontotemporal dementia
a. Change in personality
b. Hyperorality
c. Impairment in executive function, with relatively well-retained visuospatial skills
d. Loss of social awareness
D. The diagnosis of dementia must be differentiated from delirium, a disturbance in cognition that develops over a short period and is characterized by an alteration in attention that fluctuates in severity during the course of the day. Delirium may be the consequence of an acute medication condition, hospitalization, or medication/substance induced. Delirium typically may last weeks to months, with gradual improvement in cognition.

Incidence

A. Worldwide, it is estimated that there are 47.5 million people with dementia, which is expected to increase up to 75.6 million by the year 2030. Dementia is present in 5% to 20% of persons older than 65 years, and in up to 40% of those 75 years and older. It accounts for more than 50% of nursing home admissions and is the condition most feared by aging adults.

Pathogenesis

A. The most common cause of dementia is Alzheimer's disease, accounting for 60% to 80% of cases, with the other cases due to mixed causes, such as multi-infarct or vascular dementia being the second most common cause. A number of other diseases alter cerebral metabolism resulting in dementia such as Huntington's chorea and Parkinson's disease (PD). A variety of diseases that can produce or mimic dementia may be arrested or reversed. These are classified as pseudodementia, such as hypothyroidism or depression. Dementia is caused by damage to brain cells.

Predisposing Factors

A. Definite risks
1. Advanced age
2. Atrial fibrillation
3. Depression
4. Family history
5. Down syndrome

B. Possible risks
   1. Delirium
   2. Head trauma
   3. Heavy smoking

Common Complaints

Interview the patient, family members, and/or friends/caretakers who spend quality time with the patient to assess for social, neurologic, and cognitive changes experienced by the patient.
A. Memory impairment
B. Change in behavior and inability to perform normal activities of self-care

Other Signs and Symptoms

A. Disoriented to date and/or place
B. Naming difficulties (anomia)
C. Impaired recent recall
D. Decreased insight
E. Impaired judgments
F. Social withdrawal
G. Problems managing finances; inability to pay bills and to balance checkbook; spending money in usual ways
H. Getting lost in familiar environments
I. Lack of safety awareness; leaving the stove on, taking medications incorrectly, increased vulnerability to strangers

Impairment of remote memory carries a graver prognosis than the loss of recent memory alone.

Subjective Data

A. Elicit onset and duration of symptoms; commonly, this information comes from family members.
B. Question the family members and/or caregivers regarding personality changes in the patient, or any changes in personal hygiene.
C. Review the patient's history for sexually transmitted infections.
D. Is there a loss of interest in things the patient used to find important?
E. Review medications, specifically those medications with anticholinergic side effects, including over-the-counter (OTC) products such as diphenhydramine.
F. Evaluate the patient's history for any recent major life events such as the death of a spouse, a move to a new living environment, or loss of purpose following retirement.

Physical Examination

A. Evaluate blood pressure, pulse, respiration, and weight.
B. Inspect
   1. Observe general appearance; note grooming, interest in conversation, and apathy.
   2. Note the presence of slurred speech and slowed body movements.
   3. Inspect the nail beds and mucous membranes for anemia.
C. Ausculate
   1. Heart
   2. Lungs
   3. Abdomen
D. Palpate
   1. Thyroid
E. Neurologic examination
   1. Perform a complete neurologic examination, including cranial nerves, gait, motor function, and cerebellar function.
   2. Note facial asymmetry, distal weakness, and any focal neurologic findings.
   3. Complete a mental status examination with instrument of choice. See "Diagnostic Tests" section.
   4. Assess functional status. May use a functional assessment tool such as Physical Self-Maintenance Scale, Instrumental Activities of Daily Living Scale, or Reisberg Functional Assessment Staging (FAST) scale. Available at geriatrics.uthscsa.edu/tools/FAST.pdf
   5. Complete depression screening with instrument of choice:
      a. Geriatric Depression Scale (GDS). Available at https://consultgeri.org/try-this/general-assessment/issue-4.pdf
      b. Patient Heath Questionnaire (PHQ)-9. Available at www.phqscreeners.com
      c. Beck Depression Inventory. Available at www.bmc.org/Documents/Beck-Depression-Inventory-BDI.pdf

Diagnostic Tests

A. Mini-Mental State Examination (MMSE). Available at www.uml.edu/docs/Mini%20Mental%20State%20Exam _tcm18-169319.pdf
B. Pfeiffer's Short, Portable, Mental Status Questionnaire or other mental examination of choice. Pfeiffer's mental status questionnaire is available at geriatrics.stanford.edu/culturemed/overview/assessment/assessment_toolkit/spmsq.html
C. The clock-draw test (CDT) may also be administered and used as a screening tool. The CDT is available at www.rehabmeasures.org (see Section II: Procedures).
D. Rule out possible reversible causes of dementia; not all are required, so use discretion.
   1. Thyroid function tests, to rule out either hypothyroidism or hyperthyroidism
   2. Complete blood count (CBC)
   3. Vitamin B_{12} level: Anemia or B_{12} deficiency
   4. Serum chemistry profile: Hyponatremia
   5. Toxicology screen or serum drug screen: Toxicity or intoxication
   6. Venereal Disease Research Laboratory (VDRL), fluorescent treponemal antibody absorption (FTA-ABS), or microhemagglutination assay for antibody to *Treponema pallidum* (MHA-TP; cerebrospinal fluid [CSF]) to confirm syphilis
   7. HIV-1 antibody titer: AIDS–dementia complex
   8. Liver function tests: Liver disease
   9. CT scan or MRI: Vascular dementia, tumor, chronic subdural hematoma (SDH), normal pressure hydrocephalus, and AIDS–dementia complex

10. EKG: Creutzfeldt–Jakob disease
11. Neuropsychological evaluation

The history is the key to the diagnosis of dementia. The physical examination may be normal. Dementia is not a normal part of aging; normal aging intelligence scores decrease by only about 10% by age 80 years. A thorough search for a potentially reversible cause is required.

Differential Diagnoses

A. Completely reversible dementia, rarely
B. Depression and adverse reactions to medications are the most common reversible causes of dementia.
Use the DEMENTIA mnemonic

D: Drugs or depression
E: Emotional upset
M: Metabolic, for example, vitamin B_{12} deficiency or hypothyroidism
E: Ear or eye impairment or sensory impairment
N: Normal pressure hydrocephalus
T: Tumors or masses, for example, SDH
I: Infection or sepsis
A: Anemia

C. Alzheimer's disease
D. Dementia with Lewy bodies
E. Parkinson's disease (PD) with dementia
F. Vascular dementia
G. Frontotemporal dementia

Plan

A. General interventions
1. The goal is to treat identifiable abnormalities.
2. Supportive care for the family and patient should be arranged.
3. Caring for patients with dementia can be overwhelming. Caregivers need support when caring for these patients as well.
4. Encourage healthy behaviors including regular exercise, healthy diet, and stress management.
5. Maintain brain function through involvement in stimulating social activities.
6. Consider driving evaluation for safety if the patient is still driving.
7. Recommend the use of a safe-return bracelet.
8. Evaluate the home for safety features.
9. Arrange for supportive care for the family and patient.
10. Information regarding support groups for caregivers and family is helpful.

B. Patient/family teaching
1. *See Section III: Patient Teaching Guide for this chapter, "Dementia."*
2. Educate the family and the patient regarding the diagnosis, disease process, and progression.
3. Discuss advance directives and planning for future care needs.
4. Encourage patient and family caregivers to become involved in dementia support groups.
5. Avoid medications such as anticholinergic medications, including diphenhydramine, hydroxyzine, tricyclic antidepressants (TCAs), and oxybutynin.
6. Recommended handbooks for the family include:
a. *The 36-Hour Day: A Family Guide to Caring for People Who Have Alzheimer's Disease, Related Dementias and Memory Loss* (Mace & Rabins, 2012).
b. *Guidelines for Dignity* and *Family Guide*. Both books can be ordered through the Alzheimer's Disease and Related Disorders Association or its local chapters. The national headquarters can be contacted at the following address:
Alzheimer's Disease and Related Disorders Association
919 North Michigan Avenue
Suite 1000
Chicago, IL
60611–1676
800-272-3900

C. Pharmaceutical therapy
1. There are not any medications that have been found to decrease the rate of decline in cognitive behavior. However, studies have shown that patients can be treated with medications for agitation, hallucinations, and depression and to improve mental alertness. Studies indicate that patients with a diagnosis of mild to moderate Alzheimer's disease, vascular dementia, Lewy body dementia, and Parkinson's dementia may trial and benefit from a cholinesterase inhibitor.
a. Donepezil (Aricept): Start 5 mg daily at bedtime for 4 weeks, then 10 mg at bedtime.
b. Rivastigmine (Exelon): Start 1.5 mg twice daily, then increase by 1.5 mg every 4 weeks to maximum dose of 6 mg twice a day.
c. Exelon patch: Start 4.6 mg topical patch daily; increase to 9.5 mg topical patch daily after 4 weeks.
d. Galantamine (Razadyne): Start 4 mg twice a day for 4 weeks, then 8 mg twice a day. Maximum dose 12 mg twice a day.
2. Patients with moderate to severe Alzheimer's disease:
a. Memantine (Namenda): Namenda XR 7 mg daily, titrate by 7 mg/wk to recommended dose of 28 mg daily.

Follow-Up

A. Routine follow-up in 1 month to evaluate patient's status, response to medication, and side effects.
B. Patients and families have an ongoing need for education and support in learning to deal with the diagnosis.
C. Subsequent follow-up visits can be scheduled every 3 to 6 months.

Consultation/Referral

A. Refer the patient to a neurocognitive specialist if diagnosis is unclear.

B. Refer patients and families to support groups in the community.
C. Geriatric psychiatry may be appropriate for management and treatment of behavioral and psychological symptoms of dementia.
D. Refer to social services or geriatric case management for assistance with respite care and placement options.

Individual Considerations

A. Pediatrics: A patient who presents at a young age with dementia requires a thorough workup to evaluate the cause of the symptoms.
B. Geriatrics: Irreversible dementia or Alzheimer's disease begins in the fourth to fifth decade of life and is characterized by loss of recent memory, inability to learn new information, language problems, mood swings, and personality changes.

Resources

Alzheimer's Association: www.alz.org
Alzheimer's Disease Education and Referral Center: www.nia.nih.gov/alzheimers
Frontotemporal Dementia: National Institute of Neurological Disorders and Stroke: www.ninds.nih.gov
Lewy Body Dementia Association: www.lbda.org

Guillain–Barré Syndrome

Cheryl A. Glass and Julie Adkins

Definition

A. Guillain–Barré syndrome (GBS) is an acute immune-mediated polyneuropathy of the peripheral nervous system. GBS often follows an infection.
B. GBS is the most common cause of acute flaccid paralysis in healthy infants and children.
C. GBS in not contagious, and there is no known cure.
D. GBS usually presents with ascending, progressive, multifocal, symmetric muscle weakness, and paresthesia. The first symptom of GBS is weakness or tingling sensations of the legs. Most people reach the stage of greatest weakness within the first 2 weeks after symptoms appear. By the third week of the illness, 90% of all patients are at their weakest.
E. GBS is considered monophasic and remits spontaneously, but may also recur in 3% of patients. Twenty to thirty percent of patients will have persistent disability measured by tools such as the Overall Disability Sum Score (ODSS; see Table 19.1). An electronic version of the ODSS is available online at farmacologiaclinica.info/scales/overall-disability-sum-score. This application grades the arm (range 0–5) and the leg (range 0–7) to provide an overall range score. A total score of 0 equals no disability and a total score of 12 equals maximum disability.
There are several variants of GBS.

1. Miller Fisher syndrome (MFS) often follows an infection, especially *Campylobacter jejuni* gastroenteritis.
2. Acute inflammatory demyelinating polyradiculoneuropathy (AIDP): Approximately two thirds occur after an infection including *C. jejuni*, cytomegalovirus (CMV), *Mycoplasma pneumonia*, or influenza virus.
3. Acute motor axonal neuropathy (AMAN)
4. Acute sensorimotor axonal neuropathy (AMSAN)
5. Acute panautonomic neuropathy (rare)
6. Bickerstaff's brainstem encephalitis (BBE)

Incidence

A. The incidence of GBS is 1/100,000 adults.
B. GBS occurs in all age groups. GBS is more common in older adults with people older than 50 years at the greatest risk.
C. The incidence of GBS in children is 0.6 to 2.4 cases per 100,000.
D. 80% to 90% become nonambulatory during the illness.
E. Relapses are not uncommon in adults who have been treated with intravenous immunoglobulin (IVIG) and plasma exchange.
F. Approximately 30% have a residual weakness after 3 years.
G. GBS severe enough to require mechanical ventilation is associated with both incomplete recovery and up to 20% mortality.
H. Approximately 5% of patients with GBS die from medical complications such as sepsis, pulmonary emboli, and cardiac arrest related to dysautonomia.
I. GBS is reported throughout the world.

Pathogenesis

A. GBS is believed to be an immune-mediated response linked to an antecedent infection wherein a patchy demyelination of the motor component of multiple peripheral nerves occurs. This causes a failure of neuromuscular transmission and leads to abrupt, distal weakness and symmetrical onset of paresthesias. The sensory disturbance is quickly followed by a rapid progressive limb weakness and sometimes paralysis. Most patients are able to identify a specific date of onset of sensory and motor symptoms.

Predisposing Factors

A. Illness
1. Up to two thirds of patients with GBS have experienced a viral upper respiratory infection (URI) or gastroenteritis 10 to 14 days before onset.
2. *C. jejuni* gastroenteritis
3. CMV (CMV is the second most common reported infection preceding GBS)
4. Epstein–Barr virus (EBV)
5. *Mycoplasma pneumonia*
6. HIV
7. *Haemophilus influenzae*
8. Enteroviruses
9. Hepatitis A and B
10. Herpes simplex
11. *Chlamydophila* (formerly *Chlamydia*) pneumonia
12. Zika virus

B. Trauma
C. Surgery
D. Parturition
E. Immunization
1. In 1976, there was a small increase in GBS following the flu vaccine formulated to protect against swine flu.

TABLE 19.1 **Overall Disability Sum Score (ODSS) for Guillain–Barré Syndrome (GBS)**

Area of Body	Activities	Functional Ability Scale for Each Activity	Disability Scale Grade
Arm disability	A. Dressing upper part of body (excludes buttons/zippers) B. Washing and brushing hair C. Turning a key in a lock D. Using a knife and fork (use of spoon applies if never used a fork/knife) E. Doing/undoing buttons and zippers	Not affected; affected, but does not prevent activity; prevents activity	0 = Normal function for all activities 1 = Minor signs/symptoms (S/S) in one or both arms, but does not affect the activity 2 = Moderate S/S in one or both arms affecting, but not preventing, any activity 3 = Severe S/S in one or both arms preventing at least one, but not all, activities 4 = Severe S/S in both arms preventing all functions; purposeful movements still possible 5 = Severe S/S in both arms preventing all purposeful movements
Leg disability	A. Do you have any problems walking? B. Do you walk with a walking aid? C. How do you get around for 25 feet (10 m)? 1. Without aid 2. With one stick or crutch or holding someone's arm 3. With two sticks or crutches or one stick and a crutch and holding someone's arm 4. With a wheelchair D. If you use a wheelchair, can you stand and walk a few steps with help? E. If you are restricted to bed most of the time, are you able to make some purposeful movements?	No; yes; does not apply	0 = Walking is not affected 1 = Walking is affected, but does not look abnormal 2 = Walks independently, but gait looks abnormal 3 = Usually uses unilateral support (stick, crutch, one arm) to walk 25 feet (10 m) 4 = Usually uses bilateral support (stick, crutch, two arms) to walk 25 feet (10 m) 5 = Usually uses a wheelchair to travel 25 feet (10 m) 6 = Restricted to wheelchair, unable to stand and walk a few steps with help, but able to make some purposeful leg movements 7 = Restricted to wheelchair or bed most of the day, preventing all purposeful movements of the legs (e.g., unable to reposition legs in bed)

Source: Adapted from Merkies, Schmitz, van der Meché, Samihn, and van Doorn (2016).

2. Rabies vaccine is prepared from infected brain tissue.

F. There is no genetic factor for GBS.

Common Complaints

A. The classic clinical features
1. Progressive, fairly symmetric muscle weakness
    a. Difficulty walking
    b. Nearly complete paralysis, including
        i. All extremities, generally starts in the proximal legs
        ii. Facial muscles/oropharyngeal weakness
        iii. Respiratory muscles
        iv. Bulbar (ocular) muscles
2. Accompanying absent or depressed deep tendon reflexes (DTRs)

B. Acute weakness in hands, dropping things, trouble picking up small objects or buttoning buttons, inability to feel textures

C. Acute onset of persistent tingling or pins and needles "crawling-skin" sensation in feet, possibly in hands, inability to feel pain

D. Prominent severe lower back pain

Other Signs and Symptoms

A. Sinus tachycardia or other arrhythmias

B. Bilateral generally symmetric muscle weakness not improved by rest

C. Urinary retention

D. Ileus-gastric motility disorders

E. Severe residual fatigue that may persist for years

F. Loss of sweating

G. Facial or pharyngeal weakness

Subjective Data

A. Ask the patient about any dyspnea. If there is shortness of breath (SOB), assess the need to go immediately by ambulance to a hospital.

B. Elicit information regarding the onset and duration of symptoms.

C. Question the patient regarding change or progression of symptoms.

D. Ascertain if the patient has had recent URI, flu, gastroenteritis, other infections, recent trauma, or surgery: Determine if there was an associated fever.

E. Look for paresthesias preceding weakness by approximately 24 to 48 hours.
F. Look for recent exposure to environmental hazards: Lead, pesticides, volatile solvents, or ticks.

Physical Examination

A. Check temperature, pulse, respiration, and blood pressure (persistent hypotension, hypertension alternating with hypotension, or orthostatic hypotension). Hypertension is seen in about one third of patients with GBS and can be labile or followed by hypotension.
B. Inspect
- **1.** Observe overall appearance.
- **2.** Look for gait disturbance.
- **3.** Assess for difficulty with breathing or respiratory distress.

C. Auscultate
- **1.** Note heart rate and rhythm: Tachycardia is common; bradycardia and other arrhythmias may be noted.
- **2.** Auscultate the lung fields.
- **3.** Abdomen assessment for bowel sounds/dysfunction. Gastrointestinal motility disorders occur in 15% of severely affected GBS patients.

D. Palpate
- **1.** Palpate the extremities.
- **2.** Note muscle tone and normal muscle bulk.
- **3.** Assess DTRs, muscle strength, areflexia (lack of reflexes), or hyporeflexia (diminished).
- **4.** Look for symmetric weakness. Incidence of weakness in the ankle and knee is greater than in biceps and triceps.
- **5.** Palpate the abdomen: Assess urinary retention.

E. Neurologic examination
- **1.** Perform complete neurologic examination: Generally, no sensory deficits to touch or pinprick are noted. Decreased proprioception or vibration may be seen. In approximately 50% of clients, GBS may progress rapidly, sometimes within hours, to severe respiratory muscle weakness and respiratory failure. The knee-jerk reflex is usually lost.

Diagnostic Tests

Prompt treatment mandates that the clinician make the diagnosis of GBS solely on history and examination. Testing done in the inpatient setting includes:
A. Lumbar puncture (LP)
- **1.** The LP primarily rules out other infectious diseases.
- **2.** Most GBS patients have elevated cerebrospinal fluid (CSF) protein levels with normal CSF cell counts.

B. Needle electromyogram (EMG)
C. Nerve conduction studies used to confirm the presence, pattern, and severity of neuropathy
D. Antibody testing
E. Serum blood testing: Electrolytes, liver function tests, creatine phosphokinase (CPK), and erythrocyte sedimentation rate (ESR)

Differential Diagnoses

A. GBS
B. Myasthenia gravis (MG)
C. Poliomyelitis
D. Acute intermittent porphyria
E. West Nile encephalomyelitis
F. Tick paralysis: Lyme neuroborreliosis
G. Diphtheria
H. HIV
I. Cervical myelopathy
J. Sarcoidosis
K. Poisoning
- **1.** Heavy metal poisoning (arsenic, lead, thallium)
- **2.** Hexacarbon abuse (glue sniffing neuropathy)
- **3.** Organophosphate poisoning
- **4.** Botulism

L. Zika virus

Plan

A. General interventions
- **1.** Early diagnosis is crucial to appropriate management. A possible diagnosis of GBS requires *immediate* hospitalization at a facility with intensive care unit (ICU) capabilities and consultation with a neurologist who has experience managing GBS. The most critical part of treatment consists of keeping the patient's body functioning during recovery.

B. Patient teaching
- **1.** Educate the patient and family regarding what "Guillain-Barré syndrome" is.
- **2.** Inform the patient and family that there is not a cure for GBS; however, there are several treatments and therapies that may lessen the symptoms and speed up recovery time.
- **3.** Recovery period may take several weeks or months. Reinforce the critical nature of the syndrome, which may include hospitalization in the ICU for paralysis and severe complications.
- **4.** Along with physical impairments/weakness, the patient may also experience emotional problems from the sudden onset of the syndrome requiring dependence on family and friends for physical and emotional support.
- **5.** Offer professional resources for the patient and family. Resources include:
  - **a.** The National Institutes of Health's Brain Resources and Information Network (BRAIN): www.ninds.nih.gov
  - **b.** GBS/CIDP Foundation International: www.gbs-cidp.org

C. Hospital medical management
- **1.** Plasmapheresis (plasma exchange)
- **2.** Intravenous immunoglobulin (IVIG) administration
- **3.** Steroids have not been shown to be helpful and may be detrimental.
- **4.** Because of the associated autonomic instability, hypertension should be treated with short-acting intravenous agents.
- **5.** The presence of at least four of the six predictors indicate the need for support/mechanical ventilation:
  - **a.** Onset of symptoms less than 7 days
  - **b.** Inability to cough

c. Inability to stand
d. Inability to lift the elbows
e. Inability to lift the head
f. An increase in liver enzymes

6. Heparin and support/pressure stockings are used for nonambulatory patients because of the risk of deep vein thrombosis (DVT) and pulmonary embolus.

D. Pharmaceutical therapy
1. Pain therapy
a. Gabapentin (Neurontin) 15 mg/kg/d
b. Carbamazepine (Tegretol) 300 mg/d
c. Narcotics may be necessary
d. Tricyclic antidepressants (TCAs)
2. Immunizations
a. Immunizations are not recommended during the acute phase and up to approximately 1 year after the onset of GBS.
b. Influenza, tetanus, and typhoid immunizations have been most commonly associated with relapse of GBS symptoms.

Follow-Up

A. Patients generally follow up with a neurologist once they have been discharged from the hospital or rehabilitation facility.
B. Full recovery can take up to 3 years with severe cases and even 30% of patients at this point may have residual weakness and 3% of patients experience recurrence. Severe fatigue is a sequel of GBS in two thirds of adults.
C. The most critical part of treatment consists of keeping the patient's body functioning during recovery of the nervous system. Physical rehabilitation with a multidisciplinary team including occupational, speech, and physical therapists focuses on proper limb positioning, posture, orthotics, exercise, and strengthening swallowing muscles.
1. Foot and wrist drop are not uncommon and may require orthotics.
2. Joint contracture requires active and passive range of motion (ROM).
D. Psychological counseling may be required to help with adaptation.
E. The Centers for Disease Control and Prevention (CDC) has set up the Vaccine Adverse Event Reporting system (VAERS) to monitor vaccine safety. The CDC and the U.S. Food and Drug Administration (FDA) comanage the VAERS as an early-warning system about possible side effects noted following immunization.

Consultation/Referral

A. Consult with a physician if GBS is suspected.

Individual Considerations

A. Pediatrics
1. GBS is the most common cause of acute flaccid paralysis in healthy infants and children.
2. There is no evidence currently available of increased risk of GBS from the H1N1 flu vaccine.
3. The Pediatric Evaluation of Disability Inventory Computer Adaptive Test (PEDI-CAT) is designed for the assessment of children from birth to 20 years of age for physical and behavioral conditions in daily activities, mobility, and social/cognitive domains.

B. Geriatrics
1. Age greater than 55 years is a poor prognostic factor.

Resources

CDC Vaccine Adverse Event Reporting System (VAERS) website: vaers.hhs.gov
GBS/CIDP Foundation International: www.gbs-cidp.org

Headache

Cheryl A. Glass and Julie Adkins

Definition

A. Headache is a discomfort of the head that is produced from inflammation and/or tightness of the arteries, nerves, and/or muscles of the cranium. Primary headaches are a major cause for missed school and work, loss of productivity at work (presenteeism), and disability in children and adults.
B. There are multiple types of headaches: Tension-type headaches (TTHs), trigeminal autonomic cephalalgias, including cluster headaches, chronic daily headaches, and new daily-persistent headaches (NDPH; see Table 19.2). Migraines are discussed separately in this chapter under the section "Migraine Headache." Posttraumatic headaches occur within 7 days after head trauma. Tension headaches are the most frequent type, occurring as part of the postconcussive syndrome.
C. NDPHs have many similarities to TTHs and migraines. Other types of headaches, including posttraumatic headache, low cerebrospinal fluid (CSF) volume headache, raised CSF pressure headache, and headaches attributed to infection, should be ruled out. NDPH is unique in that the headache is daily and unremitting from or almost from the moment of onset, typically in individuals without a prior headache history. There are two subtypes:
1. Self-limiting, which typically resolves without therapy within several months
2. Refractory, which is resistant to aggressive treatment programs

Incidence

Headaches are very common, and their incidence depends on age, gender, and type.
A. TTHs are the most common primary headaches, affecting 31% to 74% of the population. Up to 15% of children and teens have experienced tension headaches, compared with 4% for migraines.
B. Headaches occur in 90% of school-aged children.
C. Cluster headaches have been reported in children as young as age 3 years. The prevalence of cluster headaches is in less than 1% of the population, with men affected more than women.

TABLE 19.2 International Headache Society Classification of Headaches (ICHD-II)

New Daily-Persistent Headache (NDPH)[a]	Tension-Type Headache (TTH)[b]	Cluster Headache	Medication Overuse Headache (MOH)[c]
Headache that is daily and unremitting from the moment of onset or very rapidly builds up to continuous and unremitting pain. The pain is typically bilateral, pressing, or tightening in quality and of mild to moderate intensity. There may be photophobia, phonophobia, or mild nausea.	Episodic headache lasting minutes to days. Pain is mild to moderate, typically bilateral, pressing, or tightening quality. Pain does not worsen with activity.	Episodic or chronic attacks separated by pain-free periods lasting a month or longer. Pain almost always recurs on the same side during a cluster period. May be provoked by alcohol, histamine, or nitroglycerine.	Variable headache that often has a peculiar pattern with characteristics shifting, even within the same day, from migraine-like to TTH.
Diagnostic Criteria	**Diagnostic Criteria**	**Diagnostic Criteria**	**Diagnostic Criteria**
A. Headache that fulfills criteria B–D within 3 days of onset.	A. At least 10 episodes, <1 d/mo on average and fulfills B–D criteria.	A. At least five attacks that fulfill B–D criteria.	A. Present on 15 d/mo, which fulfills B–D criteria.
B. Headache is present daily and is unremitting for >3 months.	B. Headache lasts 30 minutes to 7 days.	B. Severe or very severe unilateral orbital, supraorbital, and/or temporal pain lasting 15–180 minutes if untreated.	B. Regular overuse for 3 months of one or more drugs that can be taken for acute and/or symptomatic treatment of headaches.
C. At least two of the following pain characteristics exist: 1. Bilateral location 2. Pressing/tightening (nonpulsating) quality 3. Mild to moderate intensity 4. Not aggravated by routine physical activity such as walking or climbing	C. At least two of the following characteristics exists: 1. Bilateral location 2. Pressure/tightening, nonpulsating quality 3. Mild to moderate quality 4. No increase with routine physical activity such as walking or climbing stairs	C. Accompanied by at least one of the following: 1. Ipsilateral conjunctival infection and/or lacrimation 2. Ipsilateral nasal congestion and/or rhinorrhea 3. Ipsilateral eyelid edema 4. Ipsilateral forehead and facial sweating 5. Ipsilateral miosis and/or ptosis 6. Restlessness or agitation (usually unable to lie down and characteristically pace the floor)	C. Developed or markedly worsened during medication overuse.
D. Both of the following: 1. No more than one of photophobia, phonophobia, or mild nausea 2. Neither moderate or severe nausea nor vomiting	D. Both of the following: 1. No nausea or vomiting 2. No more than one photophobia or phonophobia	D. Attacks have a frequency from one every other day to eight per day.	D. Headache resolves or reverts to its previous pattern within 2 months after discontinuing the overused medication. Examples of medications include Ergotamine, triptans, analgesics, opioids, and combination analgesics.
E. Not attributed to another disorder	E. Not attributed to another disorder	E. Not attributed to another disorder	

[a]The patient must clearly recall and unambiguously describe the daily headache as unremitting at the moment of onset and build to continuous/unremitting pain.
[b]Previously called common, muscle contraction, stress, ordinary, or psychogenic headache.
[c]Previously called rebound, drug-induced, or medication misuse headache.
ICHD-II, The International Classification of Headache Disorders, 2nd edition.
Source: Adapted from the International Headache Society Classification of Headaches ICHD-II (n.d.-b).

D. Chronic daily headaches are more common in females than in males.
E. Medication overuse headaches (MOHs) are reported in 20% to 36% of adolescents with daily headaches.

Pathogenesis

A. Because there are different types of headaches, the origin of each type differs. Many people have a combination of the different types of headaches. Headache causes range from systemic illness such as infections; medical disorders such as tumors or hemorrhage; medications; drug use; and/or stress. Tension headaches are headaches that occur because of contracted muscles of the scalp and neck. Cluster headaches have an uncertain etiology; however, they appear to be caused by extracerebral vasodilation.
B. Review environmental/seasonal factors. Headaches may be cyclic in the spring and summer months with allergic rhinitis and in the fall and winter for carbon monoxide poisoning from gas heaters.
C. Medications commonly associated with headaches include:
  1. Nitroglycerine
  2. Nifedipine
  3. Dipyridamole
  4. Selective serotonin reuptake inhibitor (SSRI)

Predisposing Factors

A. Tension, stress
B. Cervical, or back, disorders
C. Medications (e.g., nitroglycerine)
D. Bruxism
E. Sleep disorders (e.g., snoring, insomnia)
F. Foods/caffeine/alcohol
G. Hormonal changes
H. Family history of headaches
I. Sexual activity
J. Cough
K. Exertion/exercise
L. Viral/infectious etiologies
M. Poor-fitting dentures
N. Faulty/inefficient gas heating
O. Trigeminal neuralgia
P. Valsalva maneuvers
Q. Head trauma

Common Complaints

A. Depending on type of headache, other symptoms may coexist, such as lacrimation, nasal congestion, restlessness, and visual changes.
B. Pain and location depend on the type of headache.
C. Characteristics of the headache depend on the type of headache.

Other Signs and Symptoms

A. Crying
B. Behavioral problems

Subjective Data

A. Use the following acronym for subjective information: PQRST.
  P: Provocation, or worsening of factors stimulating headaches
  Q: Quality of pain, severity of pain
  R: Region of headache
  S: Strength of pain, evaluate pain on a scale of 1 to 10
  T: Time, including onset, frequency, and duration of headaches
B. Assess whether the patient frequently has migraine headaches. Is this the first or worst headache ever experienced by the patient?
C. If recurrent headaches exist, note frequency and patterns of similar headaches.
D. Note whether the patient has ever identified potential triggers of recurring headaches such as dietary issues, stressors, and odors (e.g., perfumes, cigarette smoke).
E. Identify the location of pain, along with radiation if present.
F. Describe the type of pain: Throbbing, constant, or burning.
G. Assess the presence of associated symptoms: Nausea or vomiting, photophobia, noise sensitivity, or the presence of halos around lights.
H. Determine whether the patient experiences any neurologic symptoms and/or prodromal symptoms before a headache.
I. Review the methods used in the past to abort and/or prevent headaches and the results.
J. Inquire about past diagnostic evaluations for headaches.
K. Note a family history of headaches.
L. List current medications, including over-the-counter (OTC) medications and herbals.
M. Review the patient's medical history for head trauma, allergies, presence of a ventriculoperitoneal (VP) shunt, or other neurologic diagnoses.
N. Is the patient in the second or third trimester of pregnancy?
O. Does the patient present with a fever or have a recent history of infection?
P. Rule out gas exposure.

Physical Examination

Physical examination may be normal unless patient presents with a headache.
A. Check blood pressure, pulse, and respiration (temperature if meningeal signs are present).
B. Inspect
  1. Observe overall appearance for the presence of discomfort, photosensitivity (use of sunglasses indoors), and level of consciousness (LOC).
  2. Examine the eyes; perform funduscopic examination.
  3. Inspect the ears, nose, and throat.
C. Auscultate
  1. Listen for bruit at neck, eyes, and head for clinical signs of arteriovenous (AV) malformation.
D. Palpate
  1. Palpate the head, eyes, ears, temporomandibular joint (TMJ), sinus cavities, temporal and neck arteries.

2. Palpate cervical vertebrae, cervical muscles, and shoulder regions. Identify potential trigger areas: Occipital nerves lead halfway between the middle of the neck at the back of the neck and lateral to this area. When palpating this trigger area, pain may be reproduced with palpation.
3. Examine the spine and neck muscles.
4. Assess cervical range of motion (ROM).

E. Perform neurologic examination.
1. Extraocular movements (EOM)
2. Pupil response
3. Getting up from a seated position without any support
4. Walking on tiptoes and heels
5. Tandem gait
6. Romberg test
7. Symmetry on motor, sensory, deep tendon reflexes (DTRs), and coordination tests
8. Assess neck flexion for nuchal rigidity.

Diagnostic Tests

Tests are selected based on history and physical examination.

A. Sinus films to rule out sinusitis or a lesion
B. Sleep studies for obstructive sleep apnea
C. CT scan or MRI: Needed if headache is severe, no results are achieved with drug therapy, and/or aura is present.
D. People, especially children, with any positive neurologic signs of an intracranial process should have neuroimaging.
E. Lab tests are rarely needed for headaches, unless an infectious process is suspected.

Differential Diagnoses

A. Headache
1. Tension
2. Cluster
3. MOH
4. Migraine
5. Combination headache
6. NDPH

B. Sinusitis
C. Meningitis: Meningism, acute headache with fever, lethargy, nausea or vomiting, irritability, photophobia, and systemic infection
D. Space-occupying lesion: Subacute and progressive pain; new onset for adults older than 40 years
E. Temporal arteritis: New-onset progressive headache for adults older than 50 years, with presenting symptoms of temporal artery swelling, pain, pulselessness, visual changes, mental sluggishness, systemic symptoms (fever, anorexia, malaise), and erythrocyte sedimentation rate (ESR) greater than 50 mm/hr
F. Carotid dissection: Sudden headache with neck pain, radiating to the face, ear, or eye; onset related to neck movement or trauma, Horner's syndrome, tinnitus, ipsilateral tongue weakness, cervical bruit or tenderness, diplopia, and syncope
G. TMJ syndrome: Jaw claudication, clicking, and locking sensation, ill-fitting dentures
H. Carbon monoxide poisoning
I. Trigeminal neural
J. Pregnancy-induced hypertension (PIH)
K. Medication-induced headache: Review side effects of current medications (individual and/or combination of drugs)

Plan

A. General interventions
1. Encourage the patient to restrict associated triggers such as food, alcohol, and odors.
2. Encourage the patient to exercise daily.
3. Have the patient begin a stress management routine, including yoga, meditation, and massage.
4. Tell the patient to take medications as prescribed.
5. Advise that cluster headaches can be exacerbated by alcohol.
6. Use ice/heat for muscular tension.
7. Individual and/or family psychotherapy should be considered.
8. Complementary and alternative medicine (CAM)
   a. Nutraceutical options
      i. Magnesium 400 to 600 mg/d
      ii. Riboflavin 400 mg/d
      iii. Coenzyme Q10
      iv. Alpha lipoic acid
   b. Herbal preparations
      i. Feverfew 50 to 82 mg/d
      ii. Butternut root
      iii. Cannabis (Marijuana)
   c. Acupuncture
   d. Oxygen/hyperbaric oxygen therapy
   e. Toxic epidermal necrolysis (TENs) unit
   f. Chiropractic manipulation
   g. Physical therapy
   h. Continuous positive airway pressure (CPAP)
   i. Biofeedback
   J. Relaxation training

B. Patient teaching
1. Encourage the patient to keep a diary of headaches and associated factors to try to pinpoint headache triggers.
2. Teach patients who have menstrual headaches to avoid precipitating factors, such as alcohol, tyramine or phenylethylamine foods, missed meals, and sleeping late.
3. Discuss sleep hygiene guidelines (see Chapter 22, Psychiatric Guidelines, "Sleep Disorders" section).
4. For muscular headaches that are nonmenstrual, biofeedback, breathing exercises, and visualization are helpful. Prevention must be stressed. Encourage lifestyle changes and daily exercise.
5. When patients overuse various analgesics for headaches, paroxysmal migraines can convert into chronic daily headaches. Caution patients regarding this effect.
6. MOHs occur with the highest incidence with opioids, butalbital-containing combinations, and acetylsalicylic acid (ASA)/acetaminophen/caffeine combinations as well as triptans. Withdrawal of the overused medication is the treatment of choice for MOHs.

C. Pharmaceutical therapy: Therapy should be started at the lowest dosage and titrated up as tolerated, avoiding overuse.

1. Nonsteroidal anti-inflammatory drugs (NSAIDs)

a. ASA 650 to 1,000 mg orally; maximal dose 4 g/d

b. Ibuprofen (Advil) 400 to 800 mg every 8 hours; maximum dose 2.4 g/d

2. Combination medications

a. Acetaminophen, butalbital, and caffeine (Fioricet) with or without codeine one to two tablets every 4 hours as needed. Maximum dose is six tablets per day.

b. ASA, butalbital, and caffeine (Fiorinal) one or two tablets every 4 hours as needed. Caution the patient regarding dependency patterns.

c. Isometheptene mucate, dichloralphenazone, and acetaminophen (Epidrin or Migratine) one to two capsules every 4 hours if needed up to eight capsules in a 24-hour period for tension headaches in adults.

d. Acetaminophen, ASA, and caffeine (Excedrin) two tablets every 6 hours; maximal dose of 4 g of aspirin or acetaminophen

3. Cluster or vascular headaches

a. Verapamil is the agent of choice for prevention therapy with cluster headaches.

b. Propranolol (Inderal) or carbamazepine 80 mg daily in divided doses; maximum range 160 to 240 mg daily.

c. Oxygen 100% therapy has been effective for cluster headaches.

4. Menstrual headaches

a. Estrogen supplements or continuous cycling is used to decrease headaches. Have the patient start taking estrogen 2 days before expected migraine and use for 7 days.

b. Naproxen 275 to 550 mg every 2 to 6 hours (maximum dose 1.5 mg/d) starting 7 days as needed before menses.

c. Ibuprofen 600 mg three times daily

d. Fluoxetine (Prozac) 10 to 20 mg daily is also used for patients with premenstrual syndrome with luteal phase defect.

5. Medications may be used for preventive treatment. Medications used include: Ergot derivatives, anticonvulsants, antidepressants, tricyclic antidepressants (TCAs), muscle relaxers, antihistamines.

6. Pharmaceutical therapies for chronic daily and NDPHs combine therapy that are used for tension-type and migraine headaches.

Follow-Up

A. See the patient in 2 weeks to evaluate how therapies have worked.

B. Evaluate the patient's "headache log" to assist him or her in identifying headache triggers, if present.

Consultation/Referral

A. Consult a physician if headaches are caused by acute problems other than migraine and/or tension headaches.

B. Severe episodes need to be evaluated by a physician for opioid agonists and antagonists, narcotics, and neuroleptics.

C. If medications do not help with headaches, refer the patient to a neurologist.

Individual Considerations

A. Pregnancy

1. PIH often presents with a headache.

B. Pediatrics

1. Antihistamines are useful as a preventive agent, as are biofeedback and relaxation techniques.

2. Avoid using aspirin-containing products because of the potential of Reye's syndrome. Differentiating the causative factor is essential for this population.

3. Medication therapy is dependent on the child's age.

C. Adults: Patients who are premenopausal may see improvement when their estrogen levels are constant, instead of being cyclic.

D. Geriatrics

1. Headaches decrease with age. Serious causes of headaches increase with age. Such causes include:

a. Temporal arteritis

b. Trigeminal neuralgia

c. Sleep apnea

d. Postherpetic neuralgia

e. Cervical spondylosis

f. Subarachnoid hemorrhage (SAH)

g. Intracerebral hemorrhage

h. Intracranial neoplasm

i. Postconcussive syndrome

2. Hypnic headache occurs only in the elderly.

3. Consider imaging studies in the elderly with unusual presentations of headaches.

4. Consider chronic subdural hematomas (SDH) with patients who have frequent falls who complain of headaches; perform CT scan or MRI for evaluation.

5. Elderly patients may not exhibit any symptoms other than a headache.

6. When medicating the elderly for headaches, start dosages low and increase as tolerated.

a. Naproxen and hydroxyzine are commonly used oral rescue therapies for older adults with migraine or tension headaches.

b. Oral agents for the prevention of hypnic headaches include caffeine and lithium.

c. Consider renal function before prescribing NSAIDs.

7. Consider all contraindications when prescribing medications; many elderly patients have cardiovascular disease, which is contraindicated with ergot derivatives.

Migraine Headache

Cheryl A. Glass and Julie Adkins

Definition

A. Migraine headaches are a common medical complaint responsible for a significant disability and loss of quality of life. The economic impact involves loss of workdays, school, social interaction, and loss of productivity while at work (presenteeism). There are three types of migraines described by the International Headache Society (IHS) by type and diagnostic criteria (see Table 19.3).

B. Migraine headaches have been associated with increased risk of cerebral ischemia and an increased risk of cardiac ischemia.

Incidence

Headaches are one of the most common medical complaints. The exact incidence of migraines is unknown as patients self-treat, are underdiagnosed, and are commonly misdiagnosed. Headaches account for 10 million office visits per year. Ten to sixteen percent is the overall estimated incidence of migraines in North America and Europe; however, several subsets of migraineurs are noted in the literature. An estimated 6% of men and 15% to 17% of women in the United States have migraines, but only 3% to 5% of them receive preventative therapy. Migraines are heterogenous in frequency, duration, and disability.

A. 3% incidence in preschoolers
B. Up to 11% incidence in school-aged children
  1. Boys outnumber girls before age 7 years.
  2. Boys are equally likely to have migraines between ages 7 and 11 years.
  3. After puberty, girls have more migraines than boys.
C. 23% incidence in adolescents
D. 2% of the population has chronic migraines.
E. It is estimated that 38% of migraineurs need preventive therapy, but only 3% to 13% currently use preventive therapy.

TABLE 19.3 International Headache Society Classification of Migraines (ICHD-II)

Migraine Without Aura	Migraine With Aura (Six Subtypes)	Chronic Migraine[a]
Recurrent headache attack lasting 4–72 hours meeting the diagnostic criteria	Recurrent disorder manifesting reversible focal neurologic symptoms that usually develop gradually over 5–20 minutes and last for less than 60 minutes. Typical aura consists of visual and/or sensory and/or speech symptoms	Chronic migraine that meets the criteria for migraine without aura that occurs with a frequency of at least 15 headache days per month for longer than 3-months' duration
Diagnostic Criteria	**Diagnostic Criteria**	**Diagnostic Criteria**
A. At least two attacks that fulfill criteria B–D B. Headache attacks last 4–72 hours (untreated or unsuccessfully treated) C. Has at least two of the following: 1. Unilateral location 2. Pulsating quality 3. Moderate or severe intensity 4. Aggravated by or causing avoidance of routine physical activity D. During headache at least one of the following: 1. Nausea and/or vomiting 2. Photophobia and phonophobia E. Not attributed to another disorder	A. At least two attacks that fulfill criteria B–D B. Aura consists of at least one of the following, but no motor weakness: 1. Fully reversible visual symptoms, including positive features (e.g., flickering lights, spots, or lines) and/or negative features (i.e., loss of vision) 2. Fully reversible sensory symptoms, including positive features (i.e., pins and needles) and/or negative features (i.e., numbness) 3. Fully reversible dysphasic speech disturbance C. At least two of the following: 1. Homonymous visual symptoms (i.e., additional loss or blurring of central vision) and/or unilateral sensory symptoms 2. At least one aura symptom develops gradually over ≥5 minutes and/or different aura symptoms occur in succession over ≥5 minutes. 3. Each symptom lasts ≥5 minutes and ≤60 minutes. D. Headache fulfilling criteria B–C: Migraine without aura begins during the aura or follows the aura within 60 minutes. E. Not attributed to another disorder	A. Headache, in the absence of medication overuse headache (MOH), on ≥15 d/mo for at least 3 months B. Occurring in a patient who has had at least five attacks fulfilling criteria for migraine without aura C. On ≥ 8 d/mo for at least 3 months headache fulfills C1 and/or C2 criteria noted as follows. C1. Has at least two of the following: 1. Unilateral location 2. Pulsating quality 3. Moderate or severe pain intensity 4. Aggravation by or causing avoidance of routine physical activity *and* at least one of the following: (a) Nausea and/or vomiting (b) Photophobia and phonophobia C2; treated and relieved by triptan(s) or ergot before the expected development of C1 symptoms D. No medication overuse and not attributed to another causative disorder

ICHD-II, The International Classification of Headache Disorders, 2nd edition.
[a]A proposed alternative criteria is defined as a chronic headache for at least 4 migraine days and at least 15 total headache days, with at least 50% of headache days meeting criteria for migraine.
Source: Adapted from the International Headache Society ICHD-II (n.d.-b).

Pathogenesis

A. Migraines have broad sensory processing dysfunction, with a prominent perception of pain in the dense somatosensory innervation of intracranial vessels. Current pathophysiologic concepts of migraine and migraine aura include a possible dysfunction of neuromodulatory structures in the brainstem and cortical spreading depression (CSD). Different receptors, including calcitonin gene-related peptide (CGRP), transient receptor potential cation channel subfamily V member (TrpVI [also known as the capsaicin receptor]), and glutamate receptors, are currently being targeted for migraine therapeutics.

Predisposing Factors

A. Family history of migraines
B. Chronic use of over-the-counter (OTC) analgesics (rebound)
C. Posthead trauma
D. Food, odor, light, sound, sleep, weather changes, hormonal changes, and stress triggers
E. Menstruation
F. Obesity
G. Daily habitual snoring is a modest risk factor
H. Estrogen use

Common Complaints

A. Unilateral headache (bilateral in children)
B. Frontotemporal area (occipital in children)
C. Photophobia, or sensitivity to light (young children may cover their eyes)
D. Phonophobia, or sensitivity to sound (young children may cover their ears)
E. Osmophobia, or hypersensitivity/aversion to smells/odors
F. Nausea with/without vomiting
G. Prodrome phase: Fatigue, reduced concentration, agitation, craving, fatigue, irritability, depression, frequent yawning, or hyperexcitability hours to days before the onset of aura and headache

Other Signs and Symptoms

A. Muscle tension and neck pain
B. Cutaneous allodynia (pain from stimulus to normal skin or scalp)
C. Sinus congestion
D. Prodrome phase can last 25 hours accompanied by fatigue and a "hangover" headache
E. Abdominal pain (children)

Subjective Data

A. Use the following acronym for subjective information: PQRST.
- **P:** Provocation, or worsening of factors stimulating headaches
- **Q:** Quality of pain, severity of pain
- **R:** Region of headache
- **S:** Strength of pain, evaluate pain on a scale of 1 to 10
- **T:** Time, including onset, frequency, and duration of headaches

B. Assess whether the patient frequently has migraine headaches. Is this the first or worst headache ever experienced by the patient?
C. If recurrent headaches exist, note frequency and patterns of similar headaches.
D. Note whether the patient has ever identified potential triggers of recurring headaches such as dietary issues, stressors, and odors (e.g., perfumes and cigarette smoke)
E. Identify the location of the pain, along with radiation if present.
F. Describe the type of pain: Throbbing, constant, or burning.
G. Assess the presence of associated symptoms: Nausea or vomiting, photophobia, and noise sensitivity.
H. Determine whether the patient experiences any neurologic symptoms and/or prodromal symptoms before headache.
I. Review the methods used in the past to abort and/or prevent headaches and the results.
J. Inquire about past diagnostic evaluations for headaches.
K. Note a family history of headaches.
L. List current medications, including OTC medications and herbal products.
M. Review the patient's medical history for head trauma, infection, allergies, presence of a ventriculoperitoneal (VP) shunt, or other neurologic diagnoses.

Physical Examination

Physical examination may be normal unless the patient presents with a headache.

A. Check blood pressure, pulse, and respiration (temperature if meningeal signs are present).
B. Inspect
  1. Observe overall appearance for the presence of discomfort, photosensitivity (use of sunglasses indoors), and level of consciousness (LOC).
  2. Examine the eyes; perform funduscopic examination.
  3. Inspect the ears, nose, and throat.
C. Auscultate
  1. Listen for bruit at neck, eyes, and head for clinical signs of arteriovenous (AV) malformation.
D. Palpate
  1. Palpate the head, eyes, ears, TMJ, sinus cavities, temporal, and neck arteries.
  2. Palpate cervical vertebrae, cervical muscles, and shoulder regions. Identify potential trigger areas: Occipital nerves leave halfway between the middle of the neck at the back of the neck and lateral to this area. When palpating this trigger area, pain may be reproduced with palpation.
  3. Examine the spine and neck muscles.
  4. Assess the cervical range of motion (ROM).
E. Perform neurologic examination.
  1. Extraocular movements (EOM)
  2. Pupil response
  3. Getting up from a seated position without any support
  4. Walking on tiptoes and heels
  5. Tandem gait

6. Romberg test
7. Symmetry on motor, sensory, deep tendon reflexes (DTRs), and coordination tests

Diagnostic Tests

A. Neuroimaging, CT, and MRI are based on the history and physical examination.
1. Adults and children with stable headaches, a normal examination, and absence of seizures do not require neuroimaging.
2. Neuroimaging should be considered for children with headaches with abnormal neurologic examination and/or seizures.
3. Neuroimaging should be considered for children with severe headaches, change in headaches, or associated neurologic dysfunction.
4. An emergent noncontrast CT should be obtained when the patient complains of "the worst headache ever" or when focal neurologic findings, nuchal rigidity, or altered mental status exist.
5. The presence of personality changes, depression, and a migraine may indicate a temporal lobe tumor.
6. The presence of orbital bruit requires neuroimaging.
7. Neuroimaging is recommended for adults with onset of headache after the age of 40 years.
8. Onset of headache with exertion, cough, or sexual activity should be considered for neuroimaging.

B. A lumbar puncture may be indicated in children with altered mental status or focal findings.

C. Sinus films to rule out sinusitis or a lesion

D. Laboratory tests are not required for most patients with typical symptoms and a negative physical examination.
1. Drug screen may be indicated.
2. Complete metabolic panel (CMP)
3. Complete blood count (CBC)
4. Thyroid-stimulating hormone (TSH)
5. Sedimentation rate

Differential Diagnoses

A. Migraine
1. Migraine with aura
2. Migraine without aura

B. Other types of headaches
1. Medication overuse headaches (MOH)
2. Common headache
3. Cluster headache
4. Combination headache
5. Chronic daily headache
6. Tension headache
7. Hypnic headaches (geriatrics)

C. Sinusitis

D. Space-occupying lesion: Subacute and progressive pain, new onset for adults older than 40 years

E. Temporal arteritis: New-onset progressive headache for adults older than 50 years

F. Carotid dissection: Sudden headache with neck pain radiating to the face, ear, or eye

G. TMJ syndrome

H. Meningitis

I. Brain abscess

J. Encephalitis

K. Idiopathic intracranial hypertension

Plan

A. General interventions: There are four main approaches to migraine therapy.
1. Nonpharmacological interventions
   a. Adjust habits to maintain a routine pattern of sleeping. This is especially important to maintain on weekends and vacations.
   b. Do not skip breakfast. Eat regular meals with one or two snacks.
   c. Avoid food triggers identified by the patient's migraine diary.
   d. Encourage drinking no more than two caffeinated beverages a day.
   e. Hydration is important.
   f. Encourage at least 30 minutes of exercise 3 to 7 days a week.
   g. Cold compresses
2. Behavioral interventions
   a. Use relaxation techniques such as yoga, deep breathing, meditation, and guided imagery.
   b. Biofeedback is an adjunct to relaxation training.
   c. Cognitive behavioral therapy
   d. Psychiatric therapy
3. Complementary and alternative interventions
   a. Acupuncture
   b. Nutraceuticals, including magnesium, coenzyme Q10, and butternut root extract
   c. Vitamins: Riboflavin (B_2)
   d. Herbal (nonregulated by the U.S. Food and Drug Administration [FDA]), including feverfew and butternut root extract
   e. Physical therapy
   f. Hypnosis
   g. Toxic epidermal necrolysis (TENS), chiropractic manipulation, and occlusal adjustment are also noted in the literature.
   h. Onabotulinumtoxin A has been tested extensively and has been found to be ineffective in episodic migraines, but has been approved by the FDA in chronic headaches.
4. Pharmacological interventions: Patients should be counseled to take medications as prescribed. When patients overuse various analgesics for headaches, paroxysmal migraines can convert into chronic daily headaches.

B. Patient teaching
1. Encourage the patient to keep a headache diary; an example of a migraine diary is available at www.webmd.com/migraines-headaches/guide/headache-diary. The diary may help the patient identify triggers for the migraine headaches.
   a. Examples of food triggers are aspartame, saccharin, red wine, alcohol, chocolate, aged cheese, oranges, tomatoes, avocado, nuts, onions, tyramine, phenylethylamine, monosodium glutamate (MSG), and nitrates and nitrites found in hot dogs, luncheon meat, and sausage.

b. Examples of odor triggers include tobacco smoke, perfumes, and strong odors.

c. Examples of visual triggers include strobe lights, bright lights/sunlight, fluorescent lights, and glare.

d. Other triggers are medications, barometric weather changes, too much/too little sleep, and high altitude.

2. The 2014 American Heart Association/American Stroke Association Guidelines for the Prevention of Strokes in Women state that because of the increased stroke risk seen in women with migraine headaches with aura and smoking, it is reasonable to strongly recommend smoking cessation.

C. Pharmaceutical therapy (see Table 19.4). **The choice of drug therapy prophylactic agents depends on the patient's comorbid conditions such as cardiac, respiratory, psychiatric, sleep, and gastrointestinal disorders.**

1. Many drugs commonly used for migraines are not FDA approved for migraine therapy, including amitriptyline, nortriptyline, and selective serotonin reuptake inhibitors (SSRIs).

2. Antiepileptic medications, including valproic acid (Depakote) and topiramate (Topamax), are FDA approved for migraine prophylaxis. Topiramate should not be prescribed or discontinued for a history of kidney stones.

3. Beta-blockers are approved for migraine prophylaxis; however, they must be used with caution for patients with comorbidities such as asthma, depression, diabetes, and thyroid disease.

4. There are currently several triptans and one triptan/nonsteroidal anti-inflammatory drug (NSAID) combination. Triptans are widely used for menstrual migraines. Triptans should be used cautiously in patients with cardiovascular comorbidities, and some are not approved for children. Triptans should not be given within 24 hours of an ergot.

5. Dihydroergotamine mesylate (Migranal) is not to be used for patients during pregnancy or with heart disease, or ischemic or vasospastic circulatory disease. Use ergot derivatives selectively. These medications are not to be used on a long-term basis or more than three times per week. There is an associated risk of strokes when using these medications because of the vasoconstrictive mechanisms of the medications.

6. Ergots and triptans should not be given within 14 days of a monoamine oxidase (MAO) inhibitor.

7. Antiemetics are prescribed as needed for nausea/vomiting associated with migraines.

8. Multiple drugs are used off-label for migraines.

Follow-Up

A. See the patient in 2 weeks to evaluate how therapies have worked.

B. Evaluate the patient's headache diary to assist him or her in identifying headache triggers or patterns such as before menstruation. Use the information documented in the diary as a tool for reevaluating the need for other tests and consultations.

C. Monitor liver enzymes and CBC periodically with antiseizure medication prophylaxis.

Consultation/Referral

A. Consult a physician if headaches are caused by acute problems other than migraine and/or tension headaches.

B. If medications do not help with headaches, refer the patient to a neurologist/pediatric neurologist.

C. Send the patient to the emergency department for any neurologic, life-threatening signs.

Individual Considerations

A. Pregnancy: Many medications are contraindicated in pregnancy.

B. Pediatrics

1. Avoid using aspirin-containing products because of the potential of Reye's syndrome.

2. Differentiating the causative factor is essential for this population.

3. Adolescents may see improvement when their estrogen levels are constant instead of cyclic.

4. The choice of medication management is age dependent. Antiepileptics, antidepressants, antihistamines, calcium channel blockers, and NSAIDs are prescribed for children.

C. Geriatrics

1. Headaches decrease after the age of 50 years. Headache onset after age 50 years is associated with epilepsy, essential tremor, ischemic stroke, mood disorders, asthma, and patent foramen ovale.

2. Consider imaging studies for elderly patients who present with unusual headaches.

3. Consider chronic subdural hematomas (SDH) with patients who have frequent falls; perform CT scan or MRI for evaluation. Elderly patients may not exhibit any symptoms other than a headache.

4. Consider all contraindications when prescribing medications; many elderly patients have cardiovascular disease, which is contraindicated with ergot derivatives.

Mild Traumatic Brain Injury

Kimberly D. Waltrip

Definition

Head injury is defined as any external structural damage or functional impairment of the cranial contents (scalp, skull, meninges, blood vessels, and/or brain) secondary to a traumatic force against the head. Any of the following may occur immediately after the initial injury: Loss of consciousness or decreased level of consciousness (LOC), memory loss regarding events immediately pre- or postinjury, altered mental status, and any neurodeficits involving motor strength, balance, vision, sensation, and speech. Mild traumatic brain injury (MTBI) results in a disruption of brain function, which reflects severity of the initial injury. MTBI-related deficits are often mild without overt symptoms. Radiographic testing is

TABLE 19.4 Medications for Migraines

Medication	Class	Instructions for Adult Dosing	Acute vs. Prophylaxis
Sumatriptan (Imitrex)	Triptan	Initially 25–100 mg. May repeat in 2-hr intervals. (Maximum dose 200 mg/24 hr.) Also available subcutaneous and intranasal formulations.	Acute treatment
Sumatriptan (Alsuma)	Triptan	Initially 6 mg subcutaneous. May repeat in 1 hour. (Maximum of 12 mg/24 hr.)	Acute treatment and cluster headaches
Sumatriptan iontophoretic system (Zecuity)	Triptan	TDS that uses a low electrical current for drug delivery. Each patch delivers 6.5 mg of sumatriptan through the skin more than 4 hours. No more than two should be used in a 24-hour period. The second TDS should be applied no sooner than 2 hours after activation of the first TDS.	Acute treatment migraine with and without aura
Rizatriptan (Maxalt)	Triptan	Initially 5–10 mg. May repeat in 2-hour intervals. (Maximum dose 30 mg/24 hr.) Available in oral or disintegrating tablets.	Acute treatment
Zolmitriptan (Zomig)	Triptan	Initially 2.5–5 mg. May repeat in 2 hours. (Maximum dose 10 mg/24 hr.) Available in oral or disintegrating tablets.	Acute treatment
Naratriptan (Amerge)	Triptan	Initially 1–2.5 mg. May repeat in 4 hours. (Maximum dose 5 mg/24 hr.)	Acute treatment
Almotriptan (Axert)	Triptan	Initially 6.25–12.5 mg. May repeat in 2 hours. (Maximum dose 25 mg/24 hr.)	Acute treatment
Eletriptan (Relpax)	Triptan	Initially 40 mg. May repeat in 2 hours. (Maximum dose 80 mg/24 hr.)	Acute treatment
Frovatriptan (Frova)	Triptan	Initially 2.5 mg. May repeat in 2 hours. (Maximum dose 7.5 mg/24 hr.)	Acute treatment
Sumatriptan with naproxen sodium (Treximet)	Triptan + NSAID	1 tablet = sumatriptan 85 mg + 500 mg naproxen sodium. Initially one tablet. May repeat in 2 hours. (Maximum dose 2 tabs/24 hr.)	Acute treatment
Dihydroergotamine mesylate (Migranal)	Ergot derivative	Only available in intranasal spray. Initially 1 spray in each nostril. May repeat in 15 minutes. (Maximum 6 sprays/24 hr with a maximum of 8 sprays/wk.)	Acute treatment
Ergotamine tartrate + caffeine	Ergot derivative	Initially 2 tablets at onset. May repeat 1 tablet every half hour. (Maximum dose 6 tablets/24 hr with a maximum of 10 tablets/wk.) Also available in suppositories.	Acute treatment migraines and cluster headaches
Propranolol (Inderal)	Beta-blocker	Initially 80 mg/d. May titrate up to 240 mg/d.	Migraine prophylaxis
Timolol	Beta-blocker	10–15 mg bid: May titrate up to 30 mg/d.	Migraine prophylaxis
Topiramate (Topamax)	Antiseizure	Requires titration:	Migraine prophylaxis
		Week 1: 25 mg every bedtime.	
		Week 2: 25 mg/a.m. and 25 mg/at bedtime.	
		Week 3: 25 mg/a.m. and 50 mg/at bedtime.	
		Week 4: 50 mg/a.m. and 50 mg/at bedtime (Maximum 100 mg/24 hr.)	
Valproic acid (Depakote)	Antiseizure	500 mg/daily for 1 wk, then increase up to 1 g/d.	
Amitriptyline	Antidepressant	Initially 75 mg/d in divided doses *or* 50–100 mg at bedtime. (Maximum 150 mg/24 hr.)	Migraine prophylaxis
Nortriptyline (Pamelor)	Antidepressant	Initially 25 mg, three to four times a day. (Maximum dose 150 mg/d.)	Migraine prophylaxis
Fluoxetine (Prozac)	SSRI	Initially 20 mg/a.m. Increase if needed after several weeks. Doses >20 mg/d should be given in divided doses in the a.m. and at noon. (Maximum 80 mg/24 hr.)	Migraine prophylaxis

NSAID, nonsteroidal anti-inflammatory drug; SSRI, selective serotonin reuptake inhibitor; TDS, transdermal system.

negative for anatomic abnormalities (e.g., cerebral edema, hemorrhage). *Concussion* is a commonly used term that describes MTBI, in which a loss of consciousness may have occurred; confusion is also associated with MTBI. Ninety percent of patients with concussive injuries do not experience decreased LOC. Serious complications of MTBI include asymptomatic extradural hematomas, fatal thrombosis of the basilar artery, and hemorrhage from existing conditions such as fibrous dysplasia or essential thrombocytopenia.

The American Academy of Neurology offers the following guidelines for grading the severity of concussions.

A. Grade I: Confusion with symptoms lasting less than 15 minutes, no loss of consciousness.

B. Grade II: Symptoms persisting more than 15 minutes, no loss of consciousness.

C. Grade III: Loss of consciousness ([a] unresponsive for a number of seconds; [b] unresponsive for a number of minutes).

Incidence

A. There are approximately 1.7 million emergency department (ED) visits for evaluation and treatment of head injuries in the United States each year, with more than 750,000 hospital admissions and 52,000 deaths. Of these, an estimated 80% to 90% are considered MTBIs. Many individuals with MTBI do not seek medical attention—this is a factor to consider regarding the actual number of reported cases. Most individuals with MTBI recover fully within several days to weeks. However, approximately 10% to 15% of individuals with MTBI have persistent symptoms a year after injury.

Pathogenesis

A. Head-injured patients can potentially sustain two different types of injuries: *Primary* injury and *secondary* injury.

- **1.** A primary injury is the direct result of a head injury, occurring at the time of the initial traumatic impact or force. This type of injury is purely mechanical and may be *focal* (contusion or laceration, bone fragmentation) or *diffuse*, as in concussion or diffuse axonal injury (DAI). These injuries do not require surgical intervention.
- **2.** Secondary injury is caused by a flow-metabolism mismatch, and is therefore a complication of primary brain injury. Secondary injury includes any subsequent ischemic and hypoxic changes in the brain, cerebral edema, intracranial hemorrhage (ICH), and the effects of prolonged increased intracranial pressure (ICP), hydrocephalus, and infection. Secondary injury presents with delayed onset of signs and symptoms, occurring anytime from seconds to minutes, hours, or days.

Predisposing Factors

A. Motor vehicle accidents (MVAs)

B. Assaults

C. Sports- and recreation-related trauma

D. Male gender

E. Ages of increased incidence

- **1.** 0 to 4 years
- **2.** 15 to 19 years
- **3.** 65 years and older

F. Military occupation (i.e., exposure to blasts)

G. Falls

Common Complaints

A. Headaches that are often constant, generalized in nature; may report frontal headache pain; symptoms may persist for days or weeks.

B. Brief amnestic epoch surrounding the initial injury

C. Faintness

D. Nausea/vomiting

E. Changes in vision, often slight blurring

F. Drowsiness

G. Loss of consciousness

H. Confusion

Other Signs and Symptoms

Other presenting symptoms and complaints are identified in four categories as follows: *Physical, emotional, cognitive,* and *sleep-cycle disturbances.*

A. Physical

- **1.** Reported or observed injury to the head
- **2.** Dizziness
- **3.** Fatigue
- **4.** Impaired balance
- **5.** Photophobia
- **6.** Sensitivity to noise
- **7.** Numbness/tingling
- **8.** Seizures, delayed onset after initial injury

B. Emotional

- **1.** Irritability
- **2.** Nervousness
- **3.** Depression
- **4.** Labile mood

C. Cognitive

- **1.** Difficulty concentrating
- **2.** Impaired memory
  - **a.** Short-term memory loss
  - **b.** Repetition
- **3.** Confusion
- **4.** Slow responses/difficulty processing information
- **5.** Changes in reaction time
- **6.** Changes in speech
- **7.** Disorientation
- **8.** Fatigue

D. Sleep-cycle disturbance

- **1.** Feeling "drowsy"
- **2.** Difficulty falling asleep
- **3.** Sleeping more or less than usual

Subjective Data

A. Obtain a description of injury from the patient or witness of the traumatic event, if possible. Identify the cause of the head injury, how it occurred (direct or indirect impact), and what type of force was exerted.

B. Confirm the patient's LOC at the time of injury and afterward. Inquire about amnesia (retrograde and anterograde), which might predict increased severity of the injury. Ask about the event, whether it was observed by others, and its duration.

C. Review initial and current symptoms (refer to "Common Complaints" and "Other Signs and Symptoms" discussed earlier). Include the description, location, severity, and onset of symptoms. It is important to note what has occurred since the initial injury. It is not uncommon for patients to report symptoms that recur or worsen on exertion.

D. Obtain the patient's medical history, especially details of any previous head injuries. Learning disabilities (e.g., attention deficit hyperactivity disorder [ADHD]), developmental disorders, depression, anxiety, sleep disorders, and mood disorders should be documented because these can affect recovery.

E. Review current medications; certain medications like warfarin (Coumadin) can be predisposing factors for complications.

F. Document any recreational drug and/or alcohol history.

G. Ask family members/significant others if they have noticed any related signs or symptoms, behavioral changes, or evidence of seizure activity.

Physical Examination

A. Check pulse, respiration, and blood pressure.

B. Inspect

- **1.** Observe overall appearance. Note LOC.
- **2.** Inspect the skin and head for obvious injury. Periorbital ecchymosis ("raccoon's eyes"), postauricular/mastoid ecchymosis (Battle's sign), or evidence of a cerebrospinal fluid (CSF) leak (otorrhea, rhinorrhea) can indicate a basilar skull fracture.
- **3.** Examine the eyes for the presence of papilledema (optic disc swelling caused by increased intracranial pressure [ICP]), proptosis, and periorbital edema.
- **4.** Examine the ears (hemotympanum or possible laceration to the external canal), nose, and throat.
- **5.** Examine for facial fractures.
- **6.** Examine for any trauma (e.g., vertebral malalignment, abnormal curvature) to the cervical spine; if necessary, place the patient on spine precautions (immobilize the head and neck) and refer to orthopedics or neurosurgery for further evaluation.

C. Auscultate

- **1.** Over the globes of the eyes if warranted (bruit may indicate traumatic carotid-cavernous fistula)
- **2.** Carotid arteries bilaterally if warranted (bruit may indicate carotid dissection)
- **3.** The heart and lungs, if cardiovascular etiology is suspected
- **4.** The abdomen, if other incidental injuries are suspected (e.g., from a contact sport or MVA)

D. Palpate

- **1.** Palpate for instability of the facial bones, including the zygomatic arch—may detect a palpable step-off with orbital rim fractures.
- **2.** If appropriate, palpate the abdomen and the entire posterior spine to rule out any other incidental injuries.

E. Neurologic examination

- **1.** Assess mental status and memory. Determine whether the patient is awake, alert, cooperative, and oriented to *person*, *place*, *time*, and *situation*. Temporary impaired memory is one of the most common deficits after a head injury.
- **2.** Assess cranial nerve function.
  - **a.** Ophthalmoscopic/visual examination (cranial nerve II)
  - **b.** Pupillary response (cranial nerve III)
  - **c.** Extraocular eye movements (EOMs; cranial nerves III, IV, and VI)
  - **d.** Facial sensation and muscles of mastication (cranial nerve V)
  - **e.** Facial expression and taste (cranial nerve VII)
- **3.** Perform a motor examination on all four extremities.
- **4.** Perform a sensory examination on all four extremities.

Diagnostic Tests

A. A plain film of the skull is no longer recommended for any minor traumatic injury. If the patient has a suspected skull fracture or clinical indications for imaging, a CT scan is preferred. This type of imaging will usually reveal any linear or basilar skull fractures.

B. CT scan is indicated for patients with the following (order and perform within 1 hour):

- **1.** Decreasing consciousness during or after the injury
- **2.** Focal neurologic deficits
- **3.** Potential, penetrating, or depressed skull fractures
- **4.** Increasing or persistent, severe headache with nausea and/or vomiting
- **5.** Seizures, postinjury
- **6.** Alcohol, drug, or substance intoxication
- **7.** Posttraumatic amnesia (PTA)
- **8.** Unreliable or questionable accuracy regarding the history of the injury
- **9.** Use clinical judgment regarding certain comorbidities and conditions
  - **a.** Coagulopathy
  - **b.** Persistent alcohol, drug, or substance intoxication
  - **c.** Multitrauma or multisystem injuries
  - **d.** Concurrent medical problems
  - **e.** Age older than 65 years

C. Consider anteroposterior (AP) and lateral spine films for suspected soft tissue injury or vertebral fracture, especially if the patient has experienced an amnestic episode or is unable to recall the accident.

D. Drug screen

E. Blood alcohol level

Differential Diagnoses

A. Concussion (MTBI)

B. Contusion

C. ICH

D. Shearing injury

E. Skull fracture

F. Subarachnoid hemorrhage (SAH), traumatic

G. Subdural hematomas (SDH)

H. Epidural hematoma (EDH)

I. Vascular occlusion or dissection
J. DAI

Plan

A. General interventions

1. Initial observation for at least 4 hours, then discharge to home if the following are noted after MTBI:

- Awake, alert, oriented (AAO) × 4, demonstrating improvement after concussion
- No risk factors warranting a head CT *or* negative head CT results when risk factors are present
- No signs/symptoms or conditions indicating the need for prolonged hospital observation or admission

2. Direct admission to the hospital for decreased LOC, seizure activity, focal deficits, penetrating or depressed skull fracture, vomiting, serious facial injuries, and positive head CT findings.

3. Hospitalization may be required if the patient has an injured middle meningeal artery or if venous sinus or fractures posteriorly in the skull are suspected. Posterior fossa hematomas may present suddenly (will see a wide pulse pressure).

4. Consider possible secondary injuries including cerebral edema, cerebral infarction, cerebral hemorrhage, hydrocephalus, and infection.

5. The patient should not be impaired by alcohol or other drugs when leaving the health care area, which can affect neurologic function and potentially mask evolving deficits.

6. Hospital admission should be considered for patients without home observation/supervision.

7. Discuss suspected abuse with the patient in a private setting.

B. Patient teaching

▶ **1.** *See Patient teaching: Section III: Patient Teaching Guide for this chapter, "Head Injury: Mild."*

2. Provide instruction regarding safety and accident prevention, including the following:

a. Use safety helmets.
b. Use safety belts.
c. Never drive or operate machinery under the influence of alcohol or other substances.
d. Use age-appropriate car seats and booster seats for children.
e. Remove scatter rugs and other objects that would increase risk for falls.
f. Use nonslip mats in the shower/bathtub.
g. Install grab bars in the shower/bathtub.
h. Use safety gates at the bottom and top of the stairs in homes with small children.
i. Always keep stairs, floors, and hallways clean and clear from clutter.
j. Install handrails in stairways.
k. Wear adequate, correct protective gear specific to athletic games and work.
l. Use helmets for biking, in addition to other sports.

C. Pharmaceutical therapy

1. Analgesics: Acetaminophen, 650 mg every 6 to 8 hours as needed for headache (do not exceed 3,000 mg/d).

2. Tricyclic antidepressants (TCAs) or triptans may be used for posttraumatic migraines.

Follow-Up

A. Patients with injuries mild enough to be discharged may be observed. Patients with normal examinations in the outpatient setting generally do not require routine follow-up.

B. Assessment of driving ability in older adults should be done after MTBI from MVAs.

C. Post concussion symptoms may continue for some period of time (usually around 3 months, but possibly years in certain cases). The use of the Rivermead Post-Concussion Symptoms Questionnaire may be helpful for serial evaluation. The Rivermead tool is available at www.maa.nsw.gov.au/media/publications/for-professionals/Rivermead-Post-Concussion-Symptoms-QuestionnaireMAA218.pdf

Consultation/Referral

A. Refer all patients to the ED for the following:

1. Focal neurologic deficit(s)
2. Decreasing LOC
3. Persistent headaches, nausea, and vomiting
4. Seizures, any other evidence of skull fractures
5. Neuropsychological dysfunction

B. Refer to a neurologist for evaluation of postconcussive syndrome with continued complaints (i.e., irritability, fatigue, headaches, difficulty concentrating, dizziness, and memory problems). Further evaluation, including MRI and electroencephalographic (EEG) testing may be needed.

C. Refer to a psychologist specifically trained to perform neuropsychological testing, as indicated for patients with mild head injury. The assessment tools used will evaluate brain function in the areas of attention/concentration, initiation/planning, motor/sensory skills, visual perception, learning and memory, language, speed of processing information/reaction time, and complex problem solving.

D. Refer to a psychiatrist for evaluation and treatment of any associated disorders emerging within a month or longer after MTBI, or upon noting increased signs/symptoms (anxiety, depression, posttraumatic stress disorder [PTSD] secondary to assault or combat).

Individual Considerations

A. Pediatrics

1. Children are at risk for traumatic brain injury (TBI) caused by falls and sports injuries.

2. Teens are at increased risk for TBI caused by sports, MVAs, and at-risk behaviors.

B. Geriatrics

1. The primary risk factor for a head injury in older adults is a fall(s).

2. MVAs are the second highest risk factor for adults above age 65 years, because of vision problems, slower reaction times/reflexes, and alcohol and medication use.

3. Medications, such as aspirin and anticoagulants, increase the complications of a head injury.

Resources

Brain Injury Resource Center: www.headinjury.com
CDC Injury Prevention & Control: Traumatic Brain Injury: www.cdc.gov/headsup/youthsports/index.html
Concussion Fact Sheet for Parents: www.cdc.gov/headsup/pdfs/custom/headsupconcussion_fact_sheet_for_parents.pdf
Injury Association of America: www.biausa.org
National Collegiate Athletic Association (NCAA) has concussion fact sheets for student athletes and for coaches: http://www.ncaa.org/health-and-safety/medical-conditions/concussion-sports
TBI Resource Center: www.braininjuryresources.org
The American Academy of Neurology 2013: Evidence-Based Guideline Update for the Evaluation and Management of Concussions in Sports: www.neurology.org/content/80/24/2250.full.html

Multiple Sclerosis

Kimberly D. Waltrip

Definition

Multiple sclerosis (MS) is an autoimmune degenerative disease that damages neuronal axons and breaks down myelin. The process of inflammatory demyelination varies in progression, with recurrent relapse and remission of symptoms over time. The most common symptoms include visual disturbances, spastic paraparesis, and bladder dysfunction. The course of MS is typically intermittent with periodic exacerbations occurring in various areas of the central nervous system (CNS). MS can also present more acutely regarding the severity, progression, and variety of symptoms. Early diagnosis is difficult, but crucial to treatment. An attack or exacerbation of MS lasts at least 24 hours, without associated fever or any infectious process. Complete recovery after the first attack is common, often presenting as a *clinically isolated syndrome (CIS)*, but typically converting to MS within 5 years. Subsequent progression with exacerbations leads to diminished function over time.

The loss of myelin leads to neurologic deficits involving vision, speech, gait, writing, memory, and/or the swallowing or cough reflexes. Patients typically use the emergency department (ED) when they experience relapse; 80% present with exacerbations of previous MS-related deficits. Diagnosis is supported when at least one reported exacerbation correlates with MS-related findings obtained from the neurological examination, MRI, or visual evoked potential (VEP) studies when any visual disturbances have been noted.

MS is classified as relapsing-remitting or progressive, and further described as *active* versus *not active*, *with* or *without progression*. Progressive MS is further differentiated with the following two subtypes:

A. *Relapsing-remitting (RR)* affects approximately 85% of MS patients; exacerbations of symptoms and periodic remission occur.

B. *Primary progressive (PP)* is a less common form of MS, accounting for around 10% of MS cases; PPMS progresses slowly without periods of relapse or remission.

C. *Secondary progressive (SP)* is not unusual for patients with RRMS to progress to secondary progressive MS (SPMS) over time. Progression of the disease process continues with or without periods of remission. Symptoms do not necessarily decrease or stabilize in terms of severity.

Incidence

A. There are an estimated 2.5 million individuals with MS worldwide. In the United States, approximately 400,000 are diagnosed with MS, with prevalence estimates around 90 per 100,000. MS symptoms can present between 10 and 80 years of age, but onset usually occurs between ages 20 and 50, with the average age at 32 years. MS is one of the leading causes of disability in young adults and is difficult to accurately diagnose. There is no specific test for diagnosing MS and signs/symptoms may not be easily recognized. Therefore, the true prevalence and incidence of MS are unknown, especially when U.S. physicians are not required to report newly diagnosed cases. In 2014, the MS Prevalence Initiative was launched to determine the best method for estimating the number of MS cases in the United States. This effort, currently in progress, will use various administrative databases of patient information.

Pathogenesis

A. The cause of MS is unknown. A suspected combination of genetic predisposition and a trigger (e.g., viral infections, environmental factors, metabolic issues) may create an autoimmune disorder that facilitates the degenerative disease process. Autoimmune attacks on the myelin sheaths of nerves initiate an inflammatory response followed by eventual plaque formation and scarring, the hallmark characteristics of MS. There is a loss of saltatory conduction. Axonal death occurs during this acute inflammatory response, which explains any permanent disability. The associated inflammation and edema around an MS lesion, along with myelin and axonal loss, contribute to the associated neurologic deficit. A limited amount of remyelination and the eventual resolution of inflammation will allow a certain amount of recovery with remission. Over time, multiple plaques will continue to develop in diffuse areas of the CNS. With each attack, there is a lesser degree of recovery with subsequent decrease in function.

Predisposing Factors

A. Family history of MS

B. Female gender (two times more likely than men to develop MS)

C. Age 20 to 50 years (onset can vary from age 10 years to 59 years, regarding onset)

D. Caucasian race (Northern European ancestry)

E. Environment (living in temperate zones, e.g., Canada, northern United States, Europe).

1. A northern latitude is associated with prevalence, but no direct link has been established at this time. It is suspected that distance from the equator causes a vitamin D deficiency secondary to a lack of direct sunlight, contributing to the development of MS.

F. Previous viral infection (e.g., Epstein–Barr virus [EBV], varicella zoster) *may* increase susceptibility.

G. Smoking

Common Complaints

A. Sensory loss (e.g., paresthesia) is often reported early in the course of the disease.

B. Visual disturbances (diplopia on lateral gaze occurs in 33% of patients, blurred vision, loss of vision, eye pain)

C. Urinary incontinence, frequency, hesitancy, or urgency (more than 90% of MS patients report bladder dysfunction)

D. Fatigue (in up to 90% of MS patients)

E. Weakness in one or more extremities

F. Gait disturbance (50% will require assistance with ambulation within 15 years of the onset of MS)

Other Signs and Symptoms

A. Babinski response

B. Spasticity (usually in the lower extremities)

C. Depression (occurs in nearly 50% of MS patients; also affects memory, attention, and concentration)

D. Hyperreflexia

E. Loss of proprioception

F. Impotence (males)

G. Impaired cognition: Subjective difficulties with attention span, concentration, short-term memory, planning, and judgment; dementia is reported in 3% of patients with late-stage MS.

H. Dysarthria

I. Reduced libido (both genders)

J. Constipation

K. Pain

L. Trigeminal neuralgia (rare)

M. Dysphagia (may also have recurrent respiratory infections secondary to aspiration)

Subjective Data

A. Establish location and onset of symptoms. Is this the first time the patient has experienced the symptom in question? Was the onset acute or insidious?

B. Ask the patient to describe the quality and severity of the symptom, and how it has evolved over time, including duration. Is there an *RR* pattern? Is there progression regarding severity of the symptom?

C. Ask the patient if there are any factors that aggravate or alleviate the symptom. Does hot weather/environment (e.g., hot tubs, saunas, and overexertion) aggravate the condition? Does rest help? Did the symptom resolve on its own?

D. Establish if there have been any known viral or bacterial infections before any reported symptoms.

E. Evaluate visual complaints, including the presence of scotoma, decreased color perception, diplopia, decreased acuity, or painful extraocular eye movements (EOMs). Is visual deterioration induced by exercise, a hot meal, or a hot bath (i.e., Uhthoff phenomenon)?

Physical Examination

A. Check temperature, blood pressure, pulse, and respiration.

B. Inspect

  1. Conduct a complete eye examination (Snellen eye chart, test cranial nerves II, III, IV, and VI).

    a. Fifty percent of MS patients present with retrobulbar involvement, yet funduscopy results are negative for any related pathology.

    b. Anterior involvement causes papillitis; look for the presence of macular star.

    c. Assess pupillary response bilaterally; look for pendular nystagmus or sinusoidal involuntary oscillations of one or both eyes, and/or loss of smooth eye pursuit.

  2. Conduct a neurologic and musculoskeletal examination.

    a. Sensory: Test for perception of sharp versus dull stimulus, heat versus cold stimulus, local pain perception, proprioception; use the tuning fork to evaluate sense of vibration.

    b. Motor strength: Test all extremities and assess for any increased tone (spasticity), clonus, and/or tremors.

    c. Heel-to-toe tandem gait testing (assess for ataxia, any cerebellar involvement); Romberg test

    d. Finger-to-nose testing, heel-to-shin testing (rule out dystaxia)

    e. Check deep tendon reflexes (DTRs); assess for Babinski response, hyperreflexia.

    f. Assess mental status (orientation to person, place, time, and situation); also test short-term memory and ability to plan (impaired planning is another cognitive issue secondary to MS).

    g. Assess for pain: Location, onset, duration, timing/setting, aggravating factors, alleviating factors, and any other associated data.

    h. Assess for depression, especially with progression of MS-related symptoms.

Diagnostic Tests

A. There is no specific confirmatory test for MS.

B. MRI is the designated radiologic test to support clinical diagnosis of MS. An MRI of the head will reveal any associated plaques of MS. However, MRI cannot determine whether the identified lesions are specific to MS when other diseases may have similar findings.

  1. Transverse myelitis (TM) lesions identified with MRI may convert to MS over time.

C. Cerebrospinal fluid (CSF) analysis: Characteristics specific to MS include the presence of oligoclonal bands (in 85%–90% of MS patients), elevated immunoglobulin G (IgG; greater than 12%), and elevated white blood cells (WBCs; greater than 5%).

D. Evoked response tests (ERT) or evoked potential (EP) studies: Several different types of tests/studies evaluate brain function and the peripheral nervous system (PNS) using electroencephalogram (EEG) with nerve conduction/velocity (NCV).

  1. Brain auditory evoked response (BAER) studies can detect subtle changes in brainstem function.

  2. Visual evoked potential (VEP) studies focus on visual interpretation and perception, evaluating optical responses to strobe light and/or frequent pattern reversal (typically checkerboard patterns).

3. Somatosensory evoked potential (SSEP) studies evaluate nerve conduction from the extremities via the spinal cord to the brain.

E. Complete blood count (CBC) with differential

F. Serum glucose levels will rule out hypoglycemia and chronic hyperglycemia as potential causes of neurologic findings.

Differential Diagnoses

A. MS
B. CNS lymphoma
C. CNS infection
D. Acute disseminated encephalomyelitis (ADEM)
E. Tumor: Brainstem, cerebellar, or spinal cord
F. Amyotrophic lateral sclerosis (ALS)
G. Systemic lupus erythematosus (SLE)
H. Syringomyelia
I. Progressive multifocal leukoencephalopathy (PML)
J. Sarcoidosis
K. Sjögren's syndrome
L. Acute transverse myelitis (TM)
M. Myasthenia gravis (MG)
N. Guillain–Barré syndrome (GBS)
O. Cerebrovascular accident (CVA)
P. Diabetes mellitus
Q. Spinal cord compression (stenosis, ruptured disc)
R. Behcet's disease
S. Neuromyelitis optica (NMO)

Plan

A. Patient teaching

1. Educate on heat sensitivity and how it can aggravate symptoms: Individuals with MS must avoid hot tubs, saunas, prolonged exposure to hot/humid conditions, and choose appropriate clothing for the season.

a. Approximately 60% of individuals with MS experience heat sensitivity, facilitating a *pseudoexacerbation* in which symptoms may worsen, but do not necessarily indicate additional axon/myelin degeneration.

2. For visual disturbances, advice on resting the eyes at various times during the day may be helpful; for double vision, an eyepatch may be used temporarily.

3. Stress the importance of exercise and its effect on MS-related fatigue and spasticity; overactivity/overwork is another issue to address at this time. Rest periods are needed during exacerbations of MS.

4. Teach Kegel exercises and timed voiding (habit training) to improve bladder function; also advise individuals with MS to avoid alcohol and caffeinated beverages.

5. Advise on increasing daily water intake, dietary fiber intake, and physical activity for increased bowel motility.

6. Educate on signs and symptoms of infection, especially urinary tract infections (UTIs), and how infection can trigger exacerbations.

7. Teach self-intermittent catheterization (SIC) when necessary for urinary retention.

8. Discuss the purpose and availability of local MS support groups.

9. Discuss counseling for adaptive coping techniques, improving family dynamics/relationships with significant others, adjusting to physical disability, and addressing anticipatory grief issues.

10. Educate on all medications, including side effects and any follow-up for pertinent laboratory tests or other testing.

11. Suggest pertinent strategies for short-term memory and planning ability: Individuals with MS can benefit from writing things down, making lists, drawing pictures, and allocating more time for planning.

B. Pharmacological therapy is prescribed specifically for the type of MS and for the specific symptoms experienced. Medications may include any combination of the following:

1. Disease-modifying drugs suppress the immune system to slow progression of MS, decreasing the frequency and severity of exacerbations, and reducing MS-related plaques).

a. Injectable medications (recommended for first-line therapy)

i. Interferon beta-1a: Avonex, Betaseron, Extavia, Rebif

ii. Glatiramer acetate: Copaxone (40 mg), glatopa (a generic equivalent of Copaxone, 20 mg)

iii. Peginterferon beta-1a: Plegridy

b. Oral medications

i. Aubagio (teriflunomide): Recommended for first-line therapy

ii. Gilenya (fingolimod): Recommended for second-line therapy

iii. Tecfidera (dimethyl fumarate): Recommended for first-line therapy

c. Intravenous infusions

i. Lemtrada (alemtuzumab): Recommended for second-line therapy

ii. Novantrone (mitoxantrone): Recommended for second-line therapy

iii. Rituxan (rituximab): Off-label use for RRMS when second-line medications have been ineffective

iv. Tysabri (natalizumab): Recommended for second-line therapy

2. Short-term steroid use (e.g., methylprednisolone or prednisone for 3–5 days) may shorten a period of exacerbation. Long-term use is not recommended. IV steroids may be prescribed initially, then converted to oral steroids (prednisone, dexamethasone), and tapered off over time.

a. H.P. Acthar Gel (ACTH) is an option when individuals cannot tolerate the side effects of high-dose corticosteroids, do not respond to corticosteroid therapy, have no available IV infusion services, or when individuals have difficult/inadequate peripheral IV access.

3. Dalfampridine is an FDA-approved drug that has been shown to improve ambulation and possibly decrease fatigue in the MS population. Dalfampridine is a potassium-channel blocker that targets channels located on the outside of nerve fibers, subsequently improving nerve conduction when myelin sheaths are damaged.
4. Antivert (meclizine) may be prescribed for dizziness or vertigo.
5. Various medications (antiepileptics, antidepressants) may be considered for treatment of neuropathic or spasticity-related pain
  a. Dilantin (phenytoin)
  b. Elavil (amitriptyline)
  c. Klonopin (clonazepam)
  d. Neurontin (gabapentin)
  e. Pamelor, Aventyl (nortriptyline)
  f. Tegretol (carbamazepine)
6. MS-related spasticity may be treated with the following drugs:
  a. Baclofen
  b. Zanaflex
  c. Clonazepam, diazepam (watch for sedation, dependence)
  d. Dantrium (use only when other drugs are ineffective, as it can cause liver damage)
  e. Botulinum toxin injections
  f. Intrathecal (IT) pump placement is another option for continuous IT administration of baclofen or clonidine for spasticity.
7. Stool softeners (Colace, Pericolace), bulk-forming agents (Metamucil), and/or laxatives (milk of magnesia, MiraLAX) may be prescribed for complaints of constipation, depending on the severity of symptoms.
8. Flomax or Hytrin can be used to improve urinary flow.
9. Ditropan, Tofranil, and Detrol are several examples of medications commonly used to treat bladder spasms.
10. Options for treatment of depression include the following:
  a. Selective serotonin-norepinephrine reuptake inhibitors (SSNRIs): Cymbalta (duloxetine hydrochloride), Effexor (velafaxine)
  b. SSRIs: Prozac (fluoxetine), Zoloft (sertraline), Paxil (paroxetine)
  Individuals with protracted, painful, and/or progressive medical conditions are at risk for suicide.
11. Provigil, Symmetrel, or Prozac can be used to treat fatigue symptoms.
12. Stem cell transplantation for RRMS is emerging in the literature. Clinical trials present encouraging results that indicate reversal of symptoms while offering a way to "reset" the immune system. Stem cell transplantation shows promise as a future treatment option for RRMS.

Follow-Up

A. A neurologist who specializes in MS management should coordinate and prescribe therapies for this patient population. Nurse practitioner comanagement with a primary care physician for follow-up depends on the individual's clinical presentation, diagnosis, and therapies.

Consultation/Referral

A. Neurology referral and consultation for management of MS
B. Ophthalmology for visual disturbances, optic neuritis
C. Urology for genitourinary (GU) disturbances (impotence in males, UTIs, and other urinary symptoms of hesitancy, frequency, incontinence, and urgency)
D. Occupational therapy (OT) will address any barriers or problems with performing activities of daily living (ADLs), deficits in fine motor skills (coordination, strength in the upper extremities), and prescribe any necessary adaptive equipment.
E. Speech therapy (ST) will address any issues with language, cognition, or swallowing (including any evaluations necessary for feeding tube placement and for specific dietary recommendations).
F. Physical therapy (PT) will address gait disturbances, motor weakness, spasticity, and range of motion (ROM), and prescribe any necessary adaptive equipment for impaired physical mobility.
G. Psychiatry referral and consultation for pharmacological management of depression and/or dementia may be necessary in specific cases; also consider referrals to psychology or licensed professional counselors (LPCs) for any behavioral therapy or counseling needs.
H. Social work (SW) referrals may be necessary for assistance with insurance issues, locating community resources, applying for disability, arranging home health care, obtaining placement in a skilled nursing facility, and for counseling (individual and family).

Individual Considerations

A. Pregnancy
  1. Symptoms of MS may stabilize or remit during pregnancy, but 20% to 40% of MS patients experience relapse within 3 months postpartum.
  2. No evidence suggests that pregnancy affects the long-term course of MS. There is no acceleration in the rate of disability or disease progression over time.
  3. Neither epidural anesthesia nor breastfeeding have an adverse effect on the rate of relapse or progression of disability with MS.
  4. There are no accepted guidelines for recommending for or against pregnancy in females with MS. MS history and current neurologic deficits should be considered independently per patient.
  5. Pregnancy may affect the treatment regimen; some of the medications used to treat MS are known teratogens. For instance, glucocorticoids may cause neonatal adrenal suppression and maternal glucose intolerance.
    a. Intravenous immunoglobulin (IVIg) is an alternative to consider during pregnancy or while breastfeeding, after weighing the risks and benefits carefully before administration. The adverse effects are few, but may present complications

that can be severe (e.g., aseptic meningitis, thromboembolism).

B. Pediatrics

1. MS is rarely diagnosed in children younger than 16 years.

2. Children with MS generally have a similar clinical presentation to adults. Most diagnoses of pediatric MS are classified as RRMS.

C. Geriatrics

1. The occurrence of MS is rare in individuals older than 60 years of age.

2. Spinal infarcts are seen more often in older individuals when evaluating specific inflammatory lesions.

Resources

Multiple Sclerosis Association of America: mymsaa.org
Multiple Sclerosis Foundation: msfocus.org
National Multiple Sclerosis Society: www.nationalmssociety.org

Myasthenia Gravis

Jill C. Cash and Julie Adkins

Definition

A. Myasthenia gravis (MG) is a chronic autoimmune neuromuscular disorder that affects the neuromuscular junction and is characterized by fatigability and weakness of voluntary muscles. The hallmark of MG is muscle weakness that increases during periods of activity and improves after periods of rest.

Incidence

A. The prevalence is 0.5 to 11.5 cases per 1 million people. There are two peaks in MG incidence that are age and gender related: One is women in their 20s and 30s, and the other is men in their 60s and 70s, but can occur at any age. Cases of neonatal MG are temporary and usually disappear within 2 to 3 months after birth. MG in juveniles is uncommon.

Pathogenesis

A. MG is believed to be an antibody-mediated autoimmune attack that destroys variable numbers of acetylcholine receptors (AChR) at the postsynaptic junction. The decrease in AChRs results in weakness with repeated activities and recovery after rest. MG is often associated with thymic hyperplasia or tumors; the thymus plays an unclear role in the autoimmune process of MG. The thymus is large in infants, grows until puberty, and then gets smaller with age. In MG, the thymus gland remains large and abnormal.

Predisposing Factors

A. No predisposing factors have been identified.

B. Not inherited or contagious. Occasionally, the disease may occur in more than one family member.

Common Complaints

A. Classic triad: Ptosis, diplopia, and dysphagia

1. Fluctuating symptoms such as droopy eyelid(s)

2. Blurry or double vision

3. Sense of choking

B. Difficulty chewing

C. Slurring of speech

D. Easy fatigability

E. Symptoms are more pronounced with fatigue or in the evening.

Other Signs and Symptoms

A. Selected voluntary muscles that fatigue with activity

B. Motor function that improves with rest, but then decreases with use

C. Signs of impending MG crisis

1. Sudden onset of inspiratory distress

2. Difficulty swallowing

3. Visual difficulty

4. Tachycardia

5. Rapid onset of weakness

Subjective Data

A. Establish onset of symptoms and possible progression

B. Ask the patient what makes the symptoms better or worse: Does rest help?

C. Ask if the patient feels better in the morning, or in the afternoon, or in the evening.

D. Look for difficulties with chewing or swallowing.

E. Investigate medications the patient is currently taking or has recently taken such as antibiotics.

Physical Examination

> *Both the presentation and course of MG are highly variable; therefore MG can be very difficult to diagnose.*

A. Check temperature, pulse, respiration, and blood pressure.

B. Inspect

1. Observe overall appearance.

2. Perform complete eye examination. Subtleties of eye movement dysfunction are often key in differentiating MG from other disorders.

C. Palpate

1. Assess deep tendon reflexes (DTRs); note normal to increased reflexes.

D. Neurologic examination

1. Perform complete neurologic examination.

2. Test the following.

a. Muscle strength: Weakness is increased with repetition or sustained activity; arm raise cannot be sustained.

b. Eyes:

i. Upward or lateral gaze cannot be maintained for longer than 30 seconds.

ii. Eyes: Ptosis occurs with repetitive lid closure.

iii. Ice pack test—Fill a plastic bag or glove with ice and place over closed eyelid for 2 minutes. Remove ice and evaluate the degree of ptosis. Noted to be very sensitive with prominent ptosis.

c. Voice: Voice quality or speech changes when counting out loud to 100.

Normal coordination, normal sensory perception, and normal pupillary response are noted in MG.

Diagnostic Tests

A. Antibody titer for acetylcholine receptor (AChR-Ab) positive in 90% of patients with MG. May also perform MuSK antibody titer. Approximately 6% to 12% of patients will have negative antibody titers for both titers.
B. Cholinesterase-inhibiting drug test: Improvement in strength following injection of edrophonium (Tensilon)
C. Repetitive muscle stimulation test: Decremental response
D. Single-fiber electromyography (EMG) and/or repetitive nerve stimulation (RNS) studies are diagnostic studies performed for diagnosis.

Initial diagnostic tests may be equivocal with some negative test results, but this does not absolutely rule out MG.

Differential Diagnoses

A. MG: The most common disorder of neuromuscular transmission. **It is important to maintain a high index of suspicion and include MG in the differential diagnosis of any patient presenting with variable muscle weakness even without eye signs.**
B. Incomplete extraocular nerve palsy
C. Polymyositis
D. Brainstem transient ischemic attack (TIA)
E. Amyotrophic lateral sclerosis (ALS)
F. Brainstem vascular accident: "Dizziness" is a symptom rarely seen with MG but often associated with brainstem ischemia.
G. Guillain–Barré syndrome (GBS)
H. Brainstem tumor
I. Hyperthyroidism or hypothyroidism
J. **Cholinergic crisis: Although it is useful to distinguish myasthenic crisis (weakness from MG exacerbation) from cholinergic crisis (weakness from too much medication), both can rapidly lead to respiratory failure. Transportation to an emergency room for evaluation should not be delayed by attempts to differentiate the two.**
K. Eaton–Lambert myasthenic syndrome: Often associated with bronchogenic carcinoma but may precede detection of the carcinoma by as many as 2 years.

Plan

A. General interventions
1. MG is primarily managed by a neurologist, given the difficulty in diagnosing it, the variable course of the disease, and the highly individualized medication regimen required.
2. The course of MG fluctuates most during the first 3 to 5 years after diagnosis.
3. Autoimmune disorders, such as thyroid disease, rheumatoid arthritis, and systemic lupus erythematosus (SLE), should also be screened for inpatients diagnosed with MG.

B. Patient teaching:
1. *See Section III: Patient Teaching Guide for this chapter, "Myasthenia Gravis."* ◀
2. Patients should have a MedicAlert tag and always carry a list of their medications and dosing schedules in case of an emergency.

C. Medical and surgical management
1. Thymectomy is an early consideration; an MRI of the chest is obtained once the diagnosis is made to assess for thymic enlargement.

Thymectomy lessens the severity of MG, but rarely results in complete elimination of the need for medication.

2. Plasmapheresis, or plasma exchange to remove antibodies, is used emergently for the management of myasthenic crisis. Opinion is mixed regarding its use in the long-term management of myasthenia.
3. A myasthenic crisis occurs when the muscles that control breathing are weakened to the point of requiring ventilation. This usually is triggered by an infection, fever, or adverse reaction to a medication.

D. Pharmaceutical therapy
1. Many medications can cause worsening of myasthenic symptoms, so changes and additions of any medication require consultation with the patient's neurologist. Cholinesterase-inhibiting medications:
a. Pyridostigmine (Mestinon) 60 and 180 mg sustained release (SR) titrate as needed, with usual dose up to 600 mg/d
b. Neostigmine methylsulfate (Prostigmin) 0.25 to 0.5 and 1.0 mg/mL concentrations titrated with starting dose 0.5 mg subcutaneous (SC) or intramuscular (IM) every 3 to 4 hours
2. Steroids may be used when inpatient and then tapered on an outpatient basis, tapering every 3 days.
3. Effectiveness of medication regimen is gauged by changes in ptosis, diplopia, dysphagia, chewing ability, and muscle fatigue.
4. Care should be used with medications that may worsen symptoms of weakness.

Follow-Up

A. Patients with MG require lifelong management by a neurologist, given the variable course both of the disease and of the patient's response to treatment.
B. The patient is initially followed every 1 to 2 months, then every 3 to 4 months.

Consultation/Referral

A. If MG is suspected, consult with a physician and consider neurologic referral.

Individual Considerations

A. Pregnancy
1. MG is considered high risk for both the woman and the fetus.
a. Pregnancy requires management by the patient's neurologist and a perinatologist.
2. MG frequently manifests for the first time during pregnancy. Refer to a perinatologist.

B. Pediatrics

1. MG is associated with prematurity, and the infant may have transient neonatal myasthenia. The patient will need a neonatology consult.

2. Myasthenia is less severe and commonly remits spontaneously in children, so thymectomy is not recommended.

C. Adults

1. Oral contraceptives may worsen myasthenic symptoms.

Parkinson's Disease

Jill C. Cash and Julie Adkins

Definition

A. Parkinson's disease (PD) is an idiopathic, progressive, chronic neurologic syndrome characterized by a combination of akinesia or bradykinesia, or reduction of spontaneous activity and movement; rigidity, or increase in spontaneous muscle tone and involuntary movements; tremor; and postural instability.

Incidence

A. There are more than 200,000 new cases of PD per year. One percent of the population older than 50 years has PD. The mean age of onset is 55 to 60 years. Only 5% is seen between the ages of 21 and 40 years. There is no gender difference in prevalence. PD is seen most frequently in people of European ancestry.

Pathogenesis

A. For reasons that are unclear, degenerative changes occur in the basal ganglia and deplete the dopaminergic neurons in the substantia nigra, resulting in dopamine reduction in the striatum. This interrupts neuronal circuits and produces akinesia and rigidity. The pathophysiology of tremor is less clear, but thalamic involvement is implicated. Symptoms are caused by loss of neurons that produce dopamine. Certain nerve cells (neurons) in the brain break down or die.

Predisposing Factors

A. Antecedent encephalitis
B. Arteriosclerosis
C. Trauma
D. Toxins
E. Drugs, particularly phenothiazines
F. Familial neurodegenerative diseases in which parkinsonism is a prominent feature
G. Presence of Lewy bodies

Common Complaints

Cardinal symptoms:

A. Tremor at rest: May be intermittent, but progresses over time.

B. Rigidity: Joints are more rigid. Increased resistance to passive movement. Appears unilaterally and then progresses to the opposite side. Usually asymmetrical. Appears as decreased movement in arm swing when ambulating, stooped posture, cogwheel rigidity—resistance with tremor.

C. Bradykinesia, or slow voluntary movement, especially with daily activities such as cutting food, dressing self, and so forth. When walking, shorter steps are taken, shuffle-step, feeling of unsteadiness with walking. Postural instability.

Other Signs and Symptoms

A. Micrographia (handwriting that decreases in size when writing out name)
B. Voice changes: Fading, softness, hoarseness, and mumbling
C. Saliva escaping mouth, especially at night
D. Dysphagia
E. Neuropsychiatric changes: Cognitive impairment/dementia/memory loss, sleep disturbance, fatigue, anxiety, depression, pain, and sensory changes
F. Oily, greasy skin
G. Excessive perspiration
H. Constipation
I. Urinary hesitancy or frequency
J. Visual loss: Impaired vision, reflex, upward gaze, and convergence
K. Impaired posture and balance

Subjective Data

A. Elicit information regarding onset of symptoms. Note changes in progression of symptoms.

B. Talk with the patient and family to establish if there have been behavioral changes, problems with activities such as eating or getting out of chairs, or personality changes.

C. Determine if other family members have had similar symptoms.

D. Ascertain the patient's medical history, including current medications, both prescription and over the counter (OTC).

E. Particularly in patients younger than 55 years, investigate substance abuse and exposure to herbicides or pesticides.

Physical Examination

A. Check temperature, pulse, respiration, blood pressure, and weight: Note orthostatic hypotension.

B. Inspect

1. Observe overall appearance.

2. Note asymmetric tremor at rest.

3. Note subtle facial masking, decreased frequency and amplitude of eye blinks.

4. Note posture and gait disturbances: Festination, or shuffling, increasingly tiny steps; usually walking with arms down to side; difficulty turning; freezing, or inability to continue to move.

C. Palpate

1. Palpate extremities, noting increased tone in resting muscles.

D. Neurologic examination

1. Perform complete neurologic examination. Assess all cranial nerves. Assess deep tendon reflexes (DTRs).

2. Assess rapid alternating movements. Note difficulty with rapid alternating movements such as tapping fingers or turning palm alternately up and down.

3. Check cogwheel phenomenon, which is stepwise rigidity of movement with passive range of motion (ROM), rather than anticipated smooth movement through ROM. Best tested in wrists.

4. Perform mental status examination.

5. Assess the progression of the disease state with the scale of choice. Scales commonly used include:

a. Unified Parkinson's Disease Rating Scale: www.mdvu.org/library/ratingscales/pd

b. International Parkinson and Movement Disorder Society: This site hosts a list of rating scales and questionnaires: www.movementdisorders.org

c. Hoehn and Yahr Scale: neurosurgery.mgh.harvard.edu/Functional/pdstages.htm

d. Scales for Outcomes in Parkinson's Disease—Psychiatric Complications (nonmotor evaluation) and Nonmotor Symptom Screening Questionnaire: www.neurology.org/cgi/content/abstract/61/9/1222

Diagnostic Tests

A. There is no definitive diagnostic test for PD. Consider serum blood tests or other testing to rule out other conditions causing symptoms.

B. Urinalysis to rule out urinary tract infection (UTI) with any urinary symptoms

C. Speech therapy evaluation of dysarthria and dysphagia to assess aspiration risk

D. Brain CT scan or MRI to exclude mass lesion, multiple infarcts, or normal pressure hydrocephalus

E. MRI of cervical spine if there is increased gait disturbance after a fall.

Differential Diagnoses

A. PD

B. Essential tremor

C. Multi-infarct dementia

D. Alzheimer's disease

E. Brain tumor

F. Progressive supranuclear palsy

G. Normal pressure hydrocephalus

H. Shy–Drager syndrome

I. Hypothyroidism

J. Hereditary disease such as Huntington's chorea or Wilson's disease

K. Chorea: Not generally seen in PD; its development in a patient with PD is generally a medication side effect and should be discussed with the patient's neurologist.

Plan

A. General interventions

1. Encourage regular exercise to maintain or improve flexibility.

2. The patient should follow a diet that is high in fiber and calcium, with adequate fluid intake, to limit complications caused by constipation and osteoporosis. In some patients, protein intake may need to be timed to limit interactions with medications such as levodopa.

3. Emphasize the importance of the nonmotor symptoms being addressed and adequately treated. Encourage the family to notify the provider if these symptoms are not being controlled. Anxiety, depression, fatigue, mood changes, and behavioral issues need to be addressed and controlled for quality of life for the patient and family.

4. Home safety evaluations are recommended because the symptoms of PD place patients at high risk of falls and accidental injury.

5. Surgery, such as pallidotomy or thalamotomy, is an option for severe PD in which tremor is poorly controlled with medications.

B. Patient teaching: *See Section III: Patient Teaching Guide for this chapter, "Managing Your Parkinson's Disease."* ◀

C. Pharmaceutical therapy

1. Polypharmacy is the hallmark rather than the exception with PD. Always comanage with a neurologist.

2. Lower doses of several medications, rather than high doses of a single agent, aid in maximizing function while minimizing side effects.

3. Drug dosages are always tapered, not stopped abruptly.

4. First-line drug

a. Levodopa, combined with a decarboxylase inhibitor, is the mainstay of treatment. Sinemet is the levodopa and carbidopa combination drug most often used.

i. The dose and dosing frequency are very individualized.

ii. Patients are often on a combination of sustained release and short-acting preparations.

iii. See literature for individual dosing. Titrate dose up every 3 days for adjustments.

iv. Long-term use is often associated with adverse effects requiring careful medication dosage.

5. Second-line therapy: Dopamine agonists: Generally given in conjunction with levodopa, these allow use of lower doses of levodopa that can delay or reduce levodopa-associated problems. Examples include pramipexole (Mirapex) and ropinirole (Requip).

6. Ergot derivatives include the following:

a. Bromocriptine and pergolide are the two dopamine agonists most often used.

i. Bromocriptine mesylate (Parlodel) is initiated at 1.25 mg daily or twice a day and slowly increased to 10 to 25 mg daily.

ii. Pergolide mesylate (Permax) is initiated at 0.05 mg daily and increased slowly to 2 to 3 mg in divided doses three times a day.

b. Non ergot drugs are preferred because of fewer side effects.

i. Pramipexole (Mirapex) 0.125 mg three times daily up to 4.5 mg/d maximum is useful for tremors or ropinirole (Requip) 0.25 mg three times daily, maximum 24-hour period.

7. Neuroprotective agents: Selegiline (Eldepryl), MAO-B inhibitor 5 mg at breakfast and at lunch, may have neuroprotective effects and slow progression of symptoms.

a. Often an initial treatment, a drug is usually continued throughout the course of the disease. Maximum dose is 10 mg/d.

b. Amantadine (Symmetrel) is used as short-term monotherapy in patients younger than 60 years with mild to moderate PD in which akinesia and rigidity are more prominent than tremor.

i. Its effects tend to wane, and it should be tapered once other antiparkinsonian drugs are started.

ii. The usual dose is 100 to 300 mg twice daily. Adjust the dose gradually.

iii. Caution should be used with these medications because of the interactions with other medications and foods that can precipitate high blood pressure to dangerous levels. Advise to avoid foods high in tyramine such as some cheeses, tofu, yeast extracts, and so forth.

8. Anticholinergics: These are useful for treating resting tremor, but not akinesia or impaired postural reflexes.

a. The centrally acting drug trihexyphenidyl HCl (Artane) is the most common anticholinergic used.

i. Drug is usually started at 0.5 to 1.0 mg twice daily with food and slowly increased to 2 to 3 mg three times daily.

ii. Dosage should always be tapered, never stopped abruptly.

iii. Use is not recommended in patients older than 60 years or with dementia.

b. Benztropine mesylate (Cogentin) 0.5 to 1 mg at bedtime may also be used in PD. Maximum is 6 mg/d. Increase every 6 to 7 days.

9. Sleep disorders are common in PD and respond well to tricyclic antidepressants (TCAs), benzodiazepines, diphenhydramine, or low-dose chloral hydrate.

10. Excessive daytime sleepiness should first be evaluated as a symptom of depression before it is attributed to medications or effects of PD.

As PD progresses, patients often develop clear "on" and "off" times of medication effectiveness and functional ability; therefore, medication schedules are very carefully customized to maximize "on" times.

Follow-Up

A. PD requires lifelong management by a neurologist.

B. Frequency of appointments depends on severity of disease and response to medication. Depression and neuropsychiatric side effects of medications are often seen in patients with PD; therefore, any office visit should involve screening for these. Inquire particularly about memory loss, vivid dreams or nightmares, hallucinations, symptoms of depression or anxiety, and occurrence of panic attacks. Discuss findings with the patient's neurologist, as medication adjustments could be required.

Consultation/Referral

A. Managing PD requires referral to a neurologist to initiate and adjust medications.

B. If a PD patient requires the addition of medication for other conditions, consult the patient's neurologist to evaluate for possible serious adverse effects.

C. Involvement with a support group can be helpful for the patient and family. Information about PD and local support groups can be obtained from:

1. The American Parkinson's Disease Association, Inc.
135 Parkinson Avenue
Staten Island, New York 10305
800-223-2732 Fax 718-981-4399
apda@apdaparkinson.org
www.apdaparkinson.org

2. National Parkinson Foundation
1501 N.W. 9th Ave./Bob Hope Road
Miami, Florida 33136-1494
800-473-4636
www.parkinson.org

Individual Considerations

A. Pediatrics

1. When PD is seen in this age group, it is usually because of secondary factors.

B. Geriatrics

1. It is most commonly seen in this population.

Restless Legs Syndrome

Julie Adkins

Definition

A. Restless legs syndrome (RLS) is a neurologic disorder usually involving throbbing, pulling, creeping, or other unpleasant sensations of the legs with sometimes an overwhelming urge to move them. Symptoms occur usually at night when in a relaxing, resting position, but can increase in severity throughout the night. Moving the legs usually relieves the discomfort causing disorders of sleep. Left untreated, RLS can cause exhaustion and fatigue, which is often associated with daytime concentration, memory, and can cause depression.

Incidence

A. As much as 10% of Americans may have RLS. Moderate to severe symptoms affect 2% to 3% of adults. An additional 5% have the milder form. Children can also have RLS; almost 1 million school-age children are affected and one third have moderate to severe symptoms. RLS occurs in both men and women, but the incidence is about twice as high in women. It may begin at any age. Symptoms seem to become more frequent and last longer with age.

Pathogenesis

A. RLS is classified as a movement disorder as people are required to move their legs in order to get any relief. More than 80% of people with RLS also may experience a condition, periodic limb movement of sleep (PLMS), which involves leg twitching or jerking movements during sleep occurring every 15 to 40 seconds. Although many patients with RLS develop PLMS, most people with PLMS do not have RLS or any other cause of PLMS. Periodic limb movement disorder (PLMD) may be a variant of RLS and responds to similar treatments. The cause of RLS is unknown; however, it may have a genetic component. Evidence indicates that low levels of iron in the brain may be responsible for RLS.

B. Considerable evidence suggests that RLS is a dysfunction in the brain's basal ganglia that uses the neurotransmitter dopamine. Disruption of this pathway frequently results in involuntary movements.

C. Alcohol and sleep deprivation may aggravate or trigger RLS symptoms.

Predisposing Factors

A. Alcohol use
B. Sleep deprivation
C. Chronic diseases such as kidney failure, diabetes, anemia, and peripheral neuropathy
D. Certain medications such as antiemetic, antipsychotic drugs, antidepressants, and some cold and allergy medications
E. Pregnancy, especially during the third trimester
F. Family history of RLS

Common Complaints

A. Uncomfortable sensations in the legs with an irresistible urge to move the limb. Sensations may occur on only one side of the body, but most often affect both sides.
B. Need to keep legs in motion such as pacing the floor, moving legs while sitting, and tossing and turning in bed
C. **A classic feature of RLS is that the symptoms are worse at night with a distinct symptom-free period in the early morning.**

Other Signs and Symptoms

A. May vary day to day, in severity and frequency, and from person to person
B. Triggering factors may include long car trips; sitting for long periods of time, such as at a movie theater or long-distance flights; immobilization of a cast; or relaxation exercises.
C. Worsening of symptoms occurs with sleep deprivation.
D. In severe cases, interruption and impairment of daytime function occur.

Subjective Data

A. Ask the patient to describe the sensations (urge to move legs) that he or she is complaining of. Do sensations occur in one leg or both legs?
B. What makes symptoms worse? What makes symptoms better?
C. What does the patient do to make the sensations better?
D. Do symptoms occur during rest or activity? Is there a particular activity that usually makes the symptoms worse or better? Do they improve with movement?
E. How often are symptoms present? Do the symptoms occur during the daytime or nighttime? Daily, nightly, several times a day, once a week, and so forth?
F. Does the patient have other medical or behavioral conditions that can be attributed to the symptoms that occur?
G. Are symptoms triggered by rest, relaxation, or sleep?
H. Determine sleep patterns and disturbances.
I. Review current medications being taken and discuss chronic conditions.
J. Inquire regarding the amount of alcohol ingested each day.
K. Inquire regarding the use of tobacco.
L. If pregnant, are symptoms new during the pregnancy or has she always had the symptoms?

Physical Examination

A. Check blood pressure, pulse, respirations, and weight.
B. Inspect
  1. Overall appearance and hygiene
C. Auscultate
  1. Heart
  2. Lungs
D. Neurologic examination
  1. Perform full neurologic examination.

Diagnostic Tests

A. Laboratory tests may be performed to rule out other conditions, which include:
  1. Iron studies: Serum ferritin level
  2. Complete blood count (CBC)
  3. Vitamin B_{12} and folic acid
  4. Complete metabolic panel (CMP)
  5. Hemoglobin A_{1c} ($HgbA_{1c}$)
  6. Thyroid studies
B. Sleep study

Differential Diagnoses

A. **RLS: There is no specific test for RLS. The basic criteria for diagnosing the disorder are:**
  1. Symptoms are worse at night and are absent or negligible in the morning.
  2. A strong and often overwhelming need or urge to move the affected limb(s), often associated with parasthesias or dysesthesias
  3. Sensory symptoms that are triggered by rest, relaxation, or sleep
  4. Sensory symptoms that are relieved with movement, in which the relief persists as long as the movement continues
  5. None of the previously noted symptoms are caused by another medical condition.
B. Sleep apnea
C. Alcoholism
D. Specific vitamin deficiencies
E. Pregnancy (third trimester)
F. Parkinson's disease (PD)

Plan

A. General interventions
  1. Activities that worsen symptoms should be discontinued.

2. Medications can be prescribed and are effective for many patients.
3. Some chronic conditions may contribute to RLS, such as diabetes or peripheral neuropathy, or vitamin deficiency and should be evaluated.

B. Patient education
1. Advise patient to discontinue activities that worsen symptoms.
2. Lifestyle changes may be suggested such as discontinuing the use of alcohol, tobacco, and caffeine.
3. Bedtime rituals should be encouraged. Regular sleep patterns should be encouraged. Avoid exercise at least 1 to 2 hours before bedtime. Encourage relaxation techniques before going to bed.
4. The use of relieving techniques, such as massage or cold compresses, is encouraged.

C. Pharmaceutical therapy
1. Dopaminergic agents (increase dopamine) are recommended first-line treatment for frequent or nightly symptoms. However, caution should be used. Long-term use can lead to worsening symptoms. This is reversible with withdrawal of the medication.
   a. U.S. Food and Drug Administration (FDA)-approved non ergotamine dopamine agonists for moderate to severe RLS include:
      i. Ropinirole (Requip): 0.25 mg orally at bedtime. May increase dose every three nights, for a maximum dose of four tablets at bedtime, until symptoms are resolved.
      ii. Pramipexole (Mirapex): Initial dose: 0.125 mg one tablet at bedtime. May increase dose every three nights, for a maximum dose of four tablets at bedtime, until symptoms are resolved.
      iii. Rotigotine (Neupro) transdermal patch: 1 mg/24 hr patch; apply new patch nightly at alternating sites. May increase patch weekly to a maximum dose of 3 mg/24 hr.
   b. Levodopa formulation
      i. Levodopa/carbidopa or levodopa/benserazid: 50/12.5-mg starting dose; may increase to maximum dose of 200/50 mg.
2. Pregabalin 2 mg starting dose and my increase to a maximum dose of 300 mg until symptoms improved.
3. Analgesics, such as acetaminophen (Tylenol), nonsteroidal anti-inflammatory drugs (NSAIDs), and opioids, may be used as needed for pain.
4. Benzodiazepines, such as clonazepam 0.5 to 2.0 mg at bedtime, may be used as needed.
5. Anticonvulsants, such as gabapentin (Neurontin) 300 mg at bedtime, may increase dose every 3 to 4 nights until symptoms are controlled for a maximum dose of 1,800 mg/d, in three divided doses (600 mg three times a day).
6. Vitamin deficiencies should be treated with appropriate vitamins as diagnosed.

Follow-Up

A. Follow up in 1 to 2 weeks to evaluate effect(s) of medications.
B. Evaluate severity or minimization of symptoms.
C. Reassure patients that a diagnosis of RLS does not indicate the onset of another neurologic disorder such as PD.

Consultation/Referral

A. Consider referral to a neurologist if symptoms are not improving with treatment.

Individual Considerations

A. Pregnancy
1. Symptoms are usually worse in the third trimester.

B. Pediatrics
1. Diagnosing RLS can be difficult in children because of the child's difficulty describing symptoms such as where it hurts, when and how often it occurs, and how long symptoms last.
2. Pediatric RLS can sometimes be misdiagnosed as "growing pains" or attention deficit disorder.

C. Geriatrics
1. Symptoms progress with age. Other chronic diseases are also usually present; it can be difficult to pinpoint the diagnosis of RLS because of other chronic problems.
2. Be alert to side effects of medications used for treatment for RLS. Perform a fall risk assessment when prescribing medications for RLS.

Seizures

Cheryl A. Glass and Julie Adkins

Definition

Accurate classification of seizures is dependent on observations of witnessed seizures, full medical history, including comorbidities, and clinical findings. Epilepsy is not diagnosed until the patient has more than one seizure secondary to an underlying condition in the brain. The clinical signs and symptoms depend on the location of the epileptic discharges. Status epilepticus is a continuous state of seizure and is usually defined as 30 minutes of uninterrupted seizure activity.

A. Infantile spasms begin at 3 months to 2 years of age. They are characterized by clusters of quick, sudden movements, including the head falling forward, arm flexion, and knees drawn up to the chest.

B. Partial (focal) seizures generally only involve one portion of the brain. They are the most common type of seizure and may be accompanied by visual or auditory hallucinations.
1. Simple partial seizures (SPS) are not associated with altered consciousness or loss of consciousness.
2. Common SPS includes jerking of a limb and may be preceded by an aura, including epigastric discomfort, fear, or unpleasant smells.
3. Complex partial seizure (CPS) is notable for impaired consciousness. Confusion, fatigue, and headaches may follow a CPS.

4. A simple partial seizure may last a few seconds and develop into a CPS with symptoms that include staring, repetitive motor behaviors, clouded consciousness, and automatisms (swallowing, chewing, or lip smacking).

C. Generalized seizures are notable for electroencephalographic (EEG) changes as both hemispheres of the brain are involved. Almost all generalized seizures involve loss/impaired consciousness. There are four subtypes of generalized seizures:

1. Tonic–clonic, also known as grand mal seizures, generally last 1 to 2 minutes and are notable for falls, cries, rigidity (tonicity), jerking (clonicity), and possible cyanosis.
2. Absent seizures, also called petit mal seizures, last 2 to 15 seconds and are notable for beginning and ending abruptly. Symptoms noted include staring, eye flutters, and automatisms. First aid is not required.
3. Myoclonic seizures are characterized by rapid, brief contraction of muscles (sudden jerks or clumsiness) usually on both sides of the body, arm, or sudden jerk of a foot during sleep. First aid is generally not required.
4. Atonic seizures, also called drop seizures, are characterized by abrupt loss of muscle tone, loss of posture, or sudden collapse. These seizures tend to be resistant to medication. Protective headgear may be needed. Generally first aid is not required unless an injury occurs.

D. Lennox–Gastaut syndrome (LGS) is a rare form of epilepsy consisting of multiple seizure types. It includes cognitive impairment and drop seizures. LGS patients may require antiseizure medications, steroids or immune globulin, vagus nerve stimulation, surgical resection, and ketogenic diet.

E. Eclampsia occurs anytime in pregnancy from the second trimester to the puerperium. It is notable for the occurrence of one or more generalized convulsions and/or coma in women with preeclampsia (in the absence of other neurologic conditions).

1. Eclampsia is self-limited, and delivery is the treatment.
2. The tonic–clonic seizure generally lasts 60 to 75 seconds.
3. Fetal bradycardia lasts 3 to 5 minutes, but does not necessitate an emergent cesarean section delivery. Compensatory fetal tachycardia and transient fetal heart rate decelerations occur. Delivery should be considered for the lack of improvement in 10 to 15 minutes after maternal/fetal resuscitative interventions.
4. Seizures caused by eclampsia generally resolve within a few hours to days postpartum. HELLP (hemolysis, elevated liver enzymes, low platelets) syndrome develops in approximately 10% to 20% of women with preeclampsia/eclampsia.

F. Idiopathic seizures, gelastic seizures, dacystic seizures, posttrauma, and nonepileptic seizures are other types noted in the literature.

Incidence

A. Three million Americans are affected by epilepsy. The prevalence of active epilepsy is about 0.8%.

B. Seniors: 300,000 (most rapid population with epilepsy)

1. Stroke is the leading cause of new-onset epilepsy in adults after age 65 years.

C. Eclampsia

1. Mild preeclampsia: 0.5%
2. Severe preeclampsia: From 2% to 3%
3. Forty-eight hours postpartum: Up to 33%

D. Photosensitivity seizures are more common in children and adolescents.

Pathogenesis

A. Epilepsy is a functional disorder of the brain in which neurons signal abnormally. The exact cause of epilepsy and eclampsia is unknown.

Predisposing Factors

A. Tumors
B. Alcohol/drugs
C. Cerebral infarction/stroke
D. Hypoglycemia
E. Alzheimer's disease
F. Posttrauma (head injury)
G. Surgery
H. Pregnancy (eclampsia)
I. Febrile illness
J. Photosensitivity
K. Risk factors for recurrent seizures

1. Identifiable brain disease
2. Mental retardation
3. Abnormal neurologic examination/EEG
4. Seizures: Onset after age 10 years
5. Multiple types of seizures
6. Family history/genetics
7. Poor response to antiepileptic drugs (AEDs)/combination therapy at time of withdrawal
8. Chronic alcoholism

L. Eclampsia risk factors

1. Nulliparous
2. Pregnancy-induced hypertension (PIH)
3. Teens to lower 20s and again older than 35 years
4. Other conditions to be ruled out.
   a. Stroke
   b. Hypertensive disease
   c. Space-occupying lesion
   d. Metabolic disorders (hypoglycemia, uremia, water intoxication)
   e. Meningitis or encephalitis
   f. Drug use (methamphetamine, cocaine)
   g. Idiopathic epilepsy
   h. Thrombotic thrombocytopenia purpura (TTP)

M. Breath-holding in children

Common Complaints

A. Aura: Epigastric discomfort, fear, or unpleasant smells
B. Automatisms (swallowing, chewing, fumbling, picking clothes, or lip smacking)
C. Stiffening, then jerking of limbs

D. Staring with/without repetitive motor behaviors
E. Eclampsia
    1. Headache: Severe or persistent frontal or occipital
    2. Blurred vision
    3. Photophobia
    4. Right upper quadrant pain/epigastric pain
    5. Altered mental status
    6. Nausea and vomiting
    7. Hyperreflexia

Other Signs and Symptoms

A. Lack of memory of seizure
B. Impaired consciousness
C. Postictal
    1. Confusion
    2. Amnesia
    3. Fatigue
    4. Headaches
    5. Loss of urine or bowel control

Subjective Data

A. Obtain a history from the patient or a person who witnesses the seizure.
    1. Have the witness describe the duration, part of the body affected, and qualities of the seizure.
    2. Does the patient have a recollection of the seizure?
    3. How long did it take to feel better after the seizure?
B. Evaluate if the patient has ever had seizures, and ask whether this was an isolated event.
    1. Were there any warning symptoms before the seizure?
    2. What kind of warning was noted?
C. Did the patient have a fever or an active/recent infection?
D. Do a thorough review of the patient's medical history, including head injury, pregnancy, diabetes, and cancer.
E. Ask if there is a family history of seizures.
F. Take a full medication history, including over-the-counter (OTC) and herbal products.
    1. Is the patient on an AED?
    2. Has the patient missed any doses?
    3. When was the last blood level checked to evaluate therapeutic dosing?
G. Review alcohol intake. Alcohol interferes with the efficacy of AEDs.

Physical Examination

A. Check blood pressure, pulse, respiration, and temperature (if indicated to rule out infection).
B. Inspect
    1. Assess level of consciousness (LOC), orientation.
    2. Perform general overall examination for secondary injuries from fall or striking objects.
C. Auscultate
    1. Lungs for possible aspiration
D. Palpation (if applicable for any injuries)
    1. Elevate neck for nuchal rigidity.
E. Neurologic examination
    1. Cranial nerves testing
        a. Wrinkle forehead/raise eyebrows.
        b. Smile and show teeth.
        c. Stick out the tongue/lateral tongue movement.
        d. Ocular movements
        e. Visual field
        f. Finger-to-nose test
    2. Motor strength
        a. Shrug shoulders.
        b. Test muscle strength: Grasp hands and squeeze.
        c. Check reflexes of biceps, triceps, patellar, brachioradial, and Achilles.
    3. Sensory testing: Pinprick
    4. Gait and posture

Diagnostic Tests

A. Diagnosis is confirmed by the patient's history, witness accounts, neurologic examination, blood work, and clinical testing such as EEG.
B. EEG
C. Neuroimaging CT or MRI
D. Blood glucose
E. Drug/alcohol screen
F. Serum level of anticonvulsant
G. Lumbar puncture if indicated for signs of infection/meningitis

Differential Diagnoses

A. Seizures
B. Brain tumor
C. Central nervous system (CNS) infection
D. Drug/alcohol use
E. Stroke/transient ischemic attack (TIA)
F. Hypoglycemia
G. Trauma
H. Migraine
I. Ménière's disease
J. Syncope
    1. Cardiac arrhythmic syncope
    2. Reflex
    3. Orthostatic
K. Psychogenic
L. Breath-holding (children)

Plan

A. General interventions
    1. Emergency transport may be required. Seizures longer than 5 to 10 minutes require emergent care. If the patient has a persistent headache after a rest period, unconsciousness with failure to respond, unequal pupil size or excessively dilated pupils, or weakness of the limbs, immediate medical attention is essential.
    2. Obtain a consultation with a neurologist for a thorough evaluation.
    3. States vary on the driving requirements/restrictions for patients with epilepsy. Individual state driving requirements are noted on the Epilepsy Foundation website: www.epilepsy.com/search/site/Seizure%20Severity%20Questionnaire?f[0]=bundle%3Adriving_laws
        a. A person with epilepsy has the risk of motor vehicle accident (MVA) while driving. It is considered similar or slightly higher than in patients with

other medical conditions (diabetes, cardiovascular disease) and compares with the risk of MVA with persons with sleep apnea, alcoholism, dementia, and cellular phone use.

b. Regulatory agents, as a measure of driving risk, require having a seizure-free interval of 3 to 12 months (state dependent). In studies, the seizure-free interval was the strongest predictor of MVA.

c. Clinicians must warn patients about possible driving risks after reduction of medications or missing AED doses and must consider the patients' neurologic deficits other than seizures (e.g., cognition and visual field deficits) when making recommendations about driving. The risk factors for an MVA for persons with epilepsy are as follows.

- **i.** Medication noncompliance
- **ii.** Recent history of alcohol or drug abuse
- **iii.** Uncorrectable brain function or metabolic disorder
- **iv.** Structural brain disease
- **v.** Frequent seizure recurrence after seizure-free intervals
- **vi.** Prior crashes caused by seizures

B. Patient teaching

1. Keeping a seizure diary is extremely helpful in identifying seizure trends, maintaining drug compliance, monitoring side effects, and evaluating the need for changing the course of therapy. The frequency or time of day that seizures occur is used in the adjustment of AED dosage and timing of administration.

2. Seizure triggers

- **a.** Most common cause is missed AED and/or sudden discontinuation of meds.
- **b.** Sleep deprivation
- **c.** Alcohol/drug intake
- **d.** Stress
- **e.** Hormone fluctuations
- **f.** Pregnancy
- **g.** Photosensitivity/strobe or flashing light/intense lights
- **h.** TV and video games (flicker frequency)
- **i.** Contrasting visual patterns (grids, checkerboard, and stripes)
- **j.** Computer monitors
- **k.** Visual fire alarms
- **l.** Sunlight shimmering off water/through trees/through window blinds

3. Review the importance of medication adherence.

- **a.** Give oral and written dosing instructions.
- **b.** Refill the prescription before running out.
- **c.** Take the medication on a schedule (set a watch alarm, use a pill container, mark off the calendar). Taking an extra pill when a seizure aura occurs will not stop the seizure as it is not absorbed fast enough.
- **d.** New prescription interaction profiles should be evaluated before starting new drugs.
- **e.** Patients should not use supplements, herbals, or over-the-counter (OTC) medications without checking with their health care provider.

4. Excessive alcohol use (greater than 3 drinks/d) increases the likelihood of seizures. Patients should have no more than 1 to 2 drinks a day.

5. First aid for grand mal seizure

- **a.** Stay calm.
- **b.** Time the seizure. Call 911 if the seizure lasts longer than 5 to 10 minutes.
- **c.** Clear the area to prevent harm from surrounding objects.
- **d.** Turn the person to the side and do not put anything in his or her mouth.
- **e.** Do not hold the person down.
- **f.** Place a soft object under the head to prevent head injury.
- **g.** Cardiopulmonary resuscitation (CPR) is not necessary unless the person stops breathing after the seizure.
- **h.** Stay with the person and reassure him or her.
- **i.** Help get the person home; call family or friends.
- **j.** Immediate transport to the emergency department is necessary for known conditions such as
  - **i.** Diabetes/hypoglycemia
  - **ii.** Heat exhaustion
  - **iii.** Pregnancy
  - **iv.** Infection/high fever
  - **v.** Poisoning
  - **vi.** Head injury

6. First aid for petit mal seizures

- **a.** Stay calm.
- **b.** Guide the patient away from any dangers.
- **c.** Block access to hazards.
- **d.** Do not restrain the person.
- **e.** Stay with the person until full awareness returns.

C. Pharmaceutical therapy

1. There is controversy concerning whether to start AED therapy for the first seizure. AEDs are generally started after a second seizure.

2. The prescription of AEDs should be individually weighed with a risk-versus-benefit decision that includes factors such as age; gender; family planning/desire for pregnancy; current driver; type/recurrence of seizure; abnormal EEG; concurrent medications used for other comorbid conditions; history of depression, anxiety, suicidal ideation, and hepatic and renal disease; cost; patient preference and lifestyle issues; and side-effect profile of medications; see Table 19.5).

3. A neurological consultation should be obtained for full evaluation and prescription of AED with a neurologist or primary health care providers managing subsequent follow-up.

4. A single-agent AED is started and titrated slowly to the lowest dose that is the most effective in seizure control with the least number of side effects.

- **a.** Ideally, the patient should be maintained on one AED; however, combination therapy may be required or the first agent discontinued.

TABLE 19.5 Antiepileptic Medications

Generic (Brand Name)	Seizure Type	First-Line Treatment
ethosuximide (Zarontin)	Absence seizures	Adjunctive treatment
lacosamide (Vimpat)	Partial seizures	Adjunctive treatment
zonisamide (Zonegran)	Partial seizures	Adjunctive treatment
rufinamide (Banzel)	LGS	Adjunctive treatment
divalproex sodium (Depakote)	Absence seizures	First-line treatment
	Complex partial seizure	
phenytoin (Dilantin)	Tonic–clonic seizures	First-line treatment
	Psychomotor and neurosurgical-induced seizures	
felbamate (Felbatol)	Partial seizures LGS	Not first line in partial seizures and used as an adjunctive for LGS
tiagabine (Gabitril)	Partial seizures	Adjunctive treatment
levetiracetam (Keppra)	Partial onset seizures	Adjunctive treatment for all types of seizures
	Myoclonic seizures	
	Generalized tonic–clonic seizures	
clonazepam (Klonopin)	Absence seizures LGS	First-line treatment
	Myoclonic seizures	
lamotrigine (Lamictal)	Partial seizures LGS	First-line treatment for LGS
pregabalin (Lyrica)	Partial onset seizure	Adjunctive treatment
primidone (Mysoline)	Focal and psychomotor seizures; tonic–clonic seizures	Not first-line treatment
gabapentin (Neurontin)	Partial seizures	Adjunctive treatment
carbamazepine (Tegretol)	Partial or mixed seizures	First-line treatment
	Generalized tonic–clonic seizures	
topiramate (Topamax)	Partial onset seizures	First-line treatment and adjunctive for LGS
	Generalized tonic–clonic seizures LGS	
oxcarbazepine (Trileptal)	Partial seizures	Monotherapy or adjunct treatment
valproate	LGS	First-line treatment in LGS
magnesium sulfate ($MgSO_4$)	Eclamptic tonic–clonic seizure	First-line treatment

LGS, Lennox–Gastaut syndrome.

b. When a second AED is required, the second additional medication is started by titration, a therapeutic level is achieved, and the first AED is subsequently tapered off. During this period of time there is an increase in side effects.

c. Switching to a generic formulation has been noted to increase seizure activity.

d. Rectal diazepam gel (Diastat) may be prescribed for use at home for patients with a history of prolonged seizures.

5. Stevens–Johnson syndrome (SJS) and toxic epidermal necrolysis (TEN) can occur up to 4 months after the institution of AEDs, including carbamazepine (Tegretol), oxcarbazepine (Trileptal), phenytoin (Dilantin), and lamotrigine (Lamictal).

6. Women should be routinely prescribed folate supplements of 0.4 to 0.8 mg/d. The folic acid recommendation is 4 mg/d for 1 to 3 months before conception when the patient is on valproate or carbamazepine (Tegretol).

Follow-Up

A. Follow-up by primary health care providers is dependent on the frequency of seizures, toxicity profile of AED, and other comorbid conditions.

B. Subsequent visits include the following evaluations

1. Drug compliance

2. Seizure log/diary

a. Epilepsy.com has the Seizure Severity Questionnaire available for download for individual use for patients to describe their most common type of seizure.

3. Drug concentrations, blood counts, and hepatic and renal function

4. Premenstrual serum levels when there is an increase in seizure activity the week before menstruation
5. Yearly drug levels are required for patients on a stable dose with no seizures.

C. There is an increased risk of suicide associated with several AEDs. Evaluation of the patient 1 week after institution of therapy is prudent. Instructions should be given to notify the office concerning depression.
1. Perform serial depression/suicide screening.
2. Psychiatric comorbid conditions should be treated promptly.

D. Bone loss is noted with long-term therapy with AEDs; therefore, a dual-energy x-ray absorptiometry (DEXA) scan is warranted.
1. Vitamin D and calcium may be prescribed with AEDs.

E. Patients taking AEDs need regular dental/oral care.

F. Each state has the legal prerogative to grant driving privileges. Clinicians cannot grant or suspend driving privileges.
1. Six states require clinicians to report their patients with seizures (California, Delaware, Nevada, New Jersey, Oregon, and Pennsylvania).
2. Some states require a letter sent to the Motor Vehicle Department stating, "My patient has seizures and has been advised not to drive."
3. All states require drivers with epilepsy or seizures to report their condition.
4. Commercial driving restrictions are stricter. Restrictions for commercial vehicles involved in intrastate commerce vary among individual states.

G. Consider a sleep study to evaluate for obstructive sleep apnea.

Consultation/Referral

A. A neurology consultation is necessary for the evaluation and medication initiation and the use of a ketogenic diet.

B. A neurosurgical consultation is necessary to evaluate a vagus nerve stimulator (VNS) or surgical options.
1. The VNS has been approved for intractable epilepsy refractory to medications.

C. Refer to an obstetrician.

Individual Considerations

A. Women
1. Preconception counseling and a planned pregnancy are imperative.
a. Discuss the teratogenicity of AEDs.
i. Attempt to decrease to monotherapy.
ii. Taper doses of AEDs to the lowest possible dose.
iii. If there is an absence of seizures for 2 to 5 years, consider a complete withdrawal of AEDs.
iv. First-trimester use of one AED has been noted to have a two- to fivefold increase in major fetal anomalies such as neural tube defects, cleft lip and palate, and cardiac anomalies.
b. Increase folic acid to 4 mg/d to help prevent neural tube defects.
c. Stress the need for regular prenatal care.
d. Offer maternal alpha-fetoprotein screening test.
e. A fetal echocardiogram may be considered to diagnose cardiac defects.
f. All care providers, including nurses, pediatricians, and anesthesiologists, should be aware that the patient has epilepsy on admission.
g. Chronic hypertension develops in up to 78% of women with preeclampsia/eclampsia.
2. Oral contraceptives are less effective on AEDs. The failure rate is 0.7 to 3.1 per 100 women. Women taking enzyme-inducing AEDs should use a backup method or alternative birth control. Enzyme-inducing AEDs include:
a. Dilantin (phenytoin)
b. Phenobarbital
c. Tegretol (carbamazepine)
d. Zarontin (ethosuximide)
e. Felbatol (felbamate)
f. Topamax (topiramate)
g. Trileptal (oxcarbazepine)
3. Estrogen and progesterone act on the temporal lobe where partial seizures often begin. Seizure patterns may change during menopause.

B. Pediatrics: A ketogenic diet may be prescribed under a physician's care.

C. Geriatrics
1. Seizures are likely to begin from 60 to 80 years of age.
2. Management may be more difficult dependent on comorbidities and the use of other medications.
3. Older patients have an increase of falls and loss of independence.
4. After stroke and dementia, epilepsy is the most common serious neurologic disorder in the elderly.
5. Focus on cardiovascular and neurologic systems in the clinical physical evaluation in the elderly.
6. Commonly prescribed AEDs include the following:
a. Phenytoin
i. Most commonly prescribed AED in the elderly.
ii. Use caution as phenytoin interacts with digoxin and warfarin.
iii. Causes sedation.
b. Sodium valproate
i. Ataxia and tremor are not uncommon.
ii. Can cause reversible extrapyramidal symptoms.
c. Carbamazepine
i. Hyponatremia can occur, especially with coadministration of a diuretic.
ii. Increases warfarin metabolism.
d. Lamotrigine
i. Requires a slow titration in the elderly.
e. Levetiracetam
i. Mood and behavioral problems may occur.
f. Ginkgo biloba is the most commonly used herbal for seizures in the elderly

Seizure, Febrile (Child)

Cheryl A. Glass and Julie Adkins

Definition

Febrile seizures are the most common seizure of early childhood. The average age of onset is 18 to 22 months. Febrile seizures are of short duration, usually less than 5 minutes, and are generalized tonic–clonic convulsions; 4% to 16% have focal features. The seizures are associated with fever in the absence of central nervous system (CNS) infection, acute electrolyte imbalance, or any other defined cause for a seizure. Seizures lasting longer than 15 minutes require immediate medical attention. The majority of children with febrile seizures do not develop epilepsy.

There are three types of febrile seizures.

A. Simple seizures are brief (less than 15 minutes), generalized (without a focal component), and occur once during a 24-hour period. More than 90% of febrile seizures are simple.

B. Complex febrile seizures have at least one of the following features: Duration lasting longer than 15 minutes, multiple seizures in 24 hours, and focal features.

C. Symptomatic febrile seizure is noted with children with preexisting neurologic abnormality or acute illness.

Incidence

A. Two to five percent of the population of children up to the age of 6 years develop seizures with a febrile illness. Approximately 40% of children have recurrent febrile seizures during subsequent illnesses. It is estimated that 24% of children have a family history of febrile seizures, and 4% have a family history of epilepsy.

B. The risk of febrile seizures has been noted to increase slightly after administration of the measles, mumps, and rubella (MMR) and the measles, mumps, rubella, varicella (MMRV) vaccines. Studies show the risk is increased approximately 5 to 12 days after the first MMR is given.

C. Risk of febrile seizure has also been noted to increase the first 24 hours after receiving the inactivated influenza vaccine (IIV) at the same time as the pneumococcal 13-valent conjugate (PCV13) vaccine or the diphtheria, tetanus, acellular pertussis (DTaP) vaccine. It was not shown to occur when vaccines are given separately on different days. There has been an increased risk of seizure when giving the PCV13 alone.

Pathogenesis

A. Fever is characterized by a cytokine-mediated rise in core temperature as well as immunologic, neurologic, endocrinologic, and physiological changes. A febrile seizure is an abnormal electrical discharge of neurons in the cerebral cortex causing tonic–clonic muscular contractions, induced by fever in children.

B. Febrile seizures have been identified from a combination of genetic and environmental factors. They are to an autosomal dominant inheritance, and a few other genes and chromosomal loci have been identified.

Predisposing Factors

A. Fever
  1. Temperature of at least above 100.4°F (38.0°C). Most seizures occur with fever greater than 102.2°F (39°C).
  2. More likely to occur with the maximal rate of temperature rise
  3. May occur early or late in the course of the febrile illness.
  4. May occur before fever is apparent.

B. Family history of febrile seizures

C. Family history of seizures

D. Age
  1. It occurs between 6 months and 6 years.
  2. Median age of onset is 18 months.
  3. Fifty percent of children have febrile seizures between 12 and 30 months.

E. Recent childhood immunizations

F. Other neurologic abnormalities

G. Viral infections

H. Bacterial infections

Common Complaints

A. Fever

B. Generalized tonic–clonic seizure lasting less than 5 minutes

C. Staring and loss of muscle tone

D. Staring and muscle stiffness/rigidity

Other Signs and Symptoms

A. An altered state of consciousness after the seizure

B. Vomiting

C. Decreased feeding

Subjective Data

A. Ascertain whether the child had a fever at the time of the seizure.

B. Ask the caregiver to describe how the child appeared before the seizure: Lethargic, normal, or irritable.

C. Review what happened during the seizure: Jerky movements of one extremity, blinking, and general convulsions with loss of consciousness.

D. After the seizure, determine whether the child was very sleepy, confused, or normal.

E. Review what other symptoms, such as vomiting or diarrhea, the child has and what treatment(s) have been given before presentation.

F. Note if this has ever happened before. If so, was it the same?

G. Assess the patient's medical history and developmental course.

H. Elicit information about any family history of any type of seizures.

I. Is anyone else in the family/day care ill?

Physical Examination

A. Check temperature, pulse, respirations, blood pressure, and pulse oximetry.

B. Inspect
  1. Observe overall appearance. Observe for seizure activity and level of consciousness (LOC): Unable to

arouse? If able to arouse, is the patient having trouble staying awake?
2. Presence of difficulty breathing, grunting, and retractions
3. Presence and quality of crying: Weak, high-pitched, or continuous crying
4. Inspect the head for the presence of bulging fontanelle (if applicable).
5. Evaluate the eyes for the presence of petechiae; are they sunken?
6. Ears: Evaluate the tympanic membrane.
7. Nasal examination for signs of sinusitis and nasal flaring
8. Oral examination for dry mucous membranes, erythema, and enlarged tonsils
9. Dermal examination: Evaluate for the presence of cyanosis and pallor; check skin tone and turgor; evaluate for the presence of a rash.
10. Nails: Check for prolonged capillary refill. A capillary refill of 3 seconds or greater is an intermediate risk for serious illness such as meningococcal disease.
11. Check for nuchal rigidity/stiffness.

C. Auscultate
1. The heart
2. All lung fields for crackles and decreased breath sounds
3. All quadrants of the abdomen

D. Palpate
1. Fontanelle (if applicable for age).
2. Evaluate lymphadenopathy.
3. Palpate the abdomen for masses, tenderness, and rebound.

E. Neurologic examination: Perform a complete neurologic examination, assessing all cranial nerves. Be alert for signs and symptoms of CNS infection: Stiff neck, lethargy, and confusion are highly indicative of CNS infection. The neurologic examination should be normal. Any abnormal neurologic findings are inconsistent with febrile seizures.

Diagnostic Tests

A. Pulse oximetry
B. Complete blood count (CBC)
C. Blood chemistries are not indicated with febrile seizures unless electrolyte imbalance or other specific indications exist. Seizures that continue for more than 5 minutes should have electrolytes and glucose evaluated.
D. Urinalysis
E. Electroencephalography (EEG) is not indicated for febrile seizures; however, if neurologic signs are present or seizures are recurrent, an EEG and neurologic workup should be done.
F. Lumbar puncture is indicated if there are positive neurologic signs, especially in children 12 to 18 months and infants younger than 12 months who present after their first febrile seizure.
G. Consider chest x-ray for respiratory problems.
H. Consider stool cultures if indicated for diarrhea.
I. CT and MRI imaging are not required for children with simple febrile seizures.

Differential Diagnoses

A. Febrile seizure
B. Shaking chills from fever
C. Metabolic imbalances: Hypoglycemia, hyponatremia, and hypomagnesemia
D. Syncope
E. CNS infection: Encephalitis, meningitis, and abscess
F. Epilepsy
G. Brain tumor

Plan

A. General interventions
1. Tepid sponge baths have not been shown to be effective in the prevention of febrile seizures and are not recommended for the treatment of fever.
2. Children with fevers should not be undressed or overwrapped.
3. Support the patient with positioning to prevent aspiration; maintain airway, and administer oxygen. Do not try to pry the jaws open to place an object between the teeth.

B. Patient teaching
1. *See Section III: Patient Teaching Guide for this chapter, "Febrile Seizures (Child)."* ◀
2. Advise family that neurologic sequelae, intellectual impairment, and behavioral disorders are rare following febrile seizures.
3. Advise parents that, if a child has a seizure, to lay the child on his or her side and do not try to restrict the child's movements or convulsions. Nothing should be placed in the mouth.
4. Recommend timing the seizure to see how long the seizure lasts. Seizures that last 5 minutes or longer need immediate attention and the child should be taken to the emergency department by calling 911.
5. Never leave a child alone during a seizure.

C. Pharmaceutical therapy
1. Antipyretic agents do not prevent febrile seizures and are not used for prophylaxis. Ibuprofen (Motrin) or acetaminophen (Tylenol), using age/weight-appropriate doses every 4 hours, may be given for temperature elevation of 104°F (37.9°C).
2. Antibiotics are not indicated for a fever without an apparent source.
3. The American Academy of Pediatrics Committee on Quality Improvement and Management, Subcommittee on Febrile Seizures concluded that on the basis of the risks and benefits of effective therapies, neither continuous nor intermittent anticonvulsant therapy is recommended for children with one or more simple febrile seizures.

Follow-Up

A. See the patient for repeat seizures and as needed.
B. Seizures lasting longer than 15 minutes require immediate medical attention.

Consultation/Referral

A. Consult a neurologist for uncontrolled or repeated seizures. When no fever is present, it may signal the onset of epilepsy and should be referred. Children who have experienced prolonged febrile seizures are more likely to develop a particular type of epilepsy (temporal lobe epilepsy [TLE]).
B. When meningitis cannot be eliminated by history and physical examination, the child should be admitted to the hospital.
C. If seizures are continuous, this is a medical emergency. The patient should be sent to the hospital immediately by ambulance, and a neurologist should be consulted.

Individual Considerations

A. Pediatrics
  1. The majority of seizures occur in children between the ages of 12 to 18 months, but can occur at any age.
  2. Approximately 30% to 35% of children who have had one febrile seizure are at risk of having another seizure.
B. Geriatrics
  1. Approximately 20% to 30% of older adults have blunted or absent fever response to infection.
  2. Alteration in cognitive function, especially delirium, may be present before (or in the absence of) fever in older adults with an infection.
  3. The use of antipyretics for adults with a fever is the presence of severe coronary artery disease. Shivering is strenuous for the heart and circulatory system.
  4. Adverse consequences of fever are rare in older adults. There is little evidence that a fever increases an older adult's risk for long-term neurologic symptoms.

Transient Ischemic Attack

Cheryl A. Glass and Julie Adkins

Definition

A. Transient ischemic attacks (TIA) are brief focal brain deficits, spinal cord issues, or retinal ischemia (without acute infarction) caused by vascular occlusion. Symptoms generally last less than an hour; however, they may have permanent sequelae. TIAs are a risk factor for recurrent risk of stroke. Approximately 15% of diagnosed strokes are preceded by TIAs. TIAs can be difficult to diagnose as symptoms are transient. Assume that all stroke-like symptoms signal an emergency.
B. Presence of neurologic deficit suggests a stroke rather than a TIA.

Incidence

A. The prevalence of TIAs in the United States is between 200,000 and 500,000 per year.
B. The early risk of stroke is approximately 4% to 5% at 2 days and as high as 11% at day 7 after a TIA.
C. The risk of death from coronary artery disease and stroke is as high as 6% to 10%, depending on other risk factors.
D. More men (101/100,000) than women (70/100,000) are affected. There is an increased number of Black adults with TIAs (98/100,000) than White adults (81/100,000) affected by TIAs.

Pathogenesis

A. The pathogenesis is a neurologic event secondary to a temporary reduction of blood flow to the brain from a partially occluded vessel or related to an acute thromboembolic event.

Predisposing Factors

A. Hypertension
  1. Systolic blood pressure greater than 140 mmHg
  2. Diastolic blood pressure greater than 90 mmHg
B. Atherosclerosis
C. African American
D. Age older than 40 years
E. Hypotensive episodes
F. Oral contraceptives
G. Atrial fibrillation
H. Smoking
I. Familial hyperlipidemia
J. Diabetes mellitus
K. Valvular heart disease
L. Infective endocarditis
M. Migraine with aura
N. Medications alter bleeding time and interact with warfarin
  1. Feverfew
  2. Garlic
  3. Ginkgo biloba
  4. Ginger
  5. Ginseng

Common Complaints

Signs and symptoms depend on the affected vessel and surrounding brain tissue.

A. Acute onset of focal neurologic deficit
  1. Limb weakness or numbness
  2. Facial weakness
  3. Speech difficulty to aphasia
  4. Visual loss/blurring
  5. Ataxia
B. Acute change in level of consciousness (LOC) or confusion
C. Posterior circulation TIAs may have a headache as one of the prodromal symptoms that precedes a stroke by days or weeks.
D. Basilar artery occlusion TIAs have vertigo, nausea, and headaches that may occur as early as 2 weeks or more before the onset of stroke.

Other Signs and Symptoms

A. Dysarthria
B. Dysphagia

C. Near syncope
D. Hemiparesis
E. Temporary monocular blindness
F. Behavior changes
G. Vertigo
H. Dizziness
I. Diplopia

Subjective Data

If a TIA is suspected, call 911; symptoms of a TIA and a major stroke are not always distinguishable.

A. Ask detailed questions about symptoms before, during, and after the spell.
  1. Review the exact timing of onset of symptoms.
  2. How intense were the symptoms?
  3. What was the duration and the presence of any fluctuation of symptoms?
  4. Has there been a pattern that is becoming more frequent or escalating in symptoms?

B. Interview the patient, family members, witnesses, and emergency personnel for their description of behavior, speech, gait, memory, and movement.
C. Focus on precipitating factors and state of consciousness after the acute event.
D. Question the patient about risk factors such as hypertension, smoking, cardiac disease, and heredity.
E. Review all medications, including anticoagulants, over-the-counter (OTC), herbals, and illicit drug use such as cocaine.
F. Review the medical history.
  1. Recent surgeries, specifically carotid or cardiac surgeries
  2. Seizures
  3. Central nervous system (CNS) infection
  4. Illicit drug use
  5. Presence of any metabolic disorders
  6. Recent trauma (blunt or torsion injury to the neck)
  7. Atrial fibrillation

Physical Examination

A. Check temperature, pulse, respiration, and blood pressure, including orthostatic blood pressure and pulse and pulse oximetry.
B. General observation
  1. Observe overall appearance, LOC, ability to interact, language, difficulty swallowing, tremors, spasticity, as well as memory skills.
  2. Observe the patient walking (cerebellar system).

C. Inspect
  1. Dermal examination
    a. Overall hydration status
    b. Look for postcarotid endarterectomy scars, presence of a pacemaker, implantable cardioverter defibrillator, or other cardiac surgical scars.
  2. Check pupil size and reactivity to light.
  3. Perform a funduscopic examination to evaluate optic disc margins, retinal plaques, and pigmentation.

D. Auscultate
  1. Heart for rate, rhythm, murmurs, or rubs
  2. Lungs: Note respiratory rate and pattern.
  3. Carotid arteries for the presence of bruit

E. Palpate extremities for pulses and peripheral edema.
F. Neurologic examination
  1. Cranial nerve testing
    a. Wrinkle forehead/raise eyebrows.
    b. Smile and show teeth.
    c. Stick out the tongue/lateral tongue movement.
    d. Ocular movements
    e. Visual field
  2. Motor strength
    a. Shrug shoulders.
    b. Test muscle strength: Grasp hands and squeeze.
    c. Check reflexes of biceps, triceps, patellar, brachioradial, and Achilles.
  3. Sensory testing: Pinprick
  4. Gait and posture (cerebellar system evaluation)
    a. Ocular movements
    b. Gait
    c. Finger-to-nose test
    d. Heel-to-knee test

Diagnostic Tests

A. Pulse oximetry
B. Laboratory tests
  1. Emergent labs
    a. Glucose
    b. Serum chemistry profile, including creatinine
    c. Coagulation and hypercoagulablity testing
    d. Complete blood count (CBC)
  2. Urgent labs
    a. Erythrocyte sedimentation rate (ESR)
    b. Cardiac enzymes
    c. Lipid profile
  3. Other laboratory tests based on history.
    a. Urine drug screen
    b. Blood alcohol level
    c. Antiphospholipid antibodies
    d. Rapid plasma reagin (RPR) for syphilis

C. MRI or CT scan within 24 hours of symptom onset
D. Carotid Doppler ultrasonography identifies patients with urgent surgical needs.
E. Cardiac imaging to evaluate cardioembolic sources
F. EKG to evaluate dysrhythmias (such as atrial fibrillation)
G. Lumbar puncture to rule out infection, demyelinating disease, and subarachnoid hemorrhage (SAH)
H. EEG as indicated for seizure activity
I. Consider cardiac Holter monitor for suspected intermittent atrial fibrillation

Differential Diagnoses

A. TIA
B. Ischemia stroke
C. SAH/subdural hematoma (SDH)
D. Migraine
E. Hypoglycemia/hyperglycemia
F. Epilepsy—postictal period
G. Malignant hypertension
H. Brain tumor

I. Bell's palsy
J. Multiple sclerosis (MS)
K. Syncope
L. Drug induced
M. Concussion
N. Vertigo

Plan

A. General interventions

1. Carefully assess the patient to timely diagnose TIA.

2. Perform a full workup to determine the underlying disease process.

3. Prevent stroke by modification of risk factors.

▶ **B.** Patient teaching: *See Section III: Patient Teaching Guide for this chapter, "Transient Ischemic Attack."*

C. Medical and surgical management

1. Treat TIAs with antiplatelet drugs as soon as intracranial bleeding is ruled out.

2. Consider carotid endarterectomy.

3. Lipid control

4. Glucose control

5. Smoking cessation

6. Eliminate or reduce alcohol consumption.

7. Start exercise plan for losing weight. Recommend starting with about 30 minutes of exercise three times per week as tolerated.

D. Pharmaceutical therapy: **The mainstay of treatment for TIA is pharmacological management with antithrombotic agents.**

1. Antiplatelet therapy

a. Aspirin 50 to 325 mg/d

b. Dipyridamole (Persantine) 200 mg/d. May be given as an adjunct with warfarin therapy.

c. Aspirin + dipyridamole extended release (Aggrenox) 25/200 mg twice a day.

d. Clopidogrel (Plavix) 75 mg/d. Aspirin is not routinely recommended with clopidogrel because of the risk of hemorrhage. No dosage adjustment is necessary with clopidogrel for elderly patients or patients with renal disease.

e. Ticlopidine (Ticlid) 250 mg twice a day is a second-line antiplatelet therapy for patients who cannot tolerate or do not respond to aspirin therapy. In some circumstances, it can be an alternative to clopidogrel.

f. Warfarin (Coumadin) 5 to 15 mg; titrate for a goal international normalized ratio (INR) of 2.0 to 3.0

2. Antihypertensive therapy as indicated to maintain blood pressure below 140/90 mmHg with an angiotensin converting enzyme (ACE) inhibitor or an angiotensin receptor blocker alone or in combination with a diuretic.

3. Initiate a daily statin to a goal of low-density lipoprotein-cholesterol (LDL-C) less than 100 mg/dL.

Follow-Up

A. Rapid transfer is essential for a patient with positive symptoms for risk stratification.

B. Patients with a suspected TIA who are not admitted to the hospital should have rapid access (within 12 hours) for an urgent assessment and evaluation with CT or MRI brain scan, EKG, and carotid Doppler testing.

C. Patients managed in the outpatient setting should be fully educated about the need to return to the clinic or emergency department immediately if symptoms recur.

D. Specific follow-up depends on etiology, severity, frequency, and duration of TIAs.

E. Follow-up laboratory testing as indicated (e.g., CBC, cholesterol, INR).

F. Monitor the patient for occult bleeding if started on antiplatelet, antithrombic medications.

Consultation/Referral

A. TIA should be viewed as a medical emergency because these patients have salvageable neurologic function; consult with a physician.

B. Cardiology and neurology consultations should be obtained when cardioembolic TIAs are treated with anticoagulation therapy.

C. Ophthalmologic consultation is indicated to assess the nature of transient visual symptoms.

D. Vascular surgeon consultation is necessary for patients with significant stenosis or occlusion. Patients with symptomatic carotid artery stenosis should have a surgical evaluation immediately.

Individual Considerations

A. Children: TIA etiologies in children include

1. Congenital heart disease with cerebral thromboembolism

2. Drug abuse (e.g., cocaine)

3. Clotting disorders

4. CNS infection

5. Marfan disease

6. Tumor

B. Adults

1. TIAs that occur in the younger adult population should be evaluated for embolism.

2. Anticoagulation is not recommended for women younger than 65 years of age with atrial fibrillation who are otherwise at low risk for stroke. Antiplatelet therapy is recommended for this population.

C. Geriatrics

1. TIAs are most commonly seen in this population.

2. Screen for atrial fibrillation in women, especially older than 75 years of age.

Resources

The ABCD2 Score for TIA estimates the risk of a stroke after a TIA.

An online ABCD2 calculator is located at: www.mdcalc.com/abcd2-score-for-tia

A hard copy of the ABCD2 is available at: www.stroke.org/site/DocServer/NSA_ABCD2_tool.pdf

The National Institutes of Health Stroke Scale (NIHSS) is a stroke scale that evaluates the effect of an acute cerebral infarct. The 15-item stroke scale requires less than 10 minutes to complete.

A free online training certification course for the NIHSS is available at: www.nihstrokescale.org

A hard copy of the NIHSS is located at: www.ninds.nih.gov/doctors/NIH_Stroke_Scale.pdf

An online NIHSS calculator is located at: www.mdcalc.com/nih-stroke-scale-score-nihss

Vertigo

Jill C. Cash and Julie Adkins

Definition

A. Vertigo is the illusion of self or environmental movement, typically rotating, spinning, tilting, even a sensation that one is going to fall down. Older patients have an increased risk of falls and depression secondary to vertigo.
B. Vertigo is often classified as either central or peripheral in origin.

Incidence

A. Approximately 5% to 10% of the general population experience dizziness, vertigo, and imbalance. It reaches 40% in patients older than 40 years and decreases to 25% in patients older than 65 years.
B. It is estimated that approximately 0.5% of the population consults their primary health care provider each year regarding vertigo.
C. In 2011, approximately 3.9 million emergency department visits were seen for dizziness or vertigo.
D. Both sexes, as well as all age groups, are affected.
E. Benign paroxysmal positional vertigo (BPPV) is the most common cause of vertigo, excluding central nervous system (CNS) lesions.
  1. The prevalence of BPPV is 2.4%.
  2. BPPV rarely occurs in people younger than 35 years unless there is a history of head trauma.
  3. BPPV recurs in approximately one third of patients after 1 year and in about 50% in all patients treated after 5 years.

Pathogenesis

A. Distinguishing between peripheral and central vertigo is critical because the evaluation, treatment, and progress vary significantly. Central vertigo suggests brainstem dysfunction affecting the vestibular nuclei or their connections. This may be secondary to a structural lesion such as neoplasm or ischemia.
B. Vertigo, because of vascular insufficiency, is rarely isolated, and other symptoms of brainstem involvement are usually seen such as diplopia, dysphagia, motor weakness, or disruption in sensation. Neoplasms are usually slow growing, and the vestibular dysfunction is often insidious. Other considerations for causes of central vertigo include multiple sclerosis (MS), seizures, and migraines.
C. Vertigo of peripheral origin is more common and may be caused by dysfunction of the inner ear or vestibular nerve. BPPV is the most commonly diagnosed peripheral vestibular disorder. The cause of BPPV is unknown. The most common explanation is free otoconia within the semicircular canals that are dislodged by trauma, infection, or degeneration. The debris relocates when the head is repositioned and provokes vertigo. Causes of labyrinthine dysfunction include infection, trauma, ischemia, or toxins such as drugs or alcohol.
D. Ménière's disease causes vertigo, hearing loss, and ringing of the ears. The exact cause is unknown, but a hypothesis is a buildup of fluid in the inner ear.
E. Viral infections may lead up to vestibular neuritis (labyrinthitis). The vertigo experienced with vestibular neuritis is sudden and severe and may last days.
F. Other possible causes of vertigo are psychogenic, cardiovascular, metabolic, head trauma, and migraines.
G. Medications that cause dizziness:
  1. Anticonvulsants
  2. Antidepressants
  3. Antipsychotics
  4. Anxiolytics/sedatives
  5. Antihypertensives
  6. Nitrates
  7. Diuretics
  8. Insulin/oral hypoglycemic agents

Predisposing Factors

A. Head or body movement
  1. Rolling over in bed
  2. Getting out of bed
  3. Bending down from the waist
  4. Looking up
B. Fear or anxiety
C. Stress
D. Recent infection, usually upper respiratory in cases of vestibular neuronitis
E. Family history, especially in cases of vertiginous migraine
F. Head trauma
G. Migraines
H. Idiopathic with no cause identified
I. Hypoglycemia
J. Alcohol intoxication
K. Medication side effects
L. Cerebellar or brainstem stroke
M. Tumors
N. MS
O. Dehydration

Common Complaints

A. Dizziness with or without change in body positioning
B. Nausea/vomiting
C. Tinnitus
D. Aural fullness
E. Hearing loss

Other Signs and Symptoms

A. Central origin, including vascular insufficiencies, strokes, neoplasms, migraine, MS, seizures
  1. Double vision
  2. Dysarthria
  3. Dysphagia
  4. Paresthesias
  5. Changes in motor or sensory examination
  6. Mild to moderate vertigo
  7. Multiple episodes of vertigo lasting seconds to minutes in duration with vascular insufficiency and seizures

8. Constant complaints of vertigo with neoplasms or strokes
9. Multiple episodes of vertigo lasting hours with migraines
10. Single episodes of vertigo with MS
11. Dix–Hallpike test: Habituation common with delayed nystagmus

B. Peripheral origin, including BPPV, Ménière's disease, labyrinthitis, vestibular dysfunction, vestibular neuritis, and acoustic neuroma
1. No associated signs of brainstem dysfunction
2. Vertigo, usually described as severe
3. Multiple episodes of vertigo lasting hours with Ménière's disease
4. Single or multiple episodes of vertigo with labyrinthitis
5. Vestibular dysfunction, described as constant vertigo
6. Severe nausea or vomiting
7. Hearing loss or tinnitus; aural fullness may be present, as well as a roaring sound.
8. Triad of vertigo, tinnitus, and hearing loss is suggestive of Ménière's disease.
9. Dix–Hallpike test: No habituation: nystagmus occurs immediately.

Subjective Data

A. Elicit onset, frequency, duration, and course of presenting symptoms.
1. Is this recurrent or new?
a. Acute vertigo is seen with trauma, stroke, meningitis, otitis media, mastoiditis, drug use, vestibular neuronitis, MS, and labyrinthitis.
b. Recurrent vertigo is seen in migraines, BPPV, motion sickness, seizures, and Ménière's disease.

B. Elicit from the patient a verbal description of the sensation(s) experienced.

C. Note triggering and alleviating factors.

D. Query the patient regarding associated symptoms such as hearing loss, tinnitus, nausea, difficulty with gait, aural fullness, or other neurologic manifestations such as nystagmus.

E. Review the patient's past medical history, including recent infections; trauma; risk factors for cardiovascular disease such as smoking, diabetes, and hyperlipidemia.

F. Review over-the-counter (OTC) medications, herbal products, and medication use: Aminoglycoside, antibiotics, diuretics, antihypertensives, and antidepressants.

G. Has the patient had any previous treatments for vertigo such as an Epley procedure?

H. Has the patient had any previous testing such as:
1. Audiometric testing
2. Electronystagmogram (ENG)/videonystagmography (VNG) to evaluate balance
3. Rotational/balance platform test
4. CT or MRI
5. Computerized dynamic posturography (CDP) to evaluate postural stability/motor control

Physical Examination

A. Check temperature (if indicated), pulse, respirations, and blood pressure; note orthostatic hypotension.

B. Inspect
1. Observe overall appearance.

Generalized muscle weakness may be observed.

2. Note gait: Difficulty with tandem gait. Note global weakness.
3. Inspect the eyes: Assess for nystagmus; a few beats of nystagmus on extreme lateral gaze may be normal.
4. Ear examination: Rule out otitis media.
5. Evaluate for aphasia that may indicate a stroke.

C. Palpate extremities; note pulses and edema.

D. Neurologic examination
1. Perform complete neurologic examination.
2. Perform Rinne and Weber's test.
3. Assess cranial nerves.

Brainstem involvement is frequently seen with detailed neurologic examination. Signs of cerebellar dysfunction include difficulty with finger-to-nose testing, rapid alternating supination or pronation of hands, and gait disturbance.

4. Perform Romberg test: The patient stands with feet together and closes his or her eyes. A positive result is when the patient sways. This may be seen with vestibular disease and acoustic neuroma.
5. The Dix–Hallpike test (also called the Nylen–Bárány's maneuver test) is a provocative positional test. Perform the Dix–Hallpike: While the patient is seated on the middle third of the examination table, turn the patient's head 45° toward the affected side (problem ear). While holding the head in that position, assist the patient to the reclining position past the supine position. BPPV has a distinctive nystagmus in which there is involuntary eye movement (predominantly in a rotating fashion) starting slowly, progressing to a fast phase, and then entering a resetting phase. The nystagmus generally lasts less than 20 seconds and reverses itself upon the patient sitting upright.

The Dix–Hallpike maneuver is considered the gold standard for diagnosing BPPV. However, a negative test does not rule out BPPV if the patient is asymptomatic on the date of the test. If a positive response is observed on the initial side, no further testing is required.

6. Test for nuchal rigidity if fever is present.

E. Auscultate
1. Auscultate the heart, neck, and carotid arteries.

Physical examination may reveal cardiovascular abnormalities such as a carotid bruit.

2. Auscultate lungs—deep inspirations may cause dizziness.
3. Auscultate the abdomen.

Diagnostic Tests

A. Laboratory testing
1. Thyroid function studies: To rule out hypothyroidism
2. Venereal Disease Research Laboratory (VDRL): To rule out secondary or early tertiary syphilis, which can have symptoms similar to Ménière's disease.
3. Complete blood count (CBC): To rule out infection or severe anemia.
4. Electrolytes: To rule out hyponatremia, hypokalemia, and dehydration.
5. Urine drug screen (if indicated)
6. Cardiac panel (if indicated)
7. Urinalysis to rule out a urinary tract infection (UTI) in the elderly

B. CT scan for head trauma
C. MRI with and without contrast to assess for mass, especially if a central origin is suspected
D. Caloric test: Definitive procedure for identifying vestibular pathology
E. Electronystagmography: Most useful in chronic peripheral disorders to determine the degree and progression of vestibular deficit
F. Audiogram: Test for possible hearing loss
G. Rotating chair test: Interprets the slow component velocity of the nystagmus response with bilateral canals stimulated
H. Lumbar puncture if meningitis is suspected

Differential Diagnoses

A. Vertigo
B. Vascular insufficiencies
C. Stroke
D. Neoplasms
E. Migraine
F. MS
G. Seizures
H. BPPV
I. Ménière's disease
J. Labyrinthitis
K. Vestibular dysfunction
L. Vestibular neuritis
M. Acoustic neuroma
N. Syncope
O. Multiple sensory defects
P. Parkinson's disease (PD)
Q. Adverse reaction to medications

Plan

A. General interventions: Treatment of vertigo depends on the underlying pathology and duration of the symptoms.
1. Acute vertigo: Maintain the patient on bed rest, with the reassurance that most patients with acute vertigo recover spontaneously over a period of several weeks to months.
2. Chronic vertigo: Refer the patient for physical therapy with emphasis on vestibular rehabilitation.
a. Cawthorne Cooksey physical exercise regimen encourages eye, head, and body movements to facilitate recalibration of the vestibulo-ocular and vestibulospinal reflexes.
b. Encourage ambulation when tolerated to induce central compensatory mechanism.

3. Ménière's disease: The patient needs bed rest in the acute phase and nutritional therapy with restrictions of sodium, caffeine, alcohol, and tobacco.
4. BPPV
a. The patient needs bed rest for acute symptoms.
b. Canalith repositioning procedures (CRP) provide immediate resolution of vertigo in 85% to 95% of patients. Epley procedure: The CRP is safe, simple, inexpensive, quick, and easy to perform. It is likely to be unsuccessful in patients with bilateral positional nystagmus, and it is not recommended for patients with acute vertigo, many of whom may have vestibular neuronitis. See Section II: Procedure, "Canalith Repositioning (Epley) Procedure for Vertigo." Contraindications to performing the Epley procedure are
i. Recent neck fracture or neck instability
ii. A history of unstable carotid disease
iii. Recent retinal detachment
iv. Any physical condition that prevents the patient from lying down quickly or rolling over required for the procedure

c. Instead, meclizine may be used for 1 to 2 weeks, and then the patient is reassessed. Stop meclizine on the day the patient returns; it may suppress the positional nystagmus.
d. For patients with severe positional vertigo during the Dix–Hallpike maneuver, premedicate with a prochlorperazine (Compazine) 25 mg suppository 1 hour before performance of the CRP.
e. If the Dix–Hallpike is positive on the left, use a left-sided CRP. Conversely, if it is positive on the right, use a right-sided CRP. If the patient has bilateral disease, refer him or her to an otolaryngologist or treat the more symptomatic side first.
f. After the Epley procedures, different types of recommendations are made to prevent the otoconia from returning to their posterior semicircular canal, including
i. Wear a cervical collar for two nights after the maneuver.
ii. Stay upright for 24 hours after the procedure or have the head elevated 30° for one to two nights after the procedure.
iii. Avoid sleeping with the affected ear down.
iv. Counsel to avoid abrupt head changes for 1 week after the procedure.
v. Avoid exercise, such as yoga and sit-ups, that would make similar motions.
vi. Avoid looking up such as looking at items on the top shelves at the grocery.
vii. Symptoms may reoccur after tilting backward in dental chairs.

viii. Symptoms may reoccur after turning in the hairdresser's chair and/or tilting backward for a shampoo.

B. Patient teaching: Encourage compliance with bed rest and exercises.

C. Pharmaceutical therapy

The American Academy of Otolaryngology—Head and Neck Surgery does not recommend the use of vestibular suppressant medications to control BPPV. The American Academy of Neurology also reports that there is no evidence to support the routine use of vestibular suppressant therapy as treatment for BPPV.

1. Acute vertigo
- **a.** Metoclopramide (Reglan)
- **b.** Ondansetron (Zofran)
- **c.** Dimenhydrinate (Dramamine)
- **d.** Promethazine (Phenergan)
- **e.** Meclizine (Antivert)
- **f.** Dimenhydrinate (Dramamine)
- **g.** Diphenhydramine (Benadryl)
- **h.** Vestibular sedative
  - **i.** Cinnarizine
  - **ii.** Meclizine (Antivert)
  - **iii.** Diazepam (Valium)

2. Chronic vertigo
- **a.** Cinnarizine
- **b.** Clonazepam (Klonopin)
- **c.** Carbamazepine (Tegretol)

3. Ménière's disease
- **a.** Diuretics such as hydrochlorothiazide and triamterene (Dyazide) together will help with vertigo, but may not reduce hearing loss.
- **b.** Tricyclic antidepressants (TCAs) may be used in resistant cases.

4. Antivirals are not useful for treatment of vestibular neuritis.

5. Steroids have been used in the treatment of vestibular neuritis.

6. Vestibular migraines respond to antimigraine medications.

D. Surgery

1. Pneumatic equalization tubes

2. BPPV surgery: canal partitioning or canal plugging

3. Vestibular nerve section (vestibular neurectomy) is a treatment for intractable violent episodes of BPPV.

4. Labyrinthectomy to remove the semicircular canals, utricle, and saccule, the balance organs. This procedure is only considered when a person has already lost all hearing function in the affected ear.

5. Chemical labyrinthectomy: Gentamicin infusion destroys the vestibular hair cells.

Follow-Up

A. The American Academy of Otolaryngology—Head and Neck Surgery Foundation recommends managing patients with BPPV as follows:

1. CRP/Epley procedure should be offered unless there is a risk for impaired mobility or balance or the patient is at increased risk of falls.

2. Patients should be reevaluated in 1 month after an Epley procedure/CRP in order to confirm that the procedure resolved the symptoms of vertigo.

3. The recurrence rate after an Epley procedure is 30% to 50%.

B. Follow-up as needed according to the origin of the diagnosis and the patient's needs.

C. If indicated, transfer to the ER/call 911 for cardiovascular and cerebrovascular symptoms for treatment of stroke or cardiac events.

Consultation/Referral

A. Refer to a physician if the patient does not experience improvement in 2 to 4 weeks. If symptoms worsen, consider referring to an ear, nose, and throat specialist.

B. Refer to an otolaryngologist for testing, including

1. Audiometric testing

2. ENG to evaluate balance

3. Rotational/balance platform test

Individual Considerations

A. Pediatrics

1. The most common causes of dizziness in children are otitis media, migraine headaches, and BPPV.

2. Concussion: Nausea, vertigo, and nystagmus are classic symptoms of a concussion.

3. Drug overdoses and other poisons cause vertigo and nystagmus.

B. Geriatrics

1. Many of the medications, individually and especially in combination, used for vestibular suppression are on the American Geriatrics Society Beers Criteria list of potentially inappropriate medications for older adults.

Resources

American Speech–Language-Hearing Association (ASHA): www.asha.org
Vestibular Disorders Association: www.vestibular.org

Bibliography

Alkhawajah, N. M., & Oger, J. (2015). Treatment of myasthenia gravis in the aged. *Drugs & Aging, 32*(9), 689–697.

Alzheimer's Association. (2016). What is dementia? Retrieved from www.alz.org

American Academy of Neurology. (n.d.-a). *Guillain-Barré syndrome.* Retrieved from http://patients.aan.com/disorders/indexcfm?event=view&disorder_id=935

American Academy of Neurology Professional Association Model Policy. (n.d.-b). Canalith repositioning procedure (CRP). Retrieved from https://www.aan.com/uploadedFiles/Website_Library_Assets/Documents/3.Practice_Management/1.Reimbursement/1.Billing_and_Coding/5.Coverage_Policies/Coverage%20Policies%20-%20Canalith.pdf

American Academy of Otolaryngology—Head and Neck Surgery. (2016). Ménière's disease. Retrieved from www.entnet.org/Healthinformation/menieresDisease.cfm

American Family Physician. (2016). Headache. Retrieved from http://www.aafp.org/afp/topicModules/viewTopicModule.htm?topicModuleId=10

Annear, M. J., Eccleston, C. E., McInerney, F. J., Elliott, K. E., Toye, C. M., Tranter, B. K., & Robinson, A. L. (2016). A new standard in dementia knowledge measurement: Comparative validation of the dementia knowledge assessment scale and the Alzheimer's disease knowledge scale. *Journal of the American Geriatrics Society, 64*(6), 1329–1334.

Bergman, K., Given, B., Fabiano, R., Schutte, D., von Eye, A., & Davidson, S. (2013). Symptoms associated with mild traumatic brain injury/concussion: The role of bother. *Journal of Neuroscience Nursing, 45* (3), 124–132.

Besser, L. M., Litvan, I., Monsell, S. E., Mock, C., Weintraub, S., Zhou, X. H., & Kukull, W. (2016). Mild cognitive impairment in Parkinson's disease versus Alzheimer's disease. *Parkinsonism & Related Disorders, 27*, 54–60.

Cavazos, J. E. (2013, March 11). Epilepsy and seizures. *Medscape.* Retrieved from http://emedicine.medscape.com/article/1184846-overview

Centers for Disease Control and Prevention. (2015a, March 24). *Stroke facts.* Retrieved from https://www.cdc.gov/stroke/facts.htm

Centers for Disease Control and Prevention. (2015b, August 28). *Childhood vaccines and febrile seizures.* Retrieved from https://www.cdc.gov/vaccinesafety/concerns/febrile-seizures.html

Centers for Disease Control and Prevention. (2015c, October 16). *Guillain-Barré syndrome and flu vaccine.* Retrieved from https://www.cdc.gov/flu/protect/vaccine/guillainbarre.htm

Chawla, J. (2013, March 28). Migraine headache. *Medscape.* Retrieved from http://emedicine.medscape.com/article/1142556

Cramer, J. A. (2010). Seizure severity questionnaire v2.2 (baseline and follow-up versions). Retrieved from https://www.epilepsy.com/sites/files/atoms/files/SSQ%20BL%2BFU%20for%20academia%20use.pdf

Cruccu, G., Finnerup, N. B., Jensen, T. S., Scholz, J., Sindou, M., Svensson, P., . . . Nurmikko, T. (2016). Trigeminal neuralgia: New classification and diagnostic grading for practice and research. *Neurology, 87*(2), 220–228.

Cruse, R. P. (2013, February 1). Overview of Guillain-Barré syndrome in children. *UpToDate.* Retrieved from www.uptodate.com/contents/overview-of-guillain-barre-syndrome-in-children?topicKey=PEDS%2F6235

Cuellar, N. G., & Dorn, J. M. (2015). Peripheral diabetic neuropathy or restless legs syndrome in persons with type 2 diabetes mellitus: Differentiating diagnosis in practice. *Journal of the American Association of Nurse Practitioners, 27*(12), 671–675.

Delgado-Alvarado, M., Gago, B., Navalpotro-Gomez, I., Jiménez-Urbieta, H., & Rodriguez-Oroz, M. C. (2016). Biomarkers for dementia and mild cognitive impairment in Parkinson's disease. *Movement Disorders, 31*(6), 861–881.

Duffy, J., Weintraub, E., Hambidge, S. J., Jackson, L. A., Kharbanda, E. O., Klein, N. P., . . . DeStefano, F. (2016). Febrile seizure risk after vaccination in children 6 to 23 months. *Pediatrics, 138* (1), 1–12.

El-Chammas, K., Keyes, J., Thompson, N., Vijayakumar, J., Becher, D., & Jackson, J. L. (2013). Pharmacologic treatment of pediatric headaches: A meta-analysis. *JAMA Pediatrics, 167*(3), 250–258.

Elder, K. G., Lemon, S. K., & Costello, T. J. (2015). Increasing compliance with national quality measures for stroke through use of a standard order set. *American Journal of Health-System Pharmacy, 72*(11 Suppl. 1), S6–S10.

El-Radhi, A. S. (2015). Management of seizures in children. *British Journal of Nursing (Mark Allen Publishing), 24*(3), 152–155.

Epilepsy Foundation. (n.d.-a). Diagnosis. Retrieved from http://www.epilepsy.com/learn/diagnosing-epilepsy

Epilepsy Foundation. (n.d.-b). Driver and the law. Retrieved from http://www.epilepsy.com/search/site/driving?f[0]=bundle%3Adriving_laws

Epilepsy Foundation. (n.d.-c). Febrile convulsions (3 months to 5 years). Retrieved from http://www.epilepsy.com/information/professionals/about-epilepsy-seizures/idiopathic-epileptic-seizures-and-syndromes-1

Epilepsy Foundation. (n.d.-d). First aid for seizures. Retrieved from http://www.epilepsy.com/learn/treating-seizures-and-epilepsy/first-aid/first-aid-resources

Epilepsy Foundation. (n.d.-e). Injuries from seizures. Retrieved from http://www.epilepsy.com/get-help/staying-safe/types-injuries

Epilepsy Foundation. (n.d.-f). Photosensitivity and epilepsy. Retrieved from http://www.epilepsy.com/learn/triggers-seizures/photosensitivity-and-seizures

Epilepsy Foundation. (n.d.-g). Seizure provoking triggers. Retrieved from http://www.epilepsy.com/learn/triggers-seizures

Epilepsy Foundation. (n.d.-h). Seizures. Retrieved from http://www.epilepsy.com/learn/types-seizures

Epilepsy Foundation. (n.d.-i). Suicide risk. Retrieved from http://www.epilepsy.com/article/2014/3/antiepileptic-drugs-and-suicidality

Epilepsy Foundation. (n.d.-j). Treatment. Retrieved from http://www.epilepsy.com/learn/treating-seizures-and-epilepsy

Family Doctor. (n.d.). Headaches in elderly people. Retrieved from www.familydoctor.co.uk/node/530

Faust, K., & Jennings, C. (2016). Carpal tunnel syndrome. Retrieved from www.orthoinfo.aaos.org/topic.cfm?topic=A00005

Frishberg, B., Rosenberg, J., Matchar, D., McCrory, D., Pietrzak, M., Rozen, R., & Silberstein, S. (n.d). Evidence-based guidelines in the primary care setting: Neuroimaging in patients with nonacute headache. Retrieved from www.aan.com/professionals/practice/pdfs/gl0088.pdf

Furman, J. M. (2013). Patient information: Dizziness and vertigo (beyond the basics). *UpToDate.* Retrieved from http://www.uptodate.com/contents/dizziness-and-vertigo-beyond-the-basics?view=print

Gioia, G. A. (2014). Medical-school partnership in guiding return to school following mild traumatic brain injury in youth. *Journal of Child Neurology, 31*(1), 1–16.

Giza, C. C., Kutcher, J. S., Ashwal, S., Barth, J., Getchius, T. S., Gioia, G. A., . . . Zafonte, R. (2013). Summary of evidence-based guideline update: Evaluation and management of concussion in sports: Report of the Guideline Development Subcommittee of the American Academy of Neurology. *Neurology, 80*(24), 2250–2257.

Gullo, H. L., Hatton, A. L., Bennett, S., Fleming, J., & Shum, D. H. K. (2016). Habitual and low-intensity physical activity in people with multiple sclerosis. *Brain Impairment, 17*(1), 77–86. doi:10.1017/BrImp.2016.9

Halloran, L. (2013, April). Cognitive impairment: Pearls for practice. *Journal for Nurse Practitioners, 9*, 254–255.

Hargroves, D., & Ward, L. (2015). Anticoagulants for stroke prevention in patients with atrial fibrillation. *British Journal of Neuroscience Nursing, 11*(Suppl. 2), 31–37.

Heim, B., Djamshidian, A., Heidbreder, A., Stefani, A., Zamarian, L., Pertl, M. T., . . . Högl, B. (2016). Augmentation and impulsive behaviors in restless legs syndrome: Coexistence or association? *Neurology, 87*(1), 36–40.

Hoogwout, S. J., Paananen, M. V., Smith, A. J., Beales, D. J., O'Sullivan, P. B., Straker, L. M., . . . Champion, D. (2015). Musculoskeletal pain is associated with restless legs syndrome in young adults. *BioMedCentral Musculoskeletal Disorders, 16*, 294.

Illinois Neurological Institute. (2013). Headaches and sleep. Retrieved from www.ini.org/services/sleep-disorders/conditions-treated/headaches-and-sleep.html

International Headache Society ICHD-II. (n.d.-a). Cluster headache. Retrieved from https://www.ichd-3.org/3-trigeminal-autonomic-cephalalgias/3-1-cluster-headache

International Headache Society ICHD-II. (n.d.-b). Migraine. Retrieved from https://www.ichd-3.org/1-migraine

International Headache Society ICHD-II. (n.d.-c). New daily-persistent headache (NDPH). Retrieved from https://www.ichd-3.org/other-primary-headache-disorders/4-10-new-daily-persistent-headache-ndph

International Headache Society ICHD-II. (n.d.-d). Tension-type headache (alternative criteria). Retrieved from https://www.ichd-3.org/appendix/a2-tension-type-headache-alternative-criteria

Jamault, V., & Duff, E. (2013). Adolescent concussions: When to return to play. *Nurse Practitioner, 38*(2), 16–22; quiz 22.

Jauch, E. (2016, March). Acute management of stroke. *Medscape.* Retrieved from http://emedicine.medscape.com/article/1159752-overview#a8

Jeong, J. H., Lee, J. H., Kim, K., Jo, Y. H., Rhee, J. E., Kwak, Y. H., . . . Noh, H. (2014). Rate of and risk factors for early recurrence in patients with febrile seizures. *Pediatric Emergency Care, 30*(8), 540–545.

Kalita, J., Kohat, A. K., & Misra, U. K. (2014). Predictors of outcome of myasthenic crisis. *Neurological Sciences, 35*(7), 1109–1114.

Kang, M. Y., & Ellis-Hill, C. (2015). How do people live life successfully with Parkinson's disease? *Journal of Clinical Nursing, 24*(15–16), 2314–2322.

Khoo, T. K., Yarnall, A. J., Duncan, G. W., Coleman, S., O'Brien, J. T., Brooks, D. J., . . . Burn, D. J. (2013). The spectrum of nonmotor symptoms in early Parkinson disease. *Neurology, 80*(3), 276–281.

Klingelhoefer, L., Bhattacharya, K., & Reichmann, H. (2016). Restless legs syndrome. *Clinical Medicine (London, England), 16*(4), 379–382.

Lee, C. S., Kim, T., Lee, S., Jeon, H. J., Bang, Y. R., & Yoon, I. Y. (2016). Symptom severity of restless legs syndrome predicts its clinical course. *American Journal of Medicine, 129*(4), 438–445.

Levin, H. S., & Diaz-Arrastia, R. R. (2015). Diagnosis, prognosis, and clinical management of mild traumatic brain injury. *Lancet Neurology, 14*(5), 506–517.

Liew, W. K., & Kang, P. B. (2013). Update on juvenile myasthenia gravis. *Current Opinion in Pediatrics, 25*(6), 694–700.

Lo, A. X., & Harada, C. N. (2013). Geriatric dizziness: Evolving diagnostic and therapeutic approaches for the emergency department. *Clinics in Geriatric Medicine, 29*(1), 181–204.

Loder, E., Burch, R., & Rizzoli, P. (2012). The 2012 AHS/AAN guidelines for prevention of episodic migraine: A summary and comparison with other recent clinical practice guidelines. *Headache, 52*(6), 930–945.

Lopez, J. I. (2013, January 28). Pediatric headache treatment & management. *Medscape.* Retrieved from http://emedicine.medscape.com/article/2110861-treatment

Mace, N., & Rabins, P. (2012). *The 36-hour day: A family guide to caring for people who have Alzheimer's disease, related dementias and memory loss.* (5th ed.). Baltimore, MA: John Hopkins University Press. Retrieved from www.press.jhu.edu

Marshall, S., Bayley, M., McCullagh, S., Velikonja, D., Berrigan, L., Ouchterlony, D., & Weegar, K.; mTBI Expert Consensus Group. (2015). Updated clinical practice guidelines for concussion/mild traumatic brain injury and persistent symptoms. *Brain Injury, 29*(6), 688–700.

Mayo Clinic. (2016). Parkinson's disease. Retrieved from www.mayoclinic.org

McCarthy, C., & Thorpe, J. (2016). Some recent advances in multiple sclerosis. *Journal of Neurology, 263*(9), 1880–1886.

McCrory, P., Meeuwisse, W. H., Echemendia, R. J., Iverson, G. L., Dvorák, J., & Kutcher, J. S. (2013). What is the lowest threshold to make a diagnosis of concussion? *British Journal of Sports Medicine, 47*(5), 268–271.

MD Guidelines. (n.d.). Guillain–Barré syndrome. Retrieved from www.mdguidelines.com/guillain-barre-syndrome

Mendiola-Precoma, J., Berumen, L. C., Padilla, K., & Garcia-Alcocer, G. (2016). Therapies for prevention and treatment of Alzheimer's disease. *BioMed Research International, 2016.* Retrieved from www.hindawi.com/journals/bmri/2016/2589276

Merkies, I. S., Schmitz, P. L., van der Meché, F. G., Samihn, J. P., & van Doorn, P. A. (INCAT Group). (2016). Overall disability sum score: Overall disability scale online calculator. Retrieved from http://farmacologiaclinica.info/scales/overall-disability-sum-score/

MPR Nurse Practioners' Edition. (2013). New York, NY: Haymarket Media.

Nanda, A. (2016). Transient ischemic attack. *Medscape.* Retrieved from http://.emedicine.medscape.comarticle/1910519-overview

National Institute of Neurological Disorders and Stroke. (2013). NINDS transient ischemic attack information page. Retrieved from www.ninds.nih.gov/disorders/tia/tia.htm?css=print

National Institute of Neurological Disorders and Stroke. (2015). Restless legs syndrome fact sheet. Retrieved from http://www.ninds.nih.gov/Disorders/Patient-Caregiver-Education/Fact-Sheets/Restless-Legs-Syndrome-Fact-Sheet

National Institute of Neurological Disorders and Stroke. (2016a). Bell's palsy fact sheet. Retrieved from http://www.ninds.nih.gov /Disorders/Patient-Caregiver-Education/Fact-Sheets/Bells-Palsy-Fact-Sheet

National Institute of Neurological Disorders and Stroke. (2016b). Febrile seizures fact sheet. Retrieved from www.ninds.nih.gov/disorders/febrile_seizures

National Institutes of Health. (2016). Guillain-Barré syndrome fact sheet. Retrieved from www.ninds.nih.gov/Disorders/Patient-Caregiver-Education/Fact-Sheets/Guillain-Barré-Syndrome-Fact-Sheet

National Stroke Association. (n.d.). National Stroke Association guidelines for the management of TIA. Retrieved from www.stroke.org/site/Docserver/TIA_Guidelines_070506_sm.pdf?docID=2361

Nentwich, L. M. (2013, March 4). Transient ischemic attack. *Medscape.* Retrieved from http://emedicine.medscape.com/article/1910519-overview

Oikarinen, A., Engblom, J., Kääriäinen, M., & Kyngäs, H. (2015). Risk factor-related lifestyle habits of hospital-admitted stroke patients—an exploratory study. *Journal of Clinical Nursing, 24*(15–16), 2219–2230.

Oomens, M. A., & Forouzanfar, T. (2015). Pharmaceutical management of trigeminal neuralgia in the elderly. *Drugs & Aging, 32*(9), 717–726.

Patel, N., Ram, D., Swiderska, N., Mewasingh, L. D., Newton, R. W., & Offringa, M. (2015). Febrile seizures. *British Medical Journal (Clinical Research Ed.), 351,* h4240.

Patterson, J. L., Carapetian, S. A., Hageman, J. R., & Kelley, K. R. (2013). Febrile seizures. *Pediatric Annals, 42*(12), 249–254.

Plosker, G. L. (2015). Memantine extended release (28 mg once daily): A review of its use in Alzheimer's disease. *Drugs, 75*(8), 887–897.

Ramadan, N., Silberstein, S., Frietag, F., Gilbert, T., & Frishberg, B. (2016). Evidence-based guidelines for migraine headaches in the primary care: Pharmacological management for prevention of migraine. Retrieved from http://www.neurologiaszakvizsga.usn.hu/pdfs/71.pdf

Rose, S. C., Weber, K. D., Collen, J. B., & Heyer, G. L. (2015). The diagnosis and management of concussion in children and adolescents. *Pediatric Neurology, 53*(2), 108–118.

Roy, S., Benedict, R. H., Drake, A. S., & Weinstock-Guttman, B. (2016). Impact of pharmacotherapy on cognitive dysfunction in patients with multiple sclerosis. *CNS Drugs, 30*(3), 209–225.

Scheltens, N. M., Galindo-Garre, F., Pijnenburg, Y. A., van der Vlies, A. E., Smits, L. L., Koene, T., . . . van der Flier, W. M. (2016). The identification of cognitive subtypes in Alzheimer's disease dementia using latent class analysis. *Journal of Neurology, Neurosurgery, and Psychiatry, 87*(3), 235–243.

Silver, B. (2015). Stroke prevention. *Medscape.* Retrieved from http://emedicine.medscape.com/article/323662-overview

Suzuki, K., Miyamoto, M., Miyamoto, T., & Hirata, K. (2015). Restless legs syndrome and leg motor restlessness in Parkinson's disease. *Parkinson's Disease, 2015,* 490938. doi:10.1155/2015/490938

Sweeney, T. E., Salles, A., Harris, O. A., Spain, D. A., & Staudenmayer, K. L. (2015). Prediction of neurosurgical intervention after mild traumatic brain injury using the national trauma data bank. *World Journal of Emergency Surgery, 10,* 23.

Torkildsen, O., Myhr, K.-M., & Bø, L. (2015). Disease-modifying treatments for multiple sclerosis: A review of approved medications. *European Journal of Neurology, 23*(Suppl. 1), 18–27.

Vestibular Disorder Association. (n.d.-a). Benign paroxysmal positional vertical (BPPV). Retrieved from http://vestibular.org/understanding-vestibular-disorders/types-vestibular-disorders/benign-paroxysmal-positional-vertigo

Vestibular Disorder Association. (n.d.-b). Ménière's disease. Retrieved from http://vestibular.org/menieres-disease

Vestibular Disorder Association. (n.d.-c). Surgical procedures for vestibular dysfunction Retrieved from http://vestibular.org/understanding-vestibular-disorders/treatment/vestibular-surgery

Vestibular Disorder Association. (n.d.-d). Vestibular neuritis and labyrinthitis. Retrieved from http://vestibular.org/labyrinthitis-and-vestibular-neuritis

Vriesendorp, F. J. (2013). Treatment and prognosis of Guillain-Barré syndrome in adults. *UpToDate.* Retrieved from http://www.uptodate.com/contents/treatment-and-prognosis-of-guillain-barre-syndrome-inadults?topicKey=NEURO%2F5172

Wells, E. M., Goodkin, H. P., & Griesbach, G. S. (2016). Challenges in determining the role of rest and exercise in the management of mild traumatic brain injury. *Journal of Child Neurology, 31*(1), 86–92.

Zakrzewska, J. M. (2015). Trigeminal neuralgia: Unilateral episodic facial pain. *Journal of Pain & Palliative Care Pharmacotherapy, 29*(2), 182–184.

Zakrzewska, J. M., & Linskey, M. E. (2016). Trigeminal neuralgia. *American Family Physician, 94*(2), 133–135.

Živković, S. (2015). Intravenous immunoglobulin in the treatment of neurologic disorders. *Acta Neurologica Scandinavica, 133*(5), 84–96.

20 Endocrine Guidelines

Addison's Disease

Jill C. Cash and Mellisa A. Hall

Definition

A. Primary adrenal insufficiency resulting in glucocorticoid and mineralocorticoid insufficiency

Incidence

A. Approximately 40 to 60 cases per million people; idiopathic autoimmune disease is more common in women and children. There is no racial predilection.

Pathogenesis

A. Autoimmune dysfunction of the adrenals accounts for up to 80% of cases; 10% to 20% of cases are attributed to tuberculosis. At least 90% of the adrenal gland is destroyed, resulting in chronic cortisol deficiency, reduced aldosterone, and decreased adrenal androgens. As a result, volume and sodium depletions occur with potassium excess. The risk of death in patients with Addison's disease is twofold that of the general population due to higher rates of cardiovascular disease, cancer, and infectious disease.

Predisposing Factors

A. Other autoimmune disorders
  1. Insulin-dependent diabetes mellitus (IDDM)
  2. Pernicious anemia
  3. Thyroid disorders
B. Disseminated tuberculosis
C. Gonadal failure
D. Hypoparathyroidism
E. Vitiligo
F. Alopecia areata
G. Chronic active hepatitis
H. Metastatic disease (especially lung and breast cancer)
I. AIDS
J. Certain medications (e.g., ketoconazole, anticoagulant)
K. Fungal disease
L. Bleeding diathesis (e.g., disseminated intravascular coagulation [DIC])
M. Sepsis
N. Metabolic stress
O. Trauma
P. Bilateral nephrectomy
Q. Pituitary tumors

Common Complaints[a]

A. Weakness
B. Fatigue
C. Anorexia
D. Nausea
E. Diarrhea
F. Abdominal pain
G. Weight loss
H. Hyperpigmentation
I. Hypoglycemia (more often in children)
J. Low libido
K. Salt craving

Other Signs and Symptoms

A. Proximal muscle weakness
B. Failure to gain weight (children)
C. Muscle and joint pain
D. Reduced axillary/pubic hair in women
E. Amenorrhea
F. Hypotension
G. Anemia with
  1. Lymphocytosis
  2. Eosinophilia
  3. Neutropenia
  4. Hyponatremia
  5. Hyperkalemia
  6. Hypoglycemia
  7. Hypercalcemia
H. Positive antiadrenal antibodies
I. Low plasma cortisol or failure to rise after corticotropin (adrenocorticotropic hormone [ACTH]) administration
J. EKG changes: Decreased voltage, prolonged PR and QT intervals, and general slowed rhythm

> *Missed or delayed diagnosis can lead to acute adrenal crisis, a medical emergency evidenced by sudden low back, abdominal, or leg pain; severe vomiting or diarrhea; hypotension; and loss of consciousness.*

Subjective Data

A. Determine extent of fatigue.
B. Elicit degree and location of weakness.
C. Question the patient regarding appetite, nausea, or diarrhea.
D. Evaluate food intake.

---

[a] Usually presenting as insidious and nonspecific.

E. Determine the amount of weight loss or weight gain (children).
F. Discuss hypopigmentation or hyperpigmentation and whether it occurs on unexposed areas as well as exposed areas of the skin.
G. Note presence of abdominal, muscle, and joint pain.
H. Assess for lightheadedness and/or fainting and when it occurs.
I. Inquire about the patient's history of cancer or fungal infections.
J. Note last date of tuberculosis evaluation (purified protein derivative [PPD]) and results.
K. Determine HIV status or risk.
L. For women, discuss pubic and axillary hair distributions and note menstrual patterns.
M. Inquire about libido.
N. Inquire regarding cold intolerance.
O. Ask about recent illness and treatments.
P. Determine patient's occupation to assess safety risk if weakness or dizziness present.

Physical Examination

A. Check pulse, respirations, and blood pressure (BP); pulse and BP while seated and standing; and weight.
B. Inspect
  1. Observe overall appearance.
  2. Note hair distribution and skin pigmentation, especially sun-exposed surfaces.
C. Auscultate
  1. The heart, lungs, and abdomen
D. Palpate
  1. The abdomen
E. Musculoskeletal: Perform complete musculoskeletal examination.

Diagnostic Tests

A. Serum chemistry, electrolytes, blood urea nitrogen (BUN), creatinine, glomerular filtration rate (GFR)
B. Complete blood count (CBC)
C. PPD
D. Rapid ACTH test: Rapid ACTH stimulation test excludes or establishes adrenal insufficiency but does not differentiate between primary and secondary adrenal insufficiencies; with abnormal results (plasma cortisol less than 18–20 mcg/dL), proceed to plasma ACTH levels.
E. Plasma ACTH level
F. Serum creatinine kinase (CK) levels

Plasma ACTH level differentiates among primary (adrenal) and secondary (pituitary) or tertiary (hypothalamus) etiologies (high plasma ACTH with primary insufficiency whereas normal or low with secondary insufficiency). The clinician can use ACTH–corticotropin-releasing hormone (CRH) to distinguish between pituitary and hypothalamic etiologies.

G. Antiadrenal antibodies: A negative adrenal antibody test is observed in only 30% to 50% of persons with idiopathic Addison's disease and does not rule out adrenal insufficiency of autoimmune etiology.
H. CT scan of adrenals

Differential Diagnoses

A. Secondary adrenal insufficiency (usually after exogenous glucocorticoid therapy)
B. Hypothalamic/pituitary lesions
C. Diabetic coma
D. Salt-losing nephritis
E. Acute infections
F. Occult cancer
G. Anorexia nervosa
H. Hemochromatosis
I. Acute poisoning
J. Myasthenia gravis
K. Pigmentation due to racial/ethnic variations
L. Premature primary ovarian failure
M. Testicular failure
N. Pernicious anemia
O. Cancer
P. Iatrogenic Cushing's syndrome

Plan

A. General interventions
  1. If primary adrenal insufficiency is established, and the cause is not apparent, order adrenal CT scan to look for metastatic disease, sarcoidosis, and tuberculosis.
B. Patient teaching
  1. *See Section III: Patient Teaching Guide for this chapter, "Addison's Disease."* ◀
  2. Teach the patient regarding adrenal crisis and encourage treatment before symptoms begin.
  3. Encourage the patient to avoid contacts that predispose him or her to infections.
C. Pharmaceutical therapy
  1. Hydrocortisone (drug of choice) or prednisone in three doses (every 8 hours), or two thirds in the morning and the remainder in the afternoon or early evening; 12 to 15 mg cortisol/m^2 body surface area; most adults need a total of 20 to 30 mg/d.
  2. Increase hydrocortisone dose or add prednisone if ill; if accompanied by diarrhea, excessive sweating, or fever, the patient should double the routine dose.
  3. Simultaneously decrease fludrocortisone about 50% to avoid salt retention and elevated BP.
    a. Total daily stress dose is about 100 to 400 mg hydrocortisone.
  4. If serum aldosterone is undetectable, mineralocorticoid replacement is likely necessary in addition to glucocorticoid.
  5. Abrupt discontinuation of exogenous glucocorticoid administration after a course as short as 3 weeks may induce temporary secondary adrenal insufficiency, leading to decreased cortisol but normal or near-normal aldosterone production. This may occur up to 12 months after discontinuation of glucocorticoid therapy.
  6. Pediatrics
    a. Hydrocortisone 10 to 20 mg/m^2/d in three divided doses: With adrenal enzyme defects, 25% in morning and afternoon and 50% at night.

b. Fludrocortisone acetate typically 0.05 to 0.2 mg/d every day or two divided doses for children.

Follow-Up

A. Plasma renin activity: When less than 10 ng/mL, this is a probable indication of adequate fludrocortisone dose.
B. Serum and urinary cortisol and serum ACTH to monitor hydrocortisone dose. Urinary free cortisol greater than 70 mcg/24 hr indicates excessive hydrocortisone dose, whereas values less than 20 mcg/24 hr indicate inadequate hydrocortisone dose.
C. Monitor BP and serum electrolytes to determine fludrocortisone dose.
D. Do annual adrenal function studies.

Consultation/Referral

A. If Addison's disease is suspected, consult with a physician.
B. Consider Addison's disease in any patient with hypotension and hyperkalemia.

Individual Considerations

A. Pregnancy
 1. Due to changes in plasma cortisol, diagnosis is based on lack of rise in plasma cortisol concentration after ACTH administration.
 2. If nausea and vomiting are problems, intramuscular glucocorticoid may be necessary.
 3. Delivery requires increased glucocorticoid dose similar to surgery.
B. Pediatrics
 1. Leading causes of Addison's disease are hereditary enzymatic defects, resulting in congenital adrenal hyperplasia (CAH), as well as idiopathic causes.
 2. Although rare in pediatrics, common presentations include malaise, nausea, vomiting, and weight loss. Poor vascular tone, hyperpigmentation, hyponatremia, hyperkalemia, and ketonemia are classic findings.
 3. Medications should be adjusted with the child's growth.
C. Geriatrics
 1. Urinary excretion rate of cortisol decreases by about 25%; serum level and response to ACTH stimulation are unchanged.

> *Safety Consideration: Patients receiving long-term replacement should carry a medication card as well as wear a medical alert bracelet or necklace. Parenteral therapy is required if patients are unable to take required replacement medication orally.*

Cushing's Syndrome

Jill C. Cash and Mellisa A. Hall

Definition

A. Cushing's syndrome is a cluster of symptoms, signs, and biochemical abnormalities arising from glucocorticoid overproduction. Iatrogenically induced Cushing's syndrome is the most common cause.

Incidence

A. For endogenous cases, two to four new cases per 1,000,000 annually; it is five times more frequent in women.

Pathogenesis

The cause is exogenous (chronic glucocorticoid or ACTH administration) or endogenous (increased ACTH secretion). The endogenous type is due to either excessive pituitary or ectopic ACTH secretion (ACTH dependent), resulting in signs of androgen excess or autonomous cortisol overproduction (ACTH independent [of ACTH regulation]), as well as depressed ACTH production and absent signs of androgen excess. The etiology of spontaneous Cushing's (adults) comprises:
A. 70% to 80% pituitary ACTH hypersecretion (90% pituitary adenoma, 10% pituitary hyperplasia)
B. 10% to 15% autonomous adrenal tumor (adenoma or carcinoma)
C. 5% to 15% ectopic ACTH secretion (nonpituitary neoplasm, usually lung)
D. Less than 1% bilateral nodular hyperplasia without ACTH
E. Among children younger than 12 years, the cause is usually iatrogenic. Cortisol excess precipitates generalized protein catabolism, reduced intestinal calcium reabsorption, elevated hepatic gluconeogenesis and glycogenosis, impaired collagen production leading to atrophy of connective and fatty tissues, impaired immune and inflammatory responses, and accelerated atherosclerosis.

Predisposing Factors

A. Exogenous glucocorticoid administration
B. Excessive alcohol intake
C. Pituitary adenoma
D. Thoracic tumors
E. Adrenal neoplasms
F. Tumors of the pancreas
G. Thyroid and thymus disease
H. Pheochromocytoma

Common Complaints

A. Excessive coarse hair on face, chest, and back
B. Rapid weight gain
C. Easy bruising
D. Muscle weakness
E. Oligo- or amenorrhea
F. Impotence
G. Depression
H. Poorly controlled diabetes
I. Irregular menses

Other Signs and Symptoms

A. Cervicodorsal and supraclavicular fat pad
B. Hirsutism in women
C. Acne and/or folliculitis
D. Increased intraocular pressure
E. Purple striae
F. Increased blood pressure (BP)
G. Polydipsia/polyuria, increased serum glucose, and glycosuria

H. Osteopenia/osteoporosis
I. Mood lability/changes
J. Growth deceleration (children)
K. Delayed skeletal maturation (children)
L. Spontaneous hypokalemia
M. Erythrocytosis

Subjective Data

A. Ask whether the patient has taken exogenous glucocorticoids.
B. Determine whether the onset of complaints was acute or subacute.
C. Assess for bruising and determine if bruising was precipitated by trauma.
D. Assess for muscle weakness and, if present, whether it is proximal weakness.
E. Review the patient's menstrual history, including characteristics of menstrual periods.
F. Identify the patient's family history of similar problems.
G. Question the patient regarding any vision impairment.
H. Rule out the presence of abdominal pain.
I. Review the patient's history of neoplasms and location.
J. Identify the current pattern of sexual function.
K. Question the patient regarding mood swings or recent treatment for psychiatric disorder.
L. Identify the pattern of weight gain and effectiveness of weight-loss interventions, if implemented.
M. Assess for the presence of leg or arm pain.
N. Review the patient's history of fractures, especially if postmenopausal.
O. Determine the amount of alcohol consumed.

Physical Examination

A. Check pulse, height, and weight.
B. Inspect
  1. Inspect the skin, noting hair distribution, lesions, bruising, and striae.
  2. Observe the face and note shape.
  3. Observe the neck.

Note that a "moon-shaped" face and fat pads in posterior neck ("buffalo hump") are characteristics of patients with Cushing's syndrome.

  4. Complete a funduscopic examination. Be alert for cataracts, glaucoma, and/or signs of benign intracranial hypertension.
C. Auscultate
  1. Auscultate the heart and lungs.
  2. Hypercoagulable state should be considered with risk for pulmonary embolism.
D. Musculoskeletal
  1. Complete musculoskeletal examination. Be alert for septic necrosis of femoral and/or humeral head.
  2. Assess for kyphosis or back pain associated with osteoporosis and long-term cortisol excess.
E. Peripheral vascular
  1. Assess for deep vein thrombosis due to the hypercoagulable state.

Initial Diagnostic Tests

A. Serum electrolytes
B. Complete blood count (CBC) and glucose
C. 24-hour urine-free cortisol (at least two measurements)
D. Late-night salivary cortisol (at least two measurements)
E. Late-night serum cortisol (typically inpatient study)
F. Overnight dexamethasone suppression test, 1 mg
G. Bone density studies

The overnight dexamethasone suppression test has a false positive rate of 20% to 30%; false positives can occur with obesity, stress, depression, alcoholism, pregnancy, or medications that increase the hepatic metabolism of cortisol and dexamethasone (e.g., antiseizure drugs, estrogen, and rifampin). The false negative rate is less than 3%. Use the low-dose dexamethasone test as an alternative.

The 24-hour urinary-free cortisol is the most sensitive and specific test and is the best choice for screening.

If any of the earlier initial lab screenings are positive, the patient should be referred to endocrinology for additional evaluation.

Differential Diagnoses

A. Iatrogenically induced Cushing's syndrome
B. Depression
C. Severe obesity
D. Chronic stress
E. Familial cortisol resistance
F. Medication induced (e.g., phenytoin, phenobarbital, primidone)
G. Pituitary adenoma
H. Adrenal and other neoplasms
I. Alcoholism
J. Nephrolithiasis
K. Psychosis

Plan

A. General interventions
  1. Taper glucocorticoid dose as appropriate for the underlying disease.
  2. Begin alcohol detoxification if applicable.
  3. Consider hormone replacement therapy for postmenopausal women.
B. Patient teaching
  1. *See Section III: Patient Teaching Guide for this chapter, "Cushing's Syndrome."* ◀
C. Medical/surgical management
  1. If noniatrogenic etiology, surgery is the treatment of choice followed by irradiation and/or chemotherapy.
D. Pharmaceutical therapy
  1. Calcium 1,000 mg/d and vitamin D 400 IU/d.
  2. Mitotane (Lysodren) 2 to 5 g daily for control of adrenocortical carcinoma progression.
  3. Metyrapone inhibits adrenal steroid biosynthesis.
  4. Ketoconazole (most useful for blocking adrenal steroidogenesis) and suramin inhibit adrenal steroid biosynthesis. Ketoconazole is associated with hepatic

failure and drug–drug interactions, resulting in fatal ventricular arrhythmias. An endocrinologist should be consulted before the use of oral ketoconazole.

a. Ketoconazole should be started at a dose of 200 mg two or three times daily and increased rapidly to 400 mg three times daily; higher doses are seldom more effective. Increase every 4 to 7 days. Avoid use in pregnancy.

5. Hydrocortisone may be given in physiological doses to avoid adrenal insufficiency.

Most persons on a daily steroid program for more than 2 to 4 weeks have some degree of hypothalamic–pituitary–adrenal axis suppression.

6. Mifepristone (RU 486) is given for ectopic ACTH production or adrenal carcinoma. Mifepristone is an abortifacient.

Follow-Up

A. At the provider's discretion, 1 to 2 weeks after tests are complete, follow up to discuss results and possible therapy.

Consultation/Referral

A. If Cushing's syndrome is suspected, consult with an endocrinologist regarding treatment and therapy.

Individual Considerations

A. Pregnancy

1. Urinary-free cortisol increases in the third trimester but women still have normal 17-hydroxycorticosteroids and normal diurnal variability of serum cortisol. Dexamethasone testing is not recommended in the initial screening for Cushing's syndrome during pregnancy.

B. Pediatrics

1. It is possible to differentiate between exogenous obesity and Cushing's syndrome by the child's growth rate; exogenous obesity is characterized by normal or slightly increased growth rate.

Resource

National Adrenal Diseases Foundation: www.nadf.us/links-resources/international-adrenal-disease-groups-resources

Diabetes Mellitus

Jill C. Cash and Mellisa A. Hall

Definition

Diabetes is a group of diseases characterized by high levels of blood glucose with a defect in insulin secretion or action caused by a chronic disorder of carbohydrate, fat, and protein metabolism. There are four categories of diabetes: Type 1, type 2, gestational, and diabetes from secondary causes.

A. Type 1 diabetes, formerly referred to as insulin-dependent diabetes mellitus (IDDM) or juvenile-onset diabetes, is an endocrine condition in which there is complete destruction of pancreatic beta cells or a complete absence of insulin.

B. Type 2 diabetes, formerly referred to as noninsulin-dependent diabetes mellitus (NIDDM) or adult-onset diabetes, describes a condition in which individuals have an impairment in insulin production and/or insulin resistance.

C. Gestational diabetes is diagnosed during pregnancy. It usually disappears when the pregnancy is completed. It will increase the woman's risk of developing type 2 diabetes later in lifes.

D. Diabetes resulting from secondary causes is due to genetic defects and/or diseases of the pancreas, such as cystic fibrosis. Other causes of this type of diabetes can be drug-/chemical-induced diabetes from medications or therapies used when treating HIV/AIDS and in patients who receive treatments after organ transplantation.

E. People with diabetes are more prone to have unhealthy low-density lipoprotein cholesterol (LDL-C) and therefore are at increased risk for atherosclerotic cardiovascular disease (ASCVD). The incidence of cardiovascular disease (CVD) is two to four times higher in adults with diabetes. The risk of stroke is two to four times higher because 60% to 65% of the patients have hypertension.

Incidence

A. It is estimated that more than 29.1 million Americans have diabetes, 9.3% of the population. Diagnosed cases account for 21 million with an estimated 8.1 million who have not been diagnosed. Type 1 diabetes accounts for less than 10% of diagnosed cases. There are 1.9 million new cases reported a year, not counting people 19 years old or younger.

Pathogenesis

A. Type 1 diabetes is an inherited defect causing an alteration in immunologic integrity, placing the beta cell at risk for inflammatory damage. The mechanism of damage is autoimmune. Environmental factors that may influence the etiology of diabetes include viral illnesses: Mumps, coxsackievirus, cytomegalovirus, and hepatitis. Other factors that may influence the disease include diets high in dairy products, emotional and physical stress, and/or environmental toxins.

B. Type 2 diabetes involves impaired insulin secretion, insulin resistance, and/or an abnormally elevated glucose production by the liver. Genetics and obesity are major risk factors.

C. The severity of carbohydrate intolerance in gestational diabetes is unknown. Women identified at risk have screening done during the 24th and 28th weeks of gestation.

D. Genetic defects and medications/chemicals are thought to affect the beta-cell function and alter insulin function. Hemoglobin A_{1c} ($HgbA_{1c}$) levels may not be interpreted correctly in patients with blood disorders such as anemia/hemoglobinopathies. See www.ngsp.org/interf.asp for a complete list of laboratory methods recommended to be used to measure $HgbA_{1c}$ values for patients with hemoglobin variants (sickle cell trait, HbC, HbS, HbE, HbD trait, or elevated HbF).

Predisposing Factors

A. Body mass index (BMI) greater than or equal to 27 kg/m^2
B. Physical inactivity
C. First-degree relative with type 1 or type 2 diabetes
D. A_{1c} greater than or equal to 5.7%, impaired glucose tolerance (IGT) or impaired fasting glucose (IFG) on previous testing
E. Native American, Hispanic, Asian, African American, and Pacific Islander heritage
F. Hypertension with systolic pressure greater than 140 mmHg and diastolic pressure greater than 90 mmHg
G. High-density lipoprotein (HDL) level of 35 mg/dL or less and/or triglyceride level of greater than or equal to 250 mg/dL
H. History of giving birth to babies larger than 9 pounds or gestational diabetes
I. History of IGT or fasting glucose
J. Acanthosis nigricans or severe obesity
K. Polycystic ovarian syndrome (PCOS)
L. History of CVD
M. History of gestational diabetes
N. The United States Preventive Services Task Force (USPSTF) recommends screening for abnormal blood glucose as part of cardiovascular risk assessment in adults aged 40 to 70 years who are overweight or obese.

Common Complaints

A. Classic triad of symptoms
  1. Polyuria
  2. Polydipsia
  3. Polyphagia
B. Weight loss
C. Lack of energy
D. Recurrent infections (urinary tract, vaginal, skin breakdown that is slow to heal)
E. Asymptomatic

Other Signs and Symptoms

A. Weakness
B. Fatigue
C. Nausea and vomiting
D. Abdominal pain
E. Anorexia
F. Sexual dysfunction, including impotence or dyspareunia
G. Itching
H. Visual disturbances
I. Signs and symptoms related to nephropathy, neuropathy, and/or retinopathy

Subjective Data

A. Obtain a detailed history regarding onset, duration, and course of presenting symptoms.
B. Question the patient regarding all characteristic signs and symptoms of diabetes.
C. Determine the patient's nutritional status, 24-hour recall, weight history, and eating patterns.
D. Review the family history of diabetes or other endocrine disorders.
E. Note predisposing factors to diabetes.
F. Review the patient's social history, including smoking, alcohol, and exercise.

Physical Examination

A. Check pulse, respirations, blood pressure (BP), and weight.
B. Inspect
  1. Observe overall appearance.
  2. Perform oral examination. Diabetic patients are prone to thrush, gingivitis, plaque, and infections. A dental examination should be done every 6 months.
  3. Complete funduscopic examination. Proliferative diabetic retinopathy is the leading cause of new blindness in adults in the United States. Patients with diabetes are 25 times more at risk for blindness and have four to six times the increased risk for cataracts and twice the increased risk for glaucoma.
  4. Inspect the skin, including feet, with monofilament testing, hands, fingers, and skin folds for erythema and insulin injection sites.
C. Auscultate
  1. The heart
  2. The lungs
  3. The carotid arteries
D. Percuss
  1. The chest, abdomen, and deep tendon reflexes
E. Palpate
  1. The neck (thyroid)
  2. The abdomen
  3. The extremities for edema and assess peripheral pulses

Diagnostic Tests

A. Serum glycosylated hemoglobin A_{1c} ($HgbA_{1c}$) of 6.5% or higher
B. Fasting plasma glucose: Greater than or equal to 126 mg/dL. All patients should have a baseline fasting blood sugar (fasting for at least 8 hours) performed at 45 years of age, then repeated every 3 years. The baseline should be performed earlier if any predisposing factors exist.
C. Random plasma glucose: Greater than or equal to 200 mg/dL with symptoms of diabetes
D. Oral glucose tolerance test (OGTT): After a 75 g glucose load, a 2-hour plasma glucose greater than or equal to 200 mg/dL; IGT is a fasting plasma glucose of greater than or equal to 126 mg/dL.

> *According to the Diabetes Control and Complications Trial, an HgbA1c of 7.2% or below decreases the risk of retinopathy, neuropathy, and nephropathy by 50% to 70%.*

Differential Diagnoses

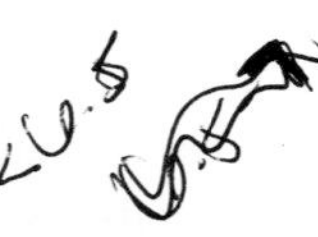

A. Diabetes mellitus (DM)
B. Benign pancreatic insufficiency
C. Pheochromocytoma
D. Cushing's syndrome
E. History of corticosteroid use
F. Stress hyperglycemia

G. Acromegaly
H. Hemochromatosis
I. Somogyi phenomenon: Early-morning hyperglycemia due to very early morning (2:00–3:00 a.m.) hypoglycemia

Plan

A. General interventions

1. Establish, review, and evaluate individual goals with the patient on a routine basis.

2. Center goals around normal metabolic control and the prevention and delay of complications while maintaining a flexible, normal, high-quality life.

3. After a new diagnosis is made and treatment has begun, be alert for an initial remission or a honeymoon phase with decreased insulin needs and better control that may last 3 to 6 months.

4. Include the following in the treatment plan:

a. Exercise plan

i. Develop a consistent, individualized exercise plan with the patient to improve insulin sensitivity, blood sugars, weight reduction, and reduction of cardiovascular complications.

ii. Evaluation by a health care provider, including a complete physical examination and EKG, must precede any exercise program.

iii. Generally, the goals for physical activity are to reduce LDL-C and non-HDL-C and to lower the BP. The exercise should be of moderate-to-vigorous intensity.

iv. Exercise should not be done if the fasting blood sugar is greater than 250 mg/dL and ketones are present in the urine or if the glucose level is greater than 300 mg/dL at any time regardless of the presence of ketones.

v. Because exercise can lower the blood sugar concentration, special precautions such as medication adjustment and meal planning should be done before and after exercise if the patient is taking insulin or a glucose-lowering medication.

b. Self-monitoring blood glucose (SMBG): The process of monitoring the patient's blood gives valuable information to the patient on a daily basis and assists the provider in identifying trends.

i. Several different meters are available with a variety of options. A certified diabetes educator can show examples of different types before the patient purchases one.

ii. Frequency of testing depends on the type of medication the patient is taking and the patient's compliance and motivation.

iii. Additional testing should be done at times of changes in medication, meal plans, and/or exercise; and during illness or stress.

iv. The Food and Drug Administration (FDA) has approved an automatic blood glucose suspend feature for continuous blood glucose monitoring that is recommended for patients with hypoglycemia unawareness or frequent nocturnal hypoglycemia.

c. Psychosocial support: It is important from the beginning of treatment to give the patient a sense of control.

i. Consistent involvement of family members will influence compliance.

ii. Assess and discuss psychosocial issues at each visit including depression.

B. Patient teaching

1. *See Section III: Patient Teaching Guide for this chapter, "Diabetes."*

2. Topics in the educational plan include the pathophysiology of diabetes, procedures for SMBG and medication therapies, recognition and treatment of hypoglycemia, and instructions for special situations such as illness and traveling.

3. Include preventive care, instructions for family members, and the importance of a MedicAlert tag available at: www.medicalert.org/product/catalog/medical-ids

4. Smoking cessation and avoidance of all tobacco products should be advised to all patients. Counseling regarding smoking/tobacco cessation methods and classes should be offered.

C. Dietary/physical activity management

1. Nutritional plan: The patient should meet with a dietitian who has experience with diabetes nutritional therapy.

2. Eating patterns and ideal percentage of calories from protein, carbohydrates, and fat should be individualized for each patient and determined along with a dietitian.

3. Involve the family to improve compliance with the individualized meal plan.

4. Overweight/obese patients are encouraged to set a goal of healthy eating strategies to enhance weight loss. Along with dietary management, exercise programs should be encouraged as soon as the primary care provider has approved that the patient is safe to perform physical exercise on a routine basis. It is recommended to perform at least 150 min/wk of moderate intensity physical exercise for at least 3 days a week, with not more than 2 consecutive days of rest. Resistance training is recommended for all patients with type 2 diabetes at least 2 days a week after authorized by the primary care provider.

D. Pharmaceutical therapy

1. Type 1 diabetes depends on exogenous insulin for treatment.

2. Type 2 diabetes is dependent on the severity of disease at the diagnosis. If the glucose is less than 300 mg/dL, a treatment is usually begun with an exercise program and nutrition plan. If glycemic goals are not reached in 2 or 3 months, monotherapy of medications is considered.

a. Monotherapy for type 2 diabetes: Metformin is the preferred oral medication for type 2 diabetes. If using monotherapy at the maximum dose and goal is not achieved after 3 months, a second oral medication should be added. Insulin may eventually be required for patients who are not controlled on oral agents.

i. Insulin should be considered initially for patients presenting with glucose levels 300 mg/dL and higher.

b. Oral combination therapies

i. Two-drug combination

1) Metformin + sulfonylurea (SU)

2) Metformin + thiazolidinedione (TZD)

3) Metformin + dipeptidyl peptidase-4 (DPP-4) inhibitor

4) Metformin + glucagon-like peptide-1 (GLP-1) receptor agonist (RA)

5) Metformin + insulin (basal) or prandial (rapid acting before meals)

ii. Three-drug combinations

1) Metformin + SU + TZD, DPP-4 inhibitor, GLP-1 RA, or insulin

2) Metformin + TZD + SU, DPP-4-I, GLP-1-RA, or insulin

3) Metformin + DPP-4 inhibitor + SU, TZD, or insulin

4) Metformin + GLP-1 RA + SU, TZD, or insulin

5) Metformin + insulin (basal) + TZD, DPP-4-I, or GLP-1-RA

iii. Complicated, uncontrolled patients on previously mentioned therapy require insulin.

c. Criteria for initiation of insulin therapy

i. Glucose level at diagnosis of type 2 diabetes is greater than 300 mg/dL

ii. $HgbA_{1c}$ greater than or equal to 10%

iii. Ketonuria

Although patients with type 2 diabetes do not depend on exogenous insulin, many will require supplemental insulin during times of stress, illness, injury, pregnancy, or routinely along with oral medication (see Tables 20.1 and 20.2).

d. Additional medications that may need to be considered:

i. Angiotensin-converting enzyme (ACE) inhibitors are the antihypertensive drugs of choice to retard renal dysfunction associated with diabetes.

ii. ACE inhibitors or angiotensin II receptor blockers (ARBs) are recommended for patients with an elevated urinary albumin excretion (30–299 mg/24 hr).

iii. Calcium channel blockers may reduce microalbuminuria and proteinuria.

iv. Aspirin therapy (75–162 mg/d) is recommended for primary prevention in patients with type 1 or type 2 diabetes with an increased risk of CVD (men older than 50 years; women older than 60 years with one or more risk factors, such as CVD, hypertension, smoking, dyslipidemia, or albuminuria). For patients who have a history of CVD with an allergy to aspirin, clopidogrel 75 mg/d should be used.

e. Some medications adversely affect diabetes.

i. Nicotinic acids affect glycemic control by increasing the insulin resistance.

ii. Beta-blockers increase the risk of hypoglycemia episodes in patients taking oral hypoglycemia agents.

iii. Thiazide diuretics increase insulin resistance.

3. In 2013, the American College of Cardiology (ACC)/American Heart Association (AHA) published guidelines on the primary prevention and

TABLE 20.1 Action Times of Insulin

Insulin	Onset	Peaks	Duration
Lispro/aspart/glulisine	10 minutes	1.5 hours	3 hours
Regular	20 minutes	3–4 hours	8 hours
NPH	1.5 hours	4–12 hours	22 hours
Lente	2.5 hours	7–15 hours	24 hours
Ultralente	4 hours	10–24 hours	36 hours
70 NPH/30 Reg	0–1 hour	Dual	12–20 hours
50 NPH/50 Reg	0–1 hour	Dual	12–20 hours
Detemir	1 hour	None	24 hours
Glargine	1 hour	None	24 hours
Afrezza (inhalation)	10 minutes	20 minutes	2.5–3 hours

NPH, neutral protamine Hagedorn.

TABLE 20.2 Diabetes Medication/Class

Drug	Brand Name	Drug Class
acarbose	Precose	Alpha-glucosidase inhibitor
pioglitazone + metformin	ActoPlus Met	Thiazolidinedione plus biguanide
glimepiride	Amaryl	Sulfonylurea
insulin glulisine	Apidra	Rapid-acting insulin
rosiglitazone + metformin	Avandamet	Thiazolidinedione plus biguanide
rosiglitazone + glimepiride	Avandaryl	Thiazolidinedione plus sulfonylurea
exenatide	Byetta	Incretin mimetic
exenatide ext. release	Bydureon	GLP-1 receptor agonist
glyburide	DiaBeta	Sulfonylurea (second generation)
pioglitazone + glimepiride	Duetact	Thiazolidinedione plus sulfonylurea
glucagon	N/A	Antihypoglycemic
metformin ext. release	Glucophage	Biguanide
glipizide ext. release	Glucotrol	Sulfonylurea (second generation)
glyburide + metformin	Glucovance	Sulfonylurea plus biguanide
glyburide micronized	Glynase Pres Tab	Sulfonylurea (second generation)
miglitol	Glyset	Alpha-glucosidase inhibitor
insulin lispro	Humalog	Rapid-acting insulin
NPH/regular insulin	Humulin 70/30 Humulin 50/50	Short- and intermediate-acting insulin Short- and intermediate-acting insulin
regular insulin	Humulin R	Rapid-acting insulin
NPH insulin	Humulin N	Intermediate-acting insulin
sitagliptin + metformin	Janumet	Dipeptidyl peptidase-4 inhibitor plus biguanide
sitagliptin	Januvia	Dipeptidyl peptidase-4 inhibitor
insulin glargine	Lantus	Long-acting insulin
insulin detemir	Levemir	Long-acting insulin
linagliptin	Tradjenta	Dipeptidyl peptidase-4 inhibitor
liraglutide	Victoza	GLP-1 receptor agonist
metformin + glipizide	Metaglip	Biguanide plus sulfonylurea
glyburide	Micronase	Sulfonylurea (second generation)
miglitol	Glyset	Alpha-glucosidase inhibitor
nateglinide	Starlix	Amino acid derivative
insulin isophane + regular insulin	Novolin 70/30	Short- and intermediate-acting insulin
insulin aspart	NovoLog	Rapid-acting insulin
insulin aspart protamine/Insulin aspart	NovoLog Mix 70/30	Short- and intermediate-acting insulin
insulin lispro protamine/insulin lispro	Humalog Mix 75/25 Humalog Mix 50/50	Short- and intermediate-acting insulin Short- and intermediate-acting insulin
nateglinide	Starlix	Insulin secretagogue
insulin isophane suspension NPH	Novolin	Intermediate-acting insulin
saxagliptin	Onglyza	Dipeptidyl peptidase-4 inhibitor
pioglitazone	Actos	Thiazolidinedione
repaglinide + metformin	Prandimet	Meglitinide analog plus biguanide meglitinide
pramlintide	Symlin	Amylin analog/amylinomimetic
repaglinide	Prandin	Meglitinide analog
rosiglitazone	Avandia	Thiazolidinedione

(*continued*)

TABLE 20.2 Diabetes Medication/Class (*continued*)

Drug	Brand Name	Drug Class
dapagliflozin	Farxiga	SGLT2 Inh SGLT2 Inh with DPP-4 Inh
empagliflozin + linagliptin	Glyxambi	SGCT2 Inh + DDP-4 Inh
canagliflozin + metformin	Invokamet	SGLT2 Inh + biguanide
canagliflozin	Invokana	SGCT2 Inh
empagliflozin	Jardiance	SGCT2 Inh
alogliptin + metformin	Kazano	DDP-4 Inh + biguanide
saxagliptin + metformin	Kombiglyze XR	DDP-4 inhibitor + biguanide
empagliflozin + linagliptin	Synjardy	SGCT2 Inh + biguanide
albiglutide	Tanzeum	GLP-1
insulin glargine	Toujeo	Long-acting (basal) insulin
insulin degludec	Tresiba	Long-acting (basal) insulin
dulaglutide	Trulicity	GLP-1
dapagliflozin	Xigduo XR Afrezza	SGLT2 Inh + biguanide Insulin for oral inhalation

DPP-4 Inh, dipeptidyl peptidase-4 inhibitor; GLP-1, glucagon-like peptide-1; N/A, not available; NPH, neutral protamine Hagedorn; SGLT2 Inh, sodium-glucose co-transporter 2 inhibitor.

treatment of cholesterol in people with DM and LDL-C of 70 to 189 mg/dL. These include:

a. Moderate-intensity statin therapy initiated or continued for adults with DM 40 to 75 years of age.

b. High-intensity statin therapy is reasonable for adults with DM 40 to 75 years of age with a greater than or equal to 7.5% estimated 10-year ASCVD risk unless contraindicated. (Use the lifetime risk calculator to define percentage of risk.)

c. In adults with DM who are younger than 40 years or older than 75 years of age, it is reasonable to evaluate the potential for ASCVD benefits and for adverse effects, for drug–drug interactions, and to consider patient preferences when deciding to initiate, continue, or intensify statin therapy.

Follow-Up

A. Determine follow-up appointments by the type of diabetes, age, patient compliance, any treatment changes, and presence of any complications related to diabetes or other health problems.

B. A glycosylated hemoglobin determination every 3 months can assist the provider in measuring the control. There are several computer software packages that print the glucometer readings for assessing the compliance; this can be done by the provider or the patient.

C. The American Diabetes Association management goals

1. Preprandial glucose 80 to 120 mg/dL

2. A glucose level of less than 180 mg/dL 1 to 2 hours after meals

3. A bedtime glucose level of 100 to 140 mg/dL

4. Hemoglobin A_{1c} ($HgbA_{1c}$) less than 7% or 7.5% in elderly

5. In 2013, the American Diabetes Association recommended the BP goal for diabetics with hypertension should be treated to a systolic blood pressure (SBP) goal of less than 140 mmHg and to a diastolic blood pressure (DBP) of less than 80 mmHg. The 2014 report from the Eighth Joint National Committee (JNC 8) recommends that in the diabetic population older than 18 years, pharmacological treatment should be initiated at a SBP greater than 140 mmHg or a DBP greater than 90 mmHg and treated to a goal of SBP less than 140 mmHg and a goal of DBP less than 90 mmHg. The JNC 8 has the same recommendation for initiation of BP medication and treatment goals for patients older than 18 years of age with chronic kidney disease.

6. Other goals are cholesterol less than 200 mg/dL, triglycerides less than 150 mg/dL, HDLs greater than 35 mg/dL, and LDLs less than 100 mg/dL and less than 70 mg/dL if heart disease is present.

D. Annual tests or examinations should include a dilated funduscopic examination by an ophthalmologist, to screen for retinopathy every 2 years, an annual EKG, monofilament foot examination, flu vaccination and other adult vaccines as recommended, thyroid studies, serum creatinine, blood urea nitrogen (BUN), glomerular filtration rate (GFR), lipid panel, urinalysis, and urine for albuminuria. Additional tests may be needed if complications develop.

Consultation/Referral

A. Refer to the physician if the patient experiences the following;

1. Diabetic ketoacidosis

2. Pediatric patients with hyperglycemia/new onset diabetes (type 1 or type 2)

3. Severe or frequent hypoglycemia that is unresponsive to conventional pharmaceutical therapy

4. Hyperosmolar hyperglycemic nonketotic syndrome

5. Pregnancy

6. Symptoms from an acute complication related to retinopathy

7. Nephropathy develops 35% to 45% of the time in type 1 and 20% of the time in type 2 diabetes; it is the leading disease requiring kidney dialysis.

8. Neuropathy: 60% to 70% of patients experience impaired sensation or pain in feet/hands, carpal tunnel syndrome; over half of all amputations of lower extremities are related to diabetes. All patients should be screened for neuropathy at the diagnosis of type 2 diabetes and at 5 years after the diagnosis of type 1 diabetes, and then annually. Early diagnosis is imperative to prevent nerve damage from occurring. Tight control of the blood glucose levels can slow down the progression of nerve damage but cannot reverse neuronal loss. The pain experienced with neuropathy can be treated with oral medications. Pregabalin and duloxetine are both FDA approved for neuropathic pain. Other medications that may be used include opioids such as tramadol and morphine, along with venlafaxine, amitriptyline, gabapentin, or valproate.

9. Persistent uncontrolled diabetes.

Individual Considerations

A. Pregnancy/preconceptual

1. Women considering pregnancy should be switched to insulin or an oral agent with safe pregnancy rating before conception and during pregnancy.

a. Fetal anomalies increase proportionally to uncontrolled diabetes.

b. $HgbA_{1c}$ goal before conception is less than 7%.

c. Gestational diabetes screening may be completed by performing the "one-step" 2-hour 75 g OGTT or a "two-step" approach with 1-hour 50 g nonfasting Glucola followed by a 3-hour 100 g OGTT for patients who test positive for the 1-hour screening.

2. Hypertensive medications may need to be changed if considering pregnancy because ACE inhibitors, beta-blockers, and diuretics are contraindicated during pregnancy.

3. Increased monitoring of blood glucose is necessary during pregnancy.

B. Pediatrics: Screening should begin at 10 years of age or the onset of puberty if younger than 10 years. Screening is recommended every 3 years. Criteria for screening for diabetes include:

1. Overweight (BMI greater than 85th percentile for age and sex, or weight for height, or weight greater than 120% for height)

2. Risk factors that include:

a. Family history of type 2 DM in a first- or second-degree relative

b. Race/ethnicity (Native American, African American, Latino, Asian American, Pacific Islander)

c. Insulin-resistance conditions (hypertension, dyslipidemia, polycystic ovarian syndrome [PCOS], acanthosis nigricans, birth weight small for gestational age)

d. Maternal history of diabetes or gestational diabetes

3. Children are encouraged to perform at least 60 minutes of physical activity on a daily basis.

4. Children diagnosed with type 1 diabetes should also be screened for celiac disease by ordering laboratory studies that include immunoglobulin A (IgA) antitissue transglutaminase or antiendomysial antibodies. If positive, the child should be referred to a rheumatologist. These children should also be screened for thyroid disease by ordering a thyroid-stimulating hormone (TSH) level test. If normal, screen every 1 to 2 years.

C. Elderly

1. Risk for hypoglycemia should be reviewed in patients using insulin or oral agents that can cause hypoglycemia. Medical alert bracelets and emergency care for hypoglycemic episodes should be reviewed during each follow-up.

2. Treatment goals for older diabetic patients should be individualized with goals equal to those of younger patients based on life expectancy.

Galactorrhea

Jill C. Cash and Mellisa A. Hall

Definition

A. The production of a milky discharge excreted from the nipple, occurring beyond the 6-month period of pregnancy and/or breastfeeding cessation.

Incidence

A. It is estimated that 1% to 50% of reproductive women will experience galactorrhea at some time in their life.

Pathogenesis

A. The pathogenesis depends on the etiology. Physiologic galactorrhea is caused by pregnancy. The anterior pituitary gland secretes prolactin, which stimulates milk production. Milk production is normal for 6 months after pregnancy and/or after breastfeeding has ceased. The majority of cases are from a benign etiology. Malignancy is responsible for 5% to 15% of cases.

Predisposing Factors

A. Reproductive women (15–50 years old)

B. Medications: Oral contraceptions, first- and second-generation antipsychotics, tricyclic antidepressants, selective serotonin reuptake inhibitor (SSRI) antidepressants, antiemetics, opioid analgesics, and antihypertensives (verapamil and methyldopa).

Common Complaint

A. Milky discharge from the nipple

Subjective Data

A. Note the onset, duration, and course of presenting symptoms.
B. Ask whether the patient has been pregnant and/or breastfed within the past 6 months. If so, how long did she nurse?
C. Review her menstrual history and pattern.
D. Ask her to describe the discharge, noting color, consistency, and/or presence of blood.
E. Determine the mechanism of production of discharge: Spontaneous or with manual expression.
F. Assess for any palpable mass in the breast.
G. Review current medications, including use of oral contraceptives.
H. Note any previous experience with galactorrhea. Discuss testing performed and treatment, if any.
I. Identify any family history of breast cancer or other tumors.

Physical Examination

A. Check pulse, respirations, and blood pressure (BP).
B. Inspect
   1. Inspect the breast and nipples for symmetry.
   2. Assess the discharge.
   3. Inspect the skin; note dimpling, retraction, and irregularities.
   4. Eyes: Complete funduscopic examination.
   5. Perform visual field testing.
C. Palpate
   1. Palpate the breasts for masses and fibrocystic changes.
   2. Squeeze the nipple to induce discharge.
   3. Palpate the axillary lymph nodes.
   4. Palpate the neck, thyroid, and lymph nodes.

Diagnostic Tests

A. Prolactin level: Normal level is 1 to 20 ng/mL.
B. Thyroid-stimulating hormone (TSH)

> *Many cases of galactorrhea are considered idiopathic. Usually endocrine studies will be normal.*

C. Beta human chorionic gonadotropin (beta hCG)
D. Hemoccult of breast discharge
E. Breast discharge for pathology
F. Periareolar ultrasound (all ages)
G. CT/MRI of sella turcica if pituitary mass is suspected
H. Mammogram in women older than 30 years if tumor is suspected
I. Breast sonography
J. Ductography /ductoscopy
K. Breast MRI
L. **Skin-punch biopsy for abnormal skin presentations**

Differential Diagnoses

A. Galactorrhea
B. Fibrocystic disease
C. Mastitis
D. Breast tumor
E. Medication induction
F. Breast cancer: Bloody nipple discharge, painless, firm fixed mass
G. Pituitary adenoma: Can produce permanent visual field loss and headaches
H. Hypothalamic disorders
I. Chiari-Frommel: Galactorrhea occurring after 6 months postpartum
J. Pregnancy

Plan

A. General interventions
   1. Treat underlying cause of nipple discharge.
   2. If induced by medications, consider stopping medications if the side effect outweighs benefits.
   3. If benign cause, no treatment is necessary with medication. Monitor symptoms. If symptoms progress, reevaluate.
B. Patient teaching
   1. Teach self-examination of the breast.
C. Pharmaceutical therapy
   1. No pharmaceuticals are advised with the exception of tapering or discontinuing medications that are causing the discharge. This is recommended only after cautious consideration of why the medication is being used (antipsychotics).

Follow-Up

A. Monitor prolactin level every 6 to 12 months.
B. Recommend yearly vision evaluation.
C. Order MRI of brain at 1 year, then every 2 to 5 years if symptoms persist.

Consultation/Referral

A. Consult a physician regardless of normal imaging results if breast tumor is suspected with bloody discharge or palpable mass noted.

Individual Considerations

A. Pregnancy
   1. Galactorrhea during pregnancy is a normal physiologic response.
   2. If galactorrhea persists after pregnancy/lactation has ceased for 6 months, a full workup evaluation is required.
B. Adults: Men: Galactorrhea is rare in men; however, it can occur with prolactinoma.

Gynecomastia

Jill C. Cash and Mellisa A. Hall

Definition

A. Gynecomastia is an enlargement of the breast tissue in males.

Incidence

A. Common in newborns; approximately 40% to 69% of adolescent boys will experience breast enlargement. It is also seen in men (between the ages of 50 and 80 years) with excessive weight gain.

Pathogenesis

A. Male breast duct proliferation occurs due to a hormonal imbalance of estrogen. Pathologic conditions such as pituitary tumors, systemic disorders, kidney disease, thyroid disorders, and liver disease can cause symptoms to occur. Medications can also induce symptoms. These medications include anti androgens, antidepressants, cimetidine, ranitidine, omeprazole, chemotherapeutic agents, amiodarone, diltiazem, nifedipine, digoxin, methyldopa, reserpine, hormones, and sedatives.

Predisposing Factors

A. Newborns
B. Puberty
C. Age (men older than 65 years)
D. Family history
E. Klinefelter's syndrome
F. Malnutrition with severe weight loss
G. Peutz–Jeghers syndrome
H. Obesity in males

Common Complaint

A. Enlargement of breast tissue with or without discomfort

Other Signs and Symptoms

A. Asymptomatic
B. Type I: Nodule present under areolar tissue area
C. Type II: Nodule palpable under and beyond areolar area
D. Type III: Breast enlargement without contour separation of tissue

Subjective Data

A. Identify when breast development first appeared.
B. Determine whether enlargement is unilateral or bilateral.
C. Review the progression of enlargement.
D. Note any pain, discharge, or masses that are palpable.
E. List current medications, drugs, and alcohol and substance abuse.
F. Review the patient's medical history.
G. Note the patient's family history of gynecomastia or breast malignancy.
H. Explore nutritional intake.
I. Discuss the patient's level of physical activity (sports, hobbies, etc.).
J. Note use of herbal products.

Objective Data

A. Inspect breasts bilaterally and surrounding nodes for enlargement or skin changes.
B. Palpate breast tissue systematically and surrounding nodes. Gynecomastia can usually be appreciated once the glandular tissue reaches 0.5 cm or larger.
C. Palpate testes for masses or atrophic changes.
D. Check body mass index (BMI).

Diagnostic Tests

A. Prolactin level
B. Thyroid-stimulating hormone (TSH)
C. Human chorionic gonadotropin (hCG)
D. Serum luteinizing hormone (LH)
E. Testosterone level
F. Estradiol level
G. Mammography for suspicious breast masses in adult males

Differential Diagnoses

A. Gynecomastia
B. Obesity: Fatty breast enlargement without glandular involvement
C. Breast cancer: Fixed, firm nodule in tissue with dimpling and/or breast discharge
D. Neurofibroma
E. Lipoma

Plan

A. General interventions
 1. Identify any pathologic condition. If none is identified, reassure the patient that normal resolution will occur over time.
B. Patient teaching
 1. Reinforce weight reduction if weight gain is a factor in the condition.
C. Pharmaceutical therapy
 1. Antiestrogens (tamoxifen)
 2. Androgens (testosterone replacement)
 3. Aromatase inhibitors (anastrozole)

Follow-Up

A. Follow-up is dependent on etiology and/or patient needs.
B. Follow up pubertal boys every 4 to 6 months for evaluation of development or regression.

Consultation/Referral

Consult a physician or refer to an endocrinologist if the male patient:
A. Is noted to have breast enlargement for longer than 2 years
B. Is a pubertal boy without genital development

Individual Consideration

A. Newborns: Commonly seen in newborns due to maternal estrogen. This breast enlargement spontaneously regresses over time.

Hirsutism

Jill C. Cash and Mellisa A. Hall

Definition

A. An excessive production of an androgenic hormone causes the development of male features in females, particularly hair distribution.

Incidence

A. Approximately 8% to 10% of women develop hirsutism after puberty.

Pathogenesis

A. The pathogenesis depends on the etiology: Excessive amounts of androgenic hormones from the ovary, adrenal gland, and/or a hormonal imbalance. The two major adrenal gland conditions responsible for hirsutism or virilism are congenital adrenal hyperplasia (CAH) and Cushing's syndrome.

Predisposing Factors

A. Females who have a family history of endocrine disorders
B. Usually occurs in the second to third decade of life
C. Southern European ancestry
D. Polycystic ovary syndrome
E. CAH
F. Ovarian tumors
G. Adrenal tumors
H. Cushing's syndrome
I. Hyperthecosis
J. Severe insulin-resistance syndrome
K. Medications
L. Obesity
M. Medications containing androgens, including oral contraceptives

Common Complaint

A. An excessive amount of hair production on the upper lip, chin, and/or chest

Other Signs and Symptoms

A. Irregular periods
B. Infertility
C. Acne
D. Virilization (temporal hair recessation, large muscle mass, deep voice)

Subjective Data

A. Note the age of onset, duration, and distribution pattern of the excessive hair growth.
B. Review any previous experiences with similar symptoms. What were the diagnosis, treatment, and results?
C. Note the patient's menstrual history. Note amenorrhea and galactorrhea. Has the patient ever had a history of infertility?

Physical Examination

A. Check pulse, respirations, and blood pressure (BP), body mass index (BMI; greater than 30 kg/m^2), central obesity pattern.
B. Inspect
   1. Look for excessive hair growth on face, breasts, abdomen, back, and shoulders.
   2. Assess for signs of virilization.
   3. Confirm expected development of secondary sexual characteristics.
   4. Assess for acne.
   5. Assess for striae acanthosis nigricans, or skin tags.
C. Palpate: Perform a pelvic examination to assess for enlarged ovaries or masses.

Diagnostic Tests

A. Total testosterone (200 ng/dL, need further workup)
B. Free serum testosterone
C. Thyroid-stimulating hormone (TSH), follicle-stimulating hormone (FSH), luteinizing hormone (LH), and prolactin levels
D. Dehydroepiandrosterone sulfate (DHEA-S)
E. 24-hour urine: 17-ketosteroid assay
F. Pelvic ultrasound
G. CT of ovaries/adrenal glands if abnormally elevated blood tests

Differential Diagnoses

A. Hirsutism: Can be secondary to primary diagnosis (idiopathic, hypothyroidism, infertility, obesity, ovarian disease, hyperprolactinemia)
B. Hypothyroidism: Elevated TSH
C. Ovarian tumor: Testosterone level greater than 200 ng/dL
D. Adrenal tumor: DHEA greater than 800 mcg/dL
E. Excessive steroid use: The patient medicates self with excessive steroids.
F. Cushing's syndrome: Centripetal obesity and muscle wasting

Plan

A. General interventions
   1. Medications are not recommended for mild cases. Hair removal by other mechanisms is recommended as the patient desires (plucking, waxing, bleaching, etc.).
   2. Moderate to severe cases require treatment with medications. Drug therapy may stop excessive hair growth. Current hair growth will not spontaneously resolve. Hair removal may also be desired until the drug shows an effect.
   3. If acne is severe, institute appropriate therapy (see "Acne Vulgaris" in Chapter 4, "Dermatology Guidelines").
B. Patient teaching
   1. If obese, reinforce weight loss management. Consider nutritional consult.
   2. Educate the patient that it may take 3 to 6 months on medication to see results.
C. Pharmaceutical therapy
   1. Use combined oral contraceptives daily if no contraindication; any brand is effective.
   2. Use high-estrogen pills to increase steroid-binding globulins if no contraindication.
   3. Use high-progesterone pills to influence the clearance of testosterone.
   4. Antiandrogens
      a. Spironolactone
      b. Cyproterone acetate
      c. Finasteride
      d. Flutamide
   5. Gonadotropin-releasing hormone (GnRH) agonists
   6. Topical therapy (Vaniqua). Topical cream to be applied twice daily to reduce growth of unwanted facial hair. Results should be noted after 4 to 6 weeks of use.

Ovarian and/or adrenal tumor must be ruled out before medication therapy is instituted.

Follow-Up

A. Follow-up depends on the treatment. If medication is used, follow up in 3 months to evaluate effectiveness.

Consultation/Referral

A. Consult a physician if abnormally elevated laboratory results exist or if Cushing's syndrome is suspected.
B. Refer to a physician if there is no improvement after 3 months of medication treatment.
C. Refer patients who have virilization and elevated testosterone levels to an endocrinologist.

Individual Considerations

A. Pregnancy
  1. If conception occurs, discontinue medications, which may be teratogenic to the fetus.
  2. If anovulation is diagnosed, fertility measures are needed if pregnancy is desired.
B. Geriatric
  1. Hirsutism may be seen in women after menopause.
  2. Hirsutism that occurs in the middle to late years in life should be closely monitored for adrenal hyperplasia and adrenal and/or ovarian tumors.

Hypogonadism

Jill C. Cash and Mellisa A. Hall

Definition

A. Hypogonadism in men is failure of the testes to produce physiological levels of testosterone and a normal number of spermatozoa.

Incidence

A. An estimated 38.7% of men older than 45 years of age have below-normal values of serum testosterone.

Pathogenesis

A. Hypogonadism in men can be the result of testicular dysfunction or nondevelopment (primary hypogonadism) or dysfunction of the pituitary or hypothalamus (secondary hypogonadism). The two clinical manifestations of impaired spermatogenesis are infertility and decreased testicular size. There are several possible clinical manifestations of testosterone deficiency, which are determined by its time of onset during reproductive development.
  1. In utero first or second trimesters: Incomplete virilization of external genitalia, incomplete development of Wolffian ducts to form male internal genitalia
  2. Third trimester in utero: Micropenis
  3. Prepuberty: Incomplete pubertal maturation, eunuchoid body habitus, poor muscle development, and reduced peak bone mass
  4. Postpuberty: Decreased energy, mood, and libido; decrease in sexual hair, hematocrit, muscle mass and strength, and bone mineral density

Predisposing Factors

A. Hypogonadism associated with Klinefelter's syndrome
B. Chemotherapy
C. Radiation therapy
D. Excessive alcohol consumption
E. Painful testicular swelling
F. Anosmia associated with Kallmann's syndrome
G. Use of medications that cause hypogonadism: Ketoconazole or extended-release opiates

Common Complaints

A. Decreased vigor and libido
B. Depression
C. Adolescent and young adult males—failure to begin or complete puberty

Other Si gns and Symptoms

A. Fatigue
B. Difficulty concentrating
C. Hot flashes
D. No change in deepening of the voice

Subjective Data

A. To patient or parent: History of known chromosomal abnormalities in family or patient
B. History of cryptorchidism
C. History of muscular weakness
D. History of varicocele unresolved within 6 months of birth
E. Known infections affecting the scrotum and testes
F. Therapeutic radiation to area
G. History of chemotherapy
H. History of long-term ketoconazole, glucocorticoid, or long-acting opiate use
I. Known testicular trauma
J. Known torsion
K. History of autoimmune disorder
L. Alcohol consumption (amount, duration, frequency)
M. Chronic illnesses including cirrhosis, chronic renal failure, or HIV
N. Decreased spontaneous erections

Physical Examination

A. Inspect
  1. Testes for appropriate size
  2. Upper and lower body musculatures
  3. Full/dense male-pattern beard
  4. Expected Tanner development for age
  5. Testes should be bilaterally descended
  6. Rule out eunuchoid appearance
  7. Gynecomastia
  8. Clinical findings of hypogonadism are more obvious after puberty and takes years to develop.
  9. Inspect penis for hypospadias.
  10. Long-term alcohol abuse: Palmar erythema, rhinophyma, telangiestasia, hand tremor
B. Palpate
  1. The scrotum and testes for masses
  2. The breasts for masses (both male and female)

Diagnostic Tests

A. Serum testosterone (morning total) repeat to confirm
B. Measurement of free testosterone if total testosterone is not near the lower limit
C. Avoid lab tests during acute illness.

Differential Diagnoses

A. Hypogonadism
B. Moderate obesity
C. Nephrotic syndrome
D. Hypothyroidism
E. Use of glucocorticoids, progestins, and androgenic steroids
F. Acromegaly
G. Diabetes mellitus
H. Hepatic cirrhosis
I. Hypopituitarism
J. Malnutrition
K. Klinefelter's syndrome
L. Depression
M. Psychological sexual dysfunction

Plan

A. General interventions
- **1.** Testosterone replacement's effect on reducing adverse health outcomes in the general population is unknown.
- **2.** Testosterone levels vary significantly with circadian rhythms, illness, and medications.
- **3.** Measurement of bone mineral density is recommended to assess fracture risk.
- **4.** Luteinizing hormone (LH) and follicle-stimulating hormone (FSH) concentrations can help distinguish between primary and secondary hypogonadism.
- **5.** Differentials for secondary hypogonadism should evaluate for pituitary neoplasia, hyperprolactinemia, hemochromatosis, obstructive sleep apnea (OSA), and genetic disorders.
- **6.** Testosterone replacement should be initiated only after a baseline prostate-specific antigen (PSA) and digital prostate examination. PSA levels should be followed routinely.

B. Patient teaching
- **1.** Both men and women with hypogonadism can lead normal lives with hormone replacement therapy.
- **2.** Hormone replacement should continue throughout life.
- **3.** Potential side effects of testosterone replacement therapy should be discussed before therapy, including gynecomastia, worsening benign prostatic hyperplasia (BPH), sleep apnea, peripheral edema, potential increased risk for myocardial infarction (MI), and cerebrovascular accident (CVA).
- **4.** Reduced sperm production and fertility is a potential side effect of testosterone replacement.
- **5.** Patients using topically absorbed testosterone gel or creams can transfer testosterone to female partners or children by direct skin-to-skin contact.

C. Pharmaceutical therapy
- **1.** Injectable testosterone: 50 up to 400 mg IM every 2 weeks
- **2.** 1% testosterone gel
- **3.** Transdermal testosterone patch
- **4.** Buccal testosterone
- **5.** Implanted subcutaneous testosterone pellets

Follow-Up

A. Patients receiving hormone replacement should be reevaluated every 6 months or more frequently, including screening for prostate cancer as recommended.
B. Testosterone replacement is contraindicated in metastatic prostate cancer and breast cancer. Routine screening should be performed.

Consultation/Referral

A. Physician consultation before initiating testosterone therapy is advised.
B. Endocrinology referral is recommended for males not responsive to the replacement therapy.
C. Patients with primary hypogonadism should be referred to an endocrinologist for initial workup and management.

Individual Considerations

A. Geriatrics: Current recommendations are *not* in favor of testosterone therapy for all older males. Providers should cautiously consider the benefits compared to the risks for older males. The benefits of testosterone replacement are unproven, and the long-term risks are unknown.
B. HIV patients: Short-term testosterone replacement should be considered for HIV men with low testosterone, weight loss, and muscular wasting.

Metabolic Syndrome/Insulin Resistance Syndrome

Jill C. Cash and Mellisa A. Hall

Definition

A. Metabolic syndrome is an association of several complex disorders: Obesity, insulin-resistant type 2 diabetes, hypertension, and hyperlipidemia. This coexistence of conditions leads to atherosclerotic cardiovascular disease. Metabolic syndrome is considered a proinflammatory and prothrombotic state. Elevated triglycerides and low high-density lipoprotein (HDL) cholesterol are strong predictors of vascular events. Triglycerides and the waist circumference are considered the strongest predictors for the development of metabolic syndrome.

The inclusion of type 2 diabetes in the definition of metabolic syndrome is debated. Currently, there is no consensus on definition for metabolic syndrome in children. The Adult Treatment Panel (ATP) III defines metabolic syndrome in adults as the coexistence of any three of five conditions (see Table 20.3).

Complications associated with metabolic syndrome include fatty liver disease, cirrhosis, chronic kidney disease, polycystic ovarian syndrome (PCOS), obstructive sleep apnea (OSA), and gout.

TABLE 20.3 Adult Treatment Panel III Criteria for Metabolic Syndrome

Metabolic Syndrome Traits	Definition
Central/abdominal obesity	Adult waist circumference: Men >40 inches (102 cm) Women >35 inches (88 cm)
	Obesity in children 6 years to <10 years: Waist circumference ≥90th percentile
	Obesity ages 10 to <16 years: ≥90th percentile ≥16 years use adult criteria
Serum triglycerides	Adults: ≥150 mg/dL *or* drug treatment for elevated triglycerides
	Children: >100 mg/dL
Serum HDL cholesterol	Adults: <40 mg/dL in men; <50 mg/dL in women; *or* drug treatment for low HDL cholesterol
	Children: ≤35 mg/dL
Blood pressure (BP)	Adults: ≥130/85 *or* drug treatment for hypertension
	Children: ≥90th percentile for age, sex, and height
Fasting plasma glucose (FPG)	Adults: ≥100 mg/dL *or* drug treatment for elevated blood glucose
	Children: ≥110 mg/dL

HDL, high-density lipoprotein.
Source: Adapted from National Institutes of Health (2015).

Metabolic syndrome is noted in the literature under other names, including insulin resistance syndrome and obesity dyslipidemia syndrome. Previously, the term "Syndrome X" was used; however, Syndrome X is noted to have normal coronary arteries and the occurrence of angina.

Incidence

A. Age-dependent increase in incidence; overall incidence is estimated at 22% of the population; however, with the increase in childhood obesity, metabolic syndrome is being diagnosed in children. The incidence in children is 4.2% to 8.4% (dependent on ethnicity).
B. Asians living in the United States and Mexican Americans have the highest age-adjusted prevalence. Among African Americans and Mexican Americans, the prevalence is higher in women than in men.
C. Ethnic background
  1. Native Americans are at the greatest risk (60% females and 45% males).
  2. Mexican Americans have the highest prevalence (31.9%).
  3. Black and Hispanic females are 1.5 times more likely than non-Hispanic White females.

Pathogenesis

A. The exact etiology is unknown; however, abdominal obesity has been associated with insulin resistance. Vascular endothelial dysfunction occurs secondary to insulin resistance, hyperglycemia, hyperinsulinemia, and adipokines. Along with high blood pressure (BP) and abnormal lipids, vascular inflammation places the individual at high risk of a cardiovascular insult.

Predisposing Factors

A. Genetic predisposition
B. Weight gain, especially central/abdominal obesity
C. Females, especially postmenopausal
D. Childhood obesity
E. Smoking
F. High-carbohydrate diet, especially soft-drink consumption
G. Lack of exercise
  1. Sedentary lifestyle
  2. Television or other electronic device use more than 2 hours per day
H. Insulin resistance

Common Complaints

A. Complaints are all related to the individual coexisting comorbid symptoms.

Other Signs and Symptoms

A. All are related to the individual coexisting comorbid symptoms.

Subjective Data

A. Review the patient's medical history related to comorbid conditions, including obesity, hypertension, and any abnormal laboratory testing (lipids, triglycerides, and glucose tolerance tests [GTTs]).
B. Review the patient's family history.
C. Review all prescription medications, over-the-counter (OTC) drugs, and herbals.
D. Review the patient's current level of exercise.
E. Review the patient's usual diet (24-hour recall) noting high fat and high glucose consumption, including fast food and processed food consumption.
F. Review the patient's reproductive history.

Physical Examination

A. Check height, weight, waist circumference, BP, pulse, and respirations.

B. Calculate the body mass index (BMI) and waist-to-hip measurement. Several Internet sites have BMI, body fat, and waist-to-hip ratio calculators. Document on a growth chart BMI results for visual teaching support for patient and parent.
C. Make general observations for acanthosis nigricans and skin tags (insulin resistance).
D. A full physical examination is guided by the patient's medical history and presenting signs and symptoms.

Diagnostic Tests

A. Fasting plasma glucose
B. Fasting lipid panel
C. Triglycerides
D. Consider thyroid function.
E. Consider C-reactive protein (CRP; optional).

Differential Diagnoses

A. Metabolic syndrome
  1. Obesity
  2. Hypertension
  3. Hyperlipidemia
  4. High-fasting plasma glucose
B. Cushing's syndrome

Plan

A. General interventions
  1. Aggressive lifestyle modification focusing on increased physical activity and weight reduction is a cornerstone for treatment.
B. Patient teaching
  1. Dietary recommendations include a low-fat, low-cholesterol and/or dietary approaches to stop hypertension (DASH) diet. Decrease simple sugar consumption, as well as saturated and trans fats and cholesterol (see Appendix B).
  2. Exercise recommendations include a minimum of 30 minutes a day of walking at a brisk pace or other activity at a moderate intensity. Start by using a pedometer, walking at breaks, or performing household work.
  3. Weight loss of 5% to 10% or more should be encouraged (gradual weight loss of 1 to 2 kg/mo). Even small losses are associated with health benefits.
  4. BP control strategies include a low-sodium diet (DASH), smoking cessation, and alcohol in moderation.
  5. Counsel on smoking cessation.
  6. Abdominoplasties do not lower the risk for coronary artery disease (CAD) or insulin sensitivity.
C. Pharmaceutical therapy
  1. Currently, the treatment for metabolic syndrome is to treat each individual component/diagnosis for the individual.
  2. Insulin-resistant patients usually are not treated by insulin.
  3. Statins are the most common classification used for elevated lipids.
  4. Low-dose aspirin may be prescribed related to the patient's risk of cardiovascular disease, with an increased risk of the patient having a prothrombotic state.
  5. Oral hypoglycemic agents used to treat type 2 diabetes are not currently recommended for the prevention of metabolic syndrome.
  6. Hypertension should be controlled with appropriate antihypertensives.

Follow-Up

A. Follow-up involves assessing patients for metabolic syndrome at a minimum of 3-year intervals for anyone with one or more risk traits. Follow-up testing includes
  1. BMI calculation
  2. Waist-to-hip calculation
  3. Fasting lipid profile
  4. Fasting glucose or other diabetic screening methods (hemoglobin A_{1c} [$HgbA_{1c}$], gamma-glutamyl transferase [GGT])
  5. BP

Consultation/Referral

A. Refer to an obstetrician/gynecologist for consultation and management for infertility/pregnancy.
B. Refer to a specialist for any comorbid condition as needed.

Individual Considerations

A. Individual considerations for pregnancy, pediatrics, and geriatrics are specific to their comorbid condition.

Polycystic Ovarian Syndrome

Jill C. Cash and Mellisa A. Hall

Definition

Polycystic ovarian syndrome (PCOS) is characterized by ovulatory dysfunction and hyperandrogenism. PCOS was previously called Stein–Leventhal syndrome. PCOS is a risk factor for metabolic syndrome, infertility, glucose intolerance, and type 2 diabetes mellitus (DM). PCOS itself is not considered a disease; instead, it is a syndrome of coexisting conditions (see Table 20.4).

The Androgen Excess Society diagnostic criteria for PCOS:
A. Hyperandrogenism
B. Ovarian dysfunction
C. Exclusion of other androgen excess or related disorders

Although obesity is one of the hallmarks of PCOS, lean women may also have insulin resistance/PCOS. The diagnosis of PCOS is based on medical history, physical examination, and laboratory tests. Aggressive lifestyle modification is the mainstay of all adolescents and women with PCOS.

Incidence

A. The incidence of PCOS is 6.5% up to 12% in the literature. It is the most common cause of infertility. It

TABLE 20.4 PCOS-Associated Symptoms

Cutaneous Signs	Hirsutism
Menstrual irregularity	Severe acne
Obesity	Alopecia
Polycystic ovaries	Oligomenorrhea
	Amenorrhea
	Dysfunctional uterine bleeding
	> inches (88 cm) waist circumference for women and adolescents ≥16 years
	≥90th percentile for ages 10 to <16 years
	Noted on pelvic ultrasound

PCOS, polycystic ovarian syndrome.

is also the most common worldwide endocrinopathy in women, with 5 to 7 million women in the United States experiencing its effects.

Pathogenesis

A. The exact etiology is unknown; however, PCOS is noted to have insulin resistance and abnormal pituitary function, as well as abnormal steroidogenesis.

Predisposing Factors

A. Obesity
B. Genetic predisposition, including Mexican American women
C. Metabolic syndrome
D. Women with oligo-ovulatory infertility
E. Type 1, type 2, or gestational diabetes
F. History of premature adrenarche
G. First-degree relatives with PCOS
H. Antiepileptic medications

Common Complaints

A. Hirsutism
B. Menstrual problems
C. Obesity
D. Infertility

Other Signs and Symptoms

A. Acne
B. Alopecia (male pattern)
C. Hyperhidrosis
D. Acanthosis nigricans
E. Seborrhea

Subjective Data

A. Review the patient's menstruation history.
- **1.** Premature puberty (younger than 8 years)
- **2.** Primary amenorrhea: Lack of menses by age 15 years
- **3.** Oligomenorrhea: Missing four periods per year
- **4.** Dysfunctional uterine bleeding (DUB): Bleeding at irregular intervals, heavy cycles, periods longer than 7 days

B. Review the patient's history of weight gain, increased waist circumference, and obesity.
C. Review the patient's history of any skin/hair changes.
D. Review the family history for the presence of diabetes, metabolic syndrome, and infertility.

Physical Examination

A. Check height, weight, waist circumference, blood pressure (BP), pulse, and respirations.
B. Calculate the body mass index (BMI) and waist-to-hip measurement. Several Internet sites have BMI, body fat, and waist-to-hip ratio calculators.
C. Inspect
- **1.** Skin
  - **a.** Evaluate hirsutism (upper lip, chin, nape of the neck, periareolar, abdomen—linea alba).
  - **b.** Pigmentation patterns for acanthosis nigricans (neck, axilla).
- **2.** Observe fat distribution.

D. Perform pelvic examination to evaluate enlarged ovaries and pelvic masses.

Diagnostic Tests

A. Fasting glucose
B. Oral glucose tolerance test (OGTT) if fasting glucose is elevated between 100 mg/dL and 125 mg/dL.
C. Thyroid function tests (thyroid-stimulating hormone [TSH], free T_4)
D. Random serum cortisol to rule out Cushing's syndrome
E. Serum luteinizing hormone (LH) and prolactin to rule out hypothalamic and pituitary diseases
F. Ultrasound to rule out ovarian pathology (as indicated: Not required for definitive diagnosis)
G. Insulin-like growth factor (IGF-I)
H. Dehydroepiandrosterone-sulfate (DHEA-S) to rule out adrenal hyperandrogenism
I. Free and total testosterone
J. Lipid profile
K. Endometrial biopsy if indicated for women without menses for 1 year
L. Pregnancy test before start of pharmaceutical therapy and history of anovulation

Differential Diagnoses

A. PCOS
B. Adrenal disorders
- **1.** Congenital adrenal hyperplasia (CAH)
- **2.** Cushing's syndrome
- **3.** Cortisol resistance

C. Hyperprolactinemia
D. Acromegaly

E. Insulin resistance (types 1 and 2 diabetes)
F. Thyroid dysfunction
G. Virilizing tumors
H. Drug induced
  1. Anabolic steroids
  2. Valproic acid

Plan

A. General interventions
  1. Aggressive lifestyle modification focusing on increased physical activity and weight reduction is a cornerstone for treatment.
B. Patient education
  1. Exercise recommendations include a minimum of 30 minutes a day of walking at a brisk pace or other activity at a moderate intensity. Start by using a pedometer, walking at breaks, or performing household work.
  2. Weight loss of 5% to 10% or more. Gradual weight loss of 1 to 2 kg/mo is recommended. Even small amounts of weight loss are associated with health benefits.
  3. Weight loss may cause a resumption of ovulation and the ability to get pregnant.
  4. High-fiber, low-fat diet and reduction of refined sugar
  5. Hair removal can be achieved with shaving, waxing, or use of depilatories. Electrolysis and laser treatment are more expensive therapies for hirsutism.
C. Pharmaceutical therapy
  1. Oral contraceptive pills (OCPs) are the most commonly used treatment for endometrial prevention and hirsutism.
    a. Due to sodium and water retention, weight reduction while on OCPs is more difficult.
    b. OCPs that contain 30 to 35 mcg of ethinyl estradiol and progestins, such as norethindrone (Ortho Micronor), norgestimate (Ortho-Tri-Cyclen), desogestrel (Desogen and Ortho-Cept), or drospirenone (Yasmin), are prescribed for PCOS.
  2. Metformin (Glucophage) is used to manage oligomenorrhea, cause weight loss, lower insulin levels, and induce ovulation for women with PCOS.
    a. Start metformin 500 mg at the evening meal. The dosage can be increased by 500 mg/wk in divided doses up to the maximum of 2,000 mg/d.
    b. Titrate slowly because of the gastrointestinal side effects (diarrhea).
    c. Check a metabolic panel before and every 3 to 6 months to evaluate for lactic acidosis.
    d. Metformin is contraindicated in patients with renal impairment; assess renal function before instituting metformin and monitor regularly.
    e. Metformin must be stopped before any procedure with radiographic dye.
  3. Medroxyprogesterone acetate (Provera) is used for a withdrawal bleed 5 to 10 mg daily for 10 days every 1 to 2 months, or micronized progesterone (Prometrium) 100 to 200 mg by mouth at bedtime for 7 to 10 days per month. This withdrawal bleeding is advised to protect the endometrium.
  4. Spironolactone (Aldactone) 100 to 200 mg twice a day is used after a 4- to 6-month oral contraceptive trial as antiandrogen therapy.
    a. Spironolactone is also a good alternative when OCPs are contraindicated. However, spironolactone can be used in combination with OCPs.
    b. Alternative methods of birth control should be used when spironolactone is used alone secondary to potential congenital defects such as abnormal development of the male fetus' external genitalia.
    c. Monitor potassium level during spironolactone therapy.
  5. Eflornithine (Vaniqa) topical may be prescribed to prevent facial hair regrowth.
  6. Clomiphene citrate (Clomid) is used to induce ovulation. Weight loss should be attempted before starting ovulation induction treatment.

Follow-Up

A. Glucose tolerance needs to be evaluated regularly for type 2 diabetes in women with PCOS (see Table 20.5).

Consultation/Referral

A. Refer to an obstetrician/gynecologist or a reproductive endocrinologist for consultation and management of
  1. Infertility/pregnancy

TABLE 20.5 Androgen Excess Society Screening and Treatment Requirements for IGT

All patients with PCOS, regardless of BMI, should be screened for IGT using a 2-hour OGTT.
Patients with a normal glucose test should be rescreened at least once every 2 years or earlier if additional risk factors are identified.
Patients with IGT should be screened annually for the development of type 2 DM.
Adolescents with PCOS should be screened for IGT using a 2-hour OGTT every 2 years. If IGT develops, the treatment with metformin should be considered.
The mainstay of treatment with PCOS and IGT is intensive lifestyle modification (diet, exercise, and weight loss).
Insulin-sensitizing agents should be considered for patients with PCOS and IGT.

BMI, body mass index; DM, diabetes mellitus; IGT, impaired glucose tolerance; OGTT, oral glucose tolerance test; PCOS, polycystic ovarian syndrome.
Source: Adapted from the 2007 Androgen Excess Society Position Statement (Salley et al., 2007).

2. Menstrual bleeding that is not controlled despite OCPs

B. An endocrinologist may be an appropriate consultation.

C. Consider a nutritional consultation for weight-loss recommendations.

Thyroid Disease: Hyperthyroidism

Jill C. Cash and Mellisa A. Hall

Definition

A. Hyperthyroidism is a condition in which thyroid hormone exerts greater than normal responses. Hyperthyroidism may be subclinical and may not be easily recognized or exhibit overt symptoms. The most common hyperthyroid conditions are Graves' disease and toxic multinodular goiter. The U.S. Preventive Services Task Force (USPSTF) does not currently recommend screening for thyroid dysfunction in asymptomatic adults who are not pregnant.

Incidence

A. Overall incidence of Graves' disease is 0.5 per 1,000. Graves' disease is responsible for 60% to 80% of cases of thyrotoxicosis.

B. Female gender
   1. 5:1 ratio higher in women than men
   2. Older women: 4% to 5% incidence
   3. Graves' disease is more common in younger women.
   4. Toxic nodular goiter is more common in older women.

C. Children
   1. Graves' disease in children 0.02% (1:5,000)
   2. Most often occurs in 11- to 15-year-olds

D. Elderly: Toxic multinodular goiter (Plummer disease) occurs in 15% to 20% of patients with thyrotoxicosis.

E. Symptomatology incidence
   1. Ophthalmopathy is more common in smokers.
   2. Atrial fibrillation 10% to 25% incidence and is more common in the elderly.
   3. Autoimmune thyroid diseases have a peak incidence in people aged 20 to 40 years.

Pathogenesis

A. Hyperthyroidism is one form of thyrotoxicosis in which an excess of hormone is excreted by the thyroid gland. The diseases that can cause hyperthyroidism include Graves' disease, toxic multinodular goiter, thyroid cancer, and increased secretion of the thyroid-stimulating hormone (TSH). Thyrotoxicosis not related to hyperthyroidism may be subacute thyroiditis, ectopic thyroid tissue, and ingestion of excessive thyroid hormone. Postpartum thyroiditis can precipitate a short-term mild hyperthyroidism, which has an onset at 2 to 6 months postpartum. Severe thyrotoxicosis of any cause is called thyrotoxic crisis or storm.

In Graves' disease, the normal feedback mechanisms that regulate hormone secretion are taken over by some abnormal thyroid-stimulating mechanism. Thyroid autoantibodies of the immunoglobulin G (IgG) class are present in more than 95% of patients with Graves' disease. The hyperfunctioning of the thyroid gland causes suppression of TSH and thyrotropin-releasing hormone (TRH). There are profound increases in iodine uptake and thyroid gland metabolism, which are believed to be the causes of the gland enlargement. The resulting increase in the level of circulating thyroid hormone is responsible for the thyrotoxic symptoms.

In the condition called toxic multinodular goiter, the thyroid gland enlarges in response to some bodily need such as puberty; pregnancy; iodine deficiency; and immunologic, viral, and genetic disorders. As TSH levels rise, the gland enlarges; when the condition demanding increased thyroid hormone resolves, TSH levels usually return to normal and the gland slowly assumes its original size.

Predisposing Factors

A. Graves' disease
   1. Women in the second through fifth decades of life
   2. Familial autoimmune thyroid disease
   3. Concomitant disorders believed to be autoimmune
   4. Increased in patients diagnosed with trisomy 21
   5. Higher incidence in persons who smoke

B. Toxic multinodular goiter
   1. Older people
   2. Recent exposure to iodine-containing medications (amiodarone and radiocontrast dye)
   3. Long-standing simple goiter
   4. Conditions such as puberty, pregnancy, iodine deficiency, and immunologic, viral, or genetic disorders

Common Complaints

A. Graves' disease
   1. Prominence/protrusion of the eye (exophthalmos)
   2. Prominent "stare"
   3. Visual changes
      a. Diplopia
      b. Photophobia
      c. Eye irritation: Gritty feeling or pain

B. Weight loss with no change in diet or an increase in appetite

C. Anorexia (may be prominent in the elderly)

D. Weakness and fatigue

E. Tachycardia

F. Decreased tolerance to heat

G. Thinning scalp hair

H. Fingernail separation from the nail bed

I. Smooth, thin skin

J. Heart palpitations (atrial fibrillation)

K. Bowel symptoms
   1. Increase in frequency and loose bowel movements (not diarrhea)
   2. Constipation (more frequent in the elderly)

L. Swelling of feet and ankles

Other Signs and Symptoms

A. Goiter: **Approximately 50% of patients will not have an enlargement of the thyroid gland.** Elderly patients are less likely to have a goiter.

B. Periorbital edema

C. Flushing, warm skin

D. Fine hand tremors
E. Dyspnea (especially elderly)
F. Exertional fatigue/exercise intolerance
G. Insomnia
H. Irritability
I. Nervousness
J. Mood swings
K. Inability to concentrate
L. Depression and apathy (elderly)
M. Hyperactivity (children)
N. Decreased menses
O. Impotence and decreased libido in men
P. Gynecomastia
Q. Galactorrhea (TSH-mediated hyperthyroidism)
R. Atrial dysrhythmias (atrial fibrillation), left ventricular dilation (common in elderly)
S. Urinary frequency and nocturia (enuresis is common in children)
T. A combination of these noted symptoms should lead to the assessment of hyperthyroidism.

Subjective Data

A. Identify when symptoms began, duration, and any change or progression.
B. Identify whether the patient has noticed enlargement of the thyroid gland, difficulty swallowing, or change in voice.
C. Assess for change in weight over the past 3 months, past 6 months, and last year. Ask the patient whether his or her appetite has changed.
D. Explore the patient's family history of thyroid problems.
E. Obtain the patient's medical history of associated diseases (especially those of autoimmune pathogenesis: Pernicious anemia, type 1 diabetes mellitus [DM], myasthenia gravis, receptor agonist [RA], ulcerative colitis).
F. Review the patient's medication history, including amiodarone, interferon alpha, levothyroxine (overdose), expectorants, and health food supplements containing seaweed.
G. Ask the patient to identify any changes in bowel habits, loose (nondiarrhea) stools, frequency of bowel movements, or constipation.
H. Ask about moods, changes in concentration, feelings of restlessness, nervousness, anxiety, and change in sleep habits.
I. Assess for any cardiac symptoms, such as palpitations, chest pain, shortness of breath, and decreased tolerance for activities previously done.
J. Ask whether the patient has noticed any swelling or puffiness anywhere.
K. Determine whether the patient has experienced changes in vision and/or eye irritation.
L. Assess for hand tremors, increase in the moistness and coolness of the skin, flushing, and blushing.
M. Ask the patient to identify any menstrual changes or whether the patient has had a recent pregnancy, or is in the postpartum period.
N. Review for a recent history of a viral infection.
O. Review recent trauma to the neck (significant trauma can cause thyrotoxicosis).

Physical Examination

A. Check temperature, if indicated, pulse (tachycardia), respirations (dyspnea), blood pressure (BP; systolic hypertension), and weight. Children: Plot height/weight on growth curve. (Accelerated growth is noted.)
B. Inspect
   1. Observe overall appearance: Does the patient have any difficulty with breathing, including dyspnea, or difficulty swallowing from tracheal obstruction secondary to a large goiter?
   2. Note eyelid retraction, lid lag, and exophthalmos. The clinician may see periorbital edema and an elevated upper eyelid, which leads to decreased blinking and a staring quality in Graves' disease.
   3. Note tremors that are best demonstrated from outstretched hands.
   4. Inspect the skin for temperature and texture.
   5. Inspect the fingernails for:
      a. Onycholysis, also known as Plummer's nails (loosening of the nails from the nail beds)
      b. Softening of the nails
   6. Inspect scalp hair.
   7. Assess Tanner stage in preadolescence/adolescence. Puberty may be delayed.
C. Auscultate
   1. The thyroid for bruits
   2. The heart and pulse rate. Patients with subclinical hyperthyroidism frequently present with atrial fibrillation.
   3. The carotid arteries for bruits
   4. Bowel sounds
D. Palpate
   1. Palpate the neck and thyroid for nodules, thrills, and enlargement. Depending on the etiology of the hyperthyroidism, the thyroid may range from normal to massive (Graves' disease or toxic multinodular goiter). Palpation of the thyroid can induce the gland to release increased hormone; be alert for signs and symptoms of thyroid storm.
   2. If the thyroid is tender and painful to palpation, granulomatous thyroiditis may be the etiology of hyperthyroidism.
   3. Palpate the heart for thrills.
   4. Palpate extremities for edema. Pretibial myxedema is noted in Graves' disease.
E. Neurologic examination
   1. Assess deep tendon reflexes (DTRs).
   2. Tests for lid lag
      a. Have the patient follow your finger as it moves up and down.
      b. Have the patient look down and observe if sclera can be seen above the iris.
   3. Have the patient stick out the tongue to observe for presence of tremors.

Diagnostic Tests

A. TSH, free thyroxine (T4), triiodothyronine (T3; see Table 20.6).
B. Radioactive iodine (131I) uptake (RAIU) if needed. If the patient has ophthalmopathy, clinical symptoms of

TABLE 20.6 Test Results in Hyperthyroidism

Disorder	TSH	Free T4	T3	RAIU and Thyroid Scan
Overt hyperthyroidism	L	H	H	H
Graves' disease	L	H	H	H
Multinodular goiter	L	H	–	H
T3 thyrotoxicosis (may be caused by antithyroid drug therapy)	L	N or H	H	N or H

H, high; L, low; N, normal, RAIU, radioactive iodine uptake; TSH, thyroid-stimulating hormone.

hyperthyroidism, and a diffusely enlarged thyroid gland, the RAIU test is not necessary to confirm Graves' disease. Pregnancy and breastfeeding are absolute contraindications to radionuclide imaging.

C. Consider additional laboratory testing.

1. Complete blood count (CBC; may have normochromic, normocytic anemia).

2. Serum ferritin (may be high).

D. If T4 and T3 are high, but TSH is normal or high, an MRI of the pituitary should be ordered to look for a pituitary mass.

E. An echocardiogram should be considered whether an irregular heart rate and signs of heart failure are noted on examination.

Differential Diagnoses

A. Hyperthyroidism

1. Graves' disease

2. T3-toxicosis

3. T4-toxicosis

4. Thyroid adenoma

5. Drug-induced hyperthyroidism, that is, iodine-rich amiodarone

6. Subclinical hyperthyroidism

7. TSH-induced hyperthyroidism (TSH-secreting pituitary adenoma)

8. Hyperthyroidism during pregnancy

9. Hashitoxicosis (combination of Hashimoto and thyrotoxicosis), rare autoimmune thyroid disease

B. Cardiovascular disease such as coronary artery disease (CAD) and heart failure

C. Gastrointestinal disorders such as irritable bowel syndrome (IBS), ulcerative colitis, and Crohn's disease

D. Cancer: Testicular germ cell tumors

E. Neurologic disorder

F. Hydatidiform mole (molar pregnancy)

G. Psychological disorder

Plan

A. General interventions

1. Carefully assess for complications of hyperthyroidism—cardiac, ophthalmologic, gastrointestinal, musculoskeletal, and psychological—and address each area identified.

2. Patients with tachycardia, palpitations, tremors, anxiety, and eyelid lag can be treated with a beta-adrenergic antagonist for some relief from those symptoms until they become euthyroid.

3. For infiltrative dermopathy over the lower extremities, the use of occlusive wraps on the affected side is recommended.

4. Only 5% of patients with Graves' disease develop severe ophthalmopathy. An initial ophthalmologic examination is recommended as baseline, with follow-up determined by the ophthalmologist.

B. Patient teaching

1. Patients taking propylthiouracil (PTU) or methimazole (MMI) should be instructed to immediately report any side effects, including rash, hives, fever, jaundice, abdominal pain, and clay-colored stools.

2. Less than 1% of patients develop agranulocytosis, but all patients should be instructed to call the provider immediately if a fever, sore throat, or joint ache develops due to their susceptibility to serious infection.

3. Patients receiving radioactive iodine (RAI) should be informed that they most likely need to take lifelong hormone replacement after the RAI treatment is completed.

4. Teach safety measures to guard against the possibility of fractures due to bone density loss secondary to hyperthyroidism.

5. Inform patients that an episode of serious depression may follow successful treatment of hyperthyroidism.

6. No special diet is required; however, patients should be told to avoid herbal supplements and sushi that contains seaweed.

C. Medical/surgical management

1. RAI is a common choice of therapy for adults. It is administered in capsule form or in water.

a. One dose is usually sufficient; however, a second dose may be given if necessary.

b. Permanent hypothyroidism requiring lifelong hormone replacement is the only notable complication.

2. A thyroidectomy is seldom used except in limited patient conditions.

a. Pregnancy if women are noncompliant or cannot tolerate thionamides because of allergies or agranulocytosis

b. Severe hyperthyroidism in children

c. Patients who refuse RAI therapy
d. Refractory amiodarone-induced hyperthyroidism
e. Patients with unstable cardiac conditions that require quick normalization of thyroid function

D. Pharmaceutical therapy
1. Antithyroid drugs: The choice of drugs depends on clinician experience, the severity of the disease, and patient preference. Provide titration of antithyroid drug dose every 4 weeks until thyroid function normalizes and to ensure the patient does not become hypothyroid. Graves' disease may go into remission after treatment for 12 to 18 months and drug therapy can be discontinued.
a. PTU
i. Initial dose 100 to 150 mg by mouth three times daily. Dosage decrease is almost always required at 4 to 8 weeks of start.
ii. Thyroid storm: 150 to 200 mg orally every 4 to 6 hours
iii. Not a first-line agent in pediatrics
iv. Except in thyroid storm, PTU is considered a second-line drug therapy. It is reserved for use in patients who are allergic to or intolerant of MMI and in women who are in the first trimester of pregnancy or planning pregnancy.
b. MMI (Tapazole)
i. Adults: 20 to 40 mg/d or in divided twice-a-day dose. Maintenance doses are 2.5 to 15 mg/d.
ii. Pediatrics: 0.2 mg/kg/d
iii. MMI is more potent than PTU and has a longer duration of action.
iv. MMI is not recommended for use in the first trimester of pregnancy.
2. RAI therapy is one of the most common treatments in adults. It is administered orally as a single dose. RAI is contraindicated in pregnancy and lactation.
3. Beta-blockers, such as propranolol (Inderal), are also used for hyperthyroidism.
4. Atrial fibrillation treatment is directed toward restoring an euthyroid state. Other therapies include
a. Beta-blockers (unless contraindicated, including chronic obstructive pulmonary disease [COPD] and asthma)
b. Calcium channel blockers if unable to use beta-blocker
c. Oral anticoagulation (keeping the international normalized ratio [INR] between 2 and 3)
d. Antiarrhythmic drugs and cardioversion may be unsuccessful until euthyroid.

Follow-Up

A. Depending on the experience of the clinician, a specialist, such as an endocrinologist, best performs treatment and therapy, including RAI and antithyroid medication.
B. Patients receiving PTU or MMI should be seen in the office every 4 to 6 weeks for evaluation and have blood drawn for serum TSH and free T4 measurements until euthyroid state is achieved and maintained.
C. Patients are usually maintained on these drugs for 1 to 2 years, with office visits every 3 months. The drug is then gradually withdrawn and 25% to 90% of patients experience permanent remission.
D. Patients with RAI therapy should be seen in the office to monitor thyroid levels. It is anticipated that most of them will require lifelong hormone replacement medication following treatment.
E. Due to the increased risk of bone loss, perform dual-energy x-ray absorptiometry (DEXA) scans to evaluate for osteopenia/osteoporosis.
F. Consider testing for impaired glucose tolerance (IGT) in untreated patients.

Consultation/Referral

A. Ophthalmology consultation is recommended for patients with ophthalmologic involvement.
B. If surgery is the choice of treatment, refer the patient to an endocrinologist and a surgeon.
C. An experienced obstetrician or perinatologist should follow pregnant women.

Individual Considerations

A. Pregnancy
1. Pregnant patients with mild hyperthyroidism may be followed with treatment.
2. If an antithyroid drug is necessary, PTU is the drug of choice in the first trimester. MMI has been associated with congenital anomalies such as tracheoesophageal fistula and choanal atresia. After the first trimester, mothers may be switched to MMI.
3. Monitor thyroid function every 4 weeks during pregnancy.
4. RAI therapy is contraindicated during pregnancy and breastfeeding.
5. Thyrotoxicosis may improve during pregnancy; however, symptoms may relapse during the postpartum period.
6. Hyperthyroidism in the third trimester may increase the risk of low birth weight.
7. Prolonged high-dose iodine therapy can cause fetal goiter.
8. Ultrasounds should be performed to evaluate fetal hyperthyroidism such as goiter, poor growth, cardiac failure, and hydrops fetalis.

B. Pediatrics
1. Low thyroid function at birth is present in approximately half of the neonates whose mother received PTU or MMI during pregnancy.
2. Graves' disease can occur in prepubescent girls. Symptoms can be vague and include hyperactivity or slowness and fatigue.
3. Carefully assess for goiter in children who present with a variety of symptoms otherwise unexplained.
4. PTU should not be used in pediatrics unless there is allergy to, or intolerance of, MMI and other options are not available.

C. Adults: Sympathetic activation (anxiety, hyperactivity, etc.) is seen in adult years more commonly than in the elderly population.

D. Geriatrics

1. Older patents exhibit only three clinical signs (tachycardia, fatigue, and weight loss), whereas younger patients may exhibit as many as 12 symptoms.
2. Rare signs in this population include atrial fibrillation, hyperactive reflexes, increased sweating, heat intolerance, tremors, nervousness, polydipsia, and increased appetite. Goiter is much less common.
3. Elderly women with hyperthyroidism are at increased risk for accelerated bone loss.

Thyroid Disease: Hypothyroidism

Jill C. Cash and Mellisa A. Hall

Definition

A. Hypothyroidism is a condition in which the body does not produce enough thyroid hormone. In general, hypothyroidism is considered permanent, requiring lifelong therapy to restore a euthyroid state. The most common physical finding is a goiter. The most common worldwide cause of hypothyroidism is iodine deficiency, whereas the most common cause in the United States is Hashimoto thyroiditis, an autoimmune thyroid disease.

Incidence

A. Hypothyroidism occurs in 5% of the population.
B. It occurs in women more than men (five to eight times higher).
C. The incidence is higher in Whites (5.1%) and Mexican Americans than in African Americans (1.7%).
D. It may present in up to 15% of people older than 65 years.
E. In adolescents, approximately 6% have acquired hypothyroidism.
F. Approximately 10% of patients with type 1 diabetes will develop chronic thyroiditis.
G. After pregnancy, up to 10% of women develop lymphocytic thyroiditis in the postpartum period (up to 10 months postpartum).
H. Approximately 1:4,000 newborns have congenital hypothyroidism (cretinism).

Pathogenesis

Hypothyroidism is caused by an insufficient production of thyroid hormones by the thyroid gland, either by a primary or a secondary cause.

A. Primary causes include decreased hormone production caused by autoimmune thyroiditis, endemic iodine deficiency, congenital defects, or decreased thyroid activity after treatment for hyperthyroidism.
The most common cause of primary hypothyroidism is chronic autoimmune thyroiditis called Hashimoto's thyroiditis. In this disease, circulating thyroid antibodies and the infiltration of lymphocytes destroy thyroid tissue. Autoimmune thyroiditis may also be a result of an inherited immune defect.

B. Secondary causes are much less common but may include insufficient stimulation from the pituitary or hypothalamus and peripheral resistance to thyroid hormones.
Acute thyroidism is a rare cause of hypothyroidism in which the cause is an acute bacterial infection. Subacute thyroiditis, a nonbacterial inflammation of the thyroid, is often preceded by a viral infection. Both of these conditions cause inflammation of the thyroid gland by lymphocytic and leukocytic infiltration into the thyroid tissue, resulting in hypothyroidism.

Predisposing Factors

A. Iodine deficiency
B. Women older than 40 years at highest risk
C. Presence of other autoimmune disorders (diagnosed and previously undiagnosed)
D. Recent acute bacterial or viral infection
E. Treatment with radioactive iodine (RAI) for thyroid gland problems
F. Surgical removal of thyroid gland
G. Exposure to external radiation
H. Evidence of pituitary or hypothalamic disease
I. Postpartum period
J. Type 1 (autoimmune) diabetes mellitus (DM)
K. Chromosomal disorders
  1. Down syndrome
  2. Turner's syndrome
  3. Klinefelter's syndrome
L. Celiac disease
M. Drug-induced
  1. Amiodarone
  2. Interferon alpha
  3. Thalidomide
  4. Lithium
  5. Stavudine
  6. Dopamine

Common Complaints

A. Weight gain/obesity
B. Fatigue/sluggishness
C. Cold intolerance
D. Constipation
E. Dry and flaky skin
F. Coarseness or loss of hair, inability of hair to hold a curl, hair loss at eyebrows, and reduced growth of hair
G. Reduced growth of nails
H. Hoarseness
I. Memory or mental impairment, difficulty concentrating, and slowed speech or thinking
J. Periorbital edema and facial puffiness
K. Irregular or heavy menses and infertility
L. Muscle aching and stiffness
M. Children
  1. Short stature
  2. Delayed skeletal maturation
  3. Overweight
  4. Delayed puberty
  5. Some adolescents have sexual precocity.
    a. Girls: Breast development
    b. Boys: Macro-orchidism

Other Signs and Symptoms

A. Asymptomatic if subclinical hypothyroidism and have no overt symptoms
B. Delayed reflexes
C. Elevated blood pressure (BP)
D. Hyperlipidemia
E. Jaundice
F. Painful subacute thyroiditis
  1. Sudden neck pain with sore throat, radiating to jaw and ears, and pain shifting to sides of the neck
  2. Late stage: Myxedema, thick scaly skin, muscle weakness/joint pain, enlarged tongue, hearing loss, bradycardia, cardiac hypertrophy, pleural effusion, and ascites
G. Pituitary or hypothalamic failure
  1. Loss of axillary and pubic hair
  2. Cessation of menses
  3. Postural hypotension
H. Exercise intolerance
I. Carpal tunnel syndrome is a common occurrence.
J. Depression
K. Ataxia
L. Decreased concentration/memory impairment

Subjective Data

A. Note history of recent illness and/or pregnancy.
B. Evaluate the patient's medical/surgical history for any treatment of hyperthyroid, including radioactive treatment or thyroidectomy.
C. Review dietary and weight history, how much weight has been gained, and over what period of time.
D. Review any changes in health status or symptoms associated with other body systems (thyroid symptoms usually involve multiple body systems).
E. Review any history of obstructive sleep apnea (OSA).
F. Assess for pain or swelling of the neck or difficulty swallowing.
G. Inquire as to the patient's history of supervoltage x-ray therapy to the neck for nonthyroid cancer or for polio.
H. Identify family history.
  1. Does the patient have a first-degree relative with thyroid disease?
  2. Is there a family history of any endocrine problems, including thyroid, type 1 DM, and/or receptor agonist (RA)?
I. Review the patient's medication history for current medication, over-the-counter (OTC) medications, vitamins, or herbal supplements.
J. Review the patient's menstrual history or history of infertility.
K. Inquire about constipation (new onset or worsening).

Physical Examination

A. Check pulse (bradycardia), respirations, BP (decreased systolic BP and increased diastolic BP), and weight. Plot the height/weight on a growth curve for children.
B. General observation
  1. Gait problems, such as ataxia or rigidity, and spasticity of the trunk and proximal extremities
  2. Quality of the patient's voice (hoarseness)
  3. Signs of depression, decreased concentration, or memory impairment
C. Inspection
  1. Inspect the skin (dry/flaky) for presence of jaundice
  2. Inspect the hair (coarse, thin, brittle) and decrease in pubic/axillary hair pattern.
  3. Perform oral examination for evaluation of macroglossia (enlarged tongue).
  4. Inspect the face/eye for periorbital puffiness/edema.
  5. Inspect the neck for the presence of a goiter and surgical scar.
  6. Child: Assess Tanner stage of puberty.
D. Auscultate
  1. The thyroid and carotids
  2. The heart
  3. The lungs
  4. The abdomen for bowel sounds in each quadrant (hypoactive)
E. Palpate
  1. The neck, thyroid gland, and lymph nodes
  2. The abdomen for presence of abdominal distension, ascites, masses in left lower quadrant, and hepatomegaly
  3. Palpate/evaluate extremities for edema.
F. Musculoskeletal examination: Perform a detailed musculoskeletal examination.
G. Neurologic examination
  1. Check visual fields (restricted with hypothyroidism).
  2. Test hearing.
    a. Whisper words and have the patient repeat.
    b. Use a ticking watch.
    c. Use a tuning fork.
      i. Weber test: Place vibrating fork on top midline of head (sound hearing equally in both ears).
      ii. Rinne test: Place vibrating tuning fork on mastoid, begin counting, and ask the patient to tell you when he or she no longer hears; then quickly reposition 1/2 to 1 inch from the ear and ask the patient when he or she no longer hears (hearing should be twice as long as bone conduction).
  3. Check for loss or reduction of deep tendon reflexes (DTRs).
  4. Evaluate proximal muscle weakness/strength.
  5. Test for abnormal tandem gait: Have the patient walk across the room in a heel–toe, heel–toe fashion.
  6. Check for sensory loss.
    a. Evaluate the first three fingers and one half of the fourth finger on testing loss of sensation from carpal tunnel syndrome.
    b. Evaluate sensory loss of the feet/legs (generally symmetrical in a "stocking-glove" distribution).

Diagnostic Tests

A. Thyroid-stimulating hormone (TSH)
B. When a high TSH is noted, repeat the test and add a free T4.
C. T3 resin uptake
D. Thyroid antibodies (see Table 20.7)

TABLE 20.7 Test Results in Hypothyroidism

Disorder	TSH	Free T4	T3	RAIU and Thyroid Scan	Peroxidase Antibodies
Hypothyroid	H	L	Sometimes L	N or L	n/a
Hashimoto's disease	H or variable	N or L	Not helpful	Variable	Positive
Subacute hypothyroidism	L	H	H or variable	L or absent	Usually thyroiditis
Silent lymphocytic thyroiditis (usually postpartum)	L when toxic; H when hypothyroid	n/a	L when toxic	Positive	

H, high; L, low; N, normal, RAIU, radioactive iodine uptake; TSH, thyroid-stimulating hormone.

E. TSH assay (if TSH assay is elevated, it indicates hypothyroidism)
F. Thyroid scan
G. Complete blood count (CBC; anemia)
H. Lipid profile
I. Ultrasound of the neck and thyroid to detect nodules (not a first-line test)

Differential Diagnoses

A. Hypothyroidism
   1. Hashimoto's thyroiditis
   2. Subclinical hypothyroidism
   3. Hypothyroidism secondary to treatment/intervention for hyperthyroidism
   4. De Quervain thyroiditis
   5. If TSH and free T4 are both low, consider hypothyroidism secondary to pituitary or hypothalamic failure.
B. Obesity: Patients with elevated total cholesterol levels or triglyceride levels are often misdiagnosed by assuming that these symptoms are caused by obesity and high-fat diets.
C. Depression
D. Ischemic heart disease
E. Nephrotic syndrome
F. Cirrhosis
G. Side effects/adverse effects of medications
H. Constipation
I. Sleep apnea/sleep disorder
J. Fibromyalgia
K. Infectious mononucleosis

Plan

A. General interventions
   1. The American Thyroid Association clinical practice guideline for detection of both subclinical and symptomatic hypothyroidism recommends that all adults age 35 years and older be screened for hypothyroidism every 5 years to identify thyroid disease in the early stages. However, Medicare does not cover a screening TSH in an asymptomatic patient.
   2. Patients with underactive thyroids require lifelong treatment with levothyroxine.
   3. In patients with subacute thyroiditis, relatively large doses of nonsteroidal anti-inflammatory drugs (NSAIDs) or prednisone may be prescribed.
   4. For patients with enlarged thyroid glands, surgery may be recommended if the gland begins obstructing the airway.
   5. The treatment of patients with malignant thyroid nodules depends on the type of cancer.
B. Patient teaching
   1. Teach the patient about the nature and course of the disease, as well as the signs and symptoms. Frequently, patients are relieved that their perceived symptoms are real and that there is treatment. This may also improve patient compliance.
   2. Teach the patient to report any side effects of the drug:
      a. Tachycardia
      b. Palpitations
      c. Chest pain
   3. Emphasize the need for lifelong treatment with levothyroxine and the dangers of noncompliance.
   4. **Thyroid replacement should be taken on an empty stomach.**
   5. The beneficial effects of thyroid replacement occur in about 3 days to 1 week; the patient may not feel the clinical effects for several months.
   6. When switching brands or using a generic, the serum TSH should be checked in 6 weeks.
C. Pharmacological therapy
   1. **Patients requiring therapy with levothyroxine should be treated with the same brand/generic consistently because potency varies between brand and generics.**
      a. Levothyroxine (Synthroid, Levoxyl, Levothroid, Unithroid)
         i. Adults 1.6 mcg/kg/d by mouth is administered as a single dose in the morning on an empty stomach.
         ii. Elderly with comorbid coronary artery disease (CAD) or severe chronic obstructive pulmonary disease (COPD) should be started at 25 to 50 mcg/d.
         iii. Maintenance dose is 50 to 200 mcg by mouth every morning.
         iv. Pediatric dosing is age and weight dependent.
      b. Desiccated thyroid (Armour thyroid)
         i. Adult initial dosing is 15 to 30 mg/d by mouth and increased by 15 to 30 mg/d every 4 weeks.
         ii. Maintenance dose is 60 to 180 mg/d.
         iii. Pediatric dosing is age and weight dependent.

2. The medication should be titrated to the lowest dosage needed to maintain euthyroidism and a non elevated serum TSH and a normal or slightly elevated T4.
3. Elderly patients and those with cardiovascular disease should be started on very low doses (25 mcg/d) of levothyroxine; doses are increased very gradually, over 8 to 12 weeks, as tolerated. Close monitoring for the development of cardiac complications such as angina, arrhythmias, and myocardial infarction needs to be undertaken.
4. Thyroid hormones should be taken on an empty stomach in the mornings to avoid insomnia.
5. Other drugs can reduce the effectiveness/affect the absorption of thyroid hormone:
   a. Cholesterol-reducing drugs
   b. Cholestyramine interferes with absorption in the gut.
   c. Calcium carbonate
   d. Aluminum hydroxide
   e. Sucralfate (Carafate)
   f. If taking one of these drugs and levothyroxine, they should be taken 4 to 6 hours apart.
6. Dietary fiber can interfere with levothyroxine absorption. Coffee reduces the absorption of levothyroxine.
7. Pharmacological treatment of the patient with subclinical hypothyroidism is controversial. If goiter is present, treatment may be considered.

Follow-Up

A. Patients who are not treated with medication should be seen every 6 to 12 months for reevaluation.
B. When medication is instituted, monitor laboratory values and patient well-being in the office every 4 to 6 weeks.
C. After the dosage is stabilized, the patient with an elevated serum TSH level should be seen every 6 to 12 months.
   1. Undetectable TSH levels are indicative of overmedication.
   2. High TSH levels are indicative of insufficient medication or patient noncompliance.
D. After the TSH is normalized, regular annual follow-up visits are required.
E. Order dual-energy x-ray absorptiometry (DEXA) scan as indicated to screen for bone loss/osteopenia/osteoporosis.

Consultation/Referral

A. Consultation with an endocrinologist is recommended for:
   1. Children/teens younger than 18 years
   2. Patients unresponsive to therapy
   3. Pregnant patients
   4. Presence of goiter, nodule, or other structural changes in the thyroid
   5. Compression symptoms of dysphagia
   6. Any patient with myxedema, significant cardiac disease, or involvement or hypothyroidism secondary to pituitary or hypothalamic failure should be managed in consultation with a physician or should be referred to an endocrinologist for continued care.
   7. If fine-needle aspiration biopsy is required

Individual Considerations

A. Pregnancy
   1. Monitor TSH levels monthly during the first trimester.
   2. Small increases in medication dosage may be required.
   3. Some women develop postpartum thyroiditis and hypothyroidism after taking hyperthyroid medication during pregnancy or immediately thereafter.
   4. Postpartum: Monitor TSH level at 6 weeks' postpartum examination.
   5. A common cause of congenital hypothyroidism is maternal and infant iodine deficiency.
   6. Monitor the TSH to avoid overtreatment in postpartum women because excess thyroid hormone levels increase the risk of osteoporosis.
   7. Hypothyroidism in pregnancy is associated with preeclampsia, anemia, postpartum hemorrhage, cardiac ventricular dysfunction, spontaneous abortion, low birth weight, impaired cognitive development, and fetal mortality.
B. Geriatrics
   1. Some elderly patients who are actually hyperthyroid exhibit symptoms of hypothyroidism.

Thyrotoxicosis/Thyroid Storm

Jill C. Cash and Mellisa A. Hall

Definition

A. Severe thyrotoxicosis of any cause is called thyrotoxic crisis or storm.

Incidence

A. It is rare; the incidence varies, depending on the cause of the thyrotoxicosis.

Pathogenesis

A. Thyrotoxic crisis or storm usually develops in patients either undiagnosed as being hyperthyroid or those who are known to be severely hyperthyroid, are being treated insufficiently, and are subjected to excessive stress from other causes. Oversecretion of T3 and T4 is followed by a release of epinephrine. Metabolism is dramatically increased. The adrenal glands produce excessive corticosteroids, which is a response to stress.

Predisposing Factors

A. Severe, uncontrolled hyperthyroidism
B. Noncompliance with anti hyperthyroid medication
C. Inadequate preparation for thyroid surgery

Common Complaints

A. Sudden onset of
   1. Hyperthermia
   2. Tachycardia (usually atrial tachydysrhythmias)
   3. High-output cardiac failure
   4. Altered sensorium (usually agitation, restlessness, delirium)
   5. Nausea, vomiting, and diarrhea

Subjective Data

A. Elicit information regarding the onset, duration, and nature of symptoms.

B. Determine the presence of cardiac symptoms.

C. Take a complete drug history, including whether or not the patient has been taking antithyroid medication as prescribed.

D. Rule out any excessive acute stressors such as infection, pulmonary or cardiac problems, dialysis, plasmapheresis, and/or emotional stressors.

Physical Examination

A. Check temperature, pulse, respirations, and blood pressure (BP).

B. Inspect

  1. The skin

C. Auscultate

  1. The heart and lungs

D. Palpate the neck carefully for thyroid nodules and enlargement.

Diagnostic Tests

A. Serum T3 and free T4

B. Thyroid-stimulating hormone (TSH)

Differential Diagnoses

A. Thyroid storm

B. Thyrotoxic crisis

Plan

A. General interventions

  1. Closely monitor temperature, pulse, respirations, and BP.

  2. Assess the need to hospitalize the patient for supportive therapy; intravenous fluids, medication treatment, antipyretics, and/or oxygen.

B. Patient teaching

  1. See "Patient Teaching" in the "Hyperthyroidism" section.

C. Pharmaceutical therapy

  1. See "Pharmaceutical Therapy" in the "Hyperthyroidism" section.

Follow-Up

A. Following resolution of the crisis, see the patient in the office every 3 to 4 weeks for evaluation and monitoring of serum TSH and free T4 levels.

B. See "Follow-Up" in the "Hyperthyroidism" section.

Consultation/Referral

A. Refer the patient to a physician immediately for possible hospitalization.

Individual Considerations

A. Pregnancy: See "Individual Considerations" in the "Hyperthyroidism" section.

Bibliography

American Diabetes Association. (2016). Standards of medical care in diabetes—2016. *Diabetes Care, 39*(Suppl. 1) Retrieved from http://care.diabetesjournals.org/content/suppl/2015/12/21/39.Supplement_1.DC2/2016-Standards-of-Care.pdf

American Geriatric Society. (2014). GNRS: A core curriculum in advanced practice geriatric nursing. In E. Flaherty & B. Resnick (Eds.), *GNRS Geriatric Nursing Review Syllabus: A Core Curriculum in Advanced Practice Geriatric Nursing* (4th ed., pp. 506–529). New York, NY: American Geriatrics Society.

Androgen Excess and Polycystic Ovarian Syndrome Society. (2016). Polycystic ovarian syndrome. Retrieved from http://ae-society.org/sub/resources.php

Arlt, W. (2015). Disorders of the adrenal cortex. In D. L. Kasper, A. S. Fauci, S. L. Hauser, D. L. Longo, & J. L. Jameson (Eds.), *Harrison's principles of internal medicine* (19th ed.). New York, NY: McGraw-Hill.

Atkinson, M. A. (2016). Type 1 diabetes mellitus. In S. Melmed, K. S. Polonsky, P. R. Larsen, & H. M. Kronenberg (Eds.), *Williams textbook of endocrinology* (13th ed. pp. 1451–1483). Philadelphia, PA: Elsevier.

Azziz, R. (2015, August). Epidemiology and pathogenesis of polycystic ovarian syndrome in adults. *UpToDate*. Retrieved from http://www.uptodate.com

Barbieri, R. L. (2013, August). Treatment of hirsutism. *UpToDate*. Retrieved from http://www.uptodate.com

Barbieri, R. L., & Ehrmann, D. A. (2015a, January). Evaluation of premenopausal women with hirsutism. *UpToDate*. Retrieved from http://www.uptodate.com

Barbieri, R. L., & Ehrmann, D. A. (2015b, March). Treatment of polycystic ovary syndrome in adults. *UpToDate*. Retrieved from http://www.uptodate.com

Barbieri, R. L., & Ehrmann, D. A. (2015c, August). Pathogenesis and causes of hirsutism. *UpToDate*. Retrieved from http://www.uptodate.com

Bhasin, S., & Jameson, J. L. (2015). Disorders of the testes and male reproductive system. In S. Melmed, K. S. Polonsky, P. R. Larsen, & H. M. Kronenberg (Eds.), *Williams textbook of endocrinology* (13th ed. pp. 785–832). Philadelphia, PA: Elsevier.

BMI Calculator. (n.d.a). BMI calculator. Retrieved from http://www.bmi-calculator.net

BMI Calculator. (n.d.b). Waist to hip ratio calculator. Retrieved from http://www.bmi-calculator.net/waist-to-hip-ratio-calculator

Braunstein, G. D. (2014, June). Causes, evaluation, and management of gyenocomastia. *UpToDate*. Retrieved from http://www.uptodate.com

Braunstein, G. D. (2015, October). Epidemiology, pathophysiology, and causes of gynecomastia. *UpToDate*. Retrieved from: http://www.uptodate.com

Bray, G. A. (2015a, January). Obesity in adults: Overview and management. *UpToDate*. Retrieved from http://www.uptodate.com

Bray, G. A. (2015b, October). Patient information: Weight loss treatments, beyond the basics. *UpToDate Online*. Retrieved from http://www.uptodate.com

Bray, G. A. (2016a, February). Obesity in adults: Prevalence, screening, and evaluation. *UpToDate*. Retrieved from http://www.uptodate.com

Bray, G. A. (2016b, March). Obesity in adults: Drug therapy. *UpToDate*. Retrieved from http://www.uptodate.com

Bray, G. A. (2016c, March). Obesity in adults: Health hazards. Retrieved from http://www.uptodate.com

Bulun, S. E. (2016). Physiology and pathology of the female reproductive axis. In S. Melmed, K. S. Polonsky, P. R. Larsen, & H. M. Kronenberg (Eds.), Williams textbook of endocrinology (13th ed., pp. 590–663) Philadelphia, PA: Elsevier Saunders

Centers for Disease Control and Prevention. (2011). Adult BMI calculator: English version. Retrieved from https://www.cdc.gov/healthyweight/assessing/bmi/adult_bmi/english_bmi_calculator/bmi_calculator.html

Centers for Disease Control and Prevention. (n.d.-a). BMI percentile calculator for child and teen: English version. Retrieved from https://nccd.cdc.gov/dnpabmi/calculator.aspx

Centers for Disease Control and Prevention, NCHS National Center for Health Statistics. (n.d.-b). Clinical growth charts. Retrieved from https://www.cdc.gov/growthcharts

Centers for Disease Control and Prevention. (2015, December). Diagnosed diabetes. Retrieved from https://www.cdc.gov/diabetes/statistics/prevalence _national.htm

Coustan, D. R. (2016, March). Diabetes mellitus in pregnancy: Screening and diagnosis. *UpToDate*. Retrieved from http://www.uptodate.com

Donohoue, P. A. (2016, March). Treatment of adrenal insufficiency in children. *UpToDate*. Retrieved from http://www.uptodate.com

Eckel, R. H. (2015). The metabolic syndrome. In D. L. Kasper, A. S. Fauci, S. L. Hauser, D. L. Longo, & J. L. Jameson (Eds.), *Harrison's principles of internal medicine* (19th ed. pp. 2449–2454). New York, NY: McGraw-Hill.

Eckel, R. H., Jakicie, J. M., Ard, J. D., Hubbard, V. S., de Jesus, J. M., Lee, I-Min., . . . Yanovski, S. Z. (2013). AHA/ACC guideline on lifestyle management to reduce cardiovascular risk: A report of the American College of Cardiology/American Heart Association Task Force on practice guidelines. *Circulation, 129*(25 Suppl. 2), S76–S99. doi:10.1161/01.cir.0000437740.48606.d1

Ehrmann, D. A. (2015). Hirsutism. In D. L. Kasper, A. S. Fauci, S. L. Hauser, D. L. Longo, & J. L. Jameson (Eds.), *Harrison's principles of internal medicine* (19th ed.). New York, NY: McGraw-Hill.

Ervin, B. (2009). Prevalence of metabolic syndrome among adults 20 years of age and older by sex, age, race, ethnicity, and body mass index United States 2003–2006. *National Health Statistics Reports.* Number 13. Retrieved from http://www.cdc.gov/nchs/data/nhsr/nhsr013.pdf

Goff, D. C., Lloyd-Jones, D. M., Bennett, G., Coady, S., D'Agostino, R. B., Sr., Gibbons, R., . . . Wilson, P. W. F. (2013, November 12). 2013 ACC/AHA guideline on the assessment of cardiovascular risk: A report of the American College of Cardiology/American Heart Association Task Force on practice guidelines. *Circulation.* doi: 10.1161/01.cir.0000437741.48606.98

Golshan, M., & Iglehart, D. (2013, June). Nipple discharge. *UpToDate.* Retrieved from http://www.uptodate.com

Hall, J. E. (2015). Menstrual disorders and pelvic pain. In D. L. Kasper, A. S. Fauci, S. L. Hauser, D. L. Longo, & J. L. Jameson (Eds.), *Harrison's principles of internal medicine* (19th ed.). New York, NY: McGraw-Hill.

James, P. A., Oparil, S., Carter, B. L., Cushman, W. C., Dennison-Himmelfarb, C., Handler, J., . . . Ortiz, E. (2013, December 18). 2014 Evidence-based guidelines for the management of high blood pressure in adults report from the panel members appointed to the Eighth Joint National Committee (JNC 8). *Journal of the American Medical Association, 311*(5), 507–520. doi:10.1001/jama.2013.284427

Jameson, J. L., Mandel, S. J., & Weetman, A. P. (2015). Disorders of the thyroid gland. In D. L. Kasper, A. S. Fauci, S. L. Hauser, D. L. Longo, & J. L. Jameson (Eds.), *Harrison's principles of internal medicine* (19th ed.). New York, NY: McGraw-Hill.

Klish, W. J. (2014, October). Clinical evaluation of the obese child and adolescent. *UpToDate.* Retrieved from http://www.uptodate.com

Klish, W. J. (2015, November). Comorbidities and complications of obesity in children and adolescents. *UpToDate.* Retrieved from http://www.uptodate.com

Klish, W. J. (2016, March). Definition; epidemiology; and etiology of obesity in children and adolescents. *UpToDate.* Retrieved from http://www.uptodate.com

Laffel, L., & Svoren, B. (2015, March). Epidemiology, presentation, and diagnosis of type 2 diabetes mellitus in children and adolescents. *UpToDate.* Retrieved from http://www.uptodate.com

LaFranchi, S. (2015a, April). Clinical manifestations and diagnosis of hyperthyroidism in children and adolescents. *UpToDate.* Retrieved from http://www.uptodate.com

LaFranchi, S. (2015b, November). Clinical features and detection of congenital hypothyroidism. *UpToDate.* Retrieved from http://www.uptodate.com

Lee, A. (Ed). *NPPR: Nurse practitioners' prescribing reference.* (2016). New York, NY: Haymarket Media.

Levitsky, L. L., & Misra, M. (2016, March). Epidemiology, presentation, and diagnosis of type 1 diabetes mellitus in children and adolescents. *UpToDate.* Retrieved from http://www.uptodate.com

Mantzoros, C. (2015, July). Insulin resistance: Definition and clinical spectrum. *UpToDate.* Retrieved from http://www.uptodate.com

McCulloch, D. K., & Munshi, M. (2015, November). Treatment of type 2 diabetes mellitus in the older patient. Retrieved from http://www.uptodate.com

McCulloch, D. K., & Robertson, R. P. (2014, September). Pathogenesis of type 2 diabetes mellitus. *UpToDate.* Retrieved from http://www.uptodate.com

Meigs, J. B. (2015, March). The metabolic syndrome (insulin resistance syndrome or syndrome X). *UpToDate.* Retrieved from http://www.uptodate.com

National Guideline Clearinghouse. (2015, May). Screening for thyroid dysfunction: U.S. Preventative Services Task Force recommendation statement. Retrieved from http://www.guideline.gov/content.aspx?id=49227&search=thyroid+screening

National Institutes of Health. (2015). *Third report of the National Cholesterol Education Program (NCEP) expert panel on detection, evaluation, and treatment of high blood cholesterol in adults (ATP III): final report.* Bethesda, MD: Author. Retrieved from https://www.nhlbi.nih.gov/sites/www.nhlbi.nih.gov/files/Circulation-2002-ATP-III-Final-Report-PDF-3143.pdf

Nieman, L. K. (2014a, May). Causes and pathophysiology of Cushing's syndrome. *UpToDate.* Retrieved from http://www.uptodate.com

Nieman, L. K. (2014b, December). Diagnosis of adrenal insufficiency in adults. *UpToDate.* Retrieved from http://www.uptodate.com

Nieman, L. K. (2014c, December). Treatment of adrenal insufficiency in adults. *UpToDate.* Retrieved from http://www.uptodate.com

Nieman, L. K. (2015a, June). Establishing the diagnosis of Cushing's. *UpToDate.* Retrieved from http://www.uptodate.com

Nieman, L. K. (2015b, July). Epidemiology and clinical manifestations of Cushing's syndrome. *UpToDate.* Retrieved from http://www.uptodate .com

Polonsky, K. S., & Burant, C. F. (2016). Type 2 diabetes mellitus. In S. Melmed, K. S. Polonsky, P. R. Larsen, & H. M. Kronenberg (Eds.), *Williams textbook of endocrinology* (13th ed., pp. 1386–1450) Philadelphia, PA: Elsevier Saunders.

Powers, A. C. (2015). Diabetes mellitus: Diagnosis, classification, and pathophysiology. In D. L. Kasper, A. S. Fauci, S. L. Hauser, D. L. Longo, & J. L. Jameson (Eds.), *Harrison's principles of internal medicine* (19th ed. pp. 2399–2424). New York, NY: McGraw-Hill.

Prescriber's Letter. (2015). Appropriate medication use in older adults: 2015 Updated. *Beer's Criteria, 22*(12), 311218. Retrieved from http://prescribersletter.therapeuticresearch.com

Rosenfield, R. L. (2014a, October). Treatment of polycystic ovary syndrome in adolescents. *UpToDate.* Retrieved from http://www.uptodate.com

Rosenfield, R. L. (2014b, October). Definition, clinical features, and differential diagnosis of polycystic ovary syndrome in adolescents. *UpToDate.* Retrieved from http://www.uptodate.com

Ross, D. S. (2015a, February). Hypothyroidism during pregnancy: Clinical manifestations, diagnosis, and treatment of hyperthyroidism during pregnancy. *UpToDate.* Retrieved from http://www.uptodate.com

Ross, D. S. (2015b, February). Thyroid storm. *UpToDate.* Retrieved from http://www.uptodate.com

Ross, D. S. (2015c, December). Diagnosis and screening for hypothyroidism in non-pregnant adults. *UpToDate.* Retrieved from http://www.uptodate.com

Ross, D. S. (2016, February). Treatment of hypothyroidism. *UpToDate.* Retrieved from http://www.uptodate.com

Rubin, D. I. (2015, April). Neurologic manifestations of hyperthyroidism and Graves disease. *UpToDate.* Retrieved from http://www.uptodate.com

Salley, K. E. S.., Wickham, E. P., Cheang, K. I., Essah, P. A., Karjane, N. W., & Nestler, J. E. (2007). POSITION STATEMENT: Glucose intolerance in polycystic ovary syndrome—A position statement of the Androgen Excess Society. *The Journal of Clinical Endocrinology & Metabolism, 92*(12), 4546–4556. Retrieved from http://press.endocrine.org/doi/pdf/10.1210/jc.2007-1549

Skelton, J. A. (2016, November). Management of childhood obesity in the primary care setting. *UpToDate.* Retrieved from http://www.uptodate.com

Snyder, P. J. (2015, January). Clinical features and diagnosis of male hypogonadism. *UpToDate.* Retrieved from http://www.uptodate.com

Stewart, P. M., & Newell-Price, J. D. (2016). The adrenal cortex. In S. Melmed, K. S. Polonsky, P. R. Larsen, & H. M. Kronenberg (Eds.), *Williams textbook of endocrinology* (13th ed. pp. 490–556.). Philadelphia, PA: Elsevier.

Stone, N. J., Robinson, J., Lichtenstein, A. H., Bairey Merz, C. N., Lloyd-Jones, D. M., & Blum, C. B. (2013, November 7). 2013 ACC/AHA guidelines on the treatment of blood cholesterol to reduce atherosclerotic cardiovascular risk in adults: A report of the American College of Cardiology/American Heart Association Task Force on practice guidelines. *Journal of the American College of Cardiology, 63*(25), pii: S0735–1097. Retrieved from https://circ.ahajournals.org/content/early/2013/11/11/01.cir.0000437738.63853.7a.full.pdf

U.S. Department of Health and Human Services. (2015a, March). Screening for abnormal blood glucose and type 2 diabetes mellitus: U.S. Preventive Services Task Force recommendation statement. Retrieved from http://www.guideline.gov/content.aspx?id=49928#Section420

U.S. Department of Health and Human Services. (2015b, May). *2014 National Diabetes Statistics report.* Centers for Disease Control and Prevention. Retrieved from http://www.cdc.gov/diabetes/data/statistics/2014statisticsreport.html

U.S. Department of Health and Human Services. (2015c, October). 2015 Recommendations for physical activity. Retrieved from https://www.nhlbi.nih.gov/health/health-topics/topics/phys/recommend

Wjjeyaratne, C. N., Udayangani, S. A. D., & Balen, A. H. (2013). Ethnic-specific polyovarian syndrome. Epidemiology, significance, and implications. *Expert Review in Endocrinology and Metabolism, 8*(1), 71–79.

21 Rheumatological Guidelines

Ankylosing Spondylitis

Jill C. Cash

Definition

A. Ankylosing spondylitis (AS) is a chronic, inflammatory joint disease that causes chronic joint pain/swelling, which primarily affects the spine and sacroiliac joints (SI); however, larger peripheral joints can also be affected.

Incidence

A. AS occurs in approximately 1% to 2% of the general population.
B. Prevalence rates differ between races. AS occurs in approximately 0.04% to 0.06% of non-Caucasians and in approximately 0.1% to 1.4% of Caucasians.

Pathogenesis

A. Inflammation occurs at the entheses (insertion site of the ligaments and tendons of the bone) throughout the body. Primary sites of involvement include the lower back, SI joint, and lower extremities. Inflammatory cells invade the joint and erode the bone and fibrocartilage of the joints. The body responds by trying to repair the tissue, in which fibrous scar tissue is formed. The structure is replaced by theossified scar tissue, which causes fusion of the joint; in return, flexibility of the joint is lost. The eroded joint tries to repair itself by osteoblast formation in building new bone tissue. This results in the production of new enthesis that deposits itself on top of the existing enthesis. Calcification of the spinal ligaments also occurs and the appearance of the vertebral bodies looks more "square" and distinct. This is referred to as a "bamboo spine."

Predisposing Factors

A. Gender (men > women, 3:1 ratio)
B. Race (Caucasians more prevalent, occurring more in the northern European countries)
C. Age: Onset of symptoms usually occurs during the early 20s. However, diagnosis usually is made several years after the onset of symptoms, more into the late 20- to 30-year range. AS rarely occurs after the age of 50.
D. Family history of AS
E. Thought to have a genetic predisposition: Serum human leukocyte antigen (HLA)-B27 positive. Approximately 90% to 95% of patients with AS have a positive HLA-B27. However, only 5% of patients with a positive HLA-B27 develop any type of spondyloarthropathy.

Common Complaints

A. Gradual onset of low back pain with initial onset of symptoms occurring in the early 20s.
B. SI joint pain
C. Joint pain occurring for more than 3 months, with morning stiffness
D. Low back pain/joint pain that improves with activity, worsens with rest
E. Dactylitis (sausage digits of the fingers/toes)
F. Enthesitis (inflammation/pain at insertion site of the tendon or ligament to the bone)

Other Signs and Symptoms

A. Peripheral joint pain and swelling
B. Decreased range of motion in joints/back/neck
C. Extra-articular features such as anterior uveitis or iritis
D. Fatigue
E. Weight loss
F. Shortness of breath (SOB)
G. Psoriasis

Subjective Data

A. Ask the patient when back pain/joint pain began. Have symptoms been present for several months/years? At what age did pain initially begin?
B. Is pain intermittent or constant?
C. Does pain improve or worsen with activity? Inflammatory back pain improves with activity and worsens with rest.
D. Does patient have complaints of other joint pain?
E. Has the patient noted any weight gain/loss, fatigue, or fevers?
F. Any history of psoriasis or other skin rashes?
G. Any gastrointestinal (GI) changes or chronic problems such as Crohn's disease, ulcerative colitis, or diarrhea?
H. Any pulmonary problems such as SOB, difficulty breathing, or SOB with activity?
I. Any cardiac changes or problems?
J. Any history of amyloidosis?

Physical Examination

A. Check vital signs, blood pressure (BP), pulse, respirations, and temperature as indicated.

B. Inspect

1. Assess the cervical spine. Ask the patient to stand straight and assess the degree of cervical change. Ask the patient to perform flexion, extension, lateral flexion, and rotate the head.

2. Inspect the thoracic and lumbar spine. Note degree of chest expansion of thoracic spine. Assess lumbar spine noting the range of motion (ROM) with flexion/extension. Have the patient bend to the right and left side and note any difference in flexion.

3. Assess gait. If abnormal gait, assess for hip pain/involvement.

4. Inspect hands/feet for sausage digits.

5. Inspect joints in hands/wrists/feet/knees for tender, swollen joints.

C. Auscultate

1. Heart

2. Lungs

D. Palpate

1. Examine the SI joints by palpating the SI joint while lying supine and while lying on the side. Have the patient flex one knee while lying supine, and externally rotate the hip. Assess for pain at the SI joint area while pressure is applied on the knee.

2. Assess for pain at the entheses site. Assess Achilles tendon and plantar fascia areas where the tendon attaches to the calcaneus.

Diagnostic Tests

A. Serum blood work:

1. HLA-B27 commonly positive

2. Rheumatoid factor usually negative

3. C-reactive protein (CRP)

4. Erythrocyte sedimentation rate (ESR)

5. Complete blood count (CBC)

6. Comprehensive metabolic panel (CMP)

7. Creatinine kinase

8. Alkaline phosphatase

9. Complement levels (C3, C4)

B. Radiographic studies

1. X-ray of cervical/thoracic/lumbar spine and pelvis

a. In AS, the spine is noted to have "squaring" of the vertebral bodies.

b. Sclerosis of the SI joint: Sacroiliitis grade 2 or above (grade 2 is bilateral sacroiliitis).

2. X-ray of peripheral joints: Erosions noted in the larger joints, loss of joint space, sclerosis

3. MRI of SI joints

4. Bone mineral density screening: High incidence of osteoporosis noted in patients diagnosed with AS.

Differential Diagnoses

A. AS

B. Reactive arthritis

C. Psoriatic arthritis

D. Spondylitis associated with inflammatory bowel disease

E. Rheumatoid arthritis (RA)

Plan

A. General interventions

1. Treatment for AS includes nonpharmacological and pharmacological interventions.

2. Osteoporosis screening and treatment are recommended for these patients.

3. Systemic steroids are not routinely prescribed; however, for severe symptoms of pain and swelling, joint injection may be considered.

B. Patient teaching

1. Encourage a healthy, active lifestyle. Activity improves symptoms. Regular exercises are recommended as tolerated. Physical therapy and/or structured exercises recommended most days of the week.

2. Medications prescribed should be used on a routine basis.

3. Fall prevention should be reviewed with the patient. The home should be modified to prevent falls. Suggestions include installing grab-bars in the bathroom tub/shower, removing loose rugs in the house, keeping walkways in the home clear and clutter free.

4. Seat belts should always be worn properly.

5. For persons with severe spinal involvement, contact sports and high-impact exercises/sports should be avoided.

C. Pharmaceutical therapy

1. Nonsteroidal anti-inflammatory drugs (NSAIDs) are first-line therapy for pain/symptoms produced from AS. All medications should not be used longer than 4 weeks.

a. Ibuprofen 400 mg every 4 to 6 hours as tolerated

b. Naproxyn 500 mg twice a day (bid) as tolerated

c. Celecoxib (Celebrex) 100 to 200 mg daily to bid as tolerated

d. Indomethacin 75 mg one to two times per day

e. Meloxicam 7.5 to 15 mg daily

f. Diclofenac 50 mg every 8 hours

2. Nonopioid analgesic

a. Acetaminophen 325 to 650 mg every 4 to 6 hours or 1,000 mg three times a day (tid)

3. Tumor necrosis factor alpha antagonists (anti-TNF) medications may be prescribed by a rheumatologist after failed NSAID use.

Follow-Up

A. Patients treated with NSAIDs should have routine follow-up at 2 weeks following initial diagnosis or sooner if not improving with treatment.

B. Patients treated with NSAIDs should be followed every 3 months with close monitoring of kidney and liver function.

Consultation/Referral

A. Patients diagnosed with AS should be referred to rheumatology for evaluation and treatment.

Individual Considerations

A. Adults

1. Young adults, typically during the 20- to 30-year range, are diagnosed with AS. Patients commonly present to the office with complaints of low back pain and are treated for noninflammatory chronic back pain. These patients may go years without the proper diagnosis and treatment. Therefore, delayed diagnosis is not uncommon in these patients.

2. Standard precautions should be followed for NSAIDs for patients with renal insufficiency and patients taking anticoagulants, systemic glucocorticoids, and other interacting medications.

B. Geriatrics

1. Not commonly diagnosed in this group of patients.

Fibromyalgia

Jill C. Cash

Definition

Fibromyalgia syndrome is a clinical condition characterized by generalized aching and stiffness, associated with the finding of numerous tender points in characteristic locations.

A. The most current guidelines for diagnosis are presented by the American College of Rheumatology (Wofle et al., 2010). The criteria for diagnosis include characteristic symptoms of pain at specific trigger point locations that are displayed by the patient for the past 3 months when there is no other reason or explanation for the associated pain.

B. Trigger point locations are found primarily in the back, neck, jaw, shoulders, chest, abdomen, arms, hips, and legs.

C. Somatic symptoms are also assessed for and present with fibromyalgia. Somatic complaints may include cognitive problems, sleeping difficulties, fatigue, headaches, and other associated symptoms. These criteria can be found at the ACR website: www.rheumatology.org

Areas palpated are considered positive if the patient verbalized the area as being "painful" when palpated.

Incidence

A. Fibromyalgia affects females more than males at a ratio of 10:1 and patients with an average age of 47 years; 5% of the population is affected with fibromyalgia. Usual onset is between 20 and 50 years; however, it has also been diagnosed in the young as well as the elderly. Often patients have symptoms for longer than 5 years before finally being diagnosed. The prevalence of fibromyalgia in rheumatology practice is 20%.

Pathogenesis

A. The cause is unclear. Studies of sleep physiology, neurohormonal function, muscular function, and psychological factors support a central mechanism for the disorder linked to depression. Other research suggests a pathophysiologic and psychological disorder.

Predisposing Factors

A. Life stress
B. Depression
C. Female gender
D. Age: Mid-30s and older

Common Complaints

A. Common complaints are multifocal pain present longer than 3 months; moderate to extreme fatigue; morning stiffness; nonrestorative sleep; pain worsening with stress; exposure to cold; inactivity or overactivity; sensitivity to touch, light, and sound; cognitive difficulties; and changes in barometric pressure.

Other Signs and Symptoms

A. Numbness
B. Swelling
C. Reactive hyperemia of skin
D. Raynaud's phenomenon
E. Irritable bowel syndrome (IBS) and bladder symptoms
F. Headaches
G. Restless legs syndrome (RLS)
H. Anxiety/depression

Subjective Data

A. Determine onset, duration, and course of complaints.
B. Does fatigue interfere with the patient's daily activity?
C. Note sleep quality. Does the patient feel rested after sleeping?
D. Do exacerbations of discomfort occur with stress, activity, and cold?
E. Has the patient experienced stress and/or depression in the past?
F. Does the patient have a family history of rheumatoid disease?
G. Has the patient ever been diagnosed with chronic fatigue syndrome, Lyme disease, or thyroid disease?

Physical Examination

A. Check temperature if indicated, pulse, and blood pressure (BP).

B. Inspect

1. Observe overall appearance.
2. Observe the nails, skin, mucous membranes, eyes, joints, and spine. If clubbing is noted and tender points are minimal, consider hypertrophic osteoarthropathy.

C. Palpate the muscles as outlined in the aforementioned criteria for classification of fibromyalgia. Note the following when palpating for tender points:

1. Pressure should be insufficient to produce pain in normal patients or at uninvolved sites in affected patients.
2. Pain on digital palpation must be present in at least 11 of 18 tender point sites.
3. "Positive pain reaction" is related to the patient stating that palpation causes pain. Tenderness is not to be considered as pain.
4. Painful points must be differentiated from trigger points of myofascial syndrome, which produce referred pain on compression.
5. Control areas not expected to be tender in fibromyalgia, such as middle of the forehead and fingertips, should be examined to exclude psychological pain or malingering.

D. Auscultate

1. Heart
2. Lungs

Diagnostic Tests

A. Antinuclear antibody (ANA)
B. Sedimentation rate
C. Thyroid-stimulating hormone (TSH)
D. Creatinine phosphokinase
E. Lyme titer if history of rash, arthritis, or deer tick exposure is present

Differential Diagnoses

A. Fibromyalgia
B. Rheumatoid arthritis (RA)
C. Osteoarthritis (OA)
D. Polymyalgia rheumatica
E. Ankylosing spondylitis
F. Myositis
G. Lupus erythematosus
H. Hypothyroidism
I. Chronic fatigue syndrome

Plan

A. General interventions: Routine follow-up is recommended. Multiple therapies may be beneficial for controlling symptoms. Stress importance of daily exercises and therapy to control pain. Support groups are beneficial for patients and families.

▶ **B.** Patient teaching: *See Section III: Patient Teaching Guide for this chapter, "Fibromyalgia."* Teach the patient that fibromyalgia is a recognizable syndrome that does not progress or cripple and does not warrant further testing. Patients can be assured it is not "all in their head."

- **1.** Exercise: Encourage the patient to exercise daily, including stretching programs along with walking, low-impact cardiovascular conditioning such as cycling, and low-impact aerobics. Initially, pain may increase with the first 2 weeks of exercise; then it improves with a routine exercise program.
- **2.** Pain control: Pain may improve with exercise, hot baths, heating pads, warm weather, and stress reduction.

C. Pharmaceutical therapy

- **1.** Amitriptyline 10 to 50 mg at bedtime for sleep
- **2.** Cyclobenzaprine 10 to 40 mg daily or other muscle relaxants
- **3.** Nonsteroidal anti-inflammatory drugs (NSAIDs) such as ibuprofen 200 to 600 mg every 4 to 6 hours. Maximum dose is 1.2 g/d.
- **4.** Analgesics such as acetaminophen (Tylenol) as needed
- **5.** Selective serotonin reuptake inhibitors (SSRIs) if depression is present.
- **6.** Pregabalin (Lyrica) 75 mg twice a day to 150 mg twice a day; maximum dose of 450 mg/d
- **7.** Duloxetine Hcl (Cymbalta) 30 to 60 mg once a day
- **8.** Milnacipran (Savella) titrated dose 12.5 mg on day 1; 12.5 mg twice a day for 2 days; 25 mg twice a day from days 4 to 7; then 50 mg twice a day (recommended dose). Maximum dose is 100 mg twice a day. Withdraw gradually. Precautions with renal impairment.
- **9.** Current guidelines suggest guarded use of opioids chronically in nonmalignant pain. Opioids have not been studied in randomized controlled trials and should be considered only after all other medicinal therapies have been exhausted. Tramadol, a centrally acting analgesic with atypical opioid and antidepressant-like activity, is moderately effective in treating fibromyalgia pain.
- **10.** Neurontin (Gabapentin) is approved for use in the treatment of neuropathic pain but not for fibromyalgia.

Follow-Up

A. Schedule regular visits in initial 2 to 4 weeks to evaluate how therapy is helping. Educate the patient each visit, and stress positive reinforcement and supervision of treatment regimen. Visits may then be scheduled every 3 months to monitor progress.

Consultation/Referral

A. Consult with a physician if the patient has abnormal laboratory results.
B. Consult or refer the patient to a physician if depression is suspected and current medication therapy is unsuccessful.

Individual Considerations

A. Geriatrics

- **1.** Fibromyalgia is common in the elderly and can be more painful for this population because of other coexisting conditions such as OA.

Gout

Jill C. Cash

Definition

A. Gout is an acute, sudden inflammatory disease of the joint, caused by high concentrations of uric acid in the joints and bones.
B. Three stages of gout

- **1.** Acute gouty arthritis: Acute attack exhibiting severe pain, redness, and swelling of a joint, which may last from days to weeks, even if left untreated.
- **2.** Intercritical gout: Period without flares
- **3.** Chronic/tophaceous gout: The progression of gout that has been inadequately treated, resulting in urate crystal deposits (tophaceous deposits) in the joints that can cause deformity and disability of the joint.

Incidence

A. Gout is most common in men from ages 30 to 60 years. Women become increasingly susceptible to gout after menopause. It is estimated that gout occurs in approximately 3% of the adult population in the United States.

Pathogenesis

A. Primary: High levels of uric acid result from either increased production or decreased excretion rates of uric acid.
B. Secondary: Hyperuricemia results from primary disease processes such as hypertension, renal failure, kidney disorders, and so forth. See the following section "Predisposing Factors."
C. Medications/toxins can also cause hyperuricemia.

Predisposing Factors

A. Chronic conditions: Hyperuricemia, chronic kidney disease, hypertension, diabetes mellitus, ischemic cardiovascular disease, hyperlipidemia, obesity
B. Gender (men older than 30 years)
C. Medications that alter uric acid level (diuretics, acetylsalicylic acid, alcohol, nicotinic acid, ethambutol, pyrazinamide)
D. Dietary factors (high intake of beer and meat/fresh seafood products)

Common Complaints

A. Redness, swelling, warmth, and/or pain in the joint (usually one joint only)—podagra (big toe). The pain is likely to be the most severe in the first 12 to 24 hours.
B. History of having severe joint pain with inflammation in other joints, followed by pain-free episodes.

Other Signs and Symptoms

A. Tophi are seen from several years of untreated gout.
B. Fever may be present in acute stages.

Subjective Data

A. Note when initial symptoms began.
B. Review patient history of gout.
C. Determine what makes the symptoms worse or better.
D. List medications/therapies used and the result of the different therapies used.

Physical Examination

A. Check temperature, pulse, respirations, and blood pressure (BP).
B. Inspect
  1. Inspect the joints.
  2. Note the presence of tophi on other joints.
C. Palpate the joints for tenderness, pain, and increase in temperature of skin.

Diagnostic Tests

A. Joint fluid aspiration for urate crystals is the gold standard in diagnosing gout. Inspect fluid with a polarized light microscopy to identify uric acid crystals.
B. Complete blood count (CBC): White blood cell count elevated
C. Erythrocyte sedimentation rate (ESR): Elevated in gout
D. Serum uric acid level: Uric acid greater than 6.8 mg/dL. Serum uric acid level may be normal during acute attacks. Perform test at least 2 weeks after acute attack or when flare has resolved.
E. Rheumatoid factor (RF) titer
F. X-ray or MRI: Identify bone cysts/gout tophi.

Differential Diagnoses

A. Gout
B. Infectious arthritis
C. Rheumatoid arthritis (RA)
D. Hyperparathyroidism
E. Pseudogout (calcium pyrophosphate deposition disease) commonly occurs in the knee, wrist, or other joints.
F. Bursitis
G. Cellulitis

Plan

A. General interventions
  1. Rest the joint area; no heavy lifting or weight-bearing activity.
  2. Aspirin products should not be used.
B. Patient teaching
  1. Increase fluid intake to at least eight glasses of water daily.
  2. Avoid alcohol intake and excessive meat and seafood products that trigger flares.
  3. Medication treatment and compliance of taking the prescribed medications can be very effective in preventing the development of the chronic tophaceous gout stage.
  4. *See Section III: Patient Teaching Guide for this chapter, "Gout."* ◄
C. Pharmaceutical therapy
  1. Analgesia
    a. Nonsteroidal anti-inflammatory drugs (NSAIDs)—most effective if started within 48 hours of presenting symptoms
      i. Indocin 50 mg every 8 hours for eight doses, then 25 mg every 8 hours until pain free for 1 to 2 days. Normal course is 5 to 7 days.
      ii. Naproxen, 750 mg initially, followed by 500 mg every 12 hours
      iii. NSAIDs are contraindicated for patients with the diagnosis of renal insufficiency, heart failure, ulcer disease, NSAID allergy, and anticoagulation therapy.
    b. Colchicine (Colcrys) is most effective if started within 12 to 24 hours of presenting symptoms: 1.2 mg initial dose, followed by 0.6 mg 1 hour later. Continue 0.6 mg one to two times daily until symptoms resolve. Medication may be stopped after the patient is free from symptoms after 2 to 3 days. Cochicine may also be used to prevent attacks. Colchicine warnings: Be aware of contraindications. Caution regarding drug interactions. Intolerable side effects of colchicine include nausea, vomiting, and diarrhea. Be cautious with use in patients with kidney/liver impairment.
    c. Corticosteroids may be used for patients who cannot tolerate oral medications. Intra-articular steroid injection of methylprednisolone acetate may be given. Oral steroids may also be prescribed for patients who cannot take NSAIDs or colchicine and who cannot tolerate intra-articular steroid injection. Prednisone is safe. Be aware of rebound effects.
  2. For hypersecretion of uric acid, long-term therapy is needed to decrease uric acid production: Allopurinol (Zyloprim) is the drug of choice. Starting dose 100 mg/d and titrate up over several weeks to a maximum of 300 mg/d. The goal is to keep the uric acid level less than 6.0 mg/dL. Febuxostat (Uloric) is also used to lower blood uric acid levels. The recommended dose is 40 mg/d with or without food; maximum dose is 80 mg/d. Initial laboratory studies include liver enzymes before beginning Uloric.

Common side effects include liver problems, nausea, gout flares, joint pain, and rash.

3. For reduced excretion rates of uric acid, consider probenecid (Benemid) 250 mg by mouth twice a day for 1 week, then increase to 500 mg by mouth twice a day. Increased consumption of fluids must be encouraged.

4. Chronic gout: If patients have three or more attacks per year, consider long-term therapy, low dose of NSAIDs, or allopurinol for 2 to 12 months.

5. Alternative medications for intolerance, renal insufficiency, and extensive tophi include oxypurinol, febuxostat, and uricase. Refer to rheumatology specialist.

Follow-Up

A. The patient should be contacted within 24 hours for evaluation.

B. Schedule follow-up visit in 1 month to reevaluate status.

C. Chronic gout: Obtain yearly uric acid levels; before initiating long-term therapy, obtain baseline blood urea nitrogen (BUN), serum lipid profile, and CBC and periodic liver enzymes.

Consultation/Referral

A. Consult and refer to physician or rheumatologist for aspiration of joint fluid and newer treatment options.

Individual Considerations

A. Pregnancy: Colchicine not recommended

B. Pediatrics

1. Colchicine not recommended
2. If gout is seen in this population, consider underlying primary cause (i.e., inborn error of metabolism).

C. Geriatrics

1. Reformation in joint areas may be seen in patients who have a history of gout from the uric acid deposits.
2. Complications for chronic gout include nephrolithiasis and chronic urate nephropathy.
3. Avoid Indocin in elderly patients because of the increased risk of adverse effects with other medications when compared with other NSAIDs.
4. NSAIDs are not recommended in the elderly with a history of heart failure, gastrointestinal (GI) ulcers/disease, and renal impairment.
5. Individual considerations must be given in this population regarding GI, cardiac, renal, and liver disease.
6. Glucocorticoids are generally well tolerated in this population and a safer alternative if NSAIDs or colchicine may increase the risks for the patient.

Osteoarthritis

Jill C. Cash

Definition

A. Osteoarthritis (OA), formerly known as degenerative joint disease, is a chronic noninflammatory disease that affects the movable joints. OA is characterized by destruction of the cartilage with resultant decrease in the joint spaces and bony overgrowth. OA is considered to be primary when there are no underlying conditions, and secondary to conditions such as trauma, septic arthritis, inflammatory arthritis, metabolic disorders, or congenital or acquired joint abnormalities.

Incidence

A. It is estimated that up to 12% of the general population between the ages of 25 and 74 years have OA. The incidence clearly increases with age as up to 85% of the general population older than 65 years of age have radiographic changes suggestive of OA.

Pathogenesis

A. Damage to the articular cartilage and subchondral bone may be because of local trauma and results in chondrocyte injury.

B. Chondrocytes release proteolytic enzymes that assist in repair of the cartilage.

C. In OA, the remodeling process of chondrocytes and release of enzymes is impaired and results in a loss of strength and greater trauma and destruction of the subchondral bone. The end result is joint destruction and bony overgrowth.

Predisposing Factors

A. Increasing age: Among patients older than 55 years

B. Gender: Women are more commonly affected and exhibit greater disease severity.

C. Genetic predisposition; distal interphalangeal (DIP) joint involvement

D. Trauma such as previous fractures, ligamentous injuries, or occupationally related repetitive stress

E. Altered joint anatomy or instability

F. Obesity: Mechanical injury in the knee may increase OA.

G. Secondary inflammation such as infections, inflammatory arthropathies, and metabolic disorders

Common Complaints

A. Unilateral joint pain frequently involving the joints of the hands, neck, lower back, knees, and hips

B. Morning stiffness lasting less than 1 hour

Other Signs and Symptoms

A. Unilateral joint pain involving the DIP and proximal interphalangeal (PIP) joints, first carpometacarpal joint, hips, knees, cervical and lumbar spine, and first metatarsophalangeal joint

B. Mild OA, or early disease, pain that increases with joint use and decreases with rest

C. Severe OA, or late disease, pain that is present with rest

Subjective Data

A. Elicit the patient's age at onset of pain.

B. Has the pain gradually gotten worse over the months or years?

C. How long does the pain last in the morning? Does the pain get worse with joint use and better with rest?

D. What joints are involved?

E. Is the joint pain described as "aching"?
F. What does the patient take to relieve the pain?
G. Is there any joint deformity, redness, swelling, or warmth?
H. Is there any decrease in range of motion (ROM) of the joint?
I. Is there any family history of OA?

Physical Examination

A. Check pulse and blood pressure (BP).
B. Inspect the joints for enlargement, edema, and erythema.
C. Palpate
  1. Palpate the joints, noting temperature, edema, and tenderness. Joints are cool; bony enlargement may be present in the PIP (Bouchard's nodes) or DIP joints (Heberden's nodes) and other weight-bearing joints.
  2. Palpate extremities. Perform assisted and active ROM exercises. With examination, limited ROM of the joint and/or pain on palpation may be present, along with crepitus.

Diagnostic Tests

A. Erythrocyte sedimentation rate (ESR): OA does not cause an increase of the ESR.
B. Chemistry profile
C. Complete blood count (CBC)
D. Rheumatoid factor (RF)
E. Routine radiography: Confirms disease severity and presence of joint narrowing
F. CT scan or MRI: Considered with nerve impingement syndrome (spine) or spinal stenosis

Differential Diagnoses

A. OA
B. Rheumatoid arthritis (RA)
C. Gout or pseudogout
D. Septic arthritis
E. Bursitis or tendonitis
F. Systemic lupus erythematosus
G. Fracture or trauma

Plan

A. General interventions
  1. Confirm diagnosis.
  2. Provide the patient with support and education to improve patient well-being and reduce discomfort.
  3. Physical therapy and/or occupational therapy should be initiated, if indicated.
B. Patient teaching
  ▶ **1.** *See Section III: Patient Teaching Guide for this chapter, "Osteoarthritis."*
  2. Reinforce the importance of joint protection; avoid repetitive stress or trauma.
  3. Encourage daily exercises and strengthening.
  4. Encourage weight loss if the patient is obese.
C. Pharmaceutical therapy
  1. First-line agents: The goal of treatment is to preserve joint mobility. First-line agents should be used in a stepwise approach.
    a. Acetaminophen up to 1 g four times daily; in early disease, this may be given on an as-needed basis.
    b. Nonsteroidal anti-inflammatory drugs (NSAIDs) if acetaminophen has failed to control the pain. Use with caution. Consider renal function and risk factors for peptic ulcer disease (PUD) and cardiovascular disease.
      i. Naproxen 220 to 375 mg one to two times daily.
      ii. Inflammatory OA: Consider naproxen 375 to 500 mg twice a day. Recommend taking this medication for 2 to 4 weeks for maximum effects.
      iii. Ibuprofen 200 to 400 mg, three times a day, may also be considered. Doses may be increased at a gradual pace for maximum benefit as tolerated. If one NSAID does not work consider other NSAIDs.
        1) Cox-2 inhibitors, such as celecoxib (Celebrex), may also be considered. Celebrex 200 mg daily to twice a day as tolerated.
        2) Meloxicam (Mobic) 7.5 to 15 mg daily.
    c. For high-risk patients, an H_2 receptor blocker may decrease gastritis and be helpful in preventing duodenal ulcers. Consider Arthrotec 50: One tablet three times a day.
    d. Misoprostol may be considered in patients who are at high risk of gastric ulcers. It should not be used by pregnant women. It is considered high risk for fetal death and possible congenital abnormalities.
    e. Topical creams
      i. Diclofenac gel (Voltaren gel) may be applied to affected area; recommended for patients with severe pain who are not able to tolerate oral NSAIDs.
      ii. Capsaicin cream may be applied to the affected area. Capsaicin creams may cause local burning at the site of application for the first several days.
  2. Second-line agents: Second-line agents, such as intra-articular corticosteroid injections, may prevent some joint erosion and decrease pain. The same joint should not be injected more than three to four times a year in 3-month intervals. If the joint is injected at this frequency for more than 1 year, alternative options, such as surgery, should be considered. Narcotics may provide relief from more severe OA pain, but they carry a risk of dependence.
  3. The use of glucosamine and chondroitin has not been established and is not recommended for patients. There does not appear to be any risks associated with using glucosamine and chondroitin. If the patient

does not notice any relief within the first 6 months of use, then recommendations are to discontinue this product.

4. Physical therapy to create an individualized exercise regimen to strengthen muscles, increase ROM, and reduce pain

5. Lubrication injections (Hyalgan or Synvisc) may also be considered. Referral to the rheumatologist should be considered for this treatment.

Follow-Up

A. Follow-up is based on disease severity and therapeutic treatment. If the patient is treated with first-line agents, follow up on pain control, nonpharmocological interventions, and possible side effects of medications within 2 to 4 weeks.

Consultation/Referral

A. Referral to an orthopedic surgeon may be considered for moderate to severe pain as indicated.

Individual Considerations

A. Pregnancy: NSAIDs should not be used in pregnancy unless clearly indicated. Misoprostol should be used with great caution in women of childbearing age because of its potential for fetal abnormalities and abortive properties.

B. Adults and geriatrics: Patients on chronic NSAIDs should be monitored closely for toxicity such as renal insufficiency, gastritis, and PUD. Elderly patients and those with preexisting gastrointestinal (GI) disease, diabetes, congestive heart failure, and cirrhosis should be monitored closely.

Osteoporosis/Kyphosis/Fracture

Jill C. Cash

Definition

A. Osteoporosis is a condition of reduced bone mass resulting in bone fragility and fracture. The World Health Organization (WHO) has defined it as "spinal or hip bone mineral density (BMD) of 2.5 standard deviations or more below the mean for healthy, young women (T-score of –2.5 or below) as measured by dual energy x-ray absorptiometry." BMD is performed on the lumbar spine, hip, and/or forearm.

B. Clinical diagnosis of osteoporosis can also be defined as having a fragility fracture of the spine, hip, wrist, pelvis, rib, and/or humerus without evidence of a BMD.

C. Osteopenia is defined as low bone mass of the spinal or hip BMD between 1 and 2.5 standard deviations below the mean as evidenced by the T-score (T-score between -1.0 and -2.5).

D. Kyphosis (dowager's hump) is the forward curvature of the thoracic spine. It is estimated that kyphosis occurs in approximately 20% to 40% of patients older than 60 years of age. Kyphosis may occur because of many different causes, including vertebral fractures, muscle weakness, degenerative disk disease, postural changes, and genetic/metabolic changes. Kyphosis is associated with other conditions such as decreased pulmonary function, back pain, increased risk of fracture of the spine, limited mobility, and an increase in mortality.

E. Osteoporotic fracture occurs from a fall while standing at normal height or less, without any type of trauma and/or while performing daily activities. A vertebral compression fracture is the most common type of osteoporotic fracture.

F. Vertebral fractures: There are three primary types of vertebral fractures:

1. Biconcave deformity
2. Wedge fracture
3. Compression fracture

Incidence

A. There are approximately 25 million people in the United States diagnosed with osteoporosis; 80% of those are women. Women are diagnosed with osteoporosis six to eight times more often than men and this is thought to be related to hormone deficiency (estrogen). The peak incidence of fractures in men occurs 10 years later in life than for women, averaging at 70 years of age.

B. Approximately 50% to 60% of 50-year-old women sustain osteoporosis-related fractures during their remaining life. Spinal fractures occur in 25% of White women by age 65 years, causing pain, deformity, and disability. Most common fractures include 25% at distal radius (Colles' fracture), 50% in vertebrae, and 25% in the hip.

C. Approximately 33% of all women and 17% of men suffer a hip fracture before age 90 years, and 20% of those who sustain a fracture die within 3 months of the event.

Pathogenesis

A. Osteoporosis occurs because of bone reabsorption being greater than bone formation.

Predisposing Factors

A. Hypogonadal states, particularly menopause
B. Small body frame, low body weight (less than 127 lbs)
C. Cigarette smoking
D. Low calcium intake
E. Lack of weight-bearing exercise
F. Family history of hip/pelvic fracture
G. Excessive alcohol intake
H. Asian or Caucasian
I. Advanced age
J. Previous fracture
K. Secondary causes
   1. Hyperparathyroidism
   2. Hyperthyroidism
   3. Cushing's syndrome
   4. Multiple myeloma
   5. Thyroid replacement therapy
   6. Corticosteroid therapy
   7. Renal disease

Common Complaints

A. Loss of height
B. Kyphosis, or dowager's hump
C. Back pain as a result of a compression fracture

Other Signs and Symptoms

A. Cervical lordosis
B. Fracture with little or no trauma
C. Crush fracture of vertebra
D. Pain

Subjective Data

A. Explore history of the following:
  1. Loss of height. Ask patient to compare current height with height written on the driver's license if height unknown.
  2. Low initial bone mass
  3. Early menopause, oophorectomy, postmenopause, or amenorrhea
  4. European or Asian family origin
  5. Family history of spinal fractures and osteoporosis
  6. Sedentary lifestyle with little weight-bearing activity
  7. Endocrine disorders
  8. Review medications taken in the present and past, including over-the-counter (OTC) and herbal supplements, with attention to medications such as corticosteroids, barbiturates, heparin, and thyroid hormone.
  9. Dietary review for low calcium and vitamin D intake
  10. Increased alcohol, caffeine, and protein intake
  11. Renal disease/dialysis
B. Determine onset, duration, location, and characteristic of back pain if present.
C. Has the patient had any recent falls?

Physical Examination

A. Check pulse, blood pressure (BP), height, and weight.
B. Inspect
  1. Compare present height with previous height.
  2. Observe presence of dorsal kyphosis.
  3. Observe physical abnormalities that interfere with mobility.
C. Palpate the joints and over the back for pain.

Diagnostic Tests

A. Laboratory studies
  1. Women: Comprehensive metabolic panel (CMP; calcium, phosphorus, albumin, total protein, creatinine, liver enzymes, alkaline phosphatase, electrolytes), thyroid-stimulating hormone (TSH), and 25-hydroxyvitamin D level
  2. Men: CMP (calcium, phosphorus, albumin, total protein, creatinine, liver enzymes, alkaline phosphatase, electrolytes), TSH, 25-hydroxyvitamin D level, and testosterone level
  3. Complete blood count (CBC), erythrocyte sedimentation rate (ESR), and serum protein electrophoresis to rule out multiple myeloma and leukemia if concerned.
B. BMD or dual-energy x-ray absorptiometry (DEXA) scan.
  1. The DEXA scan measures bone density of the lumbar spine and/or hip. Medicare will reimburse for this test to be performed every 2 years. If the spine is compressed or has severe scoliosis, BMD values may not be valid for the lumbar spine. Consider assessing the forearm for radial interpretation.
  2. The result of this procedure is read in "T-scores" or "Z-scores." T-scores are evaluated for postmenopausal women and older men. A T-score is a number given to identify the amount of bone present when compared with other healthy adults. Z-scores are recommended for premenopausal women. A Z-score is a score given to identify the amount of bone present when compared with other people of the same age, gender, and weight.
  3. The WHO Fracture Risk Assessment Tool (FRAX) was developed to determine the absolute fracture risk of breaking a bone in the next 10 years. This tool may be used with the BMD results to determine who needs to be treated with medication for prevention of fracture when treatment is unclear. FRAX should be used on women who have not previously been treated with antiresorptive therapy when T-scores are between −1.5 and −2.5. The FRAX tool can also be used on patients who have been treated with prior antiresorptive medications if they have been off these medications for more than 2 years. FRAX scoring is not recommended for patients currently being prescribed antiresorptive medications.
C. Radiography: X-ray the lumbar and thoracic spine for suspected vertebral fracture and/or for height loss greater than 2 in. Consider a CT to assess for instability of a wedge fracture. An MRI is recommended to assess for the extent of a compression fracture and/or possible malignancy.

Differential Diagnoses

A. Osteoporosis
B. Osteoarthritis (OA)
C. Secondary causes
  1. Thyroid disease
  2. Glucocorticoid therapy
  3. Malabsorption syndromes
  4. Renal or collagen disease
  5. Vitamin D deficiency
  6. Metastatic cancer
  7. Multiple myeloma

Plan

A. General interventions: Lifestyle changes should be introduced to the patient.
B. Patient teaching
  1. Educate the patient regarding calcium and vitamin D intake in diet.
    a. Calcium intake:
      i. Men younger than 50 years up to 69 years: 1,000 mg/d
      ii. Men older than 70 years: 1,200 mg/d
      iii. Women younger than or equal to 50 years: 1,000 mg/d
      iv. Women older than 50 years: 1,200 mg/d
      v. Food sources high in calcium include salmon or sardines with bones, low-fat yogurt and skim milk, green vegetables, and cheese

b. Vitamin D intake:

i. Men younger than 50 years of age: 400 to 800 IU/d

ii. Men 51 to 69 years: 800 to 1,000 IU/d

iii. Men older than 70 years of age: 800 to 1,000 IU/d

iv. Women younger than 50 years of age: 400 to 800 IU/d

v. Women 50 years of age and older: 800 to 1,000 IU/d

vi. Food sources high in vitamin D include: Vitamin D-fortified milk and cereals, fish liver oils, cod liver oil, mushrooms, herring, catfish, salmon, sardines, egg yolks, cheese, and beef liver.

2. Encourage the patient to eliminate alcohol and caffeine from diet.

3. Encourage the patient to eliminate cigarette smoking.

4. Prescribe regular moderate exercise, such as 30 minutes of walking at least three times per week. Walking 50 to 60 minutes three times per week provides optimal benefits.

5. Fall prevention: Advise the patient to avoid medications that may cause drowsiness and precipitate falls. Use extra light at night in the bathroom to help prevent falls. Remove all loose rugs and clutter from the home. Install hand rails on steps.

6. Discuss safety issues and fall prevention with the patient and family.

C. Pharmaceutical therapy

1. Calcium supplements

Calcium supplements may be contraindicated in patients who have a history of renal stones.

a. Calcium carbonate (Os-Cal) 500 mg is given orally one to three times per day, or Tums 1 tablet orally two to three times a day. See the section "Plan" discussed earlier for recommendations.

2. Vitamin D supplements: See the section "Plan" discussed earlier for recommendations. Patients diagnosed with vitamin D deficiency should ingest an increased dosage, according to the deficiency.

3. Biphosphonates: First-line therapy recommended for osteoporosis

a. Acts by reducing bone resorption and bone loss by preventing osteoclast activity

b. May be given daily, weekly, or monthly

i. Alendronate sodium (Fosamax): Available in 5, 10, 35, 40, and 70 mg tablets; 70 mg liquid; 70 mg tablet + 2,800 IU vitamin D tablet

ii. Risedronate (Actonel): Available as 5 mg daily, 35 mg weekly, or 150 mg monthly

iii. Zoledronic (Reclast): 5 mg/100 mL (intravenous [IV]) infusion once yearly as 15-minute infusion. Check serum creatinine and calcium before infusion.

c. Instruct the patient to take medication with 6 to 8 ounces of water one-half hour before breakfast or any medication for the day. Advise standing or sitting upright after taking medication. No food should be ingested for 30 minutes after taking the medication. Precautions should be used for patients who have upper gastrointestinal (GI) side effects.

d. Studies support the efficacy of treatment with bisphosphonates for up to 5 years. After 5 years of treatment, reassess the treatment options. Treatment beyond 5 years of bisphosphonate therapy is highly individualized.

4. Receptor activator of nuclear factor kappa B ligand (RANKL)

a. Acts by inhibiting osteoclast formation, decreasing bone resorption, reducing bone fracture, and increasing bone density.

i. Denosumab (Prolia) 60 mg subcutaneous injection once every 6 months. Patients with chronic kidney disease and/or a risk of hypocalcemia should have a serum calcium level checked 10 days after the administration.

5. Selective estrogen receptor modulator (SERM)

a. Raloxifene (Evista): 60 mg orally daily

b. For postmenopausal women, it prevents osteoporosis, is cardio-protective, and appears to decrease estrogen-recepted breast cancer by 65% more than 8 years (National Osteoporosis Foundation, n.d. -a, -b). Patient may note side effects of increased vasomotor symptoms and increased risk of venous thromboembolism.

6. Calcitonin

a. Intranasal calcitonin (Miacalcin): 200 IU one puff in alternating nostrils daily

b. Calcitonin injections (Calcimar): 100 IU by subcutaneous injection three times per week at bedtime

c. Fortical (Calcitonin-salmon) 200 U/spray: Nasal spray; one spray in nostril daily; alternate nostrils

7. Parathyroid hormone (PTH)

a. Recombinant human PTH rebuilds bone density and increases strength of bone. Approved for severe osteoporosis for postmenopausal women and men with the diagnosis of osteoporosis who have failed antiresorptive therapy and are not able to tolerate bisphosphonates. See package insert for contraindications.

b. Teriparatide (Forteo) 20 mcg prefilled, 28 day pen/syringe; subcutaneous injection daily. Taken for a maximum of 2 years. Check calcium and renal function before prescribing. Contraindicated for patients with a history of kidney stones and prior history of radiation therapy. See package insert.

8. Hormone replacement therapy (HRT)

Estrogen therapy and estrogen/progesterone therapy are available as tablets or transdermal patches and come in a wide variety of doses. HRT is approved for prevention of bone loss, but not approved for the treatment of osteoporosis.

Follow-Up

A. If the patient is on calcium supplements, check urinary calcium excretion two times per year. If it is below 250 mg/d, nephrocalcinosis and the risk of renal stones are decreased.
B. Bone density test is recommended every 2 years to evaluate effectiveness of medical plan.

Consultation/Referral

A. If fracture is suspected, consult with a physician.

Individual Consideration

A. Geriatrics: Assessment and treatment for osteoporosis must be performed routinely to prevent the risk of fracture, which may increase the risk of morbidity and mortality rates in this population.

Polymyalgia Rheumatica

Jill C. Cash

Definition

A. Polymyalgia rheumatica (PMR) is an inflammatory condition, with an insidious or abrupt onset, that causes morning muscle stiffness, pain, and decreased range of motion (ROM), primarily in the hips, shoulders, and neck.

Incidence

A. PMR occurs in all racial groups; however, it is rarely seen in the African American and Latino populations. It is commonly seen in adults older than 50 years, with an increased incidence in the 70- to 80-year-old population. Women are affected two to three times more often than men. PMR is occasionally associated with giant cell arteritis. Approximately 15% of diagnosed patients with PMR will also have giant cell arteritis. Approximately half of patients diagnosed with giant cell arteritis will be diagnosed with PMR.

Pathogenesis

A. The cause of PMR is unknown. Environmental and genetic factors have been shown to play a role in PMR. Studies speculate that environmental triggers, such as viruses, may cause the onset of symptoms. There are common similarities between PMR and giant cell arteritis.

Predisposing Factors

A. Age (older than 50 years)
B. Gender (women are affected two to three times more often than men)
C. Ethnicity (those of Northern European origin have a higher rate of PMR)

Common Complaints

A. Early morning joint stiffness and pain, lasting for approximately 20 to 30 minutes after waking for at least 2 weeks
B. Stiffness and pain commonly occur in the shoulders, hips, and neck
C. Decreased range of motion (ROM) of joints
D. Muscle pain
E. Weakness of joints and muscles

Other Signs and Symptoms

A. Fever
B. Fatigue
C. Malaise

Potential Complications

A. Difficulty performing daily activities, such as getting up out of a chair, dressing, and bathing
B. Decreased activity
C. Overall a decrease in general health because of limitations

Subjective Data

A. Ask the patient if there was an activity that brought about or preceded the episode of joint pain.
B. Has the patient had any recent illness or injury?
C. Ask the patient to describe the onset, duration, and intensity of pain, noting what particular joints are involved.
D. How long does pain and stiffness last in the morning?
E. Does the patient notice a decrease in ROM? Are there activities that the patient is not able to perform?
F. Ask the patient to list all medications currently being taken, particularly substances not prescribed and over-the-counter (OTC) products. What medications improve pain?
G. Has the patient noticed a problem with sleeping since the symptoms began?

Physical Examination

A. Vital signs: Check temperature, pulse, respirations, and blood pressure (BP).
B. Inspect
  1. Hands, wrists, elbows, shoulders, hips, and neck for erythema and synovitis
C. Palpate
  1. Palpate joints for swelling and pain. Marked swelling is not usually seen in patients with PMR.
  2. Assess ROM of the shoulders, hips, back, and neck. Perform passive ROM of the shoulders and hips.
  3. Assess trigger points for tenderness, assessing for symptoms of fibromyalgia.
  4. Assess muscle strength of upper and lower extremities and neck.
  5. Assess temporal arteries for signs of inflammation.
D. Auscultate
  1. Heart
  2. Lungs

Diagnostic Tests

A. Complete blood count (CBC)—normocytic anemia common
B. Erythrocyte sedimentation rate (ESR)—elevation
C. C-Reactive protein (CRP), noncardiac—elevation
D. Rheumatoid factor (RF)—negative
E. X-rays or MRI of the affected joints

Differential Diagnoses

A. Polymyalgia rheumatica
B. Rheumatoid arthritis (RA)

C. Giant cell arteritis
D. Fibromyalgia (symptoms will have been present for years)

Plan

A. General interventions
1. Treat the patient with steroid therapy to improve symptoms, starting at an adequate dose to resolve symptoms. Treatment will include slowly tapering the steroids over a period of weeks/months to keep the patient symptom free until off of steroids.
B. Patient teaching
1. *See Section III: Patient Teaching Guide for this chapter, "Polymyalgia Rheumatica."*
2. Educate the patient and family that PMR is primarily a self-limiting condition that will improve slowly over time.
3. Treatment will include several weeks/months of low-dose prednisone therapy, tapering slowly until completion of steroid therapy. Tapering slowly and patience will prevent recurrent attacks and rebound flares.
C. Pharmaceutical therapy
1. Low-dose prednisone is used to treat the symptoms. Steroids should be given to relieve symptoms (starting dose may be 10–20 mg orally [po] daily) and then will be tapered slowly over the next 6 months. Gradually decreasing the steroid dose by very small increments over time has the best results, minimizing the possibility of relapse.

Follow-Up

A. A follow-up appointment is recommended 2 weeks after the initial appointment.
B. If symptoms are improving with the steroid therapy, a follow-up appointment is recommended every 1 to 2 months until there are not any flares of symptoms and the patient has completed the steroid therapy. This treatment may take several months and even up to greater than 1 year.

Individual Considerations

A. Another condition to consider with the symptoms is remitting seronegative symmetrical synovitis With pitting edema. This condition presents with hand and distal extremity swelling, noting marked pitting edema in extremities. It is commonly seen in patients older than 50 years of age with an acute onset of swelling and pain. Symptoms respond quickly to the use of low-dose steroids. Laboratory testing for RA is negative.
B. Patients on long-term steroids should have a bone mineral density (BMD) performed to evaluate for osteoporosis.

Pseudogout

Jill C. Cash

Definition

A. An acute inflammatory condition primarily affecting the larger joints in which crystal deposits of calcium pyrophosphate dihydrate (CPP) occur in the connective tissues.

Incidence

A. Acute attacks occur more often in men than in women.
B. Women diagnosed with osteoarthritis with CPP have a higher incidence of occurrence.
C. Approximately 50% of cases occur in patients older than the age of 84 years, 36% occur during the ages of 75 to 84 years, and 15% occur in those from 65 to 74 years old.
D. Joints affected: The knee is affected approximately 50% of the time; other joints affected include wrists, shoulders, ankles, feet, and elbows.

Pathogenesis

A. Pseudogout occurs from the crystal formation in the cartilage that is shed into the synovial joint. Excessive cartilage pyrophosphate production leads to calcium pyrophosphate production and CPP crystals are formed and deposited in the joint.

Predisposing Factors

A. Older adults
B. Joint trauma
C. Hospitalization/illness
D. Familial chondrocalcinosis
E. Endocrine/metabolic disorders
1. Gout
2. Hyperparathryroidism
3. Hemochromatosis
4. Hypophosphatasia
5. Hypothyroidism
6. Hypomagnesemia
7. Gitleman's syndrome
8. Hemosiderosis

Common Complaints

A. Asymptomatic (may be visible on x-ray)
B. Acute attack of pain and swelling of affected joint, commonly a large joint
C. Erythema
D. Decreased range of motion (ROM) secondary to severe pain; inability to bear weight

Other Signs and Symptoms

A. Fever
B. Pain, swelling, and redness in several joints

Subjective Data

1. Ask the patient about the onset, progression, and duration of symptoms.
2. How many joints are affected?
3. Is this the first time this has occurred, or is this a chronic problem?
4. Ask the patient to describe the onset of symptoms, in the order of occurrence.
5. In addition to today, has this occurred in other joints?
6. Does the patient have a history of rheumatoid arthritis (RA), osteoarthritis (OA), or other types of arthritis?
7. Any previous injury to the joint?
8. What has the patient used for pain or fever?

Physical Examination

A. Check vital signs, temperature as indicated.

B. Inspect

1. Inspect the affected joint for erythema, edema, and synovitis.

2. If erythema is present, note location of erythema and evaluate if erythema extends beyond joint area.

3. While examining the joint, note facial grimaces, guarding with examination.

4. If weight-bearing joint is affected, note if the patient is able to bear weight.

C. Auscultate

1. Lungs and heart

D. Palpate

1. Palpate affected joint, noting pain and swelling in the joint.

2. Assess ROM in joint if possible.

Diagnostic Tests

A. Complete blood count (CBC)

B. Erythrocyte sedimentation rate (ESR)

C. Serum C-reactive protein (CRP)

D. Comprehensive metabolic profile (CMP)

E. Magnesium level

F. Thyroid-stimulating hormone (TSH)

G. Iron studies (iron, total iron-binding capacity, ferritin level)

H. Joint aspiration for synovial fluid: Microscope: Synovial fluid evaluation for crystals

I. X-ray of joint: Results may demonstrate linear and punctate calcifications in articular hyaline or fibrocartilage, also known as chondrocalcinosis.

Differential Diagnoses

A. Pseudogout: Joint aspiration of synovial fluid recommended for diagnosis. Diagnosis made by crystals identified by polarized light microscopy or radiographic changes of CPP crystals noted in the tissue or synovial fluid.

B. Gout

C. Septic arthritis

D. RA

E. OA

Plan

A. General interventions

1. Acute attacks should be treated with rest, immobilization, and education.

2. Differentiate between acute and chronic attacks and treatment.

3. Recurrent attacks should have long-term management.

B. Patient teaching

1. For acute attacks, encourage rest and elevation of affected joint.

2. Encourage no weight bearing until symptoms subside. Suggest the use of crutches or cane for assistance.

3. Warm, moist compresses may be used as needed for comfort.

4. As symptoms improve, suggest ROM exercises for affected joint.

5. Once symptoms have improved, weight-bearing activities may resume.

6. Symptoms should continue to improve over the next 7 to 10 days. Full recovery should be expected.

C. Pharmaceutical therapy

1. For acute attack, with one to two joints affected and no signs of infection:

a. Large joints (knees/shoulders): Joint aspiration and glucocorticoid steroid injection: Triamcinolone acetonoid 30 to 40 mg mixed with 1% procaine, 1 to 2 mL. Smaller joints require less steroid.

2. If not meeting the criteria discussed earlier, the next treatment option recommended is the use of nonsteroidal anti-inflammatory (NSAID) medications:

a. Naproxen (Naprosyn) 500 mg twice a day with food

b. Indomethacin (Indocin) 50 mg three times a day with food (not recommended in high-risk patients with heart failure, gastrointestinal [GI] effects, or decreased renal function)

c. Sulindac 200 mg twice a day with food.

3. If NSAIDs are contraindicated, use colchicine 1.2 mg within 24 hours of attack, followed by 0.6 mg 1 hour later, then 0.6 mg bid.

4. If injection and use of NSAIDs are contraindicated, use oral prednisone 30 to 50 mg daily until flare begins to resolve, then taper prednisone over the next 7 to 10 days.

5. Recurrent attacks (more than three attacks in 1 year) should be treated with colchicine. Monitor liver and kidney function. Consult with physician and/or refer to rheumatologist.

Follow-Up

A. The patient should return to the office in 48 to 72 hours after diagnosis and treatment.

B. Patient follow-up in 1 week is recommended for continued care.

C. If symptoms are not improving or are worsening, patient should return to the clinician's office or present to the emergency department for further evaluation and treatment.

Consultation/Referral

A. Refer all patients who appear to have a septic joint to the emergency department for evaluation and treatment. Refer to an orthopedic surgeon for consult.

B. Consider referring patients with pseudogout to rheumatology for evaluation and continued care.

Individual Considerations

A. Adults

1. Most commonly seen in adults older than 60 years.

2. Precautions should be used in treating patients with long-term NSAIDs. Active GI ulcers or history of GI disease should avoid NSAID use.

3. Patients on blood thinner medications should avoid the use of NSAIDs.

4. All precautions for the use of NSAIDs in adults should be considered, including chronic kidney disease.

5. Patients diagnosed with diabetes who are prescribed oral or injection steroids should be advised that steroids may increase blood sugar and to monitor blood sugar values at home as indicated.

B. Geriatrics

1. Most common in the older adult

2. Precaution should be used with using NSAIDs in the older adult.

3. Monitor renal function.

Psoriatic Arthritis

Jill C. Cash

Definition

A. Psoriatic arthritis (PsA) is a systemic inflammatory condition that occurs in the joints that presents with symptoms of joint pain, stiffness, and swelling around the tendons and ligaments. Other symptoms include psoriasis and inflammatory back pain. PsA is a chronic disease; and when left untreated, it can cause irreversible joint damage.

B. Five different types of psoriatic arthritis:

1. Symmetrical polyarthritis

2. Asymmetric oligoarthritis (fewer than four joints involved)

3. Distal interphalangeal (DIP) joint involvement

4. Arthritis mutilans (destructive and deforming, causes resorption of the phalanges)

5. Axial arthritis (spondyloarthritis)

C. The 2006 Classification of Psoriatic Arthritis (CASPAR) was developed to assist in diagnosing patients with PsA. The patient must score at least three points from the following list:

1. Skin psoriasis:

Present: 2 points

Previous history of skin changes: 1 point

Family history of psoriasis if patient not affected: 1 point

2. Nail lesions (onycholysis, pitting): 1 point

3. Dactylitis (present or past): 1 point

4. Rheumatoid factor (RF) negative: 1 point

5. X-ray evidence of new bone formation near a joint: 1 point

Incidence

A. Occurs in approximately 1% to 2% of the U.S. population.

B. It is estimated to occur in approximately 4% to 30% of patients diagnosed with psoriasis.

Pathogenesis

A. Individuals are genetically susceptible to PsA. It is thought that the immune system is triggered by something in the environment, which may include infection and/or trauma. The immune system is stimulated, activating T-cells that produce inflammatory cytokines and mediators that attack the joints, causing inflammation, pain, and/or erosions that can potentially destroy the joint. This response occurs in the joint and causes damage to the ligament or tendon attachment area (enthesium), (bone spurs), skin, and/or nails.

Predisposing Factors

A. Gender: Men and women are affected equally.

B. Commonly seen in adults ranging from 30 to 55 years of age.

C. The patient has a first-degree relative with psoriasis.

D. More common in Caucasians than African American and Native American populations.

Common Complaints

A. Pain and stiffness in joints, usually lasting longer than 30 minutes in the morning after wakening

B. Pain and stiffness that usually improves with activity

C. Enthesopathy (pain and inflammation at the ligament or tendon attachment site of the bone, commonly seen on the Achilles tendon, plantar fascia, or tibial tuberosity area)

Other Signs and Symptoms

A. Skin and nail psoriasis, nail pitting

B. Uveitis

Subjective Data

A. Does the patient have a history of skin rash, plaques, and so forth? If present, ask the patient when psoriasis began. What treatments have been used, including topical, light therapy, oral, and subcutaneous treatments?

B. Does the patient complain of photosensitivity?

C. Ask the patient to describe joint changes, such as swelling, pain, redness, and so forth. What joints are affected with pain and swelling?

D. Have any treatments used for psoriasis improved joint pain?

E. What medications or treatments are being used for the joint pain and swelling? What is the result of medications/treatments being used?

F. Does the patient have a history of back pain? If so, when did symptoms begin? Ask the patient to describe his or her back pain. Does pain improve or worsen with physical activity?

G. Does the patient have a history of frequent infections or high fevers?

H. Any history of frequent eye infections?

Physical Examination

A. Check vital signs and temperature as indicated.

B. Inspect

1. Inspect the skin for plaques or rash.

2. Inspect the nails for pitting.

3. Inspect the joints for inflammation, synovitis, and erythema.

4. Inspect the eyes for erythema and injection.

C. Auscultate

1. Auscultate the heart.

2. Lungs

D. Palpate
   1. Palpate all joints (hands, wrists, feet, elbows, ankles, knees, and shoulders) for synovitis/pain
      a. Dactylitis (swelling of the entire finger/toe that appears as a "sausage digit") occurs in approximately 50% of patients diagnosed with PsA.
      b. Enthesopathy is commonly seen in the Achilles tendon, plantar fascia, or tibial tuberosity.
   2. Note range of motion (ROM) of all joints.
   3. Palpate lumbar/thoracic spine.
   4. Palpate sacral/iliac joint for tenderness.

Diagnostic Tests

A. Erythrocyte sedimentation rate (ESR): May be elevated or normal.
B. C-Reactive protein (CRP): May be elevated or normal.
C. Complete blood count (CBC)
D. RF: Commonly negative in these patients; only 2% to 16% of patients with PsA will have a positive RF.
E. X-rays of affected joints

Differential Diagnoses

A. PsA
B. Rheumatoid arthritis (RA)
C. Ankylosing spondylitis (AS)
D. Osteoarthritis (OA)
E. Gout
F. Reactive arthritis

Plan

A. General interventions
   1. Early identification is necessary to prevent irreversible joint damage.
B. Patient teaching
   1. Nonpharmacological treatment options include the following:
      a. Exercise on most days of the week. ROM exercises are encouraged for joint stiffness.
      b. Heat application for stiffness and ice to affected joint for swelling may be used.
      c. For extended joint stiffness/pain, recommend physical therapy for assessment and treatment.
C. Pharmaceutical therapy
   1. First-line treatment: The European League Against Rheumatism (EULAR) recommends the use of nonsteroidal anti-inflammatory drugs (NSAIDs) for first-line treatment. Precautions should be given for all patients using NSAIDs (cardiovascular, renal, and gastrointestinal [GI] risks should be considered). NSAIDs are used for mild symptoms.
   2. Second-line treatment: Disease-modifying antirheumatic drugs (DMARDs), such as methotrexate (MTX), sulfasalazine, and leflunomide, are used. These medications should be prescribed by a rheumatology specialist.
   3. Third-line treatment: Biological tumor necrosis factor (TNF) inhibitors (adalimumab, certolizumab pegol, etanercept, golimumab, and infliximab). These medications should be prescribed by a rheumatology specialist.

Follow-Up

A. Follow-up is recommended in 2 weeks if prescribing NSAIDs for treatment of early disease.
B. Recommend follow-up every 3 months if not referred to rheumatology.

Consultation/Referral

A. Patients diagnosed with PsA who are not controlled with NSAIDs or who have evidence of joint changes should be referred to a rheumatology specialist for evaluation and treatment. NSAIDs do not prevent joint damage and prevention of irreversible joint damage is imperative.
B. Patients presenting with uveitis should be referred to an ophthalmologist for evaluation and treatment.
C. Patients diagnosed with severe joint damage should be referred to orthopedics for evaluation and treatment options (surgery).
D. Patients diagnosed with severe skin psoriasis should be referred to dermatology for evaluation and treatment.

Individual Considerations

A. Adults
   1. The use of oral steroids is not recommended for patients with PsA. Oral steroids have not been found to be effective; they also present a high risk of skin psoriasis flare when tapering the steroid dose.
   2. Patients diagnosed with PsA are at higher risk for cardiovascular disease and should be screened and monitored annually.
B. Geriatrics
   1. When prescribing NSAIDs, monitor renal, cardiac, and GI systems for adverse events with use.

Raynaud's Phenomenon

Jill C. Cash

Definition

Raynaud's phenomenon (RP) is an idiopathic disease in which an exaggerated vascular response occurs in extreme circumstances (heat, cold, and stress. It is manifested by bilateral blanching of the skin that is well demarcated, discomfort in the fingers, then by cyanosis, then erythema after warming the digits.

Cold hands and feet are very common complaints. RP involves both cutaneous color change and cool skin temperature. Although the hands are the most common area of attacks, RP also can occur in the toes, ears, nose, face, knees, and nipples. A Raynaud attack typically begins in a single finger and spreads symmetrically; however, the thumb is often spared.

RP may be either primary or secondary. Spontaneous remission may occur with primary RP.

A. Criteria for diagnosis of primary RP
   1. Symmetric episodic attacks
   2. No evidence of peripheral vascular disease
   3. No tissue gangrene, digital pitting, or tissue injury
   4. Negative nailfold capillary examination
   5. Negative antinuclear antibody (ANA) test
   6. Normal erythrocyte sedimentation rate (ESR)

B. Indications of secondary RP
  1. Age of onset older than 40 years
  2. Painful severe attacks with signs of ulceration/ischemia
  3. Ischemic signs/symptoms proximal to the fingers or toes
  4. Asymmetric attacks
  5. Abnormal laboratory, suggesting vascular or autoimmune disorders

Incidence

A. 3% to 20% in women
B. 3% to 14% in men
C. 3% in African Americans
D. Wide global differences from the United States

Pathogenesis

A. Primary RP: Occurs alone, without any other disease process. Speculated theories include digital microvascular vasospasm because of increased response of alpha 2-adrenergic receptors and a high sympathetic vascular tone.
B. Secondary RP: Symptoms occur as a secondary manifestation from other diseases or products such as autoimmune disorders (connective tissue disorders, systemic sclerosis, systemic lupus erythematosus, rheumatoid arthritis [RA], vasculitis, Sjögren's syndrome, dermatomyositis, polymyositis, etc.), atherosclerotic diseases, hematologic disorders (polycythemia, cryofibrinogenemia, etc.), metabolic/endocrine disorders (diabetes mellitus, pheochromocytoma, myxedema), neoplastic syndromes (lymphoma, leukemia, polycythemia, monoclonal/type 1 cryoglobulinemia), infections (hepatitis B, hepatitis C, mycoplasma infections), environmental exposures/neurologic changes (frostbite, vibratory injuries from use, lead exposure, vinyl chloride exposure, arsenic exposure, organic solvents [xylene, toluene, acetone, chlorinated solvents], carpel tunnel syndrome), and some medications/drugs (cyclosporines, antineoplastics, oral contraceptives, narcotics, ergot alkaloids, bromocriptine, beta-adrenergic blocking agents, and nicotine). Symptoms may be unilateral and may affect only one or two fingers. Secondary RP usually has a poorer morbidity than the primary disease.

Predisposing Factors

A. Primary RP
  1. Female
  2. Onset of symptoms after menarche (15–30 years)
  3. Smoking
  4. Emotional stress
B. Secondary RP
  1. Onset after age 40 years
  2. Male gender
C. Family history: Multiple family members
D. Frostbite
E. Vascular trauma (distal ulnar artery)
F. Vibration-induced/occupation exposure (jackhammers, pneumatic drills, weed eaters)
G. Medication-associated RP (see Table 21.1).

TABLE 21.1 Drugs That Induce Raynaud's Phenomenon

Amphetamines	Clonidine	Interferon-Alpha
Beta-blockers	Cocaine	Nicotine
Bleomycin	Cyclosporine	Vinblastine
Cisplatin	Ergot	Vinyl chloride

Common Complaints

A. Paleness of the fingertips after exposure to cold temperatures, followed by redness and discomfort after warming fingers
B. "White attack": Sharp, demarcated color of skin pallor
C. "Blue attack": Cyanotic skin
D. White or blue attack, usually lasting 15 to 20 minutes
E. Age of onset between 15 and 30 years

Other Signs and Symptoms

A. Paresthesias and numbness
B. Clumsiness of the aching hand/finger
C. Loss of pulp in pads of fingers (severe cases)

Subjective Data

A. Determine the age of onset, time, duration, and course of presenting symptoms.
B. Question the patient regarding location and symptoms, noting blanching, followed by erythema and pain after hands are warm.
C. Note frequency of attacks.
D. Review the presence of any other skin alterations that have occurred. Does patient also note skin mottling of the arms and legs? Livedo reticularis is a lilac or violet mottling or reticular pattern that occurs during a cold response.
E. Ask the patient to identify any events that precipitate occurrences and what makes symptoms worse or better.
  1. Air-conditioning
  2. Grocery cold/freezer food sections
  3. Cold weather
  4. Cold water
  5. Emotional stress
  6. Sudden startling
F. Identify any other symptoms that occur at the same time such as migraine headaches.
G. Review the patient's health history for underlying disorders such as hypothyroidism and autoimmune disorders/connective tissue disease.
H. Review current or past occupation (especially those that include the use of vibratory tools).
I. Review current medications, stimulants, herbals, and over-the-counter (OTC) medications.

Physical Examination

A. Check pulse, respirations, and blood pressure (BP).
B. Inspect

1. Dermal examination: Note malar/petechial rash, telangiectasias, digital pallor, or erythema. Examine for any ulceration or signs of ischemia.
2. Inspect joints for swelling or redness and overall ischemic changes.
3. Examine several fingernails using a microscope or ophthalmoscope; examine capillaries at nailfold.
   a. Normal: Fine red capillaries, lined in the same direction
   b. Abnormal: Capillaries dilated, tortuous, and irregularly spaced; avoid using the index finger for evaluation.

C. Auscultate
1. Auscultate the heart.
2. Auscultate the lungs.

D. Palpate
1. Palpate the joints for tenderness and peripheral pulses bilaterally

E. Neurologic examination: Sensory function
1. Sensory discrimination (hot/cold, sharp/dull)
2. Location of sensation (proximal/distal to previous stimuli)
3. Vibratory sensation with tuning fork (distal to proximal joints)
4. Graphesthesia (draw a number or letter in the palm of the hand with a blunt object, such as a pencil, applicator stick, or pen and have the patient identify the letter/number)

Diagnostic Tests

A. There is no gold standard diagnostic test.

B. History alone is accepted as diagnostic as no office test application consistently triggers an attack. A history of at least two color changes, pallor, and cyanosis after cold exposure is adequate for the diagnosis of RP. Ask the patient to take a picture when symptoms occur and bring it into the office for evaluation.

C. The cold water challenge test is no longer recommended.

D. Tools to assess vascular response (usually not readily available)
1. Nailfold capillaroscopy
2. Videomicroscopy
3. Thermography
4. Angiography
5. Laser Doppler
6. Direct measures of the skin temperature and local blood flow

E. Laboratory tests
1. ANA
2. ESR
3. Thyroid profile if hypothyroidism is suspected
4. Other tests are used, depending on suspected etiology; testing should be guided by results of history and physical examination.
   a. Complete blood count (CBC)
   b. Chemistry profile with renal and liver function
   c. Urinalysis
   d. Rheumatoid factor (RF)
   e. Complement (C3 and C4)
   f. ANA

Differential Diagnoses

A. RP (primary vs. secondary)
B. Scleroderma
C. Systemic lupus erythematosus
D. Occupational trauma
E. Medication induced
F. Peripheral vascular disease
G. Neurovascular processes (diabetes, atherosclerosis, thromboangitis obliterans)

Plan

A. General interventions
1. If ulcerations are present, monitor for secondary infections. Consider topical/systemic antibiotics if secondary infection. Debridement may be necessary.
2. Biofeedback and relaxation techniques are frequently used for treatment.

B. Patient teaching
1. Stress the importance of not smoking.
2. Keep the body warm.
   a. If in extreme temperatures, wear extra clothing (thermal underwear) to maintain temperature.
   b. Wear mittens instead of gloves to protect hands and keep them warm.
   c. Wear a hat to conserve heat.
3. If possible, stop all medications that could be inducing symptoms. Other drugs that should be avoided include:
   a. Decongestants
   b. Herbs that contain ephedra
   c. Medications used for migraine headaches; for example, serotonin agonists such as sumatriptan, or caffeine plus ergotamine.
4. If vibrator injury is present, stop the repetitive activity that induces symptoms. Consider alternative methods of work. If unable to totally stop the activity, decrease time spent using the vibratory equipment.
5. Emotional stress can be a trigger because of the vasoconstriction of the sympathetic nervous system being triggered. Counsel the patient regarding controlling the stress in his or her life and treatment (nonpharmacological/pharmacological) options that may be beneficial.

C. Surgical therapy (only recommended for patients resistant to initial therapies)
1. Temporary sympathectomy involving a local chemical block with lidocaine or bupivacaine (without epinephrine) relieves the pain.
2. Chemical and cervical sympathectomy may be used for severe cases with digital ischemia for temporary measures.
3. Vascular reconstruction is an option.

D. Pharmaceutical therapy
1. Therapy may be required only during the winter months.
2. Long-acting calcium channel blockers are used. Doses may be adjusted every 4 weeks or as tolerated.

Monitor by side effects: Headaches, dizziness, flushing tachycardia, and edema.

a. Nifedipine 30 to 180 mg/d

b. Amlodipine 5 to 20 mg/d

3. Low-dose aspirin antiplatelet therapy 75 to 81 mg/d may be considered in secondary RP with a history of ischemic ulcers or other thrombotic events.

4. Vasodilators (sildenafil) and endothelin receptor antagonists (bosentan) may be useful in refractory cases with associated digital ulcers/infarcts. However, these medications are not FDA approved for this is treatment.

Follow-Up

A. Follow up in 1 month or as needed by patient symptoms.

Consultation/Referral

A. Consult a physician if signs of ischemia are present and/or if refractory symptoms are present.

B. Refer to a rheumatologist if there is a moderate/high suspicion of secondary RP.

C. Refer for surgical therapies.

Individual Considerations

A. Pediatrics: RP is commonly seen in children with systemic lupus erythematosus and scleroderma.

B. Adults: The onset of RP after age 40 years is commonly associated with an underlying disease.

Rheumatoid Arthritis

Jill C. Cash

Definition

Rheumatoid arthritis (RA) is a chronic systemic disease that involves articular inflammation of the joints. The disease is generally insidious, and symmetrical involvement of synovial joints is a characteristic feature. Typically, the interphalangeal joints of the fingers and thumbs are noted; however, other joints involved include the elbows, shoulders, ankles, knees, and toes. Left untreated, the patient is at high risk of joint deformity and disability. Treatment goals of RA include remission, preventing functional decline of the patient, and halting progression of the disease.

RA is not limited to the joints; extra-articular features of RA include anemia, pleuropericarditis, neuropathy, myopathy, splenomegaly, Sjögren's syndrome, scleritis, vasculitis, and renal disease. Most patients with extra-articular symptoms also have the classic RA joint symptoms. Patients with RA are at increased risk of development of carpal tunnel syndrome, stroke, an osteoporotic fracture, and renal disease (secondary to drug toxicity).

The American College of Rheumatology (ACR) criteria for RA require that an algorithm be used to assess for criteria to meet the diagnosis for RA. A score of greater than or equal to 6/10 is recommended for the patient to be diagnosed with RA based on the working algorithm. Patients who should be screened for RA include those who have had at least one swollen joint, with the joint swelling not being caused by any other known etiology. Scoring for the algorithm may be found at: www.rheumatology.org/Portals/0/Files/ACR%202015%20RA%20Guideline.pdf

A. Classification criteria for screening for RA:

1. Duration of symptoms for more than 6 weeks

2. Joint swelling involvement (synovitis)

3. Serology: Rheumatoid factor (RF) and/or anti-citrullinated peptide/protein antibody (CCP)

4. Acute-phase reactants: C-reactive protein (CRP) and erythrocyte sedimentation rate (ESR)

B. Four stages of RA

1. Stage 1: No symptoms or signs; normal activity; RF and/or CCP antibody is present.

2. Stage 2: Morning stiffness, warmth at joint, normal activities of daily living (ADLs), minimal limitation in joint use; increased T-cells, B-cells, antibody production, and synovial cells are observed.

3. Stage 3: Morning stiffness, warmth at joint, and extra-articular manifestations; marked limitation in ADL. Increased T-cells, B-cells, antibody production, and synovial cells are observed.

4. Stage 4: Same as stage 3 plus proliferating synovial membrane involved, causing injury to the bone, tendons, and cartilage. Patient is now incapacitated or confined to a wheelchair.

Incidence

A. It is estimated that RA occurs in approximately 1.5 million adults in the United States. RA occurs at twice the rate in women compared with men. The prevalence of RA is approximately 1.06% in women compared with 0.61% in men.

Pathogenesis

A. The cause is unknown. Articular inflammation results in joint destruction. Antibody formation in the joint area results in inflammation and pain in the joint area.

Predisposing Factors

A. Family history, including 15% prevalence in monozygotic twins

B. Female gender

C. Ages 20 to 50 years

D. Recent systemic illness or trauma

Common Complaints

A. Joint pain

B. Morning stiffness in joints for at least 1 hour that has been present for more than 6 weeks.

C. Swelling and warmth in at least three joints or more for at least 6 weeks. Common joints affected include the wrists and hands, the metacarpal phalangeal (MCP) joints, and the proximal interphalangeal (PIP) joints.

Other Signs and Symptoms

A. Fatigue

B. Malaise

C. Subcutaneous nodules

D. Joint deformities

1. Proximal interphalangeal joints: Boutonniere deformities

2. Fingers: Swan-neck contractures, ulnar deviation

3. Wrists: Loss of extension

4. Hips: Loss of internal rotation, followed by flexion contractures
5. Knees: Suprapateller pouch distension
6. Elbows: Decreased extension, olecranon bursitis
7. Shoulders: Limited range of motion (ROM) movement
8. Cervical spine: Subluxation rare
9. Temporomandibular joint: Pain with biting

E. Depression
F. Low-grade fever
G. Weight loss
H. Myalgia
I. Anemia
J. Carpal tunnel syndrome

Subjective Data

A. Review when joint pains began and identify the joints involved. Is pain and stiffness worse in the morning? How long does it last? Is it symmetrical?
B. Elicit the patient's description of pain and a description of how the pain interferes with ADL (walking, climbing stairs, using the toilet, getting up from a chair, opening a jar).
C. Review the family history of RA.
D. Has the patient ever had any type of injury to the specific joint area? Rule out recent injuries.
E. Identify what makes the pain worse and alleviating factors. In patients with RA, activity typically alleviates symptoms, which is indicative of inflammation.
F. Review list of medications, including herbal and over-the-counter (OTC) medications. What therapies have specifically been used, and what were the results?
G. Review the patient's history for recent infections.
H. Does the patient use any assistive devices, including cane, crutches, walker, wheelchair/power mobility device, kitchen devices/grips, and so forth?

Physical Examination

A. Check temperature, if indicated, pulse, respirations, blood pressure (BP), and weight.
B. General observation
   1. Observe the patient getting up and down in the chair.
   2. Observe the patient walking (may have a tendency to bear weight on heels and hyperextend toes secondary to tenderness to the metatarsophalangeal joints).
   3. Observe the patient handling objects in his or her hands.
   4. Observe for signs of depression.
C. Inspect
   1. Inspect all joints, noting deformities, erythema, and temperature. (Heat and redness are not prominent features of RA.)
   2. Evaluate for pitting edema in the hand (may have a "boxing glove" appearance).
   3. Inspect for subcutaneous rheumatoid nodules (elbow is the most common site).
   4. Evaluate skin for ulcerative lesions (secondary from venous stasis and neutrophilic infiltration), skin atrophy and ecchymoses from glucocorticoids, and petechiae (side effect from medications causing thrombocytopenia).
   5. Eye examination
      a. Episcleritis: Acute redness and pain without discharge
      b. Scleritis: Deep ocular pain with dark red discoloration
D. Auscultate
   1. Auscultate the heart.
   2. Auscultate the lungs (at risk of infectious complications from immunosuppression and pulmonary toxicity from methotrexate [MTX] if currently being treated with medications)
E. Percuss
   1. Perform a patellar tap to evaluate synovial thickening/effusion of the knee.
F. Palpate
   1. Palpate the lymph nodes.
   2. Perform oral examination to palpate the salivary glands (may have lymphocytic infiltration).
   3. Palpate all joints to evaluate for tenderness with pressure, pain with movement of the joint, and "bogginess" of the joint (synovial thickening).
   4. Palpate the popliteal fossa for evidence of a popliteal (Baker's) cyst.
   5. Examine abdomen for splenomegaly.
G. Musculoskeletal examination
   1. Assess grip (a reduced grip is a useful parameter in evaluating disease activity and progression). Is the patient able to close fingers to make a fist?
   2. Assess the strength of the extremities.
   3. Assess the ROM (active and passive) and flexion.

Diagnostic Tests

A. Complete blood count (CBC) and platelets
B. ESR
C. CRP
D. Rheumatoid factor (RF), quantitative
E. CCP antibody
F. Uric acid level
G. Synovial fluid (optional)
H. Plain film radiography of the hands, wrists, and feet as a baseline and to monitor disease progression

Differential Diagnoses

A. RA
B. Osteoarthritis (OA)
C. Psoriatic arthritis (PsA)
D. Crystalline arthritis (gout and pseudogout)
E. Polyarthritis
F. Reactive arthritis
G. Acute viral/infectious process
   1. Lyme disease
   2. Hepatitis B
   3. Hepatitis C
   4. Parvovirus B19
H. Sjögren's syndrome: Keratoconjunctivitis sicca, splenomegaly, and lymphadenopathy

I. Sarcoidosis
J. Polymyositis

Plan

A. General interventions

1. Focus on exercise and joint mobility to maintain functional abilities.

2. Encourage smoking cessation, especially among females on glucocorticoids because of the risk of increased bone loss/fracture.

B. Patient teaching

1. Once diagnosed, it is recommended that treatment with medications begin to prevent joint damage. First-line medications include disease-modifying antirheumatic drugs (DMARDs). Depending on what medication is used, educate the patient regarding benefits, risks, side effects, and precautions for medications. If MTX is used, educate the patient that alcohol should be avoided to prevent hepatotoxicity.

2. Stress the importance of returning for laboratory follow-up while on DMARDs.

3. Discuss vaccinations, especially pneumonia and influenza vaccines. Emphasize the importance of keeping all vaccinations up to date. Most treatment medications suppress the immune system and increase the risk of infections.

C. Pharmaceutical therapy

1. Early disease

a. Daily nonsteroidal anti-inflammatory drugs (NSAIDs) and pain-relieving medications

i. Ibuprofen 600 to 800 mg every 6 to 8 hours as needed

ii. Naproxen 500 mg orally every 12 hours as needed

iii. Celecoxib (Celebrex) 200 mg by mouth daily

iv. Acetaminophen (Tylenol) 500 to 1,000 mg orally every 4 to 6 hours as needed

b. Comorbid conditions, such as a history of heart failure, renal disease, and peptic ulcers, should be considered before starting NSAID therapy.

c. Be aware of other medications the patient is prescribed by other providers and consider possible drug-to-drug interactions. Examples include NSAIDs, antacids, anticoagulants, oral hypoglycemic agents, antihypertensive/diuretics, lithium, MTX, and diphenylhydantoin (Dilantin).

2. Moderate to severe RA disease

a. Oral glucocorticoids, prednisone 5 to 10 mg/d, may be added for active joint inflammation. Prednisone may be used up to 6 months, but shorter courses are recommended because of the consequence of long-term steroid use. Steroids should be tapered over a period of a few months and then completely discontinued if possible.

b. Intra-articular long-acting glucocorticoid injections are used for the reduction of synovitis in inflamed joints.

c. DMARDs are recommended by AMR if early RA manifestations have been present for less than 6 months. Adding DMARDs depends on the number of inflamed joints, severity of inflammation, functional impairment, and the number of poor prognostic signs (bony erosions and extra-articular disease). The benefits, risks, and side effects of all medications should be explained to the patient before beginning therapy. Recommended blood work monitoring should also be followed according to the medication recommendations.

i. MTX is given on a weekly basis starting with 7.5 mg/wk and is increased as tolerated to control symptoms. Titration: Increase the dose after 4 weeks at a rate of 2.5 mg/wk to a maximum of 25 mg/wk. MTX should not be given to patients who desire to become or who are pregnant or patients with liver disease.

ii. Sulfasalazine (Azulfidine) 500 to 1,000 mg a day is given initially.

iii. Hydroxychloroquine (Plaquenil) 200 to 400 mg is given daily. Before starting patients on hydroxychloroquine, the patient must be counseled regarding the possible risks of the medication, including retinal damage that can lead to blindness. A baseline eye examination must be performed, followed by eye examination every 6 months to monitor for retinal changes.

iv. Leflunomide (Arava) 10 to 20 mg/d; monitoring blood work every 3 months is recommended.

d. If response is not adequate, biological agents, tumor necrosis factor (TNF) alpha inhibitors, and other classes of drugs may be instituted. Because of the associated side effects, rheumatology consult is recommended for treatment of these medications.

i. Examples of TNF inhibitors:

1) Infliximab (Remicade) 3 to 10 mg/kg every 4 to 6 weeks; IV infusion

2) Adalimumab (Humira) 0.8-mL (40 mg) subcutaneous injection into abdomen or thigh every 2 weeks

3) Etanercept (Enbrel) 50-mg subcutaneous injection into the abdomen or thigh weekly

4) Golimumab (Simponi) 50-mg subcutaneous injection monthly

5) Certolizumab pegol (Cimzia) 200-mg subcutaneous injection every other week

ii. Janus kinase inhibitor:

1) Tofacitinib citrate (Xeljanz) 5 mg orally twice a day (po bid) or 11 mg po daily

iii. Interleukin-6 (IL-6) inhibitor

1) Tocilizumab (Actemra) 162-mg subcutaneous injection is given every 1 to

2 weeks or 4 to 8 mg/kg IV infusion every 4 weeks.

iv. T-cell depletion

1) Abatacept (Orencia) IV infusion is given every 4 weeks or subcutaneous injection weekly; dosage is based on weight.

v. B-cell depleting therapy

1) Rituximab (Rituxan) 1,000-mg IV infusion is given at week 0 and week 2, and then repeated approximately every 6 months or as indicated.

e. Patients may also use combination therapy. Examples of this include using MTX plus a TNF inhibitor or sulfasalazine, and so forth.

f. Patients receiving treatment with pharmacological agents should be evaluated at routine intervals, every 3 months, regarding their functional status to identify whether treatment therapies are improving the symptoms. There are several functional forms that are available for use. The Stanford Health Assessment Questionnaire (HAQ) is a well-known questionnaire that is recommended for use.

g. Drug monitoring, by performing serum blood work, is also recommended at routine intervals when prescribing pharmacological agents to avoid adverse effects of the medications being prescribed.

Follow-Up

A. Follow-up will be guided by medication therapy. Disease activity and response to therapy should be reassessed every 4 to 6 weeks.

B. Follow laboratory values with certain medications, including MTX with liver function testing, albumin, CBC with differential, platelets, and urinalysis monthly.

C. Assume all patients with RA are at risk of osteoporosis. DEXA scan is used to evaluate bone loss secondary to glucocorticoid-induced osteopenia. Initiate bisphosphonate therapy as indicated for signs of bone loss. Use a low threshold for starting in postmenopausal women with RA.

D. Anti-TNF agents are contraindicated in patients with an active infection and those who are at high risk of reactivation of tuberculosis. A tuberculosis (TB) skin test is required before administration. Patients with a positive skin test should be treated with prophylactic antituberculosis therapy 1 month before therapy with anti-TNF agents.

E. Patients should receive a baseline ophthalmologic examination before starting antimalarial drugs, such as plaquenil, and then follow-up examinations every 6 to 12 months while on therapy.

Consultation/Referral

A. Refer all patients with early inflammatory arthritis to a rheumatologist if RA is the suspected. Early intervention may prevent bone destruction of the joints and improve the long-term outcome for the patient.

B. Patients with a history of chronic swelling and pain of the joints should be referred to a rheumatologist.

C. Refer all patients to the rheumatologist, orthopedist, or emergency room if a septic joint is suspected.

Individual Considerations

A. Pregnancy

1. RA activity improves substantially in pregnancy.

a. Approximately 70% to 80% of patients will have symptoms improve during pregnancy.

b. Approximately 90% of women will have a flare in the postpartum period. Flares usually occur within the first 3 months postpartum.

2. Leflunomide, etanercept, adalimumab, and infliximab are contraindicated in pregnancy and while breastfeeding.

3. Pregnancy should be avoided with the use of MTX and Arava. Women need to have one normal menstrual cycle following discontinuation of MTX before attempting pregnancy. Men should wait at least 3 months after discontinuing MTX before attempting to conceive.

4. Therapy during pregnancy should be coordinated with the perinatologist and the rheumatologist.

B. Pediatrics

1. In children, consider juvenile-onset RA.

2. If suspected, consider referral to a pediatric rheumatologist for evaluation and diagnosis.

C. Geriatrics

1. Use NSAIDs with caution. Consider the patient's age, weight, and chronic conditions when prescribing NSAIDs. NSAIDs are not recommended in patients with renal conditions.

Systemic Lupus Erythematosus

Jill C. Cash

Definition

Systemic lupus erythematosus (SLE) is a chronic, inflammatory autoimmune disorder. It may affect multiple organ systems. The body's immune system forms antibodies that attack healthy tissues and organs. The clinical course is marked by spontaneous remission and relapses. Severity varies from a mild episodic disorder to a rapidly fulminating fatal disease. The three types of lupus are as follows:

A. Discoid lupus erythematosus (DLE) affects the skin, causing a rash, lesions, or both.

B. SLE attacks body organs and systems, such as joints, kidneys, brain, heart, and lungs. SLE is usually more severe than DLE and can be life-threatening.

C. Drug-induced lupus symptoms usually disappear when medication is discontinued.

Incidence

A. The incidence of SLE in relation to gender, ancestry, and familial history has been repeatedly documented. About 85% of patients with SLE are women; it affects mainly young women after menarche and before menopause. The majority of patients who develop SLE during childhood or after age 50 years are also women. SLE occurs in 1:1,000 Caucasian women and 1:250 African American women. The disorder is concordant in 25% to 75% of identical twins. The risk of developing the disease if a mother has SLE is 1:40 for a daughter and 1:250 for a son. Positive antinuclear antibody (ANA) is seen in asymptomatic family members, and the prevalence of other rheumatic diseases is increased among close relatives of patients. There is a high frequency of specific genes in SLE. Ten percent of DLE patients go on to develop SLE.

Pathogenesis

A. The exact cause of SLE is unknown, but clinical manifestations of SLE are secondary to the trapping of antigen–antibody complexes in capillaries of visceral structures, or to autoantibody-mediated destruction of host cells such as thrombocytopenia. SLE is commonly precipitated by recent exposure to illness, infections, ultraviolet light, surgery, pregnancy, and stress.

Predisposing Factors

A. Female gender
B. African American, Asian, Hispanic ancestry
C. Childbearing age
D. Positive family history of SLE
E. Drug use
- **1.** Procainamide
- **2.** Hydralazine
- **3.** Isoniazid

Common Complaints

A. Joint pain: Joint symptoms occur in 90% of patients.
B. Fever
C. Loss of appetite
D. Fatigue
E. Weight loss
F. Oral or nasal ulcers
G. Hair loss
H. Photosensitive skin rash and skin lesions over areas exposed to sunlight
I. Relapsing polychondritis

Other Signs and Symptoms

A. DLE
- **1.** Rash: Erythematosus, round, scaling papules 5 to 10 mm in diameter, appearing as "butterfly" shape across bridge of nose
- **2.** Rash, commonly on the trunk, extremities, scalp, external ear, and neck
- **3.** Photosensitivity

B. SLE: The 1997 Updated American College of Rheumatology (ACR) Criteria for diagnosis must include four or more of the first 11 of the following criteria:
- **1.** Malar rash
- **2.** Discoid rash
- **3.** Photosensitivity
- **4.** Oral ulcers
- **5.** Arthritis (generally bilateral, symmetric, especially in hands and wrists)
- **6.** Serositis
- **7.** Renal disorder: Chronic renal problems as indicated by proteinuria (greater than 0.5 g/d of protein or greater than 3+ protein) or cellular casts
- **8.** Neurologic disorder (seizures or personality changes, psychosis)
- **9.** Hematologic disorder
- **10.** Immunologic disorder
- **11.** ANA; abnormal titer of ANA
- **12.** Other signs and symptoms:
  - **a.** Weight loss
  - **b.** Fatigue
  - **c.** Acute abdominal pain
  - **d.** Alopecia
  - **e.** Tendon involvement
  - **f.** Urinalysis: Active urine sediment (blood or protein without urinary tract infections [UTIs])
  - **g.** Fever and malaise
  - **h.** Lymphadenopathy
- **13.** Other complications

(Probable SLE: Have two or three of the first 11 ACR guidelines criteria, along with one other feature.)
Possible SLE: Have one of the first 11 ACR guidelines criteria, along with one other feature.)
  - **a.** Hashimoto's thyroiditis
  - **b.** Hemolytic anemia
  - **c.** Thrombocytopenia purpura
  - **d.** Arterial and venous thrombosis in the presence of antiphospholipid antibodies
  - **e.** Recurrent pleurisy
  - **f.** Pleural effusion, pneumonitis
  - **g.** Pulmonary embolism
  - **h.** Pericarditis, endocarditis, myocarditis
  - **i.** Hypertension
  - **j.** Splenomegaly
  - **k.** Recurrent miscarriages in the presence of antiphospholipid antibodies
  - **l.** Relapsing polychondritis

C. Central nervous system (CNS) problems
- **1.** Chronic headaches (migraine)
- **2.** Seizures or epilepsy
- **3.** Personality changes, chronic brain syndrome

D. Decreased hemoglobin (Hgb), white blood cells (WBC), and platelets

Subjective Data

A. Determine systemic features and onset, course, and duration of symptoms (see Other "Signs and Symptoms" section).
B. Obtain medication history (see "Predisposing Factors" section).
C. Determine family history of rheumatoid diseases or other autoimmune disorders.
D. Review the patient's recent history for possible allergen exposure.

Physical Examination

A. Check temperature, pulse, respirations, and blood pressure (BP).
B. Inspect

1. Observe general overall appearance and generalized movement of extremities.
2. Conduct dermal examination for color, petechiae, rashes, lesions, and hair loss.
3. Conduct funduscopic examination; note photosensitivity.

Funduscopic examination: Cotton–wool exudates are the most common eye lesion.

4. Examine mouth and nose for oral lesions/ulcers.
5. Observe for pericardial lifts and heaves.
6. Inspect joints for subluxation of the metacarpal phalangeal joints and swan neck deformities of the hands.

C. Palpate
1. The back for tactile fremitus; palpate the heart for lifts, heaves, and thrills
2. The neck for thyroid enlargement
3. The neck, axilla, and groin for lymphadenopathy
4. The abdomen for organomegaly, masses, and tenderness; palpate suprapubic area for suprapubic tenderness and assess back for costovertebral angle (CVA) tenderness.

D. Percuss
1. The chest, anterior and posterior lung fields, for consolidation
2. The abdomen for splenomegaly

E. Auscultate
1. Heart
2. Lungs
3. Abdomen

F. Musculoskeletal examination
1. Examine for bone or joint swelling, tenderness, and increased warmth.
2. Check lower extremities for evidence of phlebitis, asymmetrical swelling, calf tenderness, and palpable cord.

G. Neurologic examination: Complete neurologic examination with mental status examination

Diagnostic Tests

A. Complete blood count (CBC) with differential
B. Platelets
C. ANA: Indirect immunofluorescence assay (IFA) positive. In patients with SLE, the ANA will typically be positive with a high titer ANA. Note pattern associated with positive ANA. A negative ANA by the IFA method dramatically decreases the risk of SLE.
D. Complement levels (decreased C3 and C4)
E. Rheumatoid factor (RF) can be positive in patients with SLE.
F. Thyroid profile
G. Anti-DNA antibodies, seen in approximately 30% of patients with renal disease.
H. Antiphospholipid antibodies: Lupus anticoagulant immunoglobulin A (IgA), immunoglobulin G (IgG), and immunoglobulin M (IgM) anticardiolipin antibodies; IgA, IgG, and IgM anti-beta-2-glycoprotein
I. Erythrocyte sedimentation rate (ESR)
J. Urinalysis (check for hematuria, proteinuria, and cellular casts) and urine culture
K. Collection of 24-hour urine for protein and creatinine clearance
L. Skin biopsy
M. Follow-up Coombs' test: Positive
N. Microhemagglutination assay for *Treponema pallidum* antibodies (MHA-TP) to confirm reactive syphilis for positive rapid plasma reagin (RPR): False positive serologic test for syphilis needs follow-up.
O. Chest x-ray film may show changes.
P. X-ray of joints for nondestructive arthritis

Differential Diagnoses

A. SLE
B. DLE
C. Undifferentiated connective tissue disease
D. Drug-induced lupus
E. Rheumatoid arthritis (RA): Lupus can resemble RA, especially early in the course of SLE. Unlike RA, the arthritis is nonerosive: There is no joint destruction.
F. Vasculitis
G. Scleroderma
H. Chronic active hepatitis
I. Acute drug reactions
J. Polyarteritis
K. Infection
L. Influenza
M. Rosacea
N. Neoplasm

Plan

A. General interventions: After diagnosis, refer the patient to a rheumatologist and comanage with a physician.
B. Patient teaching: *See Section III: Patient Teaching Guide for this chapter, "Systemic Lupus Erythematosus."* ◀
C. Pharmaceutical therapy
1. Nonsteroidal anti-inflammatory drugs (NSAIDs) for arthritis symptoms
2. Prednisone 40 to 60 mg initially for the control of thrombocytopenic purpura, hemolytic anemia, myocarditis, pericarditis, convulsions, and nephritis
3. Always give the lowest dose that controls the condition.
4. Corticosteroids can usually be tapered to low doses, 10 to 15 mg/d, during disease inactivity.
5. Antimalarial drug, hydroxychloroquine sulfate, every day may help treat lupus rashes and joint symptoms that do not respond to NSAIDs. Do not exceed 400 mg/d. *Consult with a rheumatology specialist.*
6. Alternative drug therapy: Immunosuppressive agents, such as cyclophosphamide, chlorambucil, and azathioprine, are used in cases resistant to corticosteroids. The exact role of immunosuppressive agents is controversial.

Follow-Up

A. Very close follow-up by a physician specialist is needed when immunosuppressants are employed.

B. If fever is present on examination, explore cause of fever to rule out infection. Monitor the patient for infections, especially with opportunistic organisms.
C. Preventive heart care is important because of the presence of premature atherosclerosis seen in these patients.
D. Up-to-date immunizations
E. Osteoporosis screening

Infections are the leading cause of death secondary to the depression of WBCs, followed by active SLE, chiefly because of renal or CNS disease.

Consultation/Referral

A. After diagnosis, refer the patient to a medical specialist, a rheumatologist.
B. Referral to a specialist for a biopsy of the skin or kidney may be necessary to confirm the diagnosis.

Individual Considerations

A. Pregnancy
  1. Infertility: 25% of patients have a problem getting pregnant.
  2. Patients with SLE experience frequent miscarriages and stillbirths.
  3. Patients are considered high risk when consultation and management with a perinatologist are needed.
  4. Approximately 33% of patients have an antibody (anticardiolipin) that is associated with early failure of the placenta.
  5. Approximately 10% have a related antibody (lupus anticoagulant) that allows early pregnancy, but compromises fetal growth as the placenta fails.
  6. It is estimated that 25% of the remaining pregnancies deliver prematurely.
  7. Family planning
    a. Barrier methods or intrauterine devices (IUDs) are best and safest.
    b. Oral contraceptives may exacerbate lupus. Avoid use of estrogen birth control pills with active SLE. Consider alternate methods of birth control.
  8. Exacerbations of lupus are sometimes caused by pregnancy.
B. Pediatrics
  1. Prematurity is the greatest danger of lupus's effects on the baby.
  2. There are no known congenital abnormalities related to lupus.
  3. Three percent of all lupus patients have a baby with neonatal lupus. This is a syndrome, not SLE, and it is transient.
C. Geriatrics: Males are affected more than females.

Temporal Arteritis/Giant Cell Arteritis

Jill C. Cash

Definition

A. Temporal arteritis, also known as giant cell arteritis (GCA), is a vascular illness that can affect the entire body; however, it primarily affects the blood vessels. There is inflammation of the arteries that begins in the aortic arch and branches out to the cranial arteries.

Incidence

A. GCA occurs in approximately 1 in 500 individuals older than 50 years. GCA rarely occurs in individuals younger than 50 years and is more commonly seen during later years (older than 70 years). It can also be seen in patients diagnosed with polymyalgia rheumatica (PMR). Approximately 50% of patients diagnosed with GCA will also have PMR.

Pathogenesis

A. The cause of GCA is unknown. The immune system attacks the body and causes inflammation of the medium and large arteries, which causes thickening of the arterial walls and narrowing of the lumen. When these changes occur, the result is a decrease in blood flow that can potentially cause an occlusion in the artery, leading to ischemia. Arteries commonly involved include the temporal artery, medium and large vessels, and the vessels of the eyes. Blindness is the major acute morbidity with GCA.

Predisposing Factors

A. Age (older than 50 years)
B. Ethnicity (Scandinavian) Northern European descent
C. Gender (women > men)

Common Complaints

A. Abrupt onset of headaches
B. Visual impairment
C. Joint pain (PMR)

Other Signs and Symptoms

A. Fever
B. Anemia
C. Jaw or arm claudication
D. Fatigue
E. Weight loss

Potential Complications

A. Visual loss, blindness
B. Joint pain

Subjective Data

A. Have the patient describe the presenting complaints. What makes it better or worse?
B. Ask the patient when presenting symptoms began. Discuss the course of new-onset symptoms. Note systemic symptoms such as fever, weight loss, fatigue, headache, vision changes, jaw/arm pain.
C. Ask the patient to describe pain, for example, crushing, stabbing, or burning.
D. Have patient rate pain on a scale of 1 to 10, with 1 being the least painful.
E. What has the patient taken to relieve the pain or symptoms?
F. Has the patient noted any visual disturbance or changes? Is vision change constant or does it occur when headache is present? What makes the headache worse? What makes the headache better?

Physical Examination

A. Vital signs: Check temperature, pulse, respirations, and blood pressure (BP; take BP in both arms and note discrepancies).

B. Inspect

1. Inspect overall general appearance. Patients with GCA usually appear chronically ill.

2. Perform funduscopic examination, looking for a pale disc and blurred margins of the disc. Assess pupils equal and reactive to light and accommodation (PERLA), extraocular muscles (EOMs), and visual acuity.

C. Palpate

1. Palpate pulses (carotid, brachial, radial, pedal, and femoral pulses).

2. Perform range of motion (ROM) of all joints (shoulders, neck, hips, and extremities), noting limitations because of pain and/or swelling.

3. Assess joints for swelling and pain. (Note symptoms of PMR.)

D. Auscultate

1. Heart for murmurs

2. Carotid, brachial, femoral arteries for bruits

3. Abdomen noting any bruits

Diagnostic Tests

A. Serum laboratory studies (erythrocyte sedimentation rate [ESR], complete blood count [CBC], C-reactive protein [CRP], and comprehensive metabolic profile [CMP])

B. Temporal artery biopsy. Any patient suspicious of having temporal arteritis should have a temporal artery biopsy performed. This is the gold standard for diagnosing GCA. Recommended sample size of the artery for biopsy should be greater than or equal to 4 cm. False negative biopsy results may be up to 20%.

Differential Diagnoses

A. Temporal arteritis/GCA

B. Vasculitis

C. **PMR**

Plan

A. General interventions

1. Educate the patient and family regarding the disease process of GCA.

B. Patient teaching

1. Educate the patient and family that common symptoms of GCA include headaches, vision change, and jaw/arm joint pain.

2. Teach the patient that GCA causes inflammation of the blood vessels in the head and neck, but not the blood vessels in the brain.

3. Advise the patient that PMR may also occur in some patients, in which joint pain may be present.

4. Medications commonly used for GCA are steroids. Steroids will improve the inflammation, which in return will improve pain. The steroids are commonly used for the duration of treatment and will be tapered down over several months. Steroids are the only medication that has proven to prevent blindness. Any side effects or problems should be reported to the primary provider.

5. A baby aspirin is commonly used daily.

6. Any vision changes should be immediately reported to the primary provider. Vision loss/blindness is one of the greatest risks of GCA.

C. Pharmaceutical therapy

1. If GCA is suspected, consult with collaborating physician and begin steroids immediately. Prednisone 40 to 60 mg daily. Do not wait for biopsy results. Steroids are used to suppress the manifestations of symptoms and decrease the risk of blindness. Steroids will eventually be tapered when symptoms begin to improve, commonly after 1 month or so.

2. Aspirin 81 to 325 mg/d is recommended.

Follow-Up

A. Follow up with physician rheumatologist/surgeon as recommended.

Consultation/Referral

A. Consultation with the collaborating physician or surgeon should be obtained regarding any patient with the suspicion of having temporal arteritis.

B. Refer all patients to a rheumatologist within 1 week of diagnosis to manage the patient with GCA.

C. All patients suspicious of having temporal arteritis should be referred to a general surgeon for a temporal artery biopsy within 2 to 3 days after beginning steroids.

D. Refer the patient to the ophthalmologist for evaluation and treatment.

Individual Considerations

A. Pediatrics

1. Vasculitis is rare in children. It is estimated to occur in 12 to 50 per 100,000 children younger than 17 years.

B. Geriatrics

1. Most commonly seen in older patients. Symptoms may occur after the age of 50 years; however, GCA is most commonly seen in patients older than 70 years.

Vitamin D Deficiency

Jill C. Cash

Definition

A. Vitamin D deficiency is defined as having a serum 25-hydroxyvitamin D (25[OH]D) level lower than 15 ng/mL. Vitamin D insufficiency is defined as having a serum 25-(OH)D level lower than 30 ng/mL. Recommended vitamin D levels range between 30 and 40 ng/mL.

Incidence

A. Vitamin D deficiency is seen in all ages. It is highest in the elderly, institutionalized, and/or hospitalized patients. It is found to be more common in women than in men (83% vs. 48%), the difference most likely being less skin exposure to the sun. There is a higher incidence in the winter months, again because of less sun exposure during the winter months.

Pathogenesis

A. The best source of vitamin D is direct sunlight exposure to the skin. It is also absorbed by ingesting foods that are rich in vitamin D. The liver is responsible for breaking vitamin D down. The liver hydroxylates the vitamin D to storage form, 25[OH]D, which then breaks down into the bioactive form in the kidney, 1,25-dihydroxyvitamin D (1,25[OH]2D). The 1,25(OH)2D is regulated by the parathyroid hormone and causes calcium absorption to occur in the intestine, which in return affects bone metabolism and muscle function. When any part of this cascade is interrupted, the cascade is broken and vitamin D deficiency occurs.

Predisposing Factors

A. Race (darker skin population)
B. Age: Elderly population highest risk
C. Long-term institutionalized individuals (nursing home)
D. Obese individuals
E. Decreased sun exposure (individuals who spend very little time outdoors in the sun)
F. People with serious nervous or digestive disorders (chronic kidney disease and malabsorption problems)
G. Medications: Drugs, such as dilantin, phenobarbital, and rifampin, induce hepatic p450 enzymes and accelerate catabolism of vitamin D.

Common Complaints

A. Complaints vary from none to severe.
B. Chronic muscle aches/pain/fatigue/weakness
C. Joint pain and bone pain

Other Signs and Symptoms

A. Fracture of bone
B. Frequent falls and muscle weakness
C. The most severe form of vitamin D deficiency can cause nutritional rickets.

Subjective Data

A. With patients presenting with complaints, assess onset, duration, and course of complaints.
B. Assess daily nutritional habits. Does the patient get enough calcium and vitamin D in current diet?
C. Does the patient live in the home or an institution? Is the patient allowed to spend time outdoors in sunlight? What time of the season/year is it? Is 20 to 30 minutes in the sun without sunscreen reasonable?
D. Is the patient currently taking any vitamin supplements? If so, review vitamin and ingredients in that particular vitamin.
E. Review the patient history and determine if the patient has a chronic condition, malabsorption condition, chronic kidney condition, or medications interfering with absorption. If there is no current diagnosis of a gastrointestinal (GI) problem, inquire regarding food intolerances, stool patterns, constipation, and diarrhea history.
F. Does the patient currently take a vitamin D and/or calcium supplement?
G. Has the patient had a recent vitamin D level drawn?
H. Inquire regarding the patient's fatigue level.
I. Assess for muscle weakness and frequent falls, especially if a pattern of more falls in the winter months is noticed.
J. Has the patient been diagnosed with osteoporosis? If so, the patient needs to be screened for vitamin D deficiency.

Physical Examination

A. Check pulse and blood pressure (BP).
B. Inspect
  1. Observe the patient walk in the room and assess for stability.
  2. Observe the skin color and overall appearance and type of skin texture.
  3. Note any deformities in the spine.
    a. Kyphosis
    b. Bowing of the legs
    c. Waddling of gait
C. Palpate
  1. Joints or areas of complained tenderness that the patient presented with.
  2. The abdomen if intestinal absorption problems are suspected and workup is needed
D. Auscultate the heart and lungs.

Diagnostic Tests

A. Serum 25(OH)D: Normal (30–80 ng/mL)
B. Parathyroid hormone: Normal (14–72 pg/mL)
C. Calcium level: Normal (8.5–10.2 mg/dL)

Differential Diagnoses

A. Vitamin D deficiency
B. Osteoporosis
C. Rickets
D. Cystic fibrosis
E. Malabsorption syndrome
F. Chronic kidney disease

Plan

A. General interventions
  1. Educate the patient regarding the importance of calcium and vitamin D for the body.
  2. Vitamin D levels should be monitored. Vitamin D levels should range between 30 and 60 ng/mL.
B. Patient teaching
  1. Educate the patient about vitamin D deficiency and the importance of getting vitamin D into the diet on a daily basis.
  2. Suggest eating foods that are higher in vitamin D in the diet. These foods include fish oil, cod liver, salmon, and foods fortified with vitamin D such as milk and cereals.
  3. Discuss how inadequate sun exposure can increase the risk of vitamin D deficiency. Recommend 20 to 30 minutes of sunlight during summer months without use of sunscreen, if this is not contraindicated to other chronic conditions.
  4. Foods higher in calcium should also be included in the diet on a daily basis.
C. Pharmaceutical therapy
  1. Vitamin D-level recommendations:
    a. For vitamin D levels less than 20 ng/mL: Vitamin D_2 or D_3: 50,000 IU weekly for

8 weeks and recheck vitamin D level. If still less than 30 ng/mL at that point, repeat the dose for another 8 weeks and recheck when second course is finished.

b. Vitamin D levels between 20 and 30 ng/mL: Vitamin D_3 600 to 800 IU daily.

c. Cholecalciferol (vitamin D_3) is preferred to ergocalciferol (vitamin D_2) for supplementation when available.

2. Calcium levels should be maintained with a recommended dietary intake of 1,000 to 1,200 mg/d.

D. For malabsorption problems, refer to a GI specialist for workup.

Follow-Up

A. Follow-up should be performed according to recommendations based on laboratory results. Initial laboratory results should be repeated in 8 weeks with initial treatment. As soon as vitamin D levels are stable, repeat lab work routinely to confirm that levels remain within enormal range. If levels continue to fall, refer to a specialist.

Consultation/Referral

A. Consult with a physician or refer the patient to a gastroenterologist for those who consistently have low vitamin D levels or if malabsorption problems are diagnosed.

Individual Considerations

A. Pregnancy: No contraindications for treatment during pregnancy. The same prescribing dose is safe for pregnancy and breastfeeding patients.

B. Pediatrics

1. The American Academy of Pediatrics recommends infants fed exclusively by breast milk should have vitamin D supplementation.

2. Up to 1 year of age: Vitamin D_2 or D_3: 1,000 to 2,000 IU/d with calcium supplementation is recommended for 6 weeks then followed by 400 IU/d.

3. Ages 1 to 18 years: 50,000 IU vitamin D_2 is recommended every week for 6 weeks, then 600 to 1,000 IU/d.

C. Geriatrics

1. Vitamin deficiencies are commonly seen in this population.

2. All patients diagnosed with osteoporosis should be assessed for vitamin D deficiency.

3. Patients with a serum 25(OH)D level of less than 10 are at risk for developing osteomalacia.

Bibliography

Aletaha, D., Neogi, T., Silman, A. J., Funovits, J., Felson, D. T., Bingham, C. O., . . . Hawker, G. (2010). 2010 rheumatoid arthritis classification criteria: An American College of Rheumatology/European League Against Rheumatism collaborative initiative. *Arthritis and Rheumatism, 62*(9), 2569–2581.

American College of Rheumatology. ACR-endorsed criteria for rheumatic diseases. Retrieved from http://www.rheumatology.org/Practice-Quality/Clinical-Support/Criteria/ACR-Endorsed-Criteria

Angeline, M. E., Gee, A. O., Shindle, M., Warren, R. F., & Rodeo, S. A. (2013). The effects of vitamin D deficiency in athletes. *American Journal of Sports Medicine, 41*(2), 461–464.

Bartels, C. (2015). Systemic lupus erythematosus. *Medscape.* Retrieved from www.emedicine.medscape.com/article/332244-overview

Becker, M. A. (2016). Clinical manifestations and diagnosis of gout. *UpToDate.* Retrieved from http://www.uptodate.com/contents/clinical-manifestations-and-diagnosis-of-gout

Becker, M. A. (2016). Prevention of recurrent gout: Pharmacologic urate-lowering therapy and treatment of tophi. *UpToDate.* Retrieved from http://www.uptodate.com/contents/prevention-of-recurrent-gout-pharmacologic-urate-lowering-therapy-and-treatment-of-tophi

Becker, M. A. (2016). Treatment of acute gout. *UpToDate.* Retrieved from www.uptodate.com/contents/treatment-of-acute-gout

Behnam, B., Moghimi, J., Ghorbani, R., & Ghahremanfard, F. (2013). The frequency and major determinants of depression in patients with rheumatoid arthritis. *Turkish Journal of Rheumatology (Turkish League Against Rheumatism/Turkive Romatizma Arastima VeSavas Dernegi), 28*(1), 32–37.

Cakir, T., Evcik, F. D., Subasi, V., Gokce, I. Y., & Kayuncu, V. (2014). The effectiveness of aquatic exercises in the treatment of rheumatic arthritis. *Turkish Journal of Osteoporosis/Turk Osteoporoz Dergisi, 20*(1), 10–15.

Carter, S. C., Patty-Resk, C., Ruffing, V., & Hicks, D. (2015). *Core curriculum for rheumatology nursing* (1st ed.). Greenville, SC: Rheumatology Nurses Society.

Centers for Disease Control and Prevention. (2015a). Fibromyalgia. Retrieved from www.cdc.gov/arthritis/basics/fibromyalgia.htm

Centers for Disease Control and Prevention. (2015b). Gout. Retrieved from www.cdc.gov/arthritis/basics/gout.htm

Centers for Disease Control and Prevention. (2015c). Osteoarthritis (OA). Retrieved from www.cdc.gov/arthritis/basics/osteoarthritis.htm

Centers for Disease Control and Prevention. (2015d). Systemic lupus erythematous (SLE or lupus): Prevalence and incidence. Retrieved from www.cdc.gov/arthritis/basics/lupus.htm

Chang, S. F., Hong, C. M., & Yang, R. S. (2014). The performance of an online osteoporosis detection system: A sensitivity and specificity analysis. *Journal of Clinical Nursing, 23*(13–14), 1803–1809.

Chasset, F., Francès, C., Barete, S., Amoura, Z., & Arnaud, L. (2015). Influence of smoking on the efficacy of antimalarials in cutaneous lupus: A meta-analysis of the literature. *Journal of the American Academy of Dermatology, 72*(4), 634–639.

Correia, L. C., Sodré, F., Garcia, G., Sabino, M., Brito, M., Kalil, F., . . . Noya-Rabelo, M. M. (2013). Relation of severe deficiency of vitamin D to cardiovascular mortality during acute coronary syndromes. *American Journal of Cardiology, 111*(3), 324–327.

Cosman, F., de Beur, S. J., LeBoff, M. S., Lewiecki, E. M., Tanner, B., Randall, S., & Lindsay, R. (2014). Clinician's guide to prevention and treatment of osteoporosis. *Osteoporosis International, 25*(10), 2359–2381. Retrieved from www.Springerlink.com

Curtis, E. M., Moon, R. J., Dennison, E. M., Harvey, N. C., & Cooper, C. (2015). Recent advances in the pathogenesis and treatment of osteoporosis. *Clinical Medicine (London, England), 15*(Suppl. 6), s92–s96.

Dawson-Hughes, B. (2014). Vitamin D deficiency in adults: Definition, clinical manifestations, and treatment. *UpToDate.* Retrieved from http://www.uptodate.com/contents/vitamin-d-deficiency-in-adults-definition-clinical-manifestations-and-treatment

Dewing, K. A. (2015). Management of patients with psoriatic arthritis. *Nurse Practitioner, 40*(4), 40–46; quiz 46.

Di Lorenzo, A. L. (2015). HLA-B27 syndromes. *Medscape.* Retrieved from http://emedicine.medscape.com/article/1201027-overview#a1

Farford, B., Balog, J., Jackson, K. D., & Montero, D. (2015). Osteoporosis: What about men? *Journal of Family Practice, 64*(9), 542–552 , 549–552.

Fonseca, R., Bernardes, M., Terroso, G., de Sousa, M., & Figueiredo-Braga, M. (2014). Silent burdens in disease: Fatigue and depression in SLE. *Autoimmune Diseases, 2014.* Article ID: 790724. doi:10.1155/2014/790724

Fontenot, H. B., & Harris, A. L. (2014). Pharmacologic management of osteoporosis. *Journal of Obstetric, Gynecologic, and Neonatal Nursing, 43*(2), 236–245; quiz E20.

Fujita, T., Kutsumi, H., Sanuki, T., Hayakumo, T., & Azuma, T. (2013). Adherence to the preventive strategies for nonsteroidal anti-inflammatory drug- or low-dose aspirin-induced gastrointestinal injuries. *Journal of Gastroenterology, 48*(5), 559–573.

Gota, C. E., Kaouk, S., & Wilke, W. S. (2015). Fibromyalgia and obesity: The association between body mass index and disability, depression, history of abuse, medications, and comorbidities. *Journal of Clinical Rheumatology, 21*(6), 289–295.

Hansen-Dispenza, H. (2015). Raynaud phenomenon treatment & management. *Medscape.* Retrieved from http://emedicine.medscape.com/article/331197-treatment

Hunder, G. G. (2014). Clinical manifestations of giant cell (temporal) arteritis. *UpToDate.* Retrieved from http://www.uptodate.com/contents/clinical-manifestations-of-giant-cell-temporal-arteritis

Ikdahl, E., Rollefstad, S., Olsen, I. C., Kvien, T. K., Hansen, I. J., Soldal, D. M., . . . Semb, A. G. (2015). EULAR task force recommendations on annual cardiovascular risk assessment for patients with rheumatoid arthritis: An audit of the success of implementation in a rheumatology outpatient clinic. *BioMed Research International, 2015,* doi:10.1155/2015/515280.

Jordan, S., Maurer, B., Toniolo, M., Michel, B., & Distler, O. (2015). Performance of the new ACR/EULAR classification criteria for systemic sclerosis in clinical practice. *Rheumatology (Oxford, England), 54*(8), 1454–1458.

Kado, D. M. (2014). Overview of hyperkyphosis in older persons. *UpToDate.* Retrieved from http://www.uptodate.com/contents/overview-of-hyperkyphosis-in-older-persons

Kalunian, K. C. (2014). Diagnosis and classification of osteoarthritis. *UpToDate.* Retrieved from http://www.uptodate.com/contents/diagnosis-and-classification-of-osteoarthritis

Kalunian, K. C. (2015a). Nonpharmacologic therapy of osteoarthritis. *UpToDate.* Retrieved from www.uptodate.com/contents/nonpharmacologic-therapy-of-osteoarthritis

Kalunian, K. C. (2015b). Treatment of osteoarthritis resistant to initial pharmacologic therapy. *UpToDate.* Retrieved from www.uptodate.com/contents/treatment-of-osteoarthritis-resistant-to-initial-pharmacologic-therapy

Kim, S. J., & McMahon, M. (2013). Diagnosis and treatment of systemic lupus erythematosus. *Journal of Clinical Outcomes Management, 20*(2), 85–95.

Kinkade, S. (2007). Evaluation and treatment of acute low back pain. *American Family Physician, 75*(8), 1181–1188.

Klippel, J. H. (2008). *Primer on the rheumatic diseases* (13th ed.). New York, NY: Springer.

Lalani, S., Pope, J., de Leon, F., & Peschken, C. (2010). Clinical features and prognosis of late-onset systemic lupus erythematosus: Results from the 1000 faces of lupus study. *Journal of Rheumatology, 37*(1), 38–44.

Liedberg, G. M., & Björk, M. (2014). Symptoms of subordinated importance in fibromyalgia when differentiating working from non-working women. *Work: A Journal of Prevention, Assessment and Rehabilitation, 48*(2), 155–164.

Mackey, P. A., & Whitaker, M. D. (2015). Osteoporosis: A therapeutic update. *Journal for Nurse Practitioners, 11*(10), 1011–1017.

Marcus, D. M. (2015). Herbal remedies, supplements & acupuncture for arthritis. Retrieved from www.rheumatology.org/i-am-a/patient-caregiver/treatments/herbal-remedies-supplements-acupuncture-for-arthritis

Martin, G. M., Thornhill, T. S., & Katz, J. M. (2015). Total knee arthroplasty. *UpToDate.* Retrieved from www.uptodate.com/contents/total-knee-arthroplasty

Mayo Clinic. (2013). Gout. Retrieved from http://www.mayoclinic.org/diseases-conditions/gout/basics/definition/con-20019400

Miller, M. L., & Viegels, R. A. (2016). Clinical manifestations of dermatomyositis and polymyositis in adults. *UpToDate.* Retreived from www.uptodate.com/contents/clinical-manifestations-of-dermatomyositis-and-polymyositis-in-adults

Moerman, R. V., Bootsma, H., Kroese, F. G., & Vissink, A. (2013). Sjögren's syndrome in older patients: Aetiology, diagnosis and management. *Drugs & Aging, 30*(3), 137–153.

Montes, R. A., Mocarzel, L. O., Lanzieri, P. G., Lopes, L. M., Carvalho, A., & Almeida, J. R. (2016). Smoking and its association with morbidity in systemic lupus erythematosus evaluated by the Systemic Lupus International Collaborating Clinics/American College of Rheumatology damage index: Preliminary data and systematic review. *Arthritis & Rheumatology (Hoboken, N.J.), 68*(2), 441–448.

National Institute for Health and Care Excellence. (2014, February). *Osteoarthritis. Care and management. Clinical Guideline, No. 177* (p. 36). London, United Kingdom: Author

National Osteoporosis Foundation. (n.d.-a). Medications to prevent & treat osteoporosis. Retrieved from https://www.nof.org/?s=osteoporosis+prevention

National Osteoporosis Foundation. (n.d.-b). Prevention: Vitamin D. Retrieved from https://www.nof.org/?s=osteoporosis+prevention

Neogi, T., Jansen, T. L., Dalbeth, N., Fransen, J., Schumacher, H. R., Berendsen, D., . . . Taylor, W. J. (2015). 2015 Gout classification criteria: An American College of Rheumatology/European League Against Rheumatism collaborative initiative. *Annals of the Rheumatic Diseases, 74*(10), 1789–1798.

Painter, J. T., & Crofford, L. J. (2013). Chronic opioid use in fibromyalgia syndrome: A clinical review. *Journal of Clinical Rheumatology, 19*(2), 72–77.

Palmer, D., & El Miedany, Y. (2014). Rheumatoid arthritis: Recommendations for treat to target. *British Journal of Nursing (Mark Allen Publishing), 23*(6), 310–315.

Quéméneur, T., Mouthon, L., Cacoub, P., Meyer, O., Michon-Pasturel, U., Vanhille, P., . . . Hachulla, E. (2013). Systemic vasculitis during the course of systemic sclerosis: Report of 12 cases and review of the literature. *Medicine, 92*(1), 1–9.

Ramos-Casals, M., Brito-Zerón, P., Seror, R., Bootsma, H., Bowman, S. J., Dörner, T., . . . Vitali, C. (2015). Characterization of systemic disease in primary Sjögren's syndrome: EULAR-SS Task Force recommendations for articular, cutaneous, pulmonary and renal involvements. *Rheumatology (Oxford, England), 54*(12), 2230–2238.

Raza, K., Klareskog, L., & Holers, V. M. (2016). Predicting and preventing the development of rheumatoid arthritis. *Rheumatology (Oxford, England), 55*(1), 1–3.

Rosen, H. N., & Walega, D. R. (2014). Osteoporotic thoracolumbar vertebral compression fractures: Clinical manifestations and treatment. *UpToDate.* Retrieved from http://www.uptodate.com/contents/osteoporotic-thoracolumbar-vertebral-compression-fractures-clinical-manifestations-and-treatment

Sam Lim, S., Rana Bayakly, A., Helmick, C. G., Gordon, C., Easley, K. A., & Drenkard, C. (2014). The incidence and prevalence of systemic lupus erythematosus, 2002–2004: The Georgia Lupus Registry. *Arthritis & Rheumatology, 66*(2), 357–368.

Schur, P. H., & Moreland, L. W. (2016). General principles of management of rheumatoid arthritis in adults. *UpToDate.* Retrieved from http://www.uptodate.com/contents/general-principles-of-management-of-rheumatoid-arthritis-in-adults

Seetharaman, M. (2015). Giant cell arteritis (temporal arteritis) workup. *Medscape.* Retrieved from http://emedicine.medscape.com/article/332483-workup

Sholter, D. E., & Russell, A. S. (2016). Synovial fluid analysis. *UpToDate.* Retrieved from www.uptodate.com/contents/synovial-fluid-analysis

Shur, P. H., & Wallace, D. J. (2014). Diagnosis and differential diagnosis of systemic lupus erythematosus in adults. *UpToDate.* Retrieved from www.uptodate.com/contents/diagnosis-and-differential-diagnosis-of-systemic-lupus-erythematous-in-adults

Singh, J. A., Saag, K. G., Bridges, S. L., Akl, E. A., Bannuru, R. R., Sullivan, M. C., . . . McAlindon, T. (2016). 2015 American College of Rheumatology Guideline for the treatment of rheumatoid arthritis. *Arthritis & Rheumatology (Hoboken, N.J.), 68*(1), 1–26.

Smith, W. M. (2013). Gender and spondyloarthropathy-associated uveitis. *Journal of Ophthalmology, 2013.* Article ID: 928264. doi: 10.1155/2013/928264

Solomon, D. H. (2014). Overview of selective COX-2 inhibitors. *UpToDate.* Retrieved from http://www.uptodate.com/contents/overview-of-selective-cox-2-inhibitors

Tunnicliffe, D. J., Singh-Grewal, D., Kim, S., Craig, J. C., & Tong, A. (2015). Diagnosis, monitoring, and treatment of systemic lupus erythematosus: A systematic review of clinical practice guidelines. *Arthritis Care & Research, 67*(10), 1440–1452.

Varga, J. (2014). Diagnosis and differential diagnosis of systemic sclerosis (scleroderma) in adults. *UpToDate.* Retrieved from www.uptodate.com/contents/diagnosis-and-differential-diagnosis-of-systemic-sclerosis-scleroderma-in-adults

Varga, J., & Steen, V. (2015). Pulmonary arterial hypertension in systemic sclerosis (scleroderma): Definition, classification, risk factors, screening and prognosis. *UpToDate.* Retrieved from www.uptodate.com/contents/pulmonary-arterial-hypertension-in-systemic-sclerosis-scleroderma-definition-classification-risk-factors-screening-and-prognosis

Wolfe, F., Clauw, D. J., Fitzcharles, M. A., Goldenberg, D. L., Katz, R. S., Mease, P., . . . Yunus, M. B. (2010). The American College of Rheumatology preliminary diagnostic criteria for fibromyalgia and measurement of symptom severity. *Arthritis Care & Research, 62*(5), 600–610.

Yurdakul, F. G., Bodur, H., Sivas, F., Başkan, B., Eser, F., & Yilmaz, O. (2015). Clinical features, treatment and monitoring in patients with polymyalgia rheumatica. *Archives of Rheumatology, 30*(1), 28–33.

22 Psychiatric Guidelines

Anxiety

Moya Cook and Alyson Wolz

Definition

A. Generalized anxiety disorder (GAD) is a condition exhibited by excessive worry, tension, apprehension, and uneasiness from anticipated danger that is not controlled on most days of the week for at least 6 months. It is the "fight-or-flight" response that is part of the survival instinct. Anxiety is distinguished from fear in that fear is a response to consciously recognized external danger. The source of anxiety is largely unknown or unrecognized.

Normal anxiety allows us to get in touch with developmental learning that is part of our human growth. Anxiety in its chronic form is maladaptive and is considered a psychiatric disorder. Many cases of anxiety disorder in late life are chronic, having persisted from younger years. In its pathologic form, anxiety interferes with developmental learning because it infers significant distress.

When a patient presents with anxiety, it is often comorbid with other psychiatric disorders, particularly depression. Anxiety may act as a predispositional factor to early-onset depression (before age 26 years) and to increased frequency of depressive episodes. Patients also present clinically with only anxiety, in one of its many forms, such as GAD, posttraumatic stress disorder (PTSD), obsessive-compulsive disorder (OCD), adjustment disorder with anxious mood, phobic disorders, acute anxiety, or panic disorder, with or without agoraphobia.

Incidence

A. Anxiety disorders are the most common mental illness in the United States, affecting approximately 18% of the adult population. Although highly treatable, only about one third of individuals suffering from anxiety seek treatment. Anxiety is present in many medical illnesses and must be distinguished to treat it appropriately. GAD and panic disorder are associated with frequent suicide attempts.

Pathogenesis

A. Some degree of familial transmission of GAD, as well as panic disorder, has been noted. Unconscious conflict is thought to be the underlying cause of anxiety, which signals the ego to be careful expressing unacceptable impulses. Behavioral anxiety is considered a conditioned response to a stimulus associated with danger.

Clinically, however, identifying specific anxiogenic stimuli is difficult. The onset of GAD is also thought to be the cumulative effect of several stressful life events. Many studies have found that phobic/anxiety symptoms predated clinical alcoholism by a number of years. *t*-Aminobutyric acid–benzodiazepine receptor complex, the locus coeruleus–norepinephrine system, and serotonin are three neurotransmitter systems implicated in the biological basis of anxiety. These systems are thought to mediate "normal" anxiety and pathologic anxiety.

Predisposing Factors

A. Young to middle-aged women; onset usually at 20 to 30 years of age
B. Non-White
C. Single
D. Lower socioeconomic status
E. A childhood overanxious disorder
F. Excessive worrying
G. Unresolved unconscious conflict

Common Complaints

A. Inability to control worrying
B. Motor tension
C. Autonomic hyperactivity vigilance
D. Sleep disturbance

> *Statements concerning self-medication with alcohol to help with sleep may indicate a coexistent alcohol abuse/dependence diagnosis that must be treated concomitantly.*

E. Shortness of breath
F. Increased heart rate and respirations
G. Feelings of apprehension
H. Dizziness
I. Abdominal disturbances/nausea
J. Increased perspiration
K. Trembling

Other Signs and Symptoms

A. According to the *Diagnostic and Statistical Manual of Mental Disorders* (5th ed.; *DSM-5*; American Psychiatric Association [APA], 2013), other symptoms include excessive worry out of proportion to the likelihood or impact of the feared events that occurs for a period of 6 months or longer, during which the person has been bothered more days than not by these concerns.

B. At least three of the following six symptoms are present:

1. Muscle tension

2. Restlessness or feeling keyed up or on edge

3. Easy fatigability

4. Difficulty concentrating or "mind going blank" because of anxiety

5. Trouble falling or staying asleep

6. Irritability

C. If another Axis I disorder is present, such as depression, or bipolar affective disorder, the anxiety may be in response to fear of

1. Being embarrassed in public in the presence of a social phobia

2. Being contaminated in the presence of OCD

3. Gaining weight in the presence of anorexia nervosa

4. Having an illness (as in hypochondriasis or somatization disorder)

D. Impaired social or occupational function. The anxiety, worry, or physical symptoms significantly interfere with the person's normal routine or usual activities or cause marked distress.

Subjective Data

A. Review the onset, course, and duration of symptoms. How often does the anxiety occur (e.g., every day, week, and month)?

B. Review any history of anxiety and age of onset. If treated, how was the previous anxiety treated and what was the success of the treatment?

C. Determine whether there is a history of suicide attempts. Does the patient have a current plan or vague ideas of suicide? Ask the patient, "Have you ever thought of hurting yourself or others?" If there is any concern regarding suicide/homicide, immediately refer the patient to a psychiatrist.

D. Review drug history for prescription, over-the-counter (OTC) medications, and recreational/illicit drug use, and the patient's use of caffeine, which precipitates anxiety symptoms.

E. Review the patient's history of alcohol consumption. Mild or moderate alcohol withdrawal presents primarily with anxiety symptoms. In patients who have developed tolerance to the effects of alcohol or benzodiazepines, abrupt cessation of these agents may produce heightened anxiety over baseline, as well as a risk of seizure.

F. Review the patient's history for major stressors. Are these stressors new or chronic? If chronic problems, ask what made the patient come in today.

G. Determine how the patient has been coping with stress up until today (exercise, medication).

H. Review the patient's history of other medical problems.

I. Does anyone else in the family have the same problem? How are they treated?

Physical Examination

A. Check pulse, respirations, blood pressure, and weight.

B. Inspect

1. Observe general appearance; note grooming, dress, ability to communicate, body movements, nail biting, playing with hair, and inability to sit still.

C. Administer mental examination of choice.

1. *DSM-5* Diagnostic Criteria for Generalized Anxiety Disorder available from the APA (2013)

2. Beck Anxiety Scale

D. Physical examination as indicated by somatic complaints

Diagnostic Tests

A. Blood alcohol

B. Thyroid profile

C. Blood glucose

D. Medication level (e.g., theophylline, etc.) if applicable

E. Urine drug screen

F. Additional testing related to suspected physical pathology

Differential Diagnoses

A. Substance/medication-induced anxiety disorder

B. Psychiatric syndrome

1. Mood disorders such as depression or bipolar disorder

2. Psychotic disorders

3. Somatoform disorders (characterized by physical complaints lacking known medical basis or demonstrable physical finding in the presence of psychological factors judged to be etiologic or important in the initiation, exacerbation, or maintenance of the disturbance)

4. Personality disorders

5. Alcoholism and drug abuse/dependence

6. Attention deficit hyperactivity disorder (ADHD)

C. Medical conditions. Anxiety syndromes mimic many medical illnesses, including intracranial tumors, menstrual irregularities, hypothyroidism, hyperparathyroidism and hypoparathyroidism, postconcussion syndrome, psychomotor epilepsy, and Cushing's disease.

1. Consider hypoglycemia if anxiety is chronic.

2. Hypothyroidism

3. Hyperthyroidism: Rapid-onset anxiety could be a symptom of hyperthyroidism.

4. Tumor

5. Cushing's disease

Plan

A. General interventions

1. Treat medical conditions as appropriate.

2. Refer the patient for cognitive behavior therapy. Counseling is effective for learning new techniques to help with alleviating symptoms. Cognitive behavior therapy may be effective alone and/or may also be used as adjunct to medication treatment.

3. Encourage the patient to perform self-calming techniques at home, such as deep breathing/relaxation techniques and exercise.

B. Patient teaching: *See Section III: Patient Teaching Guide for this chapter, as appropriate: "Sleep Disorders/Insomnia" and "Alcohol and Drug Dependence."*

C. Pharmaceutical therapy

1. Selective serotonin reuptake inhibitors (SSRIs) or selective serotonin norepinephrine reuptake inhibitors (SNRIs)

a. Fluoxetine (Prozac), 5 to 10 mg/d orally initially; usual dose 20 to 80 mg a day. Long half-life; alters metabolism of cytochrome P-450 2D6-cleared agents. Use caution.

b. Paroxetine (Paxil), 10 mg/d orally initially; usual dose 25 to 50 mg a day

c. Sertraline (Zoloft), 25 to 50 mg/d orally initially; usual dose 50 to 200 mg a day

d. Escitalopram (Lexapro), 10 mg/d initially; usual dose 10 to 20 mg/d. Caution: Use 10 mg for geriatric patients. Use with caution in patients with severe renal impairment.

e. Citalopram (Celexa), 5 to 10 mg/d orally initially; usual dose 20 to 40 mg/d. *Caution*: Risk for QT prolongation, contraindicated in patients with congenital long QT syndrome and should not exceed 20 mg daily if prescribed to patients also taking CYP2C19 inhibitors (cimetidine, fluconazole, omeprazole).

f. Venlafaxine (Effexor), 37.5 mg/d orally initially; usual dose 75 to 300 mg a day

g. Duloxetine (Cymbalta), 30 mg/d for 1 week, then usual dose 40 to 60 mg/d. Maximum dose is 120 mg/d. *Caution*: Do not use in patients with severe renal impairment, chronic liver disease, or cirrhosis.

h. These medications can take 4 to 6 weeks to take effect.

i. Warn patients that they should not stop these medications abruptly; they should taper off gradually.

2. Nonbenzodiazepine anxiolytic

a. Buspirone (Buspar), 7.5 mg twice a day

b. May increase by 5 mg/d orally every 2 to 3 days

c. Usual range: 20 to 30 mg orally every day, maximum 60 mg orally every day

d. Not recommended for children younger than 18 years

e. Therapeutic effects delayed from 1 to 4 weeks

3. Short-acting benzodiazepines

a. Alprazolam (Xanax), 0.25 mg to 0.5 mg orally two to three times daily

b. Clonazepam 0.25 to 0.5 mg orally one or two times daily, titrated up to 1 mg two to three times daily as needed

c. Lorazepam (Ativan), 0.5 to 2 mg, up to 6 mg orally every day in divided doses. Maximum dose of 10 mg/d in divided doses

i. Use for initial short-term stabilization while simultaneously prescribing buspirone because therapeutic effects of buspirone are delayed from 1 to 4 weeks.

ii. Limit use to several weeks to a few months to prevent dependence.

Follow-Up

A. Follow up in 1 to 2 weeks to assess the patient's status.

B. Follow up every 2 to 4 weeks after that to check the patient's progress.

C. Assess suicide potential with every office visit.

Consultation/Referral

A. Refer to a psychiatric clinician for complex medication management and psychotherapy after initial assessment.

B. If the patient expresses suicidal thoughts, immediately refer to the emergency room (in-patient therapy) or psychiatric specialist for continuing psychotherapy.

Individual Considerations

A. Pregnancy

1. Caution should be used in prescribing medications for anxiety during pregnancy; the benefits must be weighed against the risks.

2. If the patient becomes pregnant while taking these medications, taper the medication dose instead of ceasing abruptly.

B. Pediatrics

1. Children with suspected anxiety disorders should be immediately referred to a pediatric psychiatrist.

C. Geriatrics

1. Anxiety is often unrecognized and inadequately treated in this population because of concomitant medical illness; overlap with cognitive disorders; and comorbid depression, ageism, and cohort effects.

2. Start with the lowest dose of medication and increase slowly.

D. Partners

1. If available in the community, provide resources for partners, such as the National Alliance on Mental Illness (NAMI).

2. Psychotherapy for the patient and partner is often helpful.

Attention Deficit Disorder/Attention Deficit Hyperactivity Disorder

Moya Cook and Alyson Wolz

Definition

A. Attention deficit/hyperactivity disorder (ADHD) is a syndrome that consists of a cluster of behaviors that emerge early in a child's life and persist over time. Excessively high levels of motor activity, problems with attention span, concentration, and/or impulsivity characterize ADHD. Up to 50% of patients with ADHD also have other psychosocial disorders such as oppositional defiant disorder (ODD), depression or bipolar disorder (develops in 25% of children with ADHD), posttraumatic stress disorder (PTSD), or Tourette's syndrome.

B. The diagnostic criteria for ADHD include symptoms of inattention and symptoms of hyperactivity/impulsivity as published by the American Psychiatric Association (APA), in the *DSM-5* (2013). These criteria are available at www.cdc.gov/ncbddd/adhd/diagnosis.html

Incidence

A. 3% to 5% of all school-aged children and 2.5% in adults
B. Occurs in all races and socioeconomic groups
C. Boys are more likely than girls to have symptoms by a ratio of 2:1
D. Not uncommon for this disorder to persist into adulthood
E. Approximately 33% of children with learning disabilities also have ADHD

Pathogenesis

A. Unknown, but several studies suggest a biochemical basis involving deficits in the availability of neurotransmitters to the frontal–orbital circuits of the neurobehavioral regulatory systems of the brain. ADHD may also be inherited.
B. Associated problems with ADHD include academic, social, and emotional problems.

Predisposing Factors

A. A close relative with a mood disorder, anxiety, or ADHD
B. Brain trauma
C. Selective therapeutic regimens, such as intrathecal chemotherapy
D. Recent studies have suggested a possible link to maternal smoking, alcohol abuse, or other toxins during pregnancy.
E. Some perinatal influences have been theorized to be connected to ADHD, including fetal distress, prolonged labor, prematurity, and perinatal asphyxia.

Common Complaints

A. Hyperactivity, impulsivity, and/or inattentiveness
B. Poor school performance
C. Poor peer relationships

Other Signs and Symptoms

A. Inattentive and easily distracted when completing tasks: Daydreams, does not finish work, loses things, has difficulty concentrating
B. Impulsive: Risk taking, impatient, very emotional
C. Hyperactivity/overactivity: Speech and motor skills overactive
D. Difficulty with learning, poor performance in school/work

Subjective Data

A. Determine the presenting symptoms and ascertain when symptoms first began.
B. Note duration of symptoms.
  1. Have they been present for at least 6 months?
  2. Ask regarding specific behaviors as listed in the diagnostic criteria.
C. Review settings in which symptoms are present (home, school, day care).
D. Discuss the child's past medical history.
E. Discuss the child's developmental history; did he or she meet all of the developmental milestones?
F. Review the child's family, social, and school histories.
G. Review all current medications, including any over-the-counter (OTC) medications and herbals. Specifically review medication history for theophylline, prednisone, and albuterol.
H. Review the child's diet, eating habits, and sleeping habits.
I. Review the child's routines and habits: Stimulation may come from TV, video, and computer.

Physical Examination

A. Check temperature, pulse, respirations, blood pressure, weight, and height.
B. Inspect
  1. Observe overall appearance. Note behavior and interactions with others.
  2. Inspect the skin, eyes, ears, nose, and throat.
C. Auscultate the heart, lungs, and abdomen.
D. Palpate the neck, thyroid, chest, and abdomen.
E. Perform neurologic examination.
  1. Hearing/vision evaluation: Evaluate constant, involuntary movement of the eyes (nystagmus).
  2. Evaluate coordination difficulties/impaired motor skills.
  3. Evaluate visual-motor control problems (hand–eye coordination).

Diagnostic Tests

A. Complete blood count (CBC) to rule out iron-deficiency anemia
B. Lead level
C. Thyroid studies to rule out other organic problems
D. CBC with differential (if indicated)
E. Administer the National Institute for Children's Health Quality (NICHQ) Vanderbilt Assessment Scale available at www.nichq.org/~/media/files/resources/nichq vanderbiltassessment-full.ashx. See *DMS-5* criteria for diagnosing the type of ADHD. Criteria are available at www.cdc.gov/ncbddd/adhd/diagnosis.html
F. Refer for testing for psychological tests to measure IQ, social/emotional adjustment, and presence of learning disabilities.
G. EEG may be considered.
H. MRI may be considered to rule out organic diagnoses.

Differential Diagnoses

A. Oppositional defiant disorder (ODD)
B. Autism spectrum disorder
C. Hyperthyroidism/hypothyroidism
D. Lead poisoning
E. Other behavioral/psychological disorders (pervasive developmental delay, mood disorders, anxiety, or personality disorder)
F. Learning disorders
G. Seizure disorder, nonconvulsive
H. Impaired hearing related to chronic or recurrent otitis media
I. Adverse reactions to medications (theophylline, prednisone, or albuterol)
J. Substance use/abuse disorder (caffeine, alcohol/drugs)

Plan

A. General interventions

1. Multimodal and multidisciplinary approach is imperative and includes parent education regarding the nature of ADHD. Effective behavioral management, appropriate educational placement and support, and family and/or individual therapy are strongly encouraged.

2. It is important to obtain written reports (which consist of a standardized rating, such as the Connors Tool and/or the Vanderbilt Screening Tool of ADHD) from teachers, parents, and other adults who have regular contact with the child. The Vanderbilt Assessment Scale for Parent and Teacher may be found at www.nichq.org/-/media/files/resources/nichqvanderbiltassessment-full.ashx

3. The primary care provider, school nurse, school psychologist, and/or parent may function as the case manager to coordinate services.

B. Patient teaching

▶ **1.** *See Section III: Patient Teaching Guide for this chapter, "ADHD: Tips for Caregivers of a Child With ADHD" and "ADHD: Coping Strategies for Teens and Adults."*

2. Provide ADHD resources for parents, children, teens, and adults.

C. Pharmaceutical therapy

1. Begin with short-acting stimulants. Advance dose as needed for desired result.

2. Consider adding a long-acting agent to a short-acting agent if needed.

3. Long-acting agent may also be used alone.

D. First-line agents: Rapid onset with short duration

1. Methylphenidate (Ritalin, Methylin)

2. Dextroamphetamine (Dexedrine, ProCentra, Zenzedi)

3. Amphetamine-dextroamphetamine (Adderall)

4. Dexmethylphenidate (Focalin)

E. Rapid onset with long duration

1. Methylphenidate (Concerta, Ritalin LA, Ritalin SR, Daytrana patch, Metadate CD, Metadate ER, Methylin ER, Quillivant XR)

2. Amphetamine-dextroamphetamine (Adderall XR): Duration 10 hours

3. Dexmethylphenidate (Focalin XR): Duration 12 hours

4. Lisdexamfetamine (Vyvanse): Duration 13 to 14 hours

F. Medications to use if substance abuse is a concern

1. Vyvanse

2. Bupropion

3. Strattera

G. Medications recommended for comorbidity of depression

1. Bupropion (Wellbutrin, Wellbutrin SR, Wellbutrin XL)

2. Venlafaxine (Effexor, Effexor XR)

H. Medication doses

1. Methylphenidate (Ritalin) starting dose: 0.3 to 0.6 mg/kg/dose; short half-life (3–6 hours) necessitates two to three doses per day. Children: Not recommended for younger than 6 years of age. Greater than or equal to 6 years: 5 mg before breakfast and 5 mg before lunch. Increase dose by 5 to 10 mg weekly. Maximum dose 60 mg/d. Adults: 10 to 60 mg in two or three divided doses before meals.

2. Methylphenidate HCl (Ritalin LA): Swallow whole. Do not crush. Not recommended in children younger than 6 years. Children 6 years or older: 20 mg in morning; may increase dose 10 mg weekly, maximum dose 60 mg/d

3. Methylphenidate HCl liquid (Quillivant XR): Children: Not recommended for children younger than 6 years of age. Starting dose: 10 to 20 mg orally in morning. Increase the dose weekly by 10 to 20 mg. Maximum daily dose 60 mg/d

4. Methylphenidate HCl (Concerta): Children: Not recommended for children younger than 6 years; 6 to 12 years: 18 mg/d. Increase dose in 18-mg increments weekly as needed. Maximum is 54 mg daily. Adolescents/adults: 18 mg/d with maximum 72 mg daily; increase by 18-mg increments weekly as needed. Contraindicated with severe anxiety.

5. Dexmethylphenidate HCl (Focalin XR): Children: Not recommended for children younger than 6 years of age. Starting dose: 5 mg/d in morning. Titrate weekly in 5-mg increments. Maximun dose for children: 30 mg daily in morning, adults: 40 mg daily in morning.

6. Lisdexamfetamine dimesylate (Vyvanse) pediatric dose: Children 6 to 12 years old: 30 mg daily in a single dose in the morning. May be increased by 10 mg/d. Maximum dose of 70 mg daily in the morning

7. Atomoxetine (Strattera): Not a controlled substance. Weight less than 70 kg: Less than 0.5 mg/kg/d (maximum 1.4 mg/kg/d). Weight greater than 70 kg: 40 mg/d (maximum 100 mg/d). Increase dose after 3 days as needed, then after 2 to 4 weeks for maximum dose. May take a few weeks to see the full effect. Should be taken daily at the same time every day to avoid serotonin norepinephrine reuptake inhibitor (SNRI) effects. Federal Drug Administration (FDA)-approved indication for adults.

8. Side effects of these medications include anorexia, insomnia, stomach pain, growth suppression, and tics. If weight loss occurs, give medication after meals.

9. If psychostimulants are not effective, other medications used include antihistamines, clonidine, carbamazepine (Tegretol), divalproex (Depakote), beta-blockers, and antidepressants.

10. Be cautious when prescribing other medications concurrently.

Follow-Up

A. At 1 month: Inquire about improvements in each area of life and duration of the medication's actions.

B. Medication frequency may need to be altered.
C. Consider adding a third dose if the duration of action is very short and the child needs better afternoon or evening coverage to successfully complete homework or participate in other extracurricular activities.
D. When medication schedule is stable, subsequent visits can be every 3 months.

Consultation/Referral

A. Consult with the psychiatrist to help coordinate the medications.
B. Consult with the school psychologist if indicated for additional data.
C. Refer the patient for individual and/or family therapy if indicated.

Individual Considerations

A. Pediatrics
   1. The overall goal of ADHD therapy is to build the child's sense of competence and performance.
   2. Not all behavior issues are ADHD. The diagnosis must be carefully and cautiously established according to the diagnostic criteria of the APA.
   3. Individualize medications, preparations, and timing; 80% of children respond positively to stimulants.
   4. Instituting routine drug holidays should be done with caution. It is important to occasionally stop medication to compare treated and untreated states. The child's ability to concentrate and manage behavior at all times is critical. Not instituting drug holidays may prevent a "yo–yo" behavior experience for the patient.
   5. Use caution when medicating children with a personal or family history of Tourette's syndrome. Tics may worsen in these children.
   6. When prescribing psychostimulants to children with seizure disorders who are already on anticonvulsants, closely monitor plasma levels of both medications.
   7. Treat the child, not the parents, teachers, day-care personnel, or coaches.
B. Adults
   1. Up to half of the affected children have some symptoms of ADHD that persist into adulthood. Adults tend to outgrow the "hyperactivity" aspect; however, they may still require treatment for the ADD. Teens and adults benefit from specific coping strategies for ADD.

Resources

Attention Deficit Disorder Association: http://www.add.org

CHADD (Children With ADD): CHADD National Office
8181 Professional Place
Suite 150
Landover, MD 20785
Phone: 301-306-7070
Fax: 301-306-7090
http://www.chadd.org

Bipolar Disorder

Alyson Wolz

Definition

A. Bipolar disorder, commonly called manic-depressive disorder, is a psychiatric disorder that causes changes in moods, thoughts, and behaviors. These changes may range from mania (excessive energy, euphoria, racing thoughts, decreased need for sleep, grandiosity, pressured speech, and impulsive behavior) to depression (low energy, sadness, diminished interest and pleasure in most activities, recurrent thoughts of death, changes in sleep patterns, cognitive impairment, and difficulty carrying out daily activities).
B. There are four types of bipolar disorder:
   1. Bipolar I disorder: Individual meets the diagnostic criteria for a manic episode, which may have been preceded or followed by a hypomanic or depressive episode.
   2. Bipolar II disorder: Individual has a pattern of depressive episodes and hypomanic episodes (no mania). Often symptoms of depression and hypomania, especially agitation, irritability, and verbal impulsivity, are displayed in the same episode (mixed).
   3. Cyclothymic disorder: A chronic pattern of hypomanic and depressive symptoms that do not meet the full criteria for hypomania or depressive episodes. Symptoms occur for at least 2 years (1 year in children and adolescents).
   4. Unspecified bipolar and related disorder: This category applies to situations in which there are symptoms that are characteristic of bipolar disorder, but do not meet the full criteria. There may be insufficient information to make a diagnosis, or underlying medical conditions or substance use contributing to the condition.

Specific criteria for bipolar disorder as published by the American Psychiatric Association (APA; *DSM-5*, 2013) are available at the National Institute for Mental Health website: www.nimh.nih.gov/health/topics/bipolar-disorder/index.shtml

Incidence

A. 5.7 million or 2.6% of adults ages 18 years or older in the United States.
B. Median age of onset is 25 years, although can range from childhood to late onset (50s).
C. Occurs in all races and socioeconomic groups.
D. Men may present with symptoms of mania earlier than women. Women are more likely to present with symptoms of depression and experience more rapid cycling.
E. Bipolar disorder is the sixth leading cause of disability in the world.
F. Results in 9.2 years reduction in expected life span. One in five individuals diagnosed with bipolar disorder will die by suicide.

Pathogenesis

A. No specific biological markers for bipolar disorder have been identified to date; however, studies indicate a significant genetic component. Individuals with a first-degree relative with bipolar disorder are seven to ten times more likely to develop the disorder.

Predisposing Factors

A. A family history of bipolar disorder or schizophrenia
B. Periods of high stress
C. Drug or alcohol abuse
D. Major life changes such as the death of a loved one or a traumatic experience.

Common Complaints

A. Frequently seek treatment for depressive episodes
B. Poor work or school performance; unfinished tasks
C. Mood swings, irritability, or anger episodes
D. Social problems
E. Sleep disturbance

Other Signs and Symptoms

A. Mania: Symptoms last at least 1 week and may include inflated self-esteem, grandiosity, decreased need for sleep, talkative, racing thoughts, distractibility, increase in goal-directed activity, impulsive behavior (buying sprees, sexual indiscretions, poor business decisions). Symptoms cause marked impairment in functioning and may require hospitalization.
B. Hypomania: Symptoms last at least 4 days. Symptoms same as mania, but are not severe enough to cause marked impairment. Person frequently displays irritability and agitation.
C. Depression: Symptoms last for at least 2 weeks. Depressed mood most of the day; diminished interest in pleasure; changes in weight; sleep disturbance; restlessness or low energy; fatigue; feelings of worthlessness, guilt, and burdensomeness; cognitive changes; and thoughts of death.
D. Patients in primary care settings are more likely to present for symptoms of depression, which may look like a depressive disorder. It is important to rule out bipolar disorder before initiating treatment. Screening tool for bipolar symptoms is as follows:

The Mood Disorder Questionnaire (Hirshfeld et al., 2000). www.dbsalliance.org/pdfs/MDQ.pdf

Note: During a manic episode, individuals often do not perceive that there is anything wrong, and will often refuse treatment or become angry with those who are trying to intervene.

E. Impulse control: Patient may present as extremely happy and sociable. May have rapid mood changes, such as irritability or aggression when wishes are denied, especially if using substances.
F. Suicidal or homicidal thoughts or acts. Any statements made by the patient, such as "Life isn't worth living, I wish I were dead, I don't deserve to be alive, I can't deal with this," should be taken seriously. Refer the patient for counseling and assessment and treatment.

Subjective Data

A. Review the onset, duration, and course of presenting symptoms.
B. Review any previous history of depression, mania, or mood disorders.
C. Determine how the previous mood disorder was treated, if applicable.
D. Evaluate the patient's suicide potential. Ask: "Have you ever thought of hurting yourself or others?" Does the patient have a current suicide plan or vague ideas of suicide? Has the patient had any previous history of suicide attempts? If so, evaluate how life-threatening they were.
E. Review the patient's medical history.
F. Review the patient's drug history for prescription, over-the-counter (OTC), and recreational/illicit drug use (how much, how long, how often), and review his or her history of alcohol consumption (how much, how long, how often).
G. Assess patient's compliance with prescribed medications.
H. Review the patient's history for recent major life changes such as pregnancy, death, divorce, or any loss that may be normal throughout the stages of life. The *patient's perception* of the loss is what is important.
I. Review dietary intake since the symptoms have begun.
J. Establish usual weight, review weight gain/loss, and note in what time span.
K. Review the patient's activities of daily living. Does the patient get up and dress daily, perform daily hygiene, put on makeup?
L. Review how many hours of sleep and quality of sleep per day.
M. Review the disruption of usual activities: Return to work, return to school, exercise. Has the patient been engaging in activities outside the norm?
N. Assess mood patterns, rate of cycling, seasonal changes.
O. Review occupational/home exposure to neurodegenerative products.
P. Review any exposures to infectious diseases, including Lyme disease. Does anyone else, such as family, friends, or coworkers, have similar symptoms?
Q. If female, review for symptoms of menopause (sleep disturbances, irregular menses/amenorrhea, hot flashes, vaginal dryness, dyspareunia).

Physical Examination

A. Check pulse, respirations, blood pressure, and weight.
B. Inspect
   1. Observe overall appearance; note grooming, tone of voice, eye contact, conduct of patient during communication, and breath (smell of alcohol).
   2. Complete neurologic examination with screening tool of choice.
   3. Complete dermal examination for signs of substance use (refer to "Substance Use Disorders" section).
C. Palpate
   1. Palpate the neck and thyroid; note goiter if present.

2. Palpate the axilla and groin for lymphadenopathy (infectious etiology).
3. Check the joints for swelling and arthritis and range of motion (ROM; rule out musculoskeletal cause).

D. Auscultate
1. Heart, lungs, and abdomen (as applies to physical complaints)

E. Neurologic examination
1. Complete the Mental Status Examination (MSE), including appearance, affect/mood, thought content, perception, suicide/self-destruction, homicide/aggression, judgment/insight, and cognition.

Diagnostic Tests

A. Complete blood count (CBC) to rule out iron-deficiency anemia
B. Urine/serum drug screen
C. Thyroid studies to rule out other organic problems
D. Comprehensive metabolic panel (CMP)
E. Erythrocyte sedimentation rate (ESR)
F. Liver and lipid panel
G. Refer for psychological testing to confirm diagnosis, rule out other mental health disorders, assess for social/emotional adjustment, and for the presence of learning disabilities.
H. Electrocardiogram (EKG)
I. Electroencephalogram (EEG) may be considered.
J. CT scan or MRI may be considered to rule out organic diagnoses.

Differential Diagnoses

A. Bipolar disorder
B. Substance-induced mood disorder, including caffeine, alcohol/illicit drugs
C. Head trauma
D. Hyperthyroidism/hypothyroidism
E. Lead poisoning
F. Other behavioral/psychological disorders (pervasive developmental delay, oppositional defiant disorder, seasonal affective disorder, anxiety disorder, schizoaffective disorder, schizophrenia, and personality disorder)
G. Posttraumatic stress disorder
H. Attention deficit/hyperactivity disorder (ADHD)/learning disorders (in children)
I. Seizure disorder, nonconvulsive
J. Medical conditions (menopause, neurosyphilis, multiple sclerosis, Lyme's disease)
K. Adverse reactions to medications (theophylline, prednisone, albuterol, Levequin, and antidepressant medications (may induce mania).

Plan

A. General interventions
1. Keep the patient safe from self-harm.
2. Treat physical/laboratory findings. Recommend dietary change, iron supplements, and hormone replacement therapy per findings (see related chapters).

B. Patient teaching
1. Encourage the patient to take medications as prescribed. Educate the patient that some medications may take time to get into the system to work and time should be allowed to see the effects of the medication. Review side effects.
2. Encourage the patient to express feelings or worsening of symptoms if this occurs before next appointment. Have the patient make a client contract with you that he or she will not cause harm to self or others and if the patient begins having these thoughts, the patient will contact you or go to the nearest emergency department.
3. Encourage exercise on a daily basis for 20 to 30 minutes to increase energy and enhance a feeling of well-being.
4. Encourage the patient to get at least 7 to 8 hours of sleep each night. If sleep is a problem, address this issue with the client.
5. Avoid caffeine at night and/or watching TV late at night.
6. Encourage the patient to seek counseling with a professional counselor. Refer to the appropriate site (psychologist, psychiatrist, group therapy, etc.). Offer local resources to the patient.
7. Advise patient to participate in activities to enhance interpersonal relationships and build self-esteem. Include family and friends in recommended therapies and advise them to encourage the patient to participate in activities to enhance self-esteem.
8. Once the patient is feeling better, encourage continued use of medication, activities, and resources.

Bipolar disorder is a chronic condition requiring long-term, continuous treatment. Untreated, episodes of mania and depression may become more severe and more difficult to treat over time.

C. Pharmaceutical therapy
Medication choice depends on the current episode: Mania/depression.
1. Mood stabilizers
   a. Divalproex sodium (Depakote, Depakote ER)
      i. Indicated for mania.
      ii. Initial dose of 25 mg/kg/d mg daily in divided doses.
      iii. Increase as quickly as possible to achieve target plasma concentrations of 50 to 125 mcg/mL.
      iv. Maximum concentration achieved within 14 days.
      v. Maximum recommended dose is 60 mg/kg/d.
      vi. Drug–drug interactions: May increase concentrations of clonazepam, diazepam, lamotrigine, and carbamazepine. Aspirin increases Depakote blood levels.
      vii. Labs: Check valproic acid level, liver function test (LFT), and complete blood count

(CBC) after 1 week, then at 1 to 2 months, then every 6 to 12 months thereafter.

viii. Side effects: Dizziness, sedation, nausea, tremor, thrombocytopenia, elevated liver enzymes, polycystic ovarian syndrome, and hepatotoxicity (rare)

ix. Monitoring: Serum drug levels during treatment initiation; monitor weight and menstrual history every 3 months for the first year, then annually

b. Carbamazepine ER (Equetro)

i. Indicated for mania and mixed episode.

ii. Initial dose of 200 mg twice daily

iii. Adjust dose in 200-mg increments.

iv. Capsules may be taken whole or opened and sprinkled on food.

v. Do not use with monoamine oxidase inhibitors (MAOIs) or within 14 days of using an MAOI.

vi. Side effects include dizziness, somnolence, dry mouth, constipation, aplastic anemia, agranulocytosis, rash, toxic epidermal necrolysis (TEN), and Stevens–Johnson syndrome (SJS); patients of Asian ancestry have a 10-fold greater risk of TEN/SJS.

vii. Monitoring: Serum drug levels during treatment initiation and as clinically indicated. CBC, LFT, electrolytes, blood urea nitrogen (BUN), creatinine monthly for 3 months, then annually

c. Lithium

i. Indicated for mania and maintenance.

ii. **Lithium workup** before initiating the medication: EKG, BUN/creatinine, urinalysis, CMP, and thyroid-stimulating hormone (TSH)

iii. Initial dose of 300 mg twice daily

iv. Lithium levels drawn two times per week with dose adjustments in 300 mg increments until target serum levels are reached: Target serum levels 0.6 to 1.2 mEq/L. Levels should be drawn 12 hours after last dose.

v. Lithium toxicity: Nausea, vomiting, diarrhea, muscular weakness, lack of coordination, giddiness, and large output of dilute urine; may involve multiple organs and organ systems

vii. Monitoring: Serum drug levels every 3 to 6 months once stable. Electrolytes, BUN, creatinine every 3 to 6 months to exclude renal impairment. TSH, calcium, and weight after 6 months, then annually

d. Lamotrigine (Lamictal)

i. Indicated for maintenance therapy

ii. Must titrate slowly due to risk of rash/Stevens–Johnson syndrome.

iii. Initial dose:

1) Weeks 1 and 2: 25 mg daily

2) Weeks 3 and 4: 50 mg daily

3) Week 5: 100 mg daily

4) Week 6: 200 mg daily

5) Target dose of 200 to 400 mg

iv. Titration dose adjustments required if patient is on Depakote (slower titration) or carbamazepine (faster titration).

v. Side effects: Nausea, insomnia, somnolence, rash, leg cramps, aphasia, and **Stevens–Johnson syndrome.**

e. Topiramate (Topamax)

i. Off-label use as adjunctive treatment for bipolar disorder.

ii. Side effect: Weight loss

2. Atypical antipsychotics

Potential Side Effects for All Atypical Antipsychotics

- *Extrapyramidal and/or withdrawal symptoms in neonates with third-trimester exposure*
- *Lower seizure threshold*
- *Leukopenia, neutropenia, and agranulocytosis*
- *Metabolic changes including hyperglycemia/diabetes, dyslipidemia, and weight gain*
- *Orthostatic hypotension*
- *Tardive dyskinesia*
- *Cognitive and motor impairment*
- *Increased risk of stroke in elderly patients with dementia-related psychosis; elderly patients with a history of cerebrovascular accident (CVA) treated with antipsychotic medications are at an increased risk of death.*
- *Suicidal thinking*
- *Neuroleptic malignant syndrome (NMS): High fever, stiff muscles, confusion, sweating, changes in pulse, heart rate, and elevated blood pressure*
- **Laboratory tests: Monitor body mass index (BMI), waist circumference, hemoglobin A1c (HbA_{1c}), fasting plasma glucose, and fasting lipid panel at baseline, 3 months, and then annually.**

a. Aripiprazole (Abilify)

i. Indicated for mania, mixed episodes, and maintenance.

ii. Initial dose: 15 mg daily (10–15 mg if using in addition to a mood stabilizer). Once daily with or without meals.

iii. Available in tablets, orally disintegrating tablets, oral solution, and injectable 9.75 mg/1.3 mL single-dose vial.

iv. Maximum recommended dose is 30 mg daily.

v. Drug/drug interactions: Known CYP2D6 poor metabolizers, strong CYP2D6 *or* CYP3A4 inhibitors: ½ dose, known CYP2D6 poor metabolizers *and* strong CYP3A4 inhibitors: ¼ dose.

vi. Common side effects: Akathesia (restlessness), weight gain, nausea, constipation, headache, dizziness, and stuffy nose

b. Ziprasidone (Geodon)

i. Indicated as monotherapy for mania and mixed episodes and as an adjunct to lithium or valproate for maintenance.

ii. Initial dose: Mania: 40 mg twice daily, with increase to 60 to 80 mg twice daily on day 2 of treatment. **Giving oral doses with food increases absorption up to twofold.**

iii. Available in capsules and injectable 20 mg/mL single-dose vial.

iv. Maximum recommended dose: 60 to 80 mg twice daily with food

v. Drug/drug interactions: Do not give with other medications known to cause QT prolongation.

vi. Side effects: QT prolongation. Do not use in patients with recent heart failure, recent heart attack, or arrhythmias. Other more common side effects include akathesia (restlessness), sleepiness, weight gain, nausea, constipation, headache, dizziness, and stuffy nose. Less common: Severe cutaneous adverse reactions (SCAR) such as Stevens–Johnson syndrome

c. Risperidone (Risperdal/Risperdal Consta)

i. Indicated as monotherapy for mania and mixed episodes, and as an adjunct to lithium or valproate for maintenance therapy.

ii. Dosing:

1) Risperidone: 2 to 3 mg daily with titration in 1 mg increments at intervals of 24 hours or greater. Target dose of 1 to 6 mg daily. Max dosing 6 mg/d. Once or twice daily with or without meals. Available in tablets, orally disintegrating tablets, and oral solution 1 mg/mL.

2) Risperdal Consta: 25 mg intramuscular (IM) q 2 weeks with dose increase in 4-week intervals. Max dosing 37.5 to 50 mg IM q 2 weeks. Oral dose of risperidone should be used along with the first injection of Risperdal Consta, and continued for 3 weeks. Available in dose strengths of 12.5, 25, 37.5, or 50 mg.

3) Drug/drug interactions: CYP2D6 enzyme inducers (carbamazepine), may need to increase dose up to double the patient's usual dose. CYP2D6 enzyme inhibitors (paroxetine, fluoxetine), dose of risperidone should be titrated slowly and dose may need to be decreased.

4) Side effects: Dizziness, drooling, nausea, tiredness, weight gain, akathesia, tremor, blurred vision, QT prolongation, increased prolactin levels. Dose adjustment recommended for patients with severe renal or hepatic impairment. Monitor prolactin levels along with other recommended labs.

d. Asenapine (Saphris): Dissolvable

i. Indicated as monotherapy for mania and mixed episodes, and as an adjunct to lithium or valproate for maintenance therapy.

ii. Initial dose: 5 to 10 mg sublingually twice daily

iii. Available in sublingual tablets only.

iv. Maximum recommended dose: 10 mg twice daily

v. Drug/drug interactions: Antihypertensive drugs: Saphris may cause hypotension. Paroxetine (CYP2D6 substrate and inhibitor): Reduce paroxetine dose by ½ when used in combination with Saphris.

vi. Common side effects: Orthostatic hypotension, syncope, akathesia (restlessness), weight gain, nausea, constipation, headache, dizziness, and stuffy nose. Contraindicated in patients with severe hepatic impairment.

e. Quetiapine (Seroquel/Seroquel XR)

i. Indicated as monotherapy for bipolar mania, mixed, and depressive episodes, and as an adjunct to lithium or valproate for maintenance therapy.

ii. Dosing:

1) Quetiapine:

Mania: 50 mg twice daily. Dose adjustments in increments of 100 mg daily up to total of 400 mg. Further dose adjustments up to 800 mg/d should be in increments of no greater than 200 mg/d. Target dose: 400 to 800 mg daily. Maximum recommended dose: 800 mg/d.

Depression: Administer once daily at bedtime. Initial dose of 50 mg at bedtime. Increase to 100 mg on day 2 with further increases of 100 mg daily up to 300 mg/d. Target dose: 300 mg/d. Maximum daily dose: 300 mg.

2) Quetiapine extended release: Bipolar mania/mixed episode:

Initial dose of 300 mg daily in evening without food or with light meal. Target dose 400 to 600 mg daily. Max dosing 600 mg daily. Bipolar depression: 50 mg daily in evening without food or with a light meal. Target dose: 300 mg daily. Maximum recommended dose: 300 mg daily.

3) Drug/drug interactions: Dose should be increased up to fivefold of the original dose when used in combination with a potent CYP3A4 inducer. Titrate dose based on clinical response and tolerability. Dose should be reduced to 1/6 of the original dose when used in combination with a potent CYP3A4 inhibitor. Quetiapine may cause hypotension, thus enhancing the effects of antihypertensive medications.

4) Side effects: Somnolence, dry mouth, dysarthria, increased appetite, weight gain, nausea, constipation, dizziness, stuffy nose, joint pain, QT prolongation, hypotension.

f. Olanzapine (Zyprexa, Zydis)

i. Indicated for mania, mixed episodes, and maintenance monotherapy.

ii. Initial dose: 10 to 15 mg once daily with or without meals, with dose adjustments of 5 mg daily.

iii. Available in tablets, orally disintegrating tablets, and injectable 10 mg/2.1 mL single-dose vial.

iv. Maximum recommended dose 20 mg daily

v. Drug/drug interactions: Coadministration with diazepam may potentiate orthostatic hypotension. Known CYP1A2 inducers, such as carbamazepine, increase the clearance of olanzapine. Titrate dose based on clinical response and tolerability. When used in combination with CYP1A2 inhibitors, such as fluvoxamine, lower doses of olanzapine should be considered.

vi. Side effects: Postural hypotension, akathesia (restlessness), increased appetite, weight gain, somnolence, nausea, constipation, headache, dizziness, stuffy nose, and tremors

g. Olanzapine/fluoxetine combination (Symbyax)

i. Indicated for bipolar depression.

ii. Initial dose: 6 mg/25 mg capsule daily in the evening (mg equivalent olanzapine/mg equivalent fluoxetine). Dose adjustments as needed and tolerated. Target dose within the approved dosing range of 6/25, 6/50, 12/25, 12/50 mg.

iii. Maximum recommended dose: 18 mg/75 mg daily in evening.

iv. Drug/drug interactions: Same as with olanzapine and fluoxetine individually.

v. Common side effects: Akathesia (restlessness), increased appetite, fatigue, somnolence, peripheral edema, blurred vision, weight gain, nausea, constipation, headache, dizziness, stuffy nose

h. Chlorpromazine (Thorazine)

i. Indicated for mania/mixed episode.

ii. Initial dose: 25 mg orally three times daily with gradual increase until effective dose is reached. Target dose: 400 to 500 mg daily in divided doses.

iii. Available in tablets, spansule/sustained release, single and multidose vials for IM injection, and suppositories.

iv. Maximum recommended dose: 1,000 mg daily.

v. Drug/drug interactions: Multiple drug/drug interactions, alpha blockers, anticholinergic/antispasmodic drugs. Avoid use with other medications that may cause QT prolongation or respiratory depression.

vi. Side effects: Drowsiness, postural hypotension, akathesia (restlessness), dystonia, tremor, weight gain, nausea, constipation, headache, dizziness, stuffy nose, QT prolongation

3. Antidepressants

a. Use of traditional antidepressants to treat bipolar depression is controversial and not Food and Drug Administration (FDA) approved.

b. Using antidepressants alone to treat bipolar depression is not recommended due to the potential to cause hypomania, mania, and rapid cycling.

c. According to the International Society for Bipolar Disorders (ISBD), antidepressants may be used in combination with another medication, typically a mood stabilizer, when there is a history of a positive response to antidepressants or if the patient relapses into a depression after an antidepressant is discontinued.

d. Do not prescribe an antidepressant during manic or mixed episodes.

4. Electroconvulsive therapy (ECT)

a. Short-term treatment for severe manic or depressive episodes, especially when suicidal or psychotic symptoms are present, or when medication intervention is ineffective or not well tolerated.

b. ECT is among the safest treatments for severe mood disorders and is effective in up to 75% of patients.

Follow-Up

A. Initially, monitor patients closely to assess for response to treatment, need for medication dose adjustment, side effects, and changes in level of functioning.

B. Monitor for emergence of suicidal thoughts, psychosis, mania, or depression.

C. As appropriate, order lab work to monitor serum blood levels of medications and assess for potential side effects, such as metabolic changes, elevated liver enzymes, decreased kidney functioning, cardiac changes, and blood dyscrasias.

D. After initial stabilization, follow-up appointments should be made every 1 to 3 months.

E. Patient teaching related to importance of self-care and medication compliance.

Consultation/Referral

A. If the patient is experiencing suicidal/homicidal ideations, refer immediately to the nearest emergency department to be evaluated by a mental health professional for possible emergency admission.

B. Consult with the psychiatric provider to help coordinate care.

C. Refer the patient for individual and/or family therapy if indicated.

Individual Considerations

A. Pregnancy

1. Some of the medications used to treat bipolar disorder can potentially lower the effectiveness of hormone contraception. Women should be counseled on the use of additional methods of pregnancy prevention.

2. Medications, such as mood stabilizers cause an increased risk of birth defects in the first trimester. Women of childbearing age should be counseled on planned pregnancy to allow for medication adjustment and initiation of supportive therapy/close monitoring.

3. Stopping bipolar medications during pregnancy puts a woman at high risk of relapse during the pregnancy and developing postpartum depression. Some bipolar medications pass through the breast milk. Risk versus benefits of medication use during pregnancy and breastfeeding should be discussed with the patient and significant other, if appropriate. Refer to a psychiatric specialist for consultation.

B. Pediatrics

1. Bipolar disorder in children/adolescents is difficult to diagnose and does not present with the same clinical picture as adults. Children and adolescents with suspected bipolar disorder should be referred to a pediatric mental health specialist.

C. Partners/family

1. Provide educational materials and information on local support resources to partners and family members. The National Alliance on Mental Illness provides family support groups and online resources in many rural and urban areas. Information may be accessed at: www.nami.org

D. Geriatrics

1. Dementia and delirium are common in the elderly. Rule out underlying medical conditions and possible medication-induced mood/cognitive changes.

2. Caution should be used in the treatment of bipolar mania/mixed symptoms in geriatrics. Atypical antipsychotic medications increase the risk of stroke and death in elderly patients with a history of CVA and dementia-related psychosis.

Depression

Moya Cook and Alyson Wolz

Definition

A. Depression is a mental health disorder that interferes with a person's daily life. Depression may be mild or severe, depending on signs and symptoms expressed, as well as the length of time symptoms are present. Depression affects multiple body systems and may impact one emotionally, cognitively, physically, as well as one's behavior. Symptoms of depression may include difficulty sleeping, depressed mood, inability to function at work, change in appetite, and inability to enjoy activities that bring one pleasure. There are many forms of depression, and treatment varies depending on the specific diagnosis. Types of depression include (a) Major depression, single episode, or recurrent (mild, moderate, or severe with or without psychotic features); (b) persistent depressive disorder (dysthymia); (c) premenstrual dysphoric disorder; (d) postpartum depression; (e) seasonal affective disorder (SAD); and (f) bipolar disorder. Depression is frequently a concomitant diagnosis with other physical or mental disorders.

Incidence

A. One in 10 adults experiences one or more episodes of depression during his or her lifetime. Depression can occur at any age. The median age of depression occurs between 25 and 32 years of age. The lifetime risk is estimated to be as high as 30%. Women have a twofold to threefold higher rate of reported depression than men. Estimated rates of major depression in the elderly are 3% to 5% for those living in a community dwelling; 15% to 30% for those living in an institutional setting; and 13% for those living in nursing homes.

B. Only 10% to 25% of people with depressive disorders seek treatment. There is a high mortality from suicide if untreated (see "Suicide" section that follows).

C. No single causal factor has been identified. Depressive syndromes are so varied in course and symptomatology that a single cause is unlikely. Several factors appear to contribute, including genetics; neurochemical abnormalities (reductions in adrenergic or serotonergic neurotransmission); electrolyte disturbances; and neuroendocrine abnormalities such as hypothalamic, pituitary, adrenal cortical, thyroid, and gonadal functions. Depression is frequently a concomitant diagnosis with other physical or mental disorders. Personality and psychodynamic factors of depression include low self-esteem, self-criticism, and interpersonal loss. A childhood history of emotional, physical, and/or sexual abuse can also contribute to adult-onset depression.

Predisposing Factors

A. Age (between 25 and 32 years and the elderly)

B. Lack of social support/living alone

C. A history of early parental loss

D. Female gender

1. Most common in childbearing years from ages 25 to 45 years

2. Premenstrual

3. Perimenopausal

4. Postpartum

E. Family history of depression

F. Frequent exposure to stressful events

G. Nutritional disorders

1. Vitamin B_{12} deficiency

2. Pellagra (niacin deficiency)

H. Personality characteristics that include absence of hardiness factors in response to stress (lack of resilience, flexibility, and optimism)

I. Anger not dealt with and turned in on the self

J. Negative interpretation of one's life experiences

K. Poor physical health

L. Postsurgical diagnosis of cancer

M. Chronic pain

N. Chronic medical problems such as hypothyroidism and hyperthyroidism, Cushing's syndrome, hypercalcemia, hyponatremia, diabetes mellitus, lupus erythematosus, fibromyalgia, rheumatoid disease, and chronic fatigue syndrome

O. Neurologic disorders such as stroke, subdural hematoma, multiple sclerosis, brain tumor, Parkinson's disease, epilepsy, dementias, and Huntington's disease

P. Alcoholism/drug abuse or dependence/withdrawal

Q. Infectious etiology such as mononucleosis and other viral infections, syphilis, HIV, and Lyme disease

R. Side effect of prescription drugs, such as methyldopa, antiarrhythmic, benzodiazepines, barbiturates/central nervous system (CNS) depressants, beta-blockers, cholinergic drugs, corticosteroids, digoxin, H_2-blockers, and reserpine.

Common Complaints

A. Lack of interest in pleasurable activities

B. Digestive problems

C. Chronic aches and pains that are not otherwise explained

Other Signs and Symptoms

A. Vegetative
- **1.** Changes (increased or decreased) in sleep, appetite, and weight
- **2.** Changes in appearance: Poor grooming and hygiene
- **3.** Poor eye contact, staring downward, flat affect
- **4.** Loss of energy
- **5.** Decreased interest in sex
- **6.** Psychomotor retardation or agitation

B. Cognitive
- **1.** Sense of guilt, worthlessness, low self-esteem
- **2.** Problems with attention span, concentration or memory, frustration tolerance, negative distortions, mild paranoia, and psychosis

C. Impulse control
- **1.** Suicidal or homicidal thoughts or acts. Any statements made by the patient, such as "Life isn't worth living, I wish I were dead, I don't deserve to be alive, I can't deal with this," should be taken seriously. Refer the patient for counseling and assessment and treatment.

D. Behavioral
- **1.** Depressed mood, anxiety, and irritability
- **2.** Isolation, decreased motivation, fatigability, and anhedonia (unable to derive gratification from pleasurable activities)

E. Physical symptoms
- **1.** Digestion problems, nausea, constipation, diarrhea (less common), and dry mouth
- **2.** Fatigue, but difficulty sleeping
- **3.** Physical pain, chronic aches, and pains that cannot be explained
- **4.** Recurrent headaches, backaches, or stomachaches that have no cause
- **5.** Migrating pain that disappears when depression lifts
- **6.** Increased muscle tension

Subjective Data

A. Review the onset, duration, and course of presenting symptoms.

B. Review any previous history of depression (such as postpartum depression).

C. Determine how the previous depression was treated.

D. Evaluate the patient's suicide potential. Ask: "Have you ever thought of hurting yourself or others?" Does the patient have a current suicide plan or vague ideas of suicide? Has the patient had any previous history of suicide attempts? If so, evaluate how life-threatening they were.

E. Review the patient's medical history (see "Predisposing Factors" section).

F. Review the patient's drug history for prescription, over-the-counter (OTC) medications, and recreational/illicit drug use (how much, how long, how often), and review his or her history of alcohol consumption (how much, how long, and how often).

G. Review the patient's history for recent major life changes such as pregnancy, death, divorce, or any loss that may be normal throughout the stages of life. The *patient's perception* of the loss is what is important.

H. Review dietary intake since the symptoms have begun.

I. Establish usual weight, review weight gain/loss, and note in what time span.

J. Review the patient's activities of daily living. Does the patient get up and dress daily, perform daily hygiene, put on makeup?

K. Review how many hours of sleep and quality of sleep per day.

L. Review the disruption of usual activities: Return to work, return to school, exercise.

M. Review the amount of crying per day, for what length of time (days, weeks).

N. Assess whether the depression is cyclic/seasonal (starts in the fall, ends in the spring).

O. Review occupational/home exposure to lead and lead-based products.

P. Review any exposures to infectious diseases, including Lyme disease (refer to Chapter 16, "Infectious Disease Guidelines" for specific questions). Does anyone else, such as family, friends, or coworkers, have similar symptoms?

Q. If female, review for symptoms of menopause (sleep disturbances, irregular menses/amenorrhea, hot flushes, vaginal dryness, dyspareunia).

Physical Examination

A. Check pulse, respirations, blood pressure, and weight.

B. Inspect
- **1.** Observe overall appearance; note grooming, tone of voice, conduct of patient during communication, and breath (smell of alcohol).
- **2.** Complete neurologic examination and Mini-Mental Status Examination (MMSE) available for download at www.uml.edu/docs/Mini%20Mental%20State%20Exam_tcm18-169319.pdf

3. Complete dermal examination for signs of substance use (refer to "Substance Use Disorders" section in Chapter 2).

C. Palpate
  1. Palpate the neck and thyroid; note the goiter.
  2. Palpate the axilla and groin for lymphadenopathy (infectious etiology).
  3. Check the joints for swelling and arthritis and range of motion (ROM); rule out musculoskeletal cause.

D. Auscultate
  1. The heart, lungs, and abdomen (as applies to physical complaints).

Diagnostic Tests

A. Complete blood count (CBC) with differential
B. Electrolytes, serum calcium, and phosphorus
C. Thyroid profile
D. Liver profile
E. Vitamin D_{25} hydroxy
F. Vitamin B_{12}/folate
G. Lead level
H. Follicle-stimulating hormone/luteinizing hormone (FSH/LH)
I. Viral cultures
J. Blood alcohol
K. Urine drug screen
L. Monospot
M. CT and MRI scans
N. Dexamethasone suppression test
O. Perform mental state examination with depression rating scale of choice:
  1. Beck Depression Inventory Scale (Beck, Ward, Mendelson, Mock, & Erbaugh, 1961): www.beckinstitue.org/getinformed/tools-and-resources/professionals/patient-assessment-tools/
  2. Geriatric Depression Scale (GDS): Short version (Yesavage, 1988): www.dementia-assessment.com.au/depression/geriatric_depression_scale_short.pdf

Differential Diagnoses

A. Mood disorder due to another medical condition
B. Adjustment disorder with depressed mood
C. Chronic untreated anxiety disorders such as generalized anxiety disorder (GAD), posttraumatic stress disorder (PTSD), or obsessive-compulsive disorder (OCD)
D. Personality disorders
E. Schizoaffective disorder
F. SAD
  1. Seasonal pattern: Starts in the fall, linked to lack of light exposure
  2. Women more than men
  3. Age typically in the 20s
G. Alcoholism and drug abuse/dependence
H. Early dementia
I. Endocrine etiologies (see "Predisposing Factors")
J. Infectious etiologies (see "Predisposing Factors")
K. Menopause
L. Side effect of medication (see "Predisposing Factors")
M. Cancer: 50% of patients with tumors, particularly of the brain and lung, and carcinoma of the pancreas develop symptoms of depression before the diagnosis of tumor is made.
N. Heavy metal poisoning
O. Nutritional deficit (see "Predisposing Factors")

Plan

A. General interventions
  1. Keep the patient safe from self-harm.
  2. Treat physical/laboratory findings. Recommend dietary change, iron supplements, hormone replacement therapy per findings.

B. Patient teaching
  1. Encourage the patient to take medications as prescribed. Educate the patient that some medications may take time to get into the system to work and time should be allowed to see the effects of the medication. Review side effects.
  2. Encourage the patient to express feelings or worsening of symptoms if this occurs before next appointment. Have the patient make a client contract with you that he or she will not bring harm to self or others and if he or she begins having these thoughts, the patient will contact you or go to the nearest emergency room.
  3. Encourage exercise on a daily basis for 20 to 30 minutes to increase energy and enhance a feeling of well-being.
  4. Encourage the patient to get at least 7 to 8 hours of sleep each night. If sleep is a problem, address this issue with the client.
  5. Avoid caffeine at night and/or watching TV late at night.
  6. Encourage the patient to seek counseling with a professional counselor. Refer to appropriate site (psychologist, psychiatrist, group therapy, etc.). Offer local resources to the patient.
  7. Advise patient to participate in activities to enhance interpersonal relationships and build self-esteem. Include family and friends in recommended therapies and advise them to encourage the patient to participate in activities to enhance self-esteem.
  8. Once the patient is feeling better, encourage continued use of medication, activities, and resources for at least 6 months after the patient has started feeling better to prevent relapse.

C. Pharmaceutical therapy: Table 22.1 presents dosage information.
  1. Drugs of choice: SSRI antidepressants. Caution should be used when coadministering SSRIs with drugs that have a narrow therapeutic window, such as carbamazepine (Tegretol), warfarin, tricyclic antidepressants (TCAs), antiarrhythmics, and some antipsychotic medications (risperidone, haloperidol, and phenothiazine), and other drugs including diazepam (Valium) and monoamine oxidase (MAO) inhibitors.
    a. Most antidepressant therapy takes 3 to 4 weeks for onset of action to elicit visible changes.

TABLE 22.1 **Dosages for Common Antidepressant Drugs**

Generic (Brand Name)	Adults Aged 18–60 Years	Elderly >60 Years or Renal or Hepatic Patients
fluoxetine hydrochloride (Prozac) Therapeutic onset occurs in 1–4 weeks. Serum levels peak in 4.5–8.5 hours.	20 mg daily in a.m., dosage increased according to patient response. May be given bid—in the morning and at noon. Maximum dosage is 80 mg/d.	10–20 mg daily in a.m. with clinical response monitored q 1–2 weeks. Gradual dose increases q 6 week until optimal therapeutic response is obtained.
paroxetine hydrochloride (Paxil) Therapeutic onset occurs in 1–4 weeks. Serum levels peak in 2–8 hours.	10 mg daily in a.m., p.m., or @ HS. May increase 10 mg/d increments at weekly intervals. Maximum dosage is 50 mg/d.	10–20 mg daily in a.m., p.m., or @ HS with clinical response monitored q 1–2 weeks and gradual increase.
sertraline hydrochloride (Zoloft) Therapeutic onset occurs in 2–4 weeks. Serum levels peak in 4.5–8.5 hours.	50 mg daily in a.m. May increase to 100 mg. Dosage adjustments should be made at intervals of no less than 1 week. Maximum dosage is 200 mg/d.	25–50 mg daily in a.m. with clinical response monitored q 1–2 weeks and gradual increase.
citalopram hydrobromide (Celexa) Therapeutic onset occurs in 2–4 weeks. Serum levels peak in 4 hours.	20 mg daily in a.m., p.m., or @ HS. May increase 10 mg/d increments at weekly intervals. Maximum dosage is 40 mg/d (due to potential for QT prolongation at higher doses).	20 mg daily in a.m., p.m., or HS with clinical response monitored q 1–2 weeks and gradual increase.
escitalopram oxalate (Lexapro) Therapeutic onset occurs in 1–2 weeks. Serum levels peak in 5 hours.	10 mg daily in a.m. May increase in 5–10 mg/d increments at weekly intervals. Maximum dosage is 20 mg/d.	5 mg daily in a.m., with clinical response monitored q 1–2 weeks and gradual increase.
vortioxetine (Trintellix/Brintellix) Therapeutic onset occurs in 2–4 weeks. Serum levels peak in 7–11 hours.	5–10 mg daily in a.m. or p.m. May increase in 5 mg/d increments at weekly intervals. Maximum dosage is 20 mg/d.	10–20 mg daily in a.m., p.m. with clinical response monitored q 1–2 weeks and gradual increase.
vilazodone hydrochloride (Viibryd) Therapeutic onset occurs in 2–4 weeks. Serum levels peak in 4–5 hours.	10 mg daily in a.m. or p.m., with food. May increase 10 mg/d increments at weekly intervals. Maximum dosage is 40 mg/d.	10–20 mg daily in a.m. or p.m., with food, clinical response monitored q 1–2 weeks and gradual increase.
venlafaxine (Effexor) Therapeutic onset occurs in 1–4 weeks. Serum levels peak in 2 hours. (Effexor XR) Therapeutic onset occurs in 2–4 weeks. Serum levels peak in 8 hours.	75 mg daily in divided dose. May increase 75 mg/d increments at 4-day intervals. Maximum dosage is 375 mg/d in divided doses q 8-12 hr. 37.5–75 mg daily in a.m. or p.m. May increase by 75-mg/d increments at 4-day intervals. Maximum dosage is 225 mg daily.	75–225 mg daily in divided doses q 8-12 hr with clinical response monitored q 1–2 weeks and gradual increase. 75–225 mg daily dose with clinical response monitored every 1–2 weeks and gradual increase.
desvenlafaxine (Pristiq) Therapeutic onset occurs in 1–2 weeks. Serum levels peak in 7.5 hours.	50 mg daily in a.m. or p.m. May increase to 100 mg after 1–2 weeks, although there is no evidence of increased efficacy over 50 mg dose. Maximum dosage is 100 mg/d.	25–50 mg daily in a.m. or p.m. with clinical response monitored q 1–2 weeks and gradual increase.
duloxetine delayed-release (Cymbalta) Therapeutic onset occurs in 2–4 weeks. Serum levels peak in 6–10 hours.	30 mg daily in a.m. or p.m. with increase to 60 mg after 1 week daily dosing or bid. May increase 30-mg/d increments at weekly intervals. Maximum dosage is 120 mg/d.	40–120 mg daily in a.m., p.m., single dose, or bid, with clinical response monitored q 1–2 weeks and gradual increase.
nortriptyline hydrochloride (Pamelor) Therapeutic onset occurs in 2–4 weeks or longer. Serum levels peak in 7–8.5 hours.	25 mg tid or qid initially, gradually increase to maximum dose 150 mg qd.	30–50 mg daily tid or qid or in 1 day's dose.

(*continued*)

TABLE 22.1 Dosages for Common Antidepressant Drugs *(continued)*

Generic (Brand Name)	Adults Aged 18–60 Years	Elderly >60 Years or Renal or Hepatic Patients
desipramine hydrochloride (Norpramin) Therapeutic onset occurs in 2–4 weeks or longer. Serum levels peak in 4–6 hours.	100–200 mg po in single or divided dose.	25–100 mg daily in divided doses, increase gradually to maximum of 150 mg qd.
amitriptyline (Elavil) Therapeutic onset unknown—thought to take several weeks. Serum levels peak 2–12 hours.	75 mg po in divided doses initially or 50–100 mg HS. Dose not to exceed 150 mg/d.	10–20 mg po tid and 20 mg HS daily.

Paxil works well for patients who have a component of anxiety to their depression. **Monitor prothrombin time for patients taking warfarin, sertraline, and paroxetine.**
bid, twice a day; HS, at bedtime; po, by mouth; q, every; qd, every day; qid, four times a day; tid, three times a day.

b. Never prescribe more than a week's supply or a total of 2 g of a TCA if there is a risk of suicide.
c. Medication should not be changed until a trial of 6 to 8 weeks has been given to measure the progress.
d. Before concluding that the antidepressant is ineffective, verify that the patient is taking the medication correctly.
e. First-line therapy in the elderly is SSRIs, which have significantly fewer side effects than the traditional TCAs. Paroxetine and sertraline have short half-lives and can be withdrawn quickly.
f. Antidepressant therapy should be continued for 6 months to 1 year (up to 5 years if necessary) because of the risk of recurrence of depression.
g. Taper the medication off instead of abruptly withdrawing.

2. TCAs: Avoid administration after acute myocardial infarction. **Men with prostatic hypertrophy do best with a nonsedating TCA that has a mild anticholinergic activity, such as desipramine (Norpramin) or nortriptyline (Pamelor).**

3. Adrenergic modulators: A weak inhibitor of norepinephrine, dopamine, and serotonin reuptake: Bupropion hydrochloride (Wellbutrin).
- **a.** For patients older than 18 years
- **b.** No dosage established for the elderly
- **c.** Therapeutic onset in 1 to 3 weeks
- **d.** Serum level peak within 2 hours
- **e.** Initially 100 mg twice a day for at least 3 days
- **f.** If well tolerated, increase to 375 or 400 mg daily.
- **g.** After 3 days more, 450 mg daily in four divided doses at least 4 hours apart
- **h.** Maximum single dosing 150 mg, maximum 450 mg daily
  - **i.** Avoid bedtime dosing.
  - **ii.** Do not give to patients with predisposition to seizures.
  - **iii.** Give reduced dose to patients with renal or hepatic impairment.

4. Dual reuptake inhibitors: Blocks the reabsorption of the norepinephrine and serotonin into the neurons in the CNS. When this occurs, higher levels of norepinephrine and serotonin remain and improve the nerve transmission in the brain, which then improves mood.
- **a.** Venlafaxine hydrochloride (Effexor)
  - **i.** With hepatic impairment, reduce dose by 50%.
  - **ii.** Withdraw gradually over 2 weeks when discontinuing medication.
  - **iii.** Interacts with MAO inhibitors. Do not start venlafaxine within 14 days of discontinuing an MAO inhibitor.
- **b.** Duloxetine (Cymbalta) also blocks reuptake of serotonin and norepinephrine.
  - **i.** Avoid use in patients with chronic liver disease or cirrhosis.
  - **ii.** Patients should be warned about stopping the medication abruptly; have them taper down slowly.
  - **iii.** Duloxetine is also helpful in treating the physical pain that accompanies some depression symptoms as well as patients with chronic musculoskeletal pain and fibromyalgia.

5. MAO inhibitors should be prescribed only by a psychiatrist.

Follow-Up

A. Follow up in 1 to 2 weeks to assess patient's status, drug effectiveness, and adverse reactions.
B. Patients can become suicidal after the depression is treated and they begin to have more energy to act on the suicidal ideation. **Assess suicidality with every office visit.**

C. Follow up every 2 to 4 weeks afterward to check patient's progress.
D. Once positive change is seen, the patient can be seen monthly.
E. Refer to other applicable medical diagnoses for the follow-up recommendations.

Consultation/Referral

A. If there is any potential for suicidal/homicidal behavior, refer patient immediately to a psychiatrist for possible emergency admission.
B. Consult with the physician, comanage with the physician, or the patient may need immediate referral/consult for continuing psychotherapy.
C. Patients who fail to respond to antidepressants after 1 to 2 months of appropriate antidepressant therapy should have a psychiatric consultation.

Individual Considerations

A. Pregnancy
  1. A woman with a history of depression or previous postpartum depression is at a high risk of postpartum depression (recurrent). Caution should be used in prescribing antidepressants during pregnancy. Review the benefits versus risks.
  2. Refer to Chapter 13, "Obstetrics Guidelines," for the section, "Postpartum Depression."
B. Pediatrics
  1. Children with depression are more difficult to diagnose and do not necessarily meet adult criteria. The clinical picture can be completely different, that is, acting-out behavior. Children suspected to be depressed should be referred to a child psychiatrist.
C. Adolescence
  1. Teens are at risk for suicide after recent losses from death (especially if one of their friends/family commits suicide). Recent loss includes breaking up with a boyfriend or girlfriend.
  2. If a teen has had a depressive episode, he or she may be at a higher risk for suicide if he or she is suddenly happy and things are "just fine." He or she may have decided on a suicide plan and may be experiencing a sense of relief because plans have been made.
D. Partners
  1. If available in the community, provide resources for partners, such as the National Alliance on Mental Illness (NAMI; listed in most telephone books).
  2. Frequently, partners will take too much responsibility for the depressed patient's state of mind and, over time, also become depressed. Relating to other people with depressed partners will assist them in dealing with their significant other's depression.
E. Geriatrics
  1. Dementia masked as "pseudodepression" is common in the elderly. Check for memory impairment and disorientation because delirium can often be mistaken for depression.
  2. Elderly patients who are depressed may experience agitation rather than retardation in psychomotor function.
  3. White men, aged 80 years, have the highest rate of suicide of any age group in the United States.
  4. Look for depression in caretakers of patients with Alzheimer's disease.

> *Elderly patients who are suicidal may present with atypical symptoms of depression and may not express their distress directly. Three identified behaviors include impaired ability to communicate, intractable tinnitus, and feelings of helplessness.*

Failure to Thrive

Moya Cook and Alyson Wolz

Definition

Failure to thrive (FTT) is an abnormality in growth in which an individual fails to gain weight or grow. FTT is a manifestation of an underlying problem, whether the problem be mental, physical, or psychological.
A. Children: In a growing child, a child measuring below the third to fifth percentile on the growth curve, or exhibiting a drop greater than two percentiles on the growth curve in the past several months, is referred to as FTT.
B. Adults: FTT is also seen in adults who have a weight less than 80% of the ideal average body weight for the adult.
C. Geriatrics: FTT in the geriatric population is defined as a deterioration in functional status disproportional to their disease burden. Signs are decreased appetite, weight loss of greater than 5% of their weight, decreased physical activity, along with dehydration, depression, and compromised immune status.

Incidence

A. Depends on the population; however, it is estimated that FTT is seen in 5% to 10% of low-birth-weight children and children who live in poverty. In the elderly population, it is estimated to occur in 5% to 35% of the elderly population, with nursing home residents having an occurrence rate of 25% to 40%.

Pathogenesis

A. Organic causes for FTT
  1. Gastrointestinal (reflux, celiac disease, Hirschsprung's disease, and malabsorption)
  2. Cardiopulmonary (cardiac diseases, congestive heart failure)
  3. Pulmonary (asthma, bronchopulmonary dysplasia, cystic fibrosis)
  4. Renal (diabetes insipidus, renal insufficiency, urinary tract infections)
  5. Endocrine (hypothyroidism, adrenal diseases, parathyroid disorders, thyroid disorders, pituitary disorders)

6. Neurologic (mental retardation, cerebral hemorrhages)
7. Metabolic disorders (inborn errors of metabolism)
8. Congenital (congenital syndromes such as fetal alcohol syndrome, chromosomal abnormalities, perinatal infections)
9. Infectious (gastrointestinal infections, tuberculosis, HIV)

B. Inorganic (or psychosocial) causes pertain to family dynamics among the parents, siblings, and the patient. It is common to see both organic and inorganic problems as causative factors for FTT.

C. Geriatric population

1. Feel fuller with less food; this may be an endorphin response that decreases the adaptive relaxation of the fundus of the stomach.
2. Increased number of cytokines, which contributes to anorexia
3. Diminished sense of smell or taste
4. Dysphagia
5. Medications
6. Depression, delirium, dementia
7. Alcohol or substance abuse

Predisposing Factors

A. Children: Low birth weight, prematurity
B. Geriatrics: Dementia, comorbidities (cancer, chronic infections, malabsorption syndromes, psychiatric disorders), limited mobility, despair
C. Poverty
D. Organic conditions with the major organs noted earlier
E. Parents with psychosocial disorders
F. Altered family processes

Common Complaints

A. Failure to grow and gain weight
B. Weight loss

Patients do not always present for this problem. Many patients are diagnosed at a routine examination in the ambulatory setting.

Other Signs and Symptoms

A. No growth in height
B. Loss of subcutaneous fat tissue
C. Muscle atrophy
D. Alopecia
E. Dermatitis
F. Marasmus
G. Kwashiorkor

Subjective Data

A. Obtain detailed history of the patient's diet. Note the differences between foods offered and foods eaten. If formula is used, note type, frequency, amount taken each feeding, spits, and so forth.

B. Assess quality of nutrients offered to the patient. Consider knowledge deficit of care provider if inadequate.

1. Children: If breastfeeding, note frequency, duration, milk supply, medications, or foods that would alter breast milk.
2. Geriatrics: Is patient able to chew and swallow food offered? Are supplements being offered?

C. Query regarding financial resources, and, if needed, does the family participate in low-income opportunities (Women, Infant, and Children [WIC], food stamp programs, etc.)?
D. Evaluate whether religious or unusual dietary beliefs/habits contribute to the food preparation, if inadequate.
E. For infants and children, obtain a detailed perinatal history, noting complications with mother or baby.
F. For infants and children, determine whether the formula is being prepared correctly (powder, concentrate, ready-to-feed).
G. Rule out any difficulty in swallowing or retaining ingested food.
H. Note regular bowel/bladder habits.
I. Note any recent illness, chronic or acute.
J. Query regarding lead exposure.
K. Rule out family history of cystic fibrosis or lactose intolerance.
L. Note whether a short/small stature runs in the family history.
M. Geriatrics: Evaluate nutritional screening using the Mini Nutritional Assessment.

Physical Examination

A. Check temperature, pulse, respirations, blood pressure, height, and weight.

1. Measure head circumference in children.

B. Inspect

1. Observe overall appearance.
2. Observe oral pathology; for geriatrics, check for ill-fitting dentures, dental and gum condition.
3. Note muscle tone, strength, and movement.
4. Note social interactions among family members.
5. Note social skills of the patient.
6. Perform Denver Developmental II on children.

Note any changes in growth curve, especially if crossing over percentiles, and if height and weight are not concordant. If premature, adjust for gestational age as appropriate.

C. Palpate

1. Abdomen, back, and extremities

D. Percuss

1. The abdomen

E. Auscultate

1. The heart and lungs

Diagnostic Tests

A. Complete blood count (CBC), urinalysis, electrolytes
B. Thyroid panel if indicated

C. Lead screen
D. Sweat test if indicated
E. X-rays if appropriate
F. Serum albumin in geriatrics
G. Mental status examination
H. Purified protein derivative (PPD)
I. HIV, rapid plasma reagin (RPR)
J. MRI

Differential Diagnoses

A. FTT inorganic versus organic etiology
B. Weight loss
C. Depression
D. Impaired physical function
E. Cognitive impairment
F. Depression
G. Malnutrition related to malabsorption (e.g., bariatric surgery)

Plan

A. General interventions
 1. The plan is based on the cause of FTT. Children with organic etiologies need follow-up regarding the specific problem.
 2. Severe malnutrition requires hospitalization.
 3. Geriatrics: Obtain nutritional consult to evaluate the dietary needs for protein, iron, and other nutrients.
B. Patient teaching
 1. Reinforce positive eating habits and encourage dietary meal planning.
 2. Offer nutrition counseling with dietitian.
 3. Educate the patient and family about the importance of meeting the dietary requirements for protein, iron, calcium, and other nutrients to prevent weight loss, loss of muscle and bone mass, and to prevent infection and other complications that can stress the body.
C. Dietary management
 1. Meal suggestions: Offer adequate time for meals (20–30 minutes), offer solid food before drinks/juices, and provide a pleasant environment for eating.
 2. Encourage all family members to sit down and eat at least one meal a day together. This time will also enhance family social interactions.
 3. Provide handout for high-calorie foods (peanut butter, cheese, whole milk, etc.).
 4. Consider exercise sessions for geriatrics to stimulate appetite.
 5. Encourage patients to attend centers where meals are served as a group or have meals delivered to the home.
 6. Encourage small frequent meals with snacks between meals and before bedtime.
D. Pharmaceutical therapy
 1. High-calorie supplements are recommended for some patients (Polycose, Carnation Instant Breakfast, Pediasure, Ensure).

> *Weight gain with high-calorie supplements is commonly seen with patients who have psychosocial etiology of FTT.*

 2. Geriatrics: Short-term aggressive caloric replacement has been shown to be effective in reversing FTT. Severe malnutrition may require hospitalization with total parental nutrition. Medications used to increase appetite.
  a. Megestrol 400 or 800 mg daily with meal
  b. Antidepressants such as selective serotonin reuptake inhibitors (SSRIs), tricyclic antidepressants (TCAs), and mirtazapine (Remeron) have been shown to be beneficial to help stimulate appetite and increase weight.

Follow-Up

A. Two-week evaluation for weight/height measurements and to evaluate compliance with regimen at home. Routine visits recommended every 2 to 4 weeks to monitor progress.
B. Reevaluate patient in 1 to 2 months. After 2 months, if no improvement or further loss is noted, refer to a specialist.

Consultation/Referral

A. Consult with a physician if height/weight measurements are noted below the third percentile on a graphic chart.
B. For the majority of patients, a nutrition consultation is needed to assist the parents or food provider in providing adequate resources/calories for the patient.
C. Consider social service and visiting nurses for outpatient assistance in the home.

Individual Considerations

A. Pediatrics
 1. The prognosis for inorganic etiologies of children in the first year of life is ominous due to the poor brain growth. These children will be at high risk for developmental delay, poor cognitive and emotional developments, and social/emotional problems.
 2. Approximately 10% of children are normally small children by genetic makeup. These children are not diagnosed with FTT. FTT is most commonly seen in children younger than 3 to 5 years.
 3. Consider keeping small children on formula past the 12-month age mark if FTT is diagnosed.
 4. Early intervention programs should be considered for children.
B. Geriatrics
 1. FTT in the elderly may lead to a decline in physical and mental functions. Aggressive treatment should be employed to improve the nutritional status of these patients.
 2. FTT increases the risk of morbidity and mortality.
 3. FTT increases the risk of depression and social isolation in the elderly.

Grief

Moya Cook and Alyson Wolz

Definition

A. Grief is defined as the normal, appropriate emotional response caused by a loss. This feeling of loss is a response that has been caused by a particular event in one's life. It is unique to the individual experiencing it, and there is no general timetable for completing it. Grief is commonly seen following the death of a loved one, but grief also follows other losses (e.g., loss of independence, loss of affection, or loss of body parts, pain, and distress). Mourning is defined as the process by which grief is resolved. Mourning is individual and helps in reaching acceptance of a loss.

B. The process through which one resolves grief usually follows a typical course that can be viewed in five stages.

1. Denial: Denial occurs when one refuses to accept the circumstance that has occurred. It is a natural defense mechanism that occurs to protect the body.
2. Anger: Pain, tears, anxiousness, anger, and feelings of guilt may be seen.
3. Bargaining: In this stage, the person tries to negotiate alternatives that will make him or her feel better.
4. Depression: One begins to understand what has happened and may show feelings of sadness and fear.
5. Acceptance: One begins to rebuild one's life and think about the past with pleasure. In this phase, one regains interest in activities and forms new relationships.

C. It is important to distinguish between the normal grief reactions of pathologic grief and major depression. Approximately 10% to 15% of individuals experience a severe grief reaction. Often, depressive symptoms are a pervasive part of the grief response, and a clear delineation of grief versus depression is not always possible.[a]

Incidence

A. Grief is a universal emotional response. Approximately 5% to 9% of the population will lose a close family member or friend each year. Grief is a normal emotional response that will follow this loss for an individual.

Pathogenesis

A. Grief is a normal emotional response to the loss of a loved one, pain, and/or distress. Abnormal, pathologic grief can occur if the mourner is not encouraged to grieve losses. Normal grief resolution begins to subside at approximately 6 months but may sometimes take longer.

Predisposing Factors

A. Sudden or terrible deaths

B. Excessive dependency on the deceased and feelings of ambivalence

C. Traumatic losses earlier in life

D. Social isolation

E. Actual or imagined responsibility for "causing" the death

F. Avoidance of grief and denial of loss

G. Survived a traumatic experience that killed the deceased

Common Complaints

A. Angry feelings at God or medical personnel for not doing more, anger at oneself for not seeing the warning signs, anger at the deceased for not taking better care of himself or herself. Common feelings of being left alone and not making proper financial/legal preparations may also occur.

B. Sleeping all the time or inability to sleep without medication

C. Change in eating habits with significant weight loss or gain

D. Fatigue, lethargy, or lack of motivation

E. Decreased concentration and memory, forgetfulness

F. Increased irritability

G. Unpredictable bouts of crying

H. Fears

1. Of being alone or with people
2. Of leaving the house
3. Of staying in the house

Other Signs and Symptoms

A. Normal grief

1. Protest, disbelief, shock, and denial
2. Profound sadness and survivor guilt
3. Multiple somatic symptoms without actual organic disease
4. Sense of unreality and withdrawal from others
5. Disruption of normal patterns of conduct, with restlessness and aimlessness
6. Preoccupation with memories of the deceased, dreams of the deceased, hallucinations, fear of going crazy, and transient psychotic symptoms
7. Response to support and ventilation improves over time.

B. Complicated or prolonged grief

1. Persistence of denial with delayed or absent grief
2. Depression with impaired self-esteem, suicidal thoughts, and impulses with self-destructive behavior
3. Actual organic disease and medical illness
4. Progressive social isolation
5. Persistent anger and hostility, leading to paranoid reactions, especially against those involved in medical care of the deceased, or suppression of any expression of anger and hostility
6. Continued disruption of normal patterns of conduct, often with a persistent hyperactivity unaccompanied by a sense of loss or grieving
7. Continued preoccupation with memories of the deceased to the point of searching for reunion (sustained depressive delusions)
8. Conversion symptoms similar to the symptoms of the deceased

[a] Based on the Grief Cycle model first published in *On Death and Dying,* Elisabeth Kübler-Ross, 1969. Interpretation by Alan Chapman 2006–2009. Retrieved from www.ekrfoundation.org/five-stages-of-grief

9. Self-blame
10. Prolonged grief longer than 6 months is commonly linked to complications and impairment for the next 1 to 2 years.

Subjective Data

A. Review onset, duration, and course of presenting symptoms. Review the mourner's grief symptoms.
B. Obtain an in-depth personal history of the mourner and his or her relationship to the identified loss or with the deceased.

Understanding the bereaved's history is critical to understanding the individual's loss.

C. Identify anniversary dates pertinent to the mourner's relationship with the deceased/loss.
D. Determine whether the mourner has suicidal ideation (especially with a plan). **Be sure to ask: "Have you ever thought of hurting yourself or others?"**
E. Assess whether the mourner experiences self-blame.
F. Review the mourner's appetite.
G. Establish usual weight, review weight gain/loss, and in what time span.
H. Review the mourner's activities of daily living. Does the mourner get up and dress daily and perform daily hygiene?
I. Review the mourner's sleep quality.
J. Review the mourner's daily routines: Return to work, return to school, and exercise.
K. Review the mourner's amount of crying per day, for what length of time (days, weeks).
L. Review the mourner's drug and alcohol consumption since the loss.

Statements suggesting self-medication with alcohol to facilitate sleep could indicate a coexistent alcohol abuse-dependence diagnosis.

M. Review the mourner's usual medical problems and how the loss/grief has affected these problems.

Physical Examination

A. Check temperature, pulse, respirations, blood pressure, and weight.
B. Inspect
  1. Observe overall appearance. Note grooming habits, dress, and appearance.
  2. Note social interactions among family members.
  3. Note social skills of the patient.
C. Auscultate
  1. The heart and lungs

Diagnostic Tests

A. As indicated to rule out other pathology
B. Blood glucose
C. Thyroid studies
D. If depression is suspected, perform Beck's Depression Inventory. See "Depression" section.

Differential Diagnoses

A. Grief
B. Depressive disorder
C. Posttraumatic stress disorder (PTSD)
D. Somatoform disorders (characterized by physical complaints lacking known medical basis or demonstrable physical findings in the presence of psychological factors)
E. Alcoholism and drug abuse/dependence

Plan

A. General interventions
  1. Evaluate the nature of the grief and any accompanying psychiatric symptoms.
  2. Treat physical/laboratory findings as indicated.
  3. Encourage the patient to eat a healthy diet, exercise daily, maintain normal sleep habits and activities.
  4. Encourage support by family and friend.
  5. Offer counseling with professional psychologist or group sessions.
  6. Assess for depression at each office visit and treat accordingly.
B. Patient teaching: *See Section III: Patient Teaching Guide for this chapter, "Grief."* ◀
C. Pharmaceutical therapy: Antidepressants should not be prescribed for acute grief, but reserved for a possible subsequent major depression. Clinical data suggest that selective serotonin reuptake inhibitors (SSRIs) may assist the patient with mobilizing the energy necessary to assist him or her through the grieving process.

Resist sedation of individuals suffering from acute grief because this tends to delay and prolong the mourning process. Refer to the "Depression" section for pharmaceutical therapy.

  1. Drug of choice: Sedative to help sleep
    a. Sedative anxiolytic hypnotics may be prescribed for **no more than 2 weeks at a time.** Try initially for 1 week to establish a sleep pattern. If insomnia continues, refer the patient to a specialist.
    b. Temazepam (Restoril) 7.5 to 30 mg at bedtime *or* flurazepam (Dalmane) 15 to 30 mg at bedtime
    c. Zolpidem (Ambien) 5 to 10 mg at bedtime (not to be used for more than 1 month)
  2. Sedating antihistamines
    a. Hydroxyzine HCl (Atarax) 50 to 100 mg at bedtime.
    b. Hydroxyzine pamoate (Vistaril) 50 to 100 mg at bedtime **(not to be used for more than 4 months)**
  3. Antidepressant with sedating properties
    a. Trazodone HCl (Desyrel) 50 to 100 mg at bedtime
    b. Paroxetine (Paxil) 10 to 20 mg is given at bedtime
    c. Mirtazapine (Remeron) 15 mg every day at bedtime. Increase at 1 to 2 weeks: Usual range is 15 to 45 mg every day at bedtime.

Follow-Up

A. Follow up in 1 week to assess the patient's status and symptoms.
B. Then follow up every 2 weeks to assess the patient's progress.
C. Assess for depression and suicide at every office visit.
D. Once positive change is seen, the patient can be seen monthly.

Consultation/Referral

A. Provide immediate referral/consult for continuing psychotherapy for severe depression and/or suicidal threats.
B. Consult with a physician for evaluation of pharmacologic agents versus referral.

Individual Considerations

A. Pregnancy
  1. Miscarriage, stillbirth, and neonatal death should be considered a major loss and treated as a grief reaction.
  2. Grief is also seen in pregnancy termination. The woman who terminates a pregnancy (regardless of gestational age and reason for termination) may exhibit a major response to this loss.
  3. Hospitals often provide photographs, footprints, and identification bracelets and connect families with perinatal grief support groups.
  4. Use the baby's name when discussing feelings about the loss of a child.
  5. Suggest that friends and family not put away the baby clothes and bedroom furniture. The couple should do this as part of their closure process.
B. Pediatrics
  1. Grief in children may be delayed or difficult to identify.
  2. Children who suddenly experience behavioral problems not present before the death of a significant person should be immediately referred to a child psychiatrist.
  3. Children should not be told the deceased person is "asleep" or died because they were "sick"; this may connote fears of falling asleep and becoming sick themselves.
  4. Use proper terms: Heart attack, stroke, "Your baby brother had a congenital heart defect." Use the correct terms and draw pictures to help explain.
  5. Young children do not understand death is forever and may continue to ask to see the deceased.
C. Adults: Grief responses vary from among individuals. Look for behaviors outside the norm.
D. Geriatrics: Grief in the elderly should be closely assessed to rule out medical diagnoses.
E. Partners: Involvement in grief/loss psychotherapy groups is extremely helpful.

Sleep Disorders

Moya Cook and Alyson Wolz

Definition

Insomnia disorders are categorized as situational, persistent, or recurrent.
A. In normal sleepers, transient insomnia occurs in those who have traveled to another time zone (i.e., "jet lag"), are under situational stress, or are sleeping in unfamiliar surroundings. Treatment is not required in these situations because time takes care of the problem. With short-term insomnia, the normal sleeper experiences difficulty sleeping that does not resolve within a few days. This can be the result of stress, such as financial difficulty and/or divorce. These patients may require short-term symptomatic relief of insomnia.
B. Long-term insomnia is persistent and disabling. Studies suggest that 40% to 50% have an associated psychiatric disorder, especially depression, an associated drug use/abuse/withdrawal problem, or an associated medical disorder.

Incidence

A. Difficulties with sleep are among the most common complaints of medical patients and affect a large percentage of the population. One third of adults express sleep-related complaints they consider to be serious. Sleep disorders also can affect proper mental functioning (53% of chronic insomniacs complain of memory difficulties). Sleep disorders are also implicated in decreased work efficiency, impaired industrial productivity, and increased risk of traffic accidents. They also seem to enhance the propensity for cardiovascular disease and increase the risk of death. Insomniacs are also at increased risk for the development of depression and anxiety disorders. Patients with obstructive sleep apnea (OSA) syndrome have significant performance impairments on complex motor tasks.

> *The risk of depression increases with time if insomnia is left untreated.*

Pathogenesis

A. Other than situational stress, jet lag, and sleeping in unfamiliar surroundings, difficulty with sleep can be related to psychiatric illness or medical problems. It is most frequently due to chronic depression and/or anxiety. Antisocial and obsessive-compulsive features are also common among these patients. Patients may self-medicate, which produces more insomnia.

Predisposing Factors

A. Alcohol use: Initially assists with sleep but produces fragmented sleep
B. Hypnotic medications can produce tolerance, which causes sleep disruption and rebound insomnia with withdrawal from the medication

C. Substances such as caffeine, nicotine cigarettes, amphetamines, steroids, methylphenidate; hallucinogens, aminophylline, ephedrine, decongestants, bronchodilators, weight loss/diet pills, thyroid preparations, monoamine oxidase (MAO) inhibitors, and anticancer agents
D. Women with fibromyalgia syndrome
E. Women experiencing menopausal symptoms
F. Upper respiratory symptoms
G. OSA disorders such as nasal obstruction, large uvula, low-lying soft palate, craniofacial abnormalities, excessive pharyngeal tissue, pharyngeal masses (tumors, cysts), macroglossia, tonsillar hypertrophy, and vocal cord paralysis
H. Obesity
I. Hypothyroidism
J. Acromegaly
K. Chronic pain
L. Urinary frequency possibly due to prostatism, diabetes, diuretics, and infection

Common Complaints

A. Statements regarding impaired sleep pattern
- **1.** Inability to fall asleep
- **2.** Restless throughout the night
- **3.** Early morning awakening with inability to fall back to sleep
- **4.** Difficulty concentrating during the daytime hours
- **5.** Feels fatigued after 8 hours of sleep, no energy
- **6.** Partner complains of the patient's snoring

Other Signs and Symptoms

A. Excessive daytime sleepiness
B. Feels tense, irritable, and agitated
C. Heightened anxiety and aggressiveness (occasionally)
D. Reports of prolonged pauses in respiration during sleep
E. Weight gain
F. Frontal headaches on awakening
G. Difficulty with short-term recall

Subjective Data

A. Review the onset, course, and duration of problems and symptoms.
B. Take a thorough history of the sleep problem, including the 24-hour sleep–wake cycle: Sleep–wake habit history, sleep hygiene history, meal and exercise times, ambient noise, and light and temperature.
C. Identify the pattern: Trouble falling asleep, trouble staying asleep (frequent awakenings), and early morning awakenings.
D. Inquire about life stresses, drug and alcohol use, and marital and family problems.

> *Statements suggesting self-medication with alcohol to facilitate sleep could indicate a coexistent alcohol abuse/dependence diagnosis. In patients who have developed tolerance to alcohol or sleep medications, abrupt cessation of these agents may produce increased insomnia and anxiety.*

E. Determine whether the insomnia is simply normal sleep. Some "insomniacs" get ample sleep (pseudoinsomnia), and the problems are psychological.
F. Review the patient's smoking and caffeine intake history.
G. Review all medications, including prescribed and over-the-counter (OTC) medications, recreational drug use, and weight-loss medications.
H. Review the patient's medical history: Thyroid problems, hypertension, steroid use, diabetes, and cancer.
I. Conduct an interview with the patient's bed partner to provide information about snoring, breathing pauses, and unusual body positions or movements. Is the partner concerned/frightened about the apneic pauses?
J. Review cardiopulmonary dysfunction: Orthopnea, paroxysmal nocturnal dyspnea, or nocturnal angina.
K. If female, establish last menses to rule out pregnancy or menopause. Is there regular menses, vaginal dryness, and/or hot flashes?
L. If male, review for signs of prostatism (greater than age 50 years, hesitancy, dribbling, nocturia, frequency, incomplete emptying, and so on.) *See Section III: Patient Teaching Guide, "Prostatic Hypertrophy/Benign".*

Physical Examination

A. Check pulse, respirations, blood pressure, and weight.
B. Inspect
- **1.** Observe general overall appearance; note grooming and behaviors during interview.
- **2.** Evaluate eyes: Pupil dilation/constriction (may indicate recent medication/nonprescription drug use).
- **3.** Inspect nasal mucosa for erythema, edema, discharge, and nasal patency; look for septal deviation and polyps. Transluminate sinus (if indicated).
- **4.** Inspect the mouth for erythema, the teeth for uneven surfaces (grinding), and the retropharynx for abnormality.

C. Auscultate
- **1.** Heart
- **2.** Lungs
- **3.** Abdomen

D. Palpate
- **1.** Conduct a neurologic examination.
- **2.** Palpate the neck and thyroid; note goiter.
- **3.** Check the joints for swelling, arthritis, and range of motion (ROM) to rule out musculoskeletal cause.
- **4.** Rectal examination if indicated for men with prostate symptoms.
- **5.** Perform speculum/bimanual examination if indicated to evaluate menopausal atrophy and bladder complaints.

Diagnostic Tests

A. Complete blood count (CBC) with differential
B. Electrolytes
C. Thyroid-stimulating hormone (TSH) or full thyroid profile, follicle-stimulating hormone (FSH), luteinizing hormone (LH)
D. Prostate-specific antigen (PSA) for men

E. Serum creatinine and blood urea nitrogen (BUN)
F. Urinalysis: Check hematuria.
G. Urine culture (if indicated)
H. Glucose tolerance test
I. Urine drug screen
J. Sinus x-rays
K. Urodynamics tests if bladder issues suspected
L. Postvoid residual (catheterization or ultrasound)
M. Nocturnal polysomnography or actigraphy
N. Psychiatric evaluation if indicated

Differential Diagnoses

A. Insomnia/sleep disorder

1. Inadequate sleep hygiene: Habitual behaviors that harm sleep, such as delaying morning awakening time or napping

2. Insufficient sleep syndrome: Curtailing time in bed in response to social and occupational demands over long periods of time (shift work, circadian rhythm sleep–wake disorder)

3. Adjustment sleep disorder: Acute emotional stressors (job loss or hospitalization) resulting in difficulty falling asleep because of tension and anxiety

4. Psychophysiologic insomnia: Anticipatory anxiety over the prospect of another night of sleeplessness and the next day of fatigue

5. Narcolepsy: Persistent daytime sleepiness with brief naps accompanied by vivid dreams

a. Cataplexy or abrupt paralysis or paresis of skeletal muscles following anger, surprise, laughter, or physical exercise

b. Hypnagogic hallucinations (vivid and often frightening dreams that occur shortly after falling asleep or on awakening)

c. Sleep paralysis, a transient global paralysis of voluntary muscles that occurs shortly after falling asleep and lasts a few seconds or minutes

d. Disturbed and restless sleep

B. Alcoholism and drug abuse/dependence
C. Major depressive disorder
D. Acute psychosis, mania, and hypomania
E. Medical problems such as chronic pain, anxiety, depression, hyperthyroidism, epilepsy, general paresis, diabetes, benign prostatic hypertrophy, urinary problems related to age/diuretic use, cardiopulmonary dysfunction, and menopause

Plan

A. General interventions

1. Identify cause of insomnia.

2. Treat physical/laboratory findings if underlying condition exists. Treat condition according to diagnosis made, that is, hormone replacement therapy, thyroid medications, diabetes, and so forth, as indicated.

B. Patient teaching

1. Have the patient record a 2-week log for sleep–wake habits. A sleep diary is available from the National Sleep Foundation at https://sleepfoundation.org

2. Advise the patient to avoid alcohol, caffeine, and stimulating agents during the evening hours.

3. Avoid exercising before going to bed.

4. Encourage smoking cessation. Avoid smoking in the evening hours. *See Section III: Patient Teaching Guide, "Nicotine Dependence."* ◀

5. Encourage regular sleep habit/hygiene. Recommend going to bed the same time every night and waking up the same time every day.

6. Recommend keeping the bedroom cool, quiet, and dark while sleeping.

7. Encourage relaxation exercises before going to bed.

8. If stress/anxiety contributes to sleeping disorder, recommend counseling with psychologist or counselor to identify and deal with issues.

9. *See Section III: Patient Teaching Guide for this chapter, "Sleep Disorders/Insomnia."* ◀

C. Pharmaceutical therapy

1. Eliminate prescription medications (when possible) and OTC products as part of your management plan *before writing another prescription.*

2. Only after making the assumption that the insomnia cannot be adequately treated by addressing the underlying medical problem responsible for causing the insomnia should medications for sleep be prescribed.

> *Do not prescribe medications for sleep to patients with alcohol/drug or depressive disorders.*

3. Use short-term pharmaceutical therapy.

4. Drug of choice: *Sedative anxiolytic hypnotics:* Try initially for 1 week to establish a sleep pattern.

> *If insomnia continues for more than 1 month, refer the patient to a physician or specialist.*

a. Temazepam (Restoril) 7.5 to 30 mg at bedtime (1–2 weeks)

b. Flurazepam (Dalmane) 15 to 30 mg at bedtime (1–2 weeks)

c. Zolpidem (Ambien) 5 to 10 mg at bedtime (4 weeks maximum)

d. Zolpidem XR (Ambien XR) 6.25 to 12.5 mg at bedtime

e. Eszopiclone (Lunesta) 2 to 3 mg at bedtime; start with 1 mg in the elderly

f. Ramelteon (Rozerem) 8 mg by mouth 30 minutes before bedtime; do not take with meals

g. Suvorexant (Belsomra) 10 to 20 mg by mouth 30 minutes before bedtime

> *Anxiolytic agents, such as diazepam (Valium) and alprazolam (Xanax), tend to increase the duration and frequency of sleep apneas and are contraindicated for patients with possible/undiagnosed apnea spells.*

5. Sedating antihistamines are not recommended for use over 4 months.

a. Hydroxyzine HCI (Atarax) 50 to 100 mg at bedtime

b. Hydroxyzine pamoate (Vistaril) 50 to 100 mg at bedtime

6. Antidepressants with sedating properties

a. Trazodone HCI (Desyrel) 50 to 100 mg at bedtime

b. Paroxetine (Paxil) 10 to 20 mg at bedtime

Follow-Up

A. Follow up for 1 week to assess the patient's status.

B. Then, follow up every 2 weeks to check the patient's progress.

C. Once positive change is seen, the patient can be seen monthly as needed.

D. Assess the patient's potential for suicide with every office visit.

E. If coexisting medication conditions exist, refer to medical diagnosis for follow-up recommendations.

Consultation/Referral

A. Refer to a psychiatric clinician for medication management and psychotherapy after initial assessment if psychiatric differential diagnosis is made.

B. Refer for psychological testing.

C. If insomnia continues for more than 1 month, refer to a physician if the patient requires a sedative anxiolytic hypnotic for more than 4 weeks.

Individual Considerations

A. Pregnancy: Sleep difficulties are more prevalent in second and third trimesters of pregnancy because of the growing size of the uterus and difficulty finding comfortable sleeping positions. Treat with comfort measures.

B. Pediatrics

1. Children normally require about 10 hours of sleep.

2. Children younger than 18 years with sleep problems should be referred to a pediatrician or pediatric psychiatrist, depending on clinical findings.

C. Adults

1. The "right" amount of sleep results in optimal daytime alertness and a sense of mental efficiency and well-being.

2. Daytime naps often interfere with the quality of night sleep. Encourage eliminating naps during the day.

3. Nocturia and disturbed sleep are the symptoms that cause older men to seek medical help with prostatism.

D. Geriatrics

1. With aging, it is normal for sleep time to decrease (less than 7 hours), with a tendency toward sleep fragmentation and an increase in the frequency of awakenings and brief arousals. Explain this to older adults to avoid "worry over sleeplessness."

2. Always assess for depression in elderly patients.

3. Start with the lowest dose of pharmaceutical agents.

4. Chronic pain is a leading cause for sleep disruption in elderly persons with degenerative joint pain.

5. Review elderly patients' medications and dosage for insomnia because of known side effects or as a medication toxicity.

6. Gastroesophageal reflux is commonly seen in geriatric patients at nighttime and causes them to wake up at night. Correcting the reflux with sleeping position, avoiding late night meals and spicy food, prescribing medications (proton pump inhibitors [PPIs]), and making possible weight-loss interventions could improve sleep disturbance in these patients.

7. Patients with end-stage renal disease may have nocturnal leg movement disorders and anemia due to renal failure. Improving the anemia will improve the insomnia and will decrease the leg movements.

E. Partners: Those who find it necessary to sleep in another room because of their partner's snoring should refer the snorer to the primary care physician/advanced practice nurse to rule out an OSA syndrome.

Resource

National Sleep Foundation: www.sleepfoundation.org

Suicide

Moya Cook and Alyson Wolz

Definition

A. Suicide is defined as the intentional destruction of one's own life. It is the most critical consequence of mental illness and occurs in all diagnostic psychiatric categories. Therefore, knowing the risk factors for suicide and eliciting key clinical features that differentiate the truly suicidal patient from the attention seeker are of utmost importance. **Symptoms are often missed because they can be very subtle. Because there are important legal, social, and religious implications to suicide, the general health care practitioner should not attempt to treat these high-risk patients. This section focuses on identifying the suicidal patient for immediate referral to a psychiatrist or psychiatric inpatient facility.**

Incidence

A. Approximately **15%** with recurrent depressive illness commit suicide.

B. There are approximately **75%** of suicides due to depressive illness (jumps to 90% if other mental illnesses and substance abuse are included).

C. It is estimated that **75%** of people who attempt suicide have seen their primary care provider within the 6 weeks prior to the attempt.

D. Suicide is the **10th leading cause of death** in the United States; for young people between the ages of 15 to 24 years it is the second leading cause of death.

The United States averages 13 suicides per 100,000 population annually. Every year more than 38,000 people take their own lives, not including those individuals who die as a result of fatal accidents due to impaired concentration and attention, and death due to illnesses that may be sequelae (e.g., alcohol abuse).

According to the World Health Organization (WHO), by the year 2020, depression will be the number 2 cause, worldwide, of individuals losing healthy years of their lives. Estimates associate 16,000 suicides in the United States annually with depressive disorder. Fifteen percent of those hospitalized for major depressive disorder attempt suicide. Fifteen percent of patients with severe primary major depressive disorder of at least 1 month's duration eventually commit suicide.

The rate of suicide in young adults has more than doubled since 1950. Midlife suicide rates tend to be highest among White men, although female suicide rates peak in midlife. Males are three to four times more likely to complete suicide, but females are three times more likely to attempt suicide. Whites are twice as likely as non-Whites to commit suicide, although in the 25- to 34-year age group they are equal. Rates for widowed, divorced, or separated individuals are higher than for those who are married. Rates are highest in Protestants, intermediate in Jews, and lowest in Catholics.

Pathogenesis

A. Recent studies confirm that some changes in the noradrenergic system along with reduced serotonin levels are associated with suicide. In recent studies independent of psychiatric diagnoses, one researcher identified a suicidality syndrome consisting of hopelessness, ruminative thinking, social withdrawal, and lack of activity as core symptoms.

B. Familial, genetic, early life-loss experiences, and comorbid alcoholism may be causal factors. In adolescence, depression is the largest single risk factor for suicidal behavior, although family relationship difficulties make a significant independent contribution to this. Environmental stressors in the presence of psychiatric disorders may also be responsible for initiating the impulsive behavior, leading to suicide. The risk of suicidal behaviors is higher in those with mental disorders than those with mood disorders.

Predisposing Factors

A. ***SAD PERSONAS***

- **S** = sex
- **A** = age
- **D** = depression
- **P** = previous attempts
- **E** = ethanol abuse
- **R** = rational thinking loss
- **S** = social support loss
- **O** = organized plan
- **N** = no spouse
- **A** = availability of lethal means
- **S** = sickness

Also, consider gender, race and ethnicity, medications, and other medical conditions.

Common Complaints

A. Overt or indirect suicide talk or threats: "You won't be bothered by me much longer."

Any mention of dying or ending one's life must be taken seriously.

B. Depressed or anxious mood due to depression

Every depressed patient must be assessed for suicide risk.

C. Significant recent loss such as spouse, job, or self-esteem

D. Unexpected change in behavior such as making a will, intense talks with friends, and giving away possessions

E. Unexpected change in attitude such as suddenly cheerful, angry, or withdrawn

F. Atypical symptoms of depression in the elderly such as impaired ability to communicate, intractable tinnitus, and feelings of helplessness

Other Signs and Symptoms

Indications for hospitalization of suicidal patients

A. Psychosis

B. Intoxication with drugs or alcohol that cannot be evaluated and treated over a period of time in the emergency department

C. No change in affect or symptoms despite the intervention of the physician, family, and friends

D. Command hallucinations

E. Lack of access to, or low availability of, outpatient resources

F. Family exhaustion

G. Escalating number of suicide attempts

H. Uncertainty about the risk of suicide

I. Severe psychic anxiety, anxious ruminations, and global insomnia are acute risk factors.

Subjective Data

A. Ascertain the patient's intention. Ask why he or she wants to die?

1. Asking the patient about suicide does not give the patient any ideas about suicide.

B. Determine whether the patient has thought of a suicide plan. The more specific the plan, the more likely the act. A well-worked out, realistic, and potentially lethal plan suggests great risk.

C. Rule out the presence of psychiatric or organic factors such as psychotic depression, thought disorder, or sedative self-medication.

D. Determine whether the precipitating crisis is resolving satisfactorily to the patient.

E. Take an "inventory of loss." Determine the losses the patient has incurred in the last several months or years.

F. Review the patient's plans for the future.

G. Determine whether the patient thinks he or she is going to commit suicide.

H. Evaluate whether the patient has a caring family or other support systems.

Physical Examination

A. Check pulse, respirations, blood pressure, and weight.

B. Inspect

1. Observe overall appearance; note grooming, tone of voice, conduct of patient during communication.
2. Complete dermal examination. Check for physical evidence of suicidal behavior such as wrist lacerations or rope burns around the neck. Look for signs of substance use.

C. Palpate
1. The neck and thyroid; note the goiter
2. The axilla and groin for lymphadenopathy (infectious etiology)

D. Auscultate
1. The heart, lungs, and abdomen (as applies to physical complaints).

E. Neurologic examination
1. Complete mental status review: Specific concern exists when patient displays a flat affect when discussing thoughts or plans for suicide.
2. Assess for thought disorder: Is the patient having command hallucinations telling him or her to harm or kill him- or herself? Is the patient having delusions or a strong sense of "burdensomeness," thinking that others will be better off without him or her?
3. Is the patient exhibiting obsession with taking his or her own life?

Diagnostic Tests

A. Complete blood count (CBC) with differential
B. Electrolytes, serum calcium, and phosphorus
C. Thyroid profile
D. Liver profile
E. Blood urea nitrogen (BUN), creatinine
F. Blood alcohol
G. Urine drug screen
H. EKG
I. Rapid plasma reagin (RPR)
J. CT and MRI scans
K. Perform the Mini-Mental State Examination to rule out dementia/delirium.
L. Perform suicide assessment using an assessment tool such as the Suicide Behavior Questionnaire-revised (SBQ-R) available at: www.integration.samhsa.gov/images/res/SBQ.pdf

Differential Diagnoses

A. Mood disorder due to another medical condition
B. Adjustment disorder with depressed mood
C. Personality disorders
D. Psychotic disorder
E. Alcoholism and drug abuse/dependence
F. Dementia/delerium
G. Side effect of medication (antidepressants, antipsychotics)

Plan

A. General interventions
1. If the patient is suicidal, refer immediately. Make sure there is someone with the patient at all times.
2. If the patient came to the office alone, call a family member or friend to accompany the patient to the hospital emergency room or treatment center.
3. If you are fearful the patient will try to escape or leave unaccompanied, call an ambulance to escort the patient to the hospital emergency room where commitment papers for involuntary hospital admission can be completed.

Documentation is critical. Make sure all statements are recorded and the decision-making process followed.

Be sure to advise the hospital staff of your concerns regarding the patient's suicidal status.

B. Patient teaching
1. Educate patient and family regarding treatment with medication for depression. Discuss benefits/risks of medication and side effects.
2. Encourage the patient to enroll in counseling with a psychologist/therapist to discuss current problems/needs.
3. Determine whether social services need to be contacted for patient to provide support services.
4. Provide local resources for counseling and social services as appropriate.
5. If the patient is not hospitalized, make sure that family or friends are aware of the patient's status and that he or she has someone to talk to and monitor his or her condition until the next office appointment.

C. Pharmaceutical therapy
1. See this chapter for sections on depression and/or bipolar disorder for complete pharmacological interventions for specific mood disorders.
2. Antidepressants such as serotonin reuptake inhibitors (SSRIs), serotonin norepinephrine reuptake inhibitors (SNRIs), and antianxiety medications can help to reduce symptoms of depression and severe anxiety, which may help the patient to feel less suicidal.
3. Clozapine is a Food Drug Administration (FDA)-approved medication for reduction of suicidal behavior in patients with schizophrenia.
4. Quetiapine and lithium have been shown to prevent suicide in patients with bipolar depression.

Follow-Up

A. After emergency admission for suicidal ideation or threats, patients should be closely observed, especially in the first year after the serious suicide attempt.
B. With each visit, question the patient regarding suicidal ideation or a plan (see "Subjective Data" section for important questions to ask).

Consultation/Referral

A. Consult with the patient's psychiatric practitioner. Obtain a release of information from the patient.

B. Be sure the patient continues to follow up with psychiatric counseling and medication management (see "Depression" section).

Individual Considerations

A. Pregnancy: A woman with a history of depression or previous postpartum depression is at high risk for postpartum depression (recurrent) (see "Postpartum Depression" section in Chapter 13, "Obstetrics Guidelines").

B. Adolescents

1. Teens are at risk after recent losses from death (especially if one of their friends/family commits suicide). Recent loss includes breaking up with a boyfriend or girlfriend.

2. If a teen has had a depressive episode, he or she may be at a higher risk if he or she suddenly seems happy and things are "just fine." The teen may have decided on a suicide plan and is experiencing a sense of relief because he or she has made plans.

C. Geriatrics

1. Suicide is the eighth leading cause of death in males older than 65 years.

2. Older persons use the usual means for suicide as well as a slower plan, including not eating, stopping prescription drugs or overmedicating, increasing alcohol intake, and refusing treatment.

3. The elderly population is more susceptible to the adverse effects of medications.

4. Antidepressants should be started at the lowest doses and slowly increased for the elderly. The SSRIs are considered the first line of antidepressant therapy in the elderly population (see "Depression" section in this chapter).

Resource

National Alliance on Mental Illness. (2016). NAMI family support group: https://www.nami.org/Local-NAMI/Programs?classkey=72e2fdaf-2755-404f-a8be-606d4de63fdb

Bibliography

American Psychiatric Association. (2013). *Diagnostic and statistical manual of mental disorders* (5th ed.). Arlington, VA: American Psychiatric Publishing.

Anxiety and Depression Association of America. (2014). Facts and statistics. Retrieved from http://www.adaa.org/about-adaa/press-room/facts-statistics

Beck, A. T., Ward, C. H., Mendelson, M., Mock, J., & Erbaugh, J. (1961). An inventory for measuring depression. *Archives of General Psychiatry, 4*, 561–571.

Beck Institute for Cognitive Behavior Therapy. (2013). Identifying suicide risk. Retrieved from https://www.beckinstitute.org/identifying-suicide-risk

Brandt, N. J., & Piechocki, J. M. (2013). Treatment of insomnia in older adults: Re-evaluating the benefits and risks of sedative hypnotic agents. *Journal of Gerontological Nursing, 39*(4), 48–54.

Buysse, D. J. (2013). Insomnia. *Journal of the American Medical Association, 309*(7), 706–716.

Centers for Disease Control and Prevention. (2013, 2011). *Web-based Injury Statistics Query and Reporting System (WISQARS)* [Online]. National Center for Injury Prevention and Control, CDC (producer). Retrieved from https://www.cdc.gov/injury/wisqars/index.html

Chan, D., Livingston, G., Jones, L., & Sampson, E. L. (2013). Grief reactions in dementia carers: A systematic review. *International Journal of Geriatric Psychiatry, 28*(1), 1–17.

Crum, R. M., Anthony, J. C., Bassett, S. S., & Folstein, M. F. (1993). Population-based norms for the Mini-Mental State Examination by age and educational level. *Journal of the American Medical Association, 269*(18), 2386–2391.

Depression and Bipolar Support Alliance. (2015). Peer support. Retrieved from http://www.dbsalliance.org/site/PageServer?pagename=education_statistics_bipolar_disorder

Dhekney, K., Faghih, S., & Secord, El. (2013). Fever and failure to thrive in toddler. *Contemporary Pediatrics, 30*(1), 35–40.

Hampton, T. (2015). Epidemiology and pathogenesis of bipolar disorders. Retrieved from http://www.medpagetoday.com/resource-center/bipolar-resource-center/epidemiology_pathogenesis/a/44242

Hardy, S. (2013). Prevention and management of depression in primary care. *Nursing Standard (Royal College of Nursing (Great Britain): 1987), 27*(26), 51–56; quiz 58.

Lewiecki, E. M., & Miller, S. A. (2013). Suicide, guns, and public policy. *American Journal of Public Health, 103*(1), 27–31.

McCarney, S. B., & Bauer, A. B. (1995). *Parent's guide to attention deficit disorders: Intervention strategies for the home* (2nd ed.). Columbia, MO: Hawthorne Educational Services. Retrieved from http://www.hawthorne-ed.com/pages/adhd/ad3.html

National Committee for the Prevention of Elder Abuse. (2008). Elder abuse. Retrieved from www.preventelderabuse.org/elderabuse

National Initiative for Children's Healthcare Quality. (2014). Scoring instructions for NICHQ Vanderbilt Assessment Scales. Retrieved from www.aap.org/en-us/Documents/sodbp_vanderbilt_scoringinstructions.pdf

National Initiative for Children's Healthcare Quality. (2002). NICHQ Vanderbilt Assessment Follow-up: Teacher Informant. Retrieved from http://www.copakids.com/Follow%20Up%20Vanderbilt%20Teacher%20Form.pdf

National Initiative for Children's Healthcare Quality. (2002). NICHQ Vanderbilt Assessment Scale—PARENT Informant. Retrieved from www.nichq.org/childrens-health/adhd/resources/vanderbilt-assessment-scales

National Initiative for Children's Healthcare Quality. (2002). NICHQ Vanderbilt Assessment Scale—TEACHER Informant. Retrieved from www.nichq.org/childrens-health/adhd/resources/vanderbilt-assessment-scales

National Institute on Drug Abuse. (2011). Commonly abused drugs charts. Retrieved from https://www.drugabuse.gov/drugs-abuse/commonlyabused-drugscharts

National Institute of Mental Health. (2016). *Bipolar disorder*. Retrieved from https://www.nimh.nih.gov/health/topics/bipolar-disorder/index.shtml

National Sleep Foundation. (n.d.). National Sleep Foundation sleep diary. Retrieved from https://sleepfoundation.org/search/node/sleep%20diary

NCPEA National Committee for the Prevention of Elder Abuse. (n.d.-a). Domestic violence. Retrieved from http://www.preventelderabuse.org/elderabuse/domestic.html

NCPEA National Committee for the Prevention of Elder Abuse. (n.d.-b). Financial abuse. Retrieved from http://www.preventelderabuse.org/elderabuse/fin_abuse.html

Osman, A., Bagge, C., Guitierrez, P., Konick, L., Kooper, B., & Barrios, F. (2001). The Suicidal Behaviors Questionnaire—Revised (SBQ-R): Validation with clinical and nonclinical samples. *Assessment, 8*(4), 443–454. Retrieved from http://www.integration.samhsa.gov/images/res/SBQ.pdf

Patterson, W. M., Dohn, H. H., Bird, J., & Patterson, G. A. (1983). Evaluation of suicidal patients: The SAD PERSONS scale. *Psychosomatics, 24*(4), 343–345, 348.

PDR.net. (2016). Physicians' desk reference. Retrieved from http://www.pdr.net/browse-by-drug-name

RXList. (2016). The Internet drug list. Retrieved from http://www.rxlist.com/script/main/srchcont_rxlist.asp?

Smith, M. D. (2013). America's health care problems? The solutions exist. Interview by John Marcille. Managed Care (Langhorne, Pa.), 22(1), 32–35.

Suicide Awareness Voices of Education. (2003–2013). Suicide facts. Retrieved from http://www.save.org/about-suicide/suicide-facts

Wendell, A. D. (2013). Overview and epidemiology of substance abuse in pregnancy. *Clinical Obstetrics and Gynecology, 56*(1), 91–96.

World Health Organization. (2013). Gender and women's mental health. Retrieved from http://www.who.int/mental_health/prevention/gender women/en

World Health Organization. (2016). Suicide fact sheet. Retrieved from http://www.who.int/mediacentre/factsheets/fs398/en

Yesavage, J. A. (1986). The use of rating depression series in the elderly. In L. W. Poon (Ed.), *Clinical memory assessment of older adults*. Washington, DC: American Psychological Association.

Yesavage, J. A. (1988). Geriatric Depression Scale. *Psychopharmacology Bulletin, 24*(4), 709–711.

23 Assessment Guide for Sport Participation

Student athletes who plan to participate in sport activities are required by most states to have a preparticipation sports physical examination. The primary goals of this examination include (a) to assure that the student is safe to participate in the specified sport; (b) to assess the growth and development of the person, evaluating maturation and size of the athlete; (c) to identify any congenital or new anomalies/conditions that would pose a threat of injury with activity; (d) to assess the preparticipation condition of the athlete that would put the athlete at risk while participating in the sport; and (e) to eliminate any unnecessary barriers that would restrict the student's participation in the identified sport.

Ideally, the examination should be performed several weeks (typically 6 weeks) before season activity. In the event that any conditions need to be addressed, this time frame would allow adequate time for evaluation and resolution, if possible, of the problem before participation in the sport. There is controversy regarding the frequency of these sports examinations; however, many states address this frequency and/or resort to an annual physical examination. The annual examination would suffice for each sport that the athlete is engaged in throughout the academic year.

The physical examination may be performed by the primary care provider or by attending an arranged multistation setting. These settings are frequently arranged by schools, in which multiple providers in a specialty will perform an assessment on a particular part of the body. The evaluation includes: vital signs (B/P, pulse, respirations, height, weight, body mass index [BMI]), vision, dental and physical examination, musculoskeletal examination, nutrition, flexibility/strength, speed/agility, and balance. A lead primary care provider will then evaluate the results from each substation and determine the clearance of the athlete. The American Academy of Pediatrics (AAP) has developed four forms to use for completing the athlete history and physical examination.

The sports physical forms are available on the AAP website at: www.aap.org

1. Preparticipation Physical Evaluation History Form
2. Preparticipation Physical Evaluation Physical Examination Form
3. Preparticipation Physical Evaluation Clearance Form
4. Preparticipation Physical Evaluation of the Athlete With Special Needs: Supplemental History Form (used with permission from American Academy of Family Physicians, American Academy of Pediatrics, American College of Sports Medicine, American Medical Society for Sports Medicine, 2010)

A thorough medical history is imperative to identify potential risk factors for the athlete. A complete review of systems should be discussed with the athlete to identify possible risks. Prior personal conditions/injuries should be reviewed and assessed such as previous head concussions. See "Mild Traumatic Brain Injury" in Chapter 19, Neurologic Guidelines Section for assessment and treatment guidelines. The morbidity rate increases with repetitive head concussions and new guidelines are emerging regarding assessment and clearance for these athletes with a history of head concussions.

Dizziness or syncope episodes should be evaluated. There are many causes for these symptoms; however, cardiac conditions can present with these symptoms and an in-depth cardiac evaluation should be performed. There are conflicting recommendations on routine cardiac screening for all athletes because of the poor sensitivity and high false-positive rates of the EKG. At this time, the American Heart Association recommends a screening history and physical examination, unless further screening is warranted. A thorough family history should also be obtained. A family history of conditions, such as exercise-related deaths or heart attacks before the age of 50 years, should be further evaluated.

Previous injuries, illnesses, fractures, or other trauma should be evaluated for complete resolution and healing. Prior history of heat illness poses a higher risk for reccurrence. Prior surgery or other procedures need to be assessed to document that the athlete has been released by the surgeon and there is no risk involved with participation in the sport.

Flexibility and endurance should also be evaluated and are commonly performed by sport trainers. There are several techniques available to assess flexibility and endurance. Flexibility may be assessed by having the athlete perform range of motion of extremities and comparing the left side to the right side. A goniometer is an instrument that is useful to measure the motion of specific joints. Active and passive range of motion can be used to assess the joints. Normal degrees of range of motion of particular joints can be found at: http://highered.mheducation.com.

Lower extremity range of motion can be assessed by a "sit-and-reach" test. Examples of the "sit-and-reach" and other methods of evaluation can be found at: www.topendsports.com/testing/tests/sit-and-reach.htm

Endurance can be evaluated by having the athlete perform a timed test such as measuring the distance run in a 12-minute period. Routine blood work is not recommended at this time.

Clearance for sport participation is determined once the history and examination are completed. There are different levels of clearance depending on the sport as there are different levels of contact during participation. AAP has developed two classifications of participation, depending on the level of contact in each sport. The athlete may be cleared for all sports without restriction or may be cleared for all sports without restriction with further evaluation or treatment for the particular condition diagnosed at the time of examination. An example of this may be an athlete with a history of well-controlled exercise-induced asthma. Clearance may be denied at the time of examination and the athlete given further recommendations.

Common conditions in which the athlete may be disqualified for clearance to participate in the sport include the following: dizziness with exercise, asthma history, musculoskeletal abnormality, heart murmur, visual impairment, elevation in blood pressure, and/or BMI outside of normal parameters.

If concerns regarding the medical history or examination are present and the athlete is unsure of clearance status, the AAP guidelines for clearance for sports participation can be accessed at www.aap.org.

This time spent with the athlete during the physical examination also provides an opportunity to discuss prevalent risk behaviors and issues he or she may be experiencing at that time. In addition, this is an ideal time to review preventive health strategies to help the athlete achieve his or her optimal health and participate at his or her fullest ability. Topics to consider discussing include:

1. Preventive care: Discuss the use of proper gear for each particular sport. Safety equipment such as mouth guards, goggles, proper fitting head gear/helmets, and so forth, are an important aspect of the education for the athlete to prevent injury and enhance the best performance by the athlete.

2. Injury prevention: Techniques of stretching, warming up, and cooling down should be encouraged before every practice and sport. Stretching properly can prevent musculoskeletal injuries.

3. Chronic conditions: Use of proper medications for chronic conditions, such as asthma, is imperative to prevent complications. Proper use of the rescue inhaler before exercise should be reinforced. Proper administration of the inhaler should also be reviewed. See Chapter 9, Respiratory Guidelines, "Asthma" for assessment and treatment. ◀ *See Patient Teaching Guides in Section III, "Asthma: Action Plan and Peak Flow Monitoring"* and *"Asthma: How to Use a Metered-Dose Inhaler"* for educational material.

4. Substance abuse: Education about abstinence regarding substance abuse (drugs, alcohol, and tobacco). See Chapter 2, Public Health Guidelines, "Substance Use Disorders" for screening questions and treatment. Discuss the detrimental effects of each substance on the body and the way studies show that athletes who use these substances have decreased performance. Long-term risks, such as dependence, cancer, and death, should also be discussed.

5. Depression: Screening for depression should be incorporated into the examination. See Chapter 22, Psychiatric Guidelines, "Depression" for screening questions and treatment.

6. Domestic violence: Assess for domestic violence by observing bruising, scars, cigarette burns, and so forth. See the section "Children" under "Violence" in Chapter 2, Public Health Guidelines for assessment and treatment guidelines.

7. Bullying: Bullying is very common in school-age children. Assess the athlete for being the perpetrator or the victim. The consequence of bullying greatly impacts the overall well-being of the student. Assist the student in ending this cycle by offering counseling services for the student and interventions to end the problem.

8. Nutrition: Eating disorders are commonly seen in this population. See the Section "Nutrition" in this chapter for assessment and education for the athlete. Discuss and stress the importance of hydration during the sporting event to prevent dehydration and explain the ways this can affect the body and performance.

Bibliography

American Academy of Family Physicians, American Academy of Pediatrics, American College of Sports Medicine, American Medical Society for Sports Medicine. (2010). *Preparticipation physical evaluation* (4th ed.). Elk Grove Village, IL: American Academy of Pediatrics. Copyright © 2010 American Academy of Pediatrics. Reproduced with permission. Retrieved from https://www.aap.org/en-us/professional-resources/practice-support/Documents/Preparticipation-Physical-Exam-Form.pdf

Hergenroeder, A. C. (2016). Sports participation in children and adolescents: The preparticipation physical evaluation. *UpToDate*. Retrieved from www.uptodate.com/contents/sports-participation-in-children-and-adolescents-the-preparticipation-physical-evaluation

Roberts, W. O., Löllgen, H., Matheson, G. O., Royalty, A. B., Meeuwisse, W. H., Levine, B., . . . Pigozzi, F. (2014). Advancing the preparticipation physical evaluation: An ACSM and FIMS joint consensus statement. *Clinical Journal of Sport Medicine: Official Journal of the Canadian Academy of Sport Medicine, 24*(6), 442–447.

II Procedures

- Canalith Repositioning (Epley) Procedure for Vertigo
- Cervical Evaluation During Pregnancy: Bimanual Examination
- Clock-Draw Test
- Cystometry
- Cystometry: Bedside
- Foreign Body Removal From the Nose
- Hernia Reduction (Inguinal/Groin)
- Intrauterine Device Insertion
- Neurologic Examination
- Nonstress Test
- Oral Airway Insertion
- Pap Smear and Maturation Index Procedure
- Pregnancy: Estimating Date of Delivery
- Prostatic Massage Technique: 2-Glass Test
- Rectal Prolapse Reduction
- Sprain Evaluation
- Tick Removal
- Trichloroacetic Acid/Podophyllin Therapy
- Wet Mount/Cervical Cultures Procedure

Canalith Repositioning (Epley) Procedure for Vertigo

Jill C. Cash and Cheryl A. Glass

Description

A. Benign paroxysmal positional vertigo (BPPV) occurs with changing position, and rapid head movement causes imbalance, disorientation, and nausea. Vertigo develops when there is a disturbance of the crystals that are normally evenly distributed in the fluid-filled semicircular canal and they become clumped together. Often the imbalance can be corrected by performing canalith repositioning (Epley maneuver) to redistribute the crystals in the vestibule.

Indications

A. BPPV

Contraindications

A. Testing should never be done in the case of head injury or suspected or confirmed cervical spine injury.

Equipment Required

A. Examination table
B. Stool at the head of the table for the practitioner

Procedure

A. Explain the procedure (see Figure II.1).
B. Have the patient sit on the examination table (position 1).

1. Reposition the patient to sitting in the center of the table.
2. The edge at the head of the table should be at the patient's shoulder height (head will hang off the table).
3. Your position will be at the head of the examination table, and you will use the stool for comfort while holding the patient's head with your hands.

C. Rapidly lay the patient down (position 2).

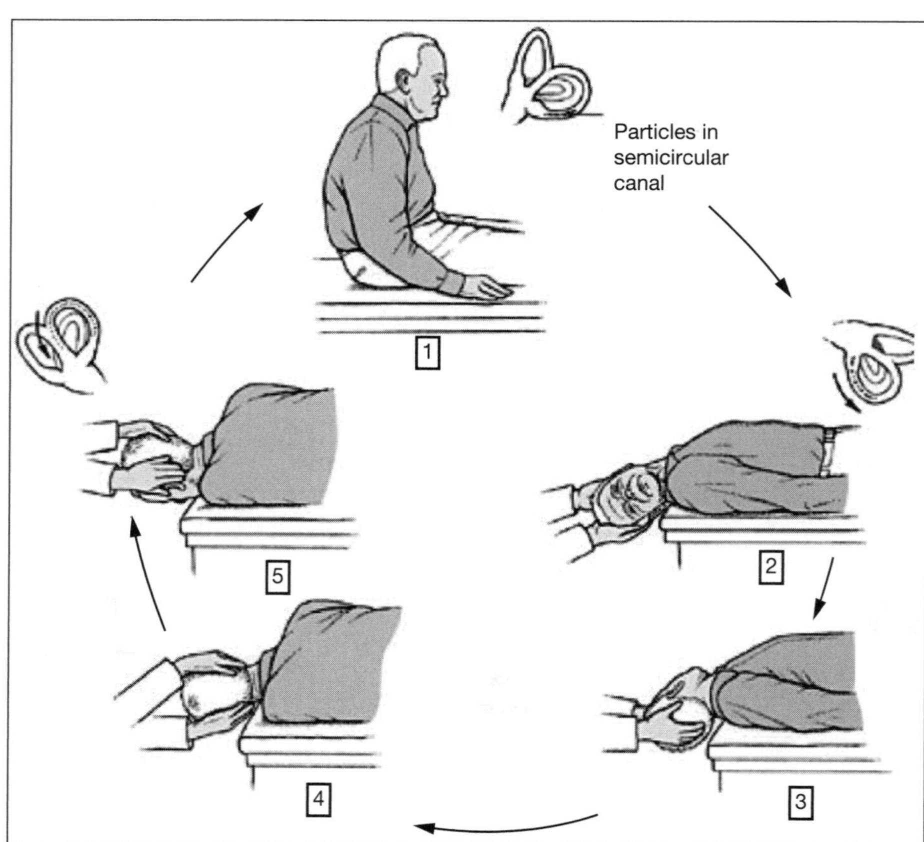

FIGURE II.1 Epley procedure for vertigo.

Source: From the *Merck Manual Consumer Version* (Known as the Merck Manual in the United States and Canada and the MSD Manual in the rest of the world), edited by Robert Porter. Copyright 2016 by Merck Sharp & Dohme Corp., a subsidiary of Merck & Co, Inc, Kenilworth, NJ. Retrieved from http://www.merckmanuals.com/consumer.

1. The patient's head should be hanging over the table in a slightly downward tilt, supported by both of your hands.

2. The patient should be instructed to keep his or her eyes open and try to focus on a stationary object on the wall throughout the positions on his or her back and sides.

3. The patient's head is turned to the same side as the affected ear with the provider supporting the head.

a. If the patient has vertigo affecting both inner ears, turn the patient's head to the dominantly affected side.

b. As an alternative to just turning the head, the patient may quickly turn and lie down on the affected side while you support the head with both of your hands.

4. After a few minutes the patient will be ready to be repositioned as evidenced by his or her lack of nystagmus (rhythmic side-to-side eye movement) and confirmation that the dizziness has stabilized.

D. Turn the patient's head in the opposite direction while you continue to support the head (position 3). Again, the head should be in a slightly downward tilt.

1. If the patient was using the side-lying position, have him or her turn to his or her back.

2. Have the patient continue to keep the eyes open and focus on a stationary object on the wall.

3. Again, the time lapse to repositioning is evidenced by the lack of nystagmus and subjective confirmation that the dizziness has stabilized or abated.

E. Ask the patient to roll from his or her back to the opposite side (or from the back to the opposition side; position 4). The patient's head should be parallel to the floor.

F. With the patient side-lying (position 5), have him or her quickly turn only his or her face to the floor, while you are supporting the head.

G. After the patient verbalizes that the dizziness has abated from side-lying (position 5)

1. The patient is to swing the legs to the edge of the table and quickly sit up.

2. He or she will continue to feel vertigo at this point.

H. Assist the patient off the examination table.

I. The patient should be instructed to be in a sitting position or with the head no farther back than a 45-degree angle for the next 24 hours.

J. The Epley does not immediately stop the vertigo. The patient may begin to feel better within a few days.

K. If the Epley procedure needs to be repeated, allow 1 week between attempts.

Cervical Evaluation During Pregnancy: Bimanual Examination

Jill C. Cash and Rhonda Arthur

Description

A. The bimanual examination is a digital evaluation of the cervix with the index and middle fingers of the examiner's hand.

Indications

A. To assess cervical dilation, effacement, presentation of the fetus, and position and station of fetal presenting part.
B. The cervix may be assigned a Bishop score to evaluate cervical change and to determine difficulty/ease with induction of labor. There is an inherent subjective difference among examiners; however, the Bishop score can be used to evaluate preterm labor cervical changes over time (see Table II.1).

Precautions

A. Bimanual examination should never be performed when there is suspicion of or history of documented placenta previa. Vaginal bleeding in second or third trimester of pregnancy should be treated as placenta previa until this is ruled out.
B. Suspicion of ruptured membranes with preterm contractions: First perform sterile speculum examination to assess for rupture. Then, if membranes are intact, proceed with bimanual examination.
C. If membranes are ruptured in the absence of active labor, avoid bimanual examination until frequent, painful uterine contractions are present.

Equipment Required

A. Gloves (nonsterile if membranes are intact; sterile if suspicion of or documented ruptured membranes)
B. Water-soluble lubricant (sterile lubricant required if membranes are ruptured)
C. Examination table or bed

Procedure

A. Stand at the foot of the examination table or sit near the foot of the bed and face the patient.
B. Place the patient in the lithotomy position, or have the patient draw knees up and allow knees to drop to opposite sides.
C. Suggest relaxation techniques to reduce discomfort. If the patient is in active labor, the cervix will be tender.
D. Place lubricant on the index and middle fingers of the examining hand.
E. Inform the patient of each step before performance: Touch inner thigh first, then touch posterior portion of introitus and introduce gloved fingers into the vagina. Encourage the patient to relax pelvic muscles (a deep breath will often encourage relaxation).
F. Palpate the cervix and lower uterine segment evaluating (see Figure II.2):

1. Dilatation
2. Effacement
3. Station
4. Consistency (softness)
5. Anterior versus midposition versus posterior placement of the cervix
6. In cases of preterm uterine contractions, it is helpful to assess the development of the lower uterine segment. A well-developed lower uterine segment (even

TABLE II.1 Bishop Scoring

Score	0	1	2	3
Dilation	0	1–2	3–4	5–6
% Effacement	0%–30%	40%–50%	60%–70%	80% or more
Station	–3	–2	–1 to 0	+1 to +2
Consistency	Firm	Medium	Soft	–
Position	Posterior	Mid	Anterior	–

Total score: 0 to 5 = difficult induction; ≥6 = easy induction.

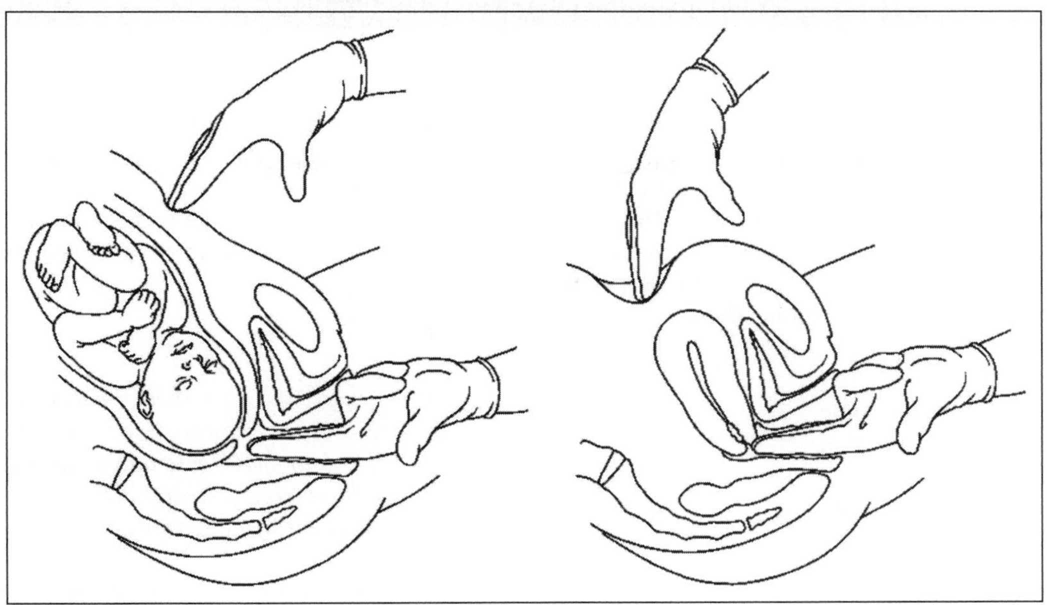

FIGURE II.2 Bimanual examination.

in the absence of cervical dilation or effacement) is often a sign of preterm labor.

7. Note fetal presentation and station of the presenting part. Use ischial spines as landmarks to determine fetal descent through the pelvis.

8. If the fetus is sufficiently descended into the pelvis, determine the position of the presenting part.

9. If present, note bag of amniotic membranes. A bulging bag, known as a "forebag," may be present, even in the presence of documented ruptured membranes.

G. Following the examination, note if blood or vaginal discharge is on gloves.

Clock-Draw Test

Cheryl A. Glass

Description

The clock-draw test is a quick screening tool to assess cognitive dysfunction. The tool can be used by itself or as a complement to other screening tests. The test is a component of the "7-Minute Neurocognitive Screening Battery." It can be administered repeatedly over time to evaluate deterioration of function. The clock-draw test evaluates:

A. Orientation
B. Conceptualization of time
C. Visual spatial organization
D. Visual memory
E. Auditory comprehension
F. Numeric knowledge
G. Concentration
H. Frustration tolerance

Indications

A. Evaluation of dementia
B. Evaluation of delirium
C. Evaluation of neurologic insult
  1. Head trauma
  2. Stroke
  3. Alcohol and drug
D. Evaluation of psychiatric illness
  1. Schizophrenia
  2. Psychotic state

Administering the Clock-Draw Test

A. A number of variations can be used in administering the clock-draw test.

This is not a timed test. There is no limitation to administration time; however, the test generally takes 1 to 2 minutes.

General Information

A. Provide the patient with an 8.5- by 11-in. blank sheet of paper and a pencil.

Setup

A. Equipment required includes a blank sheet of paper, a sheet of paper with a clock on one side, a pen, and a chair or table for ease of drawing.

Patient Instructions

A. The following instructions are given (Rouleau, Salmon, Butters, Kennedy, & McGuire, 1992):

> I would like you to draw a clock, put in all the numbers, and set the hands for 10 after 11.

Following this condition, the patient should be instructed to copy, as accurately as possible, a clock from a model. The model should contain all the numbers on the clock, be 3 in. in diameter, and be located on the upper part of an 8.5- by 11-in. sheet of paper. The hands on the model should be set for 10 after 11. The patient is then instructed to copy the model on the lower part of the same sheet of paper.

A. Instructions can be repeated if necessary.
B. Patients may use their nondominant hand for drawing the clock.

Scoring

> *There are several variations on scoring the clock-draw test. The quickest scoring involves dividing the clock into four quadrants and counting the numbers in the correct quadrant. More complex assessment evaluates up to 20 traits or categorizes errors.*

A. The placement of the arms of the clock is the most abstract feature and is useful in evaluating the early dementing process.

B. A normal clock suggests that multiple functions are intact and contributes to the assessment of the patient's ability to continue independently. This is a "normal" clock draw:

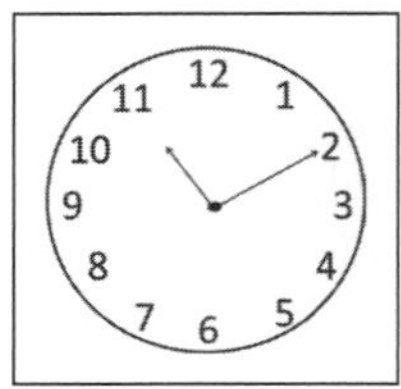

C. A grossly abnormal clock is an indicator of potential problems that require attention:

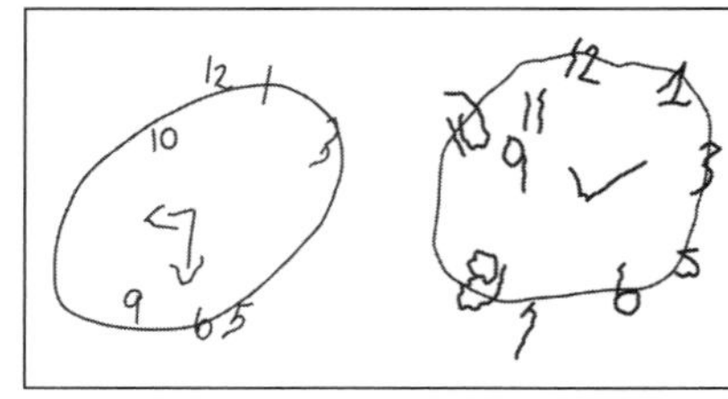

D. There are several scoring systems for evaluating the clock-draw test results. The most basic involves awarding 1 point for each of the following:

- 1 point for the clock circle
- 1 point for the numbers placed in the correct position
- 1 point for the clockface numbers placed in their proper order around and inside the clockface
- 1 point for the presence of the two clock hands
- 1 point for the correct time as instructed

A normal score is 4 or 5 points.

Note: The next two pages may be used for serial testing.

Name: ______________________________ Date: ______________________________

Draw a clock with all the numbers, and set the hands for 10 after 11.

Name: ____________________ Date: ____________________

Copy this clock.

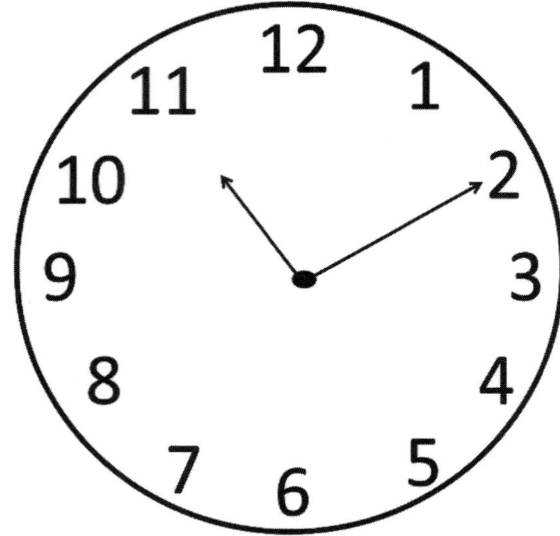

Reprinted from the Rehabilitation Measures Database (http://www.rehabmeasures.org), by Allen Heinemann, PhD, and Jennifer Moore, PT, DHS, NCS. Original instrument instructions published by Rouleau et al. (1992).

Cystometry

Cheryl A. Glass

Description

A. Cystometry testing is an office procedure to determine bladder capacity, postvoid residual (PVR), any fluid leak with stress maneuvers, or inhibited bladder capacity. Cystometry measures the intravesical bladder pressure during bladder filling. Many times cystometry is performed in conjunction with uroflowmetry. Cystometry of a female patient is described.

Indications

A. Patients presenting with complaints of urinary incontinence, stress incontinence (leaking), overactive bladder (OAB), and urinary retention (inability to empty bladder) are candidates for cystometry testing.

Before the Procedure

A. A thorough urogynecologic history should be taken and a physical examination should be performed, including a digital rectal examination.

Precautions

A. Rule out the presence of a urinary tract infection as a cause of the incontinence before cystometry testing.

B. Use universal precautions. This is a sterile procedure and is contraindicated when infection or inflammation is present.

C. Risks of the procedure

- **1.** Discomfort
- **2.** Bleeding
- **3.** Infection
- **4.** Autonomic dysreflexia (AD) from bladder instrumentation and bladder distension
    - **a.** Flushing
    - **b.** Hypertension
    - **c.** Reflex bradycardia
    - **d.** Severe headache

Equipment Required

A. Sterile straight catheter (12–14 French catheter)

B. Catheter insertion kit

C. 60 mL sterile syringe

D. 1,000 mL sterile water (CO_2, saline, or contrast medium may also be used)

E. Sterile measurement container

F. Urine collection device

G. A vaginal or rectal pressure catheter or insertion of a second catheter with a manometer to measure pressures

H. Light source for catheterization

I. Gown and drape for the patient

Procedure

A. Explain the procedure.

B. Obtain verbal and written consent.

C. Ask about any latex or Betadine allergies.

D. Throughout the procedure, ask the patient to speak to his or her sensation of the feeling of the bladder filling, any discomfort, when he or she has the urge to void, and bladder fullness. Sensations noted by the patient are subject to the rate of bladder filling and temperature of the fluid.

E. During the initial physical examination, have the patient bear down and/or cough to evaluate urinary incontinence.

F. Have the patient void, measure the urine, and collect the specimen for urinalysis.

- **1.** The measurement of the urine flow rate also screens abnormalities of micturition.
    - **a.** A simple way to measure the flow rate is to time the duration of urination and measure the volume voided. A woman usually voids in a continuous flow rate until the bladder is empty. Intermittent flow patterns indicate dysfunction with voiding.
- **2.** The evaluation of urine speed and flow rate may be measured by uroflowmetry equipment using a special toilet with a computer to record the flow rates.

G. Catheterize, using sterile technique.

- **1.** Measure urine drained from the catheter inserted postvoiding; this amount is the PVR.
    - **a.** Normal: Less than 100 mL PVR
    - **b.** Abnormal: More than 100 mL PVR
    - **c.** Differential diagnostic evaluation: Overflow incontinence secondary to retention

H. Attach the 60 mL syringe to the catheter.

- **1.** Observe if there was any difficulty passing the catheter.
    - **a.** Normal findings: Catheter passes with ease.
    - **b.** Abnormal findings: Catheter difficult or impossible to pass
    - **c.** Differential diagnostic evaluation: Overflow incontinence possibly due to obstruction

I. Place the rectal or vaginal catheter to measure intra-abdominal pressure and involuntary/voluntary detrusor contractions.

J. Using gravity, fill the bladder slowly through the catheter/syringe with sterile water (saline or contrast medium).

- **1.** Avoid instilling the sterile water too quickly; instill approximately 30 to 50 mL amounts at a time.
- **2.** Measure the amount of water instilled when the patient has the urge to void, different degrees of filling, and pain during filling.
    - **a.** Normal: Bladder capacity usually at 300 mL when urge is sensed.
    - **b.** Abnormal: Urge at less than 200 mL
    - **c.** Differential diagnostic evaluation: Urge incontinence due to small capacity
- **3.** Continue to fill, noting if there is any fluctuation of the sterile water in the syringe during filling.
    - **a.** Normal: Contractions or fluctuations occur around 200 to 250 mL from bladder into syringe (detrusor muscle contraction).
    - **b.** Abnormal: Fluid moving into the syringe

c. Differential diagnostic evaluation: Urge incontinence related to bladder spasm

4. The rectal/vaginal probe measures detrusor activity/overactivity and notes phasic pressure increases associated with symptoms of urgency or urge incontinence, indicating detrusor overactivity.

5. During the procedure, ask the patient to cough or bear down to help elicit involuntary bladder contractions. The Valsalva maneuver or cough assesses the sphincter competence.

6. The instillation of sterile water should be stopped when the patient reports a full bladder. Measure the bladder capacity; that is, the patient reports a perception that voiding can no longer be delayed.

7. If the patient has not reported a full bladder before the instillation of 600 mL, the test should be discontinued.

8. The urodynamic test is done until the point of leakage.

a. Have the patient cough or strain; observe for leaking, clamp catheter.

b. Normal: Normal capacity 400 mL, no leaking with cough

c. Abnormal: Urge before 400 mL, or leaking with pressure

d. Differential diagnostic evaluation: Urge incontinence due to small capacity and/or stress incontinence due to leakage with pressure

e. Coughing and straining during the procedure are also done to evaluate bladder pressure changes. The manometer also measures the pressure inside the bladder when leakage occurs.

9. Remove the catheter after the bladder is filled to capacity (strong urge to void); have the patient cough.

a. Normal: No leakage

b. Abnormal: Leakage of fluid

c. Differential diagnostic evaluation: Stress incontinence associated with weak pelvic muscles

10. Have the patient void; measure output, compare with amount instilled.

a. Normal: Return with a maximum of 100 mL retained (PVR)

b. Abnormal: Greater than 100 mL retained after voiding

c. Postprocedure, while the patient is emptying the bladder, the manometer measures the bladder pressure and flow rate. Then remove the vaginal/rectal probe.

d. Differential diagnostic evaluation: Overflow incontinence either from obstruction or an atonic bladder

K. Discuss treatment options, including pharmaceutical therapy and/or consultation with the urologist.

L. Postprocedure instruction and when to report problems are discussed.

1. Expect some discomfort; it should lessen over time.

2. Blood during urination may be expected after the procedure. The amount of blood lessens over time and with urination.

3. Drinking additional fluids (noncaffeinated and noncarbonated beverages) will increase urination and ease discomfort and passage of blood.

4. An antibiotic may be prescribed (per protocol).

5. Anti-inflammatories, such as ibuprofen, may be discussed.

6. Have the patient report

a. Chills and fever

b. Any abdominal pain

c. Continued bloody urine 1 day post-procedure

Cystometry: Bedside

Cheryl A. Glass

Description

A. Bedside cystometry testing is an office procedure to determine bladder capacity, postvoid residual (PVR), any fluid leak with stress maneuvers, or inhibited bladder capacity. Urodynamic testing is still considered the gold standard test; however, the cystometry is a good and sensitive screening tool.

Indications

A. Patients presenting with complaints of urinary incontinence, stress incontinence (leaking), overactive bladder (OAB), and urinary retention (inability to empty bladder) are candidates for cystometry testing.

Precautions

A. A thorough history should be taken and a physical examination should be conducted.
B. Rule out the presence of a urinary tract infection as a cause of the incontinence before cystometry testing.
C. This is a sterile procedure, not to be done when infection or inflammation is present.

Equipment Required

A. Sterile straight catheter (12–14 French catheter)
B. Catheter insertion kit
C. 60 mL sterile syringe
D. 1,000 mL sterile water
E. Sterile measurement container
F. Urine collection device

Procedure

A. Explain the procedure.
B. Obtain written and verbal consent to perform the procedure.
C. Have the patient bear down and/or cough to evaluate urinary incontinence.
D. Have patient void, measure the urine, and collect the specimen for urinalysis.
E. Catheterize using sterile technique.
- **1.** Measure urine drained from the catheter inserted postvoid; this amount is the PVR.
  - **a.** Normal: Less than 100 mL PVR
  - **b.** Abnormal: More than 100 mL PVR
  - **c.** Differential diagnostic evaluation: Overflow incontinence secondary to retention

F. Attach the 60 mL syringe to the catheter.
- **1.** Observe if there was any difficulty passing the catheter.
  - **a.** Normal findings: Catheter passed with ease.
  - **b.** Abnormal findings: Catheter difficult or impossible to pass.
  - **c.** Differential diagnostic evaluation: Overflow incontinence possibly due to obstruction

G. Using gravity, fill the bladder slowly through catheter/syringe with sterile water.
- **1.** Avoid instilling the sterile water too quickly; instill approximately 30 mL amounts at a time.
- **2.** Measure the amount of water instilled when the patient has the urge to void.
  - **a.** Normal: Bladder capacity usually at 300 mL when urge sensed
  - **b.** Abnormal: Urge at less than 200 mL
  - **c.** Differential diagnostic evaluation: Urge incontinence due to small capacity
- **3.** Continue to fill, noting if there is any fluctuation of the sterile water in the syringe during filling.
  - **a.** Normal: Contractions or fluctuation occur around 200 to 250 mL from bladder into syringe (detrusor muscle contraction)
  - **b.** Abnormal: Fluid moving into the syringe
  - **c.** Differential diagnostic evaluation: Urge incontinence related to bladder spasm
- **4.** The instillation of sterile water should be stopped when the patient reports a full bladder.
- **5.** If the patient has not reported a full bladder before the instillation of 600 mL, the test should be discontinued.
  - **a.** Have patient cough, observe for leaking, and clamp catheter.
  - **b.** Normal: Normal capacity 400 mL, no leaking with cough
  - **c.** Abnormal: Urge before 400 mL, or leaking with pressure
  - **d.** Differential diagnostic evaluation: Urge incontinence due to small capacity and/or stress incontinence due to leakage with pressure
- **6.** Remove catheter after bladder is filled to capacity (strong urge to void); have the patient cough.
  - **a.** Normal: No leakage
  - **b.** Abnormal: Leakage of fluid
  - **c.** Differential diagnostic evaluation: Stress incontinence associated with weak pelvic muscles
- **7.** Have the patient void; measure output, compare with amount instilled.
  - **a.** Normal: Return with a maximum of 100 mL retained (PVR)
  - **b.** Abnormal: Greater than 100 mL retained after voiding
  - **c.** Differential diagnostic evaluation: Overflow incontinence either from obstruction or an atonic bladder

H. Discuss treatment options, including pharmaceutical therapy and/or consultation with a urologist.

Foreign Body Removal From the Nose

Cheryl A. Glass

Description

A. This is the technique for removing a nasal foreign body (NFB) that is anterior to the pharynx and can be visualized with a nasal speculum.

Indications

A. Patients with retained NFB often present with unilateral, foul rhinorrhea, nosebleeds, or the request for foreign-body removal. This is most commonly seen toddlers.

Precautions

A. Try to identify the type of object: organic or inorganic.
  1. Organic foreign objects include food items (e.g., peas and beans), sponges, or rubber.
  2. Inorganic foreign objects include a rock, pearl, battery, or small toy parts.

B. If you cannot identify the object, do not irrigate the nares before removal.
  1. Vegetable matter will swell if hydrated, so remove it in a dry environment when possible.
  2. Small "button" batteries from toys are common and should not be irrigated due to the destruction from the low-volt current and potential spread of alkaline content.

C. When the object is too far into the nasal turbinate/cavity or when in doubt, do not attempt the procedure and refer to an otolaryngologist.
  1. The procedure may need to be done under sedation.
  2. The object may need to be removed in a surgical setting utilizing sedation.

Equipment Required

A. Proper lighting (headlight or head mirror)
B. Nasal speculum
C. Topical anesthetic for use before procedure (topical 1% lidocaine with 0.5% phenylephrine)
D. Fogarty suction and several suction tips
E. Other equipment should be available, depending on the type of foreign body: Wire loop or curette, alligator or Hartman forceps, bayonet forceps, right-angle hooks, a Foley catheter, and Fogarty suction.

Procedure

A. Determine the type of object in the nostril during history taking in order to determine the best approach for removal.
B. Explain the procedure to the patient.
C. Obtain the patient's consent for removal.
D. To best visualize the nasal cavity, have the patient lie down or sit erect with the head slightly tilted.
E. Visualize the nostril with the nasal speculum.
F. If tissue edema is present in the nares, you may use a topical anesthetic with vasoconstrictor to the affected nares to help prevent bleeding.
G. If the patient is willing, have him or her dislodge the foreign body with forceful nose blowing while occluding the unaffected nostril and keeping the mouth closed.
H. The patient should be supine or with a slight elevation of the head with assistance to stabilize the patient's head.
I. If forceful blowing is not successful, attempt to remove the foreign object using the most appropriate instrument or technique (wire loop or curette, alligator or Hartman forceps, bayonet forceps, right-angle hooks and suctioning). The choice of instrument for removal is dependent on the type of object, location, and how well the patient is able to cooperate during the procedure.
J. Use of a catheter involves lubricating the tip, inserting catheter past the foreign body, and inflating the balloon. Gentle withdrawal will pull the foreign object out.
K. Simple external pressure should be applied to prevent bleeding.

Evaluation/Results of Procedure

A. Evaluate the other nares and ears if one foreign object is found.
B. Bleeding is common after the removal of a foreign object. Pressure should be applied to stop the bleeding.
C. Follow up in 2 days to evaluate the mucosa.
D. Consult a physician if you are unable to dislodge or remove the object. Button batteries require prompt removal and inspection due to alkaline-induced liquefactive necrosis to the mucosa.

Hernia Reduction (Inguinal/Groin)

Cheryl A. Glass

Description

A. A hernia reduction may be done by a manual technique used for external replacement of the bowel (occasionally omentum) from the hernia back into the abdomen/groin.

Indications

A. Herniation of bowel contents occurs secondary to pregnancy, straining, hard physical labor, or congenital defect.

Precautions

A. *Do not try to reduce a strangulated hernia.* This is a surgical emergency and should be referred immediately to a surgeon for evaluation and treatment. This can cause gangrenous bowel to enter the peritoneal cavity. Strangulation symptoms include tenderness, discoloration, edema, fever, and signs of bowel obstruction.

Equipment Required

A. Gown/drape for the patient
B. Nonsterile gloves

Procedure

A. After doing a complete assessment, explain the reduction procedure to the patient, discussing each step just before performing it.
B. Obtain consent if required by protocol.
C. Ask the patient to void.
D. Apply the gloves.
E. Have the patient lie supine with slight flexion of the hips to relax abdominal muscles or in Trendelenburg position.
F. Ask the patient to take deep, slow, relaxing breaths. Hernia reduction should cause minimal discomfort.

1. *Males*: Gently invaginate the scrotal skin, and replace the herniated contents back through the external/internal inguinal or femoral rings.
2. *Females*: Gently invaginate the herniated bowel contents back through the external/internal inguinal or femoral rings.

G. Hernias should be easily reducible. Do not force any contents back into the abdominal wall defect.
H. After the reduction, ask the patient to cough and strain to evaluate successful reduction before discharge.

Evaluation/Results of Procedure

A. Consult a physician if unable to reduce the hernia. The hernia may be strangulated.
B. Have the patient return in 1 week for reexamination or sooner if needed.
C. Tell the patient not to strain with bowel movements, lift heavy objects, or exercise strenuously.
D. Review symptoms of obstruction or strangulation of entrapped bowel: Pain, nausea, and vomiting. Warn the patient to seek immediate medical attention for strangulated bowel.
E. Recurrent hernias and congenital defects eventually require surgical repair. Hernias secondary to pregnancy may not require surgery.

Intrauterine Device Insertion

Rhonda Arthur

Note: Only trained health care providers who carefully reviewed the selected device's manufacturer's package insert for indications and use as well as specific insertion instructions should place intrauterine devices (IUDs).

Description

A. The IUD is a long-acting method of contraception that is inserted into the uterine cavity.

   1. Copper T 380 A (ParaGard)
      a. T-shaped bound in fine copper wire
      b. Approved for 10 years
      c. Clear or white knotted double string
   2. Levonorgestrel (Mirena®)
      a. T-shaped polyethylene frame with levonorgestrel reservoir coating
      b. Approved for 5 years
      c. Dark monofilament strings
      d. Indications also include use for treatment in women who have heavy menstrual bleeding and choose IUD for contraception.

Indications

A. To provide a long-acting method (5–10 years) of contraception
B. The Mirena IUD has been therapeutic with severe dysmenorrhea and severe menorrhagia.

Precautions

A. Pregnancy must be ruled out before insertion.
B. Risks at the time of insertion include uterine perforation and/or infection and a vagal response.
C. Small amounts of progestins pass into breast milk with Mirena.
D. To minimize the risk of expulsion, it is advisable to insert an IUD when the woman is *not* on her menstrual cycle.
E. An existing IUD should be removed during the menstrual cycle.
F. Consent(s) is required by the manufacturer and by individual institutional protocols. The patient should know the type of IUD device and when it should be replaced.

Contraindications

A. Women who have a history of sexually transmitted disease and/or currently have more than one sexual partner may not be good candidates for IUD use.
B. Uterine anomaly
C. Cervical stenosis (unable to pass a uterine sound)
D. Nulliparous (especially teens) are also not good candidates for the IUD.
E. Active pelvic infection (recent, acute, or subacute)
F. Purulent cervicitis
G. History of ectopic pregnancy (strong relative risk)
H. Abnormal Papanicolau (Pap) smear/endometrial hyperplasia/cervical intraepithelial neoplasia (CIN)/cancer (review last recent Pap results); uterine or cervical neoplasm.
I. Concern for future fertility.
J. Allergy to copper (ParaGard) or allergy to component of Mirena as applies.
K. Valvular heart disease.

> *Insertion of an IUD may theoretically increase the woman's susceptibility to systemic bacterial endocarditis (SBE). No current evidence supports this. Optional therapy: Some clinicians require antibiotics for valvular coverage. High-risk patients may receive IV ampicillin and gentamicin, and moderate-risk patients may receive oral amoxicillin 2 g before insertion or removal.*

L. Acute liver disease (Mirena)
M. Known or suspected breast carcinoma (Mirena)

Equipment Required

A. IUD
B. Speculum
C. Iodine solution
D. Tenaculum
E. Uterine sound
F. Scissors
G. Sterile gloves (two pair)
H. Urine pregnancy test kit
I. Atropine 0.5 mg should be available at the time of insertion for severe vasovagal response.

> *Backup staff should be available for complications such as vasovagal response and perforation of uterus.*

Procedure

A. Perform a urine pregnancy test.
B. Perform a baseline blood pressure and pulse.
C. Obtain the patient's verbal and written consent after full history and review of last Pap smear; discuss alternative methods, pros and cons of each method, procedure, side effects, and complications of IUD insertion and device.
D. Perform a bimanual examination to determine uterine position and size.
E. Apply sterile gloves.
F. Cleanse the vagina and cervix with iodine solution.
G. Use the tenaculum to grasp the anterior lip of the cervix approximately 1.5 to 2.0 cm from the os.

   1. Atropine should be readily available for severe vasovagal response.
   2. Lidocaine (Xylocaine) gel or benzocaine (Hurricane Spray) can be used to decrease discomfort with the application and use of the tenaculum.

H. Insert the uterine sound into the cervix/uterus slowly and gently.

1. Moisture mark on the sound will indicate the depth of insertion for the IUD. (Depth less than 6 cm is contraindication.)

I. Change sterile gloves.

J. Load the IUD as directed by manufacturer.

K. Set indicator for depth of insertion as guided by the uterine sound.

L. While maintaining gentle traction with the tenaculum, insert the IUD gently to the predetermined mark on the guide sheath.

1. Spasm of the internal cervical os may occur and will resolve by waiting a few minutes.

M. Gently push the IUD through the guide into position. Excessive pain or bleeding is often a sign of perforation. Consult a physician immediately (most common perforation sites: Fundus, body of uterus, and cervical wall).

N. Remove the guide sheath.

O. Remove the tenaculum.

P. Cut the IUD strings to approximately 1-inch length past the cervix.

Q. Remove the speculum.

R. Check the patient's blood pressure and pulse to rule out vasovagal potential.

S. Recommend a prostaglandin inhibitor if cramping occurs/persists (Motrin 400 mg by mouth four times a day).

T. Prophylactic antibiotics may be used for *systemic bacterial endocarditis* (SBE) prophylaxis. Amoxicillin is used unless there is an amoxicillin/penicillin allergy; then erythromycin or clindamycin may be prescribed. Amoxicillin 3.0 g by mouth 1 hour before the procedure, then 1.5 g by mouth 6 hours later.

1. Erythromycin (EES) 800 mg by mouth 2 hours before the procedure, then 400 mg by mouth 6 hours later.

2. Clindamycin 300 mg by mouth 1 hour before the procedure, then 150 mg 6 hours later.

U. Instruct the patient regarding string location and periodic checks. The patient should not have vaginal intercourse or use a tampon for 7 days (decreasesinfection).

Evaluation/Results of Procedure

A. See the patient after first menses to check for expulsion.

B. If the patient has missed two or more periods, perform a beta human chorionic gonadotropin (HCG) test.

1. Rule out ectopic pregnancy.

2. Explore the canal for IUD.

3. Consider ultrasound to rule out pregnancy/expulsion.

4. Consider flat plate of abdomen.

5. Consult a physician.

C. Yearly evaluation with Pap smear/annual checkup

D. Consider hemoglobin for reports of heavy bleeding with ParaGard.

1. If hemoglobin (Hgb) is less than 9, remove the IUD, provide an alternative method of contraception, and prescribe iron supplement for 2 months.

2. Repeat Hgb in 1 month.

IUD Removal Procedure

A. Remove only during menses (cervix is more dilated).

B. Apply gentle, steady traction; remove slowly.

C. Consider uterine embedding if unable to remove, needs consultation.

Patient Should Call the Office for

A. A missed period

B. Abdominal pain (severe)

C. Temperature 100.4°F not associated with other problems (sinus infection, urinary tract infection [UTI])

D. Foul vaginal odor/discharge, especially if bloody or greenish color

E. Heavy bleeding with clots

Neurologic Examination

Cheryl A. Glass

Description

A. Performance of the neurologic examination is a diagnostic component of many physical examinations. Examination of all cranial nerves is not necessary for every patient; it should be performed based on patient-focused presenting complaints. The purpose of this support tool is to review the cranial nerves and the equipment needed for a neurologic examination.

A neurologic examination identifies dysfunction and assists in accurate diagnosis (see Table II.2).

Components of the Neurologic Examination

A. Thorough history
B. Assessment of mental status
C. Assessment of cranial nerve function
D. Assessment of motor function
E. Assessment of sensory function
F. Assessment of gait
G. Assessment of reflexes

Equipment Required

A. Multiple mental examinations are available. The clock-draw test and the Mini-Mental Examination are two examples.
B. Penlight/ophthalmoscope: Light source
C. Ophthalmoscope
D. Snellen chart/Rosenbaum pocket card
E. Items to taste (salt, sugar)
F. Items to smell (vanilla, cinnamon)
G. Tongue depressor
H. Tuning fork
I. Ticking watch/clock
J. Cotton or soft tissue
K. Pin or other sharp object
L. Reflex hammer

TABLE II.2 Cranial Nerve Function

Cranial Nerve Number	Cranial Nerve	Functional Test
I	Olfactory	Smell reception and interpretation: Assess patency of one nostril at a time. Occlude one nostril, have person close eyes, ask person to sniff item on hand, such as vanilla or cinnamon, and report name of substance.
II	Optic	Vision: Assess acuity and visual fields, using Snellen chart.
III	Oculomotor	Motor: Eye/lid movement up, pupil constriction, visual accommodation. Ask patient to look at the object far away, then place the object in close proximity, noting pupillary constriction at near object. Holding finger in front of face, move finger closer to the nose, noting convergence of eyes when moving closer to nose.
IV	Trochlear	Eye movement up/down: Using penlight, ask patient to follow penlight with eyes, without moving head. Move penlight upward, downward, sideways, and diagonally.
V	Trigeminal	Chewing, jaw opening and clenching, facial sensation: Palpate temporal and masseter muscles as person clenches teeth closed, resisting examiner's attempt to open jaw. Corneal, forehead, eyes, nose/mouth mucosa, teeth, tongue, and ears: Ask person to close eyes: (a) Using light sensation, brush cotton ball across forehead to see if patient feels sensation. (b) Using blunt/sharp object, assess deep sensation alternating blunt/sharp object on skin for sensation.
VI	Abducens	Lateral gaze/eye movement: Holding penlight in front of person's eyes, ask person to follow movements of penlight with eyes without moving head, while examiner performs testing for the six cardinal fields of gaze.
VII	Facial	Corneal reflex, facial expression, taste to the lateral two thirds of tongue, and sensation to pharynx, parasympathetic secretion of tears and saliva: Look for facial symmetry: Ask person to smile, frown, close eyes tightly while resisting attempt for examiner to open eyes. Show all teeth, close mouth, and puff cheeks out. Note symmetry of cheeks.
VIII	Acoustic (vestibulocochlear)	Hearing and equilibrium: Assess hearing by whispered voice, or ticking watch. May use tuning fork for Weber and Rinne tests. Ask patient to walk across room and return, noting gait stability.
IX	Glosso-medulla or glossopharyngeal	Gag reflex, cough, swallow, taste on posterior third of tongue, parasympathetic secretion of salivary glands, and carotid reflex: Using tongue blade, depress tongue, ask the person to say "Ahh." Watch soft palate and uvula rise midline, tonsils move medially. Gag reflex may be elicited by depressing back of tongue with tongue depressor.

(*continued*)

TABLE II.2 Cranial Nerve Function (*continued*)

Cranial Nerve Number	Cranial Nerve	Functional Test
X	Vagus	Laryngeal muscles—muscles of phonation, swallowing, sensation behind ear and part of external canal, parasympathetic secretion of digestive enzymes/peristalsis, as well as involuntary action of heart and lungs. Ask patient to swallow and speak, noting hoarseness in voice if present representing vocal cord abnormality.
XI	Spinal accessory	Head and shoulder movement: Have patient shrug shoulders against resistance from examiner.
XII	Hypoglossal	Tongue movement/muscles, swallowing, and sound articulation: Ask person to stick tongue out and move tongue from side to side.

Source: Adapted from Seidel, Ball, Dains, and Benedict (1991).

Nonstress Test

Jill C. Cash

Description

A. The nonstress test (NST) is a noninvasive test to assess fetal well-being. A fetus with an intact central nervous system with adequate oxygenation will demonstrate transient fetal heart rate (FHR) accelerations in response to fetal movement. Results of the NST must be evaluated with consideration of gestational age. It is not uncommon for a neurologically intact fetus between the ages of 24 and 28 weeks gestation to have a nonreactive NST.

Indications

A. Patients at risk of adverse perinatal outcome
 1. Maternal indications
  a. Hypertension
  b. Maternal cardiac disease
  c. Diabetes (including gestational diabetes)
  d. Renal disease
  e. Hyperthyroidism
  f. Collagen vascular disease
  g. Sickle cell disease
  h. Previous stillbirth
 2. Fetal indications
  a. Intrauterine growth restriction (IUGR)
  b. Postdates (greater than 41 weeks)
  c. Decreased fetal movement

B. Frequency of testing: One must consider prognosis for neonatal survival and severity of maternal disease. In general, most high-risk pregnant women should begin testing by 32 to 34 weeks estimated gestational age (EGA). In case of multiple or severe high-risk conditions, testing may begin at 26 to 28 weeks. Frequency may be weekly or biweekly. If clinical deterioration is noted, reducing the testing interval is prudent.

Precautions

A. A reactive NST is reassuring. However, the significance of abnormal results is less clear. Loss of FHR reactivity may be benign, or it may be a sign of the metabolic consequences of hypoxemia.

Equipment Required

A. Electronic FHR monitor (EFM)
B. Reclining chair or bed/stretcher
C. Sphygmomanometer
D. Vibroacoustic stimulator (protocol dependent)

Procedure

A. Place the patient in the semi-Fowler's position in a recliner or on a stretcher. Optimal positioning includes the patient tilted to the left or right side to avoid vena caval compression. The patient is preferably nonfasting and has not recently smoked.
B. Measure the patient's blood pressure.
C. Apply EFM on the maternal abdomen.
D. Record FHR for 20 to 40 minutes. Ask the mother to record fetal movements with a marker button, if available. However, all accelerations may be counted as they probably have the same significance whether or not they occur in response to the fetal movement felt by the mother.
E. Interpret FHR tracing as reactive or nonreactive (see the following).
F. If the fetus is suspected to be in a sleep state, a vibroacoustic stimulation device may be applied, placed on the maternal abdomen, and used for a 3-second stimulation in an attempt to awaken the fetus.

Evaluation/Results of Procedure

A. Reactive NST: Baseline FHR 110 to 160 beats per minute (bpm) with two or more accelerations of greater than or equal to 15 bpm amplitude that last at least 15 seconds or more, within a 20-minute period. **(Note: Before 32 weeks of gestation, accelerations are defined as two accelerations or more greater than 10 bpm amplitude that last at least longer than 10 seconds over a 20-minute period.)** If these criteria are met before 20 minutes, the test may be declared reactive. The FHR tracing may be continued for at least 40 minutes to account for the typical fetal sleep–wake cycle.
B. Nonreactive NST: The aforementioned criteria are not met within the 40-minute time frame.

Treatment

A. If the NST is a reactive, reassuring test, continue obstetrical prenatal care. Further testing is required for maternal and fetal indications as previously noted.

Consultation/Referral

A. Further evaluation is mandatory for a nonreactive NST. Consult with a physician. Depending on the situation, the patient could be given juice or sent to eat and return later for a repeat NST. She may undergo a modified NST, which includes a single 1- to 3-second sound (vibroacoustic) stimulation applied to the maternal abdomen plus the assessment of amniotic fluid and/or biophysical profile (BPP). She may also be sent to the hospital for another NST, modified NST, BPP, or a contraction stress test (CST).

The CST should only be performed in a setting where immediate delivery could occur if indicated for fetal distress.

Oral Airway Insertion

Cheryl A. Glass

Description

A. An oropharyngeal airway is a semicircular device used to hold the tongue away from the posterior wall of the pharynx. To insert this device, the mouth and pharynx should first be cleared of secretions, blood, or vomit, using suction tip catheter (if available).

Indications

A. Oral airway insertion can be used to help control the airway, suction, ventilate, and provide oxygenation of the unconscious victim.

Precautions

A. If the victim is conscious, airway insertion may stimulate vomiting and laryngospasm. Oral airways should be inserted only if the victim is unconscious, unresponsive, and has no gag reflex.
B. If the airway is too long, it could press the epiglottis against the entrance of the larynx and produce a complete airway obstruction.
C. If the airway is not inserted properly, it can push the tongue posteriorly and worsen an upper airway obstruction.
D. If the tongue and/or lips are between the teeth, trauma will result.
E. Oral airways should not be inserted if the victim has sustained oral trauma or has recently had oral surgery.

Equipment Required

A. An oropharyngeal airway (selection/measurement of the airway size is measured from the earlobe to the corner of the mouth)
B. A tongue blade
C. Gloves
D. A suction tip and canister (if available)

Procedure

A. Place head/neck in the correct position (see Figure II.3).
B. The best way to insert an oral airway is to turn it backward (upside down) as it enters the mouth.

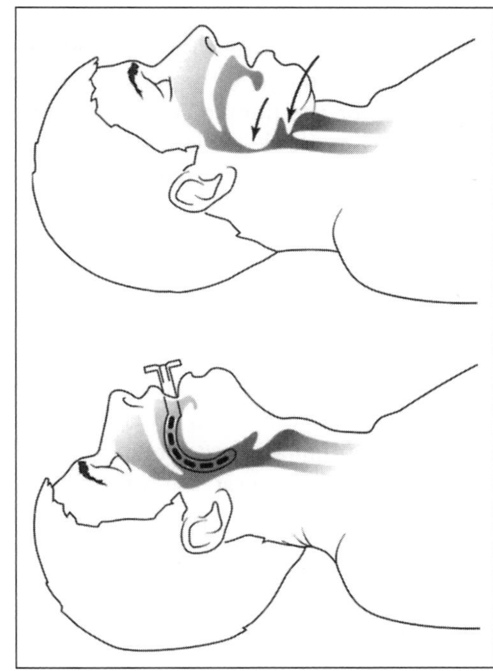

FIGURE II.3 Insertion of an oral airway.

C. As the airway transverses the oral cavity and approaches the posterior wall of the pharynx, rotate it into the proper position.
D. Open the victim's mouth using a cross-finger technique. An alternate method is to move the tongue out of the way with a tongue blade before insertion of the airway.
E. The end flared flange of the airway should rest on the victim's lips.
F. Suction if necessary.

Evaluation/Results of Procedure

A. The airway is in the proper position and of the proper size when you hear clear breath sounds on auscultation of the lungs during ventilation.

Pap Smear and Maturation Index Procedure

Rhonda Arthur

Description

A. A Papanicolaou (Pap) smear is a cytologic *screen* that is performed to detect the presence of cancerous and precancerous lesions of the uterine cervix. The procedure involves procuring a sample of both the ectocervix and endocervix. The maturation index (endocrine assessment) is a tool to evaluate atrophic vaginitis/estrogen deficiency.

Indications

A. According to the American Cancer Society (ACS) and the U.S. Preventive Task Force (USPTS) guidelines, all women should begin cervical cancer screening at 21 years. From 21 to 29 years, screen with conventional or liquid-based cytology every 3 years; from 30 to 65 years, screen with conventional or liquid-based cytology every 3 years, or to extend testing time you can use conventional or liquid-based cytology *plus* human papillomavirus (HPV) cotest every 5 years. HPV cotesting should not be used in women younger than 30 years. Stop screening at age older than 65 years with adequate screening history. Screening is not indicated for women who have had a total hysterectomy for benign indications.

A Pap smear may be obtained in pregnancy, or at the end of a period in the menses flow if light. If the patient is having a heavy menstrual flow, the procedure should be rescheduled.

A maturation index is obtained to evaluate decreased estrogenization of the vagina. Both liquid-based and conventional methods for collecting cervical cytology are acceptable.

Precautions

A. Ask the woman not to douche, use any antifungals or spermicides, or have intercourse the night before the procedure so that there will be nothing to interfere with obtaining a good sample.

B. Practitioners should be aware that some women experience discomfort during the Pap smear procedure and should be sensitive to this possibility.

C. In order to procure an adequate Pap smear, care must be taken to obtain a sample from the entire squamocolumnar junction of the cervical portio. (The squamocolumnar junction is more prominent in teens and women on oral contraceptives.)

D. Blood may obscure an adequate cytology interpretation. It is advisable, therefore, to obtain the endocervical sample following the ectocervical sample. Bleeding from the endocervix is common, particularly if a cytobrush is used. A cytobrush is recommended for sampling the endocervix as more cells are retrieved using this tool as compared to a Q-tip.

Equipment Required

A. Speculum (size appropriate for teen/woman)

B. Warm water for lubrication (excessive K-Y jelly may interfere with the smear and reading)

C. Spatula (wooden or plastic)

D. Q-tip or cytobrush

E. Glass slide (two if maturation index)

F. Container for slide(s)

G. Cytology fixative

Procedure (Conventional Method)

A. With the patient draped in a lithotomy position, insert the lightly lubricated speculum and visualize the cervix.

B. With the spatula, sample the entire (360-degree sweep) squamocolumnar junction using gentle pressure applied directly to this area (if visualized). The goal of the technique is to scrape exfoliated cells or those cells held loosely on the surface of the cervix. Vigorous scraping that abrades the cervix yields tissue that is virtually uninterpretable in the cytology smear.

C. Insert the cytobrush or Q-tip until the brush or cotton swab is no longer visible. It is not necessary to insert further to obtain an adequate sample. A fiber-tipped swab should be introduced in the canal and rotated clockwise several times to obtain cells. A cotton-tipped swab should first be moistened with saline to prevent cells from adhering to the cotton; a synthetic fiber swab is nonabsorbent and can be used without moistening. Pap smears taken with a brush have been found superior in containing endocervical cells.

D. Wipe the sample from the spatula and roll and twist the brush of the cytobrush or the Q-tip on the glass slide as quickly as possible. The cytobrush sample can be rolled through the spatula sample. It is not necessary to separate these two areas or obtain two slides.

E. Spray the slide with cytology fixative held at a distance of approximately 12 inches to avoid "blasting" the cells from the slide. If held too far away, inadequate spray reaches the slide and drying distortion could result.

1. Allow the slide to dry before covering in transport container.
2. To obtain a cytology specimen from the vaginal cuff (posthysterectomy), use a spatula (rounded end) to scrape the upper lateral third of the vaginal wall. Spread on a slide and fix the slide with cytology fixative.
3. Vaginal pool specimens for a maturation index are often recommended in perimenopausal women; sampling is done by scraping the posterior fornix with the spatula. Spread on a separate slide from the Pap smear and fix the slide.

Procedure (Liquid-Based Cytology)

A. With the patient draped in a lithotomy position, insert the lightly lubricated speculum and visualize the cervix.

B. With the spatula, sample the entire (360-degree sweep) squamocolumnar junction using gentle pressure applied directly to this area (if visualized). The goal of the technique is to scrape exfoliated cells or those cells held

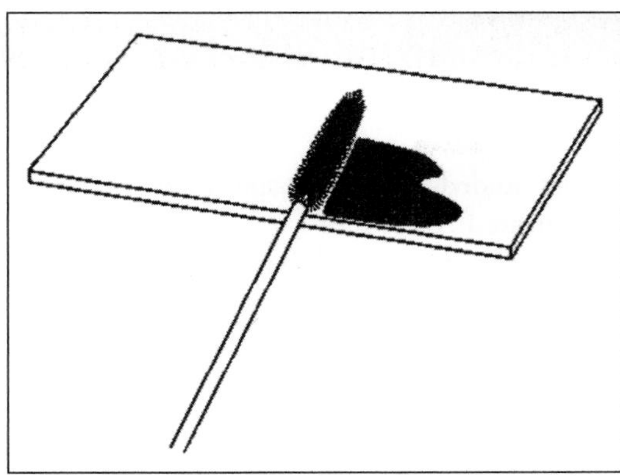

FIGURE II.4 Pap smear cytology brush.

loosely on the surface of the cervix. Rinse the spatula as quickly as possible in the solution by swirling vigorously 10 times and discard the spatula.

C. Insert the cytobrush until only the bottom-most fibers are visible. Rotate slowly one half-turn in one direction (do not overrotate). Rinse the brush quickly by rotating the brush against the container wall and swirling. Place the cap on the specimen container and label properly (see Figure II.4).

D. Alternatively, you may use the broom device instead of the cytobrush. If so, insert the central bristles of the broom device into the endocervical canal (deep enough for the short bristles to contact the ectocervix) and rotate clockwise five times. Rinse the broom by quickly pushing against the bottom of the specimen container and swirling 10 times.

Evaluation/Results of Procedure

A. A Pap smear may be classified as "inadequate" if no endocervical cells are present for interpretation (unless the patient has had a hysterectomy).

B. Pap smear adequacy may be compromised if the slide is allowed to air dry before spraying with cytology fixative.

C. A Pap smear reading may be compromised due to the presence of blood, lubricant, or certain vaginal infections creating an increase in vaginal discharge.

D. See Pap Smear Interpretation and American Society for Colposcopy and Cervical Pathology Consensus guidelines on the management of women with abnormal cervical cancer screening tests algorithms on the Internet at www.asccp.org/asccp-guidelines

Pregnancy: Estimating Date of Delivery

Cheryl A. Glass

The first 12 weeks of pregnancy are vital as the fetal organ systems are developing. Early diagnosis of pregnancy:

A. Allows counseling about potential risks to the developing fetus.
B. Enables the woman contemplating elective abortion to consider her options.
C. Affords diagnosis/intervention in an ectopic pregnancy.
D. Fosters early entry into prenatal care, which in turn may provide early identification of pregnancy complications.

Obtain Menstrual History

A. Obtain sexual history.
B. Obtain fertility history.
- **1.** Length of cycles
- **2.** Regularity of cycles. Regularity of menstruation is influenced by
  - **a.** Recent previous pregnancy and cycles that have not yet reestablished themselves
  - **b.** Breastfeeding
  - **c.** Oral contraceptive pills
  - **d.** Intramuscular contraceptive
  - **e.** Polycystic ovarian syndrome (PCOS)
  - **f.** Comorbid medical conditions

C. Is this a planned pregnancy? If so, how long did it take to conceive?
D. Has the patient been pregnant before? If so, what was the outcome of each pregnancy (miscarriage, stillbirth, live birth), delivery method, and fetal and/or pregnancy complications for each pregnancy?

Initial Assessment/Diagnosis of Pregnancy

A. Is the exact date of the last menstrual period (LMP) known, using the first day of the last period?
B. Was the LMP a normal period? If not, when was the most recent normal period?
C. Is there a known isolated sexual incident that could pinpoint a possible conception date?
D. Does the patient know when conception may have occurred?

Pregnancy Testing

Testing includes analysis of maternal blood or urine for the presence of human chorionic gonadotropin (HCG), a hormone produced by the trophoblastic cells of the developing placenta. **Positive testing is not diagnostic of a normal intrauterine pregnancy.**

A. Maternal blood: HCG
- **1.** Most accurate
- **2.** Earliest to become positive
- **3.** Negative test should be repeated in 2 weeks.

B. Urine
- **1.** More commonly used
- **2.** Accurate 4 to 7 days following conception
- **3.** Available over the counter
- **4.** First-voided morning specimen is best (most concentrated).
- **5.** Negative test should be repeated in 1 week to ensure that the first test was not done too early to detect urine HCG. HCG production decreases after 60 to 70 days, and thereafter declines below the sensitivity of some tests.

Presumptive Signs of Pregnancy

A. Amenorrhea
B. Has experienced pregnancy before and feels pregnant now
C. Nausea/vomiting: Nausea is not limited to “morning sickness.”
D. Fatigue
E. Breast tenderness
F. Urinary frequency
G. Enlarging abdomen
H. Unexplained weight gain
I. Constipation

Probable Signs of Pregnancy

A. Positive Chadwick’s sign: Purplish coloration of vagina and cervix; may be seen on speculum examination.
B. Positive Hegar’s sign: Softening of the lower uterine segment; may be palpated on bimanual examination.
C. Uterine enlargement
- **1.** 8 weeks gestation = 2 times nonpregnant size
- **2.** 10 weeks gestation = 3 times nonpregnant size
- **3.** 12 weeks gestation = 4 times nonpregnant size, uterine fundus (size of orange) palpable at symphysis pubis
- **4.** 16 weeks gestation = uterine fundus midway between symphysis pubis and umbilicus (size of grapefruit)
- **5.** 20 weeks gestation = uterine fundus at umbilicus (size of large honeydew melon)

D. Increased skin pigmentation (face [chloasma], nipples, abdomen [linea nigra])
E. Striae gravidarum: “Stretch marks”

Positive Diagnostic Signs

A. Fetal heart tones (FHTs)
- **1.** 10 to 12 weeks with ultrasonic Doppler (fetal doptone)
- **2.** If unable to hear FHTs with Doptone at 12 weeks (by size and dates), have the patient return at 14 weeks.
- **3.** If unable to hear FHTs at 14-week gestation repeat visit, the patient needs ultrasound examination to confirm fetal viability. Consult with physician if abnormal ultrasound results.
- **4.** 18 to 20 weeks with fetoscope (helps verify estimated date of delivery [EDD])

B. Fetal movements palpated by the mother or health care provider

C. Ultrasound examination

1. Gestational sac visualized by 6 weeks
2. Fetal pole visualized by 8 weeks
3. Fetal cardiac activity visualized by 8 weeks

EDD/Estimated Date of Confinement (EDC)

A. 280 days (40 weeks) after LMP

B. 266 days (38 weeks) from last ovulation (in a 28-day cycle)

C. **Naegele's rule** for establishing EDC: First day of the LMP plus 7 days minus 3 months plus 1 year = EDC.

D. Gestational calculator (in the form of a wheel) may be used to determine EDC. *Gestational wheels are based on a 28-day cycle.*

E. An online calculator is located at www.perinatology.com/calculators/Due-Date.htm

Prostatic Massage Technique: 2-Glass Test

Cheryl A. Glass

Description

A. Obtaining prostatic fluid by prostate massage using the 2-glass test known as the Nickel pre-massage and post-massage test. The Meares-Stamey, 4-glass test is considered too time-consuming and is rarely used by urologists.

Indications

A. Expressed prostatic secretion (EPS) is used to distinguish chronic prostatitis from acute prostatitis or urinary tract infection.

Precautions

A. Do not perform in patients with acute prostatitis (swollen, tender, boggy prostate); may cause septicemia.

Equipment Required

A. Clean-catch specimen cups (2)
B. Labels (2) marked:
   1. Pre massage
   2. Post massage
C. Sterilized towelette

Procedure

A. Collection of a clean-catch midstream urine specimen for male patients: The patient should retract the foreskin (if applies) and cleanse the glans penis with a sterilized towelette in order to avoid contamination.
B. The patient should collect a midstream flow of urine by starting the flow of urination, then catch at least 10 mL urine specimen in the first clean-catch specimen cup marked "pre-massage." The patient should be instructed to then stop the flow of urine.
C. The patient is asked to lean over the examining table for a digital rectal examination. With a lubricated index finger, gently enter the rectum. The prostate should be massaged by stroking it from the periphery toward the midline several times on each side (similar to a windshield wiper).
D. Following the massage, ask the patient to provide more urine in the second clean-catch specimen cup labeled "post-massage."
E. Send both the pre massage and post massage urine specimens for urine cultures.

Treatment

A. See Table II.3.

TABLE II.3 Evaluation and Results of Prostatic Secretions

Diagnosis	Microscopic Evaluation	Treatment
Urethritis	WBC, bacteria in VB_1; in no other specimens	<40 years, probably sexually transmitted infection (STI) Rx: Rocephin and doxycycline
		>40 years, probably coliform bacteria Rx: Bactrim/Septra DS po bid × 5–7 days
Cystitis	WBC, RBCs, bacteria in VB_2	Bactrim DS po bid × 5–7 days
Acute prostatitis	WBC, bacteria in VB_2 and/or EPS, VB_3	Bactrim DS po bid for 3–4 weeks
		Alternative: Quinolones: Cipro 500 mg bid for 3–4 weeks
		May need hospitalization for IV antibiotics
Chronic prostatitis	Bacteria in EPS and/or VB_3, but not in VB_1 or VB_2	Bactrim DS po bid *or* Cipro 500 mg bid for 3–4 months

bid, twice a day; EPS, expressed prostatic secretion; IV, intravenous; po, per os; RBC, red blood cell; Rx, prescription; STI, sexually transmitted infection; VB1, first void urine; VB2, midstream urine; WBC, white blood cell.

Rectal Prolapse Reduction

Cheryl A. Glass

Description

There are three types of rectal prolapse:

A. *Internal*: Patient complains of a protrusion, but no protrusion is noted on examination.

B. *Partial*: Anus is inverted; rectal mucosa protrudes 1 to 3 cm out of rectal sphincter.

C. *Complete*: All layers of rectum have intussuscepted through the anus. (Rare in adults; most often seen in children and the elderly.)

Indications

A. Diagnosis of rectal prolapse is made by inspection. Several populations are at risk for rectal prolapse, including infants, multiparous women, and the elderly. Other factors associated with rectal prolapse include malnutrition, severe constipation, severe chronic diarrhea, obstetrical injuries, rectal intercourse, and multiple sclerosis, as well as other neuromuscular diseases.

Hemorrhoids, mucosal prolapse, polyps, and cancer must be ruled out. Conditions associated with rectal prolapse include cystic fibrosis, ulcerative colitis, intussusception, and Hirschsprung's disease.

Precautions

A. Refer patients with complete prolapse to a physician for evaluation and treatment. After a rectal prolapse reduction by proctoscope, follow-up testing by a barium enema or endoscopy is indicated.

B. Surgery may also be indicated, depending on the degree of prolapse, recurrence, and risk of strangulation. **Children need further assessment for sexual abuse and cystic fibrosis.**

C. Patients with a history of surgery for rectal prolapse should be evaluated and assessed for hemorrhage, bowel obstruction, pelvic abscess, fecal impaction, and recurrent prolapse.

D. Instruct the patient on a high-residue diet, and warn him or her to avoid straining to induce a bowel movement.

Equipment Required

A. Sterile gauze
B. Normal saline
C. Anoscope
D. Water-soluble lubricant
E. Gloves
F. Chux pads and tissue
G. Light source
H. Examination table

Procedure

A. Explain the procedure to the patient and discuss all steps just before performing. Explain that during the procedure relaxation of the anal sphincter is key.

B. Obtain the patient's consent.

C. Ask the patient to void. (Urinary stress incontinence is common during the procedure.)

D. Apply gloves.

E. As the procedure is being done, give the patient and/or caregiver instructions on how reduction is done in the event of another prolapse.

1. Provide the patients with gloves and lubricant for future need.
2. Prolapses may also reduce spontaneously without any manual reduction.

F. Have the patient lie in the left lateral position and give extra tissues for urinary incontinence.

G. Ask the patient to strain (perform Valsalva's maneuver). This allows the practitioner to fully evaluate the prolapse through the anal sphincter. If this does not produce the prolapse, have the patient squat and/or sit on the toilet to strain.

H. With a good light source, do a detailed visual examination to rule out hemorrhoids versus a complete/partial prolapse.

1. Thrombosed hemorrhoids appear as blue, shiny masses.
2. A normal hemorrhoid appears as a painless, flaccid skin tag.
3. Anoscope reveals internal hemorrhoids as bright red to purplish bulges.
4. Rectal prolapse looks like a pink doughnut or rosette; a complete prolapse involving the muscular wall is larger, red, and has circular folds.

I. After visual inspection/evaluation, reposition the patient into a knee–chest position. This allows the bowel to be pulled back into the anus.

J. If, after changing positions, the prolapse does not reduce with gravity, place a saline-soaked 4-by-4 gauze over the prolapse to prevent drying.

K. Apply gentle pressure with the saline gauze, and replace the rectal prolapse/protrusion back through the anus.

L. Using a lubricated gloved hand, perform a rectal examination to evaluate sphincter tone at rest and with some straining. This rectal examination should be painless. Pain raises suspicion for other pathology, such as incarceration or an unrelated lesion.

M. Apply lubricant to anoscope and slowly insert it anteriorly into the rectum. Remove inner cannula of anoscope, and slowly withdraw it to evaluate and identify any lesions. It is rare to see a polyp or carcinoma. Usually, erythema and edema will be noted.

Evaluation/Results of Procedure

A. If reduction of rectal prolapse occurs with minimal discomfort, have the patient return in 1 week to assess sphincter function.

B. If unable to reduce prolapse, send the patient for *immediate* evaluation by a physician. Keep prolapse covered with saline-soaked gauze during transport.

C. If prolapse was partial or complete, refer the patient to a physician after reduction.

D. Further evaluation may include a sigmoidoscopy, barium enema, or biopsy.

E. Presence of pain may indicate an incarceration with impending strangulation and requires *immediate* referral.

F. All patients need to follow a high-fiber diet and have instructions on avoiding straining. Stool softeners are recommended daily.

Sprain Evaluation

Julie Adkins

McMurray Test for Knee Sprains

A. Explain the procedure.
B. Ask the patient to lie down on his or her back (supine).
C. The affected leg, right or left, should have hip flexed 60 to 70 degrees.
D. The injured knee is flexed 45 degrees.
E. Hold the foot in one hand and place the fingers of the other hand on the joint line.
F. Evaluate the patient's pain level when palpating the joint when the knee is flexed.
G. Apply valgus force by holding the femur steady and slowly move the lower leg laterally while still applying the valgus stress.
H. Then flex the knee to 135 degrees and switch to varus stress.
I. Finally, extend the knee in the varus position.
J. If the test is positive, a meniscus click or pop can be felt, which is characteristic of an anterior cruciate ligament tear or relocation.

Anterior Drawer Test for Evaluation of Lateral Ankle Sprain

A. Explain the procedure.
B. Perform this test on the uninjured ankle first, then repeat on the injured ankle.
C. Ask the patient to position the affected foot in the plantar flexion position (foot slightly at rest).
D. Grasp the lower portion of the uninjured leg for bracing. Use one hand at the shin and attempt to draw the heel anteriorly (forward) with your other hand.
E. Repeat the test on the injured ankle.
F. Anterior drawer test is positive for an ankle sprain if the talus at the injured point slides 4 mm or more than the same bone in the other joint.

Talar Tile Test for Evaluation of Lateral Ankle Sprain

A. Explain the procedure.
B. Perform this test on the uninjured ankle first, and then repeat on the injured ankle.
C. To perform the talar test, grasp the lower heel with one hand while adducting or inverting the foot with your other hand.
D. The test is positive if the tilt is 5 to 10 degrees greater around the injured joint.

Tick Removal

Cheryl A. Glass

Description

A. Ticks are vectors for Lyme disease and Rocky Mountain spotted fever. Ticks should be removed as soon as possible because they pass.

Indications

A. There are several populations at risk of tick-borne transmission diseases, including hunters, campers, landscapers, persons in contact with dogs and other animals with ticks, and those in contact with heavy, brushy vegetation.

Equipment Required

A. Tweezers
B. Antiseptic or rubbing alcohol
C. Gloves, nonsterile may be used
D. Office setting: Scalpel if the tick head remains embedded

Procedure

A. Use gloves.
B. To remove the tick, care should be taken to avoid squeezing the body of the tick.
  1. Tick should be grasped with fine-tip tweezers close to the skin.
  2. Remove by gently pulling the tick upward straight out without using any twisting motions (see figures).
  3. Do not crush the tick during removal.
C. Examine for the entire head and body removal; if the head is embedded, a small incision may be required for the removal.
D. Cleanse the skin with antiseptic or rubbing alcohol.
E. Save the tick for identification. Write the patient's name, date of removal, and date of the tick bite on a piece of paper. Place the paper and the tick in a resealable bag and place it in the freezer.

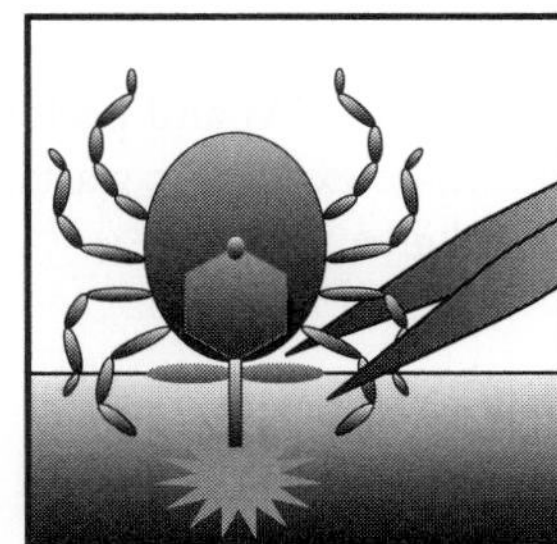

Grasp the tick's body as close to the skin as possible using a fine-tip tweezers. Avoid squeezing the body.

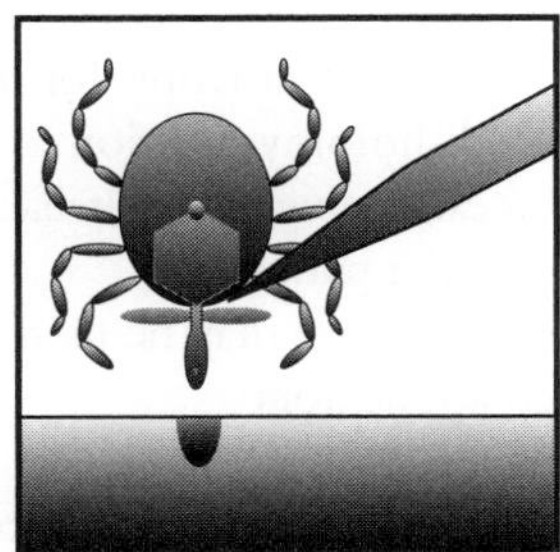

Remove by pulling the tick straight upward without using twisting motions.

Evaluation/Results of Procedure

A. Examine the rest of the body for other ticks.
B. Try to determine the length of time the tick was on the skin.
C. Assess for symptoms of Lyme disease and Rocky Mountain spotted fever.
D. Serum laboratory studies, medications, and consultants as applicable. See Chapter 16: "Infectious Disease Guidelines," "Lyme Disease" for assessment, diagnosis, and treatment guidelines.

Trichloroacetic Acid/Podophyllin Therapy

Rhonda Arthur

Description

A. Trichloroacetic acid (TCA) and podophyllin are substances used to eliminate exophytic warts on the external genitalia and perianal area.

Indications

A. External genitalia and perianal warts

Precautions

A. Podophyllin use is contraindicated in pregnancy.
B. Either substance should be applied sparingly to avoid contact with unaffected skin.

Equipment Required

A. Examining table with stirrups for positioning the female client in the lithotomy position
B. Light source for examining the genitalia and perianal area
C. Gown/drape for the patient
D. Gloves: Nonsterile glove may be used.
E. Cotton-tipped applicators
F. Petroleum jelly
G. Sodium bicarbonate (baking soda) or powder with talc
H. Plastic medicine cups
I. TCA 80% to 90% *or*
J. Podophyllin 10% to 25% in compound tincture of benzoin

Procedure

A. Assist the female client to the lithotomy position; assist the male client to a sitting or supine position on the examination table.
B. Inspect the external genitalia and perianal areas for exophytic warts.
C. Pour small amount (0.5–1.0 mL) of solution (TCA or podophyllin) to be used in a plastic medicine cup.
D. Use the cotton-tipped applicator to apply petroleum jelly on unaffected skin surrounding areas identified for therapy.
E. Use the wooden end of the cotton-tipped applicator to apply a small amount of solution (TCA or podophyllin) to warts.
F. If TCA is used, apply sodium bicarbonate or powder with talc to absorb unreacted acid.
G. If podophyllin is used, instruct the client to thoroughly wash off the solution in 1 to 4 hours.
H. Repeat weekly if necessary. If warts persist after six applications, consider other therapeutic methods.
I. Advise the client that mild to moderate pain or local irritation may occur after treatment.

Wet Mount/Cervical Cultures Procedure

Jill C. Cash and Cheryl A. Glass

Description

A. The wet mount procedure is a technique used to identify vulvovaginitis commonly caused by trichomoniasis, bacterial vaginosis, and vulvovaginal candidiasis. Any patient complaining of vaginal discharge, irritation, vaginal pain, and/or a vaginal odor should have a wet mount performed to aid in identifying the organism to assist in the diagnosis.

Indications

A. Vaginal discharge
B. Vulvar/vaginal irritation or pain
C. Vaginal discharge with an odor
D. Before the examination: Take a thorough history before the physical examination to determine if other testing needs to be performed.
E. Presenting complaints (refer to Table II.4 for a comparison of bacterial vaginosis, candidiasis, and trichomoniasis).

1. Bacterial vaginosis—complaints of a thin off-white "grayish" discharge, as well as a musty "fishy" amine odor. The odor increases after intercourse.
2. Vulvovaginal candidiasis—thick, white "cottage cheese" discharge with no odor is observed, as well as pruritus and some dysuria.
3. Trichomoniasis (parasite *Trichomonas vaginalis*)—copious, frothy, yellow gray to green-colored, malodorous vaginal discharge, pruritus, and vaginal irritation. *The patient may also be asymptomatic.*

Precautions

A. Use universal precautions when obtaining specimens.
B. All specimens need to be disposed of as biohazard waste.

Equipment Required

A. Examining table with stirrups for positioning the patient in the lithotomy position
B. Light source for examining the cervix
C. Gown/drape for the patient
D. Gloves, two pairs (nonsterile)
E. Speculum: Always have several different types and sizes of speculums on hand for appropriate sizing, visualization, and comfort.
F. Condoms available if needed
G. Q-tip/cotton-tipped applicators
H. Gen-probe, or other collecting tubes for *Neisseria gonorrhoeae* and *Chlamydia* specimens
I. Small test tube/plastic collection tube
J. Normal saline (NS) and 10% potassium hydroxide (KOH)
K. Glass slides (2): One marked "KOH" and one marked "NS"
L. Cover slips for slides (2)
M. Nitrazine pH test tape
N. Microscope with ×10 and ×40 objectives

Procedure

A. After the patient has voided and changed into a gown, assist the patient into the lithotomy position.
B. Apply gloves.
C. Prepare the test tube/specimen tube with 1 mm of NS. Prepare slides (one marked "KOH" and the other marked "NS"); apply one drop of each solution to a clean slide and set aside.
D. Inspect the perineum for lesions, erythema, fissures, condyloma, and lacerations.

1. Bacterial vaginosis—usually normal-appearing tissue
2. Vulvovaginal candidiasis—vulvar and vaginal erythema, edema, and fissures
3. Vulvar and vaginal edema and erythema

TABLE II.4 Vaginitis Differentiation

	Normal	Bacterial Vaginosis	Candidiasis	Trichomoniasis
Symptom presentation		Odor, discharge, itch	Itch, discomfort, dysuria, thick discharge	Itch, discharge, Merken 70% asymptomatic
Vaginal discharge	Clear to white	Homogeneous, adherent, thin, milky white; malodorous "foul fishy"	Thick, clumpy, white "cottage cheese"	Frothy, gray or yellow-green; malodorous
Clinical findings			Inflammation and erythema	Cervical petechiae "strawberry cervix"
Vaginal pH	3.8–4.2	>4.5	Usually ≤4.5	>4.5
KOH "whiff" test	Negative	Positive	Negative	Often positive
NaCl wet mount	Lacto-bacilli	Clue cells (≥20%), no/few WBCs	Few to many WBCs	Motile flagellated protozoa, many WBCs
KOH wet mount			Pseudohyphae or spores if non-*albicans* species	

KOH, potassium hydroxide; NaCl, sodium chloride; WBCs, white blood cells.

E. Gently insert the speculum into the vagina. Do not use lubricant as this may interfere with the quality of the specimen. Use warm water for lubrication.
F. While inserting the speculum, visualize the vaginal vault, walls, and cervix. Note any irregularities, such as lesions, masses, and lacerations.
G. If the lateral sidewalls collapse and decrease visualization of the cervix, withdraw the speculum. Apply a condom to the speculum and cut the condom tip. Reinsert the condom-covered speculum to visualize the cervix.
H. Observe for vaginal discharge, noting the amount, color, consistency, and odor.

1. Bacterial vaginosis—discolored discharge with odor, homogeneous discharge that adheres to the vaginal walls
2. Vulvovaginal candidiasis—thick, white discharge that adheres to the vaginal walls
3. Frothy, purulent discharge and a "strawberry" cervix can be identified.

I. Collect a sample of discharge with the two Q-tips.

1. Place one Q-tip into a prefilled test tube/specimen tube and make your slide later *or*
2. Collect a sample of discharge with the Q-tip and roll the Q-tip into the NS-prepared slide, then cover with a cover slip.
3. *Then* roll the Q-tip into the KOH-prepared slide.
4. Note any "musty/fishy" amine odor before placing the cover slip on the slide. (Whiff test is positive if amine odor is noted.)

Wet Mount/Cervical Cultures Procedure

A. Using the second Q-tip, roll it over a strip of nitrazine test tape to evaluate pH.
B. Using the Gen-probe, insert the tip onto the cervical os and rotate the tip in the os several times to obtain an adequate specimen (sample for a minimum of about 30 seconds).
C. Withdraw the Gen-probe applicator and place in the appropriate specimen container.
D. Gently remove the speculum and perform a bimanual examination, assessing for cervical motion tenderness and pain.
E. After completing this examination, take the specimens to the lab area for evaluation (while the patient is dressing).
F. Prepare your slides (if you did not follow steps I.1–I.4).

1. Slide 1: Place one drop of NS on the slide; roll the Q-tip and apply cover slip.
2. Slide 2: Place one drop of KOH on the slide and roll the Q-tip; note any "musty/fishy" amine odor from the slide before placing the cover slide.

G. Observe the NS slide first under the microscope. Start on low power, 10×, and adjust the focus until the specimen is clearly seen under the microscope.
H. Observe the entire field and note the number of squamous cells.
I. Switch to the high-powered field, 40×, making sure the light source and the visual focus are adequate.
J. Observe the slide for

1. Vaginal squamous epithelial cells: Appear flat, with clear edges. Red blood cells (RBCs), sperm, polymorphonuclear neutrophils (PMNs) may also be identified (see Figure II.5).
2. Clue cells: Epithelial cells with irregular borders and a granular appearance; may see the presence of coccobacilli bacteria (not present on slide; see Figure II.6).
3. Bacteria
4. *Lactobacilli*: Appear as rods (see Figure II.7).
5. White blood cells (WBCs): Note, a large number of WBCs is not normal.
6. Trichomonads: Appear as ovoid mobile organisms that dart around on the slide (see Figures II.8 and II.9).
7. *Candida*: Appear as branching pseudohyphae or budding yeast (best seen under the KOH slide; see Figure II.10).

Treatment

A. Refer to specific chapters for treatment recommendations and medication dosages.

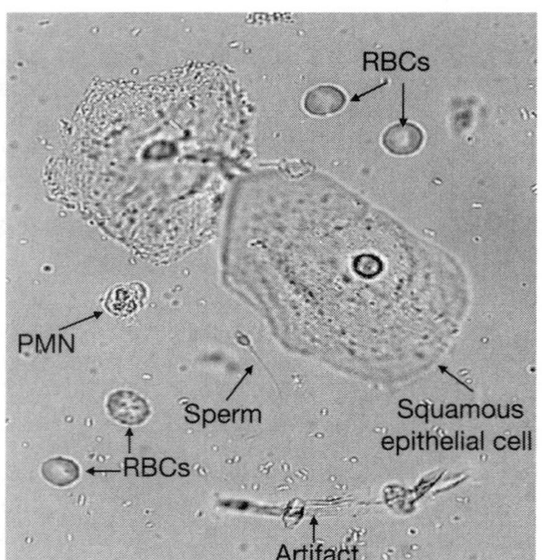

FIGURE II.5 Epithelial cells.
PMN, polymorphonuclear neutrophils; RBC, red blood cell.
Source: Reprinted with permission from the University of Washington STD Prevention Training Center.

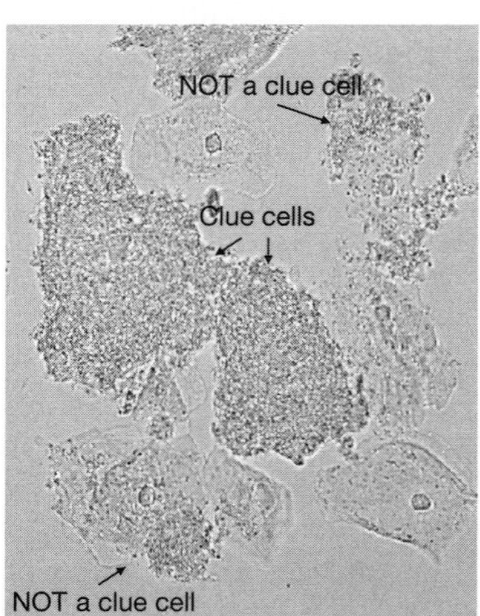

FIGURE II.6 Clue cells.
Source: Reprinted with permission from the University of Washington STD Prevention Training Center.

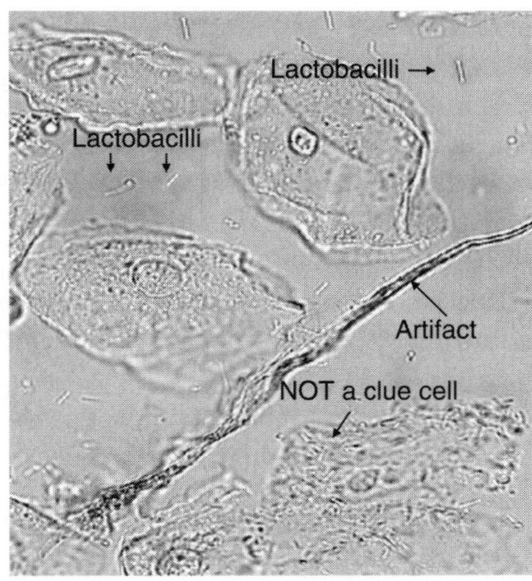

FIGURE II.7 *Lactobacilli.*
Source: Reprinted with permission from the University of Washington STD Prevention Training Center.

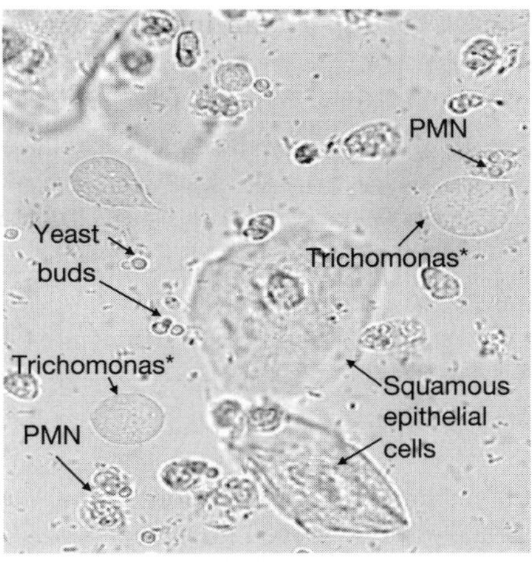

FIGURE II.9 *Trichomonas* (1,000×).
PMN, polymorphonuclear neutrophils.
Note: Organism is enlarged.
Source: Reprinted with permission from the University of Washington STD Prevention Training Center.

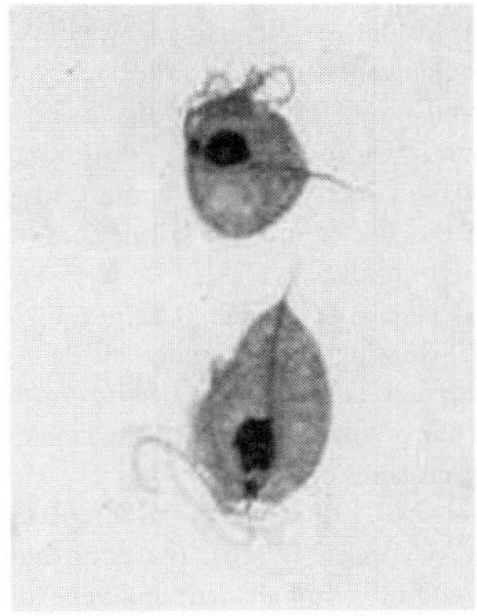

FIGURE II.8 *Trichomonas vaginalis.*
Source: Reprinted with permission from the University of Washington STD Prevention Training Center.

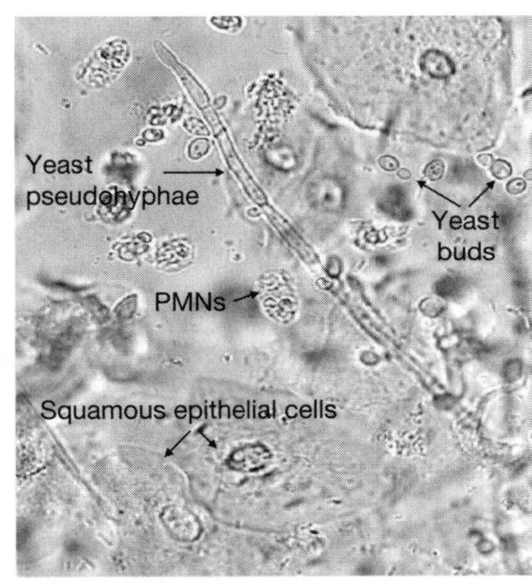

FIGURE II.10 Budding yeast cells, pseudohyphae, and septate hyphae and spores.
PMN, polymorphonuclear neutrophils.
Source: Reprinted with permission from the University of Washington STD Prevention Training Center.

Bibliography

American Cancer Society. (2012). Cervical cancer prevention and early detection. Retrieved from http://www.cancer.org/cancer/cervicalcancer/moreinformation/cervicalcancerpreventionandearlydetection/index

American College of Obstetricians and Gynecologists. (2009, July, reaffirmed 2015). ACOG Practice Bulletin No. 106: Intrapartum fetal heart rate monitoring: Nomenclature interpretation, and general management principles. *Obstetrics and Gynecology, 114*, 192–202.

American College of Obstetricians and Gynecologists. (2010, November, reaffirmed 2015). ACOG Practice Bulletin No. 116: Management of intrapartum fetal heart rate tracing. *Obstetrics and Gynecology, 116*, 1232–1240.

American National Red Cross. (2011). Airway adjuncts. Retrieved from https://www.redcross.org/images/MEDIA_CustomProductCatalog/m4240191_AirwayAdjunctsFactandSkill.pdf

American Society for Colposcopy and Cervical Pathology. (2013). Updated consensus guidelines for the management of abnormal cervical cancer screening test and cancer precursors. *Journal of Lower Genital Tract Disease, 17*, S1–S27.

American Urological Association. (n.d.). Adult urodynamics: AUA/SUFU guideline. Retrieved from www.auanet.org/education/adult-urodynamics.cfm

Beattie, S. (2005, February 1). Placing an oropharyngeal airway. *Modern Medicine.* Retrieved from www.modernmedicine.com/node/40231

Blumenfeld, H. (n.d.). Neuroanatomy through clinical cases: Extraocular movements (CN III, IV, VI). Retrieved from http://www.neuroexam.com/content.php?p=20

Cheuck, L. (2012, June 22). Diagnostic prostatic massage technique. *Medscape.* Retrieved from http://emedicine.medscape.com/article/1948091-technique#2aab6b3b2

Collins, C. W., & Winters, J. C.; American Urological Association; Society of Urodynamics Female Pelvic Medicine and Urogenital Reconstruction. (2014). AUA/SUFU adult urodynamics guideline: A clinical review. *Urologic Clinics of North America, 41*(3), 353–362, vii.

Da Costa Andrade, S., Chianca da Silva, F., dos Santos Oliveira, S., Souza Leite, K., Ferreira da Costa, T., & Lacet Zaccara, A. A. (2014). Microbiological agents of vulvovaginitis identified by Pap smear. *Journal of Nursing UFPE/Revista De Enfermagem UFPE, 8*(2), 338–345.

Davis, R., Jones, J. S., Barcocas, D. A., Castle, E. P., Lang, E. K., Leveillee, R. J., . . . Weitzel, W. (2012). Diagnosis, evaluation, and follow-up of asymptomatic microhematuria (AMH) in adults: AUA guideline. *American Urological Association (AUA).* Retrieved from https://www.auanet.org/education/guidelines/asymptomatic-microhematuria.cfm

Dickey, R. P. (2014). *Managing contraceptive pill patients* (15th ed.). Fort Collins, CO: E.M.I.S. Medical Publishing.

Dubey, P. K. (2016). Another method for the removal of spherical nasal foreign bodies in pediatric patients. *Journal of Emergency Medicine (0736-4679), 50*(1), 125–126.

The Epley Maneuver: A Simple Cure for a Common Cause of Vertigo. (2010–2013). In R. Porter (Ed.), *The Merck manual home health handbook.* Whitehouse Station, NJ: Merck Sharp & Dohme Corp., Retrieved from http://www.merckmanuals.com/home

Family Practice Notebook.com. Orthopedics Book. (n.d.a). Ankle anterior drawer test. Retrieved from http://www.fpnotebook.com/Ortho/Exam/AnklAntrDrwrTst.htm

Family Practice Notebook.com. Orthopedics Book. (n.d.b). McMurray test. Retrieved from http://www.fpnotebook.com/Ortho/Exam/McmryTst.htm

Family Practice Notebook.com. Orthopedics Book. (n.d.c) Talar tilt. Retrieved from http://www.fpnotebook.com/Ortho/Exam/TlrTlt.htm

Fetzer, S. (2015). Advance practice nursing guide to the neurological exam. *Nursing News, 39*(3), 14.

Fundakowski, C. E., Moon, S., & Torres, L. (2013). The snare technique: A novel atraumatic method for the removal of difficult nasal foreign bodies. *Journal of Emergency Medicine, 44*(1), 104–106.

Hatcher, R. A., Trussell, J., Nelson, A. L., Cates, W., Kowal, D., & Policar, M. S. (Eds.). (2011). *Contraceptive technology* (20th ed.). New York, NY: Ardent Media.

Hubbard, E. J., Santini, V., Blankevoort, C. G., Volkers, K. M., Barrup, M. S., Byerly, L., ... Stern, R. A. (2008). Clock drawing performance in cognitively normal elderly. *Archives of Clinical Neuropsychology, 23*(3), 295–327.

Interstitial Cystitis Association. (2013). Urodyamics: What, when, why. Retrieved from www.idhelp.org/page.aspx?pid=990

Jørgensen, K., Kristensen, M. K., Waldemar, G., & Vogel, A. (2015). The six-item clock drawing test—Reliability and validity in mild Alzheimer's disease. *Neuropsychology, Development, and Cognition. Section B, Aging, Neuropsychology and Cognition*, *22*(3), 301–311.

Kennard, C. (2013). Clock drawing test. *About.com Alzheimer's/Dementia.* Retrieved from http://alzheimers.about.com/od/diagnosisissues/a/clock_test.htm?p=1

Krause, R. S. (2011, July 15). Reduction of rectal prolapse. *Medscape Reference.* Retrieved from http://emedicine.medscape.com/article/80982-overview

Lab Tests Online. (2013, May 9). Vaginitis and vaginosis. Retrieved from http://labtestsonline.org/understanding/conditions/vaginitis/start/2

Lowe, S., & Saxe, J. (1998). *Microscopic procedures for primary care providers.* Philadelphia, PA: Lippincott, Williams & Wilkins.

Miller, M. (2014). Recurrent vulvovaginitis: Tips for treating a common condition. *Contemporary OB/GYN, 59*(8), 22–27.

National Kidney and Urologic Diseases Information Clearinghouse (NKUDIC). (2014, January). Urodynamic testing (NIH Publication No. 12–5106). Retrieved from http://kidney.niddk.nih.gov/kudiseases/pubs/urodynamic/index.aspx

Peters, R., Beckett, N., Pereira, L., Poulter, R., Pinto, E., Ma, S., ... Bulpitt, C. (2015). The clock drawing test, mortality, incident cardiovascular events and dementia. *International Journal of Geriatric Psychiatry, 30*(4), 416–421.

Rehabilitation Institute of Chicago. (n.d.). The clock draw test. Retrieved from www.rehabmeasures.org

Ricci, M., Pigliautile, M., D'Ambrosio, V., Ercolani, S., Bianchini, C., Ruggiero, C., ... Mecocci, P. (2016). The clock drawing test as a screening tool in mild cognitive impairment and very mild dementia: A new brief method of scoring and normative data in the elderly. *Neurological Sciences, 37*(6), 867–873.

Rouleau, I., Salmon, D. P., Butters, N., Kennedy, C., & McGuire, K. (1992). Quantitative and qualitative analyses of clock drawings in Alzheimer's and Huntington's disease. *Brain and Cognition, 18*, 70–87.

Sand, P. K. (2008). Diagnostic procedures in the evaluation of female urinary incontinence and voiding dysfunction. In S. Arulkumaran (Ed.), *The global library of women's medicine.* Carlisle, United Kingdom: The Foundation for The Global Library of Women's Medicine. Retrieved from www.glowm.com/section_view/heading/DiagnosticProceduresintheEvaluationofFemaleUrinaryIncontinenceandVoidingDysfunction/item/55. Update currently under review due 2016.

Seattle STD/HIV Prevention Training Center at the University of Washington.

Young, B. K. (2013, January 9). Antepartum fetal heart rate assessment. *UpToDate.* Retrieved from www.uptodate.com/contents/antepartum-fetal-heart-rate-assessment?source=search_result&search=antepartum+fetal+heart+rate+assessment&selectedTitle=1~72

Zasler, N. D. (2015). Validity assessment and the neurological physical examination. *NeuroRehabilitation, 36*(4), 401–413.

III Patient Teaching Guides

- Abdominal Pain: Adults
- Abdominal Pain: Children
- Acne Rosacea
- Acne Vulgaris
- Acute Otitis Media
- Addison's Disease
- ADHD: Coping Strategies for Teens and Adults
- ADHD: Tips for Caregivers of a Child With ADHD
- Adolescent Nutrition
- Alcohol and Drug Dependence
- Allergic Rhinitis
- Amenorrhea
- Ankle Exercises
- Aphthous Stomatitis
- Asthma
- Asthma: Action Plan and Peak Flow Monitoring
- Asthma: How to Use a Metered-Dose Inhaler
- Atherosclerosis and Hyperlipidemia
- Atrial Fibrillation
- Atrophic Vaginitis
- Back Stretches
- Bacterial Pneumonia: Adult
- Bacterial Pneumonia: Child
- Bacterial Vaginosis
- Basal Body Temperature Measurement
- Bell's Palsy
- Bipolar Disorder
- Bronchiolitis: Child
- Bronchitis, Acute
- Bronchitis, Chronic
- Cerumen Impaction (Earwax)
- Cervicitis
- Chickenpox (Varicella)
- Childhood Nutrition
- Chlamydia
- Chronic Obstructive Pulmonary Disease
- Chronic Pain
- Chronic Venous Insufficiency
- Colic: Ways to Soothe a Fussy Baby
- Common Cold
- Conjunctivitis
- Constipation Relief
- Contraception: How to Take Birth Control Pills (for a 28-Day Cycle)
- Cough
- Crohn's Disease
- Croup, Viral
- Cushing's Syndrome
- Deep Vein Thrombosis
- Dementia
- Dermatitis
- Diabetes
- Diarrhea
- Dysmenorrhea (Painful Menstrual Cramps or Periods)
- Dyspareunia (Pain With Intercourse)
- Eczema
- Emergency Contraception—Levonogestrel
- Emergency Contraception—Ulipristal Acetate
- Emphysema
- Endometritis
- Epididymitis
- Erythema Multiforme
- Exercise
- Eye Medication Administration
- Febrile Seizures (Child)
- Fibrocystic Breast Changes and Breast Pain
- Fibromyalgia
- Folliculitis
- Gastroesophageal Reflux Disease
- Gestational Diabetes
- Gonorrhea
- Gout
- Grief
- Head Injury: Mild
- Hemorrhoids
- Herpes Simplex Virus
- Herpes Zoster, or Shingles
- HIV/AIDS: Resources for Patients
- Human Papillomavirus
- Infant Nutrition
- Influenza (Flu)
- Insect Bites and Stings
- Insulin Therapy During Pregnancy

- Iron-Deficiency Anemia (Pregnancy)
- Irritable Bowel Syndrome
- Jaundice and Hepatitis
- Kidney Disease: Chronic
- Knee Exercises
- Lactose Intolerance and Malabsorption
- Lice (Pediculosis)
- Lichen Planus
- Lyme Disease and Removal of a Tick
- Lymphedema
- Mastitis
- Menopause
- Migraine Headache
- Mononucleosis
- Myasthenia Gravis
- Nicotine Dependence
- Nosebleeds
- Oral Thrush in Children
- Osteoarthritis
- Osteoporosis
- Otitis Externa
- Otitis Media with Effusion
- Parkinson's Disease Management
- Pelvic Inflammatory Disease
- Peripheral Arterial Disease
- Pernicious Anemia
- Pharyngitis
- Pityriasis Rosea
- Pneumonia, Viral: Adult
- Pneumonia, Viral: Child
- Polymyalgia Rheumatica
- Postpartum: Breast Engorgement and Sore Nipples
- Premenstrual Syndrome
- Preterm Labor
- Prostatic Hypertrophy/Benign
- Prostatitis
- Pseudogout
- Psoriasis
- Respiratory Syncytial Virus
- RICE Therapy and Exercise Therapy
- Ringworm (Tinea)
- Rocky Mountain Spotted Fever and Removal of a Tick
- Roundworms and Pinworms
- Scabies
- Seborrheic Dermatitis
- Shortness of Breath
- Sinusitis
- Skin Care Assessment
- Sleep Apnea
- Sleep Disorders/Insomnia
- Superficial Thrombophlebitis
- Syphilis
- Systemic Lupus Erythematosus
- Testicular Self-Examination
- Tinea Versicolor
- Tinnitus
- Toxoplasmosis
- Transient Ischemic Attack
- Trichomoniasis
- Trigeminal Neuralgia
- Ulcer Management
- Urinary Incontinence: Women
- Urinary Tract Infection (Acute Cystitis)
- Urinary Tract Infection During Pregnancy: Pyelonephritis
- Vaginal Bleeding: First Trimester
- Vaginal Bleeding: Second and Third Trimesters
- Vaginal Yeast Infection
- Varicose Veins
- Warts
- Wound Care: Lower Extremity Ulcers
- Wound Care: Pressure Ulcers
- Wound Care: Wounds
- Wound Infection: Episiotomy and Cesarean Section
- Xerosis (Winter Itch)
- Zika Virus Infection

ABDOMINAL PAIN: ADULTS

PROBLEM

Problems relating to abdominal organs may range from simple gas to appendicitis. Acute pain is pain that has started recently; recurrent pain is present on three or more separate occasions over at least a 3-month period.

It is important that you call the health care provider if you have pain that lasts 3 hours or longer, have fever, vomiting, or pain that is unusually sharp or intense.

CAUSE

Pain may result from inflammation, ischemia (poor blood supply), distension, constipation, or obstruction. Gastroenteritis is the most common cause of acute pain, and chronic stool retention (constipation) is the most common cause of chronic pain. Urinary tract infections (UTIs) can also cause abdominal pain.

A. Males: Torsion of the testicles or a strangulated inguinal hernia may cause abdominal pain.

B. Females: If you have missed a period or suspect you are pregnant, tell your health care provider; ectopic pregnancies are a medical emergency.

PREVENTION/CARE

The following suggestions can prevent abdominal pain from constipation:

A. Go to the bathroom as soon as you have the urge to have a bowel movement (BM).

B. Establish a regular toilet time such as after breakfast; 15 to 20 minutes after breakfast provides a good time, because spontaneous colonic motility is greatest during that period.

TREATMENT PLAN

Do not take laxatives, use enemas, take drugs, food, or liquids (including water) until consulting your health care provider for suspected abdominal pain and the following:

A. Increased or odd-looking vomit or stools

B. Hard, swollen abdomen

C. Lump in scrotum, groin, or lower abdomen

D. Missed period or suspected pregnancy

Activity: Engage in activity as tolerated. Abdominal pain with nausea and vomiting, with fever, or pain that lasts more than 3 hours and makes you stop doing daily activities should be reported.

Diet: Eat regular foods as tolerated. Do not eat food or drink liquids until you see a health care provider if you have pain with nausea and vomiting, with fever, or pain that lasts longer than 3 hours.

Medications:

You Have Been Prescribed: ______________________________

You Need to Take: ______________________________

You Need to Notify the Office If You Have:

A. Any change in first symptoms that brought you to the office

B. Fever higher than ______________________________ degrees

C. Other: ______________________________

Phone: ______________________________

ABDOMINAL PAIN: CHILDREN

PROBLEM

Pain in your child's "tummy" may range from simple gas to appendicitis. It is important to call the health care provider if your child has abdominal pain that lasts 3 hours or longer, has a fever, vomiting, or pain that is unusually sharp or intense. Signs that your child has abdominal pain include: lying down and drawing the his or her knees into the stomach; crying when you try to touch his or her stomach; or pointing to an area, such as the navel, when crying.

CAUSE

Pain may result from inflammation, distension, constipation, or obstruction. A gastrointestinal (GI) stomach bug (gastroenteritis) is the most common cause of acute pain. Chronic pain happens if your child holds in bowel movements, which causes constipation. Urinary tract infections (UTIs) can cause abdominal pain, and often the child with a bladder infection does not complain of burning on urination and having to go to the bathroom more often.

PREVENTION/CARE

There is no way to prevent stomach pain, but the following can prevent abdominal pain from constipation:

A. Tell your child to go to the bathroom as soon as he or she feels the urge to go.

B. If possible, set up a regular toilet time such as 15 to 20 minutes after breakfast or after school.

TREATMENT PLAN

Do not give laxatives, enemas, drugs, herbal products, food, or liquids (including water) until consulting your health care provider for suspected abdominal pain and the following:

A. Unusual cry, especially loud crying

B. Increased or odd-looking bowel movements or vomiting

C. Hard, swollen abdomen

D. Lump in scrotum, groin, or lower abdomen (tummy)

E. If you notice pain symptoms, especially if when the child bends his or her legs, draws the knees to his or her chest, and/or points to his or her navel.

Activity: Allow activity as tolerated. Children may not be able to tell you in words what is wrong with them. Children tell you they are in pain with a change in the pitch of their crying and by making faces (grimacing). For example:

A. Refusing to eat or breastfeed

B. Drawing knees to tummy when you touch the stomach

Diet: Do not give baby food or liquids until you see a health care provider if you notice a change in the pitch of your baby's crying, facial grimacing, refusal to suck, or your child draws the knees up to his or her stomach, especially after being touched.

Medications:

You Have Been Prescribed: ______________________________

You Need to Take: ______________________________

You Need to Notify the Office If You Notice That Your Child Has:

A. Any change in first symptoms that brought you to the office

B. Fever higher than ______________________________ degrees

C. Other: ______________________________

Phone: ______________________________

ACNE ROSACEA

PROBLEM

Acne rosacea is a skin condition that affects primarily the nose and face, causing redness, flushing, pimples, and bumps. The blood vessels may be more prominent on the face, causing the skin to appear reddened.

CAUSE

The cause is not known. It is thought to be caused by the blood vessels in the face being too active, causing flushing and redness of the skin.

PREVENTION/CARE

A. Avoid rubbing or massaging the face, which can irritate the skin.

B. Avoid alcoholic beverages.

C. Avoid using harsh soaps/creams on face, including cosmetics that irritate the skin.

D. Wash face with a mild soap, such as Cetaphil or Purpose soap daily. Other suggested daily cleansers are sulfa-based cleanser (Rosanil) or benzoyl peroxide cleanser.

E. Protect the skin when outdoors by wearing protective clothing, hats, and so on, to cover the face. Use a sunscreen with a sun protection formula (SPF) 30 or a zinc-based ointment, such as zinc oxide, on the skin for protection.

F. You may be prescribed an antibiotic by mouth or an antibiotic cream/gel to place on the skin. Use medications as prescribed by your provider.

G. Avoid using steroid creams on your face unless prescribed by your provider.

H. If your skin condition begins to affect your eyes, you need to notify your provider immediately. Do not apply any medications or creams on your eyes unless prescribed by your provider.

TREATMENT PLAN

A. Use antibiotics/medications as prescribed by your provider.

B. Wash face with mild cleanser daily.

Activity: As tolerated. No limitations in physical activity.

Diet:

A. Drink plenty of fluids daily.

B. Avoid alcoholic beverages.

Medications:

You or Your Child Has Been Prescribed: ______________________________

You Need to Take: ______________________________

You Need to Notify the Office If:

A. You have a reaction to any of the medications or cleansers prescribed.

B. Rash appears on your eyes or other new places.

C. Symptoms worsen, or new signs or symptoms present before your next follow-up appointment.

D. Other: ______________________________

Phone: ______________________________

RESOURCE

www.rosacea.org

PATIENT TEACHING GUIDE

ACNE VULGARIS

PROBLEM

Acne vulgaris refers to blackheads, whiteheads, or red nodules noted on the face, back, chest, and arms.

CAUSE

Accumulation of cells and bacteria clog the pores and stimulate an inflammatory response, which results in papule or pustule (pimple or blackhead) formation.

PREVENTION/CARE

A. Wash area with mild soap (Purpose or Basis soap) no more than two times per day.

B. Avoid oil-based makeup and creams. Use matte-finished makeup or pore minimizer.

C. Use facial cleansers and moisturizers such as Cetaphil and Moisturel. These prevent the skin from drying out. Benzoyl peroxide 5% lotion or gel may be used at bedtime to help open pores and kill bacteria.

D. To prevent scarring, do not pick lesions.

E. Avoid excessive sun exposure. Use oil-free sunscreen with sun protection formula (SPF) 15 or greater.

F. Do not get frustrated if lesions return. Do not stop medications without the direction of your provider.

G. Stress can influence outbreaks of lesions. Follow a routine exercise program, practice stress management tactics, and other measures that decrease stress levels in your daily routine.

TREATMENT PLAN

Activity: As tolerated. Physical activity encouraged.

Diet: Eat a well-balanced diet. Drink 8 to 10 glasses of water a day to help keep your skin well hydrated. Cocoa and chocolate do not have an effect on the development of acne vulgaris.

Medications: Antibiotics may need to be prescribed.

You Have Been Prescribed: ________________________________

You Need to Take: ________________________________

You Need to Notify the Office If:

A. You have a reaction to any of the medications prescribed.

B. You are unable to tolerate the prescribed medications.

Phone: ________________________________

ACUTE OTITIS MEDIA

PROBLEM

Acute otitis media is an infection of the middle ear that is commonly caused by bacteria. When an ear infection is present, symptoms may include swelling and pain of the ear, dizziness, and/or a decrease in hearing.

CAUSE

Bacteria or viruses may cause middle ear infections.

PREVENTION/CARE

A. Wash your child's hands often. Always wash hands before eating and after playing, especially when playing with other children.

B. **Do not smoke. Children should not be exposed to secondhand smoke. Secondhand smoke increases the risk of ear infections in children.**

C. Avoid exposure to other children/people as much as possible, especially during the first year of life. Exposure to others increases the risk of contracting a virus that may lead to getting a cold. Many ear infections occur after having a cold or upper respiratory infection.

D. If your child is bottle-fed, do not "prop" the bottle. Always hold your baby when bottle feeding.

E. Do not allow your child to have a bottle at bedtime.

F. Wean your child from the bottle by his or her first birthday.

G. Breastfeeding your baby for the first 6 to 12 months of life is highly recommended. Breastfeeding reduces the risk of ear infections because breast milk contains antibodies that fight against ear infections.

H. Childhood immunizations are encouraged to be given at the recommended ages. Some immunizations, such as the flu vaccine and pneumococcal vaccine, may protect your child from getting ear infections.

TREATMENT PLAN

Follow up with a health care provider as instructed to avoid complications of otitis or permanent hearing loss.

Activity: Your child may not play as much when he or she is sick. Activity is encouraged as tolerated.

Diet: Your child may not eat well when he or she is sick. No change in diet is recommended. Encourage fluids for hydration.

Medications:

A. Children's Tylenol and/or ibuprofen may be used for fever or pain.

B. **Do not use aspirin for children.**

C. Antibiotics may be prescribed for you or your child. Give as prescribed.

You Have Been Prescribed: ______________________________

You Need to Take: ______________________________

Your child needs to finish all of the antibiotics, even though he or she may start to feel better.

You Need to Notify the Office If You Have:

A. Continued fever or no improvement in symptoms in 48 hours

B. A child who acts as if he or she has a stiff neck, headache, or other new symptoms

C. Continual crying or not being able to console your child

D. Rash while taking medicine

E. Other: ______________________________

Phone: ______________________________

ADDISON'S DISEASE

PROBLEM

Addison's disease has many symptoms, including weakness and fatigue, fainting or dizziness, poor appetite, weight loss, nausea, vomiting, diarrhea, abdominal discomfort, skin discoloration, and low blood pressure, as well as cravings for salty foods.

CAUSE

Addison's disease is most commonly caused by your body's unusual ability to attack its own tissues, called autoimmunity. This results in inadequate amounts of cortisol and/or aldosterone produced by the adrenal glands.

TREATMENT PLAN/CARE

A. Wear your identification band stating that you have Addison's disease and that lists treatment, as well as your health care provider's name and phone number.

B. Increased medication dosage will be required during any significant illness, especially with vomiting and/or diarrhea, before dental extractions, and before major surgical procedures. **These issues need to be discussed with your health care provider so you will know the correct dosage of medication to take.**

C. Have injectable cortisol available for emergencies when you are unconscious or otherwise unable to take pills.

Activity: As tolerated, avoid overexertion.

Diet: High-sodium, low-potassium, high-protein diet.

Medications:

You Have Been Prescribed: ______________________________

You Need to Take: ______________________________

You Need to Notify the Office If:

A. You have a reaction to your medications.

B. You cannot tolerate the prescribed medications.

C. You are having dental procedures or surgery to discuss adjusting your medicines.

D. You are sick with nausea and vomiting to discuss adjusting your medicines or coming into the office.

E. Other: ______________________________

Phone: ______________________________

RESOURCES

National Adrenal Diseases Foundation (NADF): www.nadf.us

You can build your own identification bracelets or neck chains from American Medical ID: www.americanmedical-id.com

ADHD: COPING STRATEGIES FOR TEENS AND ADULTS

PROBLEM

Attention deficit/hyperactivity disorder (ADHD) is a common mental health problem in which a person has difficulty paying attention, has a short attention span, and frequently gets in trouble because of behavior issues. The patient may show signs of hyperactivity, difficulty with concentrating, reacting without thinking first, and may also have anger issues.

CAUSE

The cause of ADHD is unknown. However, it may be hereditary.

TREATMENT PLAN/PREVENTION CARE

A. Identify coping skills. Identify what things help you to control your behavior and prevent outbursts.

B. Counseling and therapy are commonly encouraged to help you learn new coping skills to help with your problem. Make sure you keep all appointments with your counselor/therapist.

C. Make sure to clarify all assignments and tasks.

D. Keep simple lists of your chores for the day.

E. Attach reminder notes to logical items; for example, put a self-adhesive note on your bathroom mirror to remind yourself to do something.

F. Organize your things in a logical way. For example, put your medication bottle with your toothbrush so you will be sure to take it in the morning.

G. Establish a daily routine and stick to it.

H. Keep your environment as quiet and peaceful as possible. Seek out work and study sites that are quiet and peaceful.

I. Be good to yourself: Eat well, get enough rest, and exercise.

J. Take your medications as prescribed. If you feel that your medication is not improving your behavior, notify your parent and/or care provider so this can be evaluated.

RESOURCES

Children and Adults With Attention Deficit Hyperactivity Disorder (CHADD): www.chadd.org
The National Attention Deficit Disorder Association: www.add.org
National Resource Center for ADHD: www.help4adhd.org

ADHD: TIPS FOR CAREGIVERS OF A CHILD WITH ADHD

A child with attention deficit hyperactivity disorder (ADHD) may not respond to your direction and discipline as easily as other children. Here are a few ways you can organize your home and your child to try to help him or her.

A. Accept your child's limitations. Understand that his or her activity and inattention are intrinsic. Be as tolerant, low key, and patient as you can possibly be.

B. Provide an outlet for the release of excess energy, such as active games, especially outdoors or in open spaces.

C. Keep your home well organized. Have routines for the usual activities for the day. This will help your child to anticipate activities. Eliminate extraneous noise and clutter, such as having the TV on or piling your kitchen table high with newspapers.

D. Be sure your child gets plenty of rest and good nutrition.

E. Avoid formal gatherings or other places where you and your child will have added stress to behave well.

F. Establish discipline that is firm, reliable, and nonphysical.

G. Stretch your child's attention span by quietly and regularly reading to or playing with him or her. Praise whenever possible.

H. Medications may be very helpful. *Often* they will allow your child to attend to his or her schoolwork; school performance and experience may be much improved.

I. Be active with your child's school. *You* are his or her most interested advocate.

J. Make sure that his or her school placement and program are appropriate. Enlist the support of the school nurse, school psychologist, or principal if needed.

K. Most important, enjoy your child as much as possible. Try to take breaks whenever possible.

ADOLESCENT NUTRITION

A. Adolescents need a well-balanced diet. However, requirements vary depending on the build and gender of the adolescent.

B. Adolescents go through a growing spurt and require extra nutrients during this time.
   1. Girls have a growth spurt generally between 10 and 14 years of age.
   2. Boys have a growth spurt generally between 12 and 15 years of age.

C. To help prevent obesity, it is important to set a good example.
   1. Limit junk foods.
   2. Limit sugary sodas.
   3. Limit fast food.
   4. Serve regular portions, not "super-sized."
   5. Teens need snacks between meals.
   6. Buy fresh vegetables and fruits for snacking.
   7. Many teens do not get enough vitamins from their regular diet and may need a vitamin supplement.

D. Enhance your diet with foods that are a good source of calcium and vitamin D.
   1. Dairy products are an excellent source of calcium and support the bones, making them healthy and stronger. Strong bones decrease the risk of the development of osteoporosis.
   2. Dairy products also provide potassium and maintain and support a healthy blood pressure.
   3. Dairy products fortified with vitamin D are also recommended to support bone health.

E. Choosing foods that are lower in saturated fats and cholesterol will also help to keep cholesterol levels low and decrease the risk of developing high cholesterol and heart disease.

F. Since body image is important to teens, making good decisions for weight control and participating in daily exercises will help reduce the risk of obesity.

Note: If you are concerned about your child's eating habits, eating too much, "bingeing," or not eating enough to control his or her weight, "anorexia," you need to notify our office.

G. A use resource is the U.S. Department of Agriculture Food Pyramid: www.ChooseMyPlate.gov

Suggested Number of Servings of Food Groups Per Day

Food Group	Number of Servings Per Day
Milk/dairy	3
Meat	2–3
Fruits	3–4
Vegetables	4–5
Grains (breads and cereal)	9–11

ALCOHOL AND DRUG DEPENDENCE

PROBLEM

Dependence on alcohol or drugs is a disease with signs and symptoms and a progressive course that requires treatment, just like diabetes or cancer.

CAUSE

Factors that contribute to dependence on alcohol and drugs may include inherited traits, the environment, occupation, socioeconomic status, family and upbringing, personality, life stress, and emotional stress. These factors vary among individuals, but no one factor can account entirely for the risk.

PREVENTION/CARE

The only way to prevent alcohol and/or drug abuse and dependence is not to start. Warning signs for needing help are not always dramatic. The following questions can help identify dependence.

A. **Are you or someone you know experiencing any of the following:**
   1. Steadily drinking or using more at a time or more often?
   2. Setting limits on how much, how often, when, or where you will drink or use other drugs and repeatedly violating your limits?
   3. Keeping a large supply on hand or becoming concerned when you run low?
   4. Drinking or using other drugs before going to activities where they won't be available (e.g., class or work)?
   5. Drinking or using other drugs alone? Drinking or using other drugs every day?
   6. Spending more money than you can afford on alcohol or other drugs?
   7. Doing or saying things when you are under the influence that you regret later or do not remember?
   8. Lying to friends and family about your drinking or other drug use?
   9. Becoming accident prone when you are under the influence (spilling, dropping, or breaking things)?
   10. Regularly hung over the morning after drinking?
   11. Worrying about your drinking or other drug use?
   12. Having work or school problems, such as tardiness or absenteeism?
   13. Reducing contact with friends, or experiencing increasing problems with important relationships?

B. **If you answered "yes" to any of these questions, it suggests your drinking or drug use may be a problem.**

TREATMENT PLAN

A. There are no "quick cures" for alcohol and drug dependence, but early intervention is of utmost importance because it helps avoid the harmful effects of long-term alcohol or other drug use.

B. Your health care provider will be suggesting a plan of action for you to consider. You are strongly encouraged to follow the recommendations.

C. Do not hang around your drinking/drug-using friends. Instead, go to new areas, play new sports, and develop new hobbies.

D. Talk to your provider about seeking professional rehab treatment.

E. Ask about a support group in your area.

Activity: Daily exercise is helpful in alleviating the craving for alcohol and drugs. Walking daily and increasing your tolerance for distance are recommended.

Diet:

A. Avoid caffeine and nicotine, if possible.

B. Try to eat three meals a day and three snacks.

C. You may be given vitamin supplements to help restore the vitamins and minerals that have been depleted as a result of your alcohol or drug dependence.

Medications: Usually, medications are not prescribed because they may make the problem worse. If you are prescribed any medications, take them exactly as directed by your health care provider.

(*continued*)

ALCOHOL AND DRUG DEPENDENCE *(continued)*

You Have Been Prescribed: ______________________________

Vitamins/Minerals: ______________________________

You Need to Take: ______________________________

You Need to Notify the Office If You Have:

A. Severe craving and the urge to use alcohol or drugs

B. Any thoughts of hurting yourself or others

C. Impulsive feelings, like you might do something you will later regret

Phone: ______________________________

RESOURCES

Al-Anon Family: 888-4AL-ANON: www.al-anon.alateen.org
Alcohol Help Line 24 hours a day, 7 days a week: 800-345-3552: www.adcare.com
American Council for Drug Education: 800-488-3784 (DRUG): www.health.gov/nhic
Cocaine Anonymous: 310-559-5833: www.ca.org
Cocaine Hotline 24 hours a day, 7 days a week: 800-262-2463: www.acde.org
Families Anonymous: 800-736-9805: familiesanonymous.org
Mothers Against Drunk Driving (MADD) 24 hours a day, 7 days a week: 877-ASK-MADD: www.madd.org
New Life (Women for Sobriety): 215-536-8026: www.womenforsobriety.org
The Phoenix House: 1-888-286-5027

ALLERGIC RHINITIS

PROBLEM

Allergic rhinitis is a chronic or recurrent condition. Common symptoms are nasal congestion, sneezing, and clear nasal discharge. It is not contagious; therefore, you cannot catch it from anyone, and you cannot spread it to others.

CAUSE

You are having an allergic response after being exposed to an allergen.

PREVENTION/CARE

A. The best prevention is to avoid things you know you are allergic to, for example, smoke (cigarette, cigar, wood smoke); pollens and molds; animal dander; dust mites; and indoor inhalants, such as hair spray and other aerosol spray products.

B. Target your bedroom as "allergy-free" by removing carpets, damp mopping floors weekly, hanging washable curtains instead of blinds, removing books and stuffed animals, using foam pillows, and encasing the pillows and mattress in plastic.

C. Do not blow your nose too frequently or too hard. It may cause your eardrum to perforate (tear). Blow through both nostrils at the same time to equalize the pressure.

D. Use tissues when you blow your nose. Dispose of them and then wash your hands. If no tissue is available, do the "elbow sneeze" into the bend of your arm (away from your open hands). Always wash your hands.

TREATMENT PLAN

A. Use the air conditioner in your house and car to decrease exposure to pollens.

B. Use an air filtration system in your house or buy a small one for your bedroom.

C. Dust your house often, using a cloth and cleaner or polish to keep dust from flying.

D. Allergy testing may need to be done if you have had allergies for a long time. Ask your health care provider about a consultation with an allergist.

Activity: There are no activity restrictions. However, you may want to exercise indoors during the spring, summer, and fall when pollen counts are high.

Diet: Eat well-balanced meals. Drink at least six to eight glasses of liquid a day.

Medications: Common medications used include antihistamines, decongestants, and nasal sprays.

Antihistamines: Some antihistamines may cause drowsiness. Use with caution. You may consider using a different antihistamine during the day that does not cause drowsiness.

Decongestants: Decongestants may increase blood pressure and may also interact with other medications. Please consult with your provider before using these medications.

Nasal Sprays: Nasal saline spray is safe to use in the nose several times a day. Nasal decongestant sprays may be used for a short period of time. Do not use longer than 3 days to prevent causing rebound side effects from this medication. Consult with your provider if using a nasal decongestant spray.

You Have Been Prescribed: ______________________________

You Need to Take: ______________________________

You Need to Notify the Office If:

A. You experience trouble breathing or catching your breath.

B. You have asthma; call if your symptoms are worse.

C. Your symptoms are not any better after using the medications for 3 complete days.

D. Your nasal discharge changes to a greenish color.

E. Other: ______________________________

Phone: ______________________________

AMENORRHEA

PROBLEM

For some reason that we do not fully understand, you have stopped ovulating, or putting out an egg each month, and you have stopped having menstrual periods. This is a very common problem.

It is not immediately dangerous for you. However, it is not good for you to let this go on for a long period of time because the inside lining of your uterus is still being stimulated by estrogen, and over a long period of time, this could become cancerous.

CAUSE

Although the cause is usually unknown, amenorrhea is often associated with low thyroid activity, excessive exercise such as that of an athlete or dancer, or excessive weight loss.

PREVENTION/CARE

There is no specific prevention. However, if you notice a decreased frequency of menstrual periods or absence of menstrual periods when you increase your exercise, you should decrease the intensity of exercise. If you lose too much weight, you could stop having periods. Try to gain some weight.

TREATMENT PLAN

Decrease exercise, increase weight, and replace progesterone.

Activity: Decrease intensity of exercise. Take at least 2 days off each week, and decrease the amount of time during each exercise session.

Sexual Activity: You may have a return of fertility without warning. If pregnancy is undesired, be sure to use an effective birth control prevention method, such as condoms and foam, to prevent unintended pregnancy.

Diet: Increase calories and try to put on 5 pounds if you have lost a lot of weight.

Medications: Your health care provider will prescribe progesterone to replace what your ovaries are not making at the present time. Progesterone may be prescribed in the form of birth control pills.

You Have Been Prescribed: ____________________

You Need to Take: ____________________

You Need to Notify the Office If:

A. You have any new symptoms.

B. You have problems taking your medication.

C. You think you might be pregnant.

D. Other: ____________________

Phone: ____________________

ANKLE EXERCISES

A. Education
   1. Exercise in your bare feet or in stocking feet.
   2. Count slowly (1,001, 1,002, etc.) when you must hold a position and count.
   3. Do each exercise 10 times the first day, and increase the repetitions by 5 each following day until you reach a maximum of 30, unless otherwise instructed.
   4. Repeat prescribed exercises three times a day.
   5. Exercise slowly and get the greatest stretch possible.
   6. Stop any exercise that causes new, unusual, or intense pain.
   7. You need to perform daily stretching exercises and toning to speed your recovery.
   8. It takes months to adequately heal these types of injuries. Therefore, do not be discouraged that it takes time for your ankle to heal.
   9. Sports to avoid: Stop-and-go activity, basketball, running, and impact aerobics.
   10. You may need to wear a velcro ankle brace or high-top tennis shoes for support.

B. Toe and foot bend (floor)
   1. Sit on the floor or bed with legs out straight.
   2. Bend the injured foot back toward the head and curl toes.
   3. Then point the injured foot away and bend the toes back.

C. Toe rise and foot slide (chair)
   1. Sit in a chair with knees bent at a right angle and feet flat on the floor.
   2. Raise all toes on the injured foot and slide the foot back 3 to 4 inches.
   3. Relax.
   4. Continue the sliding and toe raising until the heel can no longer be kept on the floor.

D. Toe and foot bends (chair)
   1. Sit in a chair with knees bent at a right angle and feet flat on the floor.
   2. Slide the foot on the injured side forward as far as possible while keeping the toes and heel in contact with the floor.
   3. From the straight-leg position, bend the foot toward the head as far as possible.
   4. Lower your foot back onto the floor.
   5. Bend the foot back and forth from the straight-leg position.

E. Heel-cord stretch
   1. Stand straight and face a wall with feet together, arms straight out, and palms flat against the wall.
   2. Lean toward the wall, bending the elbows, to stretch the cords above the heels.
   3. Continue leaning to a count of 5 and then straighten up again.

F. Inner-tube stretch
   1. Sit with feet dangling side by side at a right angle to your legs.
   2. Tie stretch bands around your feet until they are snug.
   3. Keeping ankles together, move the toes as far apart as possible.
   4. Hold the stretch for a count of 5.

G. Inner-tube stretch
   1. Sit with feet dangling.
   2. Cross your feet at the ankles.
   3. Tie bands snugly around feet.
   4. Move toes as far apart as possible.
   5. Hold the stretch for a count of 5.

APHTHOUS STOMATITIS

PROBLEM

Aphthous stomatitis describes tender ulcers in the mouth that recur.

CAUSE

The cause is unknown. Possible causes include diet (lack of iron, zinc, or B vitamins), menstrual or hormonal changes, and viruses.

PREVENTION/CARE

A. Preventing ulcers in the mouth can be difficult when the cause is unknown. Some suggestions of prevention include the following:

1. Avoiding trauma/injury to the inside of your mouth (biting cheek, etc.)
2. Avoiding toothpastes and mouth rinses that include sodium lauryl sulfate.
3. Avoiding certain foods that tend to trigger the onset of an ulcer (spicy foods, nuts, cheese, coffee, acidic food, etc.)
4. Maintaining a healthy diet in vitamin B12, folate, iron and/or zinc.
5. Avoiding stress.

TREATMENT PLAN

A. Use an over-the-counter gel such as Anbesol or Orajel four times daily.

B. You may be prescribed a mouthwash made of diphenhydramine (Benadryl), Maalox, and lidocaine or fluocinonide gel to "swish" in your mouth two to four times daily.

Activity: No restrictions are required.

Diet:

A. Avoiding spicy, salty, or hot foods may help.

B. Using a straw when drinking may decrease pain.

C. Cold foods may be easier to tolerate.

D. Avoid hard or sharp food.

E. Use a soft toothbrush.

Medications:

You Have Been Prescribed: ____________________

You Need to Take: ____________________

You Need to Notify the Office If You Have:

A. Worse symptoms than seen at the office visit today

B. Ulcers that do not heal in approximately 1 to 2 weeks

C. Other: ____________________

Phone: ____________________

ASTHMA

PROBLEM

Asthma is a chronic condition with wheezing, coughing, breathlessness, and chest tightness.

CAUSE

The most common cause is inflammation that results from exercise or exposure to environmental irritants, allergens, furry animals, cockroaches, dust mites, pollens and molds, cold air, or viral respiratory infections.

PREVENTION/CARE

Those with asthma are encouraged to get the flu vaccine every year.

You may be able to prevent frequent recurrences of asthma by following these asthma trigger avoidance strategies:

A. *Dust mite allergens:* Wash bedding weekly in hot water and dry it in a hot dryer. Encase pillows and mattresses in airtight covers. Remove carpets, especially from your bedroom. Avoid use of fabric-covered furniture, especially for sleeping.

B. *Cockroach allergens:* Clean your house thoroughly. Use poison bait or traps. Do not leave food or garbage exposed.

C. *Animal fur allergens:* Avoid keeping house pets, or at least do not allow them in sleeping areas.

D. *Smoke allergens:* Avoid all of the following: Smoking, contact with tobacco smoke, smoke from wood-burning stoves or fireplaces, and unvented stoves or heaters.

E. *Outdoor pollens and molds:* Keep windows closed when pollen or mold counts are high.

F. *Indoor mold:* Reduce dampness in your home by using a dehumidifier. Clean damp areas often. Remove carpets that are laid on concrete.

G. *Other irritants:* Avoid perfumes, cleaning agents, and sprays.

TREATMENT PLAN

See the Patient Teaching Guides “Asthma: Action Plan and Peak Flow Monitoring” and “Asthma: How to Use a Metered-Dose Inhaler.”

Activity:

A. If cold air causes symptoms, wear a scarf over your mouth and nose if you must go outside during the winter.

B. Avoid vigorous exercise if this causes asthma symptoms. Learn to recognize activities that trigger your breathing problems.

C. Make an asthma action plan to follow. Copy the plan and place it on the refrigerator door, take a copy of your action plan to school, and give each coach a copy of your asthma action plan.

D. Color code your inhalers with tape or markers, for example, use green tape for quick-relief inhalers, and blue tape for long-acting inhalers.

Diet: There are no diet restrictions unless you have found a food that causes an allergic reaction resulting in trouble with breathing.

Medications: Cough medicines should not be used for asthma symptoms.

You Have Been Prescribed: ____________________

You Need to Take: ____________________

You Need to Notify the Office If You Have:

A. A peak flow reading below 60% of your personal best number that does not return to the yellow or green zone after taking your medication

B. Other: ____________________

Phone: ____________________

ASTHMA: ACTION PLAN AND PEAK FLOW MONITORING

A peak flow meter is a device that measures how well air moves out of your lungs. This measurement is referred to as your "peak expiratory flow," or PEF.

HOW TO USE A PEAK FLOW METER

A. Place the indicator at the bottom of the numbered scale.

B. Stand up.

C. Take a deep breath, filling your lungs as deeply as possible.

D. Place the mouthpiece in your mouth and close your lips around it. Do not put your tongue inside the hole.

E. Blow into the mouthpiece as hard and fast as you can. It is important to give this your best effort.

F. Write down the number on the indicator. If you cough or make a mistake, do not record that number—do it over again.

G. Repeat steps A through F two more times.

H. Write down the highest number of the three attempts. This is your PEF.

CALCULATING YOUR PERSONAL BEST PEAK FLOW NUMBER

This number is the highest peak flow number you can achieve over a 2- to 3-week period when your asthma is under good control (when you do not have any symptoms). To find this number, take peak flow readings:

A. Twice daily for 2 to 3 weeks

B. When you wake up and between noon and 2 p.m.

C. Before and after taking your quick-relief medication

D. Or as directed by your health care provider

THE PEAK FLOW ZONE SYSTEM

Once you have determined your personal best peak flow number, your health care provider can give you the numbers that let you know what medications to take based on your PEF. The numbers are set up like a traffic light system (red, yellow, and green).

Green Zone (80%–100% of your personal best number): Signals *good control.* No asthma symptoms are present, and you should take your medication as usual.

Yellow Zone (50%–80% of your personal best number): Signals *caution.* You may be having an episode of asthma that requires an increase in your medications.

Red Zone (below 50% of your personal best number): Signals a *medical alert.* You must use your "fast" inhaler to help open up your airways right away and call your health care provider immediately if your peak flow number does not return to the yellow or green zone and stay there.

Use the following "Asthma Action Plan," which specifies what medications you should take when you are in each zone and also use the self-assessment diary provided in the table.

ASTHMA ACTION PLAN

A. My personal best PEF is ______________________________

B. When I am in the *green zone,* PEF above ______________, I should continue to take my regularly scheduled asthma medications. They are:

1. ______________________________
2. ______________________________
3. ______________________________

(*continued*)

ASTHMA: ACTION PLAN AND PEAK FLOW MONITORING *(continued)*

Asthma Diary Self-Assessment

Symptom Codes: Rate Your Symptoms 1 (Mild), 2 (Moderate), or 3 (Severe)							
My Personal Best PEF Is ______							
Date	**PEAK FLOW ZONES** ***Green*** **= Good Control** ***Yellow*** **= Caution** ***Red*** **= Emergency**			**Symptoms (Use Codes)** **W = Wheeze** **C = Cough** **S = Shortness of Breath**	**Quick-Relief Medication (Include the Number of Times Needed for Relief)**	**Anti-Inflammatory Medication**	**Additional Medications or Activity**
Monday	A.M.	P.M.	ZONE				

PEF, peak expiratory flow.

C. When I am in the ***yellow zone,*** PEF between ______ and ______, I should add the following to my regularly scheduled medications:

1. ______
2. ______
3. ______

D. When I am in the ***red zone,*** PEF below ______, I should immediately take the following rescue medication and contact my health care provider:

1. Rescue Medication: ______

E. Other Directions: ______

______

______

ASTHMA: HOW TO USE A METERED-DOSE INHALER

USING AN INHALER

To receive the proper dose from your inhaler, you must use good technique. Your health care practitioner may provide you with a drug-free practice inhaler. Practice the following steps until you are comfortable administering your inhalant:

A. Shake the inhaler well immediately before each use.

B. Using a spacer helps to deliver more medication.

C. Remove the cap from the mouthpiece. Hold the inhaler upright. Make sure the medication canister is firmly inserted into the plastic holder (actuator).

D. The first time you use your new inhaler (or if it has been 1 month or longer since the last use), test spray four times into the air.

E. Breathe out through your mouth to the end of a normal breath.

F. Position the mouthpiece about 1 to 2 inches in front of your open mouth. Or you may close your lips in a tight seal around the mouthpiece.

G. Open your mouth widely (unless you are using the closed-lip method), and position your head in a neutral position.

H. While breathing in slowly and deeply, firmly depress the container once.

I. Continue breathing in slowly until your lungs are full.

J. Once you have breathed in fully, hold your breath for 10 seconds or as long as you can.

K. If you need a second puff of the same medication, wait a minimum of 1 minute before repeating steps A through J. If you are using a different inhaler for the second puff, wait at least 5 minutes before using the second inhaler.

OTHER TIPS

A. If you are taking a steroid inhalant, rinse your mouth and throat with water after each dose.

B. When you are short of breath, use your bronchodilator ("rescue medicine") first; then wait about 5 minutes before using your steroid inhaler. The rescue inhaler opens your airways so more of the steroid medication reaches your lungs.

C. Keep the inhaler clean. Once a week, remove the medication canister from the actuator and wash the actuator in warm, soapy water. Rinse and allow to air dry. Replace the medication canister in the holder and recap the mouthpiece.

D. Always check the expiration date on your inhaler and make sure to refill your prescription before the medication expires.

E. Color code your inhalers with tape or markers; for example, use green tape for quick-relief inhalers, and blue tape for long-acting inhalers.

ATHEROSCLEROSIS AND HYPERLIPIDEMIA

PROBLEM

Hyperlipidemia (excess lipids in the blood) is called "hardening of the arteries." The excess lipids increase your risk of developing heart disease and heart attacks.

CAUSE

Elevated blood cholesterol levels lead to plaque formation in the walls of the major arteries in the body. The higher the level of low-density lipoprotein (LDL), or "bad" cholesterol, the greater the chance of getting heart disease. On the other hand, the higher the level of high-density lipoprotein (HDL), or "good" cholesterol, the lower the risk of heart disease.

PREVENTION

Lowering your risk of heart disease involves the following:

A. Diet changes to lower your bad cholesterol (LDL) and raise your good cholesterol (HDL).

B. Lose weight. Start with losing 5 to 10 lb.

C. Start or increase your physical activity. Walking is a good exercise to start getting active.

D. Other ways to modify your risk factors:
   1. Stop smoking.
   2. Control your blood pressure.
   3. If you are a diabetic, control your blood sugar level.

TREATMENT PLAN

Activity:

A. Regular exercise, such as walking vigorously for 30 minutes three times a week, increases your good cholesterol levels, lowers blood sugar, and promotes weight loss.

Diet: Follow the dietary approaches to stop hypertension (DASH) and low-fat/low-cholesterol diet:

A. Decrease total fat calories and cholesterol.

B. Decrease total saturated fats, and replace with monounsaturated fats such as canola oil, olive oil, and margarine.

C. Increase fiber with oatmeal, bran, or fiber supplements.

D. Increase daily intake of fruits and vegetables.

E. Try garlic, soy protein, and vitamin C to help lower LDL cholesterol.

Medications: You may be prescribed a medicine to lower your cholesterol. You will need to come into the doctor's office to have your blood drawn to monitor your liver and cholesterol levels.

You Have Been Prescribed: ______________________________

You Need to Take: ______________________________

You Need to Notify the Office If You Have:

A. Chest pain

B. Shortness of breath or trouble breathing while exercising

C. Abdominal pain

D. Muscle pain or weakness

E. Other: ______________________________

Phone: ______________________________

ATRIAL FIBRILLATION

PROBLEM

Atrial fibrillation is the condition that causes the upper chambers of the heart (the atria) to beat faster and irregularly (also called fibrillation). The upper chambers of the heart do not beat at the same time as the lower chambers (the ventricles). When atrial fibrillation occurs, blood clots can form in the heart and then travel to the brain, causing a stroke.

CAUSE

Atrial fibrillation is caused by a malfunction of the heart's pacemaker. Many things can cause the heart's pacemaker to malfunction, including excessive alcohol intake, emotional stress, physical stress, recent heart surgery, medication side effects, and a long list of medical conditions. These medical conditions include coronary artery disease, leaky heart valves, high blood pressure, heart failure, heart attack, thyroid disease, infections, inflammation around the heart, sleep apnea, obesity, and lung diseases such as chronic obstructive pulmonary disease, bronchitis, asthma, and emphysema.

PREVENTION/CARE

A. Stop smoking. Discuss smoking cessation with your health care provider.

B. Reduce or eliminate intake of alcohol and caffeine.

C. Lose weight. Discuss losing weight with your health care provider.

D. Make a list of your current medical conditions and current medications. Keep an updated copy in your wallet.

E. When traveling:
   1. Always travel with enough of your medication to last through your vacation plus an additional 3 days.

TREATMENT PLAN

A. Take your medications as ordered by your health care provider.

B. Effectively manage all other medical conditions, paying special attention to cholesterol, blood pressure, thyroid disease, sleep apnea, and any lung diseases.

C. Follow up with your primary health care provider and/or cardiologist on a regularly scheduled basis.

Activity:

A. Get regular exercise, after discussing the type and frequency of exercise that is safe for you with your health care provider.

Diet:

A. Eat a balanced, low-fat, and low-salt diet in addition to dietary guidelines suggested by your health care provider.

B. If you are taking the blood thinner Coumadin, you will be given a list of foods that are high in vitamin K. These foods can interfere with how the blood thinner works. Please discuss these foods further with your health care provider.

Medications:

You Have Been Prescribed: ____________________

You Need to Take: ____________________

You Need to Notify the Office If:

A. You have any of the following symptoms:
   1. Palpitations or a fluttering in your chest
   2. Chest pain
   3. Weakness or extreme tiredness
   4. Shortness of breath at rest or with activity
   5. Dizziness
   6. Disorientation
   7. Confusion

(continued)

ATRIAL FIBRILLATION *(continued)*

8. Passing out or losing consciousness
9. Severe headache
10. Frequent urination or a compelling urge to urinate
11. Anxiety or panic symptoms

B. Vomiting or other illness causes you to miss more than one dose of your medications.

C. Other: ______________________________

Phone: ______________________________

RESOURCES

American Heart Association: www.heart.org
National Heart, Lung, and Blood Institute: www.nhlbi.nih.gov

ATROPHIC VAGINITIS

PROBLEM

You have been diagnosed with atrophic vaginitis. This means that the cells lining your vagina are thinner, less pliable, and less lubricated and so are more prone to tears and abrasion. This is a natural part of aging, and it is also very common with teens and with breastfeeding.

CAUSE

Atrophic vaginitis is caused by an alteration in estrogen either from premature ovarian failure, delayed puberty, breastfeeding, or naturally occurring menopause.

PREVENTION/CARE

A. This is a physical problem, *not* an emotional problem.
   1. If you are a preadolescent girl, the symptoms will decrease as puberty approaches.
   2. If you are breastfeeding, your symptoms will resolve after weaning the baby.
   3. If you are menopausal or have premature ovarian failure, your symptoms will get better after starting a hormone replacement pill or using a hormonal vaginal cream.

B. You also can help your symptoms by doing the following:
   1. Use good hygiene; wipe yourself from front to back with every urination and bowel movement.
   2. Avoid perfumed hygiene sprays, talcs, and harsh soaps.
   3. Wear cotton underwear.
   4. Sleep without underwear.
   5. Use a water-soluble vaginal lubricant with sexual intercourse, such as K-Y jelly or Astroglide. **Do not use Vaseline.** Vaseline can contribute to infections.
   6. Regular sexual activity or masturbation facilitates the natural production of lubricating secretions of your body.
   7. Kegel exercise (using the muscles that start and stop the flow of the urine stream) improves the muscle tone and elasticity of the vagina.
   8. The female-superior “on top” or side-lying position for sexual intercourse gives you the ability to control the depth of thrusting with the penis, and this may make sex more comfortable.
   9. Yogurt douches or acidophilus tablets by mouth or inserted into your vagina can help maintain the vaginal pH to prevent vaginitis.

TREATMENT PLAN

A. Vitamin E oil may be used for vaginal dryness.

B. Use K-Y jelly or other water-soluble lubricants for intercourse.

C. You may be prescribed an estrogen cream or hormone replacements for menopause.

D. If you still have your uterus, hormones need to be balanced with estrogen and progesterone to prevent the lining of the uterus from overgrowing. Follow your hormone therapy instructions.

E. You still need regular Pap smears, even if you do not have a period.

Activity: Increase foreplay for increased lubrication. Try the previous suggestions on sexual positions for greater comfort and control.

Diet: As tolerated.

Medication:

You Have Been Prescribed: ____________________

You Need to Take It/Use It: ____________________

(*continued*)

ATROPHIC VAGINITIS (*continued*)

You Need to Notify the Office If You Have:

A. No relief of symptoms after following the aforementioned instructions
B. No relief of symptoms after beginning the hormonal replacements
C. Vaginal bleeding after intercourse
D. A change in your symptoms
E. Other: ______________________________

Phone: ______________________________

BACK STRETCHES

You have been approved to do back-stretching exercises to help with your low back pain. Follow the instructions, starting slowly to build your strength.

EQUIPMENT

Use a mat or a towel on the floor for extra padding and comfort.

A. In the lying position
   1. Lie on your back with knees bent. Cross your arms over your chest.
   2. Raise your head and shoulders and curl your trunk upward, no more than 6 inches.
   3. Keep the small of your back pressed against the mat.
   4. Exhale during the curl up.
   5. Hold ____________ seconds; do ____________ repetitions ____________ times a day (see Figure 1).

B. In the standing position
   1. Stand with your back against the wall.
   2. Place your feet shoulder width apart and 18 in. from the wall.
   3. Slowly slide down the wall until you are in the "chair" position.
   4. Hold for 10 seconds and relax, then slide back up the wall to a standing position.
   5. Do ____________ repetitions ____________ times a day (see Figure 2).

C. In the lying position
   1. Bring your right knee slowly to your chest, holding it in place with your hands on your knee.
   2. Relax the buttock and your back muscles.
   3. Hold ____________ seconds, then relax with your right knee down.
   4. Repeat with your left knee.
   5. Now that you have stretched both legs, pull both of your knees up, holding them in place with your hands on your knees.
   6. You will be curled in the fetal position.
   7. Hold ____________ seconds, then relax with your knees down.
   8. Do ____________ repetitions, ____________ times per day (see Figure 3).

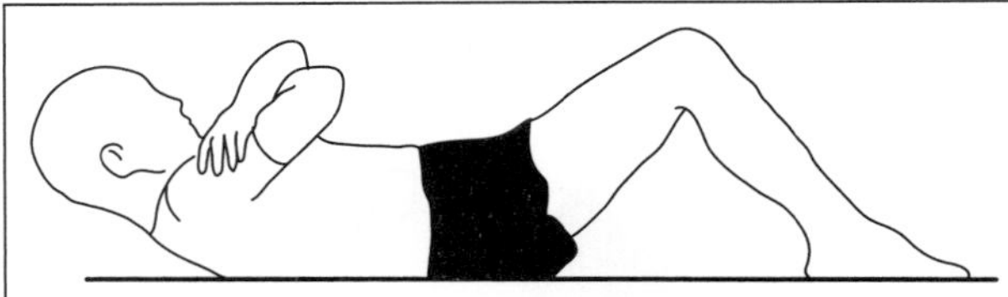

FIGURE 1 Lie on a mat or towel. Raise head and shoulders as demonstrated.

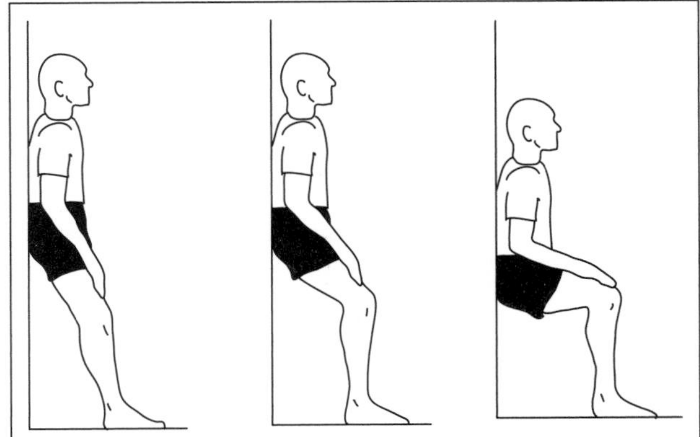

FIGURE 2 Place your feet shoulder width apart. Slide down against the wall to the "chair" position.

(*continued*)

BACK STRETCHES *(continued)*

D. In the lying position
  1. Lie on your back with your knees bent.
  2. Tighten your abdominal muscles and squeeze. As you squeeze the buttock muscles, flatten your back toward the mat/towel (as shown in Figure 4). Relax.
  3. Tighten your buttock muscles and lift your abdomen or "tummy" toward your knees while arching your back. Relax.
  4. Hold __________ seconds; do __________ repetitions __________ times a day (see Figure 4).

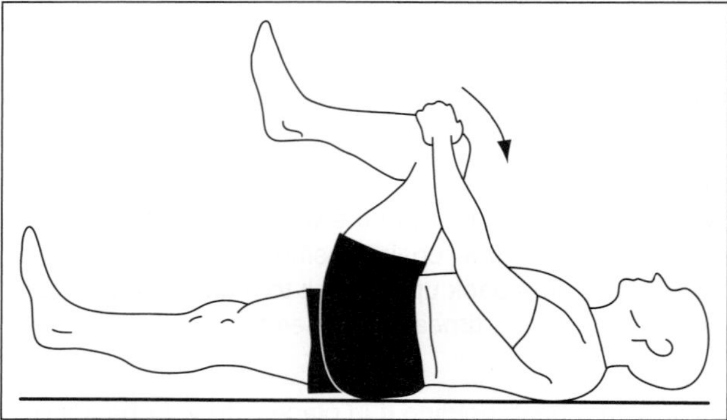

FIGURE 3 Pull your left knee toward your chest to stretch; repeat with your right knee as demonstrated.

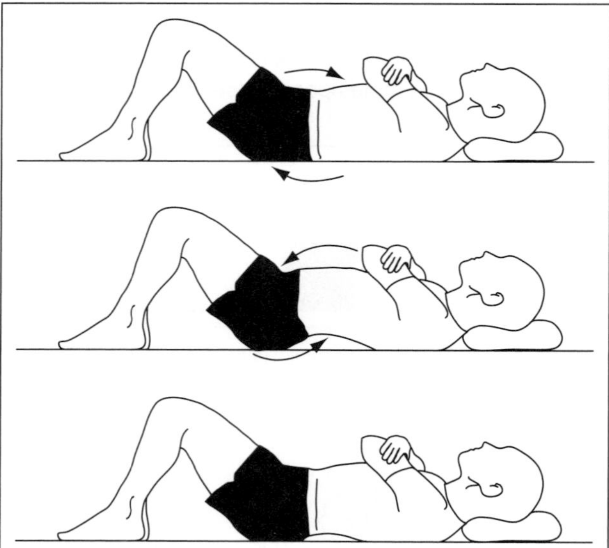

FIGURE 4 Lie with knees bent, flatten your back, and then lift your tummy toward knees with back arched.

BACTERIAL PNEUMONIA: ADULT

PROBLEM

Pneumonia is a lung infection that causes fluid to collect in the air sacs. You may have a fever, cough, or trouble breathing.

CAUSE

Respiratory bacteria or viruses cause pneumonia.

PREVENTION/CARE

People older than 65 years and younger people with severe lung disease may receive a vaccine to prevent pneumococcal pneumonia.

The flu vaccine is recommended to be taken every year.

TREATMENT PLAN

A. Use a cool-mist humidifier. Clean the humidifier daily.

B. Do not smoke, and avoid smoke-filled rooms.

C. Cover your mouth when you cough and cover your nose when you sneeze.

D. Use tissues when you blow your nose. Throw away tissues as soon as they are used. If no tissue is available, do the "elbow sneeze" into the bend of your arm.

E. Wash your hands frequently with soap and water.

Activity: Rest during the early phase of the illness.

Diet: Eat a nutritious diet. Drink 8 to 10 glasses of water a day.

Medications:

A. Do not use cough suppressants if your cough produces sputum. Use them only for a dry, nonproductive cough.

B. Acetaminophen (Tylenol) may be used for fever or body aches.

C. Antibiotics are given for pneumonia that is caused by bacteria. Take your medication as directed.

D. Finish all of your antibiotics even though you may feel better.

You Have Been Prescribed: ______________________________

You Need to Take: ______________________________

You Need to Notify the Office If You Have:

A. Increased difficulty breathing

B. Fever after 48 hours on an antibiotic

C. Blood in your sputum

D. Worsening discomfort or fatigue

E. Other: ______________________________

Phone: ______________________________

BACTERIAL PNEUMONIA: CHILD

PROBLEM

Bacterial pneumonia is a lung infection that causes fluid to collect in the air sacs. Your child may have a fever, cough, or trouble breathing.

CAUSE

Respiratory bacteria cause pneumonia.

PREVENTION/CARE

A. Keep your children away from people with respiratory illnesses.

B. The flu vaccine is recommended every year.

TREATMENT PLAN

A. Encourage fluids.

B. Use a vaporizer or humidifier to increase humidity in your child's room. Clean the humidifier or vaporizer daily.

C. Keep your child away from cigarette smoke.

D. Teach your child to cover his or her mouth when coughing and to cover his or her nose when sneezing.

E. Use tissues when your child blows his or her nose. Throw away all tissues as soon as they are used. If there are no tissues available, teach your child to do the "elbow sneeze" into the bend of the arm.

F. Use good handwashing with soap and water.

Activity: Have your child rest at first (during the acute phase). Children may return to school after 24 hours of antibiotic therapy and when they have no fever for 24 hours.

Diet: There are no diet restrictions with pneumonia. Your child may not be very hungry when he or she is feeling very sick. Encourage the child to drink liquids or suck on ice pops.

Medications:

A. Your child should take all of the antibiotics prescribed as directed.

B. It is very important for your child to finish the antibiotic, even though he or she may feel well.

C. Acetaminophen (Tylenol) may be given for fever. ***Children 18 years or younger should not be given aspirin.***

D. Do not give your child cough medicine; it is important that he or she can cough to break up any mucus. **The American College of Chest Physicians clinical guidelines recommend that cough suppressants and over-the-counter cough medications *not* be given to young children. Cough and cold medicines should *not* be given to children younger than 6 years.**

You Have Been Prescribed: ____________________

You Need to Take: ____________________

You Need to Notify the Office Immediately If:

A. Your child's breathing becomes faster, more labored or difficult.

B. Retractions (tugging between ribs) become worse.

C. Your child's lips become blue.

D. Grunting sounds occur when breathing out.

E. Your child starts acting very sick.

F. Other: ____________________

(*continued*)

BACTERIAL PNEUMONIA: CHILD *(continued)*

You Need to Notify the Office Within 24 Hours If:

A. Your child is unable to sleep.

B. Your child is not drinking enough.

C. Fever lasts longer than 48 hours on antibiotics.

D. You feel your child is getting worse.

E. Other: ______________________________

Phone: ______________________________

BACTERIAL VAGINOSIS

PROBLEM

You have been diagnosed with a vaginal infection, also known as bacterial vaginosis (BV). This is a very common problem that has a "fishy vaginal discharge." The odor increases after sexual intercourse, but it is not considered a sexually transmitted infection. Recurrence is common, and your partner may also need to be treated.

YOU CAN BE TREATED IN PREGNANCY

BV has been associated with premature rupture of the membranes and preterm labor.

CAUSE

BV is caused by an alteration in the normal flora of the vagina. There are many contributing pathogens and factors, including the routine use of douches, antibiotic use, menses, and pregnancy.

PREVENTION/CARE

A. Wear cotton panties or panties with a cotton crotch.

B. Do not wear tight restrictive clothes such as tight jeans.

C. Take off your underwear during sleep.

D. Limit tub bathing and the use of hot tubs or whirlpools.

E. Avoid the use of bubble bath, feminine deodorant sprays, and perfumed sanitary products (sanitary pads, tampons, and toilet paper).

F. Use good hygiene:
   1. Wipe with toilet tissue from front to back after urinating and bowel movements.
   2. Wipe from front to back using clean towels with each bath or shower.
   3. Change your tampons and pads often during your period.

G. Routine douching destroys the normal vaginal flora. Avoid douching unless you are prescribed a medicated douche.

TREATMENT PLAN

A. Try the prevention tips to decrease the recurrence of BV.

B. You may be given a prescription for pills or vaginal creams.

C. Do not use a tampon with vaginal creams because it will absorb the medication.

D. Clindamycin is an oil-based, medicated cream used to treat BV. It can weaken latex condoms for at least 72 hours after stopping the therapy.

E. All treatments (medications and douches) may be used during your period.

F. Metronidazole (Flagyl) oral tablets may be prescribed. The side effects include a sharp, unpleasant metallic taste in the mouth, furry tongue, and some urinary tract symptoms. Please remind your provider if you have a history of seizures or if you are on any blood-thinning drug.

Other Methods of Treatment

A. Vinegar and water douches: 1 tablespoon of white vinegar in 1 pint of water. Douche one to two times a week.

B. *Lactobacillus acidophilus* culture four to six tablets daily.

C. Garlic suppositories: Place one peeled clove of garlic wrapped in a cloth dipped in olive oil into your vagina overnight, and change daily for five nights. You will not smell like garlic.

Activity: As tolerated.

Diet: When taking the medicine metronidazole (Flagyl), you must **avoid alcohol during the entire week you are taking the medicine and 24 hours after your last dose.** The combination of the medicine and alcohol may cause nausea, vomiting, stomach upset, and a headache.

(*continued*)

BACTERIAL VAGINOSIS *(continued)*

Medication:

You Have Been Prescribed: ____________________

You Need to Take: ____________________

You Need to Notify the Office If:

A. You vomited your medication (Flagyl).

B. Your vaginal odor and discharge are not relieved after the medications.

C. You continue to have repeated infections after following the instructions.

D. Other: ____________________

Phone: ____________________

BASAL BODY TEMPERATURE MEASUREMENT

DEFINITION

Basal body temperature (BBT) assessment is done to determine if and when a woman ovulates. It may be used to achieve or prevent pregnancy. During the follicular phase of the normal menstrual cycle (the first 2 weeks), one follicle and the oocyte it contains mature. The normal body temperature during the follicular phase when estrogen dominates ranges from 97.2°F to 97.6°F.

At midcycle, when progesterone dominates, the ovum is extruded from the ovary and may be fertilized any time from 12 to 24 hours later. Ovulation manifests as an increase in BBT from 0.6° to 1°F above your baseline temperature. Some women have a dip in temperature just before the day of ovulation and then their temperature may rise.

Besides taking your temperature to predict ovulation (the best time to try to get pregnant or avoid sexual intercourse), another reason to take it is to check your cervical mucus.

CHECKING YOUR BBT

A. A BBT thermometer must be used. They are easily accessible in the contraceptive section of any pharmacy. If using any other type besides a basal body thermometer, such as a digital thermometer, it must be able to measure to 0.10° due to the slight changes that will be measured.

B. Record your temperature on the temperature chart provided in the thermometer packet or by a health care provider. The chart can be easily copied for as many months as needed.

C. Keeping your BBT calendar:
   1. Day 1 of the cycle is the first day of menstruation/bleeding.
   2. Mark the days of bleeding and other discharge, especially mucus, on the calendar.
   3. Mark any days that you are sick, stay up late, or sleep less than 6 hours because this will interfere with your temperature.
   4. Mark the days that you have sexual intercourse.
   5. Mark your medications on your BBT calendar.

D. Each morning, prior to arising or any activity, place the thermometer under the tongue, leaving it in for 1 minute. Take your temperature consistently at the same time every morning.

E. A temperature elevation that is 0.2°F or greater from your last 6 days of temperature (and that stays elevated) indicates an ovulatory pattern.
   1. This is the time when you are more likely to get pregnant.
      a. If pregnancy is desired, the standard recommendation is that sexual intercourse should be done 2 days before ovulation is expected and every 2 days thereafter until 2 to 4 days have passed following the rise in body temperature.
      b. If pregnancy is not desired, avoid sexual intercourse.

F. The record should be kept for 2 to 6 months minimum.

CHECKING YOUR CERVICAL MUCUS

Your cervical mucus ranges from thick and tacky feeling to thin and slippery, the consistency of egg whites. The type of mucus you have also signals the time of ovulation.

A. Your mucus can be checked daily by touching yourself on the outside or, to be the most accurate, inserting one finger in your vagina to check the cervix.
   1. Wash your hands.
   2. Sit on the toilet and gently insert your finger to feel the cervix.
   3. The cervix feels firm, like the end of your nose.
   4. Check the thickness of the mucus and note it on your BBT chart.

B. After you have your period, the cervical mucus is thick and tacky. It is more difficult to get pregnant when the mucus is thick.

C. As ovulation approaches, you will notice the mucus getting thinner.

D. When the mucus is the consistency feeling of egg whites, that signals ovulation and you are the most fertile.
   1. This is the time to have sexual intercourse/avoid intercourse.
   2. Continue until you see your BBT rise.
   3. You will notice the cervical mucus getting thicker.

BELL'S PALSY

PROBLEM

Bell's palsy is a disorder that can occur at any age, but most frequently occurs between the ages of 20 and 60 years. The disorder affects the muscles associated with expression on one side of the face, including the muscles that allow smiling, closing of the eyes, and raising of the eyebrows.

The exact cause of Bell's palsy remains unknown. Possible causes may include viral infections, a type of inflammatory process, or possibly an autoimmune disease.

PREVENTION/CARE

A. Bell's palsy is usually treated with a steroid, such as prednisone.

B. Pain is usually managed with acetaminophen (Tylenol) or another over-the-counter pain medication; for example, nonprescription anti-inflammatory medications (NSAIDs) such as ibuprofen or naproxen.

C. Sometimes it is helpful to use gentle massage or electrical stimulation of the nerve to help with the pain. Applying heat or cold packs for 15 to 20 minutes three to four times a day may also help with pain. When applying ice packs, do not directly apply ice to the skin and be cautious on skin to avoid frostbite to the area.

D. Protection of the eye is very important if there is loss of lid function. Eye drops and lubricating ointment may be recommended along with taping the affected eye while sleeping. Wearing eyeglasses and/or sunglasses is recommended to protect the eye.

E. Physical therapy may also be helpful with recovering function in the muscles that are weak.

F. Symptoms usually resolve within 3 or 4 weeks to a few months. Occasionally, patients have symptoms lasting longer than this. The degree of paralysis varies in each person. If symptoms change or worsen, notify your health care provider immediately.

TREATMENT PLAN

Activity: Engage in activities as tolerated. Use caution when performing activities requiring visual demands such as depth perception (driving, walking, etc.).

Diet: Eat a regular diet as tolerated.

Medications:

You Have Been Prescribed: ____________________

You Need to Take: ____________________

You Need to Notify the Office If You Have:

A. No relief of symptoms in 4 weeks.

B. New symptoms, such as headaches, visual changes, or other problems such as trouble walking.

C. Other: ____________________

Phone: ____________________

RESOURCE

The Bell's Palsy Network: www.bellspalsy.ws

BIPOLAR DISORDER

PROBLEM

Bipolar disorder, formerly called manic-depressive disorder, causes extreme mood changes, ranging from mania or hypomania (emotional "highs") to depression ("lows"). Mania may cause feelings of extreme happiness and increased energy. Sometimes mania causes people to behave in ways that are outside their normal behaviors such as spending too much money, arguing, or making impulsive decisions. Depression can cause feelings of sadness, low energy, low motivation, sleep disturbance, and suicidal thoughts.

CAUSE

The exact cause of bipolar disorder is unknown, but may have to do with physical changes or an imbalance in naturally occurring chemicals in the brain. Bipolar disorder is common in people who have a first-degree relative with the condition.

TREATMENT PLAN

Bipolar disorder is a long-term condition and is sometimes disruptive to daily living. By following a treatment plan and working closely with a mental health professional, mood swings can be managed. The process of finding the right medication may take some trial and error and it can take several weeks for medications to take full effect. Medication doses may need to be adjusted as symptoms change.

A. **Take your medications as prescribed**. Even when you are feeling better, do not stop or change your medication without talking to your provider.

B. **Keep your appointments with your provider.** You are the most important member of your treatment team. It is important for you to visit regularly with your medical provider to discuss your progress, keep your prescriptions current, and to check your lab work when needed. It may be helpful to take along a support person to help you remember questions, instructions, and treatment information. Be honest with your providers about how you feel and worries you may have.

C. **See a therapist or a counselor.** Your medical provider will work with you in managing your medications and your general health needs. A counselor or therapist will meet with you on a regular basis to help you learn about bipolar disorder and to work on effective ways to manage symptoms, cope with stressful situations, and make lifestyle changes that will improve your mental and physical health.

D. **Manage stress.** Stress can make you feel more anxious, worried, irritable, moody, and can get in the way of a good night's sleep. Take time to relax, get creative, spend time with friends/family, take a few deep breaths several times a day, focus on the "positives" in your life, and ask for help when you need it.

E. **Avoid drug and alcohol use.** Drugs and alcohol can alter your mood and interfere with prescribed medications.

F. **Practice good sleep habits.** Let your provider know about any changes in your sleep pattern. Problems with sleeping too much, or too little, can be an early warning sign for mania and/or depression.

Activity: Exercise regularly. Exercise naturally improves mood and gives an overall sense of well-being. Taking a brisk walk for 20 to 30 minutes on most days can help to relieve stress, improve your mood, help you feel better physically, and help to maintain a healthy weight. Check with your provider before starting any exercise program.
Diet: Eat well. Eating foods that are high in fats, sugars, salt, and carbohydrates can cause weight gain and make you feel more tired and sluggish. Eat plenty of fresh fruit and vegetables and try to avoid fried foods, soda, sweet tea, candies, and baked goods.

Medications:

You Have Been Prescribed: ______________________________

Labs Ordered:

You Need to Notify the Office If You Have:

A. Thoughts of harming yourself or someone else. If you are having suicidal thoughts, call 911 or have someone take you to the nearest emergency room.

(*continued*)

BIPOLAR DISORDER *(continued)*

B. No improvement, or worsening of your symptoms, even though you are taking your medications as directed
C. Physical symptoms that may be side effects from prescribed medications
D. Any new symptoms that you are concerned about
E. Other: ________________________________

Phone: ________________________________

Your next scheduled appointment: ________________________________

BRONCHIOLITIS: CHILD

PROBLEM

Bronchiolitis is a lung infection that causes difficulty breathing (respiratory distress), wheezing, coughing, and fever.

CAUSE

Respiratory viruses, usually respiratory syncytial virus (RSV), cause bronchiolitis.

The symptoms generally last approximately 7 to 10 days. Bronchitis usually occurs in fall, winter, and early spring.

PREVENTION/CARE

A. Isolate young infants from people with respiratory illnesses.

B. Avoid large crowds.

C. Wash your hands with soap and water frequently if you are caring for your child.

D. Wash toys and surfaces that your child touches.

E. The flu vaccine should be given to children every year.

TREATMENT PLAN

A. Use a cool-mist humidifier in your child's bedroom and clean the humidifier frequently. If a humidifier is not available, you and your child may stay in a steamy bathroom for 20 minutes two to three times a day.

B. Use warm water and a bulb syringe to clear your baby's stuffy nose.

C. Children should not be exposed to secondhand smoke.

D. Teach your child to cover his or her mouth when he or she coughs and to cover his or her nose when he or she sneezes.

E. Use tissues when your child blows his or her nose. Throw away tissues as soon as they are used.

F. Wash your child's hands with soap and water after coughing and sneezing into a tissue. If a tissue is not available, teach your child to "elbow sneeze" into the bend of his or her arm.

Activity: Children need rest during the early stages of the illness.

Diet:

A. Offer fluids, such as juice and water. Try ice pops if the child does not feel like drinking. Dilute juice for younger infants.

B. Your child may not be hungry but try to get him or her to eat small, frequent feedings.

Medications:

Antibiotics are not prescribed for viral infections. But your child may be given medicines for other symptoms.

The American College of Chest Physicians clinical practice guidelines recommend that cough suppressants and over-the-counter cough medications *not* be given to young children. Cough and cold medicines should *not* be given to children younger than 6 years of age.

You Have Been Prescribed: ______________________________

You Need to Take: ______________________________

You Need to Notify the Office Immediately If:

A. Your child's temperature is 101°F or greater.

B. Breathing becomes labored or difficult or is faster than 60 times a minute.

C. Wheezing becomes severe.

D. Retractions (tugging between ribs) become worse.

E. Your child stops breathing or passes out.

F. Lips become bluish.

(*continued*)

BRONCHIOLITIS: CHILD *(continued)*

G. Your child starts acting very sick or is difficult to arouse.

H. Other: ____

You Need to Notify the Office Within 24 Hours If:

A. Your child is unable to sleep or would not drink enough fluids.

B. Your child has symptoms of an earache such as tugging at his or her ears.

C. Your child has yellowish to green nasal discharge.

D. Fever greater than 100°F lasts more than 72 hours.

E. You feel your child is getting worse.

F. Other: ____

Phone: ______________________________

BRONCHITIS, ACUTE

PROBLEM

Acute bronchitis is a lung infection followed by a productive cough.

CAUSE

Respiratory viruses cause bronchitis.

PREVENTION/CARE

A. Avoid exposure to other people with respiratory illnesses.

B. Do not smoke, and avoid secondhand smoke and other smoke-filled environments.

C. Avoid air pollutants, such as wood smoke, solvents, and cleaners.

D. Cover your nose and mouth with your sneeze or cough.

E. Use tissues when you blow your nose. Throw away all tissues as soon as they are used. If no tissue is available, do the "elbow sneeze" into the bend of your arm.

F. Use good handwashing techniques with soap and water.

G. You are encouraged to take the flu vaccine every year.

TREATMENT PLAN

A. Humidity and mist may be helpful.

B. Always clean the humidifier daily to prevent bacteria from growing.

C. Twenty minutes several times a day in a steamy bathroom may provide relief.

Activity: Rest is important when you have been diagnosed with bronchitis; then increase activity as tolerated when the fever subsides. Children may attend school or day care without any problems after their fever subsides.

Diet: Eat a nutritious diet. Drink 8 to 10 glasses of water daily.

Medications:

A. Acetaminophen (Tylenol) may be used to relieve discomfort.

B. For a nonproductive cough, take cough suppressants if recommended. You may be prescribed a cough medicine or be told the best kind to buy in the drugstore. **The American College of Chest Physicians clinical practice guidelines recommend that cough suppressants and over-the-counter cough medications should *not* be given to young children. Cough and cold medicines should *not* be given to children younger than 6 years of age.**

C. Because a virus almost always causes acute bronchitis, **antibiotics will rarely be needed to get better.**

You Have Been Prescribed: ______________________

You Need to Take: ______________________

You Need to Notify the Office If You Have:

A. No improvement after 48 hours

B. Worsening symptoms

C. High fever, chills, chest tightness or pain, shortness of breath

D. Symptoms that last longer than 3 weeks

E. Other: ______________________

Phone: ______________________

BRONCHITIS, CHRONIC

PROBLEM

Chronic bronchitis is an upper respiratory infection followed by a productive cough. To be diagnosed with chronic bronchitis, you should have had the symptoms for 3 months for 2 years in a row.

CAUSE

Both viral and bacterial infections cause chronic bronchitis.

PREVENTION/CARE

A. Avoid exposure to others with respiratory illnesses.

B. Do not smoke, and avoid secondhand smoke and smoke-filled environments.

C. Avoid other air pollutants, such as wood smoke, solvents, and cleaners.

D. Use good handwashing techniques.

E. Use tissues for the mucus coughed up. Dispose of the tissues after use.

F. Cover your mouth when you cough. If you do not have a tissue, the "elbow sneeze" into the bend of your arm will prevent you from spreading your illness.

G. Although the flu vaccine does not prevent bronchitis, a yearly flu vaccine is recommended.

H. A pneumonia vaccine is recommended for people older than 65 years of age and for younger people with chronic respiratory conditions.

TREATMENT PLAN

A. Humidity and mist may be helpful.

B. Always clean the humidifier daily to prevent bacterial growth.

C. Twenty minutes several times a day in a steamy bathroom may provide relief.

Activity: Rest during the early stage of the illness, then increase activity as tolerated when the fever subsides. It is not uncommon to feel tired for several weeks.

Diet: Eat a nutritious diet. Drink 8 to 10 glasses of water daily.

Medications:

A. Acetaminophen (Tylenol) may be used to relieve fever and discomfort.

B. You may be prescribed an inhaler to help your breathing.

C. You may be prescribed steroids to help with the inflammation of your lungs. The steroids may be given by an inhaler or as a pill.

D. It is very important that you use the inhaler properly so that the medicine can go into your lungs. A teaching sheet on how to use an inhaler is available.

E. You may also be prescribed an antibiotic for a bacterial infection. Take all of your antibiotics, even if you feel better.

F. You may be prescribed a cough suppressant to take at night to help you rest. However, coughing up the mucus is very important to clear out your "wind pipes."

You Have Been Prescribed: ______________________________

You Need to Take: ______________________________

You Need to Notify the Office If You Have:

A. No improvement after 48 hours.

B. Worsening symptoms.

C. High fever, chills, chest tightness or pain, shortness of breath.

D. Symptoms that last longer than 3 weeks after taking all of your antibiotics.

E. Other: ______________________________

Phone: ______________________________

CERUMEN IMPACTION (EARWAX)

PROBLEM

A buildup of earwax in the external ear canal that may cause itching, pain, and temporary hearing loss.

CAUSE

Earwax production is a normal, healthy process of the gland of the ear. Earwax is produced to protect the ear from infection and trauma. The wax is continuously being produced and removed from the ear via its own mechanism. However, at times, an overproduction of wax may build up and remain in the external ear canal. With age, the normal mechanisms of the ear for removing earwax are decreased. This is called cerumen impaction. Use of cotton swabs to remove earwax can push wax further into the ear and cause problems deeper into the ear canal.

PREVENTION/CARE

Do not use cotton swabs, paper clips, or other objects to clean your ears. These can damage the ear canal and lead to an external ear infection.

TREATMENT PLAN

A. **Use Debrox, mineral oil, or olive oil, 2 to 3 drops per day, gently placed into the external ear canal for 1 week. These oils will soften up the wax for easier removal.**

B. Clean ears with a wet washcloth. The external ear that is visible to the eye is the only part of the ear that should be cleaned with a wet washcloth.

C. Return to the health care provider in 1 week for wax removal.

D. Do not try to remove the earwax on your own due to the chance of damaging your eardrum. Never stick any kind of tool into your ear. This will usually push the wax farther into your ear canal, making removal more difficult by your health care provider.

Activity: As tolerated.

Diet: As tolerated.

Medications: ______________________________

You Have Been Prescribed: ______________________________

You Need to Take: ______________________________

You Need to Notify the Office If:

A. You are unable to hear.

B. You have colored drainage or fluid draining from your ears.

C. You run a fever.

D. You have dizziness.

E. Other:______________________________

Phone: ______________________________

CERVICITIS

PROBLEM

You are being treated for cervicitis. The cervix is the lower section of the uterus that opens into the vagina. Cervicitis is an inflammation of the cervix.

CAUSE

Certain germs, such as *Chlamydia trachomatis* or *Neisseria gonorrhea*, may cause cervicitis; however, in many cases no specific germ may be identified. In these cases, inflammation may be due to douching, chemical irritants, or altered vaginal flora. In many cases, no cause may be found.

Your health care provider will perform a physical evaluation, including pelvic examination, and obtain certain tests to diagnose the cause of cervicitis. If a sexually transmitted organism is found, you and your partner will need to be treated.

PREVENTION/CARE

In cases in which cervicitis is caused by sexually transmitted organisms, use of condoms may prevent infection.
Do not douche or use any other chemically irritating products.

TREATMENT PLAN

A. You may be prescribed an antibiotic by your health care provider.

B. Depending on the cause of cervicitis, your sexual partner(s) may also need medical evaluation and treatment.

Activity: Avoid sexual activity until treatment is completed.

Medications:

You Have Been Prescribed: ______________________________

You Need to Take: ______________________________

You need to finish all of your antibiotics even though you may feel good.

You Need to Notify the Office If:

A. You are not able to take your medicine.

B. You have other new symptoms.

C. Other: ______________________________

Phone: ______________________________

CHICKENPOX (VARICELLA)

PROBLEM

Chickenpox is a virus in which a rash occurs, appearing like red, small bumps that usually occur in crops on the body. The virus can affect all ages, but usually affects children and older adults. If you have chickenpox, it may come back later as shingles.

CAUSE

Varicella-zoster virus is a herpes virus that is highly contagious. It is spread by direct person-to-person contact and sometimes by airborne means from respiratory secretions.

PREVENTION/CARE

A. Avoid contact with anyone with chickenpox.

B. If infected, stay in strict isolation until lesions are all crusted over.

C. Sores ("lesions") should be covered by clothing or a dressing until they have crusted. **Covering sores prevents spreading and helps prevent scarring.**

D. Practice good handwashing any time you touch the sores.

TREATMENT PLAN

A. Stay away from other people. Remain in strict isolation.

B. Children may return to day care or school only after all sores have dried and crusted.

C. Care for skin with daily cool-water bathing or soaks.

D. Keep fingernails short and clean; try to prevent scratching.

E. Using a cornstarch bath, baking soda, or oatmeal (Aveeno) or topical lotions, such as calamine, to help with itching.

F. Change your bed sheets and clothes often.

G. **Aspirin should never be used for a fever; it may contribute to the development of Reye's syndrome when given to children during a viral illness.**

Activity: Bed rest is not necessary. Quiet-play activity in a cool room or outside in the shade during nice weather is permitted. Keep all ill children away from others and away from school and day care until all blisters have crusted and there are no new ones.

Diet: No special foods are needed.

Medications: Acetaminophen may be administered for fever. Your child may have a medication prescribed for itching.

You Have Been Prescribed: ______________________________

You Need to Take: ______________________________

You Need to Notify the Office If You Have or Your Child Has:

A. Symptoms of chickenpox

B. Lethargy, headache, sensitivity to bright light

C. Fever over 101°F

D. Chickenpox sores that contain pus or otherwise appear infected

E. A cough that occurs during a chickenpox infection

F. Other: ______________________________

Phone: ______________________________

CHILDHOOD NUTRITION

TODDLERS

Appetite often decreases during the toddler years. Parents should monitor the child's nutrition by weekly intake instead of daily intake. Just like adults, children's appetites change, leaving them hungrier at certain times than others.

Toddlers love to be busy. Therefore, if mealtime tends to be a struggle, after the child tells you he or she is finished with the meal, let the child get up and move around, but continue to offer bites of the meal between the child's activities.

Toddlers also do best with finger foods, which are easy to pick up and eat. Finger-food snacks, such as crackers, carrots, and celery, are great choices. Snacks between meals are important for children. Fresh fruit and vegetables are excellent snacks. Try to limit the amount of sweets and fats the child consumes. Obesity can be a nutritional concern, especially in the early childhood stages. As a parent, set a good example and eat healthy foods and snacks. Toddlers and children learn by watching and eating the same foods that they see their parents and siblings eat.

FAMILY TEACHING TIPS FOR FEEDING TODDLERS

A. Serve small portions, and provide a second serving when the first has been eaten. Just 1 or 2 tablespoons is an adequate serving for the toddler. Too much food on the dish may overwhelm the child.

B. There is no *one* food essential to health. Allow substitution for a disliked food. Food jags in which toddlers prefer one food for days on end are common and not harmful. If the child refuses a particular food, such as milk, use appropriate substitutes such as pudding, cheese, yogurt, and cottage cheese. Avoid a battle of wills at mealtime.

C. Toddlers like simply prepared foods, served warm or cool, *not* hot or cold.

D. Provide a social atmosphere at mealtimes; allow the toddler to eat with others in the family. Toddlers learn by imitating the acceptance or rejection of foods by other family members.

E. Toddlers prefer foods they can pick up with their fingers; however, they should be allowed to use a spoon or fork when they want to try.

F. Try to plan regular mealtimes with small nutritious snacks planned between meals. Do not attach too much importance to food by urging the child to choose what to eat.

G. Dawdling at mealtime is common with this age group and can be ignored unless it stretches on to unreasonable lengths or becomes a play for power. Mealtime for the toddler should not exceed 20 minutes. Calmly remove food without comment.

H. Do not make desserts a reward for good eating habits. It gives unfair value to the dessert and makes vegetables or other foods seem less desirable.

I. Offer regularly planned nutritious snacks, such as milk, crackers, and peanut butter, cheese cubes, and pieces of fruit. Plan snacks midway between meals and at bedtime.

J. Remember that the total amount eaten each day is more important than the amount eaten at a specific meal.

K. Useful resources for parents and children are available at www.ChooseMyPlate.gov. This site provides daily food plans, interactive games, and teaching tools for adults and children regarding nutritional guidelines and recommendations for a healthy lifestyle.

(*continued*)

CHILDHOOD NUTRITION *(continued)*

Suggested Daily Food Guidelines for Toddlers

Food Group	Daily Amounts	Comments/Rationale
Grains: Breads, cereals; whole grain or enriched	2–3 y/o: 3–5 oz 4–5 y/o: 4–6 oz 1 oz grain = 1 slice of bread, 1 cup cereal, 1/2 cup cooked rice or pasta, or 1 tortilla (6″ round)	Provides thiamine, niacin, and, if enriched, riboflavin and iron.
Fruit juices; Canned fruit or small pieces of fruit	2–3 y/o: 1–1.5 c 4–5 y/o: 1–1.5 c 1/2 cup fruit = 1/2 cup juice, 1/2 cup fruit pieces, mashed or sliced, 1/2 medium banana, or 4–5 large strawberries	Use those rich in vitamins A and C; also source of iron and calcium.
Vegetables	2–3 y/o: 1–1.5 c 4–5 y/o: 1.5–2.5 c 1/2 cup vegetable = 1/2 cup mashed, sliced, or chopped vegetable, 1 cup raw leafy green vegetable, 1/2 cup vegetable juice, or 1 small ear of corn	Include at least one dark-green or yellow vegetable every other day for vitamin A.
Protein: Meat, fish, chicken, casseroles, cottage cheese, peanut butter, dried peas, and beans	2–3 y/o: 2–4 oz 4–5 y/o: 3–5 oz 1 oz protein = 1 oz cooked meat, poultry, or seafood, 1 egg, 1/2 cup casserole, 1/4 cup cottage cheese, 1 tbsp peanut butter, 1/4 cup cooked beans or peas	Source of complete protein, iron, thiamine, riboflavin, niacin, and vitamin B_{12}. Nuts and seeds should not be offered until after age 3 years, when the risk of choking is minimal.
Dairy: Milk, yogurt, cheese	2–3 y/o: 2–2.5 cups 4–5 y/o: 2.5–3 cup: 1/2 cup dairy = 1/2 cup milk, 4 oz yogurt, 3/4 oz cheese, or 1 string cheese	Cheese, cottage cheese, and yogurt are good calcium and riboflavin sources; also sources of calcium, phosphorus, complete protein, riboflavin, and niacin; also vitamin D if fortified milk is used.

y/o, year old.

Source: Reprinted by permission from the Mayo Foundation for Medical Education and Research. All rights reserved.

CHLAMYDIA

PROBLEM

Chlamydia is a sexually transmitted infection. Often, no problems are present, but you may notice a yellowish discharge from the penis or vagina, burning during urination, frequent and urgent urination, or pelvic pain.

Untreated chlamydia in females may lead to a condition called pelvic inflammatory disease (PID). PID is a leading cause of infertility, increased ectopic pregnancies, and chronic pelvic pain in women.

CAUSE

Chlamydia is caused by a bacterium called *Chlamydia trachomatis.* This bacterium is spread through sexual contact and may infect the eyes, throat, vagina, penis, or rectum.

PREVENTION/CARE

A. Limit sexual partners.

B. Have routine screening tests for chlamydia prior to beginning a new sexual relationship.

C. Use condoms with sexual activity.

TREATMENT PLAN

Abstain from sexual activity until you and your partner(s) have completed your prescribed medication. Your health care provider is required to report this disease to the public health department. The health department may contact you.

Diet: As desired.

Medications: Chlamydia can be cured by the prescribed antibiotics.

You Have Been Prescribed: ____________________

You Need to Take: ____________________

You need to take all of your antibiotics. It is very important that you keep your follow-up appointment with your provider in 3 months: Your appointment has been scheduled for: ____________________

You Need to Notify the Office If:

A. You are unable to take your antibiotics because of nausea, vomiting, or a reaction.

B. Other: ____________________

Phone: ____________________

CHRONIC OBSTRUCTIVE PULMONARY DISEASE

PROBLEM

Chronic obstructive pulmonary disease (COPD) is a chronic, progressive, debilitating disease of the lungs that does not have a cure. Most people with COPD have a combination of emphysema and chronic bronchitis. Persons with COPD usually have some of the following symptoms: Cough (usually productive), shortness of breath at rest or with exertion, wheezing, decreased energy level, and weight loss.

CAUSE

COPD is most commonly associated with cigarette smoking and long-term exposure to pulmonary irritants in the environment (e.g., coal dust). Repeated respiratory infections may also contribute to the development of COPD.

PREVENTION/CARE

A. Avoid smoking and exposure to secondhand smoke.

B. Avoid exposure to environmental irritants, including pollution, household cleaning products, and smoke from fires.

TREATMENT PLAN

A. Stopping smoking is one of the most important treatments. Talk to your health care provider about support for stopping.

B. Reduce your exposure to lung irritants and extremely hot and cold air temperatures.

C. Begin an exercise program with your health care provider's approval. Walking is a good aerobic exercise. Begin with a pace that is tolerable and easy to maintain; then increase the duration and intensity of the exercise as tolerated. Stop if you experience shortness of breath or chest pain. A realistic goal may be to walk 5 to 10 minutes a day, eventually increasing to 30 to 40 minutes a day.

D. Receive the influenza vaccine every fall. The pneumococcal vaccine is recommended every 5 years and may be given at the same time as the influenza vaccine.

E. Use a spacer/holding chamber to help you inhale all of your medicine. Spacers help you place more of your medicine in your lungs instead of at the back of your throat and mouth. Keep your spacer clean.

F. Use slow, deep breathing or pursed-lip breathing when you are short of breath. Breathe out like you are blowing out a candle.

G. Ask your health care provider if you are a candidate for low-flow oxygen treatment when shortness of breath occurs at night and causes insomnia and restlessness.

Activity: Group activities together such as planning shopping with going to the post office. Schedule rest periods throughout the day. Exercise programs should help increase activity tolerance.

Diet: Good nutrition is important. Six small, high-calorie meals a day are suggested. Avoid excessive intake of carbohydrates, especially simple carbohydrates like candy, soda, and potato chips. Milk and milk products do not increase the production of mucus. Ask your health care provider to refer you to a dietitian if nutritional problems persist.

Medications:

You Have Been Prescribed: ______________________________

You Need to Take: ______________________________

You Need to Notify the Office If:

A. Your mucus changes color, increases in amount, or the consistency becomes thicker.

B. After you start your medication, call if your wheezing or shortness of breath is getting worse.

C. You have trouble walking or talking due to your shortness of breath.

D. Other: ______________________________

Phone: ______________________________

CHRONIC PAIN

RESOURCES

Many patient resources on pain are available at your local library, bookstores, and on the Internet. Look for a local support group in your area to join and learn how other people are coping with your same condition.

An excellent resource for patients, families, and physicians is *How to Cope With Chronic Pain,* by Nelson Hendler, MD (Cool Hand Communications, 1993).

There are many pain organizations available to assist patients. Patients may wish to visit these websites for further information.

American Academy of Pain Medicine: www.aapainmanage.org

American Chronic Pain Association: www.theacpa.org

American Pain Society: www.americanpainsociety.org

Arthritis Foundation: www.arthritis.org

National Fibromyalgia Association: www.fmaware.org

CHRONIC VENOUS INSUFFICIENCY

PROBLEM

Chronic venous insufficiency (CVI) is a condition in which blood has difficulty flowing back to the heart from the arms or legs. This usually occurs when the valves along the inside of the veins are damaged and allow blood to flow backward. The pooling of blood leads to swelling, pain, a heavy feeling, darkening of the skin, and infections. Without treatment, CVI can lead to blood clots and serious infections that could lead to amputation.

CAUSE

Many things may increase the chance of having CVI. Some, like gender, age, or how tall you are, cannot be changed. Others can be changed; these include prolonged standing or sitting and excessive weight.

PREVENTION/CARE

A. Avoid standing or sitting for long periods.

B. If overweight or obese, lose weight. Discuss what you can do to lose weight with your health care provider.

TREATMENT PLAN

A. Take your medications as ordered by your health care provider.

B. Wear compression stockings. Put them on before getting out of bed in the morning. Take them off just before going to bed at night.

C. Raise the affected arm or leg whenever lying down to improve pain and swelling.

D. Avoid standing or sitting for long periods of time.

E. Follow up with your primary health care provider on a regularly scheduled basis.

Activity:

A. Get regular exercise. Discuss what type and frequency of exercise is safe for you with your health care provider.

B. Exercise leg muscles by pumping ankles when sitting. Rocking in a rocking chair is another option.

Diet:

A. Discuss the type of diet that best suits your needs with your health care provider: Diabetic diet, low-fat diet, low-cholesterol diet, and/or low-sodium diet.

Medications:

You Have Been Prescribed: ____________________

You Need to Take: ____________________

You Need to Notify the Office If You Have:

A. Fever greater than 101°F

B. Increased redness, pain, tenderness to touch, swelling, and/or warmth

C. Sudden shortness of breath

D. Chest pain

E. New wound or sore on the affected arm or leg

F. If you are taking a blood-thinning medication and have any of these symptoms:
   1. Vomit that is bright red or dark and looks like coffee grounds
   2. Bright-red blood in your stools or black, tarry stools
   3. Severe headache

(*continued*)

CHRONIC VENOUS INSUFFICIENCY *(continued)*

4. Sudden weakness in an arm or leg
5. Memory loss or confusion
6. Sudden change in vision
7. Trouble speaking or understanding others

G. Other: ____________________

Phone: ____________________

RESOURCE

Vascular Disease Foundation: vasculardisease.org/flyers/chronic-venous-insufficiency-flyer.pdf

COLIC: WAYS TO SOOTHE A FUSSY BABY

PROBLEM

Your baby has been diagnosed with colic if the following symptoms are noticed: Repeated episodes of excessive crying that cannot be explained. Crying may range from fussiness to screaming. Crying follows a pattern with colic:

A. It occurs at the same time of the day, usually late afternoon or evening.

B. It usually begins at 3 weeks of age and lasts through 3 to 4 months of age.

C. The baby's stomach may rumble, and then the baby may draw up his or her legs as if in pain.

D. No specific cause or disease can be found.

CAUSE

The cause of colic is unknown.

PREVENTION/CARE

There are no specific preventive measures. Remove any causes that can be identified.

TREATMENT PLAN

A. Record time when colic episodes occur. Soothe and comfort your baby before the "attack."

B. Do not feed your baby every time he or she cries. Look for a reason, such as a gas bubble, cramped position, too much heat or cold, soiled diaper, or a desire to be cuddled.

C. Make sure your baby is not overfed or underfed (see "Diet" section that follows). During an attack of gas, hold your baby securely, and gently massage his or her lower abdomen. Rocking may be soothing.

D. Feed your baby with the head up such as sitting up and use frequent burping.

E. Using a collapsible bag/bottle may help to reduce air-swallowing.

F. Do not give your baby any herbal products without a health care provider's approval.

Activity:

A. Overstimulation may cause infant upset. A quiet environment or being left alone in the crib to work off excess tension may be necessary.

B. Allow your baby to cry if you are certain that everything is all right. Colic is distressing, but not harmful.

C. Take time away from your infant to rest and recoup.

D. Try the following remedies:

1. Rhythmic rocking, use swings
2. Car rides
3. Walking the baby in a stroller
4. Running vacuum or vaporizer for calming noise
5. Giving your baby a pacifier for sucking
6. Swaddling and cuddling to soothe the baby
7. Playing music to quiet the baby

E. If you are breastfeeding, review all of your medications and any herbal products that you are taking with your health care provider.

Diet:

A. Your baby should be taking at least ______________________ ounces of ______________________ formula at each feeding. Interrupt bottle feedings halfway through the feeding and burp the baby. Burp your baby at the end of the feeding, too.

B. If breastfeeding, do not switch to formula unless you have discussed it with a health care provider. Interrupt breastfeeding every 5 minutes to burp. If breastfeeding, you should avoid eating the following foods: Chocolate, cabbage, beans, pizza, or spicy foods.

(*continued*)

COLIC: WAYS TO SOOTHE A FUSSY BABY *(continued)*

C. Allow at least 20 minutes to feed your baby. Hold your baby while he or she is feeding; do not prop the baby with a bottle for feeding.

D. Do not try a home remedy, such as feeding homegrown mint teas, to your baby.

You Need to Notify the Office If:

A. The baby has a rectal temperature of 101°F or higher.

B. You fear you are about to lose emotional control.

C. Your baby is taking a prescription drug and new unexplained symptoms develop: The drug may produce side effects.

D. You notice a change in your baby's eating patterns, or he or she has vomiting, diarrhea, or constipation.

E. You notice a change in your baby's pattern of behavior: He or she refuses to suck, has a high-pitched cry, draws the legs up when you touch the tummy, or your baby is limp with no activity.

F. Other: ______________________________

Phone: ______________________________

COMMON COLD

PROBLEM

The common cold is swelling of the mucous membranes of the respiratory tract. Most people complain of feeling tired and have a runny or stopped-up nose, a sore throat, hoarseness, and watery and/or red eyes. You may have a low-grade fever or no fever at all.

CAUSE

A virus usually causes the common cold.

PREVENTION/CARE

A. Colds are spread from one person to another through hand-to-hand contact and contact with air droplets from sneezing, coughing, and talking.

B. Practice good handwashing techniques with soap and water or hand sanitizers.

C. Do not drink from the same glass as others.

D. Cover your mouth and nose when you sneeze or cough.

E. Use tissues when you blow your nose. Dispose of them and then wash your hands. If no tissue is available, do the "elbow sneeze" into the bend of your arm (away from your open hands). Always wash your hands afterward.

F. The flu vaccine is recommended every year.

TREATMENT PLAN

A. Using a humidifier for your bedroom or inhaling steam helps keep the mucous membranes of your nose from drying.

B. Use a rubber suction bulb to clear nasal congestion in babies.

C. Discuss using saline nose drops.

D. Secondary infections of the respiratory tract (sinuses, lungs) may occur. If these do occur, then antibiotic therapy may be needed.

E. Zinc preparations are not recommended for an acute cough due to the common cold.

Activity: There are no activity restrictions. Frequent rest periods or naps can help with fatigue.

Diet: Eat well-balanced meals and snacks. Drink extra liquids (10–12 glasses a day). Warm fluids, such as tea and soups, can increase the rate of mucus flow and provide some symptom relief.

Medications: The American College of Chest Physicians clinical practice guidelines recommend that cough suppressants and other over-the-counter cough medications *not* be given to young children. Cough and cold medicines should *not* be given to children younger than 6 years.

A. Antibiotics are not prescribed for a cold, but they may be prescribed for a secondary infection.

B. All cold medications are available over the counter. Take as directed.

You Have Been Prescribed: ______________________________

You Need to Take: ______________________________

You Need to Notify the Office If:

A. Your child is listless or hard to wake up, refuses a bottle or would not drink liquids, does not want to play, has a fever, or has other symptoms such as shortness of breath.

B. You experience pain that is getting worse in your ears, sinuses, throat, neck, or chest.

C. You have green or yellow nasal drainage.

D. Your temperature is higher than 100.4°F.

E. You are a diabetic and your blood sugars are elevated, or you notice ketones in your urine while you are sick.

F. Other: ______________________________

Phone: ______________________________

CONJUNCTIVITIS

PROBLEM

You have an infection of the eye, or conjunctivitis, that causes redness, itching, drainage from the eye, and crusting on the eyelids.

CAUSE

Bacteria, viruses, or allergies can cause eye infections.

PREVENTION/CARE

A. Wash your hands frequently.

B. Avoid persons with conjunctivitis (pink eye).

C. Avoid known allergens.

TREATMENT PLAN

A. All types:
   1. Wash your hands frequently, especially after touching the eyes, to avoid spread.
   2. Use cool compresses on the eyes as needed.
   3. Wash crusting eyelids with baby shampoo daily.
   4. Wipe the eyes from the inner to outer corners.

B. *Bacterial*: Bacterial conjunctivitis is contagious until 24 hours after beginning medication.

C. *Viral*: Viral conjunctivitis is contagious for 48 to 72 hours, but it may last up to 2 weeks.

Activity: As tolerated

Diet: As tolerated

Medications: No medications are prescribed for viral infections. You will be given instructions on how to use eyedrops or eye ointment.

You Have Been Prescribed: ______________________________

You Need to Take: ______________________________

You Need to Notify the Office If You Have:

A. A reaction to your medication

B. Trouble seeing

C. New symptoms

D. Other: ______________________________

Phone: ______________________________

CONSTIPATION RELIEF

PROBLEM

Constipation is an infrequent and difficult passing of hard stools and the sensation of not emptying or having to strain.

CAUSES

There are many reasons why you have constipation. You may have just one or a combination of these common causes:

A. Not drinking enough liquids

B. Eating a low-fiber diet

C. Sedentary lifestyle, lack of exercise

D. Ignoring the urge to go to the bathroom

E. Taking drugs, including blood pressure (BP) medications, antidepressants, pain medications and antacids, or overusing laxatives

F. Depression

G. Other medical conditions

PREVENTION/CARE

A. Go to the bathroom as soon as you have the urge to have a bowel movement; do not wait.

B. Establish a regular toilet time such as after breakfast; 15 to 20 minutes after breakfast is a good time because spontaneous colonic motility is greatest during that period.

C. Use a footrest during elimination to provide support and decrease straining.

D. Do not rely on laxatives; use prune juice as a natural substitute.

E. Stimulate the intestine by drinking hot or cold water or prune juice before meals.

F. Decrease the intake of sweets, which increase bacterial growth in the intestine and can lead to gas.

G. Stop taking enemas and nonessential drugs and herbals.

TREATMENT PLAN

A. Follow the suggested prevention tips.

B. Change to a high-fiber diet.

C. Get daily exercise.

Activity: Daily exercise, such as walking, helps to maintain healthy bowel patterns.

Diet:

A. Eat a high-fiber diet.

B. Restrict cheese: It causes constipation.

C. Drink at least eight glasses of water each day.

D. Avoid refined cereals and breads, pastries, and sugar.

E. Coffee, tea, and alcohol decrease water to the colon. Limit your intake to two of these drinks per day.

Medications: You may be prescribed a stool softener or a laxative for short-term use only. You may be prescribed a bulk-forming agent to take on a regular basis to increase the bulk of your stool.

You Have Been Prescribed: ____________________

You Need to Take: ____________________

(*continued*)

CONSTIPATION RELIEF *(continued)*

You Need to Notify the Office If:

A. Constipation continues in spite of the self-care instructions, including diet and exercise.

B. You notice a change in your bowel movements. Changes in bowel patterns may be an early sign of cancer.

C. You develop fever or severe abdominal pain with your constipation.

D. Other: ____

Phone: ______________________________

CONTRACEPTION: HOW TO TAKE BIRTH CONTROL PILLS (FOR A 28-DAY CYCLE)

You have been prescribed an oral contraceptive, also known as a *birth control pill*. Most birth control pills contain a combination of synthetic estrogen and progestin.

A. Birth control pills suppress ovulation.

B. They make the lining of the uterus unreceptive for an egg to implant and grow. Birth control pills also alter the cervical mucus, making it thicker and harder for sperm to penetrate.

C. A birth control pill does not prevent any sexually transmitted infection or HIV. A condom must still be used to protect yourself from the HIV virus or other infections.

D. You will be asked to return to the office in 3 months after starting birth control pills to check your blood pressure and to check for other side effects of the pill, such as your potassium level and nausea.

E. If your blood pressure is normal and you are not having any other problems taking the pills, your prescription for birth-control pills may be written for 1 year.

F. At the end of that time, you will need another physical examination and possibly a Pap smear. Then your prescription can be refilled for another year.

You Have Been Prescribed:

A. This is a combination pill of estrogen and progestin.

1. Your packet contains 28 pills. Notice that your pills are different colors. **You must take them in the order that they come in the packet.** There are 21 "active" pills, and the last 7 are "inactive or sugar pills" to keep you in the habit of taking a pill every day.
2. You must take a pill **every day** at approximately the same time. Develop the habit of taking the pill with brushing your teeth, for example. You cannot share your birth control pills with anyone else.
3. Start your packet on the Sunday of your period. Take the pill marked "1," "start here," or "Sunday."
4. You take a pill every day for 21 days; when you start the last 7 pills, you will have a period or "withdrawal bleed."
5. Your period may not start for 1 to 2 days into the last week of pills. This is normal. You generally have a shorter, lighter period on birth control pills.
6. When you start your period, it is time to refill your prescription for your next month of pills.
7. If this is your first packet of birth control pills, you are not considered protected and may get pregnant. Use a backup method of birth control for the first packet of pills.
8. **Missed pills instructions:**
   a. I f you miss one pill: Take it as soon as you remember, then get back on your regular schedule (you can take two pills in 1 day).
   b. If you miss two pills: Take two pills as soon as you remember, then get back on schedule (you can take three pills in 1 day). You must use a **backup method of birth control** such as a condom until you finish that packet of pills. You may have spotting if you miss two pills. This is normal.
   c. If you miss three pills: You may have a period. Discard that packet of pills and start a new packet on Sunday. You must use a **backup method of birth control** such as a condom for the first 7 days of the new packet.
   d. If one or more birth control pills are missed, no backup method of contraception is used, and if you miss your period, you should do a pregnancy test.
9. If you are prescribed antibiotics while taking birth control pills, you must use a **backup method of birth control** such as a condom. You can get pregnant. Antibiotics and other medications such as those used to prevent seizures make birth control pills less effective, making it possible to get pregnant.

You Need to Notify the Office If You:

A. Vomit your birth control pills.

B. Have a severe or migraine-like headache.

C. Are depressed (cannot make yourself happy).

D. Have pain in your legs, especially if your calf hurts when walking or flexing your foot.

E. Break your leg and need to have a cast.

(*continued*)

CONTRACEPTION: HOW TO TAKE BIRTH CONTROL PILLS (FOR A 28-DAY CYCLE) (*continued*)

F. Think you are pregnant (skipped pills or are taking antibiotics).

G. Have blurred vision, loss of vision, or spots before your eyes.

H. Feel chest pain or shortness of breath.

I. Feel severe abdominal pain.

J. Have lots of swelling of the fingers, hands, ankles, or face.

K. Other: ____

Phone: ______________________________________

COUGH

PROBLEM

Coughing is an important defense mechanism your body uses to clear your airways of mucus and inhaled particles.

CAUSE

A cough is often associated with other respiratory symptoms and may be a sign of infection. Coughing is often related to environmental or chemical irritants such as smoking.

PREVENTION/CARE

A. Coughing cannot be prevented, but you do have some voluntary control over it.

B. Occasionally, medications can cause a cough. So review all medications with your health care provider.

C. The flu vaccine is recommended each year; however, the flu vaccine does not prevent a cough.

TREATMENT PLAN

A. **The American College of Chest Physicians clinical practice guidelines recommend that cough suppressants and other over-the-counter cough medications *not* be given to young children. Cough and cold medicines should *not* be given to children younger than 6 years.**

B. Stop smoking, including exposure to secondhand smoke. At the minimum, maintain a smoke-free bedroom.

C. Using a room humidifier may be helpful. Keep your humidifier clean—it can grow bacteria.

D. Change heating and air-conditioning filters often to decrease environmental irritants.

E. Coughing for several minutes may tire you, so you may need extra rest.

Activity: No activity restrictions.

Diet: Drink at least 10 to 15 glasses of liquids a day.

Medications: The American College of Physicians clinical practice guidelines recommend that cough suppressants and over-the-counter cough medications *not* be given to young children. Cough and cold medicines should *not* be given for children younger than 6 years.

You Have Been Prescribed: ______________________________

You Need to Take: ______________________________

You Need to Notify the Office If:

A. You have difficulty breathing.

B. Your child makes noises with coughing, such as wheezing, singsong sounds, or crowing sounds.

C. You cough up blood.

D. You develop other symptoms besides coughing, such as green sinus drainage and/or a sore throat.

E. You cannot sleep because of coughing.

F. You develop a fever over 101°F.

G. Other: ______________________________

Phone: ______________________________

CROHN'S DISEASE

PROBLEM

Crohn's disease (CD) is an inflammatory disorder of the gastrointestinal (GI) tract that produces ulceration, formation of fibrous tissue, and malabsorption. CD is chronic, relapsing, and incurable.

CAUSE

The cause is unknown, but it can be aggravated by bacterial infection or inflammation.

TREATMENT PLAN

A. Adequate nutrition is critical to the promotion of healing.

B. Vitamin, mineral, and folic acid supplementation are necessary for proper healing and to avoid secondary complications such as bone disease and low blood counts.

C. To relieve pain, apply a heating pad or warm compress to your abdomen.

D. Check your bowel movements (BM) daily for signs of bleeding.

E. Surgery may be required to help control symptoms.

F. There may be a support group near where you live. The Crohn's and Colitis Foundation website has an area to find a support group at www.ccfa.org/living-with-crohns-colitis/find-a-support-group

G. Take your medicine as your health care provider ordered to help prevent an attack.

Activity: During acute attacks, rest in bed or in a chair. Get up only to go to the bathroom, bathe, or eat. Between attacks, resume normal activities, as tolerated.

Diet:

A. When you have diarrhea, increase the fiber content of your diet.

B. Restricting milk products may stop the diarrhea. Stop using milk products for a short time, then try them again in a few weeks.

C. Decreasing the amount of fat and gluten in your diet may help.

D. Ensure, Sustacal, and Isocal have been found to improve symptoms.

E. Severe relapse may require you stop eating or drinking called a partial bowel rest. Contact the office for instruction.

Medications: You may be prescribed vitamins and minerals, medicine to control pain and relieve diarrhea, and a steroid to reduce the inflammation. Do not stop taking the steroid abruptly. Your health care provider can tell you how to taper the dose over several days.

You Have Been Prescribed the Following Vitamins and Minerals: ______________________

You Need to Take: ______________________

You Have Been Prescribed the Following to Relieve Diarrhea: ______________________

You Need to Take: ______________________

You Have Been Prescribed the Following Steroid: ______________________

You Need to Take: ______________________

Other medications to treat CD include pills, intravenous infusions, and injectable medications to control the severity of symptoms. Your health care provider will discuss these with you and the need for close follow-up monitoring.

(continued)

CROHN'S DISEASE *(continued)*

You Have Been Prescribed: ____________________

You Need to Take: ____________________

You Need to Return to the Office for Blood Work: ____________________

You Need to Notify the Office If You Have:

A. Black, tarry stools or blood in the stool

B. A swollen abdomen

C. A temperature of 101.0°F or higher

D. Other: ____________________

Phone: ____________________

RESOURCE

Crohn's and Colitis Foundation of America:
386 Park Avenue South, 17th Floor
New York, NY 10013
800-932-2423
info@ccfa.org
www.ccfa.org

CROUP, VIRAL

PROBLEM

Croup is a childhood illness of the respiratory system involving the voice box, vocal cords, windpipe, and bronchial tubes. Children become hoarse and have a barking cough, which usually gets worse at night. There may be a sore throat, fever, and a harsh sound with each inward breath (stridor). Infants may be irritable, sleepy, and have a poor appetite.

CAUSE

Croup is usually caused by a virus. Occasionally, it is caused by a bacterial infection.

PREVENTION/CARE

A. Isolate the child from others who are ill with respiratory symptoms.
B. The virus is most contagious during the first few days of fever.
C. Although the flu vaccine does not prevent croup, the vaccine is recommended every year.

TREATMENT PLAN

A. Cool mist has not been shown to be effective with croup.
B. Avoid hot steam because it may cause scalding.
C. Cool night air is often helpful, so open the window or take the child outdoors.
D. Croup tents are not generally recommended unless no alternative therapy is available.
E. Do not expose children to tobacco smoke and other irritants.
F. Count the child's breathing, and look for breathing problems, flaring of nostrils, or retractions (pulling in of chest wall while breathing).

Activity: Let your child rest. Handle your child as little as possible. Your child may return to day care or school when his or her temperature is normal and he or she feels better. A lingering cough is no reason to keep the child home.

Diet: Your child may have decreased appetite during the early part of the illness. It is more important to give plenty of fluids, such as juice and water.

Medications:
The American College of Chest Physicians clinical practice guidelines recommend that cough suppressants and over-the-counter cough medications *not* be given to young children. Cough and cold medicines should *not* be given to children younger than 6 years.

Antibiotics do not help viral croup. Your child may be prescribed other medications.

You Have Been Prescribed: ______________________________

You Need to Take: ______________________________

You Need to Notify the Office Immediately If:

A. Your child's breathing becomes difficult or fast, or his lips become blue.
B. Your child has difficulty swallowing or begins to drool.
C. Retractions develop.
D. Your child cannot sleep.
E. Mist from the vaporizer or bathroom does not help.
F. You feel your child is getting worse.
G. Other: ______________________________

You Need to Notify the Office Within 24 Hours If:

A. The cough becomes worse.
B. More than three episodes of labored breathing occur.
C. Your child is not drinking enough fluids.
D. Fever is greater than 104°F.
E. Other: ______________________________

Phone: ______________________________

CUSHING'S SYNDROME

PROBLEM

Cushing's syndrome has many symptoms, including weight gain, obesity, moon-shaped face, excessive hair growth, easy bruising, thin skin, muscle weakness, decreased or no menstrual periods, increased blood pressure, osteoporosis, and impaired wound healing.

CAUSE

Cushing's syndrome is caused by excessive cortisol production.

TREATMENT/CARE

A. Take medications precisely as directed.

B. Avoid excessive alcohol.

C. You may be instructed to purchase a Medic Alert bracelet or necklace for any emergencies. This can be used to list your treatment and health care provider's name and phone number.

Activity: Exercise is encouraged.

Diet: Low-sodium, high-potassium, high-calcium diet.

Medications:

You Have Been Prescribed: ____________________

You Need to Take: ____________________

You Need to Notify the Office If You:

A. Have a reaction to the medications

B. Cannot tolerate the prescribed medicines

C. Other: ____________________

Phone: ____________________

RESOURCES

NADF: www.nadf.us
You can build your own identification bracelets or neck chains from American Medical ID: www.americanmedical-id.com

DEEP VEIN THROMBOSIS

PROBLEM

You have inflammation or a blood clot in one of the veins in your body. Phlebitis is inflammation, and thrombosis means you have a blood clot. Symptoms include:

A. Pain

B. Fever

C. Swelling

D. Tenderness in the affected leg or arm

E. The vein may feel somewhat "hard" to touch.

CAUSE

Blood clots form because of bed rest, surgery, a heart attack, a severe illness, and birth control pills. A blood clot can also form after breaking a hip or leg, pregnancy, cancer, and some medications.

TREATMENT PLAN/CARE

A. If you have phlebitis, you may be given an anti-inflammatory medicine.

B. Some patients need to go to the hospital and get intravenous (IV) medicine to break up the clot.

C. You may be given blood thinners either as a pill or by self-injection.

D. Be sure to take all of the medicine as directed to help with the blood clot.

E. Do not smoke: This worsens your condition.

F. If you currently take any hormones, such as birth control pills, your health care provider may talk to you about stopping them.

G. Manage all other medical conditions, especially high blood pressure, diabetes, and high cholesterol, and try to lose any extra weight.

H. Follow up with your primary health care provider and/or cardiologist on a regularly scheduled basis.

Activity:

A. Get out of bed as soon as possible after surgery.

B. While in bed, perform range-of-motion exercises with your legs.

C. Exercise leg muscles by pumping your ankles when sitting.

D. Do not sit with your legs crossed.

E. Avoid standing or sitting for long periods of time.

F. Do not wear tight clothing such as knee-high hosiery.

G. Wear special supportive hosiery called compression stockings. Put them on before getting out of bed in the morning and take them off before going to bed at night.

H. When traveling:
   1. Try to take rest breaks on a regular basis.
   2. Continue to do the ankle pumping exercise when in the car or on the plane.
   3. Wear loose-fitting clothes that are comfortable.
   4. Avoid drinking alcohol.
   5. Drink plenty of fluids unless you are instructed not to do so by your health care provider.
   6. Ask your health care provider if you should wear compression stockings.

I. Wear a Medic Alert bracelet if you are put on blood thinners.

J. You will notice that you bruise easier while on your blood thinner.

K. You may need to come back to the office to have your labs drawn.

(*continued*)

DEEP VEIN THROMBOSIS *(continued)*

Diet:

A. Discuss the type of diet that best suits your needs: Diabetic diet, low-fat diet, low-cholesterol diet, and/or low-sodium diet.

B. If you are taking the blood thinner Coumadin, you will be given a list of foods that are high in vitamin K. These foods can interfere with how the blood thinner works. Please discuss these foods further with your health care provider.

C. Avoid alcohol.

Medications: If you currently take birth control pills, ask your health care provider if you should stop taking them. You may be prescribed a blood thinner by injection or pills. Take this medicine even if you feel better.

You Have Been Prescribed: ______________________________

You Need to Take: ______________________________

You Need to Notify the Office If You Have:

A. Increased swelling, pain, or warmth in your leg or arm with the deep vein thrombosis (DVT)

B. Fever

C. Sudden shortness of breath

D. Chest pain

E. If you are on a blood-thinner medicine, call for signs of bleeding. including:
   1. Nosebleed that will not stop with pressure
   2. Coughing up blood
   3. Vomiting that is bright red or dark that looks like coffee grounds or grape jelly
   4. Blood in your bowel movements that looks black or tarry in color
   5. Heavy periods
   6. Severe headache
   7. Sudden weakness in an arm or leg
   8. Sudden change in vision
   9. Trouble speaking or understanding others
   10. Memory loss or confusion

F. Any new symptoms not present at your last office visit

Phone: ______________________________

You can build your own identification bracelets or neck chains from American Medical ID: www.americanmedical-id.com

RESOURCES

Patient Education Center—Thromboembolism (DVT and Pulmonary Embolism): patienteducationcenter.org/articles/thromboembolism-deep-vein-thrombosis-and-pulmonary-embolism

Vascular Disease Foundation: vasculardisease.org/about-vascular-disease/2011-05-05-02-02-59/deep-vein-thrombosis-dvt

DEMENTIA

PROBLEM

Dementia is mental impairment due to a variety of disorders.

CAUSE

Dementia is caused by degeneration and loss of the gray matter from the brain; common causes of Alzheimer's disease are inadequate blood supply to the brain, alcoholism, chronic infections, inherited conditions, brain injury, or brain tumors.

PREVENTION/CARE

Early medical treatment is required for reversible causes of dementia. Prevention includes protection from head injury, eating a balanced diet, preventing alcoholism, avoiding drug abuse, and preventing atherosclerosis.

TREATMENT PLAN

A. Minimize changes in daily routines.

B. Provide simple memory reminders such as notes, calendars, and clocks.

C. Encourage social contacts.

D. Caregivers should treat the individual with respect.

E. Provide a safe environment.
   1. Remove scatter rugs.
   2. Install handrails and stairs.
   3. Discourage driving.
   4. Install stove cut-off switch.
   5. Lock closets.
   6. Lock up matches and firearms.

F. Encourage "thinking" games such as puzzles, word games, and reading.

G. Provide frequent gentle reorientation to surroundings.

Activity: Patient may engage in as much activity as possible with *supervision* and *direction*.

Diet: Eat a well-balanced diet low in saturated fat.

Medications: A variety of medications are available to treat symptoms.

You Have Been Prescribed: ______________________________

You Need to Take: ______________________________

You Need to Notify the Office If:

A. The symptoms/behaviors are getting worse.

B. You are unable to tolerate the medications because of side effects.

C. You need help with social services.

D. Other: ______________________________

Phone: ______________________

RESOURCE

Alzheimer's Association: www.alz.org
The Alzheimer's Association's website includes information on locating the closest support group; search by zip code: www.alz.org
24/7 Helpline 1-800-272-3900

DERMATITIS

PROBLEM

Inflammation of the skin that occurs from contact with an irritant substance (poison ivy, soaps, etc.).

CAUSE

Skin contact with irritating agent.

PREVENTION

A. Avoid aggravating agents.

B. Learn to recognize all plants (poison ivy, poison oak, etc.).

C. Flare-ups are common.

D. Avoid all known stimuli (poison ivy, soaps, etc.).

E. Do not wear tight, restrictive clothing.

F. When around irritating substances, wear gloves for protection.

G. For poison ivy
   1. Wash all clothes, shoes, pets, or other substances that may have come in contact with the poison ivy oil.

TREATMENT PLAN

Activity: As tolerated. Take cool baths as needed for itching. Oatmeal baths (Aveeno bath) help soothe the itching.

Diet: Regular diet.

Medications: Take Benadryl as needed for itching. Use calamine lotion as needed. Steroid creams may also be prescribed if reaction is severe. Steroid dose packs may be needed if you are not getting better.

You Have Been Prescribed: ____________________

You Need to Take: ____________________

You Need to Notify the Office If You Have:

A. Worsening symptoms

B. Sores on your face, eyes, or ears

C. More redness, swelling, pain, or drainage

D. Secondary bacterial infection

E. Fever

F. Other: ____________________

Phone: ____________________

DIABETES

PROBLEM

You have been diagnosed as having diabetes. Diabetes does not go away; you have to manage it every day. It is a condition in which your body cannot use the glucose from food properly. Some signs that your blood sugar is too high and too low are listed here.

A. *Hyperglycemia* (high blood sugar) signs/symptoms: Fruity breath odor, abnormal breathing pattern, rapid, weak pulse, confusion, or stupor.

B. *Hypoglycemia* (low blood sugar) signs/symptoms: Hunger, weakness, sweating, headache, shaking, rapid heartbeat, paleness, fainting, seizures, or coma.

CAUSE

Your body has an organ close to the stomach called a pancreas. Your pancreas is not making enough insulin or your body is not using the insulin it is making properly.

TREATMENT/CARE

A. Lifestyle changes—exercise, stop smoking, follow your diet, and lose some weight—are necessary to control your diabetes.
   1. Stop smoking. Smoking doubles your risk of developing heart or blood vessel disease.
   2. Weight loss of even 5 to 10 lb helps to control your diabetes.
   3. You need to wear an identification tag that tells others you have diabetes in case of an emergency.

B. Foot care is very important.
   1. Check feet every day.
   2. Wash with mild soap and lukewarm water.
   3. Apply lotion.
   4. File or clip nails after washing and drying.
   5. Do not tear skin around calluses.
   6. Wear clean socks daily.
   7. Wear well-fitted shoes at all times: No bare feet. You may not be able to feel or detect damage.
   8. Avoid crossing your legs.
   9. Take shoes off at every office visit.

C. Blood glucose monitoring: You will be instructed on how to check your blood sugar at home.
   Goals of Glycemia Control
   1. Fasting blood sugar: 80 to 120 mg/dL
   2. 2-Hour postprandial glucose: Less than 180 mg/dL
   3. Bedtime glucose: 100 to 140 mg/dL
   4. Hemoglobin A_{1c}: Less than 7%

D. For low blood sugar you need to follow the 15:15 rule:
   1. After having low blood sugar, you need to check your blood every 4 hours for the next 24 hours.
   2. 15:15 rule: Choose one to follow:
      a. Take three glucose tablets.
      b. Drink 1/2 cup orange juice.
      c. Drink 1/2 cup apple juice.
      d. Drink 1/3 cup grape juice.
      e. Drink 6 oz of regular coke.
   3. If your blood sugar drops less than 59, then you need to follow the 15:15 rule, drinking juice or taking glucose tablets, and then follow with 1/2 cup of milk and a starch and 1 ounce of protein.
   4. **If you have severe low blood sugar, you could pass out and go into a coma. You need to have glucagon for emergencies.**
      a. Glucagon is not glucose, but it helps the liver raise your blood glucose.
      b. Glucagon is a prescription drug and is given by injection; it usually works within 15 minutes.
      c. If you do not respond with the first shot of glucagon, your family needs to call 911.
      d. A second dose of glucagon should be given by your family if you do not awaken in 15 minutes.
      e. After receiving glucagon and you respond, you need to eat a snack.

(*continued*)

DIABETES *(continued)*

REGULAR CARE

A. You will need to come to the office at regular times to have your diabetes checked and make sure you do not have any complications. Your provider will follow national standards of care, including:
   1. Order a dilated eye examination every year.
   2. Check your blood pressure and keep it less than 140/80.
   3. Check your cholesterol at least once a year.
   4. Do a special foot examination at least once a year.
   5. Check your A1c every 3 months to see if your blood sugar is under control.
   6. Check your urine for protein/kidney problems.
   7. Give you a flu vaccine every year.
   8. If you are older, give you need a pneumonia vaccine, too.

SICK DAY RULES

You will also need a special plan in the event you are sick or have a special occasion.

A. Test blood sugar more often up to every 2 to 4 hours.

B. Increase your fluids, even if you do not feel like eating.

C. Follow a meal plan if you can.

D. Call your health care provider if your blood sugar is less than 70 or greater than 240 for two readings in a row that cannot be explained; if you are unable to retain food/fluids; and if you are spilling ketones.

E. Check your ketones if your blood sugar is greater than 240. If your ketones are negative, keep testing if your blood sugar stays up.

F. Continue to take your usual insulin dose.

G. **Do not take glucophage if you are dehydrated.**

Activity:

A. Exercise is very important in controlling your diabetes. It not only improves blood sugar by helping your insulin to work, but it also reduces your risk of heart attack and stroke and helps with losing weight.

B. Talk with your health care provider before starting an exercise plan. If you are currently doing some form of exercise, please continue; however, avoid any strenuous exercise.

C. Moderate exercise (walking, cycling, and swimming) is the best exercise. Your goal will be to develop a consistent exercise activity three to four times a week for 20 to 45 minutes. Drink plenty of fluids before and after you exercise to prevent dehydration.

D. Exercise causes a decrease in your blood sugar for up to 24 hours. Do not exercise if your fasting blood sugar is greater than 250 or your sugar at any time is over 300. Exercise is not recommended if you have ketones (burning fat instead of sugar).

Diet:

A. You will be seeing a dietitian to develop a nutritional plan that is suited for you.

B. Consistency with meal times and amounts and food from all the six major food groups is important.

C. Even though we stress carbohydrate counting, diabetes has abnormalities in carbohydrate, fat, and protein metabolism that cause hyperglycemia.

D. Dietary control includes control of fats such as cholesterol and saturated fat to help control blood lipid levels and prevent cardiovascular disease.

E. Eat a balanced diet, eat at regular times, and try not to skip meals; eat about the same amount of food at meal/snack times.

F. Use portion control, decrease the fats that you eat, and decrease fast simple sugars.

G. Decrease your alcohol consumption.

(continued)

DIABETES *(continued)*

Medications:

A. You may need a combination of medications or insulin to help control your blood sugar to prevent complications.

B. If you use insulin injections or the insulin pump, the best place to give it is your stomach.

C. The American Diabetes Association recommends that you take an angiotensin-converting enzyme (ACE) inhibitor (blood pressure medicine) to help protect your kidneys.

D. You may be told to take an aspirin every day (if you are not allergic).

You Have Been Prescribed: ______________________________

You Need to Take: ______________________________

You Have Been Prescribed: ______________________________

You Need to Take: ______________________________

You Have Been Prescribed: ______________________________

You Need to Take: ______________________________

You Need to Notify the Office If:

A. You are sick and unable to keep foods/fluids down (vomiting) or have severe diarrhea.

B. You intend to take over-the-counter medications because they could react with your diabetes medication.

C. You are using Metformin (glucophage) and are going to have x-rays using any dyes. You must stop your medicine.

D. Other ______________________________

Phone: ______________________________

Remember to carry an ID and carbohydrate source. Glucagon should be available for severe low blood glucose due to risk of aspiration and/or inability to swallow.

RESOURCES

American Diabetes Association (ADA): www.diabetes.org
You can build your own identification bracelets or neck chains from American Medical ID: www.americanmedical-id.com

DIARRHEA

PROBLEM

Diarrhea is a condition that causes loose, watery stools. Diarrhea is a symptom, not a disease. If you are a diabetic and have more than 1 day of diarrhea, please contact the office.

CAUSE

There are many causes of diarrhea, including infections caused by virus, bacteria, and even parasites.

PREVENTION/CARE

A. Avoid raw seafood and undercooked foods. Cut away any damaged or bruised areas on fruits and vegetables before eating.

B. Store food in the refrigerator within 1 hour of cooking to prevent the growth of bacteria. Store fruits and vegetables away from raw meat, chicken, and seafood.

C. Avoid buffet or picnic foods left out for several hours and food served by street vendors.

D. Wash your hands well before and after preparing foods, after going to the bathroom, and after handling diapers.

E. When traveling:
  1. Avoid local water supplies (including ice) when they are in question: Drink bottled water instead.
  2. Do not eat fresh vegetables that may have been washed in contaminated water.
  3. If possible, travel with antiseptic hand lotion and wipes.

F. When hiking or camping, do not drink from streams, springs, or untested wells. Boil all water used for drinking or cooking.

G. Do not allow people with diarrhea to handle food.

H. Do not buy turtles, iguanas, or reptiles for pets: They carry *Salmonella.*

I. Thoroughly cook eggs. Do not eat raw eggs or foods containing raw eggs, such as cookie dough. Store fruits and vegetables away from raw meat, chicken, and seafood.

J. Cook chicken, beef, and pork until the meat does not have any pink color.

K. Call your day care center if your child has diarrhea, especially if he or she has fever. Keep your child away from child-care centers if the diarrhea is too much for a diaper or if he or she is unable to get to the toilet.

TREATMENT PLAN

A. Diarrhea usually goes away in 24 to 48 hours.

B. Keep drinking liquids.

C. If you think a prescription drug is causing diarrhea, consult with the doctor before stopping the medication.

D. Clean toys and hard surfaces with soap and water. Chlorine-based disinfectants inactivate rotavirus and may help prevent the spread in child-care centers.

Activity: Decrease activities until diarrhea stops.

Diet:

A. If diarrhea is accompanied by nausea, suck ice chips.

B. Drink clear liquids frequently, such as 7-Up, Gatorade, ginger ale, broth, or gelatin, until diarrhea stops.

C. Use popsicles for added liquid.

D. After symptoms disappear, eat soft foods, such as cooked cereal, rice, baked potatoes, and yogurt, for 1 to 2 days.

E. Resume your normal diet in 2 to 3 days after the diarrhea stops.

F. Avoid fruits, alcohol, and highly seasoned foods for several more days.

(*continued*)

DIARRHEA *(continued)*

Medications:

You or Your Child Has Been Prescribed the Following Antidiarrheal Medication: ______________________

You or Your Child Need to Take: ______________________

You Need to Notify the Office If:

A. You or your child has diarrhea lasting more than 2 days or has chronic diarrhea.

B. You or your child has mucus, blood, or worms in the stool.

C. You or your child has a fever of 101.0°F or higher.

D. You or your child has severe pain in the stomach or in the rectum.

E. You or your child has dehydration symptoms, including dry mouth, wrinkled skin, excessive thirst, or little or no urine.

F. Your child:
   1. Becomes listless, refuses to eat, or cries loudly and persistently, even when picked up
   2. Has abnormal growth and development

G. Other: ______________________

Phone: ______________________

DYSMENORRHEA (PAINFUL MENSTRUAL CRAMPS OR PERIODS)

PROBLEM

Painful menstrual cramps, or dysmenorrhea, can cause occasional diarrhea, nausea or vomiting, and headache with menstrual periods.

CAUSE

A substance called prostaglandin causes most painful menstrual cramps. This substance is made in the uterus and causes the uterus to contract. Most menstrual cramps are normal and are not a sign of anything wrong. However, menstrual cramps may cause you to feel bad enough that you are unable to go to school or work. If that is the case, your health care provider can suggest medication to decrease the painful periods.

TREATMENT PLAN/CARE

A. Your health care provider may suggest a medicine such as a prostaglandin inhibitor. This medication helps decrease or eliminate the most likely substance that is causing the cramping of your uterus. The medication most often suggested is ibuprofen (Motrin IB, Advil, Nuprin, or others). Another medication is naproxen (Aleve).
   1. These are available at your local drug store, grocery store, or convenience store.
   2. Take any of these with a snack or meal to protect your stomach lining and prevent nausea.
   3. If you usually have very painful menstrual cramps, begin your medication as soon as your period begins or even the day before your period. This helps stop the production of prostaglandin.

B. If your cramps are not better using over-the-counter medications, your health care provider may write a prescription for a stronger medicine.

C. Many women take oral contraceptive pills to relieve menstrual cramps. A prescription is necessary. Notify your care provider if you are a cigarette smoker as smoking may increase your chance of side effects with oral contraceptives.

D. Some women find that exercise, such as walking, helps ease the cramps.

E. Another idea is a warm bath, shower, or a warm heating pad placed on your abdomen.

F. General health practices such as regular exercise, yoga, routine sleep habits, and regular sexual activity are beneficial.

Activity: Try to continue your usual activity. Try taking a walk, swimming, or doing yoga. Try a warm bath or shower.

Diet: Eat your normal diet. If you are nauseated, drink a clear carbonated soda (7-Up or Sprite).

Medication:

You Have Been Prescribed: ______________________________

You Need to Take: ______________________________

You Need to Notify the Office If You Have:

A. Any questions concerning your condition

B. Problems taking the medicine

C. No relief when taking the medicine, and other measures do not help

D. Any signs of infection, such as fever, chills, bad-smelling vaginal discharge, or burning sensation when you urinate

E. Other ______________________________

Phone: ______________________________

DYSPAREUNIA (PAIN WITH INTERCOURSE)

PROBLEM

As many as 60% of women complain of pain with sexual intercourse, also known as dyspareunia. Pain may occur with insertion of and/or with deep penetration of the penis into the vagina.

CAUSE

There are physical causes, such as episiotomy scars, a short vagina, and infections; musculoskeletal causes such as disc problems; hormonal causes such as the lack of estrogen in menopause; and poor communication with partners and lack of foreplay.

PREVENTION AND TREATMENT PLANS

A. Inadequate lubrication:
   1. More prolonged foreplay increases natural vaginal lubrication.
   2. Use a water-soluble lubricant such as K-Y jelly or Astroglide.
   3. Do not use Vaseline as a lubricant.
   4. Do not use contraceptive creams for lubrication; they often cause dryness (dehydration) and may worsen soreness.

B. Pain on insertion of penis:
   1. Try different positions that give you more control.
   2. Guide the penis for insertion.
   3. If menopausal, you may be prescribed estrogen cream to use on an intermittent basis.

C. Pain with deep penetration:
   1. Use a side-lying position during intercourse; this may be more comfortable so that deep penetration is limited.
   2. You may need to be referred to a gynecologist for further treatment and/or surgery if you have any masses or scar tissue noted on a physical examination.

D. If you have or suspect an infection:
   1. Inform your provider that you may have an infection.
   2. A culture will be done.
   3. Antibiotics will be prescribed for you and possibly your partner(s).
   4. Refrain from sexual intercourse until all medications are gone (unless otherwise instructed).
   5. If you have a Bartholin's duct cyst, it will be drained and you will be treated with antibiotics.

E. If you have a very narrow vaginal opening, you may be referred to a gynecologist for vaginal dilation.

F. Spasm of the muscles upon touching the vaginal area may be treated with medication, relaxation techniques, and Kegel exercises.

G. You and your partner may be referred to a sex counselor.

Medication:

You Have Been Prescribed: ______________________________

You Need to Take/Use It: ______________________________

You Need to Notify the Office If You Have:

A. No relief of your symptoms after your prescribed treatment

B. Other: ______________________________

Phone: ______________________________

ECZEMA

PROBLEM

Red, itching, scaling, and thickening of skin occurs in patches. You may have papules (bumps) with vesicles (clear fluid) that can be found especially on the hands, scalp, face, back of the neck, or skin creases of elbows and knees.

CAUSE

The cause is unknown. If it is an allergic reaction, it may be caused by foods such as eggs, wheat, milk, or seafood; wool clothing; skin lotions and ointments; soaps; detergents; cleansers; plants; tanning agents used for shoe leather; dyes; and topical medications. The risk for developing eczema increases with stress, medical history of other allergic conditions, clothing made of synthetic fabric (which traps perspiration), and weather extremes (cold, hot).

PREVENTION/CARE

A. Avoid risk factors.

B. Wear rubber gloves for household cleaning tasks.

C. Wear loose, cotton clothing to help absorb perspiration.

D. Keep fingernails short and wear soft gloves during sleep.

E. Scratching worsens eczema.

F. Bathe less frequently to avoid excessive skin dryness.

G. Use special nonfat soaps (Purpose or Basis soap) and tepid water.

H. Do not use soap on inflamed areas.

I. Lubricate the skin after bathing; avoid lubricants with alcohol in the ingredients.

J. Recommended creams include Eucerin, Keri Lotion, and Lubriderm. Steroid creams may be prescribed.

K. Avoid extreme temperature changes.

L. Avoid anything that has previously worsened the condition.

TREATMENT PLAN

Activity: No restrictions.

Diet: You may be told to try a special diet. Eliminate any foods known to cause flare-ups.

Medications:

You Have Been Prescribed: ______________________________

You Need to Take: ______________________________

You Need to Notify the Office If:

A. You have a reaction to any of the medications prescribed.

B. You cannot take the medications.

C. New symptoms develop.

Phone: ______________________________

EMERGENCY CONTRACEPTION—LEVONOGESTREL

You have indicated that you want to use an emergency contraception (EC) method. **There are several levonorgestrel emergency contraceptive pills with different brand names available** over the counter without prescription

TREATMENT PLAN

A. You must start levonorgestrel-based EC within 72 hours.

B. It is best to start within the first 12 to 24 hours.

C. Your health care provider will give you clear instructions.

D. The sooner you begin EC, the more effective it will be.

E. The levonorgestrel EC prevents pregnancy because the hormones cause the mucus in the cervix to thicken and the lining of the uterus and tubes to change.

F. You may not ovulate, but if you do ovulate, the egg will not be ready to be fertilized by a sperm.

G. EC in the form of hormonal pills will *not* interrupt an already established pregnancy.

H. Because you are taking more female hormones than you are used to, you may become sick to your stomach.

I. Your health care provider will tell you what medication to buy or give you a prescription for medicine to keep you from being sick to your stomach.

J. Take this medicine at least 1 hour before you take the hormone pills.

K. Other common side effects include breast tenderness, headache, or dizziness. These side effects go away in a day or two.

L. You should have a menstrual period a week or so after you take the pills.

M. If you have not had a period by 3 weeks, call the office.

N. It is unlikely that you would get pregnant, but if you do and choose to have a baby, the EC is *not* associated with any increased chance of birth defects.

O. Be sure to discuss reliable methods of birth control that are best suited for you.

Medication:

You Have Been Prescribed the Following EC Medication: ______________________

You Have Been Prescribed the Following Nausea Medication: ______________________

You Need to Call Us If You Have Any Questions or Problems.

You Need to Notify the Office If You Have:

A. Serious side effects of medicine

B. Severe chest pain

C. Severe abdominal pain

D. Headache

E. Vision changes

F. Shortness of breath

G. No period for 3 weeks

H. Other ______________________

Phone: ______________________

EMERGENCY CONTRACEPTION—ULIPRISTAL ACETATE

You have indicated that you want to use an emergency contraception (EC) method. **You have been prescribed ulipristal acetate.**

TREATMENT PLAN

A. You must start ulipristal acetate within 120 hours of unprotected intercourse.

B. Your health care provider will give you clear instructions.

C. The sooner you begin EC, the more effective it will be.

D. This method of EC prevents pregnancy by delaying ovulation.

E. Common side effects are headache and nausea.

F. Notify your health care provider if vomiting occurs within 3 hours of taking.

G. You should have a menstrual period a week to 3 weeks after you take the pills.

H. If your period is delayed by more than 1 week, call the office.

I. Do not take if you are breastfeeding or pregnant.

J. Do not take repeated doses in the same menstrual cycle.

K. This EC may decrease the effectiveness of hormonal contraceptives. Use a backup method (condom) for 14 days after taking this EC.

L. Do not use as routine contraception. Talk to your health care provider about birth control options that are best suited to you.

M. Seek medical attention if you experience lower abdominal pain 3 to 5 weeks after taking.

Medication:

You Have Been Prescribed the Following EC Medication: ______________________________

You Need to Call Us If You Have Any Questions or Problems.

You Need to Notify the Office If You Have:

A. Serious side effects of medicine

B. Severe chest pain

C. Severe abdominal pain

D. Headache

E. Vision changes

F. Shortness of breath

G. Menses delayed more than 1 week of expected date

H. Other ______________________

Phone: ______________________________________

EMPHYSEMA

PROBLEM

Emphysema is a chronic lung disease that is incurable. Emphysema can only be managed; the goal of treatment is to improve the activities of daily living and the quality of life by preventing symptoms and by preserving optimal lung function.

CAUSE

Cigarette smoking increases the risk of chronic obstructive pulmonary disease (COPD; another name for several lung diseases) by about 30 times. Environmental irritants have also been linked with chronic lung diseases.

PREVENTION/CARE

Emphysema cannot be prevented once lung changes have taken place.

TREATMENT PLAN

A. **Stop smoking—it causes more lung irritation, mucus/sputum production, and coughing. It is never too late to quit smoking.**

B. Eliminate other lung irritants, such as wood smoke; secondhand smoke; hair spray; and paint, bleach, and other chemicals found at home. Avoid sweeping and dusting, and stay indoors when air pollution or pollen counts are high.

C. Pulmonary rehabilitation may be ordered. Exercising is a very important component of pulmonary rehabilitation as well as learning breathing techniques.

D. Report respiratory infections to your health care provider as soon as possible.

E. Get a flu shot every year, and get a vaccination for pneumonia.

F. Use postural drainage: Lean over the side of the bed, rest your elbows on a pillow placed on the floor, and cough as someone gently pounds on your back.

G. Stay indoors during extremely hot or cold weather. If you must be outside in the cold, cover your nose and face. Use an air conditioner in hot weather.

H. Avoid people who have respiratory illnesses; also avoid crowds and poorly ventilated areas.

I. Oxygen therapy may be ordered if you have trouble breathing.

J. Use community resources such as Meals on Wheels, handicap tag, or parking stickers.

K. You may be asked to talk to a social worker.

Activity:

A. Pace yourself to avoid shortness of breath.

B. Follow a daily exercise plan. Start with three to four times a day, each lasting 5 to 15 minutes. Start at half-speed and build up.

C. Sexual dysfunction can occur because of lack of physical energy and trouble breathing. Find other ways to show affection such as kissing, hugging, or massage.

Diet:

A. If you do not have congestive heart failure, drink 3 L of fluids a day—equal to one and a half large soda bottles.

B. Avoid dairy products; they increase mucus/sputum production.

C. Eat five to six small meals a day. Big meals feel like pressure on your stomach and lungs.

D. Avoid foods that cause gas and stomach discomfort.

E. Use oxygen during meals, if necessary; take your time eating, rest between bites, and avoid hard-to-chew foods, because eating may tire you. Rest before and after eating if you have shortness of breath.

F. Eat a high-protein diet with a good balance of vitamins and minerals.

G. Avoid excessively hot or cold foods and drinks that may start an irritating cough.

H. Eat high-potassium foods such as bananas, dried fruit, orange and grape juice, milk, peaches, potatoes, tomatoes, and cantaloupe. Symptoms of low potassium include weakness, leg cramps, and tingling fingers.

(continued)

EMPHYSEMA *(continued)*

Medications:

You Have Been Prescribed: ______________________________

You Need to Take: ______________________________

Use of a spacer/chamber device improves aerosol delivery to your lungs and reduces side effects.

You Need to Notify the Office If:

A. You have trouble breathing.

B. You develop an infection (signs are fever, change in sputum, sinus drainage).

C. Your inhaler does not help your symptoms.

D. Your symptoms do not improve within 48 hours of starting medication.

E. Other: ______________________________

Phone: ______________________________

ENDOMETRITIS

PROBLEM

You have an infection of the inside of the uterus.

CAUSE

One or more types of bacteria that invaded damaged tissue following your delivery could cause endometritis. The bacteria may be from the vagina, the bowel, or the environment.

PREVENTION/CARE

A. Use careful perineal care:
   1. Wipe from front to back after voiding.
   2. Remove Peri-Pad from front to back.
   3. Change Peri-Pad at least every 4 hours.
   4. Use your squeeze bottle filled with warm water to cleanse after each time you urinate or have a bowel movement.
   5. Use good handwashing after changing your pads and the baby's diaper.

TREATMENT PLAN

A. You will need to be treated with antibiotic therapy.

B. Take your temperature three times a day for the first 3 days on the antibiotics.

C. Take Tylenol or ibuprofen as needed for fever or discomfort.

Activity: It is very important for you to increase rest with an infection. Try to get a nap when the baby is sleeping. You may continue to breastfeed on some antibiotic therapy. If you do not breastfeed while you are feeling bad, pump your breast milk to keep up your milk supply but dispose of it.

Diet: Eat well-balanced meals. Drink at least 10 to 12 glasses of liquid a day.

Medications: Continue your prenatal vitamins. Take all of your antibiotics even if you start feeling better.

You Have Been Prescribed: ____________________

You Need to Take: ____________________

You Need to Notify the Office If You Have:

A. Temperature that rises significantly or reaches 101°F

B. Foul-smelling vaginal bleeding

C. Increase in pain or tenderness

D. Other: ____________________

Phone: ____________________

EPIDIDYMITIS

PROBLEM

Epididymitis is infection of the gland that carries sperm.

CAUSE

The infection may be a urinary tract infection (UTI) or may be from a sexually transmitted disease (STD), such as gonorrhea or chlamydia.

PREVENTION/CARE

A. Prevent UTIs with good hygiene.
   1. Clean under foreskin if uncircumcised.
   2. Wash your hands after each time you go to the bathroom (both urine and bowel movements [BM]).

B. Limit your sexual partners and use a condom to prevent all types of infection.

TREATMENT PLAN

A. Antibiotics are used to kill bacteria that cause infection.

B. Try one of the following comfort measures:
   1. Intermittent cold compresses for acute swelling and pain relief
   2. Local heat or warm bath after the initial discomfort

C. Use an athletic supporter or elevate the scrotum on a small rolled washcloth.

D. Your sexual partner(s) need(s) to be treated for STD.

Activity:

A. Rest; do not engage in strenuous activity or heavy lifting.

B. Avoid sex until you finish the antibiotics.

Diet: Avoid foods that irritate the bladder: Caffeine, alcohol, and spicy foods.

Medications:

A. Antibiotics are used to kill bacteria causing infection.

B. Take all of the antibiotics prescribed for you; do not stop taking drugs after symptoms are gone.

C. Do not share your antibiotics with your sex partner(s); a full prescription of antibiotics is needed for each of you to get better.

D. Take pain medications or anti-inflammatory drugs, such as acetaminophen (Tylenol) or ibuprofen, as needed.

You Have Been Prescribed the Following Antibiotics: ____________________

You Need to Take: ____________________

Finish all of the antibiotics, even if you feel better.

You Have Been Prescribed the Following for Pain: ____________________

You Need to Take: ____________________

You Need to Notify the Office If:

A. You have a great increase in pain or swelling after going home.

B. You have worsening symptoms after starting the antibiotics.

C. You have fever greater than 101.0°F.

D. You get very constipated.

E. Other: ____________________

Phone: ____________________

ERYTHEMA MULTIFORME

PROBLEM

An acute inflammatory disorder of the skin and mucous membranes, erythema multiforme is usually self-limited and benign. A severe form is known as Stevens–Johnson syndrome or erythema multiforme majus, and the less severe form is referred to as erythema multiforme minus.

CAUSE

The cause is unknown in 50% of the cases. Erythema multiforme has been associated with viral infections, particularly the herpes simplex virus; bacterial and protozoan infections; an immunologic reaction of the skin; medications (sulfonamides, penicillins, anticonvulsants, salicylates, barbiturates), with reactions occurring up to 7 to 14 days after using the medication; pregnancy; premenstrual hormone changes; malignancy; or radiation therapy. Risk increases with previous history of erythema multiforme.

PREVENTION/CARE

A. Avoid suspected causes.

B. Seek prompt treatment of any illness or infection.

C. Prevent herpes simplex virus outbreaks by avoiding sun exposure and reducing stress.

D. Seek treatment immediately if at any time symptoms seem to be worsening or increasing.

E. Discontinue any implicated medication.

F. Apply wet dressings or soaks, with Burow's solution, or apply lotions to soothe the skin.

G. Bathe in lukewarm to cool water three times a day for 30 minutes.

H. Monitor yourself for any eye involvement and report it to your health care provider immediately.

I. If mouth sores are present, use good oral hygiene (brush two to three times a day using a soft brush) and rinse frequently with cool water.

J. Hospitalization may be required if there is extensive skin involvement.

TREATMENT PLAN

Activity: As tolerated by the extent of the symptoms. Restrict yourself to bed rest if fever is present.

Diet: Usually no special diet is necessary, although if mouth sores are present, a soft or liquid diet may be better tolerated. Increase fluid intake above the general 8 to 10 glasses per day.

Medications: May be prescribed to control symptoms and pain.

You Have Been Prescribed: ______________________________

You Need to Take: ______________________________

You Need to Notify the Office If:

A. You have an adverse reaction to or cannot tolerate any of the prescribed medications.

B. Symptoms worsen during treatment, or the rash does not clear in 3 weeks (usual course: Rash evolves over 1–2 weeks, usually clears in 2–3 weeks, but may take 5–6 weeks).

C. New or unexplained symptoms develop.

D. You have any questions or concerns.

Phone: ______________________________

EXERCISE

You have been evaluated and cleared for an exercise program. Your maximum target heart rate during exercise based on your age and physical fitness is ____________ beats per minute.

Your goal is to exercise at least three times a week (nonconsecutive days). Your target heart rate should be sustained for 20 to 30 minutes for maximal cardiovascular effect.

A. **Your exercise plan should include four components of activity:**
   1. Warm-up
      a. The warm-up phase prepares the body to increase the blood flow to the heart and decreases muscle tension. **The warm-up phase should last 10 to 20 minutes** and may include such exercises as head rotations, arm and shoulder circles, waist circles or bends, and side leg raises.
   2. Stretching
      a. Stretching prepares the major muscles for exercise. Slow stretching and holding repetitions help to prevent injury. Examples of stretching: Sitting hamstring leg stretches and holds, and arm stretches.
   3. Aerobic activity
      a. The aerobic phase of exercise should be continuous. **Your target heart rate should be maintained for 20 to 30 minutes for cardiovascular benefit.** Examples of aerobic activity: Brisk walking, running, or swimming.
   4. Cooldown phase
      a. **A cooldown period for 5 to 10 minutes finishes your exercise.** This gradual cooldown allows the body temperature to cool and slowly decreases the heart rate, preventing dizziness, fatigue, and nausea. Examples of cooldown exercise: Walking and cooldown stretches.

B. **Exercise should be discontinued if the following symptoms develop:**
   1. Marked increase in shortness of breath (inability to talk while exercising)
   2. Chest pain, including left arm and jaw pain
   3. Irregular heartbeat
   4. Nausea or vomiting
   5. Faintness or light-headedness
   6. Injury to muscle or joints (sprains, tears)
   7. Prolonged fatigue
   8. Muscle weakness

Seek immediate medical attention if you experience chest pain. If your shortness of breath or irregular heartbeat does not subside within 1 to 2 minutes of rest, seek help. Return to your health care provider for an evaluation before further exercise after you experience any other symptoms.

C. **Exercise can be easily incorporated into daily activities in other ways:**
   1. Use the stairs instead of the elevator.
   2. Park away from buildings to add extra walking distance.
   3. Use the walking path and carry golf clubs instead of using golf carts.
   4. Play outdoor games of catch, kickball, or hopscotch instead of indoor activities.
   5. Push-mow your yard instead of riding or hiring others for lawn care.
   6. Take an evening walk in your neighborhood or use the local mall for all-weather exercise.
   7. Shovel snow from the sidewalk instead of using a snow blower.
   8. Sweep the porch patio instead of using a leaf blower.
   9. Rake leaves for composting.
   10. Rent or buy an exercise video on yoga, Tai Chi, or aerobics instead of a movie.
   11. Turn on your radio and dance.
   12. Walk your dog for 20 to 30 minutes at a time.

EYE MEDICATION ADMINISTRATION

PROBLEM

You have been prescribed a medication for your eye(s). It is very important that you know the correct way to use your eye medication.

CAUSE

You have been diagnosed with

PREVENTION/CARE

The health of your eyes is important.

A. Use good handwashing and try not to rub your eyes with your fingers.

B. Clean your contacts regularly with contact cleaning solution. Do not put your contacts in your mouth to moisten.

C. Wear sunglasses in bright sunshine.

D. Use eye goggles when working and playing sports to ensure extra protection.

E. Replace your eye makeup often. Mascara, eye shadow, and eyeliner grow bacteria. Do not share makeup.

TREATMENT PLAN

A. Correct use of your medication is important.

B. You may or may not require an eyepatch or shield.

How to Apply Eye Ointment

A. Always wash your hands before placing medication in your eyes.

B. Gently pull down the lower eyelid.

C. Make a small pocket between the eyeball and the eyelid.

D. If you have someone helping to put your eye ointment in the lower-lid pocket, look up and away while he or she puts in the medicine.

E. Do not let the tube of medicine touch the eye or eyelid.

F. Squeeze a thin ribbon of the medication into the pocket of the eyelid.

G. Start at the inner fold of the eye going from the nose to the outer eye.

H. Let go of the eyelid and blink to spread the medication.

How to Instill Eye Drops

A. Always wash your hands before placing medication in your eyes.

B. Gently pull down the lower eyelid.

C. Make a small pocket between the eyelid and the eyeball.

D. If you have someone helping to put your eye drops in the lower lid pocket, look up and away while he or she puts in the medicine.

E. Do not let the bottle of medication touch the eye or eyelid.

F. Squeeze the prescribed number of drops of the medicine into the pocket of the eyelid.

G. Let go of the eyelid and blink (or tell the patient to blink) to spread the medication.

Activity: No restrictions are required unless you require eye surgery; then you will be given specific instructions about the amount of activity allowed.

Diet: No restrictions.

(continued)

EYE MEDICATION ADMINISTRATION *(continued)*

Medications:

You Have Been Prescribed: ______________________________

You Need to Take: ______________________________

You Need to Notify the Office If:

A. You are unable to put in the medication yourself or get help from others.

B. You are not better 24 to 48 hours after starting the medication.

C. Your vision is worse after using the medication.

D. You have an allergic reaction to the medicine.

E. Other: ______________________________

Phone: ______________________________

FEBRILE SEIZURES (CHILD)

PROBLEM

Convulsions or seizures may occur with an illness accompanied by a fever.

CAUSE

The cause of seizures with a febrile illness is not certain. Some families have seizures with fever that run in the family.

PREVENTION/CARE

A. Contact the office when your child gets sick with a fever.
   1. Aspirin is not given to a child because of the risk of Reye's syndrome.
   2. You may be instructed to give Tylenol or Motrin by your health care provider to help comfort your child. These medications do not prevent febrile seizures.
   3. Be sure that your child gets plenty of fluids and rest.
   4. You do not need to take your child's temperature on a strict schedule if he or she is not getting/feeling worse. For children ages 0 to 5 years, the rectum and mouth areas are *not routinely* used to measure fever.
   5. Do not use the thermometers with mercury in the glass. Use electronic/digital, infrared/tympanic, or chemical dot thermometers. The mouth, rectum, forehead (chemical dots), ears, or armpit are common areas for taking temperatures in children, depending on the age of the child. Always hold the thermometer while taking your child's temperature.

B. Care during a seizure:
   1. Make sure that your child is breathing without difficulty.
   2. Lay your child down on a safe surface and position the head to the side so that he or she does not spit up and get vomit into his or her lungs.
   3. Try not to restrain your child, but protect him or her from hurting himself or herself.
   4. Do not try to open his or her mouth or put your fingers in the mouth.
   5. Do not try to give your child any medications during a seizure.
   6. Seizures from fever generally last less than 5 minutes.
   7. If the seizure lasts longer than 5 to 7 minutes, or if your child is not breathing or looks blue, call 911 for an ambulance.
   8. After the seizure, your child may be sleepy. This is normal, and it is okay to let him or her rest.

Activity: When your child is not sick, there should be no restrictions on normal activity. When your child has a fever, try to keep him or her quiet and avoid strenuous play activity. Follow your child's day-care/school policy about when to return after having a fever/illness.

Diet: There is no special diet for a child with a fever; a regular diet is fine. Although your child has a fever, offer fluids to make sure he or she gets plenty of fluids, including formula and breast milk. Use juices or water, and, if directed, use Pedialyte. If your child is old enough, try ice pops for extra fluids.

Medications: You may be directed to use Tylenol or Motrin for your child's fever. These medications do not *prevent* febrile seizures.

Your Child Has Been Prescribed: ______________________________

Take the Medications on This Schedule: ______________________________

You Need to Notify the Office If:

A. Your child continues to have a high fever.

B. Your child is unable to keep fluids down due to nausea, vomiting, or diarrhea.

C. Other: ______________________________

Phone: ______________________________

If your child develops seizures lasting longer than 5 to 7 minutes or is having trouble breathing, *CALL 911.*

FIBROCYSTIC BREAST CHANGES AND BREAST PAIN

PROBLEM

You are being treated for breast pain or breast lumpiness that result from breast changes that are painful but not cancerous. You have probably had an extensive examination by your health care provider, perhaps a mammogram, sonogram, and/or a breast biopsy.

CAUSE

The cause is unknown. It is probably related to estrogen changes that occur with menstrual periods.

PREVENTION/CARE

None known.

TREATMENT PLAN

Be fitted for a well-fitting bra. This helps to eliminate breast movement as a source of pain. Try ice packs on your breasts for 20 minutes every few hours. Some women find that heat on the breast can also relieve discomfort.

Activity: There are no activity restrictions. When exercising, wear a good, supportive bra.

Diet: Eliminate or decrease salt in your diet to decrease water retention if you have swelling of your breasts near your period. Some women have reported decreased breast pain with reduced caffeine and nicotine intake.

Medications: Several medications have been found to relieve breast pain from fibrocystic breast changes, such as medications that decrease or stabilize estrogen (oral contraceptive pills). Ask your health care provider which is best for you.

Complementary: Recent research has shown that flaxseed may reduce cyclic pain (flaxseed 25 mg a day).

You Have Been Prescribed: ______________________________

You Need to Take: ______________________________

You Need to Call Us If You Have Any Questions or Problems.

Phone: ______________________________

FIBROMYALGIA

PROBLEM

You have inflammation or pain in the muscles and connective tissues, usually noted in the low back, shoulders, neck, chest, arms, hips, and thighs. This pain is chronic, and you may also have excessive fatigue and stiffness, difficulty with sleeping, and possibly other symptoms of anxiety, stress, and/or depression.

CAUSE

The cause is unknown. Fibromyalgia has been linked to anxiety, depression, stress, infections, and viruses.

TREATMENT PLAN/CARE

A. Get regular exercise.

B. Get adequate amounts of sleep.

C. For symptoms of discomfort, you may try applying heat to the areas of pain, such as hot showers, heating pad, and whirlpools.

D. Gentle massages by a massage therapist may help with comfort.

E. Try to eliminate the daily stress in your life.

F. Consider alternatives to relieving stress such as biofeedback, relaxation techniques, and yoga.

G. Notify your health care provider if you are having symptoms of anxiety or depression that need addressing and possible treatment with medications.

Activity: Regular exercise is recommended. Exercise at least 30 minutes, for three to five times a week, if possible. Even 5 minutes is better than no exercise. Establish a regular sleep time. Adequate and sound sleeping may decrease symptoms. You may require naps during the day.

Diet: Eat a nutritious regular diet. Increase your intake of fruits and vegetables. Avoid foods, caffeine, and alcohol that interfere with your normal sleep.

Medications: There are medications to help with your fibromyalgia. You may be prescribed one of these by your health care provider. Examples may include duloxetine (Cymbalta), milnacipran (Savella), or pregabalin (Lyrica).

You may also need to treat other symptoms accordingly:

1. Pain can be addressed with nonsteroidal anti-inflammatory drugs (NSAIDs) such as ibuprofen or naproxen.
2. Sleep disorder: Address this with your health care provider for treatment.
3. Anxiety/stress/depression: Address this with your health care provider.

You Have Been Prescribed: ____________________

You Need to Take: ____________________

You Need to Notify the Office If You Have:

A. New or unexplained symptoms that have developed

B. Fever higher than 100°F

C. Other: ____________________

Phone: ____________________

RESOURCE

The National Fibromyalgia Association: www.fmaware.org

FOLLICULITIS

PROBLEM

A bacterial (or fungal) infection of the hair follicle. Folliculitis is seen when a pustule develops, commonly on the arms, legs, scalp, and face (beard).

CAUSES

A. Bacterial: Infection commonly caused by *Staphylococcus* bacteria.

B. Fungal: May be caused by yeast infection.

PREVENTION

A. Keep skin clean and dry.

B. Avoid warm, moist conditions.

C. Healing generally occurs 10 to 14 days after proper treatment with medications.

D. Practice good handwashing technique, using antibacterial soaps.

E. Use clean razors daily.

F. Throw old razors away.

G. Do not share razors.

H. Shampoo scalp daily.

I. Folliculitis usually resolves within 4 to 6 weeks after proper treatment.

TREATMENT PLAN

Activity: As tolerated.

Diet: Regular diet.

Medications: Topical and/or oral antibiotics as prescribed.

You Have Been Prescribed: ______________________________

You Need to Take: ______________________________

You Need to Notify the Office If:

A. You notice lesions worsening or spreading, despite adequate medication treatment.

B. You have a fever higher than 101°F.

C. Your condition is not getting better.

D. You have a reaction to your medication.

E. Other ______________________________

Phone: ______________________________

GASTROESOPHAGEAL REFLUX DISEASE

PROBLEM

Relaxation of the lower esophageal (stomach) sphincter causes reflux of gastric acid or a feeling of "heartburn" and "acid brash."

CAUSE

Heartburn occurs when acidic stomach contents come back into the esophagus. Improper diet, spicy foods, alcohol, pregnancy, and nervous tension are all causes of gastroesophageal reflux disease (GERD).

PREVENTION/CARE

A. Avoid smoking.

B. Avoid things that increase abdominal pressure:
   1. Wearing tight clothes and belts
   2. Lying down or bending over for 3 hours after eating, which is when there can be a lot of reflux
   3. Coughing
   4. Straining

C. Avoid medications, such as aspirin or ibuprofen, that may irritate your stomach.

D. Avoid alcohol.

TREATMENT PLAN

A. Weight loss is advised to relieve symptoms.

B. Stop smoking.

C. You may be instructed to elevate the head of your bed on 6-inch blocks, or sleep on a wedge bolster pillow.

D. Review all of your medications, over-the-counter (OTC) medications, and herbal products with your health care provider to help identify any side effects that may cause your symptoms.

E. Take your medications at the correct times.

Activity: Postpone vigorous exercise until your stomach is likely to be empty, about 2 hours after eating.

Diet:

A. Eat a lower fat, bland diet.

B. Eat four to six small meals a day instead of three larger meals.

C. Do not eat 2 to 3 hours before bedtime.

D. Avoid chocolate, garlic, onions, citrus fruits, coffee (including decaffeinated), alcohol, highly seasoned foods, and carbonated beverages.

E. Eat slowly.

Medications: Sit or stand when taking solid medications (pills or capsules). Follow the drug with at least one cup of liquid. When OTC antacids do not make your symptoms better, please notify the office for medications that decrease gastric acid secretions. You may require lifelong therapy.

You Have Been Prescribed: ______________________________

You Need to Take: ______________________________

(*continued*)

GASTROESOPHAGEAL REFLUX DISEASE *(continued)*

You Need to Notify the Office If You Have:

A. No relief from antacids or second medication, so that the next step of medication therapy may be prescribed

B. New symptoms, such as blood in vomit

C. Other: ______________________________

Phone: ______________________________

GESTATIONAL DIABETES

PROBLEM

Gestational diabetes only develops during pregnancy because of the new hormones being produced. The hormonal influence makes you "insulin resistant," meaning you still produce insulin, but the hormones prevent it from working effectively.

Your blood sugar needs to be controlled so that the amount of sugar going to your baby is controlled, too. High blood sugar causes a big baby at delivery, increases your risk of a cesarean birth, causes the baby to have low blood sugar after delivery, increases jaundice, and causes other problems for the baby such as lung problems. It can also cause your baby to be overweight in childhood and increases the risk of developing diabetes.

CAUSE

You are producing new hormones that cause insulin resistance. The likelihood of having gestational diabetes increases with other factors, such as the mother's age, and it is more common in certain groups, such as Latin Americans and American Indians.

PREVENTION/CARE

Good control of your diet, exercise, and the possible use of medication and/or possibly insulin will help you to control your blood sugar during your pregnancy.

TREATMENT PLAN

A. You are asked to keep a record of your blood glucose values.
   1. You will be shown how to test your blood.
   2. You need to test your blood four times a day: First thing in the morning, before or after lunch, before or after dinner, and possibly at bedtime, depending on if your diabetes is diet controlled or controlled by medication.
   3. You will be given specific instructions before or after meals.
   4. Phone in your blood sugar values every week. Your insulin may be changed weekly.
   5. The goal of your fasting blood sugar before breakfast is 60 to 90 mg/dL.
   6. Your blood sugar goal before meals and 2 hours after meals is less than 120 mg/dL.

B. You need to test your urine for ketones every day.
   1. You will be shown how to test your urine.
   2. You need to test for ketones if you are unable to eat or if you have diarrhea.
   3. You need to test for ketones if you feel like you have a urinary tract infection (UTI), sinus infection, or any kind of infection.
   4. You need to test for ketones if your blood sugar is higher than 150 mg/dL.
   5. You must follow the diet given to you by the dietitian. If you have questions or do not understand what you should be eating, contact your dietitian.

Activity: Exercise lowers blood sugar—gestational diabetes control involves regular exercise. You need to walk at least 20 to 30 minutes a day. Try your local mall for a climate-controlled place to walk. Your heart rate should not get above 140 beats per minute.

Diet: You are placed on a ________ calorie diet. The amount of calories needs to be spread out over three meals and three snacks:

1. Breakfast, midmorning snack, lunch, midafternoon snack, dinner, and a snack at bedtime.
2. The time you eat is as important as what you eat. Try to keep on a regular schedule.

Medications: Depending on your blood sugar, you may require medication to control it. You will be instructed on how to take the medicine. If you are started on insulin, you will require extra testing for the rest of your pregnancy.

GONORRHEA

PROBLEM

Gonorrhea is a sexually transmitted infection. You may have the following symptoms: Burning during urination, yellowish discharge from the penis or vagina, heavier menstrual periods, or pelvic pain.

Untreated gonorrhea in females can lead to a condition called pelvic inflammatory disease (PID). PID is a leading cause of infertility, increased ectopic pregnancies, and chronic pelvic pain in women.

CAUSE

Gonorrhea is caused by an organism called *Neisseria gonorrhoeae.* This organism is spread through sexual contact and may infect the eyes, throat, vagina, penis, or rectum.

PREVENTION/CARE

A. Limit sexual partners.

B. Have routine screening tests for gonorrhea prior to beginning a new sexual relationship.

C. Use condoms when having intercourse.

TREATMENT PLAN

Your health care provider is required to report this disease to the public health department. The health department may contact you. **Abstain from sexual activity until you and your partner(s) have completed your prescribed medications.**

Diet: There is no special diet that needs to be followed.

Medications: Gonorrhea can be cured by the prescribed antibiotics.

You Have Been Prescribed: ______________________________

You Need to Take: ______________________________

It is very important that you keep your follow-up appointment that has been scheduled for you on: __________

All of the antibiotics need to be taken.

You Need to Notify the Office If:

A. You have any new symptoms.

B. You are unable to take all of the antibiotics due to nausea or vomiting or a reaction.

C. Other: ______________________________

Phone: ______________________________

GOUT

PROBLEM

Gout is caused by high uric acid deposits in the joints, which produce pain and swelling at the joint. Gout commonly occurs in the big toe; however, other joints may be affected, too. Other signs/symptoms include red, hot, and swollen joints, which may be tender to the touch. Gout also produces tophi, which are uric acid crystals that have formed under the skin, such as the edge of the ear, elbow, fingers, and toes, and near the Achilles tendon.

Gout is the result of too much uric acid production or not enough uric acid excretion from the kidney.

PREVENTION/CARE

A. The goal is to prevent recurrences of the attacks.

B. Acute attacks: You may apply warm or cool compresses to the affected areas for comfort.

C. Avoid weight-bearing objects on the affected joint.

D. Take your medication as prescribed.

Activity: When you have an attack, resting the joint is the best treatment. Drinking large amounts of water will keep your urine diluted to help prevent kidney stones.

Diet:

A. Drink 10 to 12 glasses of water a day. Avoid dehydration.

B. Refrain from alcohol (beer, wine, liquor). These will worsen your symptoms or trigger a new attack.

C. If overweight, you need to begin a weight-loss program appropriate for you.

D. Avoid crash diets. These will also precipitate an acute attack.

E. Foods to avoid: Purine-rich foods such as sardines, anchovies, red meat and organ meats (liver, kidney), dried beans, shrimp, and sweet bread.

Medications: Medications to avoid: Salicylates (aspirin). This can interfere with the kidney trying to get rid of the high uric acid levels.

You may be prescribed medications for pain such as nonsteroidal anti-inflammatory drugs (NSAIDs; ibuprofen or naproxen), steroids, pain relievers (acetaminophen), or colchicine.

You Have Been Prescribed: ______________________________

You Need to Take: ______________________________

You Need to Notify the Office If You Have:

A. Acute attacks

B. Fever higher than 101°F

C. Rash

D. Swelling of extremities

E. Vomiting/diarrhea

F. Signs/symptoms not improving within 3 to 4 days after starting therapy

G. Any adverse effects from your medication

H. Other ______________________________

Phone: ______________________________

GRIEF

PROBLEM

Normal grief resolution may take from 6 months up to as long as 2 years.

CAUSES

Grief can follow the death of a loved one, but grief also follows other losses such as a loss of independence, loss of affection, or loss of body parts after an accident.

TREATMENT PLAN

It is important that you talk about your loss and how it affects you. The more you are able to talk about your feelings related to the loss you are experiencing, the more you will be able to work through your feelings.

You may be encouraged to seek supportive therapy in the form of divorce groups, loss groups, or groups dealing specifically with death and dying.

Activity: Moderate exercise, such as daily walking, is encouraged. Vigorous, prolonged exercise, however, may precipitate anxiety attacks.

Diet: Avoid caffeinated beverages, including coffee, tea, and carbonated colas that do not specify "decaffeinated." Try to eat healthy food and avoid overeating or skipping meals.

Medications: Medications for loss and grief are usually avoided at first because the use of drugs can prolong the time it takes to work through your grief. However, your health care provider will discuss medications in more depth. If you are having signs of depression or think you may need treatment with medication, contact your health care provider.

You Have Been Prescribed: ______________________________

You Need to Take: ______________________________

Do not stop antidepressants quickly. Talk to your health care provider if you want to discontinue them.

You Need to Notify the Office If:

A. You feel like you cannot stop crying.

B. You are not eating and are losing weight.

C. You feel like you have no one to turn to and talk about your feelings.

D. You have difficulty sleeping after several weeks.

E. You have thoughts of hurting yourself or others.

F. You do not think you are getting better on the prescribed medication.

G. Other ____________________

Phone: ______________________________

Local Support Group: ______________________________

SUGGESTED BOOKS

Arnold, J. H., & Gemma, P. B. (1994). *A child dies: A portrait of family grief* (2nd ed.). Charles Press.

Fritsch, J., & Ilse, S. (1992). *The anguish of loss.* Wintergreen Press.

Ilse, S. (2008). *Empty arms: Coping with miscarriage, stillbirth, and infant death.* Wintergreen Press.

Smith, H. I. (2011). *A decembered grief: Living with loss while others are celebrating*. Kansas City, MO: Beacon Hill Press of Kansas City. (Original work published 1999)

Zonnebelt-Smeenge, S., & De Vries R. C. (2001). *Empty chair: Handling grief on holidays and special occasions*. Baker Books.

HEAD INJURY: MILD

PROBLEM

Mild head injury includes any bump, jolt, or blow to the head that affects normal brain function, possibly causing confusion or a loss of consciousness.

GUIDELINES FOR CARE AT HOME

Activity:

A. Have someone stay with you for the next 24 hours to be sure your head injury does not worsen.

B. Limit physical activity, especially sports, heavy exercise, and heavy lifting, and limit other activities that require you to concentrate or focus.

C. Slowly increase your activity. Pace yourself and stop to rest whenever you are mentally or physically tired.

D. Do not drive or operate heavy machinery during the next 24 hours.

E. You must have approval from your primary care provider before returning to work or school.

F. Coaches or trainers must be notified of any head injury.

Diet: Do not eat or drink if you feel sick to your stomach. When you feel better, you can eat or drink anything, except alcohol. You must not drink any alcoholic beverages until your primary care provider tells you it is safe to do so.

Medications: You should not take any medications, including the ones you take every day, until your primary care provider tells you it is safe to continue your medications.

INSTRUCTIONS FOR CAREGIVERS: OBSERVATION AFTER HEAD INJURY

Check the patient for signs and symptoms of worsening head injury during the first 24 hours after discharge. If he or she is sleeping through mealtimes or not awakening to go to the bathroom, awaken him or her for testing.

HOW TO TEST THE PATIENT

A. Test orientation: Ask the patient to tell you his or her name, where he or she is, the current month/day/year, and to tell you what your name is.

B. Test the patient's strength: Ask the patient to squeeze one or two of your fingers as hard as he or she can, checking both hands at the same time, and compare them. Also have the patient lift one leg at a time off the bed and hold it up for a few seconds.

C. Have the patient open both eyes at the same time and check his or her pupils to make sure they are the same size. (The pupil is the black round part in the center of the eye.)

D. If you are uncertain about these test results, repeat them in 5 minutes to be sure of what you see. *Call the primary care provider or go to the emergency room if you cannot tell what is normal or if the patient's head injury worsens.*

WARNING SIGNS

Call the primary care provider's office immediately or take the patient to the emergency room if you notice any of the following:

A. The patient cannot be easily awakened or sleeps constantly in between activities or tests for no apparent reason.

B. The patient cannot answer orientation questions correctly or becomes confused.

C. The patient has new or increasing weakness in any arm or leg, or has trouble standing or walking.

D. The patient becomes very restless, agitated, is acting unusual, or has any other change in behavior.

E. One pupil in an eye is larger than the other.

F. You cannot understand what the patient is saying or the patient cannot understand what you have said.

G. The patient complains of a severe or worsening headache.

H. The patient continues to complain of nausea or begins vomiting.

I. The patient has a fever over 100.9°F.

(*continued*)

HEAD INJURY: MILD *(continued)*

J. The patient has a convulsion or seizure, or passes out.

K. The patient has clear or blood-tinged fluid leaking from the nose or ear.

If any of the previous situations occur or if you have any questions/concerns regarding any of the tests, please call the primary care provider immediately or bring the patient to the emergency room or clinic right away.

Phone: ______________________________

WHAT TO EXPECT AFTER A HEAD INJURY

After a head injury, it is not unusual to have fatigue, headaches, irritability, dizziness, problems with sleep, trouble keeping your balance, or difficulty working in school or at your job. It is important to ***gradually*** increase your level of activity at home, school, and work. Take time to rest and schedule breaks whenever you feel physically or mentally tired. Usually, these symptoms or problems will lessen within a week and you will continue to improve over the next 3 months. Sometimes it may take longer to recover from a head injury. If you are still having symptoms or problems after 3 months, contact your primary care provider for additional treatment and advice.

HEMORRHOIDS

PROBLEM

A hemorrhoid is a varicose vein of the rectum. You can have hemorrhoids for years but not know you have them until bleeding occurs. They may cause rectal pain, itching, or a sensation that you have not emptied completely after a bowel movement. Hemorrhoids are often found after painless rectal bleeding with a bowel movement.

CAUSE

Repeated pressure in the anal or rectal veins causes hemorrhoids. They are commonly seen with obesity, pregnancy, constipation, inactive lifestyle, and liver disease.

PREVENTION/CARE

A. Avoid heavy lifting.

B. Try to prevent constipation or straining.

C. Eat a high-fiber diet.

D. Drink 8 to 10 glasses of water a day.

E. Lose weight if you are overweight.

F. Exercise regularly.

TREATMENT PLAN

A. Spend less time sitting on the toilet to reduce pressure in the veins around the anus.

B. Pat with toilet paper instead of rubbing.

C. Take sitz baths or soak in a warm bathtub three or four times a day for comfort.

D. Apply cold packs or witch hazel (Tucks) compresses for symptom relief.

E. Take a stool softener two to three times a day to prevent straining with bowel movements (BM).

F. A hemorrhoid treatment, such as ligation, freezing, or surgery, may need to be done for severe cases.

Activity: No restrictions are required. Bowel function improves with good physical activity.

Medications:

You Have Been Prescribed the Following Stool Softener: ____________________

You Need to Take: ____________________

You Have Been Prescribed the Following Local Cream: ____________________

You Need to Apply: ____________________

You Need to Notify the Office If You Have:

A. A hard lump that develops where a hemorrhoid has been.

B. Hemorrhoids that cause severe pain that is not relieved by the aforementioned treatment.

C. Excessive rectal bleeding: More than a trace or streak on the toilet paper or bowel movement. **Rectal bleeding may be an early sign of cancer.**

D. Other: ____________________

Phone: ____________________

HERPES SIMPLEX VIRUS

PROBLEM

You may experience oral or genital bumps or lesions (often painful), burning, itching, sensation of pressure, painful urination, painful lymph nodes (bumps along underwear line), or flu-like symptoms (fever, headache, muscle aches, tired feeling).

CAUSES

A. The herpes simplex virus (HSV) is spread by direct contact with the secretions of someone who has the virus.

B. Viruses cannot be cured, but the problems or symptoms caused by them can often be managed with medication.

C. It is possible for someone to have HSV and have no symptoms. The first outbreak after contact with an infected individual usually occurs within 2 to 10 days, but it may take up to 3 weeks.

D. More severe symptoms are experienced with the first outbreak of HSV. The symptoms usually peak 4 to 5 days after the onset of infection and resolve after 2 to 3 weeks without medication.

E. Medication may decrease the severity and duration of the symptoms. Recurrent outbreaks usually last 5 to 7 days.

F. The virus may be spread even when symptoms are not present. This is known as viral shedding. Medication may also decrease the time of viral shedding.

G. Often, individuals with HSV experience itching, burning, or a feeling of pressure at the site 24 to 48 hours before an outbreak. This is known as a prodrome.

H. Sexual activity should be avoided during this time because the viral shedding is occurring, which means the infection may be spread.

TREATMENT PLAN

A. Avoid sexual activity when lesions are present or when you feel the prodrome.

B. Use condoms with sexual activity.

C. Limit sexual partners.

D. Do not use any creams, lotions, or powders on lesions unless instructed to do so by your health care provider.

E. If urination is painful, pour water over the genital area while urinating.

F. Dry affected area thoroughly.

G. If you are pregnant at any time, notify your provider of your diagnosis of herpes to allow the provider to treat you accordingly prior to delivery to prevent spreading the herpes infection to your baby.

Activity: Stress is a trigger for an outbreak. Exercise may help with keeping your stress level down.

Diet: There is no special diet.

Medications: Antiviral medications are used to suppress the virus. They do not cure it but decrease the intensity of viral outbreaks.

You Have Been Prescribed: ______________________________

You Need to Take: ______________________________

You Need to Call the Office If:

A. You are unable to empty your bladder when you have an outbreak.

B. Other: ______________________________

Phone: ______________________________

HERPES ZOSTER OR SHINGLES

PROBLEM

Shingles is a reactivation of the viral infection of childhood known as chickenpox. **The virus is contagious for those who have not had chickenpox.**

CAUSE

Varicella-zoster virus is stimulated and produces a blisterlike rash, commonly seen on the chest and trunk area. The rash is commonly confined to one side of the body.

PREVENTION

Zostavax is a vaccination for the prevention of shingles. The Centers for Disease Control and Prevention (CDC) recommends this one-time vaccine for anyone age 60 years and older.

TREATMENT PLAN

A. Zostavax cannot be used to treat the shingles breakouts or the painful sensations (postherpetic neuralgia) after shingles develops.

B. The shingles rash usually lasts 2 to 3 weeks; however, symptoms may persist beyond this period.

C. The goal is to relieve the itching.

D. Apply warm soaks of Burow's solution three times a day to lesions.

E. Notify family and friends of active virus. Advise anyone who has had contact with you that you have shingles, especially pregnant women and those who have never had chickenpox.

Activity: Avoid touching the shingles. Wash your hands. Your partners should not touch the area, especially when blisters are present. Use separate bath towels.

Diet: There is no special diet for shingles.

Medications: Oral and topical medications may be prescribed to soothe the itching. Take acetaminophen (Tylenol) as needed for comfort. Antiviral medications are available to help slow down the virus if started within 48 to 72 hours after the initial outbreak. You may be prescribed medications to help with the painful sensations (neuralgia).

CDC Guidelines recommend all adults 60 years of age and older receive the Zostavax vaccine.

You Have Been Prescribed: ______________________________

You Need to Take: ______________________________

You Need to Notify the Office If You Have:

A. Severe pain at lesion sites

B. Any new symptoms relating to the shingles, such as excruciating pain, headaches, numbness, tingling sensation, or other symptoms

C. Any questions regarding the shingles

Phone: ______________________________

HIV/AIDS: RESOURCES FOR PATIENTS

AIDS HEALTHCARE Foundation
http://www.aidshealth.org

A Positive Life
Features real people telling their stories.
http://www.apositivelife.com

Centers for Disease Control and Prevention (CDC)
Provides general information on HIV.
http://www.cdc.gov/hiv/default.htm

HIVandHepatitis.com
Provides the latest information about coinfection with hepatitis B and hepatitis C.
http://www.hivandhepatitis.com

National Association of People With AIDS
POZ AIDS Services Directory is a comprehensive guide to HIV care and services.
http://directory.poz.com/napwa

Project Inform (includes Spanish resources)
Provides multiple topics, including the latest treatment options.
www.projectinform.org

The AIDS InfoNet
http://www.aidsinfonet.org

The Body
The most-visited Internet site about HIV.
http://www.thebody.com

The Well Project
Designed for HIV-positive women.
www.thewellproject.org

Treat HIV
Provides information about your treatment options.
http://www.treathiv.com

HUMAN PAPILLOMAVIRUS

PROBLEM

Human papillomavirus (HPV), also known as condyloma, or genital or venereal warts, is a sexually transmitted infection.

A. You may experience "bumps" or lesions on genitals or the perianal area. They may be raised and rough appearing or flat and smooth. They are often wartlike in appearance.

B. Lesions may appear singly or in clusters and may be small or large. They are usually soft, painless, and pale pink to grayish in color, and they may itch.

C. **It is very important to get regular Pap smears.**

D. There are several treatment options that your health care provider will discuss.

CAUSE

HPV is acquired by having genital contact or intercourse with someone who has the infection.

PREVENTION/TREATMENT PLAN

There is no cure for HPV, but the following may decrease the spread of HPV:

A. Do not have genital contact or intercourse without a condom when the lesions are present. Some people who have the infection never have symptoms (bumps or warts). It is possible to spread the infection even when no symptoms are present.

B. Limit sexual partners and openly discuss the need to use a condom.

C. Examine new partners for bumps or warts.

D. Ask your provider about receiving the Gardasil vaccine for preventing the HPV virus. It is available for males and females ranging from 9 to 25 years of age.

Medications:

You Have Been Prescribed: ______________________________

You Need to Take: ______________________________

You Need to Notify the Office If:

A. You have any new symptoms.

B. It is time for your Pap smear.

C. Other: ______________________________

Phone: ______________________________

INFANT NUTRITION

BREASTFEEDING

Breast milk is the best choice for feeding infants. Mothers are encouraged to breastfeed for at least 6 to 12 months. However, if you are unable to breastfeed for this length of time, breastfeeding for the first few weeks is highly beneficial to the newborn. If breastfeeding, you should consult with your practitioner prior to taking any medications.

Advantages of Breastfeeding

A. It allows increased contact with your baby.

B. Breast milk is digested more easily by infants than baby formula.

C. Breast milk causes fewer spit ups and stomach problems than formula.

D. There is no preparation, it is ready to feed anytime, it is always in the correct temperature.

E. It is inexpensive.

F. Babies who are breastfed have fewer allergies in childhood.

G. Antibodies in the mother's breast milk protect the newborn against infections.

H. It prevents overfeeding. Breastfed babies usually feed "on demand."

General Guidelines for Breastfeeding

A. You should breastfeed your baby when he or she is hungry. It is recommended to breastfeed your baby every 2 to 4 hours, which is approximately 8 to 12 times in a 24-hour period, during the first few days of life.

B. Babies may go through a "growth spurt" on day 3 or 4 after birth. Your baby may want to feed more frequently, every 1 to 2 hours during growth spurts.

C. After the baby is 1 to 2 weeks old, he or she will develop a routine pattern of eating every 2 to 4 hours during waking hours and possibly every 4 to 5 hours at nighttime.

D. Length of time feeding your baby at each feeding should last until the baby is full. Signs of fullness from your baby may include turning away from the breast, no longer feeding, or falling asleep.

E. It is not recommended to feed your baby water or formula in addition to breastfeeding. Some women may choose to occasionally add a supplement with formula. A soy-based formula is usually tolerated best by the baby.

F. The diet of a breastfeeding mother requires increased nutrition: 500 kilocalories above the normal diet and increased fluids are recommended.
   1. Mother's diet should exclude caffeine, chocolate, cabbage, beans, and other gas-forming foods. Alcohol and tobacco should also be avoided.

G. **Fluoride**
   1. When your child is fed solely breast milk, you should consider adding a vitamin and fluoride supplement.
   2. Fluoride supplementation may also be needed for babies who live in an area where the water is low in fluoride.
   3. Fluoride is important for prevention of dental caries.
   4. Even though your baby does not have any teeth, he or she still needs fluoride for building the developing teeth.
   5. Consult with your practitioner regarding this supplementation.

H. All medications and supplements should be avoided by the mother when breastfeeding. If these medications are necessary, please check with your health care provider to make sure the medication or supplement is safe while breastfeeding.

BOTTLE FEEDING

If breastfeeding is not an option, nutritional formulas are available. Ask your practitioner which is best suited for your baby.

A. It is best to have 6 to 8 bottles and 6 to 10 nipples prepared.

B. Formula may be purchased in powder, concentrate, or ready-to-feed forms.

C. Please read the can and be aware of the proper mixing method for each type of formula.

D. When feeding your baby, make sure the nipple is full of milk to avoid getting excess air in the baby's stomach.

E. You should never prop bottles on blankets or other objects when feeding your baby.

(*continued*)

INFANT NUTRITION *(continued)*

ROUTINE SCHEDULE OF FEEDING

A. Newborn:
   1. Give a newborn baby 1 to 2 oz of formula every 3 to 4 hours.
   2. Increase formula by 1 oz as tolerated by the baby.
   3. Give similar amounts at each feeding. The approximate total amount of formula your baby should take per day is determined by his or her weight (see table).
   4. If your baby seems dissatisfied with feedings, you may add 1/2 to 1 more ounce of formula. Be careful not to add more than this at a time, because overfeeding may cause the baby to have a "bellyache" or diarrhea.
   5. By 4 months of age, babies usually take 32 oz of formula per day. At this time, solid foods (e.g., baby cereal) are introduced.

SOLIDS

A. Solid foods are generally introduced to the baby at approximately 4 months.
   1. You may introduce new solid baby food every 3 to 5 days as tolerated by your baby.
   2. It is necessary to use this 3- to 5-day span between foods in case your baby is allergic or does not tolerate a specific food.
   3. If you have waited after trying a new food, you will be able to determine which food your baby was not able to tolerate.

B. Begin with rice infant cereal mixed with breast milk or formula.

C. Begin with 1 tablespoon. You may increase the amount to 2 to 5 tablespoons one to two times a day as tolerated by the baby.

D. Next, introduce fruits followed later by vegetables, increasing the amount as tolerated.
   1. If your baby does not like one vegetable, wait a few weeks to try to introduce it again.
   2. Some babies may be very finicky regarding the texture of solid food. Do not give up! One day the baby may accept the foods he or she used to spit out because of taste or texture.

E. Meats are usually the last food introduced and many babies do not like the texture; however, you should continue to offer them.

F. Juices are usually introduced last, at approximately 6 months.

COW'S MILK

A. It is not recommended to feed cow's milk to a baby during the first year of life.

B. Cow's milk may be introduced after your baby turns 1 year old.

HONEY

Honey is not recommended during a baby's first year of life because of the risk of infant botulism.

NUTRITIONAL INFORMATION

Beechnut Nutrition: 800-BEECH NUT or 1-800-233-2468 or www.beechnut.com
La Leche League Helpline: 800-LALECHE or 1-800-525-3243 or www.llli.org

Total Formula Needs Per Infant Weight

Infant Weight (Pounds)	Total Infant Formula Per Day (Ounces per Day in Divided Feedings)
7	19
8	21
9	24
10	27
11	30

INFLUENZA (FLU)

PROBLEM

Influenza (flu) is an acute, self-limiting, febrile illness of the respiratory tract. You are contagious for 24 to 48 hours before feeling symptoms, and you are contagious up to 7 days after symptoms begin. Coughing and sneezing spread the flu.

CAUSE

There are many flu viruses. Stress, excessive fatigue, poor nutrition, recent illness, crowded places, and immunosuppression from drugs or illness lower your resistance to these viruses.

PREVENTION/CARE

A. Although the flu vaccine neither prevents nor causes the flu, the flu vaccine is recommended for almost everyone.

B. The flu vaccine should be taken yearly (in the fall) if you are at high risk:
   1. Health care worker
   2. Immunocompromised (transplant patients, HIV-positive patients, etc.)
   3. Pregnant (after the first trimester)
   4. Elderly (older than 65 years)
   5. A child with severe asthma

C. Avoid unnecessary contact with sick persons, including in crowded areas.

D. To keep the flu from spreading:
   1. Cover your mouth when coughing or sneezing.
   2. Use tissues when you blow your nose. Dispose of them and then wash your hands.
   3. If no tissue is available, do the “elbow sneeze” into the bend of your arm (away from your open hands).
   4. Do not share drinking glasses.
   5. Wash your hands with soap and water or use hand sanitizer.

TREATMENT PLAN

A. Rest.

B. Drink lots of fluids.

C. Run a cool-mist vaporizer.

D. Take tepid sponge baths in warm water to prevent chilling and shivering.

E. Gargle with warm salt water for a sore throat.

F. Use warm compresses or a heating pad on low for aching muscles.

Activity: Stay in bed for at least 24 hours after your fever is gone.

Diet: You may not be hungry, but you do not need to be on a special diet for the flu. Drink plenty of liquids (at least 10 glasses a day).

Medications:

A. **Antibiotics do not help the flu because it is a virus.**

B. Do not use aspirin for a child because of the risk of Reye’s syndrome.

C. Special medications shorten the flu. They must be started within 2 days of contracting the flu.

You Have Been Prescribed for Your Fever: ____________________

You Need to Take: ____________________

You Have Been Prescribed for Your Respiratory Symptoms: ____________________

(*continued*)

INFLUENZA (FLU) *(continued)*

You Need to Take: ____________________

The American College of Chest Physicians Clinical Practice Guidelines recommend that cough suppressants and over-the-counter (OTC) cough medicine not be given to young children. Cough medicine should not be given to children younger than 4 years of age.

You Have Been Prescribed for Your Respiratory (Cough Suppressant) Symptoms: ____________________

You Need to Take: ____________________

You Need to Notify the Office If You Have:

A. Thick, green nasal drainage

B. Ear pain

C. Increase in fever or cough

D. Shortness of breath (SOB) or chest pain

E. Blood in your sputum

F. Neck pain or stiffness

G. New or unexplained symptoms

H. Other: ____________________

Phone: ____________________

INSECT BITES AND STINGS

PROBLEM

Skin changes and insect bites or stings that cause other reactions.

A. **Seek immediate help if you or a family member has any symptoms of allergic reaction or anaphylaxis, either immediately after the bite or in 8 to 12 hours after the bite.**

B. You may need to call 911 or your local emergency response service.

C. If you have had a previous life-threatening allergic reaction, carry an anaphylaxis kit for emergency treatment.
   1. *Local skin reactions* include red bumps on the skin that usually appear within minutes after the bite or sting, but may not appear for 6 to 12 hours. Itching and discomfort may occur at the site.
   2. *Systemic (body) reactions* include nausea or vomiting; headache, fever, dizziness, or light-headedness; swelling; or convulsions.
   3. *Allergic reactions* include itchy eyes, facial flushing, dry cough, wheezing, or chest or throat constriction or tightness.

CAUSE

Bites or stings can be caused by mosquitoes, fleas, chiggers, bedbugs, ants, spiders, bees, scorpions, and other insects. Risk increases with exposure to areas with heavy insect infestation, warm weather in spring and summer, lack of protective measures, use of perfumes or colognes, and previous sensitization.

PREVENTION/CARE

A. **Institute first-aid measures and activate emergency services if severe, life-threatening reactions occur.**

B. Avoid risk factors.

C. Wear protective clothing.

D. Use insect repellents with diethyltoluamide (DEET), avoiding the head, face, eyes, and mouth, especially with children.

E. Products containing DEET are not recommended for children under the age of 2 years.

Specific Insect Care

A. For all stingers: Remove stinger.

B. Bee, wasp, yellow jacket, or hornet stings: Rub a paste of meat tenderizer and water into the site.

C. Ant bites: Rub bite with ammonia, and repeat as often as necessary.

D. Spider and scorpion bites: Capture the arachnid if possible and seek medical attention.

E. Mites: Apply a petroleum product (Vaseline) until the animal withdraws from the skin.

F. Ticks: Remove the tick by following the instructions in Section II: Procedures "Tick Removal."

General Care for All Bites

A. Clean wound with soap and water.

B. Apply ice pack (no ice directly on skin; use towel or cloth to protect skin).

C. Elevate and rest the affected body part.

D. Immerse affected part or apply warm-water soaks to site. However, if site itches, cool water feels best.

E. For minor discomfort, you may use nonprescription oral antihistamines (Benadryl) or topical steroid preparations (hydrocortisone cream).

F. Use only low-potency topical steroid products without fluorine on the face and groin area.

G. You may be prescribed more potent, prescription medications.

TREATMENT PLAN

Activity: No restrictions.

Diet: Eat a regular diet. Maintain adequate hydration with 8 to 10 glasses of water per day.

(*continued*)

INSECT BITES AND STINGS *(continued)*

Medications: You may be prescribed an EpiPen to use for future major reactions. You need to keep this with you at all times.

You Have Been Prescribed: ______________________________

You Need to Take: ______________________________

You Need to Notify the Office If:

A. Self-care treatment does not relieve symptoms or if no improvement is noticed after 2 to 3 days.

B. A bitten area becomes red, swollen, warm, and tender to the touch; these symptoms indicate infection.

C. You have a temperature higher than or equal to 101°F.

D. You have a reaction or cannot tolerate any of the prescribed medications.

Phone: ______________________________

INSULIN THERAPY DURING PREGNANCY

You Have Been Prescribed Insulin Therapy:

A. Your insulin needs may change weekly because of the change in your hormones (you become more insulin resistant as your pregnancy progresses).

B. Insulin therapy is safe for your baby. Insulin does not cross the placenta like the sugar does.

C. The insulin lowers your blood sugar and therefore controls the amount of sugar that goes to your baby.

D. You may have been prescribed Humulin insulin, which works very much like your own body's insulin.

E. Some of the insulin therapies have a mix of short-term regular (clear) insulin with intermediate-acting (cloudy) insulin.
   1. You will be instructed in how to mix and give yourself your insulin.
   2. The first key to insulin therapy is to be able to recognize signs of too much and too little insulin. A chart is included to post on your refrigerator (see the following table).
   3. The second key is to let people know you are on insulin.
   4. You need a Medical Alert bracelet or necklace as well as information to put in your car and billfold.
   5. The third key is to have your baby and yourself evaluated more often when on insulin therapy.
      a. You need to be seen twice a week from 32 weeks gestation to delivery, or as recommended by your health care provider.
      b. You will have extra testing to make sure the baby is doing well and to make sure you are doing well, too.

F. You need to check your blood sugars four times a day. Your blood sugar target is ________________
   1. Fasting ________________
   2. Before lunch ________________
   3. Before dinner ________________
   4. Before going to bed ________________

G. You will be instructed to check your urine for ketones when you are sick or if you have high blood sugar.

Activity: It is important to continue to exercise.

Diet: Eat a good, healthy diet. You will be instructed on how many calories to eat. Eat six smaller meals a day; with insulin, it is important to eat snacks.

Signs of High and Low Blood Sugar

Blood Sugar	What to Watch for	What to Do	Causes
HYPOGLYCEMIA Low blood sugar	Excessive sweating Feeling faint Feeling shaky Headache Impaired vision Hunger Irritable feelings Personality change Trouble awakening	**Call the health care provider immediately if your blood sugar is below ________________** Take glucose tablets or eat Do not take your insulin Do not try to force any food or liquids by mouth if patient is not conscious	**Too much insulin** Not eating on time or enough food Unusual amounts of exercise
HYPERGLYCEMIA High blood sugar	Increased thirst Need to urinate more often Large amounts of sugar in your blood or urine Ketones in your urine Weakness and generalized aches Heavy, labored breathing with a fruity breath Nausea and vomiting	Test your blood sugar **Call your provider immediately if your blood sugar is ________________** Test your urine for ketones Drink extra water if able to swallow	**Too little insulin** Eating more foods and foods not on your diet Infections and fever Stress

(*continued*)

INSULIN THERAPY DURING PREGNANCY *(continued)*

You Need to Notify the Office If:

A. You have moderate ketones in your urine.

B. You are unable to eat or you have loose diarrhea stool.

C. You have insulin reactions (blood sugar is below 50 mg/dL or you feel the symptoms of low blood sugar).

D. You have blood sugars higher than 175 mg/dL for two readings.

E. You have any signs of infection.

F. You have a decrease in fetal movement or do not feel your baby moving.

G. Other: ____________________

Phone: ____________________

IRON-DEFICIENCY ANEMIA (PREGNANCY)

PROBLEM

You have a "low blood count" called iron-deficiency anemia. Iron is needed for red blood formation.

CAUSE

This is caused by a deficiency of iron in your diet, and it is very common.

PREVENTION/CARE

Anemia may be prevented by increasing iron in your diet and by taking extra iron tablets.

TREATMENT PLAN

A. You need to increase iron-rich food in your diet.

B. You will be prescribed an iron supplement.

C. Antacids for indigestion and dairy products interfere with iron absorption. Do not take your iron supplements with milk or just before or after taking an antacid.

D. You may be eligible for the Women, Infants, and Children (WIC) program, which provides supplemental foods for pregnant women and young children. Ask your health care provider for information about WIC availability in your community.

Activity: You may feel more tired than usual because of anemia. You may need to rest more than usual; however, try to continue your current exercise routine as tolerated. Alternative exercise includes walking 20 minutes a day or swimming.

Diet: You need to increase the amount of iron in your diet. Generally, the redder the meat and the greener the vegetable, the richer it is as a source of iron. You also need to make sure you have adequate intake of vitamin C (this helps increase the absorption of iron into your body). Vitamin C is found in fresh, dark-green vegetables and citrus fruits. Drink 8 to 10 glasses of liquids every day.

Medications:

You Have Been Prescribed: ____________________

You Need to Take: ____________________

Special Instructions About Iron Supplements:

A. Take the iron medication as prescribed; higher doses are not better. You may need to take the medication for a longer time. High doses of iron can be toxic to children and adults.

B. Your body only absorbs a small portion of the iron pills you take.

C. You may notice green or black bowel movements. This is normal.

D. It is best to take the iron pills on an empty stomach.

E. Try taking your iron pill with a glass of orange juice. The vitamin C in the juice helps the iron be absorbed better.

F. You may have nausea or vomiting when you take iron pills, especially during early pregnancy. If this happens, try taking the pill with food. It is better to take your iron with food than to skip your pill altogether.

G. If you are not able to tolerate the iron in the morning, try taking it in the middle of the afternoon or at bedtime.

H. You may become constipated while taking iron pills. Increase your intake of fruits, vegetables, and water to avoid constipation.

You Need to Notify the Office If You:

A. Have nausea and vomiting while taking the iron supplement even after following the special instructions.

B. Become extremely constipated even after increasing the fiber and liquids in your diet.

C. Other: ____________________

Phone: ____________________

IRRITABLE BOWEL SYNDROME

PROBLEM

Irritable bowel syndrome (IBS) is an irritative and inflammatory disorder of the intestine. You may have diarrhea, you may have constipation, or you may have problems with alternating constipation and diarrhea.

CAUSE

IBS is **not contagious,** inherited, or cancerous. It has no known direct cause, but it flares with severe stress and may also be triggered by eating.

PREVENTION/CARE

A. Try to reduce stress or modify your response to it. Keep a stress diary to avoid stress triggers.

B. Good food habits also help.

C. No specific food has been identified as responsible for all IBS symptoms. Keep a food diary to identify and avoid your food triggers.

TREATMENT PLAN

A. Quit smoking: Nicotine may contribute to the problem.

B. Apply a warm heat compress to your abdomen for comfort.

Activity: Exercise, such as walking 20 minutes a day, improves bowel function and helps reduce stress. Other stress-reduction techniques include self-hypnosis and biofeedback.

Diet:
A. Eat a high-fiber diet. Fiber is good for both diarrhea and constipation.

B. Avoid sorbitol-containing (sugar-free) candies and gum as well as lactose-containing milk products to see if this eases your diarrhea symptoms.

C. Do not eat or drink anything that aggravates your symptoms such as the following:
   1. Coffee may be a major food trigger.
   2. Avoid spicy and gas-producing foods.
   3. Avoid large meals, but eat regularly.
   4. Limit alcohol.

Medications:

You Have Been Prescribed: ______________________________

You Need to Take: ______________________________

You Need to Notify the Office If You Have:
A. Fever

B. Black or tarry-looking bowel movements (BM)

C. Vomiting

D. Unexplained weight loss of 5 pounds or more

E. Symptoms that do not improve despite changes in diet, exercise, and medication

F. Other: ______________________________

Phone: ______________________________

JAUNDICE AND HEPATITIS

PROBLEM

Jaundice is a yellow tinge of the skin or mucous membranes that line the mouth and other body cavities. Jaundice is a symptom, not a disease. It occurs when the blood contains too much bilirubin—a yellow pigment found in bile, which is a fluid secreted by the liver.

When the liver is damaged, bilirubin builds up in the body and skin, turning the skin yellow and itchy. Other symptoms that occur with jaundice are dark urine, light-colored bowel movements (BM), fatigue, fever, chills, appetite loss, nausea, and vomiting.

CAUSE

Jaundice usually comes from a liver disorder such as cirrhosis, hepatitis, or a disease of the gallbladder or pancreas. However, it can also be a symptom of other disorders such as anemia or severe heart failure. Sometimes jaundice results from taking a drug that damages the liver.

PREVENTION/CARE

Although hepatitis is considered contagious, you do not need to be confined to your home. However, to help prevent the spread of hepatitis:

A. There are vaccinations for hepatitis A and for hepatitis B. There is no vaccination for hepatitis C. The hepatitis B vaccination is recommended for all infants. It is recommended that babies get the first hepatitis B shot before leaving the hospital.

B. Do not prepare or handle food for others until cleared by your health care provider.

C. Wash your hands well after using the toilet and changing diapers.

D. If you have hepatitis A or B, avoid intimate sexual contact until cleared by your health care provider.

E. If you have hepatitis B or C, do not share razors, toothbrushes, and other personal items.

F. Never donate blood after a hepatitis B or C infection.

G. Your family and sexual partners may need an injection of immune globulin or a vaccination, depending on the type of hepatitis you have.

H. School exposure to hepatitis A does not generally pose a risk to others.

I. Risk of hepatitis B transmission in day-care centers appears to be extremely rare.

TREATMENT PLAN

Treatment for jaundice includes the following:

A. Use good hygiene with bathing, using the bathroom, and handwashing.

B. Apply anti-itch lotions such as calamine.

C. Rest.

D. Review all of the medications, over-the-counter (OTC) medications, and herbal products that you are taking. Your medications may need to be stopped or have their dose strength changed.

E. Surgery may be required to remove a gallstone or to have a procedure called lithotripsy to crush it, if a stone blocking the bile duct is causing jaundice.

F. If you have hepatitis, you may need to be referred to a specialist.

G. The public health department will be notified by your health care provider for acute hepatitis.

H. Your health care provider may discuss the need for a liver biopsy.

I. Your health care provider may discuss treatment to help treat a virus that is causing hepatitis.

J. Avoid alcohol.

Activity: Plan rest periods throughout the day. Avoid strenuous exercise. Gradually resume activities and mild exercise during the time you are getting better. You may get extra teaching about ways to protect yourself and others while having sex to prevent giving hepatitis to your partners.

(*continued*)

JAUNDICE AND HEPATITIS *(continued)*

Diet: Eat small, frequent, low-fat, high-calorie meals. You may be instructed to limit protein during acute phases of some types of hepatitis. Sit down to eat to decrease pressure on your liver. Drink 8 to 10 glasses of liquids a day.

Medications:

You Have Been Prescribed: ______________________________

You Need to Take: ______________________________

You Have Been Prescribed: ______________________________

You Need to Take: ______________________________

You Need to Notify the Office If You Have:

A. Mild confusion

B. Personality changes

C. Worsening symptoms

D. Tremors

E. Other: ______________________________

Phone: ______________________________

RESOURCES

Centers for Disease Control and Prevention: www.cdc.gov/hepatitis
Hepatitis B information is available from the Hepatitis B Foundation: www.hepb.org
Hepatitis C information is available from the American Liver Foundation: www.liverfoundation.org

KIDNEY DISEASE: CHRONIC

PROBLEM

Chronic kidney disease (CKD) means that the kidney is having trouble performing its normal function to maintain health.

Functions of a Normal Kidney

The kidney has several functions:

A. Removal and absorption of fluids to maintain balance

B. Filtration of blood to remove waste products

C. Regulation of blood pressure (BP)

D. Hormone regulation for blood production in the bone marrow

E. Regulation of hormones and minerals

F. Maintenance of healthy bones

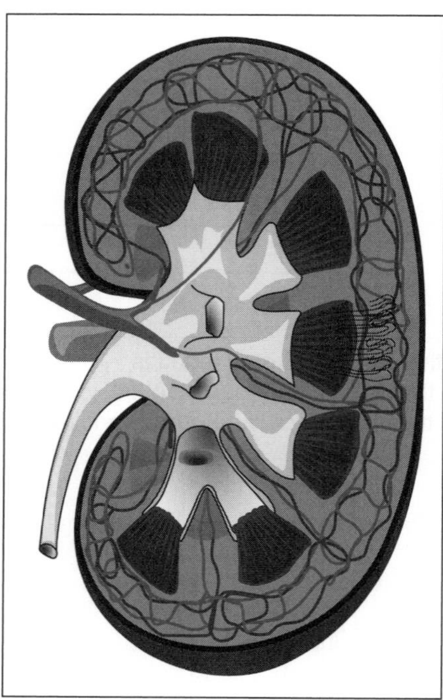

Adapted from Piotr Michal Jaworski, Wikipedia.

CAUSE

CKD has multiple causes.

A. Diabetes is the leading cause of CKD in the United States.

B. Hypertension is the second leading cause of CKD in the United States.

C. Other causes of CKD
   1. Glomerulonephritis
   2. Genetics (inherited) disease: Polycystic kidney disease and Alport's syndrome
   3. Congenital diseases
   4. Autoimmune disease
   5. Urinary tract infections (UTIs)
   6. Drugs (legal and illegal) and toxic substances

DETECTION

CKD can be detected by:

A. Blood tests: Blood urea nitrogen (BUN) and creatinine

(*continued*)

KIDNEY DISEASE: CHRONIC *(continued)*

B. Urinalysis (protein in urine and creatinine clearance)

C. Other (ultrasound, immunoassays, CT scan, biopsies, etc.)

D. Glomelular filtration rate (GFR)
   1. Normal rate: 90 or higher without protein in the urine
   2. Gets lower with age
   3. An indicator on the function of the kidney
   4. Used to determine CKD stages
   5. Is lower as the kidney function worsens

STAGES OF CKD

Stage	GFR
Stage I (with protein in the urine)	GFR: 90 or higher
Stage II (mild)	60–89
Stage III (moderate)	30–59
Stage IV (severe)	15–29
Stage V (kidney failure)	14 or less

GFR, glomelular filtration rate.

SYMPTOMS OF CKD

Symptoms can vary.

A. Usually unnoticed

B. More noticeable symptoms as CKD worsens (usually around Stage III)

C. It can include:
   1. Nausea
   2. Fatigue/weakness, no energy
   3. Decreased or lack of appetite
   4. Weight loss or rapid weight gain
   5. Shortness of breath, which may worsen with activity or at rest (when awakening in the morning)
   6. Swelling of the legs and feet, around the eyes
   7. Cloudy mind or difficulty concentrating
   8. Muscle cramps
   9. Frequent nighttime urination
   10. Difficulty sleeping or staying asleep

PROBLEMS CAUSED BY CKD

CKD can cause multiple problems.

A. Heart, including heart failure and blood vessel dysfunction
   1. High BP
   2. Cholesterol abnormalities
   3. Heart attack
   4. Stroke

B. Poor nutritional status

C. Weak and unhealthy bones

D. Anemia

E. Water retention

F. Progression to kidney failure

(*continued*)

KIDNEY DISEASE: CHRONIC *(continued)*

LIFESTYLE CHANGES TO PREVENT PROGRESSION OF CKD

Ways you may slow down the progression of CKD and cope with other effects of CKD:

A. Take charge and be proactive.
   1. Be familiar with the health care team.
   2. Provide information on beliefs and practices relating to health.
   3. Inform the health care team about herbs and other alternative medicine being used.
   4. Be involved in the treatment plan.

B. Diet
   1. Meet with a registered dietitian.
   2. Eat a well-balanced meal.
   3. Some dietary restrictions may be necessary based on kidney function and stages of CKD.
   4. Follow dietary instructions regarding protein, fats, sodium, and minerals.
      a. Dietary intake of protein is usually restricted to 0.8 to 1.0 g/kg per day.
      b. Dietary sodium should be restricted to no more than 2 g daily.
      c. Potassium should be restricted to 40 to 70 meq/d.
      d. Calories should be restricted to 35 kcal/kg/d; if the body weight is greater than 120% of normal weight or the patient is older than 60 years of age, a lower amount may be prescribed.
      e. Fat intake should be about 30% to 40% of total daily caloric intake.
      f. Phosphorus should be restricted to 600 to 800 mg/d.
      g. Calcium should be restricted to 1,400 to 1,600 mg/d.
      h. Magnesium should be restricted to 200 to 300 mg/d.
      i. Carbohydrates: The recommended normal intake is 225 to 358 g/d.

C. Exercise
   1. Moderate exercise is recommended for at least 30 minutes, five times a week.
   2. The benefits of exercise:
      a. Lowers BP
      b. Improves cholesterol
      c. Lowers hemoglobin A1c (HgA1c) in diabetes
      d. Strengthens bones
      e. Leads to weight loss
      f. Improves signs/symptoms of depression
      g. Boosts the immune system
      h. Reduces stress
      i. Provides an overall better feeling

D. Target heart and blood vessels
   1. Control blood pressure; goal is less than 130/80 mmHg.
   2. Lower your low-density lipoprotein.
   3. Weight loss
   4. Lower HgA1c level with the goal of less than 6.9% if you have diabetes.
      a. Exercise
      b. Diet: No restriction, low-saturated-fat, low-carbohydrate diet
      c. Smoking cessation is essential.
      d. Reduce or eliminate alcohol intake.
      e. Medications may be necessary for the following:
         i. Hypertension: BP medications
         ii. Hyperlipidemia: Cholesterol medications
         iii. Diabetes: Medications to control the blood sugar

E. Target bones
   1. Be familiar with your lab results (vitamin D level, calcium level, phosphorus level).
   2. Supplements: Vitamin D, calcium supplements, and phosphate binders may be necessary.
   3. Low phosphorous diet may be necessary.
   4. Exercise: Weight-bearing exercise will help strengthen bones (walking, dancing, lifting weights, etc).

(continued)

KIDNEY DISEASE: CHRONIC *(continued)*

F. Target anemia
   1. Goal of the hemoglobin should be 11 g/dL or better.
   2. Diet rich in iron
   3. Medication may be necessary (depends on the type of anemia).
      a. Erythropoeitin-stimulating agents
      b. Vitamin B_{12}
      c. Folic acid
      d. Iron

G. Target water retention
   1. Limit salt intake.
   2. Diet (avoid processed foods/fast foods).
   3. Medications may be needed (diuretics).

FOODS HIGH IN PHOSPHORUS

Below is a list of foods with the estimated amount of phosphorus in each food. Limit portions (consultation with registered dietitian is recommended).

Biscuits (mix) 1 (1 oz): 133 mg	Cheese (1 oz): 161 mg
Chocolate 1 bar (2 oz): 137 mg	Cola 1 can (12 oz): 60 mg
Cream soups (1 cup): 151 mg	Dried beans and peas (1 cup cooked): 206 mg
Hot dogs and sausage (2 each): 162/220 mg	Ice cream (1 cup): 157 mg
Liver and organ meats (3.5 oz): 400 mg	Macaroni and cheese (1 oz): 265 mg
Pancake mix 3 (4 inch pancakes): 368 mg	Peanut butter (3 tbsp): 172 mg
Pizza (1 slice): 259 mg	Pork and beans (1 cup): 266 mg
Yogurt (8 fl. oz) and pudding (½ cup): 292/280 mg	

POTASSIUM-FRIENDLY FOODS

Limit portion to half cup unless noted otherwise (consultation with registered dietitian is recommended).

Fruits	
Apple (1 small)	Canned pear
Cherries	Grapes (15 small)
Juices (apple, cranberry, grape, lemon, nectar, pear, peach, and pineapple)	Lemon (1/2)
Peach (1/2 cup canned or 1 small fresh)	Pineapple
Plum (1/2 cup canned or 1 medium)	Raspberries (blueberries, blackberries, and cranberries)
Strawberries	Watermelon (1 cup)
Vegetables	
Cabbage	Carrots (1/2 cup cooked or 1 small raw)
Celery (1 stalk)	Corn (1/2 canned or ear)
Cucumbers	Eggplant
Green (or wax) beans	Green peas
Lettuce (1 cup)	Onion
Radishes	Squash (Crookneck, Summer, and zucchini)

(continued)

KIDNEY DISEASE: CHRONIC *(continued)*

RESOURCES

A. BC Renal Agency: www.bcrenalagency.ca
   1. Shopping guide for kidney health: http://www.bcrenalagency.ca/sites/default/files/documents/files/Shopping_Guide_For_Kidney_Health_WEB_Dec_11.pdf

B. National Kidney Foundation: www.kidney.org
   1. Kidney Kitchen recipes: www.kidney.org/patients/kidneykitchen/recipes.cfm

C. American Diabetes Association: www.diabetes.org
   1. Food and Fitness: www.diabetes.org/food-and-fitness/?loc=GlobalNavFF

KNEE EXERCISES

CARE FOR YOUR KNEE

Please follow the type of exercises recommended for your knee. You may begin straight-leg raises after the pain resolves. Continue to wear your brace with activities as directed. It may take months for your knee to completely heal. You may gradually resume normal activity as directed by your provider. If you are not sure what activities you may perform, ask your provider before performing the activity.

A. Quad sets
   1. Exercise may be done while standing, sitting, or lying down.
   2. Straighten knee with intensity.
   3. Hold for 10 counts, then relax.
   4. Repeat the exercise three to four times per day.
   5. If a cast or splint is in place, straighten the knee until the front of the thigh and the cast pinch together.
   6. If the knee is bent, keep the foot planted and use the floor to push against.

B. Co-contractions
   1. Similar to quads, but the difference is to tighten the entire thigh while straightening the knee.
   2. Hold for 10 counts, then relax.
   3. Repeat the exercise approximately three to four times a day.

C. Hamstring sets
   1. Pull the leg back against the other foot, floor, or cast.
   2. Hold approximately 10 counts, then relax.
   3. Perform these sets three to four times a day.

D. Heel lifts
   1. Lie on back with support under the knee.
   2. Lift the heel while resting the knee on support.
   3. Make the knee as straight as possible.
   4. Hold for 10 counts, then relax.
   5. Do not use weights.
   6. Perform these exercises three to four times a day.

E. Straight-leg raises
   1. Straighten the knee.
   2. Lift and pause for 5 to 10 counts, then relax.
   3. Lower leg and relax, then repeat.
   4. Do three to five sets, three to four times a day. Rest between each set.
   5. Start with ________________________ pounds of ankle weight and work up to ________________ pounds.
   6. Gradually increase weight used.

F. Hip flexors
   1. While sitting, lift the knee toward the chest.
   2. Hold for 10 counts, then relax.
   3. Lower the leg and relax. Repeat.
   4. Do 10 times, three to four times a day.
   5. Start with ____________________________________ pounds of weight and work up gradually to ____________________________________ pounds.
   6. The weights should be on the knee or ankle.

G. Hamstring stretches
   1. While seated on a sturdy table with the foot of your injured leg resting on the floor, lean forward with chin directed toward the toes.
   2. Hold for at least 10 counts, then relax.
   3. The knee should be straight from your hips.
   4. **Do not do this exercise with bouncing or violent movements.**
   5. Do ___________________________ minutes, ________________________ times a day.

LACTOSE INTOLERANCE AND MALABSORPTION

PROBLEM

You have been diagnosed as having difficulty digesting milk (lactose) products or having problems with malabsorption. Lactose intolerance can cause gas, bloating, abdominal cramps, diarrhea, and nausea or vomiting. You may be able to eat small portions without problems or be unable to tolerate any foods containing lactose.

CAUSE

Lactose is the sugar present in milk. Lactose intolerance is very common; it occurs when the body is not able to appropriately digest this milk sugar content and results in diarrhea.

PREVENTION/CARE

Follow a lactose-free or lactose-controlled diet.

TREATMENT PLAN

Activity: No restrictions are required. Resume normal activities as soon as diarrhea symptoms improve. You may be sent to see a registered dietitian to assist in your dietary plan.

Diet:

A. Limit or stop eating foods that contain milk, lactose, whey, or casein.

B. Lactose-controlled diets allow up to 1 cup of milk per day for cooking or drinking, if you can tolerate it.

C. If you cannot tolerate any lactose, choose lactose-free foods with lactate, lactic acid, lactalbumin, whey protein, sodium caseinate, casein hydrolysates, and calcium compounds. Read labels carefully.

D. You may also choose kosher foods marked “pareve” or “parve,” which do not contain lactose. Read labels carefully.

E. A low-fat diet is important if you have fat malabsorption.

F. To help with diarrhea caused by malabsorption, avoid more than one serving a day of caffeine-containing drinks.

G. Beverages with high sugar content, such as soft drinks and fruit juices, may increase diarrhea. Juices and fruits with high amounts of fructose include apples, pears, sweet cherries, prunes, and dates.

H. Sorbitol-containing candies and gums may cause diarrhea.

Medications: You may need the enzyme lactase to help you digest your food. You may need vitamins and minerals if you are having problems with malabsorption/diarrhea.

You Have Been Prescribed: ____________________

You Need to Take: ____________________

You Need to Notify the Office If You Have:

A. Severe abdominal pain

B. Diarrhea causing dehydration

C. Other: ____________________

Phone: ____________________

LICE (PEDICULOSIS)

PROBLEM

A parasite called a louse has been found on your body or hair. Lice tend to live on the scalp, eyebrows, or genital area, or in warm, moist areas of your skin. You may notice you have intense itching, swelling, or reddened areas of the skin, and sometimes even enlarged lymph glands.

CAUSE

The lice bite the skin, which causes the intense itching. Lice and their eggs (called nits) may be difficult to see on the skin and shafts of hair. Lice look like small, 2- to 3-mm, tan-colored bugs. The eggs are tiny white eggs that stick to the hair shaft.

PREVENTION

You can prevent repeated episodes of lice if you bathe daily; avoid crowded living conditions; change the bed linens frequently; do not share hats, combs, brushes, or other belongings. When your children or other family members have been in contact with others diagnosed with lice, check family members closely for lice and treat as appropriate.

TREATMENT PLAN

A. Use medicated shampoo as directed.

B. Machine wash all linens, stuffed animals, or any other items with which the lice may have come in contact.

C. Wash clothes in hot, soapy water.

D. Dry all linens in a hot dryer for at least 30 minutes.

E. Items that cannot be washed must be taken to the dry cleaner or wrapped and sealed in a plastic bag for 14 days.

F. Boil all hair accessories and clean well.

G. Do not share hats and combs.

H. Spray all furniture with appropriate products that kill all nits and lice.

I. Vacuum.

Activity: There is no activity restriction.

Diet: There is no special diet.

Medications:

A. Food and Drug Administration (FDA)-approved over-the-counter products:
   1. Pyrethrins combined with piperonyl butoxide—brand names: Rid, Triple X, A-200, Pronto, R & C. Approved for children 2 years and older. Avoid if allergic to ragweed or chrysanthemums.

B. FDA approved for 2 months and older. Permethrin lotion 1%—brand name: Nix. Repeat application on day 9 of initial dose.

You Have Been Prescribed: ______________________________

A. Treat as directed on the bottle.

B. After shampooing as directed, make sure to remove each single nit from each shaft of hair. Any nits left in the hair will hatch and start the cycle over again. Comb any dead or remaining live lice out of the hair with a fine-tooth comb.

C. Repeat in 24 hours, then again in 1 week.

D. Do not use a shampoo/conditioner or conditioner before use of the lice medications. Do not wash the hair for 1 to 2 days after lice medication treatment.

You Need to Notify the Office If You Have:

A. Any questions regarding the removal of the nits and lice, or if you need any assistance. If other family members need to be evaluated, please let us know. If secondary infection occurs, please call the office.

B. Precautions: Do not overuse medications or combine different head lice medications. Use only as directed. These medications are insecticides and can be dangerous if used incorrectly.

Phone: ______________________________

LICHEN PLANUS

PROBLEM

A chronic skin eruption, lichen planus is not cancerous or contagious. It frequently appears as small, slightly raised, itchy, purplish bumps with a whitish surface. Sudden hair loss from the head may occur. Lichen planus may involve the skin of the legs, trunk, arms, wrists, scalp, or penis; the lining of the mouth or vagina; and the nail beds of the toenails and fingernails.

CAUSE

The cause is unknown, but it may be caused by a virus. In a few cases, this may be an adverse reaction to certain drugs. The risk of developing lichen planus increases with stress, fatigue, or exposure to drugs or chemicals.

PREVENTION/CARE

Currently, there are no known preventive measures.

A. The goal of treatment is to relieve symptoms.

B. Use cool water soaks to relieve itching.

C. Reduce stress; this may help to prevent recurrences. Learn relaxation techniques or obtain counseling, if necessary.

D. Speak with your health care provider if you suspect a drug to be the cause.

TREATMENT PLAN

Activity: No restrictions.

Diet: Eat a well-balanced diet; drink 8 to 10 glasses of water every day.

Medications:

You Have Been Prescribed: ____________________

You Need to Take: ____________________

You Need to Notify the Office If:

A. You have a reaction to any of the prescribed medications.

B. You are unable to tolerate the prescribed medications.

C. Hair loss or nail destruction occurs.

D. New lesions appear as old lesions resolve.

E. Other: ____________________

Phone: ____________________

LYME DISEASE AND REMOVAL OF A TICK

PROBLEM

Ticks are vectors for Lyme disease and Rocky Mountain spotted fever. You have been diagnosed with Lyme disease.

CAUSE

Lyme disease is caused by a spirochete from ticks.

PREVENTION/CARE

A. Avoid areas with large deer populations.

B. Wear light-colored clothes to make ticks easier to spot. Wear long sleeves and tuck pants into the socks to form a barrier.

C. Stick to hiking trails. Avoid contact with overgrown foliage. Ticks prefer dense woods with thick growth of shrubs and small trees as well as areas along the edge of the woods.

D. Check for ticks after each outdoor activity, especially in hairy regions of the body and beltline, where ticks often attach. Check for ticks before bathing, especially at the back of the neck, knees, and ears.

E. Remove ticks promptly.

F. Inspect pets daily and remove ticks when present.

G. Some manufacturers currently offer permethrin-treated clothing that is effective for up to 20 washings. This clothing is not recommended for children.

H. Use tick repellent with diethyltoluamide (DEET; except for small children younger than 2 years). As an alternative, picaridin and oil of eucalyptus preparations have been approved for use as repellents by the U.S. Environmental Protection Agency (EPA).

Precautions When Removing Ticks

A. Do not hold a lighted match or cigarette to the tick. Do not apply gasoline, kerosene, or oil to the tick's body.

B. Avoid squeezing the body of the tick.

C. Grasp the tick with a fine-tip tweezer close to the skin. Remove by gently pulling the tick upward straight out without using any twisting motions (see the following figures).

D. In the home, if fingers are used to remove ticks, they should be protected with facial tissue or gloves and washed after removal of the tick.

E. Do not crush the tick during removal.

F. **Save the tick for identification in case you become ill. Write the date of the tick bite on paper and place the paper and the tick in a resealable baggie and place it in the freezer.**

TREATMENT PLAN

A. Antibiotics are effective against Lyme disease.

B. If you are prescribed doxycycline, avoid exposure to the sun because a rash may develop.

Activity: As tolerated.

Diet: Eat a regular diet.

Medications:

A. Acetaminophen may be taken for body aches and any fever.

B. You may be given antibiotics for infection.

You Have Been Prescribed: ____________________

(*continued*)

LYME DISEASE AND REMOVAL OF A TICK *(continued)*

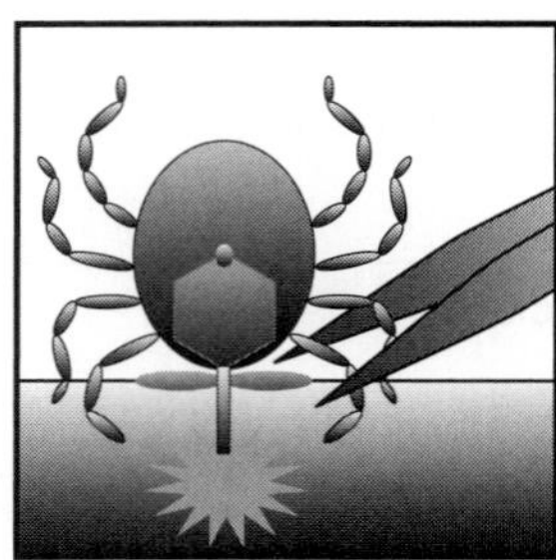

Grasp the tick's body as close to the skin as possible using a fine-tip tweezer. Avoid squeezing the tick's body.

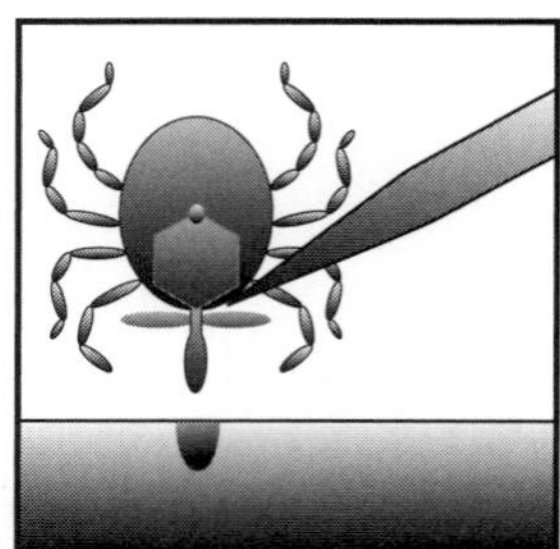

Remove by pulling the tick straight upward without using twisting motions.

You Need to Take: ______________________________

Take all of your antibiotics even if you feel better.

You Need to Notify the Office If You Have:

1. No signs of improvement with antibiotic therapy
2. Other: ______________________________

Phone: ______________________________

LYMPHEDEMA

PROBLEM

Lymphedema is the backup of fluid in the lymphatic system into an arm or leg. The fluid causes severe swelling, which restricts movement and can lead to infection and, in rare cases, a form of cancer called lymphangiosarcoma.

CAUSE

Many factors can cause lymphedema. These include a diagnosis of cancer treated with radiation, surgical removal of lymph nodes, infection, and disorders from birth that affect the structure of the lymph system.

PREVENTION/CARE

A. Protect your arm or leg while recovering from cancer treatment.

1. Avoid heavy lifting, if it involves an arm.
2. Avoid strenuous exercise.
3. Avoid heat on your arm or leg.
4. Avoid tight clothing.

TREATMENT PLAN

A. Raise the affected arm or leg whenever lying down to improve pain and swelling.

B. Wear compression stockings. Put them on before getting out of bed in the morning. Take them off just before going to bed at night.

C. Apply lotion every day to the affected area.

D. Check the affected area every day and report any skin changes to your health care provider, especially any cracks or cuts.

E. Follow up with your primary health care provider and other specialty providers on a regularly scheduled basis.

Activity:

A. Get regular exercise. Discuss with your health care provider what type and frequency of exercise is safe for you.

B. Exercise leg muscles by pumping ankles when sitting. Rocking in a rocking chair is another option.

Diet:

A. Discuss with your health care provider the type of diet that best suits your needs: Diabetic diet, low-fat diet, low-cholesterol diet, and/or low-sodium diet.

Medications:

You Have Been Prescribed: ____________________

You Need to Take: ____________________

You Need to Notify the Office If You Have:

A. Fever greater than 101°F

B. Increased redness, pain, tenderness to touch, and/or warmth in affected arm or leg

C. New pain, swelling, or warmth in an arm or leg

D. Other: ____________________

Phone: ____________________

RESOURCES

National Cancer Institute: cancer.gov/cancertopics/pdq/supportivecare/lymphedema/healthprofessional/page2
National Lymphedema Network: lymphnet.org
Patient Education Center—Lymphedema: patienteducationcenter.org/articles/lymphedema

MASTITIS

PROBLEM

You have an infection in your breast tissue, not your breast milk.

CAUSE

The most common organism causing mastitis is *Staphylococcus aureus.* The immediate source of the organism is almost always the nursing infant's nose and mouth. Mastitis often develops in the presence of breast injury, such as cracked nipples.

PREVENTION/CARE

A. Prevent injury to the breast:
   1. Avoid overdistension of the breasts; feed infant or use the breast pump frequently (every 2–4 hours).
   2. Avoid clogged milk ducts by applying moist heat to the breasts and massage.
   3. Avoid rough manipulation of the breast; pump carefully.
   4. Avoid cracking of nipples by proper positioning of the infant's mouth on the nipple during feeding. The baby's mouth should cover the entire areola (dark brown part of the nipple area).
   5. Read the Patient Teaching Guide, "Breast Engorgement and Sore Nipples" in this section.

B. Personal hygiene measures:
   1. Avoid soap on the nipples; cleanse nipples with warm water only.
   2. Avoid decrusting the nipple of dried colostrum or milk.
   3. Use purified lanolin cream after each breastfeeding for sore, cracked nipples. (If lanolin is purified, there is no need to remove it prior to the next feeding.)
   4. Use good handwashing techniques before handling the breast and before and after breastfeeding.

TREATMENT PLAN

A. Complete course of antibiotics. Be aware that antibiotics may cause a yeast infection.

B. Continue breastfeeding even on the antibiotics. It is not uncommon for your baby to develop "thrush" (looks like white patches on your baby's mouth and tongue). You may also be prescribed Nystatin cream to apply to your breasts to help prevent thrush.

C. Apply warm soaks to your breast (see the Patient Teaching Guide, "Postpartum Breast Engorgement and Sore Nipples" in this section). Breast massage may be needed, too.

D. Use Tylenol or ibuprofen for pain (see the Patient Teaching Guide, "Postpartum Breast Engorgement and Sore Nipples" in this section).

Activity: Increased rest is recommended. Try to lie down for a nap when the baby goes to sleep.

Diet: There are no dietary restrictions; continue your regular diet and avoid gas-producing foods that may upset your baby's tummy (cabbage, chocolate, beans, pizza, spicy foods). Increase fluid intake with elevated temperature. Drink at least 10 to 12 glasses of liquid a day. Use caffeine in moderation (eliminate if possible).

Medications: Continue your prenatal vitamins while breastfeeding.

You Have Been Prescribed: ______________________________

You Need to Take: ______________________________
Take all of your antibiotics even if you feel better.

You Have Been Prescribed: Nystatin cream for your breasts and nipples.

You Need to Apply It:

A. After each feeding, apply Nystatin to each nipple and areola of your breast.

B. Before feeding, wipe off the excess cream with a warm washcloth (do not use soap for your breast because it causes excessive drying and cracking).

(*continued*)

MASTITIS *(continued)*

You Have Been Prescribed ______________________________

You Need to Use It: ______________________________

You Need to Notify the Office If:

A. You have a temperature that does not decrease within 2 days and resolve within 4 days of taking the antibiotics.

B. You have pain that is not controlled with acetaminophen or ibuprofen.

C. Your baby develops thrush. Notify your baby's health care provider for medication.

D. Other: ______________________________

Phone: ______________________________

MENOPAUSE

DEFINITION

Menopause is the cessation of menses (stopping of menstrual periods) for 12 consecutive months and is generally experienced in women between 45 and 55 years of age; however, for some women menopause may be earlier or later.

A. Menopause before the age of 40 years is considered premature.

B. Induced menopause is the abrupt cessation of menses related to chemical or surgical interventions.

Perimenopause is the time preceding menopause and may last several years. The average age of onset is usually in a woman's 40s but may occur earlier. Symptoms may occur during this time period because of fluctuations in hormone levels. Owing to fluctuations in ovarian function, **pregnancy may still occur and unintended pregnancy should be avoided.**

CAUSE

Menopause can be natural or induced. Natural menopause is a normal function of aging. Surgical or chemical intervention can result in induced menopause.

SYMPTOMS

Symptom occurrence and severity vary from very mild to moderate or severe. Symptoms may include:

A. Hot flashes

B. Night sweats

C. Insomnia

D. Vaginal dryness

TREATMENT PLAN

Your care provider will work with you to develop a plan of treatment that is based on your individual symptom pattern. Inform your care provider if you have:

A. Acute liver disease

B. Cerebral vascular or coronary artery disease, myocardial infarction (MI), or stroke

C. History of or active thrombophlebitis or thromboembolic disorders

D. History of uterine or ovarian cancer

E. Known or suspected cancer of the breast

F. Known or suspected estrogen-dependent neoplasm

G. Pregnancy

H. Undiagnosed, abnormal vaginal bleeding

Activity:

A. Regular physical exercise can be beneficial for weight reduction and symptom control.

B. Dress in layers to accommodate hot flashes and avoid warm areas.

C. Avoid hot showers and baths.

D. Regular sexual intercourse is encouraged and you may find water-soluble vaginal lubricants (K-Y jelly, Astroglide, Replens) helpful for vaginal dryness.

E. Be sure to use a method of **birth control** to prevent undesired pregnancy if you have had a period within 1 year.

Diet: You need to eat a well-balanced diet (three meals). Supplement your diet to achieve calcium 1,000 to 1,200 mg/d and vitamin D 600 IU/d from age 1 year until age 70 years and then 800 IU/d for 71 years and older. Avoid alcohol, caffeine, and spicy food as they may trigger hot flashes.

(*continued*)

MENOPAUSE *(continued)*

Medication:

You Have Been Prescribed: ______________________________

You Need to Take/Use It: ______________________________

You Need to Notify the Office If:

A. You experience unexpected vaginal bleeding.

B. Your symptoms worsen.

C. You are on hormone replacement therapy and you experience calf pain, chest pain, or shortness of breath; cough up blood; or have severe headaches, visual disturbances, breast pain, abdominal pain, or yellowing of the skin.

D. Other: ______________________________

Phone: ______________________________

MIGRAINE HEADACHE

PROBLEM

You have been diagnosed with migraine headaches. There are many ways that a migraine headache is described, including pulsating, pain on one side of the head, pain behind one eye, seeing spots before your eyes, and a possible loss of vision for a short time.

Other symptoms of a migraine include nausea and vomiting; sensitivity to sound; sensitivity to light, especially to flickering lights; sensitivity to smells; and pain that gets worse with activity.

CAUSE

A. Migraines run in families; your mother or sister may also have migraines.

B. Head trauma may trigger headaches.

C. You may have a migraine headache when you start your period due to the change in your hormones.

D. Medicines, such as birth control pills and hormone replacement therapy, may cause migraines.

E. Many odors, such as smelling perfumes, cigarette smoke, scented candles, and food odors, may trigger a headache.

F. Changes in weather and high altitude may also make you have a migraine.

G. Alcohol and some foods trigger a headache.

H. Another cause of a migraine headache is a rebound from taking too much over-the-counter pain medication such as ibuprofen, Aleve, aspirin, and Excedrin products. The headache gets better with the pain products, but comes back the next day so that you take the medicine again, causing a vicious cycle.

PREVENTION/CARE

A. Keep a diary to identify foods that trigger headache. Some foods that might trigger migraines:
   1. Alcohol, especially red wine
   2. Foods such as hot dogs, ham, and bacon
   3. Aged cheese
   4. Citrus foods such as oranges, lemons, limes, and tomatoes
   5. Not eating

B. Read labels to avoid the following preservatives:
   1. Aspartame—often found in yogurt
   2. Saccharin—often found in diet drinks and artificial sweeteners
   3. Tyramine—found in aged cheese such as feta and blue cheese, pickles, and olives
   4. Phenylethylamine—often found in sugarless gum and breath mints
   5. Monosodium glutamate (MSG)—often found in Chinese food
   6. Nitrates and nitrites—found in cured meats, such as ham and hot dogs

C. Keep a diary to identify visual triggers:
   1. Strobe lights
   2. Flickering light from going from sun into shade
   3. Fluorescent lights
   4. Sunlight glare off shiny objects and water

D. Keep a diary to identify other triggers, including:
   1. Too much sleep/too little sleep
   2. Strong odors
   3. Medicines
   4. Changes in weather

TREATMENT PLAN

A. One of the first things to look at is your diary of triggers in order to avoid or modify them.

B. You may be sent to a neurologist to evaluate if you need any special testing.

C. You may be sent to have your eyes examined for glasses.

(*continued*)

MIGRAINE HEADACHE *(continued)*

D. Many medications are used to treat migraines:
   1. Over-the-counter pain medications, including ibuprofen, Aleve, aspirin, and Excedrin, may be used in limited amounts.
   2. Medications for depression are commonly used.
   3. Medications for seizures are also commonly used.
   4. Medications for blood pressure have been found to control migraines.
   5. Medications for nausea and vomiting cab be helpful.

E. A special class of drugs called triptans is used to treat the migraine when it first starts. Some of the triptans are Imitrex, Maxalt, Zomig, Amerge, Relpax, and Frova. These medicines come in pill form as well as nasal spray, and are also given as a shot.

Activity: Relaxation training, such as yoga and biofeedback, helps headaches. Physical therapy and hypnosis have also helped migraine headaches.

Diet: There is no special diet for migraines.

A. Avoid the food triggers that you identified in your migraine diary.

B. Drink plenty of liquids.

You Have Been Prescribed the Following Medication for Acute Pain to Help Stop Migraines:

You Need to Take: ____________________

You Have Been Prescribed the Following Medication to Take Every Day to Manage Migraines:

You Need to Take: ____________________

You Have Been Prescribed the Following Medication for Nausea:

You Need to Take: ____________________

You Need to Notify the Office:

A. If you feel that this is the "worst headache you have ever had."

B. If you have difficulty with speech.

C. If you have fever with a stiff neck.

D. Other: ____________________

Phone: ____________________

RESOURCES

Mayo Clinic: www.mayoclinic.org/diseases-conditions/migraine-headache/home/ovc-20202432
Migraine diaries are available for iPhones, iPod touch, and the iPad on iTunes.
National Institute of Neurological Disorders and Stroke: www.ninds.nih.gov/disorders/migraine/migraine.htm
*Web*MD Migraines & Headaches Health Center: www.webmd.com/migraines-headaches and a headache diary is located on the *Web*MD site: www.webmd.com/migraines-headaches/guide/headache-diary

MONONUCLEOSIS

PROBLEM

Mononucleosis (mono) is an acute, infectious, viral disease. Mono causes fever, sore throat, and swollen lymph glands.

CAUSE

Epstein–Barr virus causes mono and is spread to other persons by kissing, sharing food, and coughing without covering your mouth.

PREVENTION/CARE

A. Avoid contact with persons diagnosed with mono.

B. Cover your mouth and nose when you cough or sneeze to prevent the spread of infection.

C. Use tissues to blow your nose and throw them away immediately.

D. If you do not have a tissue, use the "elbow sneeze" using the bend of your arm.

E. Wash your hands or use hand sanitizer.

TREATMENT PLAN

There is no specific cure. Gargle with warm salt water for a sore throat.

Activity:

A. Mono makes you very tired; rest in bed, then gradually return to normal activity.

B. You should not do any physical activity, especially contact sports (football, soccer, basketball, etc.), unless you have been cleared by your health care provider.

Diet: Eat a high-calorie diet. Drink plenty of liquids (at least 8 glasses a day).

Medications:

A. Acetaminophen may be taken for body aches.

B. You may be given antibiotics for infection, if indicated.

You Have Been Prescribed: ____________________

You Need to Take: ____________________

Take all of your antibiotics even if you feel better.

You Need to Notify the Office If You Have:

A. Fever more than 102°F.

B. Severe pain in the upper left abdomen (rupture of the spleen is a medical emergency).

C. Swallowing or breathing difficulty from a severe throat inflammation.

D. A rash may follow the use of antibiotics.

E. Other: ____________________

Phone: ____________________

MYASTHENIA GRAVIS

PROBLEM

Myasthenia gravis or MG is a chronic disorder in which the body's immune system mistakenly attacks and destroys proteins that help muscles respond to nerve impulses. This causes people to have muscle weakness that is worse with use and better with rest.

Eye muscles and muscles that help with chewing, swallowing, and talking tend to be affected the most. MG can be treated but not cured.

People with myasthenia generally have to take medicine for the rest of their lives to control the disorder. Surgery to remove their thymus gland may be necessary.

TREATMENT PLAN/CARE

A. Wear a Medic Alert tag and keep a list of medicines and the dosing schedule, with you at all times along with the name and telephone number of your neurologist in case of emergency.

B. Dentists and any other health care providers should know that you have MG because many medicines can make your MG worse. Some examples of medicines that can be problems for people with MG are birth control pills, some antibiotics, and some local anesthetics. Many medicines can be problematic, so you should *never* start a new medicine without talking to your neurologist first, even if you took it in the past without having problems.

C. Any time you feel worse, particularly if you are having trouble with chewing and swallowing, you should contact your neurologist and plan to go to the hospital, because MG could possibly affect your breathing. You should have a plan for emergencies that includes how you will get to a hospital, child-care arrangements, and how to contact your neurologist.

D. An annual flu shot is recommended because infections can make MG worse.

E. Emotional upset and stress also can make MG worse. Your health care provider can supply you with information on handling stress effectively or assist in referring you to a counselor.

F. Surgery can make MG worse, so it should, when possible, be planned with your neurologist. Some changes in your medication schedules in the weeks before the surgery can make problems less likely.

G. Plasmapheresis may be recommended to you. This procedure is performed to remove the antibodies that make the disease process worse. This procedure is similar to donating blood. Blood is removed from a vein, the antibodies are removed, and then the blood is donated back to you in another vein. This procedure may be offered to you many times because the effects are not permanent.

Activity: It is best to plan your activities to take advantage of the peak effects of your medicine and to avoid getting overtired.

Diet: A diet high in potassium-rich foods has been found by some to be helpful because low body potassium is associated with muscle weakness.

Medications: You may be prescribed steroids or medications that improve muscle strength.

You Have Been Prescribed: ____________________

You Need to Take: ____________________

You Need to Notify the Office If:

A. You have worsening or new symptoms.

B. You are unable to tolerate your medicines due to side effects.

C. Other: ____________________

Phone: ____________________

RESOURCES

Myasthenia Gravis Foundation of America, Inc.: www.myasthenia.org
You can build your own identification bracelets or neck chains from American Medical ID: www.americanmedical-id.com

NICOTINE DEPENDENCE

PROBLEM

Cigarette smoking is one of the most **preventable causes of death and disability in the United States.** Other forms of nicotine, such as chewing tobacco and pipe tobacco, can be just as harmful. Risks of lip, tongue, mouth, and throat cancer are associated with use of nicotine. Smoking may cause bleeding in pregnancy and may be responsible for the baby not growing well. It is well documented that infants and children who are exposed to long-term smoke inhalation are at increased risk of **sudden infant death syndrome** and frequent **ear infections and chronic illnesses.**

Nicotine is addictive and so stopping smoking is difficult.

CAUSE

Seeing your parents smoke and using tobacco may be one of the reasons that caused you to start using tobacco. Peer pressure is a big reason why you may have started smoking as a teenager.

REASONS TO QUIT

A. Quitting tobacco will add years to your life.

B. You will have healthier lungs, which will decrease your risk of developing cancer and having a heart attack or stroke.

C. You will also have more energy and feel better physically and mentally.

D. Smoking cessation will also decrease the secondhand smoke exposure around your family and friends, which will also make them healthier too.

E. Secondhand smoke causes asthma attacks and other health problems.

F. Some insurance plans are more expensive if you smoke.

G. You will save a lot of money by not buying cigarettes.

H. Do not quit for yourself: Quit for someone you love.

I. You will have fewer wrinkles.

TREATMENT PLAN

A. Set a quit date within 2 to 4 weeks and get information/treatment from your provider.

B. Throw away all cigarettes, matches, lighters, and ashtrays in your home, car, and workplace.

C. Make smoking very inconvenient.

D. Ask your family/friends for support and encouragement to help you stop.

E. Stay in nonsmoking environments and avoid friends/family members who smoke.

F. If you get the urge to smoke, take deep cleansing breaths and try to occupy your time with something else, like chewing gum.

G. Leave the table and change your routine to avoid old triggers such as smoking with your coffee after meals.

H. Reward yourself often for staying smoke free.

I. It is not unusual that you will go back to smoking; it is difficult to quit. Smoking even one less cigarette counts.

J. It may take several times to finally quit for good.

Activity:

A. Exercise daily to help alleviate the craving for nicotine.

B. Avoid caffeine if possible.

C. Chew gum or suck on hard candy when you crave a cigarette.

D. Eat celery sticks or carrots in place of smoking a cigarette.

E. Drink a lot of water and other fluids to keep hydrated.

(*continued*)

NICOTINE DEPENDENCE *(continued)*

Medications:

A. Discuss options available with your health care provider to help you quit.

B. Medications are available to help you quit.

C. The nicotine patch, inhaler, and gum are available and may be right for you. Discuss these options with your health care provider because they are good steps to quitting.

D. Many of the stop-smoking medicines may be covered by your insurance.

You Have Been Prescribed: ____________________

You Need to Take: ____________________

You Need to Notify the Office If You Have:

1. Severe craving and the urge to smoke or chew tobacco even on medicines.
2. Feelings of impulsiveness, like you might do something you will later regret.
3. Started smoking again after you have stepped down while using the nicotine patch.
4. Other: ____________________

Phone: ____________________

RESOURCES

The American Cancer Society has some good tips on quitting smoking: www.cancer.org
The American Lung Association also has good guides to help stop smoking: www.lung.org

NOSEBLEEDS

PROBLEM

Most nosebleeds stop within 10 minutes. **If you have trouble breathing with a nosebleed, *call 911.***

CAUSES

Nosebleeds may be caused by several problems:

A. Trauma from nose picking or forcefully blowing the nose

B. Chronic sinus infections

C. Allergies

D. Drugs, including over-the-counter medications such as aspirin and Pepto-Bismol, or street drugs such as snorted cocaine

E. Exposure to irritants

PREVENTION/CARE

A. Avoid picking your nose. Keep fingernails trimmed short.

B. Do not blow your nose too frequently or too hard (this may also cause eardrum tearing).

C. Blow your nose through both nostrils at the same time to equalize pressure.

D. Use a humidifier in your home, or place a container of water near the radiator.

E. Use a lubricant, such as petrolatum, A & D Ointment, or a skin barrier, such as zinc oxide, applied with a Q-tip to add moisture to the inside of your nose and promote healing.

F. Avoid smoking and secondhand smoke.

TREATMENT PLAN

A. If you experience a nosebleed, take these steps:
   1. Sit up and lean forward.
   2. Apply pressure to the bridge of your nose for 10 to 15 minutes to stop the blood flow.
   3. If the bleeding continues, spray Afrin into your nostril.
   4. If the bleeding still continues, lightly soak a cotton ball with the nasal spray, insert it into your nose, and press.
   5. Apply zinc oxide, petrolatum, or A & D Ointment to prevent further drying and abrasion of the nasal septum (the partition between the two nostrils).

B. Gently blowing your nose also decreases or stops a nosebleed.

Activity: Avoid or limit the following activities for 3 to 5 days after a nosebleed:

A. Heavy lifting

B. Straining

C. Bending over from the waist

D. Very hot showers

Diet: Avoid hot, spicy foods for 3 to 5 days after a nosebleed.

Medications: Avoid medications that increase bleeding, such as aspirin and Pepto-Bismol.

You Have Been Prescribed: ______________________________

You Need to Take: ______________________________

You Need to Notify the Office If:

A. Bleeding does not stop with pressure or nasal spray applied to the bleeding site.

B. You keep having nosebleeds (more than two in a week or four in a month).

C. Other: ______________________________

Phone: ______________________________

ORAL THRUSH IN CHILDREN

PROBLEM

Oral thrush is a white patch that coats the inside of the mouth and tongue. It mainly affects bottle-fed infants, although breastfed infants and debilitated older children may also be affected.

CAUSE

Thrush is caused by a yeast called *Candida* that grows rapidly on the lining of the mouth in areas abraided by prolonged sucking. It may also occur after a course of antibiotic medication.

PREVENTION/CARE

A. Do not use large pacifiers and nipples.

B. Boil bottle nipples and pacifiers.

C. Cleanse your nipples well after breastfeeding.

TREATMENT PLAN

A. Try to remove any large plaques with a moistened cotton-tipped applicator or gauze pad.

B. Cleanse the infant's mouth before giving medication.

C. Place the medication in the front of the mouth on each side.

D. Rub it directly on the plaques with a cotton swab.

E. Feed the infant temporarily with a cup and spoon.

F. Give a pacifier only at bedtime.

Diet: Decrease sucking time until thrush clears up.

Medications: Nystatin is an oral medication used to treat thrush. Nystatin 1 mL four times a day after meals or 30 minutes before feeding. Patches should improve within 2 to 3 days of using the medication.

You Have Been Prescribed: ____________________

You Need to Take: ____________________

You Need to Notify the Office If:

A. The child refuses to eat or drink.

B. Symptoms do not improve or thrush lasts longer than 10 days.

C. Unexplained fever occurs.

D. Secondary infection occurs in the mouth (pain, tenderness, sores).

E. Other: ____________________

Phone: ____________________

OSTEOARTHRITIS

PROBLEM

Osteoarthritis (OA) is a very common disorder that affects the weight-bearing and movable joints. OA damages the cartilage tissue in the joint. The cartilage provides the cushion around the joint. If the cartilage becomes damaged, it will become inflamed and irritated and start to thin. When this occurs, there is less cushion between the bones, and you will experience more pain and swelling. The joints most commonly involved are the finger and toe joints, knees, hips, and spine.

CAUSE

There are many different causes of OA. A previous injury to the joint, repeated stress to the joint (like a bricklayer's hands), genetics, age, obesity, and other diseases (such as diabetes or infections) may cause OA.

TREATMENT PLAN

A. The goal of treatment is to prevent further joint damage.

B. Learn as much as you can about this disorder and ask your health care provider several questions.

C. Heat and massage may increase joint movement and decrease pain.

D. Physical or occupational therapy may be needed.

E. Heat or ice packs may be used for localized relief.

Activity:

Exercise:

1. Range-of-motion (ROM) exercises increase the movement of the joint.
2. Careful exercise may also strengthen the muscles around the joint.
3. Ask your provider to advise the best type of exercise for you.
4. Yoga and acupuncture have been shown to help relieve pain and stiffness.
5. Joint protection: Do not overuse a joint.
6. If you work with your hands and have OA of the fingers, take frequent rest periods. This applies to all the other joints as well.

Diet: Low-fat, low-cholesterol diet may be suggested. Losing weight may help if you have OA of the knees, hips, or spine.

Medications: Your health care provider may recommend that you take acetaminophen or an anti-inflammatory drug. This should help relieve the pain and stiffness. Special creams also sometimes help joint pain. In cases of severe OA, your health care provider may recommend an injection to the joint or surgery. *Remember* to take only the medicines prescribed for you.

You Have Been Prescribed: ____________________

You Need to Take: ____________________

You Need to Notify the Office If You Have:

A. Increased pain despite medication

B. Fever higher than 100.4°F

C. Abdominal pain or discomfort after taking medicine

Phone: ____________________

RESOURCE

Arthritis Foundation
800-283-7800
www.arthritis.org

OSTEOPOROSIS

PROBLEM

Osteoporosis is a condition in which the bone loses its normal density, mass, and strength, which makes it weak and more vulnerable to fracture (break).

CAUSE

The weakening of the bone can be caused by several factors. Some of these risk factors include:

A. Inadequate amounts of calcium, protein, and vitamin D in the diet

B. Decreased exercise

C. Some chronic diseases such as thyroid disease, diabetes, and heart failure

D. Cancer

E. Smoking

F. Low estrogen levels (menopause)

G. Excessive alcohol intake

H. Advancing age

I. Being a Caucasian and Asian woman

J. Long-term use of certain medications such as steroids, thyroid medications, seizure medications, and some cancer treatment medications

PREVENTION/CARE

A. Be sure to get adequate calcium intake daily (1,500 mg/d) and vitamin D intake (600–2,000 IU/d). Ask your health care provider for the appropriate dose of calcium and vitamin D for you.

B. Food sources of calcium are best absorbed.

C. Calcium and vitamin D supplements may also be needed to meet the daily recommendation.

D. Get daily weight-bearing exercise such as walking, jogging, or running. Avoid high-impact exercises.

TREATMENT PLAN

A. If osteoporosis is suspected, your provider may order a bone density study of your bones. Goals are to prevent the disease from occurring.

B. If you have been diagnosed with osteoporosis, you need to prevent the disease from progressing and take measures to prevent all bone fractures.

C. Use caution when walking on wet, slippery surfaces.

D. Avoid risk of falls by making your home safe. Avoid throw rugs on floors and remove small items that are easily tripped over. Use caution when pets are around to prevent falling over your pet.

Activity:

A. Physical activity is vital to maintain and prevent further bone loss.

B. Weight-bearing activity, such as walking or running, is the best activity.

C. Avoid high-impact sports and activities, such as jumping, and high-impact aerobics to prevent fracturing the bones.

D. Avoid any risk of falls.

E. Use walking devices, such as a cane or walker, if needed.

F. Bathtubs should have nonskid protection.

Diet:

A. Eat a regular well-balanced diet. Increase food sources rich in calcium, protein, and vitamin D.

B. Sources of vitamin D include milk, some fish (salmon), and drinks and cereals with added vitamin D and minerals.

(*continued*)

OSTEOPOROSIS *(continued)*

C. You can also get vitamin D from spending 20 to 30 minutes in the summer sunlight, exposing your skin to the sun without wearing sunscreen for this length of time.

D. Sources of calcium include dairy products, green leafy vegetables (broccoli), almonds, tofu, and drinks fortified with calcium such as orange juice and soy milk.

E. If you are overweight, a low-fat, low-cholesterol diet is suggested to lose weight.

Medications:

A. You may be prescribed nonprescription medications like acetaminophen (Tylenol) as needed for pain.

B. Supplements: Calcium, vitamin D, and hormone replacement for women who are menopausal.

C. If prescribed bisphosphonate, take medication with a full glass of water.

D. Wait approximately 30 to 60 minutes before reclining or consuming other medications, beverages, or food to lower the risk of regurgitation or a burning sensation.

You Have Been Prescribed: ______________________________

You Need to Take: ______________________________

You Need to Notify the Office If You Have:

A. Been experiencing any pain; you need to have your provider assess this pain.

B. Other: ______________________________

Phone: ______________________________

RESOURCES

National Osteoporosis Foundation: www.nof.org
The National Women's Health Information Center: https://www.womenshealth.gov

OTITIS EXTERNA

PROBLEM

Your practitioner has diagnosed you with a condition known as otitis externa, sometimes also referred to as "swimmer's ear." This is a common condition characterized by itching in the ear, sometimes followed by ear pain, swelling, and drainage of the ear canal. Difficulty hearing may also occur. The eardrum is rarely affected.

CAUSE

Otitis externa occurs from irritation to the external canal of the ear. The most common causes for otitis externa are long exposure to water in the ear canal after frequent swimming and too vigorous cleaning of the wax from your ears. It may involve either a bacterial or a fungal infection.

PREVENTION/CARE

You may prevent future problems with otitis externa by following these measures:

A. Clean the outer ear only as needed. Do not use cotton-tipped swabs or any other device to clean down into the ear canal. Usually, wax is just pushed deeper into the canal with this method, and the canal may be traumatized by the instrument used.

B. For swimmers or others susceptible to frequent recurrences of otitis externa, it may be helpful to dry the ear canals with a blow dryer on a low setting after exposure to water. You may also instill a solution of 50% isopropyl alcohol and 50% vinegar in the ear twice daily and after every submersion in water. Over-the-counter eardrops labeled for "swimmer's ear" may also be used as directed.

TREATMENT PLAN

For the most common bacterial infections associated with otitis externa, antibiotic/steroid eardrops are usually prescribed. In addition, you should keep water out of your ears for 4 to 6 weeks. (This means no swimming until symptoms are totally resolved. Recommendations include avoid getting water in the ear canal and only swim with water-resistant earplugs in the future.)

To bathe or shower, first coat cotton balls with petroleum jelly and use them to plug ears when bathing.

Activity: The only activity restrictions are those involving submersion in water. Bathing and hair washing are permitted as described previously.

Diet: No changes are required in your diet.

Medications:

A. Eardrops are used to treat otitis externa.

B. The drops should be applied down the ear canal's opening, moving the earlobe back and forth to help the eardrops pass downward.

C. In severe cases, antibiotics may be given.

You Have Been Prescribed: ____________________

You Need to Instill ____________ **Drops Into the Affected Ear** ____________ **Times Per Day.**

You Need to Notify the Office If You:

A. Have symptoms that have not cleared up in 3 days.

B. Have a fever over 100°F.

C. Have severe ear pain or new symptoms present.

D. Are unable to instill ear drops into the ear due to swelling of the ear canal.

E. Other: ____________________

Phone: ____________________

OTITIS MEDIA WITH EFFUSION

PROBLEM

You have inflammation of the middle ear with effusion, which is the presence of fluid in the middle ear without infection.

CAUSE

The middle ear fluid can remain behind the tympanic membrane after you have been treated for an ear infection (otitis media). The eustachian tube is blocked, and the fluid behind the ear does not drain out properly. Symptoms may include difficulty hearing and a feeling of fullness in the ear.

TREATMENT PLAN

A. Determine if you or your child is having difficulty with hearing.

B. Make accommodations for the hearing loss, such as sitting in the front of the classroom at school; speaking clearly and loudly. Reduce or eliminate external noises while having a conversation.

C. If you or your child has a buildup of fluid in the middle ear for 6 weeks up to 3 months, you should receive a hearing evaluation.

D. Follow up with a health care provider as instructed to avoid complications and/or permanent hearing loss.

Activity: There is no activity restriction.

Diet: There is no special diet.

Medications: There are not any medications that are used for fluid behind the ear. If infection is present, antibiotics are used to treat this infection.

You Have Been Prescribed: ______________________

You Need to Take: ______________________

You Need to Notify the Office If You Have:

A. Fever

B. Decreased appetite

C. Decreased activity level

D. Ear pain

E. Noticed a change in hearing loss or speech development

F. Any other new symptoms that occur

G. Other: ______________________

Phone: ______________________

PARKINSON'S DISEASE MANAGEMENT

PROBLEM

Parkinson's disease (PD) is a problem with the central nervous system that causes progressive muscle rigidity and tremors. The ability to move your muscles becomes difficult and you may also notice difficulty with walking and swallowing. Common symptoms you may experience include tremor at rest, rigidity (feeling stiff and finding it hard to start moving), bradykinesia (movements of your muscles slow down), and having a difficult time maintaining your posture, making you feel like you are going to fall down. Other symptoms may also include difficulty speaking, swallowing, drooling more, changes in mood, and sleep patterns.

CAUSE

The brain is not able to produce or use the correct amount of a chemical, called dopamine, required by the body, and therefore the nervous system reacts by producing a loss in control of your muscles and movements.

TREATMENT PLAN/CARE

A. There is no cure for PD. However, medications may relieve a lot of your symptoms. Your health care provider will share the medications that are available to you.

B. People with PD can be very sensitive to heat. During hot weather, stay outside only for very short periods of time, stay inside during the hottest part of the day, and increase your fluid intake.

C. Balance problems are common with PD and increase the risk of falls. Some ways to avoid injury are not to have loose rugs or other floor coverings; install grab bars around the tub and toilet; ensure a sturdy rail on stairs and adequate lighting so you can see where you are going; use straight-backed, firm chairs with arms.

D. Tremor increases the risk of accidents. Use sturdy plastic cups instead of glasses, use an electric razor to shave, and be cautious with sharp objects and power tools.

E. For clothes, Velcro fasteners, zippers, and snaps are easier to fasten than buttons. Loose clothing is also easier to put on and take off.

F. To avoid sleep problems, stay busy during the day and avoid naps. Discuss any problems you have with your neurologist; sometimes changes in your medication schedule can help.

G. If you have speech problems, work on ways to make your needs known. Practice speech exercises or consider speech therapy with a speech therapist.

H. Stay active in your daily work, hobbies, and other daily activities you enjoy.

I. If you are having signs of anxiety, depression, sleep problems, or other symptoms, please discuss these with your provider. These symptoms are common and can be addressed and treated with other medications.

Activity: Regular exercise helps maintain muscle flexibility and may reduce medication needs. Exercises to improve facial, jaw, and tongue movement are encouraged.

Diet: Your diet should include plenty of fluids and adequate fiber to prevent or manage constipation. Have bran cereal in the morning and eat five or more servings of fruits and vegetables throughout the day. Bananas are low in fiber and should be avoided.

Plan medication schedules so that you are functioning well at meal times. Be sure you allow plenty of time to finish your meal.

If you need help planning your meals, your health care provider can suggest a dietitian with whom you can talk about food choices.

Alcoholic beverages are discouraged as alcohol can interfere with the effectiveness of your medications.

If you are having difficulty with swallowing, let your provider know. Take your time eating meals. Sit upright. Thick liquids are easier to swallow than thin liquids.

Medications:

A. The medicines you are taking can improve your ability to carry out everyday activities, but they cannot totally eliminate your symptoms. It is important that you know why you are taking each medication as well as the possible side effects of each.

B. Check with your neurologist before starting any new medicine to be sure it does not interact with your PD medicines. Even vitamins can be a problem, so take only those recommended by your neurologist.

(*continued*)

PARKINSON'S DISEASE MANAGEMENT *(continued)*

C. In case of emergency, keep with you a list of your medicines, including the amounts you take and your schedule for taking them.

You Have Been Prescribed: ______________________________

You Need to Take: ______________________________

You Need to Notify the Office If:

A. You have a reaction to your medication.

B. You are unable to tolerate your medication because of side effects.

C. Your symptoms become worse.

D. Other: ______________________________

Phone: ______________________________

RESOURCES

National Parkinson Foundation
1501 N.W. 9th Avenue/Bob Hope Road
Miami, FL 33136-1494
1-800-473-4636
www.parkinson.org

The Michael J. Fox Foundation for Parkinson's Research
Grand Central Station
PO Box 4777
New York, NY 10163-4777
www.michaeljfox.org

Worldwide Education and Awareness for Movement Disorders: www.wemove.org
Parkinson's Disease Foundation, 1359 Broadway, Suite 1509
New York, NY 10018
212-923-4700
www.pdf.org

PELVIC INFLAMMATORY DISEASE

PROBLEM

You have been diagnosed as having pelvic inflammatory disease, also known as PID. This inflammation can involve the uterus, fallopian tubes, ovaries, broad ligament, and/or the pelvic vascular system or pelvic connective tissue.

CAUSE

Organisms that go up from the vagina and cervix into the uterus cause PID. The two most common organisms cultured from patients with PID are *Chlamydia trachomatis* and *Neisseria gonorrhoeae.* Your period increases the ability of gonococcal invasion into the upper genital tract. Infection and inflammation spread throughout the endometrium to the fallopian tubes. From there, it extends to the ovaries and peritoneal, or abdominal, cavity.

PREVENTION/CARE

A. Condoms and a spermicidal foam or cream with nonoxynol 9 is very protective against PID.

B. Condoms must be used with *every* sexual intercourse.

C. Vaginal douching may lead to an increased risk for PID.
   1. Routine douching is *not recommended;* it wipes out the normal vaginal flora.
   2. If you douche, do not douche more than once a month.

D. The more sex partners you have, the greater the chances are of contracting sexually transmitted infections.

TREATMENT PLAN

A. Your partner(s) need(s) to be evaluated and treated with antibiotic therapy, too.

B. Sexual abstinence
   1. **You should not have sexual intercourse until all of your symptoms are gone and your partner(s) has (have) completed antibiotic therapy.**
   2. If you do have sexual intercourse, you should use condoms consistently.

Activity: Limit yourself to bed rest for about 3 to 4 days, and then pursue activity as tolerated.

Diet:

A. You need to drink at least 10 to 12 glasses of liquid every day.

B. You need to eat a well-balanced diet (three meals).

C. You need to eat high-protein snacks such as peanut butter sandwiches and milk.

D. If you have been prescribed Flagyl (metronidazole), you must avoid all alcohol ingestion for at least 3 days after the last dose or you will experience severe nausea and vomiting.

Medications:

A. You will be prescribed *two or more* antibiotics; it is extremely important to **take all of the antibiotics.**

B. You may take acetaminophen (Tylenol) for fever.

C. You may be prescribed some pain medication.

You Have Been Prescribed: ____________________

You Need to Take: ____________________

Take all of your antibiotics, even if you feel better.

Your Second Prescribed Antibiotic Is: ____________________

(*continued*)

PELVIC INFLAMMATORY DISEASE *(continued)*

You Need to Take: ____________________

You need to take all of both antibiotics, even if you feel better.

You Have Been Prescribed the Following for Your Pain: ____________________

You Need to Take: ____________________

You Need to Notify the Office If:

A. Your fever does not respond to acetaminophen (Tylenol).

B. Your symptoms worsen, even while taking both antibiotics.

C. You vomit or cannot tolerate your antibiotics.

D. You must return to the office 2 or 3 days after the antibiotics have been started for a repeat examination and if you are unable to return for your follow-up office visit.

E. Other: ____________________

Phone: ____________________

Next Appointment: Date ______________ **Time** ______________

PERIPHERAL ARTERIAL DISEASE

PROBLEM

Peripheral arterial disease is a condition in which fatty deposits build up on the inside of vessels that carry blood to the hands and feet. This makes it difficult for blood to travel to hands and feet, which causes pain with activity and when resting. If these blockages increase in size, the pain will also worsen and infections can occur that could lead to amputation.

CAUSE

Many things cause these fatty deposits to build up inside arteries. Some, like age, gender, and genetics, cannot be changed. Others can be changed; these include smoking, diabetes, high cholesterol, high blood pressure, and excessive weight.

PREVENTION/CARE

A. Stop smoking.

B. To prevent injury that could progress into an infection, do the following:
   1. Wear well-fitting shoes that protect your feet.
   2. Look and feel inside your shoes before putting them on.
   3. Look at your feet daily for any signs of injury or infection.
   4. Dry feet well after bathing, including between toes.
   5. Do not trim your own toenails or shave off calluses. A health care provider should do this for you to prevent infection.
   6. Do not use a heating pad or hot water on your hands or feet to keep warm. Wear gloves or socks instead.

TREATMENT PLAN

A. Take your medications as ordered by your health care provider.

B. Effectively manage all other medical conditions, paying special attention to cholesterol, blood pressure, diabetes, and obesity.

C. Follow up with your primary health care provider and/or cardiologist on a regularly scheduled basis.

Activity:

A. Get regular exercise, after discussing with your health care provider the type and frequency of exercise that is safe for you.

Diet:

A. Discuss the type of diet that best suits your needs: Diabetic diet, low-fat diet, low-cholesterol diet, and/or low-sodium diet.

B. Follow the dietary guidelines suggested by your health care provider.

Medications:

You Have Been Prescribed: ____________________

You Need to Take: ____________________

You Need to Notify the Office If You Have:

A. Any of the following symptoms:
   1. Worsening pain in your arm or leg
   2. Fever of 101.5°F or greater
   3. Any temperature change in a hand or foot
   4. Any change in feeling of a hand or foot
   5. Any change in the color of a hand or foot
   6. Difficulty walking
   7. Vomiting or other illness that causes you to miss more than one dose of your medications
   8. Other: ____________________

Phone: ____________________

RESOURCE

Patient Education—Center-PAD: www.patienteducationcenter.org/information/peripheral-arterial-disease

PERNICIOUS ANEMIA

PROBLEM

You have been diagnosed with a condition called pernicious anemia. It is a condition in which vitamin B_{12} is not well absorbed. Vitamin B_{12} is necessary for red blood cell function.

CAUSE

Pernicious anemia is a common problem in pregnancy, with vegetarian diets, with previous stomach problems, and as you get older. Your condition may be due to the lack of a special factor in your stomach juices whereby your body cannot absorb the vitamin, or it may be from an autoimmune reaction.

PREVENTION/CARE

Pernicious anemia cannot always be prevented, but it is treatable once the cause is identified.

TREATMENT PLAN

A. You will need vitamin B_{12} injections for the rest of your life. This treatment cannot be given in pill form.
   1. After you have been on the shots for a while, the nurses can teach you or a family member to give the shot. Please ask your health care provider about this.
   2. Common side effects of vitamin B_{12} shots include:
      a. Pain and burning at the place the shot is given; this does not last very long.
      b. Some people experience diarrhea after taking the shot.

B. You may need to take iron tablets too.

C. You may be sent to see a nutritionist to help you review your diet and how you prepare foods.

Activity: Pernicious anemia may cause the loss of some senses and give you numbness and tingling, memory loss, loss of coordination, and some depression or irritability.

A. It is important to avoid extremely hot foods and drinks.

B. It is important to use caution in your home such as:
   1. Do not use loose "scatter" rugs, which can cause slips.
   2. Install shower or tub rails to help get in and out and toilet rails to get up and down easier.
   3. Use hand rails going up and down stairs.
   4. Do not use extremely hot water for bathing, showers, and doing dishes.
   5. Use nonslip surfaces in the tub and shower.
   6. **Do not use a heating pad if you do not have all your sensations.**

A home safety evaluation should be done to reduce the risk of falls. A checklist can be obtained from the National Safety Council: 1250 Eye Street, NW Suite 1000, Washington, DC 20005; www.homesafetycouncil.org

Diet: A balanced, healthy diet is important. Increase your liquids to 8 to 10 glasses a day; iron supplements tend to cause constipation. Increase the fiber in your diet.

Medication:

You Have Been Prescribed the Following Iron Supplement: ______________________________

You Need to Take It: ______________________________

Your Next Vitamin B_{12} Shot Is Due: ______________________________

You Need to Notify the Office If: ______________________________

A. You feel worse the first week after the shot or have symptoms such as chest pain and shortness of breath.

B. You have worsening symptoms such as problems with balance and walking.

C. You have leg pain, especially when you put your weight on it.

D. You would like to make arrangements for home injections.

E. Other: ______________________________

Phone: ______________________________

PHARYNGITIS

PROBLEM

Pharyngitis (sore throat) is a condition that occurs when the throat becomes inflamed.

CAUSE

The inflammation can be due to a virus, a bacterial infection, or a fungus. Other noninfectious causes include postnasal drip, allergies, mouth breathing, and trauma.

PREVENTION/CARE

A. Avoid sick people and crowds. Stay at home if you are sick.

B. Cover your mouth when coughing.

C. Do not share a drinking glass, kiss, or have close contact with anyone who has an upper respiratory infection.

TREATMENT PLAN

A. Hot tea, soup, and throat lozenges soothe your throat.

B. Use disposable tissues when sneezing. Use tissues when you blow your nose. If no tissue is available, do the "elbow sneeze" into the bend of your arm (away from your open hands). Dispose of tissues and then wash your hands.

C. Avoid smoking and secondhand smoke.

Activity: If you have strep throat, do not return to school or work until you have completed a full 24 hours of antibiotic. Rest or nap as often as possible while you are sick.

Diet: Eat a healthy diet. If swallowing is difficult, eat soft foods such as ice cream, Jell-O, pudding, and soup. Avoid salt and spicy foods. Increase your fluid intake to 10 to 12 glasses a day.

Medications: You will be prescribed antibiotics if you have a bacterial infection. If your sore throat is due to a virus, antibiotics would not help. Do not share your prescription medications with other family members who are also sick. They need a full prescription, too. Many other medications are available over the counter, such as throat lozenges, cough suppressants, and so forth.

You Have Been Prescribed: ______________________________

You Need to Take: ______________________________

If you are prescribed antibiotics, complete all of the doses.

You Need to Notify the Office If:

A. You have difficulty breathing because of the sore throat or enlarged tonsils.

B. Your symptoms are worse after 24 hours of antibiotics.

C. You are unable to keep down your antibiotic because of vomiting.

D. Your sick child refuses to eat or drink.

E. You develop a rash or itch after starting the antibiotic.

F. You are a diabetic and your blood glucose is high, or you have ketones in your urine.

G. Other: ______________________________

Phone: ______________________________

PITYRIASIS ROSEA

PROBLEM

Pityriasis rosea is a very common condition characterized by a rash that may or may not itch. You may have noticed a large, scaly patch before breaking out with the more generalized rash. **It is not known to be contagious, and you do not need to isolate yourself.**

CAUSE

The cause of pityriasis rosea is unknown.

PREVENTION/CARE

Because the cause of pityriasis rosea is unknown, there are no recommended preventive measures.

TREATMENT PLAN

Good hygiene and avoidance of scratching are recommended to prevent a secondary infection.

Activity: It is not necessary for you to limit your activity. Sunlight exposure to skin for short periods of time daily for 5 consecutive days will decrease itching and improve the rash. Care should be taken not to burn skin with short-term exposure to the sun.

Diet: No changes are required in your diet.

Medications: You may be prescribed an antihistamine medication to take by mouth and topical steroid creams to apply to the rash itself. If the itching is severe, oral steroids may be prescribed.

You Have Been Prescribed: ______________________________

You Need to Take: ______________________________

You Need to Notify the Office If You Have:

A. Any new symptoms

B. Any reaction to your medication

Phone: ______________________________

PNEUMONIA, VIRAL: ADULT

PROBLEM

Viral pneumonia is an infection of the lung that causes fluid in the air sacs. You may have fever, cough, or difficulty breathing.

CAUSE

Respiratory viruses cause viral pneumonia and bacteria.

PREVENTION/CARE

A. Avoid contact with people with respiratory illnesses.

B. Although the flu vaccine does not prevent pneumonia, a yearly flu shot is recommended.

C. The pneumonia vaccine helps prevent pneumonia caused by bacteria. If you are older than 65 years or have other chronic respiratory illness, the pneumonia vaccine is recommended.

TREATMENT PLAN

A. Use a cool-mist humidifier, and clean it daily.

B. Take deep breaths and cough frequently to clear secretions from lungs.

C. Avoid smoking and exposure to secondhand smoke.

D. Practice good handwashing techniques or use hand sanitizers.

Activity: Rest frequently during the early phase of the illness. Fatigue may continue for up to 6 weeks.

Diet: Eat a nutritious diet. Drink 8 to 10 glasses of water a day.

Medications:

A. Take acetaminophen (Tylenol) for fever, discomfort, and headache.

B. Do not take cough suppressants. It is important for you to cough and get up any mucus.

C. Antibiotics are not given for a viral infection. If you have a bacterial infection, then you may be put on an antibiotic.

You Have Been Prescribed: ______________________________

You Need to Take: ______________________________

You Need to Notify the Office If You Have:

A. Increased difficulty breathing.

B. Fever greater than 101°F, or fever that persists after 48 hours of antibiotics.

C. Worsening discomfort.

D. Shortness of breath.

E. Blood in sputum

F. Nausea, vomiting, or diarrhea

G. Other: ______________________________

Phone: ______________________________

PNEUMONIA, VIRAL: CHILD

PROBLEM

Viral pneumonia is an infection of the lung that causes fluid to collect in the air sacs. Your child may have fever, cough, or difficulty breathing.

CAUSE

Respiratory viruses cause viral pneumonia.

PREVENTION/CARE

A. Isolate young infants from people with respiratory illnesses.

B. Although the flu vaccine will not prevent viral pneumonia, children should get an influenza vaccine every year.

TREATMENT PLAN

A. Encourage fluids.

B. Use a vaporizer to increase humidity in the child's room.

C. Keep the child away from cigarette smoke.

Activity: Have your child rest during the acute phase. Your child may return to school or day care when he or she is free from fever for 24 hours.

Diet: There is no special diet for viral pneumonia. Follow a regular diet. Increase fluids.

Medications:

A. You may give your child acetaminophen (Tylenol) for fever.

B. Children should never be given aspirin due to the increased risk of Reye's syndrome.

C. **Do not give cough suppressants. The American College of Chest Physicians clinical practice guidelines recommend that cough suppressants and over-the-counter cough medications should *not* be given to young children. Cough medicines should *not* be given to any child younger than 6 years of age.**

D. Antibiotics are not used for viral infections. Your child may be given an antibiotic if he or she has any infection other than the viral pneumonia.

Your Child Has Been Prescribed: ______________________________

Your Child Needs to Take: ______________________________

You Need to Notify the Office Immediately If:

A. Your child's breathing becomes more labored or difficult, or his or her lips become blue.

B. Retractions (tugging between ribs) become worse.

C. Grunting sounds occur when the child breathes out.

D. Your child starts acting very sick.

E. Other: ______________________________

You Need to Notify the Office Within 24 Hours If:

A. Your child is unable to sleep.

B. Your child is not drinking enough.

C. Fever is over 101°F or persists after 48 hours on antibiotics.

D. Your child is getting worse.

E. Other: ______________________________

Phone: ______________________________

POLYMYALGIA RHEUMATICA

PROBLEM

Polymyalgia rheumatica (PMR) is a common disorder experienced by adults older than the age of 50 years in which complaints involve overall joint stiffness and pain. Common complaints include feeling fine one day and the following day having overall joint pain, with difficulty getting out of bed or standing up from a chair. Symptoms may occur gradually over a period of several days or weeks, or may occur abruptly overnight. Symptoms are usually worse in the morning hours. The joints most commonly affected are the upper arms, shoulders, thighs, hips, and neck.

CAUSE

A. The cause of PMR is unknown.

B. Some theories maintain that PMR may be triggered by an infection; however, research does not identify any specific infection.

PREVENTION/CARE

There is not any way to prevent the onset of PMR.

TREATMENT PLAN

A. You may be treated with low-dose steroid by mouth daily. Prednisone is a common medication used to treat this disorder. Stiffness and joint pain may quickly improve with the use of oral steroids. If improvement with steroids does not occur within 2 weeks of treatment, you should notify your provider.

B. Once improvement is noted, your provider will begin to lower the steroid dose gradually over time. This may take several weeks to months.

C. Do not change or taper your steroid dose on your own. Your provider will advise you on the tapering dose when appropriate.

Activity:

A. Once stiffness and pain have improved, you may resume normal activities. Exercise is encouraged on most days of the week.

Diet:

A. There is not any special diet to follow for this disorder.

B. Blood sugar: Side effects of the prednisone may include increased blood sugar. If you have concerns regarding your blood sugar values, or if you are diabetic, you need to discuss proper management and monitoring of your blood sugar while taking steroids.

Medications:

A. Oral steroids (prednisone) are commonly prescribed over a period. Discuss proper dosages and tapering of this medication with your provider.

You Have Been Prescribed: ______________________________

You Need to Take: ______________________________

You Need to Notify the Office If You Have:

A. Any new symptoms such as headache, jaw pain, or vision changes

B. Side effects from the prednisone or other medications prescribed

(*continued*)

POLYMYALGIA RHEUMATICA *(continued)*

C. Increase in pain, or weakness while using prednisone

D. Any other concerns

Phone: ______________________________

RESOURCES

The Arthritis Foundation: www.arthritis.org

National Institute of Arthritis and Musculoskeletal and Skin Diseases Information Clearinghouse: www.niams.nih.gov/Health_Info/Polymyalgia/default.asp

POSTPARTUM: BREAST ENGORGEMENT AND SORE NIPPLES

PROBLEM

Engorgement causes swollen, tender breasts, which may have palpable nodular areas.

CAUSE

Engorgement may develop because of inadequate suckling by your baby.

PREVENTION/CARE

A. At first, nurse your baby every 2 to 3 hours.

B. Make sure your baby latches onto the areola (darkened area around the nipple) as much as possible. The baby suckling on the tip of the nipple does not provide the stimulation necessary to let down the milk and can make your nipples sore and cracked.

C. If your baby is not well attached to the breast, detach the baby and make sure he or she opens his or her mouth wide to accommodate most of the areola.

D. Wear a supportive nursing bra (avoid underwire bras as they can exert pressure on certain areas of the breast and cause milk stasis, which is a good medium for bacterial growth and infection); make sure that your bra does not squeeze your breasts too tightly.

E. Make sure that the baby is properly attached to the nipple; this helps to avoid cracking of nipples that can predispose you to an infection of the breast called *mastitis*.

F. After the baby feeds, express some milk and apply it to the areola to keep the nipple hydrated and to avoid cracking.

G. Purified lanolin can also be very helpful for sore nipples and can prevent further cracking and infection. Apply routinely after each breastfeeding session for the first several days of nursing and longer if tender or cracked nipples occur. If the lanolin is purified, there is no need to wash it off before feedings.

TREATMENT PLAN

A. Engorgement
   1. Treatment of engorgement includes the application of heat, breast massage, and expression of milk for comfort only.
   2. A warm moist washcloth or a warm shower before massaging the breast decreases discomfort.
   3. Massage the breast by making several gentle but firm stroking movements with the fingertips along the swollen ducts, moving toward the nipple. This should be done around the entire breast.
   4. After massaging, milk should be expressed or pumped until the breast softens enough for the baby to latch well. The baby should then be allowed to nurse from both breasts.
   5. The best strategy for engorgement is frequent breastfeeding (at least every half an hour to 2 hours until engorgement resolves).

B. Sore nipples
   1. Sore nipples are usually caused by the improper positioning of the baby on the nipple.
   2. Ensure your baby is grasping the areola when sucking and not just the nipple.
   3. Continuous suction pressure at the same spot of the nipple can be painful.
   4. Change the position of the baby to change the “latching on” position of your baby’s mouth.
   5. If nipples become sore or cracked, start feeding on the less affected breast first.
   6. Apply purified lanolin to nipples after each feeding.
   7. Prevent mastitis with the following personal hygiene measures:
      a. Avoid using soap on nipples.
      b. Avoid decrusting the nipples of dried colostrum or milk.
      c. Change breast pads frequently.
      d. Wash hands before handling your breast and before breastfeeding.

Activity: As tolerated, extra rest is recommended after delivery.

Diet:

A. Breastfeeding mothers need extra liquids for milk production.

B. Drink 10 to 12 glasses of liquid a day.

(*continued*)

POSTPARTUM: BREAST ENGORGEMENT AND SORE NIPPLES *(continued)*

C. Use caffeine in moderation (eliminate if possible).

D. Continue your regular diet and add about 500 extra calories per day.

E. Avoid gas-producing foods that may upset your baby's stomach.

Medications: Continue your prenatal vitamins while breastfeeding.

You Have Been Prescribed: Acetaminophen 500 mg or ibuprofen 600 mg every 3 to 4 hours for discomfort.

You Need to Notify the Office If You Have:

A. Temperature of 100.4°F or higher

B. Pain that is not controlled with Tylenol or ibuprofen

C. Flu-like symptoms (fever, chills, malaise)

D. Red streaks on breast

E. Headache with the aforementioned symptoms

F. Other: ______________________________

Phone: ______________________________

PREMENSTRUAL SYNDROME

DEFINITION

Premenstrual syndrome (PMS) is a common problem experienced by women in their reproductive years. You may have some or all of the following symptoms:

A. Cravings for food, particularly chocolate and salty foods

B. Irritability

C. Feelings of depression; crying spells

D. Bloated stomach

E. Weight gain and water retention

F. Difficulty concentrating

G. Tiredness

H. Feelings of faintness

I. Sometimes clumsiness

J. Sore breasts

CAUSE

Although the cause is really not known, PMS is a response of your body to the changes in female hormones during the last half of your menstrual cycle.

PREVENTION/CARE

All of your symptoms probably cannot be prevented, but some of them may be made less severe.

TREATMENT PLAN

A. Keep track of your symptoms for at least 3 months so that your health care provider can determine if the symptoms always happen in the last half of your cycle.

B. Eat six small meals each day. Eat breakfast, have a morning snack like fruit or a glass of milk, eat lunch, have an afternoon snack, eat supper, and then have another evening snack. This helps keep your blood sugar even, to avoid low blood sugar.

C. Avoid candy, desserts, and other sugars. They may be associated with episodes of low blood sugar. Complex carbohydrates, such as pasta, potatoes, fresh fruit, rice, and bread, break down more slowly than sweets and keep your blood sugar steadier.

D. Stay away from salty foods such as chips, fast-food, and pickles.

E. Avoid caffeine in soda, coffee, and chocolate. Caffeine makes you irritable and nervous.

F. Exercise daily. It is a good idea to do aerobic exercises or even walking. Exercise increases chemicals in your brain that help with your mood.

G. Join a PMS group so that you can get support from other women who have similar symptoms. You may get ideas of how other women handle PMS, and you can share your ideas, too.

H. If you smoke, try to cut down or quit.

I. Get a good night's rest and take naps during the day if possible.

J. Try stress-reduction classes or yoga. Local community organizations usually have classes available.

Medications: There are a number of medications available that your health care provider may suggest for you.

You Have Been Prescribed: ____________________

(*continued*)

PREMENSTRUAL SYNDROME *(continued)*

You Need to Take: ______________________________

You Have Also Been Prescribed: ______________________________

You Need to Take: ______________________________

You Need to Notify the Office If:

A. You have questions or concerns.

B. You feel that things are not improving.

C. Other: ______________________________

Phone: ______________________________

PRETERM LABOR

PROBLEM

Premature contractions and early labor put your baby at risk of premature delivery. Babies born too soon are at risk of breathing problems, bleeding into their brain, infection, and bowel problems, to name a few. Early recognition is the key to stopping premature labor and delivery.

CAUSE

There are several predisposing factors for preterm labor, including previous premature delivery, smoking, incompetent cervix, multiple gestation (twins or triplets), and infection. In most cases, the cause of preterm labor is unknown.

PREVENTION/CARE

You can decrease your risk of preterm labor by living a healthy lifestyle with a balanced diet, proper fluid consumption, and no smoking. Please review any previous preterm labor symptoms with your health care provider. Early recognition is a key to success.

TREATMENT PLAN

Treatment depends on the clinical picture. In general, you should remember:

A. Drink at least 8 to 10 glasses of liquid a day; dehydration can increase contractions.

B. Empty your bladder every 2 to 3 hours.

C. Report any bladder infection symptoms, such as burning with urination, to your health care provider.

D. Avoid breast stimulation (including showers where the water stream is on your breasts); this can stimulate contractions.

E. Rest frequently. Rest means lying down on either side, not on your back.

F. Contractions and cramping happen more often in the evening and nighttime after activity during the day.

G. Do not have intercourse or sexual stimulation without asking your nurse practitioner, certified nurse-midwife, or doctor. If intercourse is okay, use a condom to decrease infection.

H. Try to arrange for help with housework and child care to help you maintain your bed-rest schedule.

I. Take medications to stop contractions as directed.

Activity: Activity at home is based on how strong your preterm labor has been. You should follow the following activity guidelines:

Level 1: As Tolerated

A. Avoid heavy lifting above 20 lb.

Level 2: Modified Bed Rest

A. You may be out of bed for breakfast.

B. Rest for 2 hours in the morning with only moderate activity until lunch.

C. Rest for 2 hours with only moderate activity until dinner.

D. Go to bed by 8 p.m.

Moderate activity consists of short periods of cooking, light housework (dusting and sweeping).

Level 3: Strict Bed Rest

A. You may be out of the bed only to go to the bathroom or to move to the couch.

B. You may take a shower, use the toilet, brush your teeth, then return immediately to bed.

C. You should not engage in lifting, bending, housework, or lengthy cooking.

D. You should not have sexual intercourse.

E. Perform range-of-motion (ROM) exercises as directed by your practitioner to avoid muscle weakness and blood clots in your legs. Example: Make small circles with your feet, bend and straighten your legs.

Level 4: Hospitalization

(*continued*)

PRETERM LABOR (*continued*)

Diet: Diet as tolerated, or follow your prescribed diet. Drink 8 to 10 glasses of water each day. Avoid beverages with caffeine. Eat fresh vegetables, fruits, and bran cereal to avoid becoming constipated.

Medications: Continue taking your prenatal vitamin every day.

You Have Been Prescribed: ____________________

You Need to Take: ____________________

You Need to Notify the Office If You Have:

A. Contractions or cramping more frequent than four in 1 hour

B. A gush of fluid or blood from your vagina (it is normal to have spotting after vaginal examination or intercourse)

C. Pelvic pressure or low, dull backache

D. Noticed that your baby is not moving as much as usual: Less than 10 fetal movements in 2 hours after drinking and resting on your side.

E. Chest pain or difficulty breathing

F. Other: ____________________

Phone: ____________________

PROSTATIC HYPERTROPHY/BENIGN

PROBLEM

Enlargement of the prostate causes the feeling of needing to urinate. Symptoms include having to go to the bathroom more often, especially at night; trouble starting or stopping your urine; decreased stream; and feeling that you do not empty.

CAUSE

The cause is not known, but it may be because of change in hormones with age.

PREVENTION/CARE

None.

TREATMENT PLAN

Treatment depends on how bad the symptoms are. Medications can help, but an operation to fix the obstruction may be needed. Empty your bladder on a schedule every 2 to 3 hours to prevent overfilling of the bladder.

Activity: There are no restrictions. You may need to plan schedules with access to bathrooms in mind.

Diet: Avoid spicy foods that irritate the bladder. Caffeine and alcohol act as diuretics and increase your need to urinate.

Medications:

A. Medications that help relieve the blockage may block hormones or relax the muscles that control urination.

B. Antibiotics are used if there is also an infection in your bladder or prostate.

C. Do not take over-the-counter (OTC) medications like cold medications, decongestants, antihistamines (for allergies), and diarrhea medicines; they make symptoms worse.

D. Always read labels to check for the advice: "Do not take if you have prostate enlargement."

E. Avoid drinking liquids before bedtime or before going out.

F. Double void to empty your bladder more completely.

You Have Been Prescribed: ______________________________

You Need to Take: ______________________________

You Need to Notify the Office If: ______________________________

A. You cannot urinate.

B. Your symptoms worsen.

C. You have a fever.

D. Other: ______________________________

Phone: ______________________________

PROSTATITIS

PROBLEM

Prostatitis is infection and/or inflammation of the prostate. Symptoms can be problems with urinating, increased frequency or painful urination, fever, or chills. You may have pain in the scrotum and buttocks and blood in the urine or semen. Prostatitis can be treated and does not cause impotence.

CAUSE

An infection may be caused by bacteria from the bladder or reflux of urine, or it may have started from a rectal infection.

PREVENTION/CARE

A. Prevent prostate infection with good hygiene.
   1. Clean under foreskin if uncircumcised and wash your hands after each time you go to the bathroom (urine and bowel movements [BM]).
   2. Limit your sexual partners and use a condom to prevent all types of infection.
   3. Urinate when you have the urge. Do not hold your urine for a long period.

B. Staying sexually active with ejaculation may decrease the incidence.

TREATMENT PLAN

A. You may have to be in the hospital for severe infections.

B. At home, try the following comfort measures:
   1. Use a sitz bath or sit in warm bath water or a whirlpool three times a day to provide some relief.
   2. You may find you feel more comfortable when you empty your bladder in a warm water bath when your pelvic muscles relax.

C. Your sexual partner(s) may need to be evaluated and treated too (ask your health care provider).

Activity: Rest; do not engage in strenuous physical activity or heavy lifting.

Diet: Increase fluid intake. ***Fluid Exception:*** **Decrease caffeine and alcohol, which can irritate the urethra.**

Medications: Antibiotics cure the infection by killing bacteria. You need to continue taking these drugs until the infection is completely cured (usually about 1 month). You need to take all the antibiotics even if your symptoms are gone.

You Have Been Prescribed the Following Antibiotics: ____________________

You Need to Take: ____________________

Finish all of the antibiotics even if you feel better.

Pain medications combined with anti-inflammatory drugs to decrease pain are usually taken for 3 to 7 days. Take acetaminophen (Tylenol) to bring down fever.

You Have Been Prescribed the Following for Pain: ____________________

You Need to Take: ____________________

You Have Been Prescribed the Following for Fever: ____________________

You Need to Take: ____________________

You Need to Notify the Office If You Have:

A. Symptoms that get worse or do not improve during treatment.

B. Symptoms that recur after treatment.

(continued)

PROSTATITIS *(continued)*

C. Fever higher than 101.0°F.

D. Other: ____________________

Phone: ____________________

RESOURCES

American Urological Association Foundation: www.UrologyHealth.org
National Kidney and Urologic Disease Information Clearinghouse: www.kidney.niddk.nih.gov
National Urology Health Hotline Toll Free 1-800-828-7866
The Prostatitis Foundation: www.prostatitis.org

PSEUDOGOUT

PROBLEM

Pseudogout, also known as calcium pyrophosphate deposition disease (CPPD), is a type of disorder that causes acute joint pain and swelling, primarily in the shoulder and knees. It can also occur in smaller joints, such as the ankles, feet, elbows, wrists, and hands.

CAUSE

Pseudogout is caused from calcium crystals building up in the joint, causing inflammation and pain. Having pseudogout can increase your risk of osteoarthritis (OA). OA is a common type of arthritis seen in older adults that can cause joint pain, stiffness, and sometimes swelling in the joints.

PREVENTION/CARE

There is not anything you can do to prevent this disease from occurring. However, if you are having three or more attacks per year, notify your practitioner. There are medications that can be prescribed to help prevent future attacks.

TREATMENT PLAN

Treatment depends on how many joints are affected. If you have one or two joints affected, your provider may drain the fluid from the joint and inject steroids into the joint, which will improve the pain. If you have several joints affected, you will probably be given oral medications such as nonsteroidal anti-inflammatory drugs (NSAIDs). These medications (indomethacin, naproxen, ibuprofen, etc.) will help with the swelling and pain. If you cannot take these medications because of other illnesses, please make sure your provider is aware of this. There are other medications available if you are not able to take these medications.

Activity: For acute attack, rest and elevation of the affected joint is recommended. If you are having difficulty with bearing weight on the joint, make sure your provider is aware of this; you need to stay off the joint.

Diet: No special diet is recommended.

Medications:
A. NSAIDs:

B. Steroids:

You Have Been Prescribed the Following Medication: ______________________________

You Need to Take: ______________________________

You Have Been Prescribed the Following for Discomfort: ______________________________

You Need to Take: ______________________________

You Need to Notify the Office If You Have:

A. No improvement in 1 to 2 days after being seen by your provider

B. Redness, increase in swelling, and/or pain in the affected joint

C. Redness, swelling, or pain in another new joint

D. Fever or new onset of other symptoms

E. Unable to tolerate medications prescribed by your provider today

F. Other:

Phone: ______________________________

PSORIASIS

PROBLEM

Psoriasis is a chronic, scaly, thickened-skin disorder with frequent remissions and recurrences. The skin of the scalp, elbows, knees, chest, back, arms, legs, toenails, fingernails, and fold between the buttocks may be involved.

CAUSE

The cause of psoriasis is unknown.

PREVENTION/CARE

A. There is no known prevention, but symptoms can be controlled.

B. Moving to a warmer climate might be beneficial. Severity increases with cold.

C. Maintain good skin hygiene with daily baths or showers.

D. Avoid harsh soaps.

E. Avoid skin injury, including harsh scrubbing, which can trigger new outbreaks.

F. Avoid skin dryness.

G. To reduce scaling, use nonprescription, waterless cleansers, and hair preparations containing coal tar (Zetar, T/Gel, Pentrax), emollients (Eucerin Plus lotion or cream, Lubriderm, Moisture Plus, Moisturel), or products containing cortisone (often prescription strength).

H. Expose the skin to moderate amounts of sunlight as often as possible. Avoid long periods in the sun to prevent sunburn.

I. Oatmeal baths may loosen scales. Use 1 cup of oatmeal to a tub of warm water.

J. Stress may increase outbreaks of psoriasis. Consider counseling to assist in lifestyle changes, coping, or any psychological problems caused by psoriasis.

TREATMENT PLAN

Activity: There are no activity restrictions.

Diet: Eat a well-balanced diet. You may be instructed to try a gluten-free diet. Drink 8 to 10 glasses of water per day. Avoid alcohol in your diet.

Medications: You may be prescribed the following types of medications:

A. Creams to rub on the skin
   1. Ointments containing coal tar. These may stain clothing.
   2. Salicylic acid cream, anthralin cream, or vitamin D-like cream (calcipotriene).
   3. Topical cortisone creams may also be used for short periods of time.

B. Psoralen plus ultraviolet light (PUVA; combination of a medication and exposure to ultraviolet A light)

C. Combination of tar baths with ultraviolet B light

D. Antihistamines to relieve itching

You Have Been Prescribed: ____________________

You Need to Take: ____________________

You Need to Notify the Office If:

A. You have an adverse reaction to or cannot tolerate any of the prescribed medications.

B. Symptoms recur after treatment. Notify your health care provider if, during an outbreak, pustules erupt on the skin and/or are accompanied by fever, muscle aches, and fatigue.

(*continued*)

PSORIASIS *(continued)*

C. New, unexplained symptoms develop.

D. Other: ______________________________

Phone: ______________________________

For severe cases, you may be referred to a dermatologist (specialist for skin disorders).

RESOURCE

National Psoriasis Foundation, Suite 200, 6415 SW Canyon, Ct. Portland, OR 97221, Phone: 800-723-9166, www.psoriasis.org

RESPIRATORY SYNCYTIAL VIRUS

PROBLEM

Respiratory syncytial virus (RSV) causes respiratory distress, wheezing, coughing, and fever.

CAUSE

RSV is a common respiratory virus that affects infants and children in fall, winter, and early spring.

PREVENTION/CARE

A. Isolate young infants from people with respiratory illnesses.

B. Wash hands frequently if you are a caregiver.

C. Wash toys and surfaces the child touches.

D. Although the flu vaccine does not prevent RSV, a flu vaccine is recommended every year.

TREATMENT PLAN

A. Do not smoke around the child.

Activity: The child needs rest during the early stages of the illness.

Diet: Continue to breastfeed. Offer fluids, such as juice and water, frequently. Dilute juice for younger infants. Offer small, frequent feedings.

Medications:

A. Antibiotics do not help with viruses.

B. There is a special vaccination for RSV, but your child must meet special requirements that are recommended by the American Academy of Pediatricians.

C. **The American College of Chest Physicians clinical practice guideline recommends that cough suppressants and over-the-counter cold medicines *not* be given to young children. Cough and cold medicines should *not* be given to children younger than 6 years of age.**

D. Your child may be given other medications to control other symptoms.

You Have Been Prescribed: ______________________________

You Need to Take: ______________________________

You Need to Call 911 or Call the Office Immediately If:

A. Your child's breathing gets labored, difficult, or faster than 60 times a minute.

B. Your child's lips become bluish, or he or she stops breathing or passes out.

C. Wheezing becomes severe.

D. Retractions (tugging between ribs) become worse.

E. Your child starts acting very sick and lethargic.

F. Other: ______________________________

You Need to Notify the Office Within 24 Hours If:

A. Your child is unable to sleep.

B. Your child will not drink enough fluids.

C. Your child has any suggestion of an earache, a yellow nasal discharge, or a fever over 100°F for more than 72 hours.

D. You feel your child is getting worse.

E. Other: ______________________________

Phone: ______________________________

RICE THERAPY AND EXERCISE THERAPY

RICE therapies are used for muscle injuries. RICE stands for rest, ice, compression, and elevation.

REST

A. Take it easy; eliminate abuse; reduce regular exercise or activities of daily living as needed but do not eliminate them.

B. Change activity or components of activity; for example, change running to walking.

C. Stop sports; restrict squatting, kneeling, and repetitious bending.

D. Limit weight bearing; immobilize with crutches for partial weight bearing.

ICE

A. Use cold in the acute phase of the injury (first 72 hours) to reduce pain and swelling.

B. Use cold in the form of ice in a plastic bag or even use frozen peas in a bag.

C. Apply cold four to eight times a day for 20 minutes at a time, with 45 to 60 minutes between applications.

COMPRESSION

A. Use elastic bandages, dry or wet, or open basket-weave tape.

B. Avoid trying to provide support with elastic bandages; a brace, overlap taping, or a cast may be needed.

ELEVATION

A. Elevate the joint above the level of the heart to reduce swelling.

B. Apply cold compresses while the joint is elevated.

EXERCISE THERAPY

A. Begin exercise therapy after the initial 48-hour period if pain and swelling begin to resolve.

B. Do gentle range-of-motion exercises several times a day within limits of pain for 7 to 10 days after knee ligament strain.

C. Exercise after 6 minutes of icing to take advantage of the cold's numbing effect.

D. Start with nonresistive, nonweight-bearing exercises.

E. Use exercises that improve range of motion and strength.

F. Maintain fitness of the extremity.

RINGWORM (TINEA)

PROBLEM

Ringworm is a fungal infection of the skin, which can be found on any part of the body. A worm does not cause ringworm; it gets the name because of the round ring shape that is red on the outside and normal on the inside. It is not uncommon to get more than one time. Other tinea fungal infections are:

A. Tinea pedis (athlete's foot)

B. Tinea cruris (jock itch)

C. Tinea capitis (ringworm on the head)

CAUSE

The fungus is transmitted by direct contact. It can be transmitted from objects, shoes, locker rooms, animals, and people.

PREVENTION

A. Use good hygiene, including not sharing hairbrushes and combs.

B. Keep skin cool and dry.

C. Wear shoes in locker rooms and around pools.

D. Wear loose-fitting clothing.

E. Treat pets' skin problems adequately. Ringworm is often blamed on cats, but it can come from almost any animal, including horses, rabbits, dogs, and pigs.

F. Infections of fingernails and toenails may require prescription medications.

TREATMENT PLAN

Activity: As tolerated. Some contact sports may increase contracting tinea (football and wrestling).

Diet: There is no special diet.

Medications:

You Have Been Prescribed: ____________________

You Need to Take: ____________________

You Need to Notify the Office If:

A. Your symptoms get worse.

B. Other: ____________________

Phone: ____________________

ROCKY MOUNTAIN SPOTTED FEVER AND REMOVAL OF A TICK

PROBLEM

Ticks are vectors for Lyme disease and Rocky Mountain spotted fever. You have been diagnosed with Rocky Mountain spotted fever.

CAUSE

Rocky Mountain spotted fever is caused by a bacterium from ticks.

PREVENTION/CARE

A. Avoid areas with large deer populations.

B. Wear light-colored clothes to make ticks easier to spot. Wear long sleeves and tuck pants into the socks to form a barrier.

C. Stick to hiking trails. Avoid contact with overgrown foliage. Ticks prefer dense woods with thick growth of shrubs and small trees as well as areas along the edge of the woods.

D. Check for ticks after each outdoor activity, especially in hairy regions of the body and beltline, where ticks often attach. Check for ticks before bathing, especially at the back of the neck, knees, and ears.

E. Remove ticks promptly.

F. Inspect pets daily and remove ticks when present.

G. Some manufacturers currently offer permethrin-treated clothing that is effective for up to 20 washings. This clothing is not recommended for children.

H. Antibiotic therapy to prevent Rocky Mountain spotted fever is not recommended for tick exposure. Instead, tell your health care provider if any symptoms, especially fever and headache, occur in the following 14 days.

I. Use tick repellent with diethyltoluamide (DEET; except for small children younger than 2 years). As an alternative, picaridin and oil of eucalyptus preparations have been approved for use as repellents by the U.S. Environmental Protection Agency (EPA).

Precautions When Removing Ticks

A. Do not hold a lighted match or cigarette to the tick. Do not apply gasoline, kerosene, or oil to the tick's body.

B. Avoid squeezing the body of the tick.

C. Grasp the tick with a fine-tip tweezer close to the skin. Remove by gently pulling the tick upward straight out without using any twisting motions (see the following figures).

D. In the home, if fingers are used to remove ticks, they should be protected with facial tissue or gloves and washed after removal of the tick.

E. Do not crush the tick during removal.

F. **Save the tick for identification in case you become ill. Write the date of the tick bite on paper and place the paper and the tick in a resealable baggie and place it in the freezer.**

TREATMENT PLAN

Activity: Regular activity as tolerated. Tepid sponge baths may be taken for fever.

Diet: Eat a regular diet. Drink 8 to 10 glasses of water daily.

Medications:

A. Acetaminophen (Tylenol) may be taken for body aches.

B. You may be given antibiotics for a secondary infection if needed.

(*continued*)

ROCKY MOUNTAIN SPOTTED FEVER AND REMOVAL OF A TICK *(continued)*

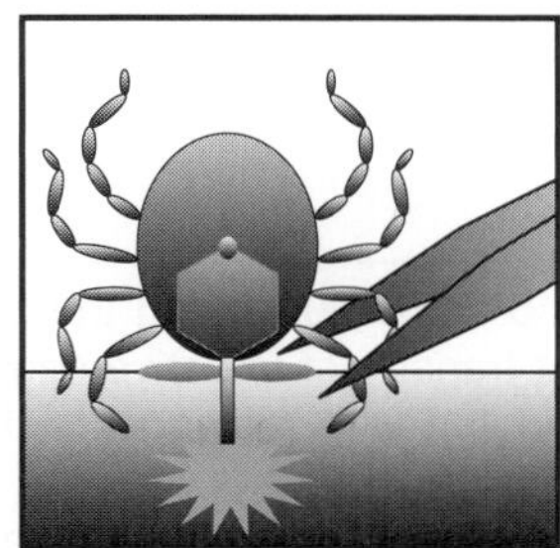

Grasp the tick's body as close to the skin as possible using a fine-tip tweezer. Avoid squeezing the tick's body.

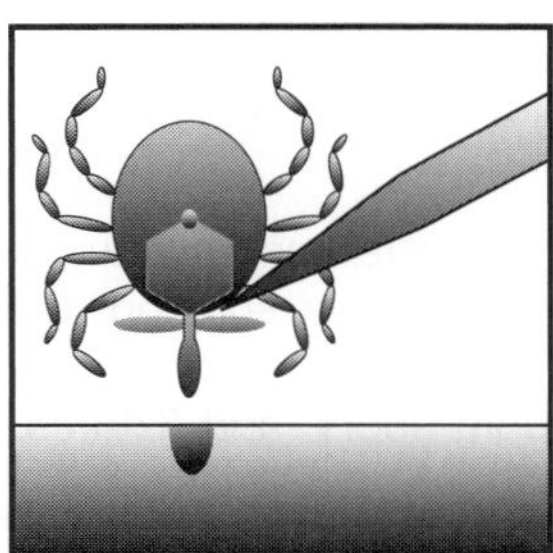

Remove by pulling the tick straight upward without using twisting motions.

You Have Been Prescribed: ______________________________

You Need to Take: ______________________________

Take all of your antibiotics even if you feel better.

You Need to Notify the Office If You Have:

A. No improvement while on antibiotic therapy

B. Decreased urinary output, or dryness of your skin or mouth

C. Other:______________________________

Phone: ______________________________

ROUNDWORMS AND PINWORMS

PROBLEM

Roundworms and pinworms are intestinal parasites. Roundworms look like earthworms; pinworms are small, white, and threadlike. Both types of worms thrive in the intestinal tract and are very common in children. They can spread to other family members, so the entire family needs to be treated.

CAUSE

Pinworms live in the human rectum or colon and come out during the night onto the skin around the anus. Pinworms are transmitted from person to person by direct transfer of infective eggs to the mouth, or by indirect transfer through clothing, bedding, food, or other items contaminated with the eggs. Nighttime itching is one of the main symptoms of pinworms.

Roundworm eggs enter the human body by drinking contaminated water or eating contaminated food or by transfer from contaminated unwashed hands.

PREVENTION/CARE

The following measures help prevent the spread of worms:

A. Remove sources of infection by treating the infected person and family members.

B. Household measures:
   1. Wash (132°F) or boil soiled bed sheets, nightclothes, underwear, towels, and washcloths used by infected persons.
   2. Soak fabrics that cannot be boiled in an ammonia solution: One cup of household ammonia to 5 gallons of cold water.
   3. After treatment, scrub toilet seats, bathroom floors, and fixtures. Vacuum rugs, and clean table tops, curtains, sofas, and chairs carefully.

C. Practice good personal hygiene. Wash hands before handling foods and eating, and after using the toilet. Wash the anus and genitals with warm water and soap at least twice a day. Rinse well and then wash your hands.

D. Take a morning bath to remove most eggs. Other people should not take a bath in the same water.

E. Keep fingers away from the mouth. Cut nails and discourage nail biting and scratching the bare anal area.

F. Clean fingernails before meals and after bowel movements.

G. Reduce overcrowding when possible.

H. For roundworms: Have pets treated, and avoid stray animals.

TREATMENT PLAN

Parasitic infection is easily treated with medication. All family members need to be treated.

Activity: Resume normal activities after treatment is complete and symptoms improve.

Diet: No special foods are needed.

Medication:

You Have Been Prescribed: ____________________

You Need to Take: ____________________

You Need to Notify the Office If You Have:

A. Reappearance of worms after treatment

B. New or unexplained symptoms. Drugs used in treatment may produce side effects.

C. Other: ____________________

Phone: ____________________

SCABIES

PROBLEM

Scabies is a common condition characterized by severe itching. You may have noticed small burrows between your fingers and in other locations, or you may have some redness and skin irritation that is aggravated by scratching.

CAUSE

Scabies is caused by an infestation of the skin by a mite. You contract scabies by coming in close contact with an individual who has the condition.

PREVENTION/CARE

You can prevent reinfection of scabies by following these measures:

A. Make sure all close contacts, sexual partners, family, and household contacts are treated.

B. All bedding and clothing that has touched infected skin should be machine washed and machine dried on the highest heat cycle.

C. Any clothing or bedding that cannot be laundered in the way previously mentioned should be placed in a plastic bag that is securely tied for at least a week. The mites cannot live this long away from human skin.

D. Coats, furniture, rugs, floors, and walls do not require any special cleaning or treatment.

TREATMENT PLAN

A. Most patients with scabies are successfully treated with only one overnight application of a cream known as a scabicide.

B. You should let your practitioner know if you are pregnant or breastfeeding.

C. You may itch for up to a week even with successful treatment.

D. If you still have symptoms after 2 weeks, you should see your practitioner, who will determine if you need a second treatment.

Activity: Affected children in day care or school can return the day after treatment is completed.

Diet: There is no special diet.

Medications: The most common medications used to treat scabies include:

A. Permethrin (Elimite cream), which is applied to all body areas from the neck down and washed off in 8 to 14 hours.

B. Lindane (Kwell cream), which is applied to all skin surfaces from the neck down and washed off in 8 to 12 hours.

C. You may be told to use Benadryl 25 to 50 mg if needed for itching.

D. Do not use near your eyes.

You Have Been Prescribed: ______________________________

You Need to Take: ______________________________

You Need to Notify the Office If:

A. You have new symptoms.

B. You have a reaction to the medication.

C. Other: ______________________________

Phone: ______________________________

SEBORRHEIC DERMATITIS

PROBLEM

Seborrheic dermatitis is a skin condition characterized by greasy or dry, white, flaking scales over reddish patches on the skin. The scales anchor to the hair shafts and may itch, but they are usually painless unless complicated by infection.

CAUSE

The cause is unknown. The risk of seborrheic dermatitis increases with stress; hot and humid or cold and dry weather; infrequent shampoos; oily skin; and other skin disorders such as rosacea, acne, or psoriasis; obesity; Parkinson's disease; use of lotions that contain alcohol; and HIV/AIDS.

PREVENTION/CARE

A. There are no specific preventive measures.

B. The goal of care is to minimize the severity or frequency of symptoms.
   1. Shampoo vigorously and as often as once a day. The type of shampoo is not as important as the way you scrub your scalp. To loosen scales, scrub with your fingernails while shampooing, and scrub at least 5 minutes.
   2. If you suffer from minor dandruff, you may use nonprescription dandruff shampoos with selenium sulfide (Selsun Blue, Exsel) or zinc pyrithione (Zincon) and lubricating skin lotion.
   3. For severe problems, shampoos that contain coal tar or scalp creams that contain cortisone may be prescribed. **Do not use coal tar products on infants or children without specific physician prescription.**
   4. To apply medication to the scalp, part the hair a few strands at a time, and rub the ointment or lotion vigorously into the scalp.
   5. Topical steroids may be prescribed for other affected parts of the skin.
   6. Be sure to dry skin folds thoroughly after bathing.
   7. Wear loose, ventilating clothing. Avoid constant cap wearing.

TREATMENT PLAN

Activity: No restrictions. Outdoor activities in the summer may help alleviate symptoms.

Diet: Eat a well-balanced diet. Drink eight to 10 glasses of water per day. Avoid foods that seem to worsen your condition.

Medications:

You Have Been Prescribed: ______________________________

You Need to Take: ______________________________

You Need to Notify the Office If:

A. You have an adverse reaction to any of the prescribed medications.

B. You are unable to tolerate any of the medications.

C. You have any secondary infection in affected area.

D. Other: ______________________________

Phone: ______________________________

SHORTNESS OF BREATH

PROBLEM

You have been diagnosed with shortness of breath. Shortness of breath may be due to different reasons, or a combination of reasons. The symptom can come on suddenly or develop slowly, over several months. Some common reasons for shortness of breath are listed subsequently.

CAUSES

A. Being overweight or out of shape

B. Heart or lung disorders

C. Asthma

D. Infections of the upper or lower respiratory systems

E. Pregnancy

F. Nervousness/excessive stress

G. Allergies

PREVENTION/CARE

A. There is no way to prevent shortness of breath that is due to an underlying cause. It can be treated, however, by treating the underlying disorder.

B. One way to help discover the cause of your shortness of breath is to keep a "diary" of what makes the symptoms worse, and how often it happens.

TREATMENT PLAN

A. You should see your health care provider to have your shortness of breath evaluated.

B. Based on the reason for your shortness of breath, a more active lifestyle may be recommended.

C. Everyone's shortness of breath is different, and discovering the cause of your symptoms is important to determine your treatment.

Activity:
A. Your recommended activity level is based on the cause of your shortness of breath.

Diet: There is no special diet for shortness of breath, unless certain foods make the symptoms worse.

Medications:
The medicines used to treat shortness of breath are chosen based on the underlying reason for the symptom.

You Need to Call the Office Immediately If:

A. Your shortness of breath comes on suddenly or has worsened.

B. Other: ______________________________

Phone: ______________________________

RESOURCES

Chronic Obstructive Pulmonary Disease, Including Emphysema: www.uptodate.com

SINUSITIS

PROBLEM

Sinusitis (sinus infection) is classified as an acute, subacute, or chronic condition. In acute sinusitis, the infection is resolved after treatment. In subacute sinusitis, there is a persistent, yellow to green nasal discharge despite treatment. In chronic sinusitis, episodes of prolonged inflammation continue longer than 3 months despite treatment.

CAUSE

Sinusitis occurs when the mucous lining in your sinus cavities becomes inflamed and infected with bacteria or an allergen. This can occur after a cold or tooth abscess.

PREVENTION/CARE

A. If you have a tooth abscess, see your dentist and finish all your antibiotics.

B. Do not blow your nose too frequently or too hard. It may cause your eardrum to perforate (tear). Blow through both nostrils at the same time to equalize pressure.

C. To prevent spreading germs to others, cover your mouth when you cough.
   1. Use tissues when you blow your nose. Dispose of them and then wash your hands.
   2. If no tissue is available, do the "elbow sneeze" into the bend of your arm (away from your open hands).

D. Always wash your hands after coughing or using tissues.

TREATMENT PLAN

A. Avoid smoking and secondhand smoke.

B. Use steam inhalation to liquefy secretions.

C. Use a room humidifier. Keep your humidifier clean—it can grow bacteria.

Activity: There are no activity restrictions; however, diving, swimming, and flying may increase the occurrence of symptoms or make them worse. Make sure to get plenty of rest each day.

Diet: Eat a healthy diet. Drink at least 8 to 10 glasses of liquid every day.

Medications: Take all of your prescribed antibiotics, even if you feel better.

Over-the-Counter Medications:

A. **Pain relievers:** Ibuprofen (Advil) or acetaminophen (Tylenol) as needed for facial pain.

B. **Antihistamines:** Some antihistamines may cause drowsiness. Use with caution. You may consider using a different antihistamine during the day that does not cause drowsiness.

C. **Decongestants:** Decongestants may increase blood pressure and may also interact with other medications. Please consult with your provider before using these medications.

D. **Nasal sprays:** Nasal saline spray is safe to use in the nose several times a day. Nasal decongestant sprays may be used for a short period of time. Do not use longer than 3 days to prevent causing rebound side effects from this medication. Consult with your provider if you are using a nasal decongestant spray.

You Have Been Prescribed: ____________________

You Need to Take: ____________________

You Need to Call the Office If:

A. Your eyelids begin to swell or droop, or you experience decreased vision.

B. You have stiffness in your neck or increased fever.

C. You have asthma, and you are getting worse.

D. You begin vomiting and are unable to keep down your antibiotic.

E. You are a diabetic and your blood sugars are elevated, or you notice ketones in your urine.

F. Other: ____________________

Phone: ____________________

SKIN CARE ASSESSMENT

PROBLEM

Skin cancer is the most common type of cancer. In 2006, the Centers for Disease Control and Prevention (CDC) noted that the rate of skin cancer varies by the state where you live. A state map is located on the Internet at www.cdc.gov/cancer/skin/statistics/state.htm.

CAUSE

Skin cancer is frequently caused by damage from the ultraviolet rays of the sun. Some people are at a higher risk of developing skin cancer. These risk factors include:

A. Fair complexion

B. Advanced age with sun-damaged skin

C. A history of severe sunburn

D. A history of spending long hours outdoors

E. Having a history of x-ray procedures for skin conditions

F. Genetic susceptibility

PREVENTION/CARE

A. Protect yourself and prevent sun exposure to your skin by staying out of the harmful rays as much as possible, especially between the hours of 11:00 a.m. and 2:30 p.m. This time frame accounts for approximately 70% of the harmful ultraviolet radiation.

B. If you are exposed to the sun, wear a sunscreen product with an SPF of 15 or greater at all times.

C. Wear hats that screen your face and neck, as well as your ears.

D. Clothing is available with sun-protective materials. Regular long shirts and long pants also help to protect your skin.

E. Sit in the shade to rest.

F. Do not use a tanning booth.

Steps to Take to Prevent Yourself From Being a Victim of Skin Cancer

A. Examine your skin monthly.
   1. Use a good light source and a mirror to see areas of your skin not clearly visible.
   2. Examine your entire body closely.
   3. Pay particular attention to areas that are frequently exposed to the sun, especially your face, lips, eyes, neck, scalp, and ears.
   4. Monthly screening allows you to familiarize yourself with birthmarks and moles. Note the size, shape, and color of these marks. Note any changes in these marks, using the "ABCDE" method:
      a. *Asymmetry:* The shape of the mark should be noted. Any change in shape or irregularity of the mark needs to be evaluated by your health care provider.
      b. *Border:* Look carefully at the border of the mark. If the border edge is ragged, notched, and not smooth, your health care provider needs to evaluate it.
      c. *Color:* Note the color of moles. If you notice any change in color, or if you notice the mole to have several colors (brown, black, tan, red, etc.), you need to alert your health care provider.
      d. *Diameter:* Measure the size of the mark and document it. Any change in size, especially if it is greater than 6 mm, should be brought to the attention of your health care provider.
      e. *Elevation:* Note elevation of the lesion, change in size, and any evolving changes of the lesion. You need to alert your health care provider if changes occur.
   5. You should also evaluate lesions on your skin for any type of change. If the lesions begin bleeding or hurting, or change in texture or in any other way, your health care provider needs to evaluate the change.
   6. Be alerted to any skin ulcers that do not heal within 1 month. Also, any new moles or lesions need to be evaluated by your health care provider for proper diagnosis of the type of lesion.

(*continued*)

SKIN CARE ASSESSMENT *(continued)*

TREATMENT PLAN

Activity: As tolerated, but protect yourself from sun exposure.

Diet: There is no special diet that will stop skin cancer.

Medications: There are no medications that prevent skin cancer.

You Need to Notify the Office If You Have:

A. Any of the skin changes mentioned previously need to be evaluated by your health care provider

Phone: ____

SLEEP APNEA

PROBLEM

You have been diagnosed with sleep apnea. During your sleep your tongue and throat relax, causing less air to go down into your lungs. When you sleep and snore you have short periods when you stop breathing and may wake up gasping for breath. Your bed partner may shake you awake because of your loud snoring or may notice that you have stopped breathing. The sleep apnea makes you very tired, leading you to take daytime naps.

CAUSES

A. Being overweight and having a "thick neck" can cause sleep apnea.

B. As you get older you are more likely to have sleep apnea.

C. After menopause, women may start having sleep apnea.

D. If you have not had your tonsils removed, they may be part of the problem as your tongue and throat relax.

E. Alcohol and some medicines cause sleep apnea.

F. Allergies may also cause some sleep apnea.

PREVENTION/CARE

A. There is no way to prevent sleep apnea once you have it.

B. One way to help your sleep apnea is to lose weight.

TREATMENT PLAN

A. Review all of your medicines and any herbal products with your health care provider.

B. You may be told to sleep with your head up on two pillows, use a tennis ball under your pillow, or even sleep with a backpack under your pillow. This raises your head up higher and prevents your tongue from making your wind pipe smaller.

C. You may also need a mouthpiece to help your tongue from relaxing when you sleep. Your dentist will need to help you find the best one.

D. You may be sent to a lung specialist to help with your treatment.

E. You may be told you need to have a sleep study to check out and measure how often you stop breathing at night.

F. After your sleep study, your lung specialist may order you to have a sleep machine called continuous positive airway pressure (CPAP) or biphasic positive airway pressure (BiPAP).
   1. The sleep machine uses nose tubing, a nasal mask, or a full face mask.
   2. The machine is small and portable.
   3. Your CPAP machine can be taken through the airport.
   4. You will have a supplier send you more tubing and breathing tubes/masks on a regular schedule.

Activity:

A. You will continue to need to sleep with your head higher, use the mouth piece, or use the sleep machine to keep from having sleep apnea.

B. Exercise; losing even a small amount of weight will help with sleep apnea.

C. Stop smoking.

D. Avoid alcohol, especially near your bedtime.

Diet: There is no special diet for sleep apnea, but losing weight helps.

Medications:

There are no medicines for sleep apnea.

(*continued*)

SLEEP APNEA (*continued*)

You Need to Notify the Office If:

A. Your bed partner complains that your snoring or sleep apnea has worsened.

B. You want to make an appointment to discuss having a sleep study.

C. Other: ____

Phone: ________________________________

RESOURCE

The National Sleep Foundation: www.sleepfoundation.org

SLEEP DISORDERS/INSOMNIA

PROBLEM

Continued loss of sleep over a long period (several days to weeks) can produce a decrease in daytime awareness and functioning, as well as work and driving impairment.

CAUSE

Most sleep difficulties are related to situational problems and are best treated without medications. Medical illness may also predispose you to a sleeping disorder.

PREVENTION/CARE

A. Practice good "sleep hygiene." Here are a few tips:
  1. Try to get to bed at the same time every night (even on weekends).
  2. Plan for 8 hours of sleep.
  3. Maintain the same waking time every morning (even on weekends).
  4. Reserve the bedroom for sleeping. Do not do your work/homework in the bed. Do not watch TV in the bedroom, unless you sit in a chair. Do not read in bed.
  5. Put your children in their own beds/bedrooms.
  6. Try a small bedtime snack.
  7. Do not drink any liquids for at least 1 hour before going to bed. This helps prevent getting up to go to the bathroom during the night.
  8. Review all of your prescription medications, over-the-counter (OTC) drugs, and herbal products with your health care provider to evaluate if the drugs are making you stay awake.
  9. Avoid alcohol and tobacco.

B. If you do not get a restful night of sleep, awaken yourself snoring, or your partner complains of your snoring, gasping, or stopping breathing, you may need to have a sleep study.

TREATMENT PLAN

A. Develop a "sleeping ritual": Wear your favorite pajamas and use your favorite pillows.

B. Keep the room dark and quiet. Try not to use a nightlight.

C. Run a small fan for background noise.

D. Arise promptly in the morning.

E. Avoid sleeping medication if possible.

F. Try some relaxation exercises, like yoga, self-hypnosis, or meditation. There are many books on these subjects that will assist you in developing good sleep hygiene. (Try your local library or bookstore.)

G. Keep a sleep diary to help identify the causes of your inability to sleep.

H. Discuss snoring and your partner's concerns about your breathing and the need for a sleep study.

Activity: Regular exercise during the day helps. (Do not exercise vigorously 1 hour before your bedtime—this could keep you awake.)

Relaxation techniques, such as progressive relaxation, biofeedback, self-hypnosis, and meditation, are helpful when done before bedtime. Avoid vigorous mental activities late in the evening.

Diet:

A. Avoid caffeinated drinks, including coffee, tea, and soda.

B. Avoid large meals in the evening.

C. Eat a nutritious balanced diet.

D. Limit your liquids to early evening. Do not drink water after 8 p.m.

Medications: Discuss the need for *short-term* medications to help you sleep.

(*continued*)

SLEEP DISORDERS/INSOMNIA *(continued)*

You Have Been Prescribed: ______________________________

You Need to Take: ______________________________

You Need to Notify the Office If You Have:

A. No relief of your symptoms and you are following the previous recommendations

B. No relief of your symptoms and you are taking your medications as directed

C. Feelings of depression or thoughts of hurting yourself or others

D. Noticeable physical symptoms that were not mentioned in your office visit or any new symptoms that you are concerned about

E. Other ______________________

Phone: ______________________________

RESOURCES

National Institutes of Health: www.health.nih.gov/topic/SleepDisorders
The National Sleep Foundation: www.sleepfoundation.org

SUPERFICIAL THROMBOPHLEBITIS

PROBLEM

Superficial thrombophlebitis occurs when a vein is irritated or injured. The portion of the vein that is affected can develop a blood clot or become infected, causing redness, swelling, and pain. If untreated, the infection and/or blood clot can progress into a life-threatening condition like sepsis, deep vein thrombosis, or pulmonary embolism.

CAUSE

Many things can cause irritation and injury to veins. These include a recent intravenous (IV) line placed during a hospital stay, infection, some medications, and pregnancy. Some risk factors cannot be changed, like genetics, while others can be changed, including inactivity and excessive weight.

PREVENTION/CARE

A. Avoid standing or sitting for long periods of time.

B. If you smoke, stop or reduce the amount you smoke.

C. If overweight or obese, lose weight. Discuss what you can do to lose weight with your health care provider.

TREATMENT PLAN

A. Take your medications as ordered by your health care provider.

B. Raise the affected arm or leg whenever lying down to improve pain and swelling.

C. Warm compresses to the affected area may improve pain.

D. Wear compression stockings. Put them on before getting out of bed in the morning. Take them off just before going to bed at night.

E. Avoid standing or sitting for long periods of time.

F. Follow up with your primary health care provider on a regularly scheduled basis.

Activity:

A. Get regular exercise. Discuss with your health care provider what type and frequency of exercise is safe for you.

B. Exercise leg muscles by pumping ankles when sitting. Rocking in a rocking chair is another option.

Diet:

A. Discuss with your health care provider the type of diet that best suits your needs: Diabetic diet, low-fat diet, low-cholesterol diet, and/or low-sodium diet.

Medications:

You Have Been Prescribed: ______________________________

You Need to Take: ______________________________

You Need to Notify the Office If You Have:

A. Fever greater than 101°F

B. Sudden shortness of breath

C. Chest pain

D. New pain, swelling, or warmth in an arm or leg

E. If you are taking a blood-thinning medication and have any of these symptoms:
   1. Vomit that is bright red or dark and looks like coffee grounds
   2. Bright red blood in your stools or black, tarry stools
   3. Severe headache
   4. Sudden weakness in an arm or leg
   5. Memory loss or confusion

(*continued*)

SUPERFICIAL THROMBOPHLEBITIS *(continued)*

6. Sudden change in vision
7. Trouble speaking or understanding others

F. Other: ______________________________

Phone: ______________________________

RESOURCES

Mayo Clinic—Thrombophlebitis: mayoclinic.com/health/thrombophlebitis/DS00223
Patient Education Center—Superficial Thrombophlebitis: patienteducationcenter.org/articles/superficial-thrombophlebitis

SYPHILIS

PROBLEM

You may have round or oval painless lesions, most commonly in the genital region, but they may occur anywhere on the body where transmission occurred.

A. You may experience a rash covering your body, including palms of hands and soles of feet.

B. **Flu-like symptoms** include fever; headache; sore throat; swollen, tender lymph nodes; and decreased appetite.

CAUSE

Syphilis is contracted by genital or oral contact with someone who has the infection. The infection is spread when lesions are present.

PREVENTION/CARE

A. Use condoms.

B. Limit sexual partners.

C. Screen new sexual partners by asking about any known infections.

TREATMENT PLAN

Do not engage in sexual activity while lesions are present. Notify all partners of the need for treatment. Keep follow-up appointments to determine if treatment has been effective.

Diet: There is no special diet.

Medications: Penicillin is the drug of choice for treating syphilis. Other antibiotics can be used if you are allergic to penicillin. Within 24 hours of receiving antibiotic treatment, you may experience a fever or headache. Aspirin, acetaminophen (Tylenol), or ibuprofen may be taken if these symptoms occur.

You Have Been Prescribed: ______________________________

You Need to Take: ______________________________

You need to finish all of your antibiotics.

You Need to Notify the Office If You Have:

A. Any new symptoms

B. Any reaction to your antibiotics

C. Any other concerns about syphilis

Phone: ______________________________

SYSTEMIC LUPUS ERYTHEMATOSUS

PROBLEM

You have been diagnosed with a condition called systemic lupus erythematosus (SLE) or lupus. Lupus is a chronic, inflammatory, autoimmune disorder. There is currently no cure for lupus; however, it can be managed and can go into remission or a dormant state. Rashes, hair loss, arthritis-like joint pain, and fatigue are very common problems with lupus.

CAUSE

Lupus causes your body to attack its own cells. The exact cause is unknown. Lupus tends to run in families, but it is not contagious.

PREVENTION/CARE

There is no known prevention, only long-term management.

TREATMENT PLAN

A. Avoid sun exposure:
   1. Many lupus patients' eyes are sensitive to light; wear sunglasses, and avoid direct exposure.
   2. Light exposure can make your rash worse.
   3. Apply a protective lotion or sunscreen to your skin while outside.
   4. Wear long sleeves and use hats.

B. You may be given steroids for your skin rashes or lesions.

C. Avoid exposure to drugs and chemicals.

D. Review all of your medications and over-the-counter (OTC) drugs with your health care provider.

E. Avoid hair sprays and hair-coloring agents.

F. Mouth ulcers may occur with lupus:
   1. Avoid hot or spicy foods that might cause irritation to ulcers.
   2. Use good oral hygiene:
      a. Get regular dental examinations.
      b. Floss your teeth daily.
      c. Brush your teeth at least twice a day.

G. Rest and drugs called nonsteroidal anti-inflammatory drugs (NSAIDs) are used for minor joint pain.

H. It is very important for you to have your eyes examined **twice** a year to monitor eye changes.

I. Talk to your health care provider if you are planning a pregnancy.

Activity: You may get tired more easily; plan rest periods. However, you should still get some exercise as tolerated. Many people gain some weight from steroids.

Diet: Eat a regular diet as tolerated; you do not need any special foods.

Medications:

You Have Been Prescribed the Following Steroid: ______________________________

You Need to Take: ______________________________

A. Do not stop taking your steroid abruptly.

B. **Steroid medication should be tapered off (decreased until you are off of it).**

You Need to Notify the Office If:

A. You are unable to tolerate your medication.

B. You have any sign of infections, sinusitis, bronchitis, flu, or urinary tract infections (UTIs).

(*continued*)

SYSTEMIC LUPUS ERYTHEMATOSUS *(continued)*

C. You are getting worse or do not feel better.

D. You are planning a pregnancy or think you are pregnant.

E. Other: ______________________________

Phone: ______________________________

RESOURCES

Lupus Foundation of America: 800-558-0121 or www.lupus.org
Lupus Research Institute: www.lupusresearchinstitute.org; 212-812-9881 e-mail: lupus@lupusny.org

TESTICULAR SELF-EXAMINATION

The testicular self-examination is easy to do and does not take very much time to perform. Checking every month is a good way to become familiar with this area of your body and will help detect testicular cancer.

Set a date for the same day every month. An easy way to remember is choosing the first day of the month, or the last day of the month, or your birth date. The best time to check your testicles is during or after a hot bath or shower. (Heat makes the testicles relax.)

Tumors can be felt. Boys and men from 15 to 35 years are at the highest risk because of hormonal activity.

PROCEDURE

A. If possible, do the self-examination in front of a mirror after a hot bath or shower.

B. Check for any swelling of the skin.

C. Support each testicle with one hand and examine it with the other hand.

D. Use both hands to feel all of the scrotal bag.
   1. With one hand, lift your penis, and check your sac with the other hand. Feel any change in shape or size.
   2. Look for red veins or veins that are bigger than they used to be.
   3. The left side may hang slightly lower than the right (this is normal).

E. Check each testicle.
   1. Place your left thumb on the front of your left testicle and your index and middle fingers behind it.
   2. Gently but firmly roll the testicle between your thumb and fingers.
   3. Then use your right hand to examine the right testicle the same way.
   4. The testicles should feel smooth, rubbery, oval shaped, and slightly tender. They should move freely.
   5. Locate the epididymis and spermatic cord. The epididymis is the irregular, cord-like structure on the top and the back of the testicle.
      a. Gently squeeze the spermatic cord above your left testicle between your thumb and the first two fingers of your left hand.
      b. Check for lumps and masses along the entire length of the cords.
      c. Repeat on the right side, using your right hand.

F. Call your health care provider if you notice:
   1. Any lumps, even small pea-sized ones
   2. Any masses, like a bag of worms
   3. A dull ache in the lower abdomen or in the groin
   4. A feeling of heaviness in the scrotum
   5. A significant loss of size in one of the testicles
   6. Pain or discomfort in a testicle or in the scrotum
   7. Any other changes since the last time you felt yourself for your examination

G. Your health care provider may refer you to a urologist for further evaluation.

TINEA VERSICOLOR

PROBLEM

A yeast infection of the skin, tinea versicolor may cause color changes of the skin, commonly on the chest, back, shoulders, arms, and trunk. During the summer, these spots usually appear pale and do not tan. During the winter, the spots may appear pinker or darker than the normal skin color.

CAUSE

Tinea versicolor is caused by an increased production of yeast on the skin, which is influenced by warm, moist conditions. It is common to have recurring episodes.

PREVENTION/TREATMENT PLAN

A. Air dry skin as much as possible.

B. Apply medication as directed.

C. Patches on skin (color changes) may take several weeks to resolve.

D. Monthly treatments may help prevent recurrences.

Activity: There are no activity restrictions with tinea versicolor.

Diet: There is no special diet.

Medications:

A. Apply Selsun Blue shampoo or other medication as directed.

B. Most medications may be washed off of skin 30 minutes after application.

C. Selsun Blue shampoo may be used daily on affected skin for 2 weeks.

D. Keep shampoo out of the eyes and genital area.

E. Leave it on skin for about 20 minutes and then rinse it off.

You Have Been Prescribed: ______________________________

You Need to Take: ______________________________

You Need to Notify the Office If You:

A. Do not see improvement, despite proper treatment

B. Develop new symptoms

C. Other: ______________________________

Phone: ______________________________

TINNITUS

PROBLEM

Tinnitus is an irritating noise or sound that is heard in one or both ears, commonly referred to as a buzzing, humming, or ringing noise.

CAUSE

Tinnitus is caused by a change in the normal hearing pathway of the ears. This can be caused from damage or irritation of the hearing pathway, which may be temporary or permanent. Damage to the nerves in the ear, fluid, wax buildup and/or a mass in the middle ear are a few causes for tinnitus.

TREATMENT PLAN

A. A hearing evaluation will be performed to determine if there is hearing loss.

B. A CT or MRI may be performed to evaluate for the cause of the tinnitus.

C. Once the cause of the tinnitus is noted, treating the cause will begin.

D. There are some medications that are used to help decrease the "ringing, buzzing" noise that you are hearing. Ask your health care provider about these medications.

E. Surgery may be considered if a mass is noted on the CT or MRI scan.

F. Rest and exercise are encouraged to reduce the amount of stress that can worsen symptoms of tinnitus.

Activity: There is no activity restriction.

Diet: Some foods may make the tinnitus worsen. Therefore, reducing the amount of caffeine (tea, coffee, soft drinks) is encouraged.

Medications: Avoid aspirin. Aspirin has been known to aggravate the symptoms of tinnitus.

You Have Been Prescribed: ______________________________

You Need to Take: ______________________________

You Need to Notify the Office If You Have:

A. Fever

B. Ear pain

C. Noticed a change in hearing loss or speech development

D. Any other new symptoms that occur

E. Other: ______________________________

Phone: ______________________________

TOXOPLASMOSIS

PROBLEM

Toxoplasmosis is an infection acquired through contact with infected cat feces or from eating raw or undercooked meat.

CAUSE

Toxoplasmosis is caused by a parasite. Cats are the primary host, and humans are the intermediate host. **You do not need to destroy your cat.**

PREVENTION/CARE

A. Avoid uncooked eggs and unpasteurized milk.

B. Wash hands after handling raw meat.

C. Meat should be thoroughly cooked at 152°F or higher, or frozen for 24 hours in a household freezer before eating (smoked meats and meats cured in brine are considered safe). Avoid tasting meat while cooking.

D. Wash fruits and vegetables before eating.

E. Wash all kitchen surfaces that come into contact with uncooked meats.

F. Avoid drinking unfiltered water in any setting.

G. Use care in gardening where cats have access.

H. Wear gloves for gardening and landscaping.

I. Wear gloves for handling kitty litter, and wash hands after contact with cats. **Change kitty litter daily.**

J. Keep outdoor sandboxes covered.

K. Domestic cats can be protected from infection by feeding them commercially prepared cat food and preventing them from eating undercooked kitchen scraps and hunting wild rodents.

L. If you are not pregnant and have toxoplasmosis, you should not get pregnant for at least 6 months.

TREATMENT PLAN

A. If you are pregnant, you may be referred to a specialist.

B. If you have AIDS, you will be referred to a specialist.

Activity: There is no activity restriction for toxoplasmosis.

Diet: There is no special diet for toxoplasmosis. Avoid uncooked eggs and unpasteurized milk. Meat should be thoroughly cooked.

Medications: Depending on your risk, you may be prescribed one or two medications. You may be required to take the medication for several weeks.

You Have Been Prescribed: ________________

You Need to Take: ________________

You Need to Notify the Office If You Have:

A. Headache, dull and constant, with no relief from acetaminophen (Tylenol)

B. Abnormal speech

C. Seizures

D. Loss of visual acuity

E. Poor concentration, forgetfulness

F. Personality changes

G. Other: ________________

Phone: ________________

TRANSIENT ISCHEMIC ATTACK

PROBLEM/CAUSE

A transient ischemic attack (TIA) is a temporary loss of brain function due to a decrease of blood flow to the brain. It is considered a mini stroke. The symptoms may last only a few minutes, but the risk for a stroke is increased over the next week.

RISK FACTORS FOR TIAs

A. High blood pressure

B. Irregular heartbeat (atrial fibrillation)

C. Smoking

D. High cholesterol

E. Being overweight

F. Diabetes

G. Obstructive sleep apnea

WARNING SIGNS OF A TIA

A. Weakness or numbness of face, arm, or leg on one side of the body

B. Trouble talking or understanding others when they talk

C. Changes in eyesight such as dimness, double vision, or loss of vision

D. Dizziness, unsteadiness, or sudden falls

E. Sudden severe headaches

If you experience any of these signs, seek medical attention (call 911) immediately.

PREVENTION/CARE

A. A full workup is necessary to decide why you are having TIAs.

B. You may be referred to a neurologist—a doctor who specializes in medical problems involving the brain.

C. Special tests or surgery may be done to evaluate your heart and blood vessels. A carotid angioplasty and carotid endarterectomy are two procedures that may be performed to insert a stent into the artery or remove a blockage from the artery. Other treatment depends on your test results.

D. Treatment starts with modifying your risk factors. Weight loss, eating a healthy diet, lowering your cholesterol, and eliminating alcohol in your diet are encouraged. If you are a diabetic, you must keep your diabetes under control to lower your risk.

E. Do not smoke or use any tobacco products.

F. Aspirin is commonly prescribed after a TIA. You may be prescribed a blood thinner. Some blood thinners require regular laboratory testing. Discuss treatment with your health care provider.

G. If you are taking a blood thinner, get a Medic Alert bracelet/necklace, or carry a card in your wallet and car in case you are in an accident. Medic Alert jewelry can be purchased at local drug stores, and there are multiple websites for ordering a Medic Alert identification. You can build your own identification bracelets or neck chains from American Medical ID: www.americanmedical-id.com

Activity: You need to exercise at least 30 minutes daily three to four times a week. Please make sure you have been released by your health care provider to begin exercising.

Diet: Eat a low-fat, low-cholesterol, and low-sodium diet.

Medications:

(*continued*)

TRANSIENT ISCHEMIC ATTACK *(continued)*

You Have Been Prescribed: ____________________

You Need to Take: ____________________

Phone: ____________________

RESOURCES

American Heart Association
7272 Greenville Avenue
Dallas, TX 75231-4596
www.heart.org

National Stroke Association
9707 East Easter Lane, Suite B
Centennial, CO 80112-3747
www.stroke.org

TRICHOMONIASIS

PROBLEM

You may experience increased vaginal discharge that is yellow-green or watery gray in color. It may have a foul odor. You may also have vaginal itching or irritation, burning during urination, discomfort during sexual intercourse, spotting or bleeding during or after sexual intercourse, or abdominal discomfort.

CAUSE

Trichomonas vaginalis is acquired by having sex with someone who has the infection.

PREVENTION/CARE

A. Use condom with each act of intercourse.

B. Limit the number of sexual partners.

C. Screen new sexual partners.

TREATMENT PLAN

Do not have sexual activity until you and your partner have both completed your medications. There are no limitations in other physical activity.

Diet: Do not drink alcohol during the use of medication and for 3 days after taking the last dose of your medicine. Alcohol use while taking this medication may result in nausea, vomiting, and severe upset stomach. You may have a metallic taste from the medicine that may slightly alter the taste of food. No other limitations in diet are required.

Medications: Metronidazole (Flagyl) is used to treat the infection.

You Have Been Prescribed: ______________________________

You Need to Take: ______________________________

Finish all of the medication.

You Need to Notify the Office If:

A. You are unable to tolerate the medicine.

B. Any new symptoms develop

C. Other: ______________________________

Phone: ______________________________

TRIGEMINAL NEURALGIA

PROBLEM

Trigeminal neuralgia is a nerve disorder of the face, causing extreme, sporadic, sudden burning or shock-like pain of the cheek area. It is most commonly caused from an irritation of the trigeminal nerve, such as a blood vessel pressing on the nerve, which carries sensation from your face to your brain. It occurs most often in people older than age 50 years, but can occur at any age. With treatment, approximately 80% of patients will become pain free. Other treatment options are available if medications do not improve symptoms.

PREVENTION/CARE

A. Irritating factors can make symptoms worse. Avoid triggers such as:
   1. Shaving
   2. Stroking face
   3. Too much pressure putting on makeup
   4. Wind exposure
   5. Vigorous washing of face
   6. Drinking too hot or cold beverages
   7. Eating tough meat or hard candies

B. If prescribed medication, take your medication as ordered and report any side effects to your primary care provider or neurologist. Avoid taking medications without provider input.

C. Pain varies and may be sudden and sporadic, affecting a small area of the face, or more widespread. Trigeminal neuralgia is unpredictable. You may have periods of being pain free for days, weeks, or months. Then it may return unexpectedly. If pain worsens, notify your health care provider immediately.

Activity: Engage in activities as tolerated, avoiding triggers as much as possible. Use caution in activities if experiencing side effects of balance impairment, drowsiness, or dizziness.

Medications: You may be treated with an anticonvulsant medication, such as carbamazepine (Tegretol), phenytoin (Dilantin), gabapentin (Neurontin), lamotrigine (Lamictal), topiramate (Topamax), valproic acid (Depakote), or others. Muscle relaxants, such as baclofen, may also be prescribed with the anticonvulsant medication for symptoms.

You Have Been Prescribed: ______________________________

You Need to Notify the Office If You Have:

A. Worsening pain

B. Side effects of medications

C. Any new symptoms

D. Other: ______________________________

Phone: ______________________________

ULCER MANAGEMENT

PROBLEM

An ulcer is a sore in the lining of the stomach or intestine that occurs in areas exposed to acid and pepsin. Complications include bleeding ulcer and perforation, and obstruction can be life threatening.

CAUSE

Although the exact cause of ulcer formation is not completely understood, the process appears to involve excess acid. A type of bacteria called *Helicobacter pylori* and certain medications have been suggested as causing ulcers.

PREVENTION/CARE

Modify your lifestyle to include health practices that prevent recurrences of ulcer pain and bleeding.

TREATMENT PLAN

A. If aspirin or a nonsteroidal anti-inflammatory drug (NSAID) causes the ulcer, eliminate the drug. If you need the drug for other health problems, discuss other options with your health care provider. You may need to stop the medicine or take a lower dose.

B. Avoid caffeine, colas, alcohol, and chocolate because they may increase acid production.

C. Stop smoking: It slows the ulcer's healing and increases its chance of coming back.

D. Be sure to tell health care providers about your history of ulcer and gastrointestinal (GI) pain if you need new prescriptions or are sent to the hospital.

E. Review all of your medications, over-the-counter (OTC) medications, and herbal products for possible causes or ulcer irritants.

Activity: Exercise daily. Plan rest periods, avoid fatigue, and learn to cope with or avoid stressful situations.

Diet:

A. Eat a well-balanced diet with high-fiber content.

B. Eat meals at regular intervals. Frequent small feedings are unnecessary. Avoid bedtime snacks.

C. Eliminate foods that cause pain or distress; otherwise, your diet is usually not restricted. Examples of foods that cause worse pain are:
   1. Peppermint
   2. Spicy food
   3. Alcohol

D. Avoid extremely hot or cold food or fluids, chew thoroughly, and eat slowly while relaxed for better digestion.

Medications:

A. Acid blockers and medicines called proton pump inhibitors (PPIs) reduce stomach acid.

B. You may need to take antibiotics to fight *H. pylori* infection.

C. Other medications may be prescribed to coat the ulcer area. Antacids can be taken during the ulcer treatment, but should not be used 1 hour before or 2 hours after the ulcer treatments because antacids can interfere with absorption.

D. Take the entire prescription: Do not stop when you feel better.

E. If you have been prescribed metronidazole (Flagyl) or clarithromycin, you may notice a metallic taste in your mouth.

F. Alcohol (including wine) should be avoided when taking Flagyl. The interaction can cause skin flushing, headache, nausea, and vomiting.

G. If you are prescribed bismuth, you may notice black bowel movements.

You Have Been Prescribed: ______________________________

(*continued*)

ULCER MANAGEMENT *(continued)*

You Need to Take: ______________________________

You Need to Notify the Office If You Have:

A. Worsening symptoms while taking your medication

B. Vomiting that is bloody or looks like coffee grounds

C. Tar-colored or "grape jelly" bowel movements. If this occurs, bring a stool sample to the office.

D. Diarrhea and/or severe pain despite treatment

E. Unusual weakness or paleness

F. Other: ______________________________

Phone: ______________________________

URINARY INCONTINENCE: WOMEN

PROBLEM

Urinary incontinence is the condition in which you are unable to hold your urine.

CAUSE

The cause depends on the type of incontinence you have.

PREVENTION/CARE

Exercise regularly, and practice pelvic floor exercises, commonly called Kegel exercises. Do not become constipated so you do not strain to have a bowel movement. Stop smoking. If you have a cough, you may need to see your health care provider to help treat it.

TREATMENT PLAN

Treatment depends on the cause and type of incontinence. Fill out the bladder diary to help figure out what kind of problem you have (see the following table).

A. Pelvic floor exercises should be done every morning, afternoon, and evening; repeat the exercise five times for each set, gradually increase to 10 times each set. To perform these exercises:
   1. Start by doing your pelvic muscle exercises lying down. When your muscles get stronger, do your exercises while sitting or standing.
   2. Do not tighten your tummy, leg, or butt muscles: Just squeeze the muscles you use to start and stop the flow of urine.
   3. Do not hold your breath or practice while you are on the toilet urinating.
   4. Pull in pelvic muscles and hold it tight for a count of 5.
   5. Repeat five times.
   6. Work up to doing 3 sets of 10 repeats.
   7. Kegel exercises take just a few minutes a day, and most women notice an improvement after a few weeks of daily exercise.

B. Empty your bladder frequently. As soon as you feel the urge to urinate, go to the bathroom.

C. You may be taught relaxation techniques to control the feeling of having to go quickly.

D. Fill out your bladder diary and return it to your health care provider.

Activity: Try to get daily exercise. Use absorbent undergarments until your bladder leaking is under control.

Diet: Eat a well-balanced diet. If you are overweight, consider a weight-loss program. Avoid drinking lots of liquids, especially caffeinated beverages and alcohol.

Medications: What you take depends on the type of bladder leakage you have.

You Have Been Prescribed: ______________________________

You Need to Take: ______________________________

You Need to Notify the Office If You Have: ______________________________

Phone: ______________________________

RESOURCES

American Urogynecologic Society: www.augs.org
American Urological Association: www.UrologyHealth.org
National Association for Continence: www.nafc.org
The Simon Foundation for Continence: www.simonfoundation.

(*continued*)

URINARY INCONTINENCE: WOMEN *(continued)*

Bladder Control Diary

Your Daily Bladder Diary

This diary will help you and your health care team figure out the causes of your bladder control trouble. The "sample" line shows you how to use the diary. Use this sheet as a master for making copies that you can use as a bladder diary for as many days as you need.

Your name: ____________________

Date: ____________________

Time	Drinks		Trips to the Bathroom		Accidental Leaks	Did You Feel a Strong Urge to Go?	What Were You Doing at the Time?
	What Kind?	***How Much?***	***How Many Times?***	***How Much Urine? (circle one)***	***How Much? (circle one)***	***(circle one)***	***Sneezing, Exercising, Having Sex, Lifting, etc.***
Sample	Coffee	2 cups	✓ ✓	(sm) med lg	sm (med) lg	Yes (No)	Running
6–7 a.m.				sm med lg	sm med lg	Yes No	
7–8 a.m.				sm med lg	sm med lg	Yes No	
8–9 a.m.				sm med lg	sm med lg	Yes No	
9–10 a.m.				sm med lg	sm med lg	Yes No	
10–11 a.m.				sm med lg	sm med lg	Yes No	
11–12 noon				sm med lg	sm med lg	Yes No	
12–1 p.m.				sm med lg	sm med lg	Yes No	
1–2 p.m.				sm med lg	sm med lg	Yes No	
2–3 p.m.				sm med lg	sm med lg	Yes No	
3–4 p.m.				sm med lg	sm med lg	Yes No	
4–5 p.m.				sm med lg	sm med lg	Yes No	
5–6 p.m.				sm med lg	sm med lg	Yes No	
6–7 p.m.				sm med lg	sm med lg	Yes No	
7–8 p.m.				sm med lg	sm med lg	Yes No	
8–9 p.m.				sm med lg	sm med lg	Yes No	
9–10 p.m.				sm med lg	sm med lg	Yes No	
10–11 p.m.				sm med lg	sm med lg	Yes No	
11–12 midnight				sm med lg	sm med lg	Yes No	
12–1 a.m.				sm med lg	sm med lg	Yes No	
1–2 a.m.				sm med lg	sm med lg	Yes No	
2–3 a.m.				sm med lg	sm med lg	Yes No	
3–4 a.m.				sm med lg	sm med lg	Yes No	
4–5 a.m.				sm med lg	sm med lg	Yes No	
5–6 a.m.				sm med lg	sm med lg	Yes No	

I used __________ pads today. I used __________ diapers today (write number).

Questions to ask my health care team: ____________________

Let's Talk About Bladder Control for Women is a public health awareness campaign conducted by the National Kidney and Urologic Diseases Information Clearinghouse (NKUDIC), an information dissemination service of the National Institute of Diabetes and Digestive and Kidney Diseases (NIDDK), National Institutes of Health.

Adapted from NKUDIC, National Institutes of Health (NIH). (www.niddk.nih.gov/health-information/health-topics/urologic-disease/urinary-incontinence-women/pages/insertb.aspx)

URINARY TRACT INFECTION (ACUTE CYSTITIS)

PROBLEM

You have a bladder infection. The symptoms include painful, frequent urination, and pain over the bladder. Your symptoms may be mild, moderate, or painful.

CAUSE

Bacteria caused the infection of the bladder. A bladder infection is more common in women and in men who have prostate problems.

PREVENTION/CARE

A. Empty your bladder often:
   1. As soon as you feel the urge to go, empty your bladder at that time. Do not hold your urine.
   2. You may need to urinate on a schedule during the day, at least every 2 to 3 hours.

B. Wash your hands after going to the bathroom (both urine and bowel movements [BM]).

C. Good hygiene for females:
   1. Wipe front to back every time you empty your bladder and especially after bowel movements.
   2. Take showers instead of baths; do not take bubble baths.
   3. Empty your bladder before and after sex.
   4. Avoid feminine hygiene sprays and douches.

D. Wear cotton underwear. Do not wear tight underwear and clothes. Take off your underwear at night while sleeping.

TREATMENT PLAN

Treatment depends on how bad (severity) the infection is. Antibiotics are used to kill bacteria that cause infections. The most important thing is to finish all of your medications even if you feel better.

Activity: Rest; avoid strenuous activity. Avoid sexual activity until you finish the antibiotics.

Diet:

A. Increase fluids; drink at least one large glass of liquid every hour.

B. Avoid foods that irritate the bladder: Caffeine, alcohol, and spicy foods.

C. Drink cranberry juice to help fight bladder infections. If you do not like plain cranberry juice, mix it with another juice such as orange juice.

Medications:

A. Antibiotics kill bacteria that cause infection. Make sure you take all of your medications, not just until you feel better.

B. Take acetaminophen (Tylenol) for fever.

C. You may be prescribed a medication to prevent bladder spasms and pain while urinating. This changes the color of your urine to orange or blue.

You Have Been Prescribed the Following Antibiotics: ______________________________

You Need to Take: ______________________________

Take all of your antibiotics, even if you feel better.

You Have Been Prescribed the Following for Discomfort: ______________________________

You Need to Take: ______________________________

(*continued*)

URINARY TRACT INFECTION (ACUTE CYSTITIS) *(continued)*

You Need to Notify the Office If You Have:

A. Worsening symptoms or symptoms not improving during treatment.

B. Fever higher than 100.4°F.

C. Blood in your urine.

D. Symptoms that come back after you finish all of your medications: painful urination, back pain, fever, chills, or nausea.

E. Other: ______________________________

Phone: ______________________________

URINARY TRACT INFECTION DURING PREGNANCY: PYELONEPHRITIS

PROBLEM

You have been diagnosed with an infection of the kidney (where urine is made). Bladder infections can spread to the kidney.

CAUSE

Bacteria from the bladder can move up to the kidney and cause a kidney infection. Other causes are blockage in the urine system or having a catheter, or tube, in the bladder.

PREVENTION/CARE

A. Urinate frequently. Do not hold urine for a long period.

B. Empty your bladder as soon as you feel it is filling.

C. Urinate before and after sexual intercourse.

D. After urinating, always wipe from front to back with toilet tissue.

E. Do not wear tight underwear or pants that can cause increased moistness and warmth in the perineal area.

F. Cotton panties are the best.

G. Wash your hands every time after going to the bathroom.

H. Do not use the same tissue that you blow your nose with to wipe after emptying your bladder: This spreads infection.

TREATMENT PLAN

Antibiotics kill the bacteria that cause infection.

Activity: Rest; do not engage in strenuous physical activity.

Diet: Increase fluids; drink at least one large glass of water every hour while you are awake. Drink cranberry juice to help fight and prevent urinary tract infections (UTIs). If you do not like the taste of cranberry juice, mix cranberry juice with another juice like grape juice.

Medications: You will be prescribed antibiotics to kill the bacteria causing infection. The drugs may be changed if your urine culture results show different bacteria. You may need mild pain relievers if you have a lot of back pain. Medications, such as Tylenol, may be used to bring down fever. You may be prescribed a medicine to stop bladder spasm and pain.

You Have Been Prescribed the Following Antibiotics: ______________________________

You Need to Take: ______________________________

Finish all of your antibiotics even if you feel better.

You Have Been Prescribed the Following for Bladder Spasms: ______________________________

You Need to Take: ______________________________

This medicine will make your urine turn a different color.

You Need to Notify the Office If You Have:

A. Symptoms that worsen or do not get better during treatment.

B. New symptoms that develop during treatment.

C. Symptoms that return after treatment when you finish all of your antibiotics.

D. Difficulty taking your medication (you break out or vomit)

E. Other: ______________________________

Phone: ______________________________

VAGINAL BLEEDING: FIRST TRIMESTER

PROBLEM

Vaginal bleeding may occur in the first trimester of pregnancy. The amount of bleeding may range from spotting to a complete miscarriage.

CAUSE

Bleeding may occur for a variety of reasons, including smoking, trauma, abnormal fetus, or other problems.

PREVENTION/CARE

In most cases, the cause of vaginal bleeding may not be prevented. If bleeding is light, it may lessen or stop. You need to avoid sexual intercourse, tampons, and douches. If you smoke, it is highly recommended that you cut down and stop smoking.

TREATMENT PLAN

Treatment depends on the cause or suspected cause of your bleeding.

Activity:

A. Many women experience less bleeding and cramping while on limited activities or bed rest. Unfortunately, activity restriction does not prevent miscarriage.

B. Avoid sexual intercourse until at least 2 weeks after the bleeding has stopped, or until your provider tells you.

C. If bed rest is prescribed, perform simple range of motion (ROM) activities as directed by the practitioner. Examples are foot circles and moving legs in bed.

D. Do not use tampons during this period. Use pads so that you can evaluate how much you are bleeding.
   1. **Scant amount:** Blood only on tissue when wiped or less than 1-inch stain on Peri-Pad.
   2. **Light amount:** Less than 4-inch stain on Peri-Pad.
   3. **Moderate amount:** Less than 6-inch stain on Peri-Pad.
   4. **Heavy amount:** Saturated Peri-Pad within 1 hour.

Diet: As tolerated. If you are on bed rest, eat fresh vegetables, fruits, and bran cereal to avoid becoming constipated.

Medications: You may not be prescribed any medications.

You Need to Notify the Office If:

A. You develop a fever with your bleeding.

B. You have a gush of blood from your vagina that is more than a period.

C. You pass blood clots or tissue from your vagina.

D. Your vaginal bleeding has a foul odor.

E. You experience abdominal pain or uterine cramping not relieved by taking acetaminophen.

F. Other: ______________________________

Phone: ______________________________

VAGINAL BLEEDING: SECOND AND THIRD TRIMESTERS

PROBLEM

Vaginal bleeding may occur during the second and third trimesters of pregnancy (more than 12 weeks). The bleeding may range from spotting of blood on your panties to bleeding like a menstrual period.

CAUSE

A small amount of bloody mucous discharge or spotting may occur for about 1 day following a pelvic examination or sexual intercourse. This is normal if it is not associated with cramping or contractions.

Other causes of vaginal bleeding may be related to the location of the placenta (placenta previa) or premature separation (abruption) of the placenta from your womb. Placental abruption can be associated with cocaine use, cigarette smoking, and trauma (injuries from car wrecks or physical violence).

PREVENTION/CARE

There is no known way to prevent most types of vaginal bleeding. If you have been diagnosed with placenta previa, you may be able to prevent bleeding by avoiding sexual intercourse and maintaining bed rest.

There is no known method of preventing placenta previa. Smoking has been associated with placental abruption and placenta previa. You should not smoke or at least you should try to cut down and stop smoking during pregnancy. When you stop smoking, it is also good for your baby's health after delivery.

TREATMENT PLAN

A. Treatment depends on the cause of your vaginal bleeding. You may be placed on bed rest.

B. Stop smoking. Ask your provider for a handout on tips to stop smoking.

C. You may need to be on a rest schedule.

D. You may need to stop working.

E. You need to arrange help for child care, grocery shopping, and housework.

Activity: The checked activity restriction(s) are prescribed by the provider.

Level 1: As tolerated, avoid heavy lifting above 20 lb.

Level 2: Modified bed rest.
You may be out of bed for breakfast; rest (lying down) for 2 hours in the morning with moderate activity until lunch; rest for 2 hours with moderate activity until dinner.
Go to bed by 8 p.m.
Moderate activity consists of short periods of cooking and light housework.

Level 3: Strict bed rest.
You may be out of the bed only to go to the bathroom or to move to the couch.
You may take a shower, use the toilet, and brush your teeth, but then return immediately to bed.
No sexual intercourse.
Perform range-of-motion (ROM) exercises as directed by your practitioner.

Diet: Eat fresh vegetables, fruits, and bran cereal to avoid becoming constipated on bed rest. Drinking extra liquids (especially water) also helps to prevent constipation.

Medications: Continue taking your prenatal vitamins every day.

You Need to Notify the Office If You Have:

A. Contractions or cramps, eight in 1 hour or four in 20 minutes

B. Bloody, mucous discharge not associated with recent sexual intercourse or a pelvic examination

C. Bright-red or dark-red vaginal spotting

D. Bleeding like a period

(*continued*)

VAGINAL BLEEDING: SECOND AND THIRD TRIMESTERS (*continued*)

E. A gush of fluid or blood from your vagina

F. Sharp, knifelike pain in your abdomen that does not go away

G. Pelvic pressure or low backache not relieved with emptying your bladder and resting on one side

H. Noticed decreased movement of the baby

I. Other: ____

Phone: ______________________________________

VAGINAL YEAST INFECTION

PROBLEM

You have been diagnosed with a vaginal yeast infection. This is an infection or inflammation of the vagina that is caused by a fungus known as yeast (*Monilia* or *Candida albicans*).

CAUSE

Yeast cells (*Monilia*) are normally present on the skin in healthy people. These cells may be found in the vagina or rectal area. However, due to a disturbance in the body's hormones and pH, an overproduction of these cells has occurred and has caused an infection. Several factors can cause this disturbance, which include menstrual periods, pregnancy, diabetes, antibiotics or other medications, increased dietary intake of sugars and alcohol, and an increase in moisture and warmth in the vaginal or rectal area by wearing tight, restrictive clothing.

PREVENTION/CARE

A. Keep the vaginal and rectal areas clean and dry.

B. Shower daily and avoid tub baths.

C. Avoid tight, restrictive clothing such as tight jeans and underwear.

D. Wear cotton panties that allow air to circulate. At bedtime, do not wear underwear with your pajamas.

E. Obesity can contribute to this problem, too. If you have gained an excessive amount of weight, try to lose these extra pounds.

F. Avoid douching because this changes the normal flora and pH of the vagina, which can contribute to causing yeast infections.

TREATMENT PLAN

A pelvic examination may have been necessary to identify the source of your infection. Practice preventive tips to speed your recovery.

Activity: Avoid excessive exercise and activities that produce excessive sweating; also avoid sexual intercourse until your infection is gone. Your partner may also need to be treated for this same infection.

Diet: Drink plenty of water and other liquids. Avoid alcohol and excessive sugars. Increase the intake of yogurt and buttermilk in your diet.

Medications: Antifungal medications may be prescribed for you.

1. Over-the-counter medications may include Monistat vaginal suppositories and cream. This is also known as miconazole nitrate, which you may find in the drug store at a much lower price and which can be just as effective.
2. You must use the full days of the over-the-counter medication. If you stop too early, the yeast can regrow.

If you have also been diagnosed with a bacterial infection of the vagina, other medications may also be prescribed. If your provider has prescribed Flagyl (metronidazole), **please do not drink any alcohol while taking this medication and for the next 3 days following this medication. The combination of this medication and alcohol can make you very sick.**

You Have Been Prescribed: ____________________

You Need to Take: ____________________

You Need to Notify the Office If:

A. Over-the-counter medications do not help your symptoms.

B. You develop other symptoms.

C. Other: ____________________

Phone: ____________________

VARICOSE VEINS

PROBLEM

Varicose veins are caused when the valves inside of veins are damaged and allow blood to flow backward instead of toward the heart. This backflow of blood increases the pressure in the vein, leading to pain and swelling, and makes them more visible. Varicose veins can worsen and increase the risk of blood clots, infection, bleeding, and changes to the skin.

CAUSE

There are many factors that increase the chance of developing varicose veins. Some cannot be changed, like age and genetics. Some can be changed; these include prolonged standing, restrictive clothing, excessive weight, and smoking.

PREVENTION/CARE

A. Avoid prolonged standing. If prolonged standing is required, shift weight from one leg to the other.

B. Do not sit with legs dependent.

TREATMENT PLAN

A. Raise the affected arm or leg whenever lying down to improve pain and swelling.

B. Wear compression stockings. Put them on before getting out of bed in the morning. Take them off just before going to bed at night.

C. Avoid standing or sitting for long periods of time.

D. Follow up with your primary health care provider on a regularly scheduled basis.

Activity:

A. Get regular exercise. Discuss with your health care provider what type and frequency of exercise is safe for you.

B. Exercise leg muscles by pumping ankles when sitting. Rocking in a rocking chair is another option.

Diet:

A. Discuss with your health care provider the type of diet that best suits your needs: Diabetic diet, low-fat diet, low-cholesterol diet, and/or low-sodium diet.

B. If you are taking the blood thinner Coumadin, ask your health care provider about which foods are high in vitamin K and whether you should limit those foods in your diet.

Medications:

You Have Been Prescribed: ______________________________

You Need to Take: ______________________________

You Need to Notify the Office If You Have:

A. New pain, swelling, or warmth in an arm or leg

B. Increased redness, pain, tenderness to touch, and/or warmth in the affected arm or leg

C. Sudden shortness of breath

D. Chest pain

E. Other: ______________________________

Phone: ______________________________

RESOURCES

Patient Education Center—Varicose Veins: patienteducationcenter.org/articles/varicose-veins

Patient Handout—Varicose Veins: nursing.advanceweb.com/sharedresources/ADVANCEfornurses/Resources/DownloadableResources/N1010504_p30handout.pdf

WARTS

PROBLEM

A wart is a raised, rough growth projecting from the skin, which can be contagious.

CAUSE

Warts are caused by a viral infection that stimulates the cells of the skin to multiply rapidly, which results in an outward growth.

PREVENTION/TREATMENT PLAN

A. Wash hands well.

B. Avoid scratching or picking warts. Warts bleed easily.

C. Some warts go away spontaneously after time without any treatment.

D. Medications may be prescribed.

To Enhance Destruction

A. Soak the wart in warm water 10 to 15 minutes a day.

B. After soaking, use an emery board to file the wart down.

C. Apply over-the-counter medication as prescribed (Compound W) to the site.

D. Duct tape may be applied over the wart. Perform these steps every night until resolved.

E. Warts may reappear at the same spot or in other areas.

F. Cryotherapy "freezing" is another treatment option. Discuss this with your health care provider.

Activity: There are no activity restrictions for warts.

Diet: There are no special diets for warts.

Medications:

You Have Been Prescribed: ____________________

You Need to Take: ____________________

You Need to Notify the Office If:

A. You develop an infection at the site of the wart.

B. Other: ____________________

Phone: ____________________

WOUND CARE: LOWER EXTREMITY ULCERS

PROBLEM

An ulcer on the body that lies on the lower extremities

CAUSE

Edema, trauma, ischemia, venous insufficiency

PREVENTION/CARE

A. Keep the area clean and free of foreign debris.

B. Dressing changes: ________________

C. You may be prescribed antibiotics; if so, take all antibiotics until they are completely gone.

TREATMENT PLAN

Activity: Do not apply direct pressure to the site of the ulcer. You may be prescribed to elevate your lower extremities.

Diet: Eat a well-balanced diet. Increase protein intake.

Medications:

You Have Been Prescribed: ____

You Need to Take: ____

You Need to Notify the Office If You Have:

A. A reaction or cannot tolerate any of the prescribed medications

B. A fever and a general ill feeling

C. Any new or unexplained symptoms related to the ulcer
   1. Increase in size
   2. New odor
   3. Increased drainage
   4. Change in color of the drainage
   5. Increased pain at the site

D. Any questions or concerns

Phone: ____

WOUND CARE: PRESSURE ULCERS

PROBLEM

An ulcer on the body that lies over a bony surface

CAUSE

Prolonged periods of pressure to the area of ulcer causing a breakdown of skin integrity.

PREVENTION/CARE

A. Keep the area clean and free of foreign debris.

B. You may be prescribed dressing changes.
   1. Remove dressing.
   2. Clean the ulcer with normal saline.
   3. Apply prescribed medication (see the following).
   4. Cover with dry dressing, change as ordered.

C. You may be prescribed antibiotics; if so, take all antibiotics until they are completely gone.

TREATMENT PLAN

Activity: Do not apply direct pressure to the site of the ulcer.

Diet: Eat a well-balanced diet. Drink 8 to 10 glasses of water per day. Increase protein intake.

Medications:

You Have Been Prescribed: ______________________________

You Need to Take: ______________________________

You Need to Notify the Office If You Have:

A. A reaction or cannot tolerate any of the prescribed medications

B. A fever and a general ill feeling

C. Any new or unexplained symptoms
   1. Increase in size
   2. New odor
   3. Increased drainage
   4. Change in color of the drainage
   5. Increased pain at the site

D. Any questions or concerns

Phone: ______________________________

WOUND CARE: WOUNDS

PROBLEM

A wound is a break in the external surface of the body.

CAUSE

Wounds are often due to an accidental or intentional injury. Wound infection is usually caused by bacterial contamination of the site.

PREVENTION/CARE

A. Prevent accidental or intentional injury.

B. Immediately after injury, cleanse the wound well with soap and water.

C. Remove all dirt and foreign material.

D. You may be prescribed antibiotics; if so, take all antibiotics until they are completely gone.

E. You may need a tetanus shot.

TREATMENT PLAN

Activity: No restrictions. If infection is present, you may need to increase rest.

Diet: Eat a well-balanced diet. Drink 8 to 10 glasses of water per day.

Medications:

You Have Been Prescribed: ______________________________

You Need to Take: ______________________________

You Need to Notify the Office If You Have:

A. A reaction or cannot tolerate any of the prescribed medications

B. A fever and a general ill feeling

C. A wound/infection that seems to worsen

D. Any new or unexplained symptoms

E. Any questions or concerns

Phone: ______________________________

WOUND INFECTION: EPISIOTOMY AND CESAREAN SECTION

PROBLEM

You have an infection of your episiotomy site or cesarean section incision.

CAUSE

The cause is one or more types of bacteria that invaded the tissue following your delivery. The bacteria may be from the vagina, the bowel, or the environment.

TREATMENT PLAN

A. Take your temperature if you have fever and chills.

B. Episiotomy:
   1. Wash hands before and after changing your sanitary pads and your baby's diaper.
   2. Wipe or pat dry from front to back after every urination or bowel movement.
   3. Apply and remove perineal pad from front to back.
   4. Change perineal pad at least every 4 hours and after each void or bowel movement (BM).
   5. Use a squeeze bottle: Position the nozzle between the legs, empty the entire bottle over the perineum, blot dry with toilet paper, and avoid contamination from the anal area.
   6. Use a blow dryer on the lowest setting to "air dry" your stitches.
   7. Wash the perineum with mild soap and warm water at least once daily.

C. Cesarean section incision:
   1. Wash hands before and after dressing change and wound care.
   2. Follow all of the aforementioned directions (except 6) for your bleeding, too.
   3. After showering, gently pat dry your abdomen.
   4. If the wound is draining, cover it with a clean dressing and call the office for instructions. Otherwise, leave it open to air.
   5. Cleanse the incision with hydrogen peroxide and cotton swab. Do not clean the same area more than once with the same swab.
   6. If your incision opens, notify your practitioner for further instructions.

Activity: Increased rest is recommended; try to lie down for a nap when the baby goes to sleep.

Diet: There are no dietary restrictions; eat well-balanced meals. Increase your fluid intake with an infection. Drink at least 10 to 12 glasses of liquid a day.

Medications: Continue your prenatal vitamins. You may take acetaminophen one to two tablets every 4 to 6 hours for your fever and/or discomfort.

You Have Been Prescribed the Following Antibiotics: ____________________

You Need to Take: ____________________
Take all of your antibiotics, even if you feel better, unless you have an adverse reaction to them. Then call the office.

You Need to Notify the Office If You Have:

A. Temperature that rises significantly or reaches 101°F

B. Foul-smelling drainage from the incision or episiotomy site

C. Increased pain or tenderness

D. Separation of wound or incision

E. Other: ____________________

Phone: ____________________

XEROSIS (WINTER ITCH)

PROBLEM

Xerosis is severely chapped skin that becomes cracked, fissured, and inflamed. It can appear on skin anywhere on the body, but it is seen most commonly on the legs.

CAUSE

Xerosis is caused by insufficient oil on the skin's surface, which allows water to evaporate through the skin. Oil in the skin decreases with aging, excessive bathing, and excessive rubbing of the skin. An environment with low humidity also promotes dryness of the skin.

PREVENTION/CARE

A. Reduce water loss from the skin.
   1. Decrease the frequency and duration of baths or showers; use tepid water.
   2. Use soap sparingly.
   3. Avoid detergent soaps.
   4. Pat skin dry rather than rubbing.
   5. Apply skin lubricants (Lac-Hydrin, Eucerin, etc.) to dry skin before chapped areas become inflamed.
   6. Use ultrasonic, cool-mist humidifiers if the air is very dry.
   7. Clean the humidifier daily.
   8. Oil (such as Nivea) in the bath water may be helpful.
   9. Apply lubricants after bathing when possible to trap additional moisture before evaporation occurs.

B. Apply hand cream four to eight times a day to hands and twice daily on the trunk and extremities.

TREATMENT PLAN

Activity: No restrictions. Avoid long-term exposure to drying environments.

Diet: Eat a well-balanced diet; drink 8 to 10 glasses of water per day.

Medications:

You Have Been Prescribed: ______________________________

You Need to Take: ______________________________

You Need to Notify the Office If You Have:

A. Severely chapped skin, and self-care does not relieve the symptoms in 1 week

B. Chapped skin that becomes inflamed or if you see any oozing

C. Any questions or concerns

Phone: ______________________________

ZIKA VIRUS INFECTION

PROBLEM

The Zika virus is a virus that is transmitted to humans by infected mosquitoes. Symptoms of the virus include low-grade fever, hand and/or foot joint pain, skin rash, headache, and/or eye discomfort or pain. The virus can spread to other humans by sexual contact with someone who is infected with the virus. A pregnant woman infected with the virus can spread the virus to her unborn baby.

CAUSE

The disease is caused by a bite from a mosquito infected with the Zika virus.

PREVENTION/CARE

Avoid traveling to countries with known cases of the Zika virus. The outbreak of this virus has been documented in Central and South America, Mexico, the Caribbean, and the Pacific Islands. It has also been documented in the United States territories of Puerto Rico, the U.S. Virgin Islands, and American Samoa.

There have been reported cases in the United States; however, the people diagnosed with the Zika virus had previously traveled to countries in which mosquitoes carry the virus.

TREATMENT PLAN

A. There is no medication or vaccination approved to treat the Zika virus.

B. Prevention of the virus is the most important thing one can do to protect from getting the virus. Avoid traveling to areas in which the Zika virus is transmitted by mosquitoes.

C. Medications, such as acetaminophen (Tylenol), may be given to improve symptoms if present such as headaches, fever, joint pain, eye pain, and muscle weakness.

D. It is thought that the Zika virus can cause another condition called Guillain–Barré syndrome, in which symptoms of severe muscle weakness can occur and even lead to paralysis. Notify your health care provider if you have any of these symptoms.

Activity:

Avoid sexual contact with any person thought to have the Zika virus.

A. Women:
  1. If you have traveled to any of the countries at risk of the Zika virus you should use condoms with sexual activity or do not have sex for at least **8 WEEKS** after your symptoms start.
  2. If you have traveled to any of the countries at risk of the Zika virus and you **DO NOT** have any symptoms, you should use condoms with sexual activity or do not have sex for at least **8 WEEKS** after returning.
  3. Avoid becoming pregnant while traveling to high-risk areas and avoid becoming pregnant up to **8 WEEKS** after travel.

B. Men:
  1. If you have traveled to any of the countries at risk of the Zika virus and you **HAVE** any of the above symptoms, you should use condoms with sexual activity or do not have sex for at least **6 MONTHS** after your symptoms started.
  2. If you have traveled to any of the countries at risk of the Zika virus and you **DO NOT** have any symptoms, you should use condoms with sexual activity or do not have sex for at least **8 WEEKS** after returning.
  3. If you have traveled to any of the countries at risk of the Zika virus and your **PARTNER IS PREGNANT** you should use condoms with sexual activity, or do not have sex, for the rest of your partner's pregnancy.

C. Precautions to use if you travel to a country with the Zika virus:
  1. Stay indoors. Mosquitoes infected with the Zika virus usually bite during the daytime, but precautions should also be taken for evening and nighttime hours.
  2. If screens in windows are not available, use a bed net to cover you while sleeping.
  3. Small children in strollers should also be covered with netting for protection.
  4. Wear loose clothing to cover most of your body (light-colored clothing, long sleeves and pants, hat) to avoid mosquito bites.
  5. Spray clothing with an insect repellant that contains permethrin when going outdoors.

(*continued*)

ZIKA VIRUS INFECTION *(continued)*

6. Apply insect repellant that contains diethyltoluamide (DEET) or a chemical called *picaridin* to skin. Precautions should be used when using the insect repellant DEET on young children.
7. Insect repellent with DEET should not be used on children younger than 2 years old.
8. Apply insect repellent after sunscreen.
9. Avoid bodies of standing water such as pools, lakes, ponds, and so forth. Empty any containers with standing water such as buckets, plants, and so on.

Diet:
No special diet will prevent or improve the virus. You need to drink plenty of fluids to stay well hydrated.

Medications:
A. Acetaminophen (Tylenol) may be used for fever, body pain, and joint pain.

B. Avoid aspirin and nonsteroidal anti-inflammatory drugs (NSAIDs; ibuprofen, naproxen) because of the risks of bleeding if other conditions are present.

C. Children younger than 18 years should not use aspirin because of the risk of Reye's syndrome.

You Have Been Prescribed: ____________________

You Need to Take: ____________________

You Need to Notify the Office If:
A. Muscle weakness occurs. Guillain–Barré syndrome is a condition that is thought to be triggered by the Zika virus. Symptoms include muscle weakness and can lead to paralysis of the muscles and even death.

B. High fever, increased joint pain, severe headache, confusion, or any other new symptoms present.

C. Other: ____________________

Phone: ____________________

Appendices

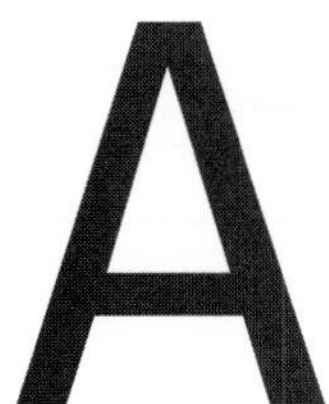

Normal Laboratory Values

Normal laboratory values are presented here. However, ranges of laboratory value differ from laboratory to laboratory. They differ because of age and gender. Different values are presented; all normal values are listed under the Females column. Values for males and children are the same unless otherwise noted. Legend: 10^6 = 1,000,000; 10^3 = 1,000.

Normal Laboratory Values

	Females	Males	Children
Complete Blood Count			
Red blood cells (RBCs)	3.8–5.1 10^6/µL	4.2–5.6 10^6/µL	3.5–5.0 10^6/µL
Hemoglobin (Hgb) ↑ Polycythemia, dehydration, ↓ blood loss, severe anemia, low production or death of blood cell	11–16 g/dL	14–18 g/dL	10–14 g/dL Newborn 15–25 g/dL
Hematocrit (Hct) ↓ Anemia, massive blood loss, ↑ dehydration or hemoconcentration with shock	34%–47%	39%–54%	30%–42%
Mean corpuscular volume (MCV) RBC size: Normocytic, microcytic, macrocytic	78–98 fL		
Mean corpuscular hemoglobin (MCH) RBC color: Normochromic, hypochromic	27–35 pg		
Mean corpuscular hemoglobin concentration (MCHC)	31–37 g/dL or %		
Reticulocyte count Measures the number of new RBCs produced by the bone marrow	33–137 × 10/µL		
White Blood Cells (WBCs)			
↑ Bacterial infections, infectious diseases (mononucleosis), ↓ stress, tissue death, leukemia, cancer, hemorrhage	3.8–11.0 million/mm	3.8–11.0 10^3/mm^3	5.0–10.0 10^3/mm^3
Differential			
Segmented neutrophils ↑ stress, trauma, inflammatory disorders, ↓ viral infections, severe bacterial infections, aplastic anemia	50%–81%		
Band neutrophils	1%–5%		
Lymphocytes ↑ chronic bacterial infection, viral infections, ↓ leukemia, AIDS, lupus erythematosus	14%–44%		
Monocytes ↑ chronic inflammatory disorders, viral infections, chronic conditions, ↓ steroid therapy	2%–6%		
Eosinophils ↑ allergies, parasite infections, leukemia	1%–5%		
Basophils ↑ leukemia ↓ allergic reactions, stress, hyperthyroidism	0%–1.0%		
Serum iron concentration of iron bound to transferrin	60–160 mcg/dL	80–180 mcg/dL	
Total iron-binding capacity (TIBC) Amount of iron transferrin can bind	250–460 mcg/dL		

(*continued*)

Normal Laboratory Values *(continued)*

	Females	Males	Children
Erythrocyte sedimentation rate (ESR)	Women <50	Males <50	
↑ Pregnancy, inflammatory conditions, ↓ sickle cell anemia	<20 mm/hr Women >50 <30 mm/hr	<15 mm/hr Males >50 <20 mm/hr	
BUN/Creatinine-Renal Function Tests			
Blood urea nitrogen (BUN)	6–23 mg/dL	0.2–0.6 mg/dL	
Creatinine (Cr)	0.6–1.5 mg/dL	3.5–7.7 mg/dL	
Creatine	0.6–1.0 mg/dL		
Uric acid	2.5–6.6 mg/dL		
Thyroid Studies			
Thyroid-stimulating hormone (TSH)	2.0–10.5 mcg/mL		
↑ Hypothyroidism, ↓ hyperthyroidism	0.8–1.1 mcg/dL		
T3 ↑ pregnancy and oral contraceptive use	5.0–13.0 mcg/dL		
Thyroxine (T4) ↑ hyperthyroidism, ↓ hypothyroidism			
Aminotransferases			
↑ Liver damage and medications	4–35 U/L	7–46 U/L	
Alanine transaminase (ALT)	6–18 U/L	7–21 U/L	
Aspartate aminotransferase (AST)			
Bilirubin (Measures Bile Salt Conjugation and Excretion)			
Direct bilirubin	0.0–0.4 mg/dL		
Indirect bilirubin	Total bilirubin minus direct bilirubin		
Total bilirubin	0.21–1.0 mg/dL 3.0 mg/dL indicates hepatic disease, jaundice is visible		

Glucose
Fasting 65–110 mg/dL
2-hr postprandial 65–140 mg/dL
Serum albumin (measures protein synthesis)
3.5–5.0 g/dL
↑ Dehydration, inflammatory illness, liver insufficiency, malnutrition, and cancer
Lipid profile—adults
Fasting cholesterol: Less than 200 mg/dL indicates low risk for coronary heart disease (CHD)
200–239 mg/dL: Borderline risk for coronary heart disease
>240 mg/dL: High risk for CHD
Triglycerides
<149 mg/dL: Low risk for CHD
150–199 mg/dL: Borderline risk for CHD
>200 mg/dL: High risk for CHD
High-density-lipoprotein (HDL): >40 mg/dL, desirable levels higher than 50 mg/dL
Low-density-lipoprotein (LDL): <100 mg/dL
100–159 mg/dL: Borderline CHD
>160 mg/dL: High risk for CHD
Triglycerides
Ages 0–9 years: <75 mg/dL; ages 10–19 years: <90 mg/dL
Ages 0–9 years: 75–99 mg/dL; ages 10–19 years: 90–129 mg/dL borderline risk for CHD
Ages 0–9 years: >100 mg/dL; ages 10–19 years: >130 mg/dL high risk for CHD
HDL: >45 mg/dL
40–45 mg/dL: Borderline risk for CHD
<40 mg/dL: High risk for CHD
LDL: <110 mg/dL
110–129 mg/dL: Borderline risk for CHD
>130 mg/dL: High risk for CHD

(continued)

Normal Laboratory Values *(continued)*

Coagulation

Prothrombin time (PT): 10–14 sec
Partial thromboplastin time (PTT): 32–45 sec
Fibrinogen: 160–450 mg/dL
Bleeding time: 3–7 min
Thrombin time: 11–15 sec
Platelets: 140,000–450,000/mL
↓ Thrombocytopenia, acute leukemia/aplastic anemia during chemotherapy, interferon, infections, and drug reactions
↑ Myeloproliferative disease, cancer, and rheumatoid arthritis (RA)

Sickle cell disease

Sickle cell hemoglobin (HgbS): Normal, none present
Homozygous HgbS: Sickle cell disease
Heterozygous HgbS: Sickle cell trait
Hemoglobin electrophoresis: Determines hemoglobin types and percentages

Hepatitis B

Hepatitis B surface antigen: Negative
Positive: Acute or chronic infection, further liver function tests needed
Hepatitis B surface antibody: Positive indicates immunity to infection (previous infection or hepatitis B vaccine)

Serum alkaline phosphatase (ALP; marks liver disease)

30–120 IU/L
Pregnancy value 30–200 IU/L
↑ Bile stones, biliary and pancreatic cancer, viral hepatitis, cirrhosis, Paget's disease, osteomalacia, bone metastasis

Urinalysis

Color: Pale yellow/straw to amber
Clarity: Clear
Specific gravity: 1.001–1.035
pH: Normal 4.6–8.0 (acidic)
Glucose: Absent
Ketones: Absent
Protein: Negative

Urine dipstick U/A

Nitrites: Negative (positive = bacteria, infection)
Leukocytes oxidase: Negative (positive = WBCs)

Arterial blood gas values

pH: 7.3–7.45
$PaCO_2$: 35–45 mmHg
HCO_3: 22–26 mEq/L
O_2 saturation: 96–100%
PaO_2: 85–100 mmHg
Base excess (BE): −2 to +2 mmol/L

Venous blood gas values

pH: 7.31–7.41
$PaCO_2$: 41–51 mmHg
HCO_3: 22–29 mEq/L
O_2 saturation: 60%–85%
PaO_2: 30–40 mmHg
BE: 0 to +4 mmol/L

HIV

ELISA: Negative
ELISA: Positive: Repeat; if second ELISA positive. Perform Western blot
Western blot negative: No evidence of HIV
Western blot positive: Evidence of HIV

Rubella

Titer: >1:10 immune
Titer: <1:8 nonimmune administer Rubella vaccine

Female hormone levels

	Follicle-Stimulating Hormone (FSH)	Luteinizing Hormone (LH)	Progesterone	Prolactin
Follicular phase	2–25 mIU/mL	5–30 mIU/mL	0.2–6.0 mIU/mL	<23 ng/mL
Midcycle phase	10–90 mIU/mL	75–150 mIU/mL	6–30 mIU/mL	<28 ng/mL
Luteal phase	2–25 mIU/mL	3–40 mIU/mL	5.7–28.1 mIU/mL	5–40 ng/mL
Postmenopausal	40–350 mIU/mL	30–200 mIU/mL	0–0.2 mIU/mL	<12 ng/mL

B Diet Recommendations

Bland Diet

Cheryl A. Glass and Jill C. Cash

You have been prescribed a bland diet. This diet provides adequate nutrition along with the treatment of gastrointestinal (GI) problems such as ulcerative conditions or inflammatory problems of the stomach and intestines. It is intended to decrease irritation in the lining of the stomach and intestines.

Food Tips

Foods to Avoid

Garlic, onions, alcohol, fatty foods, fried foods, chocolate, cocoa, coffee (even decaffeinated), dried fruits, citrus fruit and juices (orange, pineapple, and grapefruit), tomato products, peppermint, whole-grain breads and cereals, prespiced foods such as processed lunch meats and ham, pepper, and chili powder. Avoid pepper, chili powder, and cocoa spices.

General Instructions

A. Eat at least three small meals a day.
B. Avoid alcohol and beer.
C. Avoid caffeinated drinks/colas.
D. Avoid fried, greasy foods.
E. Bake or broil your foods.
F. Trim the fat from meats before cooking.
G. Bake, broil, mash, or cream potatoes.
H. Avoid raw fruits and vegetables, such as corn on the cob, and other gas-forming vegetables such as cabbage, dried beans, and peas.
I. Avoid rich desserts.
J. Avoid bedtime snacks—they may increase acid production and cause discomfort at night.
K. Avoid eating 2 hours before you go to bed.
L. Ask your health care provider if nutritional supplements are necessary.

Approved Foods by Food Group

A. Dairy products
- **1.** Whole milk
- **2.** Low-fat or 2% milk
- **3.** Skim milk
- **4.** Evaporated milk
- **5.** Buttermilk
- **6.** Cottage cheese
- **7.** Yogurt
- **8.** Cheese

B. Meat
- **1.** Beef
- **2.** Veal
- **3.** Fresh pork
- **4.** Turkey
- **5.** Chicken
- **6.** Fish (canned or fresh)
- **7.** Liver
- **8.** Egg (as a meat substitute)

C. Breads/grains
- **1.** Enriched breads (plain toast)
- **2.** Oats
- **3.** Cereal
- **4.** Tortillas
- **5.** English muffins
- **6.** Saltine crackers
- **7.** Pasta (all types)

D. Fruits/vegetables
- **1.** All vegetables
- **2.** All fruits and juices (except citrus)

E. Desserts
- **1.** Custard
- **2.** Pudding
- **3.** Sherbet
- **4.** Ice cream (except peppermint and chocolate)
- **5.** Gelatin
- **6.** Angel food cake
- **7.** Pound cake
- **8.** Sugar cookies
- **9.** Jams and jellies
- **10.** Honey

F. Drinks
- **1.** Decaffeinated tea
- **2.** Juices (except citrus)
- **3.** Caffeine-free sodas

G. Spices
- **1.** Salt
- **2.** Thyme
- **3.** Sage
- **4.** Cinnamon
- **5.** Paprika
- **6.** Apple cider vinegar
- **7.** Prepared mustard
- **8.** Lemon and lime juices

DASH Diet: Dietary Approaches to Stop Hypertension

Cheryl A. Glass and Jill C. Cash

The Dietary Approaches to Stop Hypertension (DASH) diet is based on a combination of different types of foods and is recommended to help control high blood pressure (BP). It is a food plan that is based on foods that are low in cholesterol and high in dietary fiber, potassium, calcium, and magnesium; it is moderately high in protein. DASH eating has a reduction in lean red meats, added sugar, and sugar-containing sodas. The DASH diet's dairy food portions make the diet high in calcium and vitamin D. Overall, Americans, especially African Americans, are deficient in vitamin D.

The DASH diet, along with weight loss and exercise, is used to control other health problems such as type 2 diabetes and heart disease. If your ethnic background is Hawaiian, American Indian, Eskimo, Hispanic, or African American, you are at higher risk for high BP. Following a DASH eating plan will also help lower the bad cholesterol, or low-density lipoprotein (LDL), which can reduce heart disease.

A major way the DASH diet helps lower BP is to limit the amount of salt (sodium). The recommendations are limiting sodium to 2,300 mg a day or less. If you have high BP, you may be limited to 1,500 mg or less a day. One teaspoon of salt contains 2,000 mg of sodium.

Foods high in sodium make you retain extra fluid. If you notice that your hands are swelling (rings are tight) or your feet and legs swell (sock rings or shoes feel tight), you are getting too much salt. Fluid retention is bad if you have heart failure. This diet is rich in potassium, which can help you get rid of the extra sodium and decrease the fluid retention.

Sea salt, even though it may contain less sodium, is not low enough in sodium to use as a substitute for regular salt. Salt substitutes contain potassium chloride; this can cause more fluid retention. Potassium chloride salt substitutes may also interfere with your BP medications, so check with your health care provider before using them.

Tips for Reducing Sodium

A. Slowly cut back on your salty foods and begin to use healthier products. Take the saltshaker off the table.

B. Eat fresh foods.
   1. Avoid prepackaged foods.
   2. Eat fresh vegetables instead of canned vegetables. If you use canned vegetables, choose the low-sodium option and/or rinse the vegetables.

C. Read food labels.
   1. Sodium is in almost all processed foods, including milk.
   2. Focus on the amount of sodium per food serving.
   3. Do not forget to read labels on soda and sports drink bottles.
   4. Choose your favorite food brand with low-salt or low-sodium labels on the package instead of the same product with more salt.

D. Avoid salty snacks and foods, including:
   1. Crackers, chips, and pretzels
   2. Cheeses
   3. Olives, pickles, pickled okra, and other foods
   4. Processed foods, including jerky, hot dogs, bacon, deli meats, canned fish, and canned meats, which contain a large amount of sodium.

E. Limit using soy sauce, seasoned salts, and meat tenderizers.

F. Many seasonings, including ketchup and sauces, contain a lot of sodium. Substitute with other flavors such as fresh herbs (e.g., rosemary, thyme, oregano, cilantro, and basil). Use garlic powder, lemon and lime juice, and crushed red peppers, as well as ginger.

G. Try making your own salt-free herb blend to use on your foods. Ingredients that can add flavor without adding salt include:
   1. Peppers such as cayenne, black pepper, and lemon pepper
   2. Dried herbs such as thyme
   3. Garlic powder
   4. Paprika
   5. Celery seed

H. Helpful websites for salt-free herb blend, products, and recipes are:
   1. Salt-free seasoning recipes:
      a. busycooks.about.com
      b. www.tasteofhome.com/Recipes/Salt-Free-Seasoning-Mix
   2. Websites with low-salt recipes:
      a. http://homecooking.about.com/library/archive/blhelp13.htm
      b. McCormick: www.mccormick.com
      c. Mrs. Dash: www.mrsdash.com

Tips on Eating the DASH Way

A. Start small. Make gradual changes in your eating habits, such as eating smaller portions (see Tables B.1 and B.2).

B. Center your meal around carbohydrates such as pasta, rice, beans, or vegetables.

C. Treat meat as only part of a whole meal instead of the main focus of the meal.

D. Use fruits or low-fat, low-calorie foods such as sugar-free gelatin for desserts and snacks.

E. Choose "whole" grains in breads and cereals.

F. Choose to eat vegetables without butter or sauce.

G. Choose lean cuts of meat. Use fresh poultry, for example, skinless turkey and chicken.

H. Choose ready-to-eat breakfast cereals that are lower in sodium.

I. Eat fruits for dessert. Use fruits that are canned in their own juice.

J. Add fruit to plain yogurt.

K. To increase eating vegetables, stir-fry with 2 oz of chicken and use 1½ cups of raw vegetables.

L. Snack on vegetables, bread sticks, graham crackers, or unbuttered/unsalted popcorn.

M. Drink water or club soda.

N. Table B.3 lists the number of servings suggested and Table B.4 offers an example of the caloric adjustment for 2,000 calories a day using the DASH diet.

TABLE B.1 **DASH Diet Serving Portion Sizes**

Food	Portion Size	Food	Portion Size
1 baked potato	Fist	1 cup of popcorn (unbuttered)	Baseball
1 cup of flaked cereal	Baseball	½ cup of fresh fruit	½ Baseball
1½ oz cheese	4 Dice	½ cup of pasta, rice, or potato	½ Baseball
1 tbsp of margarine	1 Die	½ cup of ice cream	½ Baseball
¼ cup of raisins	Egg	3 oz of meat, includes fish, meat, and chicken	Deck of cards
¼ cup almonds	Golf ball	1 pancake	Compact disk (CD)
2 tbsp peanut butter	Ping-Pong ball	1 piece of cornbread	Bar of soap
1 cup of salad	Baseball	3 oz of grilled or baked fish	Checkbook

Adapted from the National Heart, Lung, and Blood Institute (NHLBI), (2013).

TABLE B.2 **DASH Diet Daily Servings**

Food Group	Daily Servings	Serving Sizes	Examples and Notes	Significance of Each Food Group to the DASH Diet Pattern
Grains and grain product	6–8	1 slice bread ½ cup dry cereal ½ cup cooked rice, pasta, or cereal	Whole-wheat bread, English muffin, pita bread, bagel, cereals, grits, oatmeal, couscous	Major sources of energy and fiber
Vegetables	4–5	1 cup raw leafy vegetables ½ cup cooked vegetables 6 oz vegetable juice	Tomatoes, potatoes, carrots, peas, squash, broccoli, turnip greens, collards, kale, spinach, artichokes, beans, sweet potatoes	Rich sources of potassium, magnesium, and fiber
Fruits	4–5	6 oz fruit juice 1 medium fruit ¼ cup dried fruit ¼ cup fresh, frozen, or canned fruit	Apricots, bananas, dates, grapes, oranges, orange juice, grapefruit, grapefruit juice, mangoes, melons, peaches, pineapples, prunes, raisins, strawberries, tangerines	Important sources of potassium, magnesium, and fiber
Low-fat or fat-free milk and dairy foods	2–3	1 cup milk 1 cup yogurt 1.5 oz cheese	Skim or 1% milk, skim or low-fat buttermilk, nonfat or low-fat yogurt, part-skim mozzarella cheese, nonfat cheese	Major sources of calcium and protein
Lean meats, poultry, and fish	6 or less	1 oz cooked meats, poultry, or fish 1 egg	Select only lean; trim away visible fat; broil, roast, or boil instead of frying; remove skin from poultry	Rich sources of protein and magnesium
Nuts, seeds, and legumes	4–5 per week	1½ oz of nuts ½ oz or 2 tbsp seeds 2 tbsp of peanut butter ½ cup cooled legumes	Almonds, filberts, mixed nuts, peanuts, walnuts, sunflower seeds, kidney beans, lentils	Rich sources of energy, magnesium, potassium, protein, and fiber
Sweets and added sugars	5 or less per week	1 tbsp sugar 1 tbsp jelly or jam ½ cup sorbet or gelatin 1 cup lemonade	Fruit-flavored gelatin, fruit punch, hard candy, jelly, maple syrup, sugar	Sweets should be low in fat

DASH, dietary approaches to stop hypertension.
Source: Adapted from the National Heart, Lung, and Blood Institute (NHLBI) DASH Diet Eating Plan.

TABLE B.3 Total Number of Servings in 2,000 Calories per Day DASH Diet

Food Group	Servings
Grains	6–8
Vegetables	4–5
Fruits	4–5
Fat-free or low-fat milk and dairy foods	2–3
Lean meats, poultry, and fish	2 (6 oz)
Nuts, seeds, and legumes	1 (4–5/wk)
Fats and oils	2–3
Sweets and added sugars	1 (<5/wk)

TABLE B.4 DASH Example Menu (2,000 Calories)

Food	Amount	Servings Provided
Breakfast		
Orange juice	6 oz	1 fruit
1% low-fat milk	8 oz (1 cup)	1 dairy
Corn flakes (with 1 tbsp sugar)	1 cup	2 grains
Banana	1 medium	1 fruit
Whole-wheat bread (with 1 tbsp jelly)	1 slice	1 grain
Soft margarine	1 tsp	1 fat
Lunch		
Chicken salad	¾ cup	1 poultry
Pita bread	½ large	1 grain
Raw vegetable medley:		
Carrot and celery sticks	3–4 sticks each	1 vegetable
Radishes	2	
Loose-leaf lettuce	2 leaves	
Part-skim mozzarella cheese	1.5 slice (1.5 oz)	1 dairy
1% low-fat milk	8 oz (1 cup)	1 dairy
Fruit cocktail in light syrup	½ cup	1 fruit
Dinner		
Herbed baked cod	3 oz	1 fish
Scallion rice	1 cup	2 grains
Steamed broccoli	½ cup	1 vegetable
Stewed tomatoes	½ cup	1 vegetable
Spinach salad:	½ cup	1 vegetable
Raw spinach		
Cherry tomatoes	2	
Cucumber	2 slices	
Light Italian salad dressing	1 tbsp	½ fat
Whole wheat dinner roll	1 small	1 grain
Soft margarine	1 tsp	1 fat
Melon balls	½ cup	1 fruit
Snacks		
Dried apricots	1 oz (¼ cup)	1 fruit
Mini-pretzels	1 oz (¾ cup)	1 grain
Mixed nuts	1.5 oz (½ cup)	1 nuts
Diet ginger ale	12 oz	0

Resources

DASH Diet Calorie Adjustments for 1,200, 1,600, 2,000, and 2,400 calorie diets: http://dashdiet.org/images/calories.pdf

The DASH Diet Eating Plan: http://dashdiet.org/dash_diet_recipes.asp

DASH Diet Recipes: www.mayoclinic.com/health/dash-diet-recipes/RE00089

DASH for Health: www.dashforhealth.com/index.php

Foods to Avoid While Taking Warfarin (Coumadin, Jantoven)

Cheryl A. Glass and Jill C. Cash

Warfarin is a medication that thins the blood to prevent blood clots. Some nutrients and foods can interfere with warfarin and make the warfarin less effective or not work as well. Therefore, it is important to closely monitor the foods that you eat daily to make sure your medication is working for you the same way every day. One nutrient that causes this problem is vitamin K. Vitamin K interferes with the warfarin and can cause problems with thinning the blood. Therefore, it is important to avoid foods and nutrients that would cause this problem. It is suggested to eat foods that contain the same amount of vitamin K every day. This will help to prevent problems with thinning your blood.

The recommended intake of vitamin K for the adult man is 120 mcg and for adult women is 90 mcg.

The following is a list of foods that have a **MODERATE to HIGH level of vitamin K and should be avoided:**

1. Broccoli (cooked)
2. Brussels sprouts
3. Chard
4. Collard greens
5. Green tea
6. Kale
7. Mustard greens
8. Parsley
9. Spinach
10. Turnip greens

Some drinks can also interfere with warfarin and **should be avoided**. These drinks include:

1. Cranberry juice
2. Alcohol

Foods that have a **LOWER level of vitamin K** and are safer to eat in moderate portions include:

1. Asparagus
2. Avocado
3. Blackberries/ blueberries
4. Cabbage
5. Carrots
6. Cauliflower
7. Cucumbers
8. Lettuce, iceberg and romaine
9. Peas
10. Peppers
11. Potatoes
12. Prunes
13. Squash (summer and winter)
14. Sweet potatoes
15. Tomatoes
16. Tuna

Medications (prescribed and over-the-counter [OTC] medications, multivitamins, supplements, and herbal supplements) may also interfere with warfarin and should only be taken after discussing the medication, vitamin, or supplement with your health care provider for safety.

If you have questions about certain foods or medications, you need to discuss this with your health care provider.

Foods Rich in Vitamin K

If you are taking a blood thinner, you should be aware that certain foods are high in vitamin K.

Vitamin K can interfere with how blood thinners work.

You do not necessarily have to stop eating these foods, just be consistent and maintain your regular eating habits.

Please discuss these foods further with your health care provider.

These vitamin K-rich foods include the following:

1. Broccoli
2. Brussels sprouts
3. Collard greens
4. Endive
5. Kale
6. Mustard greens
7. Parsley
8. Swiss chard
9. Spinach
10. Turnip greens

Foods that are low in vitamin K:

1. Asparagus
2. Avocado
3. Blackberries
4. Blueberries
5. Cabbage
6. Cranberry juice
7. Green tea
8. Lettuce (iceberg & leafy)
9. Liver
10. Peas
11. Prunes
12. Tuna

Gluten-Free Diet

Cheryl A. Glass and Jill C. Cash

Gluten-Free Diet Tips

The symptoms from celiac disease are triggered from glutens in your diet. Three cereals that contain gluten are wheat, rye, and barley. Glutens are also present in other products, such as food additives, so it is very important to read all the ingredients on food labels (see Table B.5).

Dietary Recommendation for Celiac Disease

A. You may also be told to follow a lactose-free diet for a short time to help your symptoms.
B. Most bread sold in the grocery aisle is not allowed on a gluten-free eating plan.
C. All vegetables and fruits are gluten-free. However, frozen and canned fruits and vegetables may contain an additive with gluten.
D. Although you should not enjoy beer, wine is still on the menu when you go to dinner.
E. Specialty bakeries are able to make gluten-free cakes for special occasions. Plain hard candy, marshmallows, and other candies are usually gluten-free.
F. Caution should be taken when ordering any breaded foods such as chicken nuggets or breaded fish.
G. Deli meats may also contain gluten.
H. Gluten-free foods are often not fortified with vitamins and minerals. It is recommended to take a daily multivitamin.

Resources

Celiac Disease Foundation: www.celiac.org
www.celiac.com
www.chex.com/glutenfree
www.BettyCrocker.com/glutenfree
https://celiac.org/celiac-disease/understanding-celiac-disease-2/what-is-celiac-disease/
Gluten-Free Recipes: http://allrecipes.com/Recipes/Healthy-Cooking/Gluten-Free/Main.aspx

TABLE B.5 Examples of Foods That Are Allowed and Avoided on a Gluten-Free Diet

Allowed	Avoid
Fresh fruits and vegetables without any processing or additives	Wheat, wheat berry, wheat bran, wheat germ, wheat grass, whole wheat berries
Meat	Flours, bread flour
Soy, soybean, tofu	Bulgur (bulgur wheat, bulgur nuts)
Brown rice	Rye
Enriched rice/instant rice/wild rice	Barley
Buckwheat	Barley malt/barley extract
Millet	Oats, oat bran, oat fiber
Sorghum	Cereals
Alfalfa	Matzo
Almond	Beer, ale, porter, stout
Canola	Farina
Chickpea	Croutons
Corn, corn flour, cornmeal	Bran
Brown rice flour	Tabbouleh
Tapioca	Soy sauce

High-Fiber Diet

Cheryl A. Glass and Jill C. Cash

Fiber is a plant cell-wall component that is not broken down by the digestive system. An old term for fiber is roughage because it absorbs fluid and moves waste faster through the intestines in a bulky mass. The Food and Drug Administration (FDA) defines as high-fiber those products that contain 20% of the daily fiber value. High-fiber diets are used to help prevent constipation as well as diarrhea. Fiber has been used to help several medical conditions such as diabetes, diverticulosis, irritable bowel syndrome (IBS), and high cholesterol, as well as weight loss. If you have a chronic health condition, check with your health care provider about starting any new dietary change.

Fiber provides a full feeling that can help with spacing meals further apart (3–4 hours). Fiber recommendations change with your age (see Table B.6).

Tips for Increasing Fiber in Your Diet

A. Read the Nutrition Facts food label for fiber content per food serving.

- **1.** Cereals that provide 5 g of fiber per serving give you 20% of your daily fiber.
- **2.** Look for "whole grain" on the label. Just because bread is brown does not mean it is whole grain.

B. Increase fiber in your diet gradually to prevent gas. Adding too much fiber too quickly may give you abdominal pain, bloating, and constipation. Increase your fiber over several weeks so that it gives time for you to adjust.

C. As you increase fiber, it is also important to increase the amount of fluids you drink up to six to eight glasses a day, including tea, milk, fruit juices, coffee, and even soft drinks. The extra fluids that you drink along with the extra fiber makes you feel fuller, which can help control snacking.

D. Keep a food diary and review it periodically to decide on other diet adjustments that need to be made.

E. Several fiber supplements are available over the counter (OTC) to help you get your daily recommendation of fiber.

Good Food Sources of Fiber

A. Bran: Add 1 teaspoon of whole-grain bran to food three times a day, or take an OTC fiber supplement, such as psyllium (Metamucil), as directed.

B. Whole-grain cereals and breads: Eat oat, bran, multigrain, light, wheat, or rye breads rather than pure white bread or breads that list eggs as a major ingredient. Grains are not only a good source of fiber but also contain vitamins and minerals. Folic acid has been added to breads and cereals to help reduce neural tube defects.

C. Fresh or frozen fruits and vegetables: Citrus fruits are especially good sources of fiber. Eat raw or minimally cooked vegetables, especially squash, cabbage, lettuce and other greens, and beans. Leave the skin on fruits and vegetables; eating the whole fruit is better than drinking the juice. Whole tomatoes offer more fiber than peeling the skin off. The more colorful the fruit and vegetable (dark green, reds, blue, yellow), the better; they provide a good source of antioxidants that are good for the heart and the prevention of some cancers. Apples are a good source of both fiber and water.

D. Legumes (pods): Peas and beans are a good source of fiber. Add chickpeas and kidney beans to salads for extra fiber and flavor. Add baked beans as a delicious side item to your meal.

E. Coffee is another source of fiber.

F. Nuts are an excellent source of fiber. They are considered nutrient-dense and are a good source of vitamins and folic acid. Sprinkle sunflower seeds on a salad to add flavor and fiber. The amount of nuts eaten should be limited to 1 to 2 oz because they are also high in calories.

G. If you have diverticulosis: Avoid foods with seeds or indigestible material that may block the neck of a diverticulum such as nuts, corn, popcorn, cucumbers, tomatoes, figs, strawberries, and caraway seeds.

TABLE B.6 Fiber Recommendations by Age

Group/Gender	Age (Years)	Fiber Recommendations (g of Fiber Each Day)
Children	1–3	19
Children	4–8	25
Boys	9–13	31
Boys	14–18	38
Girls	9–13	26
Girls	14–18	26
Men	Younger than 50	38
Women	Younger than 50	25
Men	Older than 50	30
Women	Older than 50	21

Source: Adapted from the American Heart Association (2015).

Lactose-Intolerance Diet

Cheryl A. Glass and Jill C. Cash

Lactose is the sugar present in milk. Lactose intolerance is very common; it occurs when the body is not able to appropriately digest this milk sugar content and the result is diarrhea. You have been diagnosed as having difficulty digesting milk (lactose) products or you have problems with malabsorption. Lactose intolerance can cause gas, bloating, abdominal cramps, diarrhea, and nausea or vomiting. You may be able to eat small portions without problems, or you may be unable to tolerate any foods containing lactose (see Table B.7).

Tips for Following a Lactose-Intolerance Diet

A. Limit or omit foods that contain milk, lactose, whey, or casein.
B. Lactose-controlled diets allow up to 1 cup of milk per day for cooking or drinking, if you can tolerate it.
C. Read labels carefully. If you cannot tolerate any lactose, choose lactose-free foods with lactate, lactic acid, lactalbumin, whey protein, sodium caseinate, casein hydrolysates, and calcium compounds.
D. You may also choose kosher foods marked "pareve" or "parve," which do not contain lactose. Read labels carefully.
E. A low-fat diet is important if you have fat malabsorption.
F. To help with diarrhea because of malabsorption, avoid more than one serving a day of caffeine-containing drinks.
G. Beverages with high sugar content, such as soft drinks and fruit juices, may increase diarrhea. Juices and fruits with high amounts of fructose include apples, pears, sweet cherries, prunes, and dates.
H. "Sugarless" sorbitol-containing candies and gums may cause diarrhea.

TABLE B.7 Recommended Foods for Lactose Intolerance

Foods	Recommended	Not Recommended
Milk	Soybean milk, milk treated with lactase, nondairy creamers, whipped topping; up to 1 cup/d of buttermilk, yogurt, sweet acidophilus milk, or whole, low-fat, or skim milk	Milk products in excess of 1 cup/d, malted milk, milkshakes, hot chocolate, cocoa
Meat and protein foods	All meats, fish, poultry, eggs, peanut butter, tofu, or hard, aged, and processed cheese, if tolerated	Sandwich meat, hot dogs that contain lactose, cottage cheese, any meat prepared with milk products
Vegetables	All fresh, frozen, canned, buttered, and/or breaded vegetables	Any vegetable prepared with milk or milk products in excess of allowance (1 cup)
Fruits	All fresh, frozen, or canned fruits	Any fruits processed with lactose
Breads, cereal, and starchy food	White, wheat, rye, or other yeast breads, crackers, macaroni, spaghetti, popcorn, dry or cooked cereals	Commercial bread products (French toast, bread mixes, pancakes, biscuits), cakes/cookies containing milk or milk products
Fats and oils	Butter/margarine, salad dressing, mayonnaise, all oils, nondairy creamers, bacon	Sour cream, salad dressings with milk products in excess of 1 cup allowance
Soups	Vegetable and meat soups, broth, and bouillon	Dried soups, creamed soups made with milk
Desserts	Plain and fruit-flavored gelatins, sherbet, fruit pies, cakes, pudding, pastries, angel food cake, sponge cake	Ice cream, ice milk, cream pie, puddings, custards, cakes, and pastries with milk (unless count as day's allowance)
Beverages	Coffee, tea, soft drinks, fruit juices, carbonated and mineral waters	Beverages with milk over the 1 cup allowance
Miscellaneous condiments	Catsup, mustard, soy sauce, vinegar, steak sauce, Worcestershire sauce, chili sauce	None
Seasonings	Salt, pepper, spices, herbs, and seasonings	None
Sweets	Sugar, jelly, honey, molasses, preserves, marmalade, syrups, hard candy, baker's cocoa, carob powder, artificial sweeteners	Cream or chocolate candies containing milk or milk products (unless count as day's allowance), caramels, toffee, and butterscotch

Low-Fat/Low-Cholesterol Diet

Cheryl A. Glass and Jill C. Cash

The connection between fat in the diet and heart attack is cholesterol. Cholesterol is a fatlike substance produced by your liver and also found in many foods. Too much cholesterol causes heart attacks by clogging the arteries that deliver blood to your heart.

Exercising and following a low-fat/low-cholesterol diet can help control your blood cholesterol and reduce your risk of heart attack.

Tips

A. Read food labels. Use the ingredient list on labels to identify products containing saturated fat. High-fat ingredients may have many names. Remember: Foods can say "no cholesterol" and still be high in saturated vegetable fat and calories.

B. Train yourself to think "low fat" in your food and cooking methods.

- **1.** Bake
- **2.** Broil
- **3.** Grill
- **4.** Stir-fry

C. Eat less fried food, fast food, and baked products.

D. Eat more fruits and vegetables.

E. Organize your shopping around low-fat foods.

F. Add flavor to foods by using herbs and spices instead of butter and sauces.

G. Choose coleslaw, sliced tomatoes, or a dill pickle instead of fries and chips.

Foods to Avoid or Limit

A. Proteins/meats

- **1.** Shrimp
- **2.** Fried meats, fish, or poultry
- **3.** Fatty ground meat
- **4.** Prime or heavily marbled meats
- **5.** Bacon, sausage, high-fat deli meats, and cheeses
- **6.** Liver and organ meats

B. Breads/cereals

- **1.** High-fat baked foods, such as Danish, croissants, and doughnuts
- **2.** Fried rice, crispy chow mein noodles
- **3.** Granola bars with coconut or coconut oil
- **4.** Chips, cheese, or butter crackers
- **5.** High-fat cookies and cakes

C. Fruits and vegetables

- **1.** Coconut
- **2.** Fried vegetables such as onion rings and breaded fried pickles, mushrooms, and okra
- **3.** Cream, cheese, or butter sauces on vegetables

D. Milk/dairy products

- **1.** Whole or 2% milk
- **2.** Cream, half-and-half, nondairy creamers
- **3.** Ice cream, whipped cream, nondairy whipped toppings
- **4.** Whole-milk yogurt, sour cream
- **5.** Cheeses: Cheddar, American, Swiss, cream cheese, Brie, Muenster

E. Very high-fat foods

- **1.** Butter or margarine made with partially hydrogenated oils
- **2.** Lard, meat fat, and coconut or palm oils
- **3.** Salad dressings made with sour cream or cheese
- **4.** Chocolate
- **5.** Beef tallow
- **6.** Hydrogenated or partially hydrogenated vegetable shortening
- **7.** Cream
- **8.** Cocoa butter

Foods That Are Allowed

A. Proteins/meats

- **1.** Fish and shellfish
- **2.** Chicken and turkey cooked without the skin
- **3.** Ground turkey
- **4.** Eggs: Limited to two yolks per week
- **5.** Dried beans, lentils, tofu
- **6.** Small amounts of meat and seafood

B. Breads/cereals

- **1.** Plain bread and English muffins and bagels
- **2.** Plain pasta, rice
- **3.** Cereals, oatmeal
- **4.** Pretzels, air-popped popcorn, rice cakes, Melba toast
- **5.** Low-fat baked goods: Angel food cake, graham crackers, fruit cookies, and gingersnaps

C. Fruits and vegetables

- **1.** Eat several servings per day of high-nutrition, low-fat fruits and vegetables.
- **2.** Prepare vegetables by steaming, broiling, baking, or stir-frying.

D. Milk/dairy products

- **1.** Skim or 1% milk
- **2.** Low-fat milk, evaporated milk, nonfat dry milk powder
- **3.** Frozen yogurt, ice milk, sherbet, sorbet
- **4.** Low-fat yogurt
- **5.** Low-fat cheeses: 1% cottage cheese, skim-milk ricotta, mozzarella, and American cheeses

E. Allowed high-fat foods

- **1.** Margarine made with liquid safflower, corn, or sunflower oils
- **2.** Olive, canola, or peanut oils
- **3.** Nut snacks in moderation (high fat and calories)
- **4.** Salad dressings made with saturated oils

Nausea and Vomiting Diet Suggestions (Children and Adults)

Cheryl A. Glass and Jill C. Cash

For simple nausea and vomiting with an upset stomach, follow these steps:

Step 1: Replace Lost Fluids

A. Rest your stomach for 1 to 2 hours.
B. Infants and small children: Pedialyte or Ricelyte are recommended because children become dehydrated quickly.
C. Infants: Resume breast- or bottle-feeding as soon as possible.
D. Young children: Give very small sips every 10 to 20 minutes until they keep the fluid down.
E. Older children: Give Gatorade or Pedialyte.
F. Older child and adults
  1. After vomiting stops, take sips of clear liquids at room temperature, such as flat ginger ale, flat cola, or gelatin.
  2. Suck on lollipops or Popsicles.
  3. Gradually increase the amount of liquids. If 4 hours pass without vomiting, progress to Step 2.

Step 2: Dry Diet

The foods in this diet do not meet all daily food requirements and should be used only for a short period before adding foods or advancing to Step 3.

A. Cheerios
B. Crackers
C. Cornflakes
D. Graham crackers
E. Rice Krispies
F. Vanilla wafers
G. Toast
H. Dinner rolls

Step 3: More Advanced Carbohydrates

A. Oatmeal
B. Grits, unseasoned
C. Rice, unseasoned
D. Mashed potatoes
E. Baked potato
F. Noodles
G. Peanut butter
H. Pudding

Step 4: Bland Foods With Limited Odors

After you are able to eat dry and more complex carbohydrates, a trial of bland foods may be tried. Foods with little or no odors are more easily tolerated after experiencing nausea and vomiting (see Table B.8).

BRAT Diet

You may be told to use a BRAT diet. This is a combination of foods that make up a bland diet and help with nausea and vomiting: Bananas, rice, applesauce, and toast as tolerated.

TABLE B.8 Bland Foods With Limited Odors

Apple Juice	Canned Pears	Ice Cream
Apple sauce	Chicken noodle soup	Iced tea
Baked chicken	Cottage cheese	Low-fat milk
Baked turkey	Fresh apple	Sherbet
Canned peaches	Fresh banana	½ turkey sandwich

Vitamin D and Calcium Handout

Cheryl A. Glass and Jill C. Cash

Vitamin D–Enriched Foods

Food Source	Serving Size	Food International Units (IU)
Fish liver oils, cod liver oil	15 mL	1,360
Mushrooms	3 oz	2,700
Fortified milk	8 oz	100
Herring	3 oz	1,383
Catfish	3 oz	425
Mackerel (cooked)	3.5 oz	345
Salmon (cooked)	3.5 oz	360
Sardines (canned in oil, drained)	1.75 oz	250
Fortified orange juice	8 oz	100
Fortified cereal	1 serving	100
Fortified cheese	3 oz	100

Calcium-Rich Foods

Food Source	Serving Size	Food International Units (IU)
Yogurt	1 cup	448
Orange juice	1 cup	350
Fat-free milk	1 cup	316
Shrimp	3 oz	275
Salmon	3 oz	182
Instant oatmeal	1 packet	165
Tofu	½ cup	130
Broccoli	1 cup	94
Dried beans, cooked	½ cup	50
Cheddar cheese	1½ oz	306
Turnip greens	1 cup	197
Cereal bars, snack bars (fortified)	1 bar	200

Sunlight exposure to the skin is also recommended for approximately 20 to 30 minutes without sunscreen. Sun exposure provides an adequate source of vitamin D. Care should be taken not to burn skin.

1. Vitamin D recommendations:
   - **a.** Men and women age younger than 50: 400 to 800 IU/d
   - **b.** Men and women 50 years and older: 800 to 1,000 IU/d
2. Calcium recommendations:
   - **a.** Women 50 and younger: 1,000 mg/d; women age 51 years and older: 1,200 mg/d
   - **b.** Men age younger than 70: 1,000 mg/d; men 70 years and older: 1,200 mg/d
3. Vitamin D assists with calcium absorption into the bones.
4. Research indicates that caffeine interferes with calcium absorption and lowers bone density. Carbonated beverages appear to be worse than coffee.
5. Vitamin D and calcium deficiency contribute to bone loss, and thus, osteoporosis.

Bibliography

American Dietetic Association Reports. (2008). Position of the American Dietetic Association: Nutrition guidance for healthy children ages 2 to 11 years. *Journal of the American Dietetic Association, 108*, 1038–1047.

American Heart Association. (2015). Fiber and children's diets. Retrieved from http://www.heart.org/HEARTORG/HealthyLiving/HealthyEating/Nutrition/Fiber-and-Childrens-Diets_UCM_305981_Article.jsp#.WGagdLnT8rM

Banks, D. (n.d.). Salt: Too much of a good thing. In *University of Illinois extension: Thrifty living*. Retrieved from http://urbanext.illinois.edu/thriftyliving/tl-salt.html

Boyle, M., & Long, S. (2013). *Personal nutrition* (8th ed.). Belmont, CA: Wadsworth Cengage.

The DASH Diet Eating Plan. (n.d.a). Retrieved from http://dashdiet.org/default.asp

The DASH Diet Eating Plan. (n.d.b). The DASH diet and African American heart health. Retrieved from http://dashdiet.org/dash_diet_and_african_american.asp

The DASH Diet Eating Plan. (n.d.c). DASH diet FAQ. Retrieved from http://dashdiet.org/dash_diet_faq.asp

The DASH Diet Eating Plan. (n.d.d). Low salt, low sodium, and the DASH diet. Retrieved from http://dashdiet.org/low_salt_diet.asp

Dietary Fiber Guide. (n.d.). High fiber foods. Retrieved from http://dietaryfiberguide.com

National Heart, Lung, and Blood Institute. (2013). Serving sizes and portions. Retrieved from: http://www.nhlbi.nih.gov/health/educational/wecan/eat-right/distortion.htm

National Heart, Lung, and Blood Institute. (n.d.a). Tips for reducing sodium in your diet. Retrieved from www.nhlbi.nih.gov/hbp/prevent/sodium/tips.htm

National Heart, Lung, and Blood Institute. (n.d.b). Tips on how to make healthier meals. Retrieved from www.nhlbi.nih.gov/hbp/prevent/h_eating/tips.htm

National Heart, Lung, and Blood Institute. (2015). In brief: Your guide to lowering your blood pressure with DASH. Retrieved from http://www.nhlbi.nih.gov/files/docs/public/heart/dash_brief.pdf

National Institute of Diabetes and Digestive and Kidney Diseases. (2015). Lactose intolerance. Retrieved from https://www.niddk.nih.gov/health-information/health-topics/digestive-diseases/lactose-intolerance/Pages/facts.aspx

National Osteoporosis Foundation. (n.d.). Calcium and vitamin D: What you need to know. Retrieved from www.nof.org/articles/10

The University of Chicago Celiac Disease Center. (n.d.). Is a gluten-free diet similar to a diabetic diet? Retrieved from www.cureceliacdisease.org/?s=glutentfree+diet

C Tanner's Sexual Maturity Stages

	Sexual Maturity Stages in Females	**Sexual Maturity Stages in Males**
Stage	**Breasts**	**Penis, Testes, and Scrotum**
1	Preadolescent: Only papilla is elevated above the level of the chest wall	Preadolescent: All are the size and proportion seen in early childhood (testes 1 cm)
2	Breast budding: Breast and papilla elevated as small mound; increased diameter of areola	Slight enlargement, with alteration in color (more reddened) and texture of scrotum (testes 2.0–3.2 cm)
3	Continued breast and areola enlargement; no contour separation	Further growth and enlargement (testes 3.3–4.0 cm)
4	Areola and papilla form secondary mound	Penis significantly enlarged in length and circumference; further development of glands; enlargement of testes and scrotum with darkening of scrotal skin (testes 4.1–4.9 cm)
5	Mature: Nipple projects; areola is part of general breast contour	Genitalia of adult size (testes 5.0 cm)
Stage	**Pubic Hair**	**Pubic Hair**
1	Preadolescent: None or vellus hair in pubis area	Preadolescent: None or vellus hair in pubis area
2	Sparse, straight, lightly pigmented along medial border of labia	Sparse, straight, lightly pigmented at base of penis
3	Darker, coarser, curlier, and in increased amount	Darker, coarser, curlier, and in increased amount
4	Abundant, but has not spread to medial surface of thighs	Abundant, but less quantity than adult type
5	Adult feminine, inverse triangle, spread to medial surface of thighs	Adult distribution, spread to medial surface of thighs

Used with permission from the Child Growth Foundation (www.childgrowthfoundation.org).

D Teeth

DECIDUOUS (BABY)

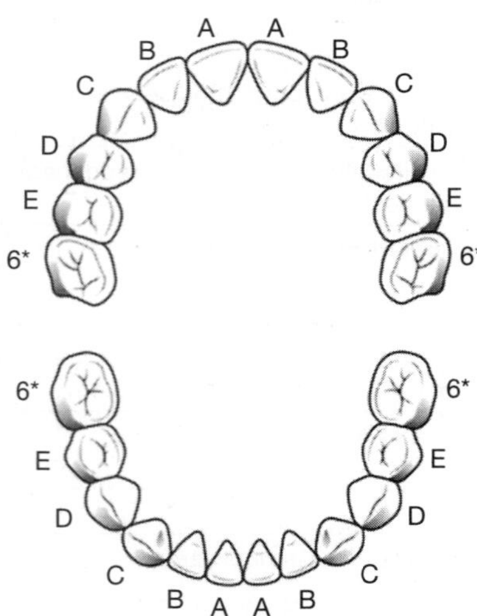

A, B: Incisors, 6 to 9 months
C: Cuspid (eyetooth), 16 months
D: First molar; 14 months
E: Second molar; 26 months

When they are lost:

A: 6 to 8 years
B: 7 to 9 years
C: 9 to 13 years
D: 8 to 12 years
E: 8 to 12 years
6*: Sixth-year molar*, first permanent tooth

Expected number of teeth up to 24 months = age of child in months – 4 (e.g., 18-month-old should have 14 teeth)

PERMANENT

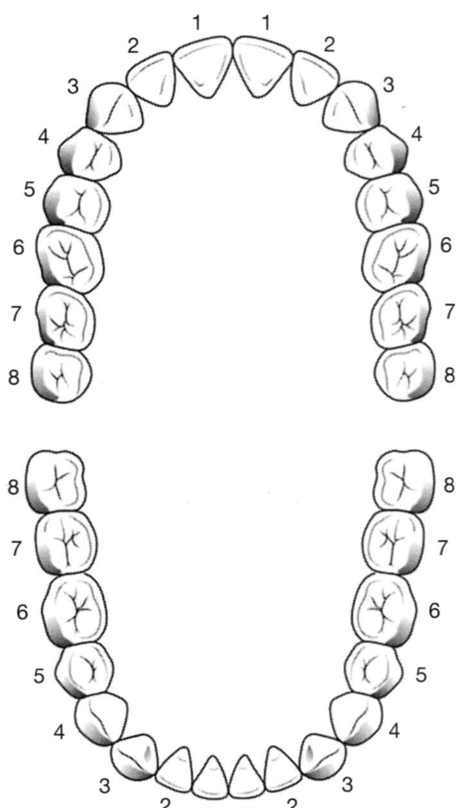

1, 2: Incisors, 7 to 9 years
3: Cuspid (eyetooth), 11 to 13 years
4: First bicuspid, 9 to 11 years
5: Second bicuspid, 10 to 12 years
6: Sixth-year molar, first permanent tooth
7: Second molar, 12 to 14 years
8: Third molar (wisdom), 16 to 20 years

Index